Notice to the Reader

Acknowledgments

We would like to extend our thanks and appreciation to Beth Williams, Nursing Editor, Delmar Publishers, for her support and assistance. Special thanks go to Marjorie Bruce, Mary Robinson, Susan Simpfenderfer, and Helen Yackel of Delmar Publishers and Joy Perry, each of whom worked especially hard to ensure that the manuscript process flowed smoothly. We would also like to extend appreciation to Seamus McCague, ICPC, Dublin, Ireland, who continues to improve the production process.

G. Spratto extends appreciation to Charles O. Rutledge, Dean of the Schools of Pharmacy, Nursing, and Health Sciences at Purdue University for his encouragement and for being supportive of the need for this project. Greatest appreciation and love go to my wife, Lynne, and sons, Chris and Gregg, who have always been supportive of the project and who continue to make many sacrifices.

A. Woods would like to thank her friends and colleagues for their support and encouragement of this endeavor. Love and appreciation to my husband, Howard, for his continued support, love, and encouragement. Special hugs and love to my babies, Katy and Nate, for trying to be patient while waiting and waiting for Mom to finish.

Preface

As with past editions, NDR-93 provides up-to-date information on the newest and most widely used prescription and over-the-counter drugs. These drugs are presented alphabetically in Chapter 3. Approximately thirty new drugs have been added to NDR-93. In addition, literally hundreds of changes were incorporated into NDR-93. Trade names of drugs marketed in both Canada and the United States are listed; trade names of drugs marketed only in Canada are designated by a maple leaf.

General information on drug classes is located in Chapter 2, which makes this information easier to locate and use. Additionally, general information concerning nursing considerations relating to each drug class is detailed in this section and referred to throughout the text to prevent lengthy repetitions. New entries have been added for ACE inhibitors, histamine H_2 antagonists, and fluoroquinolone antibiotics. Chapter 1 should be consulted first because it outlines how to use NDR-93.

A new feature for drug classes and individual drugs is the addition of symptoms of overdose, which is located at the end of the section entitled *Side Effects*. Also, treatment of overdose has been added as the last entry under *Administration/Storage*. Several features have been continued in NDR-93. The section entitled *Special Concerns* provides information of special note to the practitioner. For example, topics include the pregnancy category, whether the drug is considered safe and effective for use in children, during lactation, during pregnancy, and in the geriatric client.

As in the past, the most important feature of the text is the presentation of nursing considerations in a nursing process format. Such information provides the practitioner with a mechanism to perform assessments of the client before and after prescribed drug therapy, to initiate appropriate nursing interventions, to incorporate appropriate client/family teaching to ensure proper drug therapy, and to evaluate the effectiveness of drug therapy. A new feature is a reorganization of the evaluation process that increases clarity and provides information on the expected outcome(s) of the drug therapy. Chapter 1 should be consulted for a more thorough discussion of how nursing considerations are presented.

We have retained the appendices and other information such as commonly accepted therapeutic drug levels and the table of weights and measures as these have proven valuable supplements to the information on drugs. The appendices include a definition and listing of drugs controlled either by the U.S. Controlled Substances Act or the Canadian Controlled Substances Law (Appendix 1), definitions of the FDA pregnancy categories (Appendix 2), commonly used laboratory test values (Appendix 3), the BSA nomogram (Appendix 4), a listing of the Certified Poison Control Centers in the United States (Appendix 5), Drug Preview (Appendix 6), which describes some new FDA-approved drugs, and Medic Alert Systems (Appendix 7).

Another important new change is that the index has been arranged to facilitate drug location. The trade name has been paired with the generic name to assist in the quick, easy location of desired information.

We believe the format used for NDR-93 makes it an easy-to-use and valuable text for the latest information on drugs and the proper monitoring of drug therapy by the practitioner.

Quick Guide to the Use of *RN's NDR-93*

An understanding of the format of *RN's NDR-93* will help you reference information quickly.

- There are three chapters:
  1. Detailed information on "How to Use NDR-93"
  2. Alphabetical listing of therapeutic/chemical drug classes with general information for each, plus a list of each drug in the class covered in Chapter 3
  3. Alphabetical listing of drugs by generic name
- Each entry in Chapter 3 consists of two parts: general drug information and nursing considerations
- **General drug information** (similar to format in Chapter 2) includes these categories (not all categories may be provided for each drug):
  - **Combination Drug** heading indicates two or more drugs are combined
  - **Generic name** of drug with simplified **phonetic pronunciation**
  - **Trade name(s)** by which drug is marketed; maple leaf indicates trade names available only in Canada
  - **Drug schedule** if drug is controlled by U. S. Federal Controlled Substances Act (such as C-II, C-III)
  - **Rx** = prescription drug; **OTC** = nonprescription, over-the-counter drug
  - See also reference to classification in Chapter 2, if applicable
  - **Classification/Content**: Classification is the type of drug or drug class; Content (for combination drugs) is the generic name and amount of each drug in the combination product.
  - **General Statement**: general information and/or unusual aspects of drugs in a class; also diseases for which drugs may be used
  - **Action/Kinetics**: mechanisms by which drug achieves therapeutic effect, including rate of absorption, minimum effective serum or plasma level half-life (time for half the drug to be removed from blood), duration of action, metabolism, excretion routes and other pertinent information
  - **Uses**: applications, including any investigational uses for the drug
  - **Contraindications**: diseases or conditions for which drug should not be used
  - **Special Concerns**: considerations for use in pediatric, geriatric, pregnant or lactating clients; FDA pregnancy category, if assigned (see definition in Appendix 2)

– **Side Effects**: unwanted or bothersome effects in some clients, listed by body organ or system affected; includes **Symptoms of Overdose**

– **Drug Interactions**: drugs that may interact with one another, with increase or decrease in effect of drug; when listed for class of drugs, are likely to apply to all drugs in class

– **Laboratory Test Interferences**: effect on laboratory test values; may also appear in Nursing Considerations section

– **Dosage**: adult and pediatric dosages and available dosage forms

– **Nursing Considerations**: in nursing process format

• **Administration/Storage:** guidelines for preparing medications for administration, proper storage and, when applicable, treatment of symptoms of overdose

• **Treatment of Overdose**: under Nursing Considerations, last entry in Administration/Storage

• **Assessment:** guidelines to help nurse assess client before and after drug therapy

• **Interventions:** guidelines for appropriate nursing actions for drug therapy

• **Client/Family Teaching:** guidelines to promote education and compliance with drug therapy

• **Evaluation:** includes outcome criteria to determine effectiveness of drug therapy and client response

– **"Additional Contraindications," "Additional Side Effects,"** or **"Additional Nursing Considerations"**: information relevant to a specific drug but not necessarily to the class overall

• Index: extensively cross-referenced; **boldface** = generic drug name; *italics* = therapeutic drug class; regular type = trade name; CAPITALS = combination drugs; trade name is paired with generic name

Table of Contents

Commonly Used Abbreviations

A, aa	of each
ABG	arterial blood gas
a.c.	before meals
ad	to, up to
ad lib	as desired, at pleasure
AIDS	acquired immunodeficiency syndrome
A.M., a.m.	morning
AMI	acute myocardial infarction
aq	water
aq dest.	distilled water
a.u.	each ear, both ears
a.d.	right ear
a.l.	left ear
ARC	AIDS related complex
ASA	aspirin
ASAP	as soon as possible
AV	atrioventricular
b.i.d.	two times a day
b.i.n.	two times a night
BP	blood pressure
BUN	blood urea nitrogen
c̄	with
CA	cancer
Caps, caps	capsule(s)
CBC	complete blood count
CHF	congestive heart failure
cm	centimeter
COPD	chronic obstructive pulmonary disease
CVP	central venous pressure
d.	day
dc	discontinue
dil.	dilute
dL	deciliter (one-tenth of a liter)
dr.	dram (0.0625 ounce)
EC	extracorporeal cardiopulmonary bypass
emuls.	emulsion
elix	elixir
ext.	extract
FSH	follicle stimulating hormone
g (gm)	gram (1,000 mg)
GFR	glomerular filtration rate

GI, gi	gastrointestinal
gr	grain
gtt	a drop, drops
GU	genitourinary
h, hr	hour
HA, HAL	hyperalimentation
HDL	high density lipoproteins
HIV	human immunodeficiency virus
h.s.	at bedtime
IA	intra-arterial
ICP	intracranial pressure
IM, im	intramuscular
IV, iv	intravenous
IVPB	IV piggyback, a secondary IV line
kg	kilogram (2.2 lb)
KVO	keep vein open
L, l	liter (1,000 ml)
Ⓛ	left
LDH	lactic dehydrogenase
LDL	low density lipoprotein
LH	luteinizing hormone
MI	myocardial infarction
m., min	minim
min	minute
M	mix
M^2, m^2	square meter
mg	milligram
MAO	monoamine oxidase
max	maximum
mCi	millicurie
mcg	microgram
mEq	milliequivalent
mist, mixt	mixture
ml	milliliter
NG	nasogastric
ng	nanogram
noct	at night, during the night
non rep	do not repeat
NPO	nothing by mouth
NR	do not refill (e.g., a prescription)
NSAID	nonsteroidal anti-inflammatory drug
NSR	normal sinus rhythm
O_2	oxygen
o.d.	every day
O.D.	right eye
O.S.	left eye
os	mouth
OTC	over the counter

O.U.	each eye, both eyes
oz.	ounce
PA	pulmonary artery
PACWP	pulmonary artery capillary wedge pressure
p.c.	after meals
PCP	*Pneumocystis carinii* pneumonia
PE	pulmonary embolus
per	by, through
PO, po, p.o.	by mouth
PR	by rectum
PRN, p.r.n.	when needed or necessary
PUD	peptic ulcer disease
q	every
q.d.	every day
q.h.	every hour
qhs	every night
q2h	every two hours
q3h	every three hours
q4h	every four hours
q6h	every six hours
q8h	every eight hours
q.i.d.	four times daily
q.o.d.	every other day
q.s.	as much as is needed or required
®	right
RA	right atrium
RV	right ventricular
Rx	take, symbol for a prescription
Rept.	let it be repeated
R/T	related to
s̄	without
SA	sinoatrial
SBE	subacute bacterial endocarditis
SC, sc	subcutaneous
SCID	severe combined immunodeficiency disease
SGOT	serum glutamic-oxaloacetic transaminase
SGPT	serum glutamic-pyruvic transaminase
Sig, S.	mark on the label
SL	sublinqual (beneath the tongue)
s.o.s.	if necessary, once only
sol	solution
sp	spirits
ss	one-half
stat	immediately, first dose
SVT	supraventricular tachycardia
syr	syrup
tab	tablet
TB	tuberculosis
t.i.d.	three times daily

t.i.n.	three times nightly
T.O.	telephone order
TPN	total parenteral nutrition
μ	micron
μCi	microcurie
μg	microgram
U	unit
ung	ointment
ut dict	as directed
VLDL	very low density lipoproteins
vin	wine
V.O.	verbal order
>	greater than
<	less than
×	times, frequency
↑	increased, higher
↓	decreased, lower

CHAPTER ONE
How To Use NDR-93

NDR-93 is intended to be a quick reference to obtain useful information on drugs. An important objective is also to provide information on the proper monitoring of drug therapy by practitioners and to assist them in teaching clients and family members about important aspects of drug therapy.

Chapter 2 includes general information on important therapeutic or chemical classes of drugs. The classes of drugs are listed alphabetically. The specific drugs in the therapeutic or chemical class are found in Chapter 3 (alphabetical listing of drugs). A listing of drugs for which information is provided in Chapter 3 will be found at the beginning of the information on each therapeutic or chemical class in Chapter 2.

Information for individual drugs (and for drug classes when appropriate) is presented as follows:

Drug Names: The generic name for the drug is presented first, followed by one or more trade names. If the trade name is available only in Canada, the name will be followed by a maple leaf (✹). Also, if the drug is controlled by the U.S. Federal Controlled Substances Act, the schedule in which the drug has been placed follows the trade name (e.g., C-II, C-III, C-IV). See Appendix 1 for a listing of controlled substances.

Classification: Defines type of drug or the class under which the drug has been listed. This information is most useful in learning to categorize drugs.

General Statement: Presents information about the class of drug and/or what might be unusual about a particular group of drugs. In addition, information may be presented about the disease(s) for which the drugs are indicated.

Action/Kinetics: The action portion of this entry describes the mechanism(s) by which a drug is able to achieve its therapeutic effect, (e.g., certain antibiotics interfere with the growth of bacteria). Not all mechanisms of action are known, and some are self-evident, as when a hormone is administered as a replacement. The kinetics entry lists pertinent facts, if known, about rate of drug absorption, minimum effective serum or plasma level, biologic half-life ($t\frac{1}{2}$), duration of action, metabolism, and excretion. The time it takes for half the drug to be excreted or removed from the blood, $t\frac{1}{2}$, is important in determining how often a drug is to be administered and how long to assess for side effects. Therapeutic serum or plasma levels indicate the desired concentration, in serum or plasma, for the drug to exert its beneficial effect. More and more drug therapy is being monitored in this fashion (e.g., antibiotics, theophylline, cardiac glycosides). An additional feature is a listing of commonly accepted therapeutic drug levels on the inside front cover. Metabolism and excretion routes may be important for clients with systemic liver disease or kidney disease or both. Again, information is not available for all therapeutic agents.

Uses: Therapeutic application(s) for the particular agent. Investigational uses are also listed for selected drugs.

Contraindications: Disease states or conditions in which the drug should not be used. The safe use of many of the newer pharmacologic agents during pregnancy or childhood has not been established. As a general rule, the use of drugs during pregnancy is contraindicated unless specified by a physician.

Special Concerns: This section will list information of special concern to the practitioner. For example, whether the drug is considered safe and effective for use in children, during lactation, during pregnancy, and in the geriatric client may be listed. Also, the FDA pregnancy category (for definitions see Appendix 2) to which the drug has been assigned will be listed in this section. Situations when the drugs should be used with caution are listed in this section.

Side Effects: Unwanted or bothersome effects the client *may* experience while taking the particular agent. Side effects are listed by the body organ or system affected. This feature allows easy access to information on potential side effects of each drug. When appropriate, this section will also provide a list of the symptoms observed following an overdose of the drug. The *Treatment of Overdose* will be found as

the last entry in *Administration/ Storage* under *Nursing Considerations*.

Drug Interactions: Drugs that may interact with one another are listed under this entry. The study of drug interactions is an important area of pharmacology and is changing constantly with the influx of new drugs. The compilation of such interactions is far from complete; therefore, listings in this manual are to be considered *only* as general cautionary guidelines.

Drug interactions may result from a number of different mechanisms (additive effects, interference with degradation of drug, increased speed of elimination). Such interferences may manifest themselves in a variety of ways; however, an attempt has been made throughout the text to describe these interactions whenever possible as an increase (↑) or a decrease (↓) in the effect of the drug, followed by a brief description of the reason for the change.

It is important to realize that any side effects that accompany the administration of a particular agent may also be increased as a result of a drug interaction.

The reader should also be aware that the drug interactions are often listed for classes of drugs. Thus, the drug interaction would be likely to occur for all drugs in that particular class.

Laboratory Test Interferences: The manner in which a drug may affect the laboratory test values of the client. Some of these interferences are caused by the therapeutic or toxic effects of the drugs; others result from interference with the testing method itself. Interferences are described as false +, or (↑), values and as false ($-$), or ($\downarrow$), values. Many of the laboratory test interferences are also listed under the *Nursing Considerations* for each drug.

Dosage: The adult and pediatric doses, as well as the dosage form(s) for which the drug is available, are presented when possible and are so indicated. The listed dosage is to be considered as a general guideline, since the exact amount of the drug to be given is determined by the physician. However, one should question orders from the physician when dosages differ markedly from the accepted norm. We have tried to give complete data for drugs that are prescribed frequently.

Nursing Considerations: These will be presented in a nursing process format. The nursing considerations are designed to assist the practitioner in preparing the medications for administration, proper storage, and when applicable, treatment of symptoms of overdose. Also, guidelines to perform assessments of the client before and after prescribed drug therapy will be identified as well as nursing interventions appropriate for the prescribed drug therapy. Important client/family teaching issues related to the particular drug therapy will be addressed and specific outcome criteria will be listed to help the practitioner evaluate the effectiveness of the prescribed drug therapy. Nursing considerations that include assessments and interventions may contain specifics such as:

1. Gathering of physical data and client history.
2. Assessment of specific physiologic functions that may be affected by the drug.

3. Identification of sensitivities and conditions that may contraindicate a particular drug therapy.
4. Physiologic, pharmacologic, and psychologic effects of the drug and how these affect the nursing process.
5. Emergency situations or adverse reactions that can arise as a result of drug therapy and appropriate nursing interventions for these situations.
6. Specific nursing interventions that help relieve a client's discomfort, which may have been precipitated by a particular drug.
7. Nursing interventions that help ensure the safety of the client when receiving drug therapy.

The practitioner must also assess the client for the *Side Effects* listed for that drug. Side effects must be documented and reported to the physician. Severe side effects are generally cause for discontinuation of the drug.

Specific information on client education is provided in the *Nursing Considerations* for each drug. *Nursing Considerations,* related to client/family teaching, emphasizes the practitioner's role as he/she applies the nursing process in client education and in promoting drug compliance. Emphasis is placed on helping the client/family recognize side effects, avoiding potentially dangerous situations, and alleviating anxiety that may result from taking a particular drug. Details on administration including methods and return demonstrations have been addressed. Side effects that should be reported to the physician have been included as well as specifics on how to minimize side effects for certain medications (i.e., take medication with food to decrease GI upset) have also been noted.

The proper education of clients is one of the most challenging aspects of nursing, but the instructions must be tailored to the needs, awareness, and sophistication of each client. Some drugs and drug therapy require the active participation of clients and/or family. For example, clients who take medication to lower blood pressure should assume responsibility for taking their own blood pressure or identifying someone, a significant other perhaps, who is willing to learn how to take their blood pressure. Clients should be taught to always carry identification listing the drugs currently prescribed, to keep a written record of the drugs they take, as well as a record of their blood pressure recordings. One may suggest that this can be done in a notebook or on a calendar. Clients should be instructed to bring these records with them whenever they go for a check-up or seek medical care. These records may also be shared with the pharmacist if there is a question concerning drugs prescribed, if the client is considering taking an over-the-counter medication, or if the client has to change pharmacies. The records should be shared with the health care provider to ensure accurate evaluation of the response to the prescribed drug therapy. The practitioner should use a return demonstration teaching format to ensure understanding and compliance, and to identify early any problems or lack of client ability to comply with the prescribed therapy. They may also provide the client with a phone number to call with

any questions or concerns about the prescribed therapy.

Finally, when taking the nursing history, emphasis should be placed on the client's ability to read and to follow directions. The ability to comprehend what is written or said should not be assumed based on the client's level of education or command of language. Given the current rate of illiteracy, it is possible that persons of another era, who had limited education, may not be able to comprehend what is taught concerning their drug therapy. Clients with language barriers should be identified and appropriate written translations should be provided for these persons. In addition, client life-style and income are important factors that may affect compliance with prescribed drug therapy. The potential for a client being/becoming pregnant, and whether or not a mother is breast feeding her infant should be included in assessments as appropriate. The age of clients and their state of mental acuity, whether learned from personal observation or from discussion with close friends or family members, can be critical in determining potential relationships between drug therapy and/or drug interactions. Including these factors in the nursing assessment will assist all on the health care team to determine the type of therapy and drug delivery system best suited to a particular client and will promote the highest level of client compliance. All clients should be advised to always carry identification and a list of drugs currently prescribed and for what conditions.

An evaluation section has been included to assist the practitioner in determining the effectiveness of the prescribed drug therapy. Specific outcome criteria related to each drug have been delineated to help determine the effectiveness of the drug therapy and to assess the client's response (some of which may include ↓ blood pressure, subjective reports of symptomatic improvement in allergic manifestations, and effective pain control).

The previous points are covered for all drugs or drug classes. When drugs are presented as a group (as in Chapter 2) rather than individually, the points may be covered only once for each group. In this case the practitioner must look for the appropriate entry for the drug class. For example, the *Contraindications, Side Effects, Drug Interactions,* and *Nursing Considerations* for all the insulins are so similar that they are generally listed only once in Chapter 2, under Insulins. However, the individual drug entries are cross-referenced, with page numbers, to this general information.

Information relevant to a particular drug, and not to the whole group, is listed under appropriate headings, such as *Additional Contraindications,, Additional Side Effects,* or *Additional Nursing Considerations.* Such entries are *in addition to* and not *instead of* the regular entry, which must also be consulted.

Additional information to assist the practitioner in administering drugs and monitoring drug therapy appropriately is also found in the text. For example, commonly used laboratory test values and a list of drugs controlled by the U.S. Federal Controlled Substances Act and the Controlled Substances Law (Canada) are found in the appendices. Also, commonly used equivalents, a list of certified poison control centers, and information on the Medic Alert Systems are all included to assist the practitioner. Importantly, nomograms for computing the body surface area for children are included. Dosage based on body surface area is frequently used when calculating the dosage of potent drugs such as those used in chemotherapy to treat cancer.

You are now ready to use NDR-93. We hope that the text will be useful and assist you in your profession. Even though the material presented might, at first, appear overwhelming, remember that the effective drugs currently at the disposal of the health care team are the key to today's better, more effective, and efficient medical care. Certainly, the administration of drugs, assessment of potential interactions, and the evaluation of their effects on the client are crucial parts of the nursing process.

CHAPTER TWO

Therapeutic Drug Classifications

ADRENERGIC BLOCKING AGENTS (SYMPATHOLYTICS)

See also the following individual entries:

Acebutolol Hydrochloride
Atenolol
Betaxolol Hydrochloride
Carteolol Hydrochloride
Esmolol Hydrochloride
Levobunolol
Methysergide Maleate
Metoprolol
Nadolol
Penbutolol Sulfate
Phenoxybenzamine
  Hydrochloride
Phentolamine Mesylate
Pindolol
Propranolol Hydrochloride
Timolol Maleate
Tolazoline Hydrochloride

General Statement: As their name implies, the adrenergic blocking agents (sympatholytics) reduce or prevent the action of the sympathomimetic agents. They do this by competing with norepinephrine or epinephrine (the neurotransmitters) for the various subtypes of either alpha-adrenergic or beta-adrenergic receptor sites. For example, alpha-adrenergic blocking agents prevent the smooth muscles surrounding the arterioles from contracting, whereas beta-adrenergic blocking agents prevent the excitatory effect of the neurotransmitters on the heart. It should also be noted that several antihypertensive agents act by blocking alpha (especially in the CNS) or beta receptors.

Some of the adrenergic blocking agents also have a direct systemic cardiac effect in addition to their peripheral vasodilating effect. The fall in blood pressure accompanying their administration may trigger a compensatory tachycardia (reflex stimulation). The cardiac blood vessels of a patient with arteriosclerosis may be unable to dilate rapidly enough to accommodate these changes in blood volume, and the patient may experience an acute attack of angina pectoris or even cardiac failure.

Adrenergic blocking agents have many undesirable effects which, although not toxic, limit their use. Treatment should always be started at low doses and increased gradually.

ALPHA-ADRENERGIC BLOCKING AGENTS : These drugs reduce the tone of muscles surrounding peripheral blood vessels and consequently increase peripheral blood circulation and decrease blood pressure.

BETA-ADRENERGIC BLOCKING AGENTS : These drugs block the

nerve impulse transmission to the beta receptors of the sympathetic division of the ANS. These receptors are particularly numerous at the postjunctional terminals of the nerve fibers that control the heart muscle and reduce muscle tone. These drugs include atenolol, carteolol, metoprolol, nadolol, penbutolol, pindolol, propranolol, and timolol.

NURSING CONSIDERATIONS

Assessment

1. Note any evidence or history of peptic ulcer disease as drugs should be used cautiously in this setting.
2. Determine baseline blood pressure and pulse and monitor throughout drug therapy.
3. Document any evidence of heart disease and currently prescribed therapy.

Client/Family Teaching

1. Take with milk or meals to minimize GI upset.
2. Advise client to rise slowly from a supine position and dangle legs and feet before rising to prevent orthostatic effects.

Evaluation: Evaluate client for:
- Evidence of a ↓ blood pressure
- Reports of a reduction in anxiety
- ECG evidence of control of ventricular arrhythmias

ADRENOCORTICOSTE-ROIDS AND ANALOGS

See also the following individual entries:

Beclomethasone Dipropionate
Betamethasone
Betamethasone Acetate and Betamethasone Sodium Phosphate
Betamethasone Benzoate
Betamethasone Dipropionate
Betamethasone Sodium Phosphate
Betamethasone Valerate
Corticotropin
Corticotropin Repository
Corticotropin Zinc Hydroxide
Cortisone Acetate
Cosyntropin
Desoxycorticosterone Acetate
Desoxycorticosterone Pivalate
Dexamethasone
Dexamethasone Acetate
Dexamethasone Sodium Phosphate
Fludrocortisone Acetate
Flunisolide
Fluticasone Propionate
Halobetasol Propionate
Hydrocortisone
Hydrocortisone Acetate
Hydrocortisone Butyrate
Hydrocortisone Cypionate
Hydrocortisone Retention Enema
Hydrocortisone Sodium Phosphate
Hydrocortisone Sodium Succinate
Hydrocortisone Valerate
Methylprednisolone
Methylprednisolone Acetate
Methylprednisolone Sodium Succinate
Prednisolone
Prednisolone Acetate
Prednisolone Acetate and Prednisolone Sodium Phosphate
Prednisolone Sodium Phosphate
Prednisolone Tebutate
Prednisone

Triamcinolone
Triamcinolone Acetonide
Triamcinolone Diacetate
Triamcinolone Hexacetonide

Action/Kinetics: The hormones of the adrenal gland influence many metabolic pathways and all organ systems and are essential for survival.

The release of adrenocorticosteroids is controlled by hormones such as corticotropin-releasing factor, produced by the hypothalamus, and ACTH (corticotropin), produced by the anterior pituitary.

The natural adrenocorticosteroids play an important role in most major metabolic processes. They have the following effects:

1. **Carbohydrate metabolism.** Deposition of glucose as glycogen in the liver and the conversion of glycogen to glucose when needed. Gluconeogenesis (i.e., the transformation of protein into glucose).
2. **Protein metabolism.** The stimulation of protein loss from many organs (catabolism). This is characterized by a negative nitrogen balance.
3. **Fat metabolism.** The deposition of fatty tissue in facial, abdominal, and shoulder regions.
4. **Water and electrolyte balance.** Alteration of glomerular filtration rate; increased sodium and consequently fluid retention. Also affects the excretion rate of potassium, calcium, and phosphorus. Urinary excretion rate of creatine and uric acid increases.

According to their chemical structure and chief physiologic effect, the adrenocorticosteroids fall into two subgroups, which have considerable functional overlap.

1. Those, like cortisone and hydrocortisone, that mainly regulate the metabolic pathways involving protein, carbohydrate, and fat. This group is often referred to as *glucocorticoids*. Glucocorticoids are qualitatively similar. Differences between these agents are due to duration of action and half-life (see individual agents).
2. Those, like aldosterone and desoxycorticosterone, that are more specifically involved in electrolyte and water balance. These are often referred to as *mineralocorticoids*. Hormones with mineralocorticoid activity result in reabsorption of sodium (and therefore water retention) and enhanced potassium and hydrogen excretion. Substances such as cortisone and hydrocortisone, although classified as glucocorticoids, possess significant mineralocorticoid activity.

Therapeutically, the adrenocorticosteroids are used for a variety of purposes; a distinction must be made between physiologic doses used for replacement therapy and pharmacologic doses used to treat inflammatory and other disease states. Many slightly modified synthetic variants are available today that possess glucocorticoid but minimal or no mineralocorticoid activity.

The hormones have a marked anti-inflammatory effect because of their ability to inhibit prostaglandin synthesis. These agents also inhibit accumulation of macrophages and leukocytes at sites of inflammation as well as inhibit phagocytosis and lysosomal enzyme release. They aid the organism in coping with various stressful situations (trauma, severe illness). The immunosuppressant effect is thought to be due to a reduction of the number of T lymphocytes, monocytes, and eosinophils. Adrenocorticosteroids also decrease binding of immunoglobulin to receptors on the cell surface and inhibit the synthesis and/or release of interleukins which, in turn, decrease T-lymphocyte blastogenesis and reduce the primary immune response.

Uses: When used for anti-inflammatory or immunosuppressant therapy, the corticosteroid should possess minimal mineralocorticoid activity. Therapy with glucocorticoids is not curative and in many situations should be considered as adjunctive rather than primary therapy.

1. **Replacement therapy.** Acute and chronic adrenal insufficiency, including Addison's disease, congenital adrenal hyperplasia, adrenal insufficiency secondary to anterior pituitary insufficiency. However, not all drugs can be used for replacement therapy; some lack glucocorticoid effects, whereas others lack mineralocorticoid effects. For replacement therapy, drugs must possess both effects.

2. **Rheumatic disorders.** Rheumatoid arthritis (including juveniles), ankylosing spondylitis, acute and subacute bursitis, acute nonspecific tenosynovitis, acute gouty arthritis, psoriatic arthritis, posttraumatic osteoarthritis, synovitis of osteoarthritis, epicondylitis.

3. **Collagen diseases.** Including systemic lupus erythematosus, acute rheumatic carditis, polymyositis.

4. **Allergic diseases.** Control of severe allergic conditions refractory to conventional treatment as serum sickness, drug hypersensitivity reactions, anaphylaxis, urticarial transfusion reactions, acute noninfectious laryngeal edema.

5. **Respiratory diseases.** Including bronchial asthma (and status asthmaticus), symptomatic sarcoidosis, seasonal or perennial rhinitis, berylliosis, aspiration pneumonitis, fulminating or disseminated pulmonary tuberculosis (with appropriate antitubercular therapy), Loeffler's syndrome refractory to other treatment.

6. **Ocular diseases.** Severe acute and chronic allergic and inflammatory conditions including conjunctivitis, keratitis, herpes zoster ophthalmicus, iritis, iridocyclitis, chorioretinitis, diffuse posterior uveitis and choroiditis, optic neuritis, allergic corneal marginal ulcers, sympathetic ophthalmia, and anterior segment inflammation.

7. **Dermatologic diseases.** Including severe erythema multiforme (Stevens-Johnson syndrome), exfoliative dermatitis, mycosis fungoides, severe seborrheic dermatitis, bullous dermatitis herpetiformis, severe psoriasis, angioedema or urticaria, contact dermatitis, atopic dermatitis, pemphigus.

8. **Diseases of the intestinal tract.** To assist client through crises of chronic ulcerative colitis, regional enteritis, intractable sprue.

9. **Nervous system.** Acute exacerbations of multiple sclerosis.

10. **Malignancies.** Including leukemias and lymphomas in adults and acute leukemia in children.

11. **Nephrotic syndrome.** To induce diuresis or remission of proteinuria due to lupus erythematosus or of the idiopathic type.

12. **Hematologic diseases.** Including acquired hemolytic anemia, red blood cell anemia, idiopathic and secondary thrombocytopenic purpura in adults, congenital hypoplastic anemia.

13. **Intra-articular or soft tissue administration.** To treat acute episodes of synovitis of osteoarthritis, rheumatoid arthritis, acute gouty arthritis, epicondylitis, acute nonspecific tenosynovitis, posttraumatic osteoarthritis.

14. **Intralesional administration.** To treat keloids, psoriatic plaques, granuloma annulare, lichen simplex chronicus, discoid lupus erythematosus, cystic tumors of an aponeurosis or ganglia, lesions of lichen planus, necrobiosis lipoidica diabeticorum, alopecia areata.

15. **Miscellaneous.** Septic shock (use controversial), trichinosis with neurologic or myocardial involvement, tuberculosis meningitis with subarachnoid block or impending block (with appropriate antitubercular therapy).

Contraindications: Corticosteroids are contraindicated if infection is suspected because these drugs may mask infections. Also peptic ulcer, psychoses, acute glomerulonephritis, herpes simplex infections of the eye, vaccinia or varicella, the exanthematous diseases, Cushing's syndrome, active tuberculosis, myasthenia gravis. Recent intestinal anastomoses, congestive heart failure or other cardiac disease, hypertension, systemic fungal infections, open-angle glaucoma. Also, hyperlipidemia, hyperthyroidism or hypothyroidism, osteoporosis, myasthenia gravis, tuberculosis. Lactation (if high doses are used).

Topical application in the treatment of eye disorders is contraindicated in dendritic keratitis, vaccinia, chickenpox, or other viral disease that may involve the conjunctiva or cornea. Also tuberculosis and fungal or acute purulent infections of the eye. Topical treatment of the ear is contraindicated in aural fungal infections and perforated eardrum. Topical use in dermatology contraindicated in tuberculosis of the skin, herpes simplex, vaccinia, varicella, and infectious conditions in the absence of anti-infective agents.

Special Concerns: Glucocorticoids should be used with caution in the presence of diabetes mellitus, hypertension, chronic nephritis, thrombophlebitis, convulsive disorders, infectious diseases, renal or hepatic insufficiency, pregnancy. Chronic use of corticosteroids may inhibit the growth and development of children or adolescents. Pediatric clients are also at greater risk for developing cataracts, osteoporosis, avascular necrosis of the femoral heads, and glaucoma. Geriatric clients are more likely to develop hypertension and osteoporosis (especially postmenopausal women).

Side Effects: Small physiologic doses given as replacement therapy or short-term high-dosage therapy during emergencies rarely cause side effects. Prolonged therapy may cause a Cushing-like syndrome with atrophy of the adrenal cortex and subsequent adrenocortical insufficiency. A steroid withdrawal syndrome may occur following prolonged use; symptoms include anorexia, nausea, vomiting, lethargy, headache, fever, joint pain, desquamation, myalgia, weight loss, hypotension.

Fluid and electrolyte: Edema, hypokalemic alkalosis, hypokalemia, hypocalcemia, hypotension or shock-like reaction, hypertension, congestive heart failure. *Musculoskeletal:* Muscle wasting, muscle pain or weakness, osteoporosis, spontaneous fractures including vertebral compression fractures and fractures of long bones, tendon rupture, aseptic necrosis of femoral and humeral heads. *GI:* Nausea, vomiting, anorexia or increased appetite, diarrhea or constipation, abdominal distention, pancreatitis, gastric irritation, ulcerative esophagitis. Development or exacerbation of peptic ulcers with the possibility of perforation and hemorrhage; perforation of the small and large bowel, especially in inflammatory bowel disease. *Endocrine:* Cushing's syndrome (e.g., central obesity, moonface, buffalo hump, enlargement of supraclavicular fat pads), amenorrhea, postmenopausal bleeding, menstrual irregularities, decreased glucose tolerance, hyperglycemia, glycosuria, increased insulin or sulfonylurea requirement in diabetics, development of diabetes mellitus, negative nitrogen balance due to protein catabolism, suppression of growth in children, secondary adrenocortical and pituitary unresponsiveness (especially during periods of stress). *CNS/Neurologic:* Headache, vertigo, insomnia, restlessness, increased motor activity, ischemic neuropathy, EEG abnormalities, seizures, pseudotumor cerebri. Also, euphoria, mood swings, depression, anxiety, personality changes, psychoses. *CV:* Thromboembolism, thrombophlebitis, ECG changes (due to potassium deficiency), fat embolism, necrotizing angiitis, cardiac arrhythmias, myocardial rupture following recent myocardial infarction, syncopal episodes. *Dermatologic:* Impaired wound healing, skin atrophy and thinning, petechiae, ecchymoses, erythema, purpura, striae, hirsutism, urticaria, angioneurotic edema, acneiform eruptions, allergic dermatitis, lupus erythematosus-like lesions, suppression of skin test reactions, perineal irritation. *Ophthalmic:* Glaucoma, posterior subcapsular cataracts, increased intraocular pressure, exophthalmos. *Miscellaneous:* Hypercholesterolemia, atherosclerosis, aggravation or masking of infections, leukocytosis, increased or decreased motility and number of spermatozoa.

In children: Suppression of linear growth; reversible pseudobrain tumor syndrome characterized by papilledema, oculomotor or abducens nerve paralysis, visual loss, or headache.

PARENTERAL USE: Sterile abscesses, Charcot-like arthropathy, subcutaneous and cutaneous atrophy, burning or tingling (especially in the perineal area following IV use), scarring, inflammation, paresthesia, induration, hyperpigmentation or hypopigmentation, blindness when used intralesionally around the face and head (rare), transient or delayed pain or soreness, nystagmus, ataxia, muscle twitching, hiccoughs, anaphylaxis with or without circulatory collapse, cardiac arrest, bronchospasm, arachnoiditis after intrathecal use, foreign body granulomatous reactions.

INTRA-ARTICULAR: Postinjection flare, Charcot-like arthropathy, tendon rupture, skin atrophy, facial flushing, osteonecrosis. Due to reduction in inflammation and pain, clients may overuse the joint.

INTRASPINAL: Aseptic, bacterial, chemical, cryptococcal, or tubercular meningitis; adhesive arachnoiditis, conus medullaris syndrome.

INTRAOCULAR: Application of corticosteroid preparations to the eye may reduce aqueous outflow and increase ocular pressure, thereby inducing or aggravating simple glaucoma. Ocular pressure therefore should be checked frequently in the elderly or in clients with glaucoma. Stinging, burning, dendritic keratitis (herpes simplex), corneal perforation (especially when the drugs are used for diseases that cause corneal thinning). Posterior subcapsular cataracts, especially in children. Exophthalmos, secondary fungal or viral eye infections.

TOPICAL USE: Except when used over large areas, when the skin is broken, or with occlusive dressings, topically applied corticosteroids are not absorbed systemically in sufficiently large quantities to cause the side effects noted in the previous paragraphs. Topically applied corticosteroids, however, may cause atrophy of the epidermis, drying of the skin, or atrophy of the dermal collagen. When used on the face, the agents may cause diffuse thinning and homogenization of the collagen, epidermal thinning, and striae formation. Topical corticosteroids should be used cautiously, or not at all, for infected lesions, and in that case, the use of occlusive dressings is contraindicated. Occasionally, topical corticosteroids may cause a sensitization reaction, which necessitates discontinuation of the drug.

Symptoms of Overdose (continued use of large doses)—Cushing's syndrome: Acne, hypertension, moonface, striae, hirsutism, central obesity, ecchymoses, myopathy, sexual dysfunction, osteoporosis, diabetes, hyperlipidemia, increased susceptibility to infection, peptic ulcer, electrolyte and fluid imbalance. Acute toxicity or death is rare.

Drug Interactions

Acetaminophen / ↑ Risk of hepatotoxicity due to ↑ rate of formation of hepatotoxic acetaminophen metabolite

Alcohol / ↑ Risk of GI ulceration or hemorrhage

Amphotericin B / Corticosteroids ↑ K depletion caused by amphotericin B

Aminoglutethimide / Aminoglutethimide ↓ adrenal response to corticotropin

Anabolic steroids / ↑ Risk of edema

Antacids / ↓ Effect of corticosteroids due to ↓ absorption from GI tract

Antibiotics, broad-spectrum / Concomitant use may result in emergence of resistant strains, leading to severe infection

Anticholinergics / Combination ↑

intraocular pressure; will aggravate glaucoma

Anticoagulants, oral / ↓ Effect of anticoagulants by ↓ hypoprothrombinemia; also ↑ risk of hemorrhage due to vascular effects of corticosteroids

Anticholinesterases / Corticosteroids may ↓ effect of anticholinesterases when used in myasthenia gravis

Antidiabetic agents / Hyperglycemic effect of corticosteroids may necessitate an ↑ dose of antidiabetic agent

Asparaginase / ↑ Hyperglycemic effect of asparaginase and the risk of neuropathy and disturbances in erythropoiesis

Barbiturates / ↓ Effect of corticosteroids due to ↑ breakdown by liver

Bumetanide / Enhanced K loss due to K-losing properties of both drugs

Carbonic anhydrase inhibitors / Corticosteroids ↑ K depletion caused by carbonic anhydrase inhibitors

Cholestyramine / ↓ Effect of corticosteroids due to ↓ absorption from GI tract

Colestipol / ↓ Effect of corticosteroids due to ↓ absorption from GI tract

Contraceptives, oral / Estrogen ↑ anti-inflammatory effect of hydrocortisone by ↓ breakdown by liver

Cyclophosphoramide / ↑ Effect of cyclophosphoramide due to ↓ breakdown by liver

Cyclosporine / ↑ Effect of both drugs due to ↓ breakdown by liver

Digitalis glycosides / ↑ Chance of digitalis toxicity (arrhythmias) due to hypokalemia

Ephedrine / ↓ Effect of corticosteroids due to ↑ breakdown by liver

Estrogens / Estrogens ↑ anti-inflammatory effect of hydrocortisone by ↓ breakdown by liver

Ethacrynic acid / Enhanced K loss due to K-losing properties of both drugs

Folic acid / Folic acid requirements may be increased

Furosemide / Enhanced K loss due to K-losing properties of both drugs

Heparin / Ulcerogenic effects of corticosteroids may → ↑ risk of hemorrhage

Immunosuppressant drugs / ↑ Risk of infection

Indomethacin / ↑ Chance of GI ulceration

Insulin / Hyperglycemic effect of corticosteroids may necessitate an ↑ dose of antidiabetic agent

Isoniazid / ↓ Effect of isoniazid due to ↑ breakdown by liver and ↑ excretion

Ketoconazole / ↓ Effect of corticosteroids due to ↑ rate of clearance

Mexiletine / ↓ Effect of mexiletine due to ↑ breakdown by liver

Mitotane / Mitotane ↓ response of adrenal gland to corticotropin

Muscle relaxants, nondepolarizing / ↓ Effect of muscle relaxants

Neuromuscular blocking agents / ↑ Risk of prolonged respiratory depression or paralysis

Nonsteroidal anti-inflammatory drugs / ↑ Risk of GI hemorrhage or ulceration

Phenobarbital / ↓ Effect of corticosteroids due to ↑ breakdown by liver

Phenytoin / ↓ Effect of

corticosteroids due to ↑ breakdown by liver

Potassium supplements / ↓ Plasma levels of potassium

Rifampin / ↓ Effect of corticosteroids due to ↑ breakdown by liver

Ritodrine / ↑ Risk of maternal edema

Salicylates / Both are ulcerogenic; also, corticosteroids may ↓ blood salicylate levels

Somatrem, Somatropin / Glucocorticoids may inhibit effect of somatrem

Streptozocin / ↑ Risk of hyperglycemia

Theophyllines / Corticosteroids ↑ effect of theophyllines

Thiazide diuretics / Enhanced K loss due to K-losing properties of both drugs

Tricyclic antidepressants / ↑ Risk of mental disturbances

Vitamin A / Topical vitamin A can reverse impaired wound healing in patients receiving corticosteroids

Laboratory Test Interferences: ↑ Urine glucose, serum cholesterol, serum amylase. ↓ Serum potassium, triiodothyronine, serum uric acid. Alteration of electrolyte balance.

Dosage: Dosage is highly individualized, according to both the condition being treated and the client's response. Although the various adrenocorticosteroids are similar in their actions, clients may respond better to one type of drug than to another. It is most important that therapy not be discontinued abruptly. Except for replacement therapy, treatment should always involve the minimum effective dose and the shortest period of time. Long-term use often causes severe side effects. If corticosteroids are used for replacement therapy or high doses are used for prolonged periods of time, the dose must be *increased* if surgery is required.

For topical use, ointment, cream, lotion, solution, plastic tape, aerosol suspension, and aerosol cream are selected, depending on dermatologic condition to be treated.

Lotions are considered best for weeping eruptions, especially in areas subject to chafing (axilla, feet, and groin). Creams are suitable for most inflammations; ointments are preferred for dry, scaly lesions.

NURSING CONSIDERATIONS

Administration of Oral Corticosteroids

1. Administer oral forms of drug with food to minimize ulcerogenic effect.
2. When corticosteroids are given chronically, use the smallest dose possible that will achieve the desired effect.
3. At frequent intervals, the dose of medication should be gradually decreased to determine if symptoms of the disease can be effectively controlled by the smaller amount of drug.
4. When treating clients with conditions such as asthma, ulcerative colitis, and rheumatoid arthritis, corticosteroids, given every other day, may maintain therapeutic effects while reducing or eliminating undesirable side effects. When ordered every other day, administer in the morning to coincide with the normal body secretion of cortisol.
5. Local administration of corticosteroids is preferred over systemic therapy to minimize systemic side effects.

6. Corticosteroids should be discontinued gradually if used chronically.

7. Alternate day therapy may be beneficial in selected clients requiring chronic steroid therapy. With this therapy, twice the usual daily dose of an intermediate-acting steroid is given every other morning. This regimen provides the beneficial effect of the steroid while minimizing pituitary-adrenal suppression.

8. *Treatment of Chronic Overdose:* Gradually taper the dose of the steroid and frequently monitor lab tests. During periods of stress, steroid supplementation is necessary. Dose should be reduced to the lowest one that will control the symptoms (or discontinue the steroid completely). Recovery of normal adrenal and pituitary function may take up to 9 months. Large, acute overdoses may be treated with gastric lavage, emesis, and general supportive measures.

Administration of Topical Corticosteroids

1. Cleanse the area before applying the medication.

2. Wear gloves to apply the agent; apply sparingly and rub gently into the area.

3. When prescribed, apply an occlusive dressing to promote hydration of the stratum corneum and increase the absorption of the medication.

4. The following are two methods of applying an occlusive type dressing (Do not apply an occlusive dressing if infection is present):

- Apply a large amount of medication to the cleansed area. Cover with a thin, pliable, nonflammable plastic film, which is then sealed to the surrounding tissue with skin tape or held in place with gauze. Change the dressing every 3–4 days.

- Apply a small amount of medication to the area and cover with a damp cloth. Then cover with a thin, pliable, nonflammable plastic film and seal to the surrounding tissue with tape, or hold in place with gauze. Change dressing b.i.d.

Assessment

1. Obtain baseline data concerning the client's mental status and neurologic function and record on the client's record.

2. Check medication history for evidence of allergic reactions to corticosteroids or tartrazine, a coloring agent used in certain preparations.

3. Obtain baseline ECG, electrolytes, liver and renal function studies.

4. Document baseline blood pressure, pulse, temperature, and weight.

5. List any medication the client is taking and identify those that may interact with corticosteroids. These include antidiabetic agents, cardiac glycosides, oral contraceptives, anticoagulants, and drugs influenced by liver enzymes.

6. If the client is female, of childbearing age, and sexually active, discuss the possibility of pregnancy and notify the physician if pregnancy is determined.

Interventions

ORAL CORTICOSTEROIDS

1. When the client is first placed on corticosteroids, take the blood pressure at least twice a day until a maintenance dose has been established. Document and report any increases in blood pressure to the physician.
2. Continuously monitor for symptoms of adrenal insufficiency, which include hypotension, confusion, restlessness, lethargy, weakness, nausea, vomiting, anorexia, and weight loss.
3. Repeatedly evaluate the client for increased sodium and fluid retention. Monitor the client's weight and observe for other evidences of edema. If fluid and salt retention are noted, adjust the client's diet to one that is low in sodium and high in potassium. Weigh daily under standard conditions. Anticipate a small weight gain due to increased appetite, but sudden increases are probably due to edema and must be reported. Edema occurs most frequently with cortisone or desoxycorticosterone acetate and occurs less frequently with the new synthetic agents.
4. Assess the client for shortness of breath, distended neck veins, edema and easy fatigue. The client may be in congestive heart failure. Obtain a chest X ray and ECG and compare with the baseline studies.
5. Conduct periodic blood glucose determinations and monitor serum electrolytes and platelet counts for clients on long-term therapy. Note any complaint of unusual bleeding, bruising, the presence of petechiae and any other skin changes.
6. Assess the client's muscles for weakness and wasting as these are signs of a negative nitrogen balance.
7. Report changes in the client's appearance especially those resembling Cushing's syndrome, such as rounding of the face, hirsutism, presence of acne, and thinning of the hair and nails.
8. If the client has diabetes, monitor the blood glucose levels frequently while on corticosteroid therapy. The client may develop hyperglycemia and a change in diet and insulin dosage may be necessary.
9. Assess the client for signs of depression, lack of interest in personal appearance, complaints of insomnia and anorexia. Document on the client's record, compare with prior data, and notify the physician.
10. Discuss with female clients the potential for menstrual difficulties and amenorrhea that may be caused by long-term therapy with corticosteroids.
11. Observe the client for signs and symptoms of other illnesses during therapy with adrenocorticosteroids as these drugs tend to mask the severity of most illnesses.
12. Check the height and weight of children regularly because growth suppression is a hazard of adrenocorticosteroid therapy.
13. GI bleeding may occur. Therefore, when the client is on long-term therapy periodically test the stools for the presence

of occult blood and monitor CBC.

Client/Family Teaching

1. Review the appropriate method for administration or application and the prescribed dosing intervals.

2. Take the medication with food and report to the physician any symptoms of gastric distress. To prevent the problem of gastric irritation, discuss the use of antacids and special diets. Suggest eating frequent small meals. If the symptoms persist, diagnostic X rays may be ordered.

3. Review the symptoms of adrenal insufficiency (see #2 under Interventions) and provide a printed list of adverse drug reactions that should be reported to the physician should they occur.

4. Caution clients and family members to report any changes in mood or affect to the physician.

5. Instruct clients to monitor and record their weight, blood pressure, temperature, and pulse for evidence of physiologic changes that should be reported to the physician. Advise clients to weigh themselves daily at the same time, wearing clothing of approximately the same weight, and using the same scales. Consistent weight gain may be evidence of fluid retention.

6. Assist in identifying foods high in potassium and low in sodium content. Explain how to supplement the diet with potassium-rich foods such as citrus juices and bananas. Instruct in what to look for on labels of canned or processed foods.

7. Encourage clients to eat a diet high in protein to prevent the development of Cushing's syndrome.

8. To decrease the possibility of osteoporosis, explain the need to exercise daily and review foods high in calcium that should be included in the diet.

9. Be especially careful to avoid falls and other accidents. Steroids may cause osteoporosis, which makes the bones more susceptible to fractures. To reduce the possibility of falling and subsequent injury, advise clients to use a night light and to have a hand rail or other device for support if they get up at night.

10. Women using oral contraceptives need to be warned that corticosteroids can cause a loss of contraceptive action. Teach the client how to keep an accurate record of her menstrual periods. If pregnancy is suspected, the physician should be notified immediately.

11. Warn males that corticosteroids may have an adverse effect on the sperm production and count.

12. Review the possible effects on body image (weight gain, acne, excess hair growth, etc.) and explore coping mechanisms and support persons and groups.

13. Explain that if there is a need to withdraw the medication, the process should proceed slowly so that the client's own adrenal cortex will gradually be reactivated and take over the production of hormones. Sudden

withdrawal may be life-threatening. If adverse side effects occur, remind the client not to discontinue therapy with the idea that the changes will be reversed. Any sudden change will provoke symptoms of adrenal insufficiency.

14. If dosage of drug is reduced, provide supportive measures and reassurance to clients who are having flare-ups. Explain that these symptoms are caused by the reduction of drug dosage.

15. Explain to clients with arthritis that they should not overuse the joint once it has become painless. Permanent joint damage may result from overuse, because underlying pathology is still present.

16. If the client has diabetes, discuss the need to monitor glucose levels frequently while taking steroids. If any change is noted, report to the physician and discuss the alterations in insulin and diet that may be necessary.

17. Explain that wounds may heal slowly because steroid therapy causes a delay in development of granulation tissue. There is also an increased potential for infection. Therefore, clients should observe any healing process carefully for signs of infection and report any injury to the physician so that appropriate medical supervision can be implemented.

18. These drugs mask symptoms of infection and cause immunosuppression. Because antibody production is decreased by adrenocorticosteroids, clients are at risk for infection. Explain the need to maintain general hygiene and scrupulous cleanliness to avoid infection. Advise clients to notify the physician if they have a sore throat, cough, fever, malaise, or an injury that does not heal and to avoid contact with persons with known contagious diseases.

19. Advise the client to delay any vaccination while receiving adrenocorticosteroid therapy because there is limited immune response during therapy with steroids.

20. Clients on long-term ophthalmic therapy are prone to developing cataracts, exophthalmus, and increased intraocular pressure. Advise these clients to have routine visits to the ophthalmologist for eye examinations.

21. Assist the client in establishing a means of maintaining a supply of medication on hand to avoid running out of the drug.

22. Stress the need for regular medical supervision to have the dosage of medication checked and adjusted as needed.

23. Remind the client to carry a card identifying the drug being used, the dosage, the condition being treated, and who to contact in the event of an emergency.

24. Discuss with parents the fact that children may develop pseudotumor cerebri. Symptoms of this disorder include vertigo, headache, and convulsions. The physician should be notified immediately. These symptoms should disappear once the therapy is discontinued under medical supervision.

Interventions

TOPICAL CORTICOSTEROIDS

1. Assess for local sensitivity reaction at the site of application. Withhold the medication and report any sensitivity response to the physician.
2. Observe the client closely for signs of infections since corticosteroids tend to mask the problem. Do not apply an occlusive dressing when an infection is present. Document the site of the infection, the nature of the infection and if there is any redness, swelling, odor, or drainage present and report to the physician.
3. If the client has a large occlusive dressing, take temperature every 4 hr. If the temperature is elevated, remove the dressing and notify the physician.
4. Routinely assess the client for evidence of systemic absorption of the medication. Symptoms may include edema and transient inhibition of pituitary-adrenal cortical function as manifested by muscular pain, lassitude, depression, hypotension, and weight loss.
5. If family members are to apply the topical ointment, advise them to wash their hands and to wear gloves or to apply the medication with a sterile applicator. Instruct them concerning what to expect in response to the prescribed therapy.

Evaluation

1. Evaluate client for:
   - Clinical response to date and any need for modifications in diet, drug dosage, or length of therapy
   - Evidence of effectiveness of drug therapy as demonstrated by effective wound healing, suppression of inflammatory and immune responses in allergic reactions, autoimmune diseases, and organ transplant recipients
2. Obtain serum cortisol levels to evaluate effectiveness of replacement therapy in adrenal deficiency states.

ALKYLATING AGENTS

See also the following individual entries:

> Busulfan
> Carboplatin for Injection
> Carmustine
> Chlorambucil
> Cyclophosphamide
> Dacarbazine
> Ifosfamide
> Lomustine
> Mechlorethamine
>   Hydrochloride
> Melphalan
> Mesna
> Pipobroman
> Streptozocin
> Thiotepa
> Uracil Mustard

Action/Kinetics: Alkylating agents are highly reactive in that under physiologic conditions they donate an alkyl group (carbonium ion) to biologically important macromolecules, such as DNA. These reactions inactivate the molecule, bringing *cell division* to a halt. This cytotoxic activity is not limited to cancerous cells, but affects replication of the other cells of an organism, especially that of rapidly proliferating tissues, such as the bone marrow, intestinal epithelium, and hair follicles.

The toxic effects of the alkylating agents are usually cell-cycle non-specific. The cytotoxic effect on cell division becomes apparent when the cell enters the S phase and cell division is blocked at the G_2 phase (premitotic phase), resulting in cells having a double complement of DNA.

Resistance of cancer cells to alkylating agents usually develops slowly and gradually. The resistance seems to be the sum total of several minor adaptations and not a reaction to a single one. Such mechanisms include decreased permeability of the cells, increased production of noncancer receptors (nucleophilic substances), and increased efficiency of the DNA repair system.

NURSING CONSIDERATIONS

See *Nursing Considerations* for individual agents and *Nursing Considerations* for *Antineoplastic Agents,* p. 88.

AMEBICIDES AND TRICHOMONACIDES

See also the following individual entries:

Erythromycins
Gentian Violet
Metronidazole
Paromomycin Sulfate
Tetracyclines

General Statement: Amebiasis is a widely distributed disease caused by the protozoan *Entamoeba histolytica.* The disease has a high incidence in areas with low standards of hygiene. In the United States, the average rate of infestation is generally 1%–10% of the population; however, in certain southern localities, the incidence is as high as 40% of the population.

E. histolytica has two forms: (1) an active motile form known as the trophozoite form, and (2) a cystic form that is resistant to destruction and is responsible for the transmission of the disease.

The overt manifestations of amebiasis vary. Some clients manifest violent acute dysentery (characterized by sudden development of severe diarrhea, cramps, and passage of bloody, mucoid stools); others have few overt symptoms or are even completely asymptomatic.

Diagnosis is made on the basis of microscopic examination of fresh, or at least moist, stools by a trained examiner. More than one sample of stool must be negative before amebiasis can be ruled out.

Amoebae often migrate from the GI tract to other parts of the body (extraintestinal amebiasis). The spleen, lungs, or liver are frequently affected. The amoebae colonize in these organs and form abscesses that may rupture and thereby serve as infectious foci.

At present, no one drug can cure both intestinal and extraintestinal amebic infestations; physicians prefer to use a combination of therapeutic agents. Often the more effective but toxic agents are used initially for a short period of time, while long-term eradication or prophylaxis is carried out with less toxic agents.

Since many of the agents used in the treatment of amebiasis are also used for trichomoniasis, nursing considerations for both amebicides and trichomonacides are listed below.

Infestation with the parasite *Trichomonas vaginalis* causes vaginitis, characterized by an irritating, profuse, creamy, or frothy vaginal discharge associated with severe itching and burning. Diagnosis is made by demonstrating the presence of the trichomonad microscopically in the vaginal secretion.

Vaginitis caused by *T. vaginalis* is treated by various locally applied antitrichomonal agents—often effective amebicides—and also by the oral administration of metronidazole. This drug is usually prescribed for both sexual partners to prevent reinfection. Acid douches (vinegar or lactic acid) are a helpful adjunct to treatment.

Eradication of the infectious agent—which frequently becomes resistant—should be ascertained for 3 months after treatment has ceased. The examination usually is made after menstruation, since trichomonal infections often flare up during menstruation.

The incidence of infections by another protozoan organism, *Giardia lamblia,* is increasing in North America. The organism is transmitted in the feces. Infections are characterized by mucous diarrhea, abdominal pain, and weight loss. Drugs of choice are metronidazole and quinacrine.

NURSING CONSIDERATIONS

See also *General Nursing Considerations For All Anti-Infectives,* p. 83

AMEBICIDES

Assessment: Closely assess clients on therapy for acute dysentery or extraintestinal amebiasis because the agents of choice are highly toxic.

Interventions

1. Anticipate that clients frequently are on combination-drug therapy for amebiasis; observe for toxic reactions to compounds.

2. Be prepared to give intensive supportive nursing care to clients having acute dysentery; assist in the effort to control diarrhea, maintain fluid and electrolyte balance, skin integrity, comfort, and prevent complications caused by malnutrition. The client's activity may have to be curtailed during the acute phase of the disease.

3. Administer drugs only for the period of time ordered and allow for rest periods between courses of therapy. Advise clients against self-medication.

Client/Family Teaching

1. Carriers must continue with drug therapy; stress the benefit to themselves, their families, and their co-workers.

2. Emphasize the necessity for thorough washing of hands, especially in factories, schools, and other institutions where disease is easily spread.

3. Explain the need for food handlers to be particularly conscientious about washing hands after toileting. Emphasize the need to use soap, water, and towels.

4. Client and carriers need to have regular stool examinations to check for recurrence.

5. Instruct clients to have well water tested, as this may be the source of contamination.

6. Stress that client and carriers need to report for follow-up visits to ensure eradication of organisms.

TRICHOMONACIDES

Client/Family Teaching

1. Review the proper methods for douching and stress the im-

portance of good feminine hygiene.

2. Explain the prescribed method of administration; insufflation or insertion of vaginal suppository. Have client self-administer and be available to answer any questions or concerns.

3. Advise to wear a sanitary napkin to prevent clothing or bed linen from becoming stained by the medication in vaginal suppositories, especially if they contain iodine (which does stain). Stress that the sanitary pad must be changed frequently and immediately upon staining because it may serve as a growth medium for the infecting organism.

4. Stress that the sexual partner may be an asymptomatic carrier and may also require therapy to prevent reinfection of the woman.

5. Instruct to use condoms during sexual intercourse while undergoing treatment to prevent reinfections.

Evaluation: Evaluate client for:
- Negative laboratory culture reports and resolution of symptoms of infection
- Clinical and laboratory confirmation of successful eradication and prophylaxis of amebiasis and trichomoniasis

AMINOGLYCOSIDES

See also the following individual entries:

Amikacin Sulfate
Gentamicin Sulfate
Kanamycin Sulfate
Neomycin Sulfate
Paromomycin Sulfate
Streptomycin Sulfate
Tobramycin Sulfate

General Statement: The aminoglycosides are broad-spectrum antibiotics, primarily used for the treatment of serious gram-negative infections caused by *Pseudomonas, Escherichia coli, Proteus, Klebsiella,* and *Enterobacter.* Aminoglycoside antibiotics are distributed in the extracellular fluid and cross the placental barrier, but not the blood-brain barrier. Penetration of the CSF is increased when the meninges are inflamed.

The aminoglycosides are excreted, largely unchanged, in the urine. This makes the drugs suitable for urinary tract infections. Concomitant administration of bicarbonate (alkalinization of urine) improves the treatment of such infections. Considerable cross-allergenicity occurs among the aminoglycosides. These drugs are powerful antibiotics and can induce serious side effects. They should not be used for minor infections. Except for streptomycin, resistance of the organisms to aminoglycosides develops slowly. Whenever possible, the sensitivity of the infectious agent should be determined before instituting therapy.

Action/Kinetics: Believed to inhibit protein synthesis by binding irreversibly to ribosomes (30S subunit), thereby interfering with an initiation complex between messenger RNA and the 30S subunit. This leads to production of nonfunctional proteins; polyribosomes are split apart and are unable to synthesize protein. The aminoglycosides are usually bactericidal as a result of disruption of the bacterial cytoplasmic membrane.

The aminoglycosides are poorly absorbed from the GI tract and are therefore usually administered parenterally, the only occasional exceptions being some enteric infections of the GI tract and prior to surgery. They are also absorbed from the peritoneum, bronchial tree, wounds, denuded skin, and joints.

The aminoglycosides are rapidly absorbed after IM injection. **Peak plasma levels:** Usually attained $1/2$–2 hr after IM administration. Measurable levels persist for 8–12 hr after a single administration. **t$1/2$:** 2–3 hr. This value increases sharply in patients with impaired kidney function. Ranges of t$1/2$ from 24 to 110 hr have been observed. Excreted mainly unchanged in urine.

Uses: Gram-negative bacteria causing bone and joint infections, septicemia (including neonatal sepsis), skin and soft tissue infections (including those from burns), respiratory tract infections, postoperative infections, intra-abdominal infections (including peritonitis), urinary tract infections. In combination with clindamycin for mixed aerobic-anaerobic infections. Also, see individual drugs.

They should be used for gram-positive bacteria only when other less toxic drugs are either ineffective or contraindicated. Their use in CNS *Pseudomonas* infections such as meningitis or ventriculitis is questionable.

Contraindications: Hypersensitivity to aminoglycosides, long-term therapy (except streptomycin for tuberculosis). Use with extreme caution in clients with impaired renal function or preexisting hearing impairment. Safe use in pregnancy and during lactation not established.

Special Concerns: Premature infants, neonates, and older clients receiving aminoglycosides should be assessed closely as they are particularly sensitive to their toxic effects.

Side Effects: *Ototoxicity:* Both auditory and vestibular damage have been noted. The risk of ototoxicity and vestibular impairment is increased in clients with poor renal function and in the elderly. Auditory symptoms include tinnitus and hearing impairment, while vestibular symptoms include dizziness, nystagmus, vertigo, and ataxia.

Renal Impairment: This may be characterized by cylindruria, oliguria, proteinuria, azotemia, hematuria, increase or decrease in frequency of urination; increased BUN, nonprotein nitrogen, or creatinine; and increased thirst. *Neurotoxicity:* Neuromuscular blockade, headache, tremor, lethargy, paresthesia, peripheral neuritis (numbness, tingling, or burning of face/mouth), arachnoiditis, encephalopathy, acute organic brain syndrome. CNS depression, characterized by stupor, flaccidity, and rarely, coma, and respiratory depression in infants. Optic neuritis with blurred vision or loss of vision. *GI:* Nausea, vomiting, diarrhea, increased salivation, anorexia, weight loss. *Allergic:* Rash, urticaria, pruritus, burning, fever, stomatitis, eosinophilia. Rarely, agranulocytosis and anaphylaxis. Cross-allergy among aminoglycosides has been observed. *Miscellaneous:* Joint pain, laryngeal edema, pulmonary fibrosis, superinfection.

Symptoms of Overdose: Extension of side effects.

Drug Interactions

Bumetanide / ↑ Risk of ototoxicity

Capreomycin / ↑ Muscle relaxation

Cephalosporins / ↑ Risk of renal toxicity

Ciprofloxacin HCl / Additive antibacterial activity

Cisplatin / Additive renal toxicity

Colistimethate / ↑ Muscle relaxation

Digoxin / Possible ↑ or ↓ effect of digoxin

Ethacrynic acid / ↑ Risk of ototoxicity

Furosemide / ↑ Risk of ototoxicity

Methoxyflurane / ↑ Risk of renal toxicity

Penicillins / ↓ Effect of aminoglycosides

Polymyxins / ↑ Muscle relaxation

Skeletal muscle relaxants (surgical) / ↑ Muscle relaxation

Vancomycin / Additive ototoxicity and renal toxicity

Vitamin A / ↓ Effect of vitamin A due to ↓ absorption from GI tract

Laboratory Test Interferences: ↑ BUN, BSP retention, creatinine, AST, ALT, bilirubin. ↓ Cholesterol values.

NURSING CONSIDERATIONS

See also *General Nursing Considerations For All Anti-Infectives,* p. 83.

Administration/Storage

1. Check expiration date.
2. Warn client if the particular drug being administered stings or causes a burning sensation.
3. During IM administration
   - Inject drug deep into muscle mass to minimize transient pain.
   - Use a Z track method for thin, elderly clients.
   - Rotate and document injection sites.
4. With IV administration
   - Dilute with the appropriate compatible solution.
   - Infuse at the rate ordered to prevent excessive serum concentrations.
5. Administer for only 7–10 days and avoid repeating course of therapy unless a serious infection is present that does not respond to other antibiotics.
6. Administer around the clock to maintain therapeutic drug levels.
7. *Treatment of Overdose:* Undertake hemodialysis (preferred) or peritoneal dialysis.

Assessment

1. Assess for any history of adverse reactions and hypersensitivity to anti-infective medications.
2. Weigh client prior to administering medication to ensure correct calculation of dosage.
3. Determine baseline renal and auditory function.
4. Assess renal, auditory, and vestibular function before and regularly during drug administration.
5. Assess client for the presence and possibly source(s) of infection. Document vital signs (evidence of fever), culture reports, and wound appearance when applicable.

Interventions

1. Monitor intake and output and ensure adequate fluid intake.

2. During therapy, monitor serum drug levels and if levels are elevated, withhold drug and notify the physician. (Blood levels exceeding 30 mcg/ml of amikacin are considered toxic.)

3. Protect client with vestibular dysfunction by supervising ambulation and providing side rails if necessary. Flag chart with (potential for) fall hazard.

4. Continue to monitor for ototoxicity, because the onset of deafness may occur several weeks after the aminoglycoside has been discontinued.

5. Do not administer concurrently or sequentially with a topical or systemic nephrotoxic or ototoxic drug (e.g., potent diuretics such as ethacrynic acid or furosemide) unless physician determines that the benefits outweigh the risks.

6. Monitor for signs of ototoxicity; pretreatment audiograms may be helpful in evaluating this problem. Subjective hearing loss or loss of high tones on the audiometer is most common with kanamycin and neomycin. Also, assess for tinnitus and vertigo (signs of vestibular injury more common with gentamicin and streptomycin).

7. Observe for neuromuscular blockade with muscular weakness leading to apnea, when aminoglycoside is administered together with a muscle relaxant or after anesthesia. Have calcium gluconate or neostigmine available to reverse blockade.

8. Note the presence of cells or casts in the urine, oliguria, proteinuria, lowered specific gravity, or increasing BUN, nonprotein nitrogen, or creatinine, all of which are indicators of altered renal function.

Client/Family Teaching

1. Review goals of therapy and appropriate prescribed method of administration.

2. Discuss potential side effects and stress the importance of notifying physician if any of these occur, as drug may need to be discontinued.

3. Teach the importance of following a balanced diet and maintaining good nutrition.

4. Explain the importance of taking medications at the prescribed time intervals, around the clock, until the prescription is finished.

5. Stress that any alterations in hearing, vision, and/or ambulation should be reported immediately.

6. Review symptoms of superinfection (black, furry tongue; loose, foul-smelling stools; vaginal itching) and advise to report immediately.

Evaluation: Evaluate client for:

- A positive clinical response as evidenced by negative laboratory culture reports
- Evidence of knowledge and understanding of illness and assess response to teaching as well as compliance with prescribed therapy
- Clinical evidence and subjective reports of symptomatic improvement
- Laboratory confirmation that serum drug levels are within desired therapeutic range.

4-AMINOQUINOLINES

See also the following individual entries:

Chloroquine Hydrochloride
Chloroquine Phosphate
Hydroxychloroquine Sulfate

Action/Kinetics: Several mechanisms have been proposed for the action of 4-aminoquinolines. These include (a) an active chloroquine–concentrating mechanism in the acid vesicles of the parasite causing inhibition of growth, (b) release of aggregates of ferriprotoporphyrin IX from erythrocytes in the parasite causing membrane damage and erythrocyte or parasite lysis, (c) interference with hemoglobin digestion by the parasite, and (d) interference with synthesis of nucleoprotein by the parasite. The drugs are active against the erythrocytic forms of *Plasmodium vivax* and *P. malariae* as well as most strains of *P. falciparum*. The aminoquinolines are rapidly and almost completely absorbed from the GI tract and are widely distributed throughout the body. **Peak serum levels:** 1–6 hr. These agents are excreted extremely slowly, and the presence of some drug has been demonstrated in the bloodstream weeks and even months after the drug has been discontinued. Up to 70% may be excreted unchanged. Urinary excretion is increased by acidifying the urine; excretion is slowed by alkalinization.

Uses: Treatment or prophylaxis of acute attacks of malaria caused by *Plasmodium falciparum, P. vivax, P. ovale,* and *P. malariae*. Will cause a radical cure of vivax and malariae malaria if combined with primaquine. The drugs are effective only against the erythrocytic stages and therefore will not prevent infections. However, the drugs will completely cure infection due to sensitive strains of falciparum malaria.

Extraintestinal amebiasis caused by *Entamoeba histolytica*. Discoid or lupus erythematosus, scleroderma, pemphigus, lichen planus, polymyositis, sarcoidosis, porphyria cutanea tarda.

Contraindications: Hypersensitivity. Changes in retinal or visual field. Lactation. Use in psoriasis or porphyria only if benefits clearly outweigh risks. Not to be used concomitantly with gold or phenylbutazone or in clients receiving drugs that depress blood-forming elements of bone marrow.

Special Concerns: To be used with extreme caution in the presence of hepatic, severe GI, neurologic, and blood disorders. Infants and children are sensitive to the effects of 4-aminoquinolines. Certain strains of *P. falciparum* are resistant to 4-aminoquinolines.

Side Effects: *GI:* Nausea, vomiting, diarrhea, cramps, anorexia, epigastric distress, stomatitis, dry mouth. *CNS:* Headache, fatigue, nervousness, anxiety, irritability, agitation, apathy, confusion, personality changes, depression, psychoses, seizures. *CV:* Hypotension, ECG changes (inversion or depression of T wave, widening of QRS complex). *Dermatologic:* Pruritus, changes in pigment of skin and mucous membranes, dermatoses, bleaching of hair. *Hematologic:* Neutropenia, aplastic anemia, thrombocytopenia, agranulocytosis. *Ocular:* Retinopathy that may be permanent and may lead to blindness. Blurred vision, difficulty in focusing or in accommodation; chronic use may lead to corneal deposits or keratopathy. *Miscellaneous:* Peripheral neuritis, ototoxicity, neuromyopathy manifested by muscle weakness. *Symptoms of Overdose:* Headache, drowsiness, visual disturbances, cardiovascular collapse, seizures followed by sudden and early respiratory and cardiac arrest. Infants and children have manifested respiratory depression, cardiovascular collapse, shock, seizures, and death following overdoses of parenteral chloroquine. ECG changes include nodal rhythm, atrial standstill, prolonged intraventricular conduction, and bradycardia, which lead to ventricular fibrillation or arrest.

Drug Interactions

Acidifying agents, urinary (ammonium chloride, etc.) /
↑ Urinary excretion of antimalarial and thus ↓ its effectiveness

Alkalinizing agents, urinary (bicarbonate, etc.) /
↓ Excretion of antimalarial and thus ↑ amount of drug in system

Antipsoriatics /
4-Aminoquinolines inhibit antipsoriatic drugs

MAO inhibitors / ↑ Toxicity of 4-aminoquinolines due to ↓ breakdown in liver

Laboratory Test Interference: Colors urine brown.

Dosage: See individual drug entries.

NURSING CONSIDERATIONS

See also *General Nursing Considerations For All Anti-Infectives,* p. 83.

Administration/Storage

1. Store in amber-colored containers.
2. *Treatment of Overdose:* Undertake gastric lavage or emesis followed by activated charcoal. Seizures should be controlled prior to gastric lavage. Seizures due to anoxia can be treated by oxygen, mechanical ventilation, or vasopressors (in shock with hypotension). Tracheostomy or tracheal intubation may be required. Forced fluids and acidification of the urine may hasten excretion. Peritoneal dialysis and exchange transfusions may also help.

Assessment

1. Assess for retinopathy manifested by visual disturbances. Retinal changes are not reversible. Regular ophthalmologic examinations are mandatory during prolonged therapy.
2. Note any evidence of hepatic, neurologic, or blood disorders.

Interventions

1. Observe for acute toxicity, which may occur in accidental overdosage in children or in suicidal clients. Symptoms of acute toxicity develop within 30 min of ingestion. Death may occur within 2 hr.
2. Symptoms of acute toxicity to observe for may include headache, drowsiness, visual disturbances, cardiovascular collapse, convulsions, and cardiac arrest.
3. Monitor vital signs, intake and output, and state of consciousness at frequent intervals and document.
4. Anticipate that fluids will have

to be forced and ammonium chloride administered for weeks to months to acidify urine and promote renal excretion of the drug.

5. Check toxic effects of other drugs being used because the combination with chloroquine may intensify toxic effects.

6. For suppressive therapy, administer the drug on the same day each week. Give immediately before or after meals to minimize gastric irritation.

7. Administer with the evening meal when managing discoid lupus erythematosus.

8. Evaluate ophthalmologic examination findings to determine if any retinal damage has occurred.

Client/Family Teaching

1. Review the prescribed method for administration and time intervals at which to take the medication.

2. Provide a printed list of the signs and symptoms of drug toxicity. Instruct client to report any persistent or bothersome side effects.

3. Stress the importance of reporting for scheduled medical visits and lab studies.

4. Ensure that adequate fluid intake as well as the medications prescribed to acidify urine are taken and followed as ordered.

5. Explain that drug may discolor urine brown and not to be alarmed.

6. Keep medications in child-proof containers and warn to keep out of children's reach.

Evaluation: Evaluate client for:

• Evidence of knowledge and understanding of illness and response to therapy as well as level of compliance

• Status of pretreatment symptoms and review laboratory findings for evidence of parasites

• Reports of improvement of symptoms

• Freedom from complications or adverse drug effects

AMPHETAMINES AND DERIVATIVES

See also the following individual entries:

Amphetamine Sulfate
Benzphetamine Hydrochloride
Dextroamphetamine Sulfate
Diethylpropion Hydrochloride
Fenfluramine Hydrochloride
Mazindol
Methamphetamine
 Hydrochloride
Phendimetrazine Tartrate
Phentermine Hydrochloride
Phentermine Resin
Phenylpropanolamine
 Hydrochloride

Action/Kinetics: Response to amphetamines is individualized. Psychic stimulation is often followed by a rebound effect manifested as fatigue. Tolerance will develop to all drugs of this class. The slight differences in the pharmacologic reactions and side effects of the different anorexiants (appetite suppression, respiratory stimulation, length of action) dictate their principal use.

These drugs are thought to act on the cerebral cortex and reticular activating system (including the medullary, respiratory, and vasomotor centers) by releasing norepinephrine from central adrenergic neurons. High doses cause release of dopamine from the mesolimbic system. The stimulatory effect on the CNS causes an increase in motor activity and mental alertness, a mood-elevating effect, a slight euphoric effect, and an anorexigenic effect. The anorexigenic effect is thought to be produced by direct stimulation of the satiety center in the lateral hypothalamic feeding center of the brain. Peripheral effects are mediated by alpha- and beta-adrenergic receptors and include increases in both systolic and diastolic blood pressure and respiratory stimulation. Amphetamines are readily absorbed from the GI tract and are distributed throughout most tissues, with the highest concentrations in the brain and CSF. Duration of anorexia (PO): 3–6 hr. Metabolized in liver and excreted by kidneys.

There is a relatively wide margin of safety between the therapeutic and toxic doses of amphetamines. However, amphetamines can cause both acute and chronic toxicity. Amphetamines are excreted slowly (5–7 days), and cumulative effects may occur with continued administration.

Uses: See individual drugs.

Contraindications: Hyperthyroidism, advanced arteriosclerosis, nephritis, diabetes mellitus, hypertension, narrow-angle glaucoma, angina pectoris, cardiovascular disease, and individuals with hypersensitivity to these drugs. Use in emotionally unstable persons susceptible to drug abuse and in agitated states. Psychotic children. Lactation. Appetite suppressants in children less than 12 years of age. Within 14 days of MAO inhibitors.

Special Concerns: Pregnancy category, amphetamines: C. To be used with caution in clients suffering from hyperexcitability states; in elderly, debilitated, or asthenic clients; and in clients with psychopathic personality traits or a history of homicidal or suicidal tendencies.

Side Effects: *CNS:* Nervousness, dizziness, depression, headache, insomnia, euphoria, symptoms of excitation. Rarely, psychoses. In children, manifestation of vocal and motor tics and Tourette's syndrome. *GI:* Nausea, vomiting, cramps, diarrhea, dry mouth, constipation, metallic taste, anorexia. *CV:* Arrhythmias, palpitations, dyspnea, pulmonary hypertension, peripheral hyper- or hypotension, precordial pain, fainting. *Dermatologic:* Symptoms of allergy including rash, urticaria, erythema, burning. Pallor. *GU:* Urinary frequency, dysuria. *Ophthalmologic:* Blurred vision, mydriasis. *Hematologic:* Agranulocytosis, leukopenia. *Endocrine:* Menstrual irregularities, gynecomastia, impotence, and changes in libido. *Miscellaneous:* Alopecia, increased motor activity, fever, sweating, chills, muscle pain, chest pain.

Long-term use results in psychic dependence, as well as a high degree of tolerance.

Symptoms of Acute Overdose (Toxicity): Restlessness, irritability, insomnia, tremor, hyperreflexia, rhabdomyolysis, rapid respiration, hyperpyrexia, assaultiveness, hallucinations, panic states, sweating, mydriasis, flushing, hyperactivity, confusion, hypertension or hypotension, extrasystoles, tachypnea, fever, delirium, self-injury, arrhythmias, seizures, coma, circulatory collapse, death. Death usually results from cardiovascular collapse or convulsions.

Symptoms of Chronic Toxicity: Chronic use/abuse is characterized by emotional lability, loss of appetite, severe dermatoses, hyperactivity, insomnia, irritability, somnolence, mental impairment, occupational deterioration, a tendency to withdraw from social contact, teeth grinding, continuous chewing, and ulcers of the tongue and lips. Prolonged use of high doses can elicit symptoms of paranoid schizophrenia, including auditory and visual hallucinations and paranoid ideation.

Drug Interactions

Acetazolamide / ↑ Effect of amphetamine by ↑ renal tubular reabsorption

Ammonium chloride / ↓ Effect of amphetamine by ↓ renal tubular reabsorption

Anesthetics, general / ↑ Risk of cardiac arrhythmias

Antihypertensives / Amphetamines ↓ effect of antihypertensives

Ascorbic acid / ↓ Effect of amphetamine by ↓ renal tubular reabsorption

Furazolidone / ↑ Toxicity of anorexiants due to MAO activity of furazolidone

Guanethidine / ↓ Effect of guanethidine by displacement from its site of action

Haloperidol / ↓ Effect of amphetamine by ↓ uptake of drug at its site of action

Insulin / Amphetamines alter insulin requirements

MAO inhibitors / All peripheral, metabolic, cardiac, and central effects of amphetamine are potentiated for up to 2 weeks after termination of MAO inhibitor therapy (symptoms include hypertensive crisis with possible intracranial hemorrhage, hyperthermia, convulsions, coma); death may occur. ↓ Effect of amphetamine by ↓ uptake of drug into its site of action

Methyldopa / ↓ Hypotensive effect of methyldopa by ↑ sympathomimetic activity

Phenothiazines / ↓ Effect of amphetamine by ↓ uptake of drug at its site of action

Sodium bicarbonate / ↑ Effect of amphetamine by ↑ renal tubular reabsorption

Thiazide diuretics / ↑ Effect of amphetamine by ↑ renal tubular reabsorption

Tricyclic antidepressants / ↓ Effect of amphetamines

Laboratory Test Interference: ↑ Urinary catecholamines, ↑ plasma corticosteroid levels.

Dosage: See individual drugs. Many compounds are timed-release preparations.

NURSING CONSIDERATIONS

Administration/Storage

1. If the drug is prescribed to suppress the appetite, administer 30 min before meals.
2. The initial dose should be small, then increased gradually as necessary, for the individual.
3. Unless otherwise ordered by the physician, the last dose of drug for the day should be administered at least 6 hr before the client retires.
4. *Treatment of Acute Toxicity (Overdosage):*
   - Symptomatic treatment. After oral ingestion, induce emesis or perform gastric lavage, followed by use of

activated charcoal. Acidification of the urine increases the rate of excretion. Fluids should be given until urine flow is 3–6 ml/kg/hr; furosemide or mannitol may be beneficial.

- Adequate circulation and respiration should be maintained.
- CNS stimulation can be treated with chlorpromazine and psychotic symptoms with haloperidol. Hyperactivity can be treated with diazepam or a barbiturate. Stimuli should be reduced and the client maintained in a quiet, dim environment. Clients who have ingested an overdose of long-acting products should be treated for toxicity until all symptoms of overdosage have disappeared.
- IV phentolamine may be used for hypertension, whereas hypotension may be reversed by IV fluids and possibly vasopressors (used with caution).

Assessment

1. Obtain a complete drug history. Identify the medications the client is currently taking, the reasons, and the effectiveness of these medications in treating the problem.
2. Note any physical conditions that would contraindicate the client receiving drugs in this category.
3. Note the client's age and whether debilitated.
4. Drugs in this category are under the Controlled Substances Act. Therefore, follow appropriate policy for handling

amphetamines to restrict availability and discourage abuse.

Interventions

1. Note if the client appears agitated or complains of sleeplessness. Notify the physician and anticipate a reduction in the dosage of drug.
2. Clients who have been receiving MAO inhibitors or who have received them 7–14 days before starting amphetamine therapy are susceptible to hypertensive crisis. Monitor such clients closely. If the client develops fever, marked sweating, excitation, delirium, tremors, or twitching, document and report to the physician immediately. If the client is in the hospital, pad the side rails and have a suction machine available at the bedside.
3. Monitor vital signs and blood pressure. Assess for evidence of arrhythmias, tachycardia, or hypertension. Cardiovascular changes accompanied by psychotic syndrome usually indicate acute toxicity.
4. If the client complains of loss of appetite, somnolence, appears mentally impaired, and experiences occupational impairment, the drug should be discontinued.
5. Observe for signs of psychologic dependence and drug tolerance because, if present, the drug should be discontinued.
6. At least once a week weigh the client to detect weight loss. Clients receiving amphetamines may become anorexic. Severe and persistent weight loss should be reported to the

physician. The dosage of drug may need to be adjusted or the drug therapy may need to be changed.

7. Document growth inhibition in children through periodic determinations of height.

Client/Family Teaching

1. When anorexiants are used for weight reduction, their effect lasts only 4–6 weeks. Stress that use is short term. Therefore, clients need to follow a dietary and exercise regimen established by the physician to maintain weight loss.

2. Advise to take 1 hr before meals. Have a dietitian discuss a weight control and/or reducing diet with clients and assist them with meal planning.

3. Advise to take only as directed and never to share medications. Provide a printed list of symptoms of drug tolerance and explain that these may develop rapidly. If tolerance does develop, notify the physician and begin decreasing the dose of medication, as directed.

4. Warn that amphetamines may cause a false sense of euphoria and well being as well as mask extreme fatigue. These may impair judgment and ability to perform potentially hazardous tasks, such as operating a machine or an automobile. Using amphetamines to treat fatigue is inappropriate because rebound effects may be severe.

5. Advise clients that they should seek medical assistance if they experience extreme fatigue and depression once the drug is discontinued. Advise that periodic "drug holidays" may be ordered to assess progress and prevent dependence.

6. Avoid ingesting large amounts of caffeine in any form.

7. Advise that symptoms of drug-induced dry mouth may be decreased by frequently rinsing the mouth, chewing sugarless gum, or sucking sugarless hard candies.

8. Amphetamines may alter insulin and dietary requirements. Therefore, clients with diabetes mellitus need to be warned to monitor their blood sugar closely. Client may require a change in the dose of insulin, oral hypoglycemic agent, and/or dietary requirements.

9. Advise clients to take medication only as prescribed and remind them of the importance of keeping all appointments for regular medical follow-up.

10. Store all medications safely out of the reach of children.

Evaluation

1. Evaluate client for a positive clinical response as demonstrated by an improvement in or resolution of pretreatment symptoms, such as improved attention span, a reduction in weight, or a decreased incidence of narcolepsy.

2. Assess client for any early symptoms or evidence of drug toxicity and/or drug dependence.

ANGIOTENSIN-CONVERTING ENZYME (ACE) INHIBITORS

See also the following individual entries:

Benazepril
Captopril
Enalapril
Fosinopril
Lisinopril
Quinapril
Ramipril

Action/Kinetics: The angiotensin-converting enzyme (ACE) inhibitors are believed to act by suppressing the renin-angiotensin-aldosterone system. Renin, which is synthesized by the kidneys, is released into the general circulation where it produces angiotensin I, an inactive decapeptide derived from plasma globulin substrate. Angiotensin I is converted to angiotensin II by angiotensin-converting enzyme. Angiotensin II is a potent vasoconstrictor that also stimulates secretion of aldosterone from the adrenal cortex, resulting in sodium and fluid retention. The ACE inhibitors prevent the conversion of angiotensin I to angiotensin II. This results in a decrease in plasma angiotensin II and subsequently a decrease in blood pressure and decreased aldosterone secretion (leading to sodium and fluid loss). There may be either no change or an increase in cardiac output. Several weeks of therapy may be required to achieve the maximum effect to reduce blood pressure. Standing and supine blood pressures are lowered to about the same extent. The drugs are also antihypertensive in low renin hypertensive clients.

Uses: Alone or in combination with other antihypertensive agents for the treatment of hypertension. See also individual drug entries.

Contraindications: History of angioedema due to previous treatment with an ACE inhibitor.

Special Concerns: Pregnancy category: C (captopril); pregnancy category: D (benazepril, enalapril, fosinopril, lisinopril, ramipril). ACE inhibitors may cause a profound drop in blood pressure following the first dose; therapy should be initiated under close medical supervision. Use with caution in renal disease as increases in BUN and serum creatinine have occurred; thus, monitor carefully in clients with impaired renal function. With the exception of fosinopril (contraindicated), use with caution during lactation. Geriatric clients may show a greater sensitivity to the hypotensive effects of ACE inhibitors. For most ACE inhibitors, safety and effectiveness have not been determined in children.

Side Effects: See individual entries. Side effects common to most ACE inhibitors include the following. *GI:* Abdominal pain, nausea, vomiting, diarrhea, constipation. dry mouth. *CNS:* Sleep disturbances, insomnia, headache, dizziness, fatigue, nervousness, paresthesias. *CV:* Hypotension, palpitations, angina pectoris, myocardial infarction, orthostatic hypotension, chest pain. *Miscellaneous:* Cough, dyspnea, increased sweating, diaphoresis, pruritus, rash, angioedema, impotence, syncope, asthenia, arthralgia, myalgia.

Symptom of Overdose: Hypotension is the most common.

Drug Interactions

Allopurinol / ↑ Risk of
    hypersensitivity reactions
Antacids / Possible ↓
    bioavailability of ACE inhibitors
Digoxin / ↑ Plasma digoxin levels
Indomethacin / ↓ Hypotensive
    effects of ACE inhibitors,
    especially in low renin or

volume-dependent hypertensive clients

Lithium / ↑ Serum lithium levels → ↑ risk of toxicity

Phenothiazines / ↑ Effect of ACE inhibitors

Potassium-sparing diuretics / ↑ Serum potassium levels

Potassium supplements / ↑ Serum potassium levels

Thiazide diuretics / Additive effect to ↓ blood pressure

Laboratory Test Interferences: ↑ BUN and creatinine (both are transient and reversible). ↑ Liver enzymes, serum bilirubin, uric acid, blood glucose. Small ↑ in serum potassium.

Dosage: See individual drugs.

NURSING CONSIDERATIONS

Administration/Storage

1. ACE inhibitor therapy should not be interrupted or discontinued without consulting a physician.
2. *Treatment of Overdose:* Supportive measures. The treatment of choice to restore blood pressure is volume expansion with an IV infusion of normal saline. Certain of the ACE inhibitors (captopril, enalaprilat, lisinopril) may be removed by hemodialysis.

Assessment

1. Note any previous therapy with antihypertensive agents and the results.
2. Obtain baseline vital signs, electrolytes, CBC, and renal function studies. Assess urine for proteins.
3. List other medications client currently prescribed noting any that may interact unfavorably.

4. Document any history of hereditary angioedema especially if caused by a deficiency of C1 esterase inhibitor.
5. Evaluate the extent of client's understanding of the disease of hypertension and the therapy as prescribed.
6. Ascertain life-style changes clients may have to make to achieve and maintain the goal of lowered blood pressure.
7. Determine client's ability to take own blood pressure measurement and maintain a record as requested.

Interventions

1. Monitor CBC. Observe clients closely for evidence of neutropenia, (especially in those receiving captopril) as this is an indication to discontinue drug therapy.
2. Monitor client for any evidence of angioedema (swelling of face, lips, extremities, tongue, mucous membranes, glottis, or larynx) especially after first dose of drug. Symptoms may be relieved with antihistamines. If angioedema involves laryngeal edema, client warrants astute observation for airway obstruction. *Discontinue* drug therapy and have epinephrine (1:1000 SC) available.
3. Monitor I&O, weight, and renal function studies, reporting any increases in serum BUN and creatinine.
4. Periodically evaluate urine for any evidence of proteinuria.
5. Monitor BP closely during initiation of therapy, assessing for the development of severe hypotension.

6. For clients undergoing surgery or general anesthesia with drugs that cause hypotension, ACE inhibitors will block angiotensin II formation; thus, hypotension can be corrected by volume expansion.

Client/Family Teaching

1. Take 1 hr before meals and only as directed. Consult physician before interrupting or discontinuing drug therapy.
2. Practice birth control and advise physician if pregnancy is suspected.
3. Discuss the expected drug responses and the adverse side effects of prescribed drugs advising client to report:
   - The development of a nonproductive, persistent, chronic cough as this may be drug induced.
   - Symptoms of sore throat, fever, swelling of hands or feet, irregular heartbeat, signs of angioedema, chest pains, difficulty breathing, or hoarseness immediately.
   - Excessive perspiration, dehydration, vomiting, and diarrhea as these will cause a reduction in BP.
   - Any itching, joint pain, fever, or skin rash.
4. Review prescribed dietary guidelines and advise that salt substitutes containing potassium should not be used without consulting a physician.
5. Explain the importance of adhering to the treatment plan prescribed by the physician. Review the importance of exercise, proper diet, and rest, and of complying with the prescribed drug therapy.
6. Instruct that medication controls but does not cure hypertension. Remind client to take prescribed medication despite feeling better and not to stop abruptly.
7. Teach clients and a family member how to take blood pressure recordings and to report any changes. Explain the importance of keeping a written record to share with the health care provider so that prescribed therapy may be evaluated at each visit.
8. Do not perform activities that require mental alertness until drug effects are realized as they may cause dizziness, fainting, or lightheadedness, especially during the first few days of therapy.
9. Advise to rise slowly from a lying position and to dangle feet before standing and to avoid sudden changes in posture to minimize postural effects.
10. Teach the client and family how to accurately monitor fluid intake and output and weights. Advise to report any overt changes.
11. Avoid any OTC medications, especially cold remedies, without first consulting the physician or pharmacist.
12. Avoid excessive amounts of caffeine, tea, coffee, or cola.
13. Review additional interventions for BP control such as reducing the use of alcohol, discontinuing tobacco products, and developing methods to reduce stress.

Evaluation: Evaluate client for evidence of control of hypertension with a minimum of adverse drug effects.

ANTACIDS

See also the following individual entries:

Aluminum Hydroxide Gel
Aluminum Hydroxide Gel, Dried
Basic Aluminum Carbonate Gel
Calcium Carbonate Precipitated
Dihydroxyaluminum Sodium Carbonate
Gelusil
Gelusil-II
Maalox
Maalox Plus
Maalox TC
Magaldrate
Magnesium Hydroxide
Magnesium Oxide
Mylanta
Mylanta II
Sodium Bicarbonate

General Statement: Hydrochloric acid maintains the stomach at a pH (1–2) necessary for optimum activity of the digestive enzyme pepsin and for stimulating the release of secretin when the acid contents of the stomach pass into the duodenum. Under certain circumstances, however, people suffer adverse reactions due to gastric acidity ranging from heartburn to life-threatening peptic or duodenal ulcers. Although production of acid has an important role in the development of gastric and duodenal ulcers, other factors are also involved. These include endogenous histamine (which can stimulate gastric acid secretion), antigen-antibody reactions, and the psychologic makeup of the client. Acute and chronic GI disturbances are among the most common medical conditions requiring treatment. Various drugs and dietary measures are used for the treatment of hyperacidity states and ulcers, and the use of antacids is an important part of such regimens.

Action/Kinetics: Antacids act by neutralizing or reducing gastric acidity, thus increasing the pH of the stomach and relieving hyperacidity. If the pH is increased to 4, the activity of pepsin is inhibited. The ability of a specific antacid to neutralize acid is termed *acid-neutralizing capacity,* and antacids are selected on this basis. Acid-neutralizing capacity is expressed as mEq/ml and is defined by the HCl required to maintain an antacid suspension at pH 3 for 2 hr in vitro. Ideally, antacids should not be absorbed systemically, although substances such as sodium bicarbonate or calcium carbonate may produce significant systemic effects. The most effective dosage form for antacids is suspensions. Antacids also promote healing of peptic ulcers.

Antacids containing magnesium have a laxative effect, whereas those containing aluminum or calcium have a constipating effect. This is why patients are often given alternating doses of laxative and constipating antacids. Antacids containing aluminum bind with phosphate ions in the intestine forming the insoluble aluminum phosphate, which is excreted in the feces. This is of value in treating hyperphosphatemia of chronic renal failure. **Onset:** Depends on ability of the antacid to solubilize in the stomach and react with hydrochloric acid. The poorly soluble antacids (e.g., magnesium trisilicate) react slower with hydrochloric acid than do the more soluble compounds. **Duration of antacids:** 30 min if fasting; up to 3 hr if taken after meals.

Uses: Treatment of hyperacidity (heartburn, acid indigestion, sour stomach), gastric ulcer, duodenal ulcer, gastroesophageal reflux. Adjunct (with histamine H$_2$-receptor antagonists) in the treatment of hypersecretory conditions (e.g., Zollinger-Ellison syndrome), systemic mastocytosis, and multiple endocrine adenoma. Treatment of hypocalcemia, hypophosphatemia. Prophylaxis of renal calculi.

Contraindications: Sodium-containing products are contraindicated in congestive heart failure, hypertension, or conditions requiring a low-sodium diet. Pregnant or lactating women should not use antacids without physician approval. Children less than 6 years of age.

Special Concerns: Chronic use of aluminum-containing antacids may aggravate metabolic bone disease seen in geriatric clients; also, chronic use of aluminum-containing antacids may contribute to development of Alzheimer's disease.

Side Effects: *Aluminum-containing antacids:* Constipation, intestinal obstruction, aluminum intoxication, hypophosphatemia, osteomalacia. *Calcium carbonate, aluminum-magnesium hydroxide, magnesium oxide, soluble bismuth salts, sodium bicarbonate:* Milk-alkali syndrome, rebound hyperacidity. *Magnesium-containing antacids:* Diarrhea, hypermagnesemia in clients with renal failure.

Drug Interactions

1. *Aluminum-containing antacids:* ↑ Effect of benzodiazepines. ↓ Effect of allopurinol, corticosteroids, diflunisal, digoxin, iron products, isoniazid, penicillamine, phenothiazines, ranitidine, and tetracyclines by ↓ absorption from GI tract.
2. *Aluminum- and magnesium-containing antacids:* ↑ Effect of levodopa, quinidine, and valproic acid probably by ↓ excretion. ↓ Effect of benzodiazepines, captopril, cimetidine, corticosteroids, iron products, ketoconazole, penicillamine, phenothiazines, phenytoin, quinolones, ranitidine, salicylates, tetracyclines either by ↓ absorption from GI tract or ↑ excretion.
3. *Calcium-containing antacids:* ↑ Effect of quinidine by ↓ excretion. ↓ Effect of iron products, phenytoin, salicylates, and tetracyclines either by ↓ absorption from GI tract or ↑ excretion.
4. *Magnesium-containing antacids:* ↑ Effect of dicumarol and quinidine probably by ↓ excretion. ↓ Effect of benzodiazepines, corticosteroids, digoxin, iron products, nitrofurantoin, penicillamine, phenothiazines, and tetracyclines either by ↓ absorption from GI tract or ↑ excretion. Also, systemic antacids ↓ excretion of amphetamines leading to ↑ effect and the effect of anticholinergics is ↓ due to ↓ absorption.

Dosage: See individual drugs.

NURSING CONSIDERATIONS

Administration/Storage

1. Clients who have an active peptic ulcer should take antacids every hour during waking hours for the first 2 weeks.
2. For peptic ulcer disease, it is recommended that most ant-

acids be taken 1 hr and 3 hr after meals and at bedtime.

3. Tablets should be thoroughly chewed before swallowing and followed by a glass of milk or water.

4. Liquid preparations have a more rapid action time and greater activity than tablets.

5. Shake liquid suspensions thoroughly before pouring the medication.

6. The absorption rate of many drugs may be affected by antacids. Enteric-coated tablets may dissolve prematurely. Therefore, if other oral drugs are to be taken, it should be done at least 2 hr after ingestion of the antacid.

7. Administer laxative or cathartic dose at bedtime, as medication takes about 8 hr to be effective and the effect should not interfere with the client's rest.

Assessment

1. Determine if the client has a history of cardiac disease or hypertension. These clients often are on low-sodium diets, so prescribed antacids should also be low in sodium.

2. Note if the client has problems with diarrhea. Antacids containing magnesium may have a laxative effect, worsening this problem.

3. List other drugs the client may be taking to ascertain if any have an unfavorable interaction with the antacid ordered.

4. Note subjective reports of heartburn, indigestion, or epigastric pain. Document precipitating factors and foods as well as location, character, and duration of discomfort.

Interventions

1. Clients taking antacid preparations containing calcium or aluminum are prone to constipation. Encourage them to drink 2500–3000 cc of fluid/day, unless contraindicated and also to increase consumption of foods high in bulk.

2. If the client has renal failure, increasing fluid intake to avoid constipation is not an option. Stool softeners may be necessary.

3. If constipation persists, consult with the physician concerning either changing the antacid or using laxatives and/or enemas.

4. Clients taking antacids that contain magnesium may report having diarrhea. Document and report this to the physician. A change in antacid or alternating a magnesium-based antacid with an aluminum- or calcium-based antacid may be indicated.

Client/Family Teaching

1. Take the medication with water or milk. The liquid acts as a vehicle, transporting the medication to the stomach, where the desired drug action occurs.

2. Take the drug at the prescribed times. Some may need to be taken on an empty stomach, whereas others, such as those used to bind phosphate, may need to be taken with meals.

3. Report persistent constipation or diarrhea to the physician.

4. Avoid taking OTC preparations unless specifically ordered by the physician.

5. Avoid smoking or using alcoholic beverages.

6. Report any evidence of GI

bleeding (dark black or tarry stools, coffee ground emesis) to the physician.

7. Discuss the importance of following the specific dietary regime established as well as adhering to the medication protocol. Explain that antacids should be taken for 4–6 weeks after symptoms have disappeared as healing of the ulcer is not correlated with the disappearance of symptoms.

8. Instruct client to report to the physician if the symptoms for which they are being treated show little or no improvement.

Evaluation: Evaluate client for:
- A positive clinical response as evidenced by an improvement in or resolution of pretreatment symptoms
- Reports of a decrease in gastric pain and upset
- Evacuation of a soft, formed stool
- An increase in gastric pH

ANTHELMINTICS

See also the following individual entries:

Mebendazole
Oxamniquine
Piperazine Citrate
Praziquantel
Pyrantel Pamoate
Thiabendazole

General Statement: Helminthiasis, or infestation of the body by parasites, is a common affliction. Helminths (worms) may infect the intestinal lumen or the worm also may migrate to a particular tissue. Treatment of helminth infections is complicated by the fact that a worm may have one or more morphologic stages. Thus, it is important to ensure that therapy rids the body of eggs and larvae, as well as worms. Also, a client may be infected by more than one type of worm. Factors such as availability and cost of the drug, toxicity, ease of administration, and how long it takes to complete therapy also have a significant impact on successful treatment of helminths. Accurate diagnosis is extremely important before treatment is started because its success depends on selecting the drug best suited for the eradication of a specific infestation. Parasites that infest only the intestinal tract can be eradicated by locally acting drugs. Other parasites enter tissues and must be treated by drugs that are absorbed from the GI tract.

Since many parasitic infestations are transmitted by persons sharing bathroom facilities, the physician may wish to examine all members of the household for parasitic infestation. Treatment is often accompanied or followed by repeated laboratory examinations to determine whether the parasite has been eradicated.

Helminths can be divided into three groups: cestodes (flatworms, tapeworms), nematodes (roundworms), and trematodes (flukes). The following is a brief description of the more common helminths and the drug of choice to treat infections by that particular helminth.

CESTODES (FLATWORMS, TAPEWORMS): The more common tapeworms are the beef tapeworm (*Taenia saginata*), pork tapeworm (*T. solium*), dwarf tapeworm (*Hymenolepis nana*), and the fish tapeworm (*Diphyllobothrium latum*).

The tapeworm consists of a scolex or head that hooks into a segment of intestine. The body is that of a segmented flatworm, sections of which are found in the stools. Tapeworm infestations are difficult to eradicate but have few side effects. **Drug treatment:** Niclosamine and praziquantel.

NEMATODES: 1. **Filaria (filariasis).** Infections due to *Wuchereria bancrofti, Brugia malayi,* and *B. timori* are transmitted by mosquitoes. These parasites are tiny roundworms that migrate into the lymphatic system and bloodstream. Living and dead worms can obstruct the lymphatic system, causing elephantiasis. Mosquito control is the best means of combating this infestation.

Other filarial infections include *Loa loa,* transmitted by the bite of a horsefly, and *Onchocerca volvulus* (onchocerciasis, river blindness), which is transmitted by the bite of a blackfly. **Drug treatment:** Diethylcarbamazine. Suramin sodium (available from Centers for Disease Control) is used to treat onchocerciasis.

2. **Hookworm (uncinariasis).** Intestinal infection caused by *Ancylostoma duodenale* or *Necator americanus,* these infections cause debilitation resulting in iron-deficiency anemia, characterized by fatigue, lassitude, and apathy. **Drug treatment:** Mebendazole or pyrantel pamoate.

3. **Pinworm (enterobiasis).** These intestinal infestations are common in school-age children. Complications are rare, although heavy infestations may cause abdominal pain, weight loss, and insomnia. **Drug treatment:** Mebendazole, piperazine, pyrantel pamoate, pyrvinium pamoate, thiabendazole.

4. **Roundworm (ascariasis).** Caused by *Ascaris lumbricoides,* this infection can cause obstruction of the respiratory and GI tracts. **Drug treatment:** Mebendazole, pyrantel pamoate.

5. **Trichinosis.** Caused by *Trichinella spiralis,* these parasites are transmitted by the consumption of raw or inadequately cooked pork. The infection is serious; larvae burrow into the bloodstream and form cysts in skeletal muscle. **Drug treatment:** Corticosteroids to control the inflammation caused by systemic infestation; mebendazole, thiabendazole.

6. **Threadworm (strongyloidiasis).** This parasite (*Strongyloides stercoralis*) infests the upper GI tract. Heavy infestations can result in malabsorption syndrome, diarrhea, and general discomfort. **Drug treatment:** Thiabendazole.

7. **Whipworm (trichuriasis).** This threadlike parasite (*Trichuris trichiura*) lodges in the mucosa of the cecum. **Drug treatment:** Mebendazole.

TREMATODES: Schistosomiasis (blood flukes or bilharziasis) can be transmitted by contaminated water supplies. The organisms are *Schistosoma mansoni, S. japonicum, S. haematobium,* and *S. mekongi.* The infection is difficult to eradicate. **Drug treatment:** Praziquantel, oxamniquine (*S. mansoni* only).

Side Effects: Since the anthelmintics do not belong to any one chemical group, their side effects are related to specific compounds. However, nausea, vomiting, cramps, and diarrhea are common to most.

NURSING CONSIDERATIONS

See also *General Nursing Considerations For All Anti-Infectives,* p. 83.

Client/Family Teaching

1. Provide written instructions regarding prescribed diet, cathartics, enemas, medications, and follow-up tests when treatment is to be carried out at home.
2. Review these instructions to be sure they are understood by the person responsible for the client's treatment and care. *Good hygienic practices reduce the incidence of helminthiasis.*
3. Advise parent to notify school or institution that child is undergoing therapy.
4. Emphasize the need for follow-up examinations to check the results of treatment.
5. Specific practices are as follows:

PINWORMS

1. Instruct responsible family member how to prevent infestation with pinworms by:
   - Washing hands after toileting and before meals
   - Keeping nails short
   - Washing ova from anal area in the morning
   - Applying antipruritic ointment to anal area to reduce scratching, which transfers pinworms
2. Alert family that physician may wish all members to be examined for pinworms.
3. After the end of the treatment course, swab the perianal area each morning with transparent tape until no further eggs are found on microscopic examination for 7 consecutive days.

ROUNDWORMS: Two to 3 weeks after therapy, stools should undergo microscopic examination to determine fecal egg count. Stools must be examined daily until no further roundworm ova are found.

HOOKWORM/TAPEWORM: After administration of medication, cathartics, and enema, examine the results of the enema for the head of the worm, which will appear bright yellow.

Evaluation: Evaluate client for:
- Evidence of knowledge and understanding of illness and compliance with prescribed therapy
- Negative stool exams and perianal swabs. Check for evidence of eggs and worms and send specimens for microscopic examination to determine effectiveness of drug therapy.
- Causes for repeated infestation and need for further treatment

ANTIANEMIC DRUGS

See also the following individual entries:

Ferrous Fumarate
Ferrous Gluconate
Ferrous Sulfate
Ferrous Sulfate Exsiccated

General Statement: Anemia refers to the many clinical conditions in which there is a deficiency in the number of red blood cells (RBCs) or in the hemoglobin level within those cells. Hemoglobin is a complex substance consisting of a large protein (globin) and an iron-containing chemical referred to as heme. The hemoglobin is contained inside the RBCs. Its function is to combine with oxygen in the lungs and transport it to all tissues of the body, where it is exchanged for carbon dioxide (which is transported back to the lungs where it can be excreted). A lack of either RBCs or hemoglobin may result in an inadequate supply of oxygen to various tissues.

The average life span of a RBC is 120 days; thus, new ones have to be constantly formed. They are produced in the bone marrow, with both vitamin B_{12} and folic acid playing an important role in their formation. In addition, a sufficient amount of iron is necessary for the formation and maturation of RBCs. This iron is supplied in a normal diet and is also salvaged from old RBCs. There are many types of anemia. However, the two main categories are (1) iron-deficiency anemias, resulting from greater than normal loss or destruction of blood cells, and (2) megaloblastic anemias, resulting from deficient production of blood cells. Iron-deficiency anemia can result from hemorrhage or blood loss; the bone marrow is unable to replace the quantity of RBCs lost even when working at maximum capacity (due to iron-deficient diet or failure to absorb iron from the GI tract). The RBCs in iron-deficiency anemias (also called *microcytic* or *hypochromic anemias*) contain too little hemoglobin. When examined under the microscope, they are paler and sometimes smaller than normal. The cause of the iron deficiency must be determined before therapy is started.

Therapy consists of administering compounds containing iron so as to increase the body's supplies.

Megaloblastic anemias may result from insufficient supplies of the necessary vitamins and minerals needed by the bone marrow to manufacture blood cells. Pernicious anemia, for example, results from inadequate vitamin B_{12}. The RBCs characteristic of the megaloblastic anemias are enlarged and particularly rich in hemoglobin. However, the blood contains fewer mature RBCs than normal and usually contains a relatively higher number of immature RBCs (megaloblasts), which have been prematurely released from the bone marrow.

Iron Preparations: These agents are usually a complex of iron and another substance and are normally taken by mouth. The amount absorbed from the GI tract depends on the dose administered; therefore the largest dose that can be tolerated without causing side effects is given. Under certain conditions, iron compounds must be given parenterally, particularly (1) when there is some disorder limiting the amount of drug absorbed from the intestine or (2) when the client is unable to tolerate oral iron.

Iron preparations are effective only in the treatment of anemias specifically resulting from iron deficiency. Blood loss is almost always the only cause of iron deficiency in adult males and postmenopausal females. The daily iron requirement is increased by growth and pregnancy, and iron deficiency is, therefore, particularly common in infants and young children on diets low in iron. Pregnant women and women with heavy menstrual blood loss may also be deficient in iron.

Iron is available for therapy in two forms: bivalent and trivalent. Bivalent (ferrous) iron salts are administered more often than trivalent (ferric) salts because they are less astringent and less irritating than ferric salts and are better absorbed.

Iron preparations are particularly suitable for the treatment of anemias in infants and children, in blood donors, during pregnancy, and in clients with chronic blood loss. Optimum therapeutic responses are usually noted within 2–4 weeks of treatment.

The RDA for iron is 90–300 mg daily.

Action/Kinetics: Iron is an essential mineral normally supplied in the diet. Iron salts and other preparations supply additional iron to meet the needs of the patient. Iron is absorbed from the GI tract through the mucosal cells where it combines with the protein transferrin. This complex is transported in the body to bone marrow where iron is incorporated into hemoglobin. Absorption kinetics depend on the iron salt ingested and on the degree of deficiency. Under normal circumstances, iron is well conserved by the body although small amounts are lost through shedding of skin, hair, and nails and in feces, perspiration, urine, breast milk, and during menstruation. Iron is highly bound to protein.

Uses: Prophylaxis and treatment of iron-deficiency anemia.

Contraindications: Clients with hemosiderosis, hemochromatosis, peptic ulcer, regional enteritis, and ulcerative colitis. Hemolytic anemia, pyridoxine-responsive anemia, and cirrhosis of the liver.

Side Effects: *GI:* Constipation, gastric irritation, mild nausea, abdominal cramps, and diarrhea. These effects may be minimized by ad-ministering preparations as a coated tablet. Soluble iron preparations may stain the teeth.

Symptoms of Overdose: Symptoms occur in four stages—(1) Lethargy, nausea, vomiting, abdominal pain, weak and rapid pulse, tarry stools, dehydration, acidosis, hypotension, and coma within 1–6 hr. (2) If client survives, symptoms subside for about 24 hr. (3) Within 24–48 hr symptoms return with diffuse vascular congestion, shock, pulmonary edema, acidosis, seizures, anuria, hyperthermia, and death. (4) If client survives, pyloric or antral stenosis, hepatic cirrhosis, and CNS damage are seen within 2–6 weeks. Toxic reactions are more likely to occur after parenteral administration.

Drug Interactions

Allopurinol / May ↑ hepatic iron levels

Antacids, oral / ↓ Effect of iron preparations due to ↓ absorption from GI tract

Chloramphenicol / Chloramphenicol ↓ iron clearance from plasma and ↓ iron uptake into red blood cells

Cholestyramine / ↓ Effect of iron preparations due to ↓ absorption from GI tract

Pancreatic extracts / ↓ Effect of iron preparations due to ↓ absorption from GI tract

Penicillamine / ↓ Effect of penicillamine due to ↓ absorption from GI tract

Tetracyclines / ↓ Effect of tetracyclines due to ↓ absorption from GI tract

Vitamin E / Vitamin E ↓ response to iron therapy

Laboratory Test Interference: Iron-containing drugs may affect electrolyte balance determinations.

Dosage: See individual drugs. Most replacement iron is given orally in daily doses of 90–300 mg elemental iron. Duration of therapy: 2–4 months longer than the time needed to reverse anemia, usually 6 or more months.

NURSING CONSIDERATIONS

Administration/Storage

1. For infants and young children, administer liquid preparation with a dropper. Deposit liquid well back against the cheek.
2. *Treatment of Iron Toxicity:*
   - General supportive measures.
   - Maintain a patent airway, respiration, and circulation.
   - Induce vomiting with syrup of ipecac followed by gastric lavage using tepid water or 1%–5% sodium bicarbonate (to convert from ferrous sulfate to ferrous carbonate, which is poorly absorbed and less irritating). Saline cathartics can also be used.
   - Deferoxamine is indicated for clients with serum iron levels greater than 300 mg/dl. Deferoxamine is usually given IM, but in severe cases of poisoning it may be given IV. Hydration should be maintained.
   - It may be necessary to treat for shock, acidosis, renal failure, and seizures.

Assessment

1. Prior to administering medication, assess client and take a complete drug history, including:
   - Client use of antacids and any other drugs that may interact with these preparations

   - Any OTC drugs, such as iron compounds or vitamin E, which are being used
2. Ask client about any evidence of GI bleeding such as tarry stools or bright red blood in stool or vomitus.
3. Note any complaints of fatigue, pallor, poor skin turgor, or change in mental status, especially among the elderly.
4. Assess nutritional status and diet history through questioning as well as observation of intake if possible.
5. Pregnancy has generally been considered an indication for prescribing iron prophylactically.
6. Obtain baseline CBC, iron, and TIBC results.

Interventions

1. Establish goals for therapy with client and other members of the health care team.
2. Check for occult blood if GI bleeding is suspected, as drugs may alter stool color.
3. Encourage persons with symptoms of anemia to seek medical assistance; discourage self-medication with iron based on symptoms only.
4. Coated tablets may be prescribed to diminish effects on the GI tract such as nausea, constipation or diarrhea, gastric irritation, and abdominal cramps.
5. Be prepared to assist with treatment of clients who may develop symptoms of iron intoxication, (most likely to occur after parenteral administration). If a client has iron poisoning:
   - Stop parenteral iron administration.

- Notify physician.
- Monitor vital signs for 48 hr since a second crisis is likely to occur within 12–48 hr of the first one.
- Follow guidelines for *Treatment of Iron Toxicity*.

6. Anticipate that the medication will be discontinued if 500 mg of iron daily does not cause a rise of at least 2 mg/100 ml of hemoglobin in 3 weeks.

7. Iron will reduce the absorption of tetracycline. If a client is to receive tetracyclines as well as iron products, establish a schedule that allows at least 2 hr to elapse between administering the iron product and the tetracycline.

Client/Family Teaching

1. Many clients will be taking their medications at home and without constant supervision. Therefore, it is important to teach them to adhere to the prescribed regimen and report any problems with medication therapy immediately.

2. Take iron preparations with meals to reduce gastric irritation.

3. Taking iron preparations with citrus juices enhances the absorption of iron.

4. Unless taking ferrous lactate, advise the client *NOT* to take iron compounds with milk products or antacids as these will interfere with absorption.

5. Discuss the possibility of indigestion, change in stool color (black and tarry or dark green), and constipation.

6. Explain the possible side effects that may occur (gastric irritation, constipation or diar-

rhea, abdominal cramps) and encourage immediate reporting of these symptoms because they may be relieved by changing the medication, dosage, or time of administration.

7. Encourage clients to eat a well-balanced diet, stressing the intake of foods high in iron. When working with poor families, explore the kinds of foods they can afford to assure that the diet prescribed is one they have access to (e.g., raisins, green vegetables, and liver may be more affordable than apricots or prunes).

8. Iron preparations are extremely dangerous for children. An overdosage can be fatal so keep iron preparations out of the reach of children.

9. When administering liquid iron medications to young children, dilute well with water or fruit juice and use a straw to minimize the possibility of staining the teeth.

10. When working with pregnant women, review their need for an iron-rich diet. Also, The American Academy of Pediatrics recommends an iron supplement for infants during their first year of life.

11. Follow administration guidelines for each product to minimize side effects. Advise against self-medicating with vitamins and mineral supplements.

Evaluation

1. Evaluate client for:
   - Laboratory confirmation of resolution of anemia. Review CBC and iron levels to assess for a positive clinical response to drug therapy. Generally, if Hb has not in-

creased 1 g/100 ml in 2 weeks then the diagnosis of iron deficiency anemia should be reconfirmed.

- Evidence of improvement in exercise tolerance

2. Compare client condition against the baseline data prior to drug administration (skin pallor, color of nail beds, prior blood studies, changes in stool color, etc.) to assess client compliance with and response to the prescribed drug regimen.

ANTIANGINAL DRUGS— NITRATES/NITRITES

See also the following individual entries:

Amyl Nitrite
Erythrityl Tetranitrate
Isosorbide Dinitrate
Nitroglycerin IV
Nitroglycerin Lingual Aerosol
Nitroglycerin Sublingual
Nitroglycerin Sustained Release
Nitroglycerin Topical
Nitroglycerin Transdermal
    Systems
Pentaerythritol Tetranitrate

General Statement: Angina pectoris may occur as a result of coronary atherosclerotic disease where there is an imbalance between the demand for oxygen by the myocardium and the oxygen supply (called secondary angina). The oxygen supply is compromised due to the inability of coronary blood flow to increase proportionally to increases in myocardial oxygen requirements. Angina pectoris may also result from vasospasm of large, surface coronary vessels or one of their major branches (called primary angina). In some clients, angina is due to a combination of constriction of coronary vessels and an insufficient oxygen supply.

Three groups of drugs are currently used for the treatment of angina. These agents include the nitrates/nitrites, beta-adrenergic blocking agents, and calcium channel blocking drugs. These drugs reduce the frequency and/or severity of angina by either increasing myocardial oxygen supply and/or decreasing the oxygen demand of the myocardium.

Action/Kinetics: The main mechanism of action of nitrates is to relax vascular smooth muscle by stimulating production of intracellular cyclic guanosine monophosphate production. Dilation of postcapillary vessels decreases venous return to the heart due to pooling of blood; thus, left ventricular end-diastolic pressure (preload) is reduced. Relaxation of arterioles results in a decreased systemic vascular resistance and arterial pressure (afterload). The oxygen requirements of the myocardium are also reduced. There is also a more efficient redistribution of blood flow in myocardial tissue. Reflex tachycardia may occur due to the overall decrease in blood pressure. For nitrates, several dosage forms are available, including sublingual, topical, transdermal, parenteral, oral, and buccal. The onset and duration depend on the product and route of administration.

Uses: Treatment and prophylaxis of acute angina pectoris, treatment of chronic angina pectoris. IV nitroglycerin is used to decrease blood pressure in surgical procedures resulting in hypertension, as well as an adjunct in treating hypertension or congestive heart failure associated with myocardial infarction (MI). *Investigational:* Nitroglycerin ointment has been used as an adjunct in treating Raynaud's disease. Sublingual and topical products have been used to decrease cardiac workload in clients with acute myocardial infarction and in congestive heart failure.

Contraindications: Sensitivity to nitrites, which may result in severe hypotensive reactions, MI, or tolerance to nitrites. Severe anemia, cerebral hemorrhage, recent head trauma, postural hypotension, closed angle glaucoma, impaired hepatic function, hypertrophic cardiomyopathy, hypotension, recent MI. Oral dosage forms should not be used in clients with GI hypermotility or with malabsorption syndrome. The injection should not be used in clients with hypovolemia or with normal or low pulmonary capillary wedge pressure.

Special Concerns: Pregnancy category: C (except amyl nitrite, which is category X). Use with caution during lactation and in glaucoma. Tolerance to the antianginal and vascular effects may occur. Safety and efficacy have not been determined during lactation and in children.

Side Effects: *CNS:* Headaches (most common), restlessness, dizziness, weakness, apprehension, vertigo. *CV:* Postural hypotension (common) with or without paradoxical bradycardia and increased angina, tachycardia, palpitations, syncope, rebound hypertension, crescendo angina, retrosternal discomfort, cardiovascular collapse. *GI:* Nausea, vomiting, dry mouth, abdominal pain, involuntary passing of feces and urine. *Dermatologic:* Transient flushing, rash, exfoliative dermatitis, crusty skin lesions. *Miscellaneous:* Sweating, muscle twitching, methemoglobinemia, cold sweating, blurred vision. **Topical use:** Peripheral edema, contact dermatitis.

Tolerance can occur following chronic use. Nitrites convert hemoglobin to methemoglobin, which impairs the oxygen-carrying capacity of the blood, resulting in anemic hypoxia. This interaction is dangerous in clients with preexisting anemia.

Symptoms of Overdose (Toxicity): Severe toxicity is rarely encountered with therapeutic use. Symptoms include hypotension, flushing, tachycardia, headache, palpitations, vertigo, perspiring skin followed by cold and cyanotic skin, visual disturbances, syncope, nausea, dizziness, vomiting with the possibility of bloody diarrhea and colic, anorexia, and increased intracranial pressure with symptoms of confusion, moderate fever, and paralysis. Tissue hypoxia (due to methemoglobinemia) may result in cyanosis, metabolic acidosis, coma, seizures, and death due to cardiovascular collapse.

Drug Interactions

Acetylcholine / Effects ↓ when used with nitrates
Alcohol, ethyl / Hypotension and cardiovascular collapse due to vasodilator effect of both agents
Antihypertensive drugs / Additive hypotension
Aspirin / ↓ Effects of nitrates
Beta-adrenergic blocking drugs / Additive hypotension
Calcium channel blocking drugs / Additive hypotension, including significant orthostatic hypotension

Dihydroergotamine / ↑ Effect of dihydroergotamine due to increased bioavailability

Heparin / Possible ↓ effect of heparin

Narcotics / Additive hypotensive effect

Phenothiazines / Additive hypotension

Sympathomimetics / ↓ Effect of nitrates; also, nitrates may ↓ effect of sympathomimetics resulting in hypotension

Laboratory Test Interference:
↑ Urinary catecholamines. False (−) decrease in serum cholesterol.

NURSING CONSIDERATIONS

Administration/Storage

1. Nitrites and nitrates are available in a variety of dosage forms including sublingual, chewable, topical, transdermal, oral, inhalation, and parenteral. It is important to understand the appropriate use of each of these dosage forms.
2. Tablets and capsules should be stored tightly closed in their original container. Avoid exposure to air, heat, and moisture.
3. Inhalation products should be used with the client either lying or sitting down.
4. Inhalation products are flammable and should not be used under situations where they might ignite.
5. *Treatment of Overdose (Toxicity):*
   - Induction of emesis or gastric lavage followed by activated charcoal.
   - Maintain client in a recumbent shock position and keep warm. Give oxygen and artificial respiration if required.
   - Methemoglobin levels should be monitored.
   - Elevate the legs and administer IV fluids to treat severe hypotension and reflex tachycardia. Phenylephrine or methoxamine may also be helpful.

Assessment

1. Note any history of sensitivity to nitrites.
2. If client has a history of anemia or glaucoma, document and administer this category of drugs with extreme caution.
3. Determine client experience with self-administered medications and note if physician has ordered sublingual tablets at the bedside.
4. Assess and document location, intensity, duration, extension, and any precipitating factors surrounding client's anginal pain.

Interventions

1. If hospitalized clients are instructed to keep sublingual tablets at the bedside, instruct them so that accurate records of attacks and the extent of medication relief are noted.
2. While caring for the client in the hospital, mutually record how much drug the client requires to keep angina under control. Record:
   - How frequently the drug is given
   - The duration of the attacks
   - Whether the relief is partial or complete
   - How long it takes for relief to occur
   - Whether or not there are any side effects

3. Remind client to notify someone when the medication is consumed so that effectiveness can be determined.
4. Monitor blood pressure and pulse. Assess for symptoms of sensitivity to the hypotensive effects of nitrites. These may include the presence of nausea, vomiting, pallor, restlessness, and cardiovascular collapse.
5. Monitor for the presence of hypotension when clients are receiving additional drugs that may cause hypotension. Drug dosage adjustment may be necessary.
6. Be alert for signs of tolerance, which generally occurs following chronic use but may begin several days after treatment is started. This is manifested by absence of response to the usual dose. (Nitrites may be discontinued temporarily until such tolerance is lost, and then reinstituted. During the interim, other vasodilators may be ordered.)
7. Observe clients for nausea, vomiting, complaints of drowsiness, headache, or visual disturbances during long-term prophylaxis. These are prolonged effects and may require a change in medication.
8. Note change in client activity and response to the drug therapy. Determine if client experiences less discomfort when performing regular activity.

Client/Family Teaching

1. Oral medications should be taken on an empty stomach.
2. Always carry sublingual tablets for use in aborting an attack. Observe the expiration date on the bottle, and obtain a fresh bottle when needed.
3. The presence of a burning sensation under the tongue attests to the potency of the drug. If there is no burning sensation, the potency may have diminished and a fresh supply should be obtained.
4. Carry sublingual tablets in a *glass* bottle, tightly capped. Do not use plastic containers because drug will deteriorate in plastic; also, do not use bottles with child-proof caps since client must get to the tablets quickly.
5. If anginal pain is not relieved in 5 min by first sublingual tablet, take up to 2 more tablets at 5-min intervals. If pain has not subsided 5 min after third tablet, client should be taken to emergency room by a family member or by ambulance. Client should **not** drive.
6. Take sublingual tablets 5–15 min prior to any situation likely to cause anginal pain (e.g., climbing stairs, sexual intercourse, exposure to cold weather).
7. To prevent the occurrence of postural hypotension, take sublingual tablet while sitting or lying down. Make position changes slowly and rise only after dangling feet for several minutes.
8. Elderly clients should be encouraged to sit or lie down when taking nitroglycerin. Elderly clients are more prone to hypotensive side effects and may become dizzy and fall.
9. Do not drink alcohol. Nitrite syncope, a severe shock-like state, may occur.
10. Follow specific instructions on

how to apply topical nitroglycerin. Some practitioners prescribe removing at bedtime and then resuming on arising.

11. Prescriptions should generally be renewed/replaced every 6 months.

12. Brand interchange is not recommended due to differences in effectiveness between products manufactured by different companies.

13. Clients should be advised to wear a Medic Alert bracelet and carry identification at all times.

Evaluation: Evaluate client for:
- Reports of a decrease in the frequency and severity of anginal attacks
- Clinical evidence of an increase in activity tolerance

ANTIARRHYTHMIC DRUGS

Adenosine
Amiodarone Hydrochloride
Bretylium Tosylate
Digitoxin
Digoxin
Diltiazem Hydrochloride
Disopyramide
Flecainide Acetate
Indecainide Hydrochloride
Lidocaine Hydrochloride
Mexiletine Hydrochloride
Moricizine Hydrochloride
Phenytoin
Phenytoin Sodium
Procainamide Hydrochloride
Propafenone
Propranolol Hydrochloride
Quinidine Bisulfate
Quinidine Gluconate
Quinidine Polygalacturonate
Quinidine Sulfate
Tocainide Hydrochloride
Verapamil

General Statement: The orderly sequence of contraction of the heart chambers, at an efficient rate, is necessary so that the heart can pump enough blood to the body organs. Normally the atria contract first, then the ventricles. Altered patterns of contraction, or marked increases or decreases in the rate of the heart, reduce the ability of the heart to pump blood. Such altered patterns are called *cardiac arrhythmias*. Some examples of cardiac arrhythmias are:

1. *Premature ventricular beats* or beats that occasionally originate in the ventricles instead of in the sinus node region of the atrium. This causes the ventricles to contract before the atria and ultimately results in a decrease in the volume of blood pumped into the aorta.

2. *Ventricular tachycardia*. A rapid heartbeat with a succession of beats originating in the ventricles.

3. *Atrial flutter*. Rapid contraction of the atria at a rate too fast to enable it to force blood into the ventricles efficiently.

4. *Atrial fibrillation*. The rate of atrial contraction is even faster than that noted during atrial flutter and more disorganized.

5. *Ventricular fibrillation*. Rapid, irregular, and uncoordinated ventricular contractions that are unable to pump any blood to the body. This condition will cause death if not corrected immediately.

6. *Atrioventricular (AV) heart block*. Slowing or failure of the transmission of the cardiac impulse from atria to ventricles, in the AV junction. This can result in atrial contraction

not followed by ventricular contraction.

The effective treatment of arrhythmias depends on accurate diagnosis, changing the causative factors, and, if appropriate, selecting an antiarrhythmic drug. The various antiarrhythmic drugs are classified according to both their mechanism of action and their effects on the action potential of cardiac cells. Importantly, one drug in a particular class may be more effective and safer in an individual client. The antiarrhythmic drugs are classified as follows:

1. Type I. These drugs decrease the rate of entry of sodium during cardiac membrane depolarization, decrease the rate of rise of phase O of the cardiac membrane action potential, prolong the effective refractory period of fast-response fibers, and require that a more negative membrane potential be reached before the membrane becomes excitable (and thus can propagate to other membranes). Drugs classified as type I are further listed in subgroups as follows:

   • Type IA: Depress phase O and prolong the duration of the action potential. The drugs are disopyramide, procainamide, and quinidine.
   • Type IB: Slightly depress phase O and are thought to shorten the action potential. The drugs include lidocaine, mexiletine, phenytoin, and tocainide.
   • Type IC: Slight effect on repolarization but marked depression of phase O of the action potential. Significant

slowing of conduction. The drugs in this group are flecainide and indecainide.

2. Type II. The drugs of this type competitively block beta-adrenergic receptors. These drugs may also cause a membrane-stabilizing effect. Acebutolol, esmolol, and propranolol are type II antiarrhythmics.

3. Type III. The drugs in this group prolong the duration of the membrane action potential without changing the phase of depolarization or the resting membrane potential. Drugs in this group include amiodarone and bretylium.

4. Type IV. The drug in this group (verapamil) slows conduction velocity and increases the refractoriness of the AV node.

It is important to monitor serum levels of antiarrhythmic drugs since some drugs can cause toxic side effects which can be confused with the purpose for which the drug is used. For example, toxicity from quinidine can result in cardiac arrhythmias.

NURSING CONSIDERATIONS

Assessment

1. Assess the extent of the client's palpitations, fluttering sensations, or missed beats prior to initiating the therapy.
2. Obtain pretreatment ECG and evaluate.
3. Note client complaints of chest pains or fainting episodes.
4. Obtain client BP, pulse, apical rate, and listen to heart sounds and record findings. These should serve as baseline data against which to measure the outcome of the prescribed therapy.

5. Ensure that laboratory tests for liver and renal function and electrolytes and blood glucose levels have been completed.

Interventions

1. Attach client to a cardiac monitor if administering antiarrhythmic drugs by IV route.
2. If the client is to receive continuous drip infusion, microdrip tubing and an infusion control device or electronic infusion pump should be used.
3. Obtain specific written guidelines concerning what to do should the client develop unusual changes in heart rate or rhythm.
4. Monitor BP and pulse. A heart rate of less than 60 beats/min or greater than 120 should generally be avoided, depending on the client's baseline level. Request written parameters for BP and pulse.
5. Report any new onset of bradycardia as this may be an early indicator of approaching cardiac collapse.
6. Have emergency drugs and equipment available in the event of an adverse reaction to therapy. Be prepared to help withdraw the medication, administer emergency drugs, and use resuscitative techniques.
7. Monitor for changes in cardiac rhythm. Document with rhythm strips and report to the physician as the drug administration may need to be altered.
8. Note any depression of cardiac activity, such as the prolongation of the PR interval, widening of the QRS complex, increased AV block, or aggravation of the arrhythmia and report.

9. Monitor serum concentrations of the antiarrhythmic agent throughout initial therapy.
10. Monitor serum electrolyte levels, diet, and drug regimens to determine if the serum potassium levels are sufficient to enhance drug effectiveness.

Client/Family Teaching

1. Explain the desired effects of the drug therapy.
2. Review the signs and symptoms of adverse reactions that should be reported.
3. Advise to avoid any OTC products without physician approval.
4. Stress the importance of taking the drugs as ordered. If a dose of medication is missed the client should not double up on the next dose unless this is specifically ordered by the physician.
5. Establish a time and a method of recording that would enable clients to remember to take the medications as ordered.
6. Do not drink alcohol, as this may alter drug absorption.
7. Stress the importance of returning for follow-up visits as scheduled.
8. Remind clients to inform all health care providers that they are taking antiarrhythmic agents. An ID bracelet may be helpful.

Evaluation

1. Evaluate client/family knowledge and understanding of illness, assess response to teaching, and level of compliance with prescribed therapy.
2. Obtain ECG and compare to pretreatment ECG to determine response to therapy.

3. Evaluate serum drug concentrations to determine if levels are within therapeutic range.
4. Observe client for any evidence of adverse side effects that may be drug related.

ANTIASTHMATIC DRUGS

See   *Theophylline   Derivatives,*
p. 226.

ANTICOAGULANTS

See also the following individual entries:

Heparin Calcium
Heparin Lock Flush Solution
Heparin Sodium
Warfarin Sodium

General Statement: Blood coagulation is a precise mechanism that can be defined as follows:

1. The process of coagulation is initiated when an inactive precursor escapes from the damaged platelets and activates *thromboplastin.*
2. The activated thromboplastin helps convert the protein *prothrombin* into *thrombin.*
3. *Thrombin* mediates the formation of the threadlike *fibrin*— an insoluble protein—from the soluble *fibrinogen.* The former forms a clot, trapping blood cells and platelets. Vitamin K, calcium, and various accessory factors manufactured in the liver are essential for blood coagulation.

Once formed, the blood clot is dissolved by another enzymatic chain reaction involving a substance called fibrinolysin. Blood coagulation can be affected by a number of diseases. An excessive tendency to form blood clots is one of the main factors involved in cardiovascular disorders, and a defect in the clotting mechanism is the cause of hemophilia and related diseases. Since several of the factors that participate in blood clotting are manufactured by the liver, severe liver disease can also affect blood clotting, as does vitamin K deficiency. Drugs that influence blood coagulation can be divided into three classes: (1) *anticoagulants,* or drugs that prevent or slow blood coagulation; (2) *thrombolytic agents,* which increase the rate at which an existing blood clot dissolves; and (3) *hemostatics,* which prevent or stop internal bleeding. The dosage of all agents discussed must be carefully adjusted since overdosage can have serious consequences.The three major types of anticoagulants are: (1) dicumarol and warfarin, (2) anisindione (indanedione-type), and (3) heparin. The following considerations are pertinent to each type. Anticoagulant drugs are used mainly in the management of patients with thromboembolic disease; they do not dissolve previously formed clots, but they do forestall their enlargement and prevent new clots from forming.

Uses: Venous thrombosis, pulmonary embolism, acute coronary occlusions with myocardial infarctions, and strokes caused by emboli or cerebral thrombi. Prophylactically for rheumatic heart disease, atrial fibrillation, traumatic injuries of blood vessels, vascular surgery, major abdominal, thoracic, and pelvic surgery, prevention of strokes in clients with transient attacks of cerebral ischemia, or other signs of impending stroke.

Contraindications: Clients with possible defects in the clotting mechanism (hemophilia) or with frail or weakened blood vessels, peptic ulcer, chronic ulcerations of the GI tract, hepatic and renal dysfunction, subacute bacterial endocarditis, or severe hypertension. Also after neurosurgery or recent surgery of the eye, spinal cord, or brain, or in the presence of drainage tubes in any orifice. Alcoholism.

Side Effects: See individual drugs.

NURSING CONSIDERATIONS

See also *Nursing Considerations* for individual agents and *Nursing Considerations* for *Anticoagulants, Coumarin,* p. 59

Assessment

1. Obtain a thorough nursing history and complete drug profile prior to initiating therapy. Note any potential drug interactions.
2. Through the health history profile identify client complaints that may indicate defects in the clotting mechanism.
3. Observe for any evidence of weakened blood vessel walls (capillary fragility).
4. Review past health problems (peptic ulcer, evidence of chronic ulcerations of the GI tract, renal or liver dysfunction, infections of the endocardium, hypertension) as evidence for contraindications to this therapy.
5. Note any evidence of alcoholism as anticoagulants are contraindicated. This is particularly important when working with clients who are homeless. Also,

such evidence suggests the client may have problems with drug compliance.
6. Determine that appropriate blood tests have been conducted to serve as a baseline against which to measure response of the client to treatment.

ANTICOAGULANTS, COUMARIN

See also the following:

Warfarin Sodium

General Statement: Blood coagulation is a precise mechanism that can be defined as follows:

1. The process of coagulation is initiated when an inactive precursor escapes from the damaged platelets and activates *thromboplastin.*
2. The activated thromboplastin helps convert the protein *prothrombin* into *thrombin.*
3. *Thrombin* mediates the formation of the threadlike *fibrin*—an insoluble protein—from the soluble *fibrinogen.* The former forms a clot, trapping blood cells and platelets. Vitamin K, calcium, and various accessory factors manufactured in the liver are essential for blood coagulation.

Once formed, the blood clot is dissolved by another enzymatic chain reaction involving a substance called fibrinolysin. Blood coagulation can be affected by a number of diseases. An excessive tendency to form blood clots is one of the main factors involved in cardiovascular disorders, and a defect in the clotting mechanism is the cause of hemophilia and related diseases. Since several of the factors that participate in blood clotting are manufactured by the liver, severe liver disease can also affect blood clotting, as does vitamin K deficiency. Drugs that influence blood coagulation can be divided into three classes: (1) *anticoagulants,* or drugs that prevent or slow blood coagulation; (2) *thrombolytic agents,* which increase the rate at which an existing blood clot dissolves; and (3) *hemostatics,* which prevent or stop internal bleeding.

Action/Kinetics: These drugs act only in vivo by preventing the formation of factors II, VII, IX, and X in the liver due to inhibition of vitamin K-mediated gamma-carboxylation of precursor proteins. There is a delay in reaching full beneficial effects since circulating coagulating factors must first be removed by normal catabolism. Highly bound to albumin (99%). The drugs are metabolized by the liver and excreted through the urine.

Uses: Prophylaxis and treatment of deep venous thrombosis, pulmonary thromboembolism, thrombophlebitis. Prophylaxis of thromboembolism due to chronic atrial fibrillation or myocardial infarction. *Investigational:* Reduce risk of postconversion emboli; prophylaxis of recurrent, cerebral thromboembolism; prophylaxis of myocardial reinfarction; treatment of transient ischemic attacks; reduce the risk of thromboembolic complications in clients with certain types of prosthetic heart valves; reduced risk of thrombosis and/or occlusion following coronary bypass surgery. Heparin is often used concurrently during the therapeutic initiation period.

Contraindications: Hemorrhagic tendencies, blood dyscrasias, ulcerative lesions of the GI tract, diverticulitis, colitis, subacute bacterial endocarditis, threatened abortion, recent operations on the eye, brain, or spinal cord, regional anesthesia and lumbar block, vitamin K deficiency, leukemia with bleeding tendencies, thrombocytopenic purpura, open wounds or ulcerations, acute nephritis, impaired hepatic or renal function, or severe hypertension.

Special Concerns: The drugs should be used with caution in menstruating women, in pregnant women (because they may cause hypoprothrombinemia in the infant), during lactation, during the postpartum period, and following cerebrovascular accidents. Geriatric clients may be more susceptible to the effects of anticoagulants.

Side Effects: *CV:* Hemorrhagic accidents are the chief danger of anticoagulant therapy. Frequent prothrombin time determinations should be performed for clients on long-term therapy to ascertain that values remain within safe levels. *GI:* Nausea, vomiting, diarrhea, abdominal cramps, anorexia. *Dermatologic:* Necrosis or gangrene of the skin and other tissues, alopecia, dermatitis, urticaria. *Hematologic:* Agranulocytosis, eosinophilia, leukopenia. *Other:* Fever, delayed hypersensitivity reactions, priapism, urine that becomes red-orange in color, mouth ulcers, nephropathy, hepatotoxicity, jaundice. Blood in urine may be a first warning of impending hemorrhage. *Symptoms of Overdose:* Early symptoms include microscopic hematuria, melena, petechiae, excessive menstrual bleeding, bleeding from gums after brushing teeth, and oozing from nicks due to shaving.

Drug Interactions: These drugs are responsible for more adverse drug interactions than any other group. Patients on anticoagulant therapy must be monitored carefully each time a drug is added or withdrawn. Monitoring usually involves determination of prothrombin time. In general, a lengthened prothrombin time means potentiation of the anticoagulant. Since potentiation may mean hemorrhages, a lengthened prothrombin time warrants **reduction of the dosage of the anticoagulant.** However, the anticoagulant dosage must again be increased when the second drug is discontinued. A shortened prothrombin time means inhibition of the anticoagulant and may require an increase in dosage.

Drug Interactions

Acetaminophen / Slight ↑ in hypoprothrombinemia

Alcohol, ethyl / ↑ or ↓ Effect of oral anticoagulants

Allopurinol / ↑ Effect of anticoagulants due to ↓ breakdown by liver

Aminoglycoside antibiotics / Potentiate pharmacologic effect of anticoagulants

Anabolic steroids / Potentiate pharmacologic effect of anticoagulants

Antacids, oral / ↓ Effect of anticoagulants due to ↓ absorption from GI tract

Antidepressants, tricyclic / ↑ Effect of anticoagulants due to ↓ breakdown by liver

Barbiturates / ↓ Effect of anticoagulants due to ↑ breakdown by liver

Carbamazepine / ↓ Effect of anticoagulants due to ↑ breakdown by liver

Cephalosporins / ↑ Effect of anticoagulants due to ↑ prothrombin time

Chloral hydrate / ↑ Effect of anticoagulants by ↓ plasma protein binding

Chloramphenicol / ↑ Effect of anticoagulant due to ↓ breakdown by liver

Cholestyramine / ↓ Anticoagulant effect due to binding in and ↓ absorption from GI tract

Cimetidine / ↑ Anticoagulant effect due to ↓ breakdown by liver

Clofibrate / ↑ Anticoagulant effect by ↓ plasma protein binding

Colestipol / ↓ Effect of anticoagulants due to ↓ absorption from GI tract

Contraceptives, oral / ↓ Anticoagulant effect by ↑ activity of certain clotting factors (VII and X)

Contrast media containing iodine / ↑ Effect of anticoagulants by ↑ prothrombin time

Corticosteroids, corticosterone / ↓ Effect of anticoagulants by ↓ hypoprothrombinemia; also ↑ risk of GI bleeding due to ulcerogenic effect of steroids

Danazol / ↑ Effect of anticoagulants

Dextrothyroxine / ↑ Effect of anticoagulants

Disulfiram / ↑ Effect of anticoagulants by ↓ breakdown by liver

Estrogens / ↓ Anticoagulant response by ↑ activity of certain clotting factors

Ethchlorvynol / ↓ Effect of anticoagulants due to ↑ breakdown by liver

Glucagon / ↑ Effect of

anticoagulants by ↑ hypoprothrombinemia

Glutethimide / ↓ Effect of anticoagulants due to ↑ breakdown by liver

Griseofulvin / ↓ Effect of anticoagulants due to ↑ breakdown by liver

Haloperidol / ↓ Effect of anticoagulants due to ↑ breakdown by liver

Heparin / ↑ Effect by ↑ prothrombin time

Hypoglycemics, oral / ↑ Effect of anticoagulants due to ↓ plasma protein binding; also, ↑ effect of sulfonylureas

Indomethacin / ↑ Effect of anticoagulants by ↓ plasma protein binding; also, indomethacin is ulcerogenic and may inhibit platelet function, leading to hemorrhage

Methotrexate / Additive hypoprothrombinemia

Methylthiouracil / Additive hypoprothrombinemia

Metronidazole / ↑ Effect of anticoagulants due to ↓ breakdown by liver

Mineral oil /
↑ Hypoprothrombinemia by ↓ absorption of vitamin K from GI tract; also mineral oil may ↓ absorption of anticoagulants from GI tract

Penicillin / Penicillin may potentiate the pharmacologic effect of anticoagulants

Phenylbutazone / ↑ Effect of anticoagulants by ↓ plasma protein binding and ↓ breakdown by liver; phenylbutazone may also produce GI ulceration and therefore ↑ chance of bleeding

Phenytoin / ↑ Effect of phenytoin due to ↓ in breakdown by liver; also possible ↑ in anticoagulant effect by ↓ plasma protein binding

Propylthiouracil / Additive hypoprothrombinemia

Quinidine, quinine / Additive hypoprothrombinemia

Rifampin / ↓ Anticoagulant effect due to ↑ breakdown by liver

Salicylates / ↑ Effect of anticoagulants by ↓ plasma protein binding, ↓ plasma prothrombin, and ↓ platelet aggregation; also, ↑ risk of GI bleeding due to ulcerogenic effect of salicylates

Sulfinpyrazone / ↑ Anticoagulant effect due to ↓ breakdown by liver and inhibition of platelet aggregation

Sulfonamides / ↑ Effect of sulfonamides by ↑ blood levels; also ↑ anticoagulant effect due to ↓ plasma protein binding and ↓ breakdown by liver

Sulfonylureas / ↑ Effect of anticoagulant due to ↓ plasma protein binding; also, ↑ effect of sulfonylureas

Sulindac / ↑ Effect of anticoagulants

Tetracyclines / IV tetracyclines ↑ hypoprothrombinemia

Thyroid hormones /
↑ Anticoagulant effect due to ↑ breakdown of clotting factors

Triclofos / ↑ Effect of anticoagulants due to ↓ plasma protein binding

Xanthines / ↓ Effect of anticoagulants by ↑ plasma prothrombin and factor V

Laboratory Test Interferences: False ↓ levels of serum theophylline determined by Schack and Waxler UV method (warfarin and dicumarol). Metabolites of indanedione derivatives may color alkaline urine red; color disappears upon acidification.

Dosage: See individual drugs.

NURSING CONSIDERATIONS

See also *Nursing Considerations* for *Anticoagulants*, p. 55.

Administration/Storage

Treatment of Overdose: Coumarin-type drugs can be counteracted by oral (2.5–10 mg) or IV (5–50 mg) administration of vitamin K_1 (phytonadione). Fresh whole blood, fresh frozen plasma (200–500 ml), or factor IX complex may be required in emergencies.

Assessment

1. Take a complete drug history prior to initiating therapy and note any potential drug interactions.
2. Determine that prothrombin levels have been obtained prior to beginning therapy. This should serve as a baseline against which to evaluate the effectiveness of the therapy.
3. Through the health history profile identify client complaints that may indicate defects in the clotting mechanism.
4. Review with clients any prior problems they may have had with bleeding tendencies (e.g., ulcerative lesions of the GI tract, colitis, or history of leukemia).
5. Observe for any evidence of weakened blood vessel walls (capillary fragility).
6. Review past health problems (peptic ulcer, evidence of chronic ulcerations of the GI tract, renal or liver dysfunction, infections of the endocardium, hypertension) as evidence for contraindications to this therapy.
7. Note any evidence of alcoholism as anticoagulants are contraindicated. This is particularly important when working with clients who are homeless. Also, such evidence suggests the client may have problems with drug compliance.
8. Determine that appropriate blood tests have been conducted to serve as a baseline against which to measure response of the client to treatment.
9. Note if the client is a woman in the childbearing years and if she is sexually active. Include in the history if the woman is postpartum or is nursing a baby. In these instances, anticoagulant therapy must be used with caution.

Interventions

1. Post and advise all personnel caring for the client that client is receiving anticoagulant therapy.
2. Assist the health team in evaluating the client's ability to take medication without supervision.
3. Monitor prothrombin levels closely; anticipate dose adjustment of the anticoagulant if the client is also receiving one of the many drugs known to interact with anticoagulants.
4. Question client for evidence of bleeding (bleeding gums, hematuria, tarry stools, hematemesis, ecchymosis and/or petechiae) during initial therapy and also during therapy with a medication that increases the anticoagulant effect. If clients have discolored urine, determine cause. Determine if discoloration is from drug therapy or if it is hematuria.
5. Report the sudden appearance

of lumbar pain in clients receiving anticoagulant therapy, since this symptom may indicate retroperitoneal hemorrhage.

6. Report symptoms of GI dysfunction in a client on anticoagulant therapy, since these symptoms may indicate intestinal hemorrhage. Anticipate that a client who has a history of ulcers or who has recently undergone surgery should have frequent laboratory tests for blood in the urine and feces, as well as measurement of hemoglobin and hematocrit to assess for bleeding.

7. Have vitamin K available for parenteral emergency use.

8. Apply pressure to all venipuncture and injection sites to prevent bleeding or hematoma formation.

Client/Family Teaching

1. Establish a routine that allows the medication to be taken at the same time every day or as otherwise prescribed.

2. Discuss the possibility of bleeding and symptoms of impending hemorrhage. Clients should be encouraged to report immediately dizziness, headaches, bleeding gums or wounds, or vomiting of coffee ground material. This is particularly important when working with an elderly client.

3. Bleeding or the presence of black and blue areas on the skin, or blood in the urine, is an indication that the medication should be stopped and the physician notified for further instructions.

4. Indanedione-type anticoagulants turn alkaline urine a red-orange color. Discoloration that results from the drug can be differentiated from hematuria by acidifying urine and reevaluating its color.

5. Advise clients receiving coumarin-type therapy to carry a card with the name of the drug therapy, the client's name, and the name of the physician who is providing care so that appropriate persons may be contacted by paramedical personnel if excessive bleeding occurs or if emergency surgery is required.

6. Clients and families need to be aware of the necessity of remaining under medical supervision for blood tests and adjustment of drug dosages. If necessary, ask a reliable relative or friend of the client to report any adverse effects and to make sure that the client takes the medication and comes in for blood tests as ordered.

7. Other medications and changes in diet or physical state may affect the action of the anticoagulant. Illness should be reported to the physician promptly.

8. Check with the prescribing physician prior to taking any nonprescription drugs such as aspirin, vitamin preparations with high levels of vitamin K, mineral preparations from health food stores, or alcohol. If the physician is not available, clients should discuss this with the pharmacist from whom they receive the prescription drugs.

9. Carry vitamin K capsules at all times.

10. To prevent cuts, clients should

use an electric razor for shaving instead of a razor blade.
11. To reduce the potential of bleeding gums, use a soft bristle toothbrush.
12. Arrange furniture in the home to allow open space for ambulation. This diminishes the chance of bumping into objects that may cause bruising and bleeding.
13. When the client has severe problems with sight, teach family members that it is important that furniture not be moved from usual places. This creates confusion for someone without full vision and can cause accidents resulting in bleeding and/or bruising. Advise client to use a night light to prevent falls and bumps in the dark.
14. Clients should be warned against ingesting salicylates or alcohol in any form.
15. Review the dietary sources of vitamin K (asparagus, spinach, broccoli, brussels sprouts, cabbage, collards, turnips, mustard greens, milk, yogurt, and cheese) that should be consumed in limited quantities because these foods will alter prothombin time.
16. The client should be instructed to always wear a Medic Alert bracelet and carry identification noting prescribed drug therapy.
17. Stress the importance of follow-up visits and lab studies to evaluate the effectiveness of drug therapy and to ensure proper dosage.

Evaluation: Evaluate client for:
- Laboratory confirmation of prothrombin times (usually 1.5–2 times the control) and for cumulative effects of the

drug and to determine if the effects of the drug therapy are consistent
- Freedom from complications of drug therapy and abnormal bleeding

Special Concerns
1. Elderly people are more prone to developing bleeding complications than are other groups. Therefore, special attention must be given to this problem.
2. Unusual hair loss and itching are common problems with the elderly during drug therapy and should be reported immediately.
3. Since many elderly people use many different pharmacies to fill prescriptions, make sure that they have a printed form with the name and dosage of all drugs they are currently taking.

ANTICONVULSANTS

See also the following individual entries:

Acetazolamide
Carbamazepine
Clonazepam
Clorazepate Dipotassium
Diazepam
Ethosuximide
Magnesium Sulfate
Methsuximide
Phenobarbital
Phensuximide
Phenytoin
Phenytoin Sodium Extended
Phenytoin Sodium Parenteral
Phenytoin Sodium Prompt
Primidone
Valproic Acid

General Statement: Anticonvulsant agents are used for the control of the chronic seizures and involuntary muscle spasms or movements characteristic of certain neurologic diseases. They are most frequently used in the therapy of epilepsy, which results from disorders of nerve impulse transmission in the brain. Therapeutic agents cannot cure these convulsive disorders, but do control seizures without impairing the normal functions of the CNS. This is often accomplished by selective depression of hyperactive areas of the brain responsible for the convulsions. Therefore, these drugs are taken at all times (prophylactically) to prevent the occurrence of the seizures. There are several different types of epileptic disorders; the International Classification of Epileptic Seizures is as follows: I. Partial seizures which usually involve one brain hemisphere at onset. Seizures are either simple (where consciousness is not impaired) or complex (where consciousness is impaired). Simple seizures may be accompanied by motor symptoms (Jacksonian, adversive), somatosensory (or other sensory) symptoms, autonomic symptoms, or psychic symptoms. Complex seizures may be manifested by simple partial seizures at onset (followed by impaired consciousness) or impaired consciousness at onset. Either simple or complex seizures may evolve to generalized tonic-clonic seizures. II. Generalized seizures which involve both hemispheres of the brain at onset and where consciousness is usually impaired. Generalized seizures are further categorized as (a) absence (typical or atypical), (b) myoclonic, (c) clonic, (d) tonic, (e) tonic-clonic, or (f) atonic. III. Localization-related (focal) which are categorized as either idiopathic (benign focal epilepsy of childhood) or symptomatic (chronic progressive epilepsia partialis continua, temporal-lobe, or extratemporal). IV. Generalized epilepsy which is further categorized as (a) idiopathic (benign neonatal, childhood absence, or juvenile myoclonic convulsions) or (b) cryptogenic or symptomatic (infantile spasms–West syndrome, early myoclonic encephalopathy, Lennox–Gestaut syndrome, progressive myoclonic epilepsy). V. Special syndromes which includes febrile seizures. No single drug can control all types of epilepsy; thus, accurate diagnosis is important. Drugs effective against one type of epilepsy may not be effective against another. Anticonvulsant therapy must be individualized. Therapy begins with a small dose of the drug, which is continuously increased until either the seizures disappear or drug toxicity occurs. If a certain drug decreases the frequency of seizures but does not completely prevent them, another drug can be added to the dosage regimen and administered concomitantly with the first. Often a drug is ineffective and then another agent must be given. Failure of therapy most often results from the administration of doses too small to have a therapeutic effect or from failure to use two or more drugs together. If for any reason drug therapy is discontinued, the anticonvulsant drugs must be withdrawn gradually over a period of days or weeks to avoid severe, prolonged convulsions. This guideline also applies when one anticonvulsant is substituted for another; the dosage of the second drug is slowly increased at the same time that the dosage of the first drug is being reduced. With appropriate diagnosis and selection of drugs, four out of five cases of epilepsy can be controlled adequately, but it may take the physician some time to find the best drug or combination of drugs with which to treat the client.

Dosage: Dosage is highly individualized. However, trauma or emotional stress may necessitate an increase in drug dosage requirements (e.g., if the client requires surgery and starts having seizures). For details, see individual agents.

NURSING CONSIDERATIONS

Administration/Storage

1. Oral suspensions of drugs should be shaken thoroughly before pouring to ensure uniform mixing.
2. Drug therapy must be individualized according to the needs of the client.
3. Medication should not be discontinued abruptly unless the physician advises it. Withdrawal should occur over a period of days or weeks to avoid severe, prolonged convulsions.
4. If there is reason to substitute one anticonvulsant drug for another, the first drug should be withdrawn slowly at the same time the dosage of the second drug is being increased.
5. Be prepared, in case of acute oral toxicity, to assist with inducing emesis (provided the client is not comatose) and with gastric lavage, along with other supportive measures such as administration of fluids and oxygen.
6. *Treatment of Overdose:* Anticipate that peritoneal dialysis or hemodialysis may be instituted in the treatment of acute toxici-

ty for barbiturates, hydantoins, and succinimides (hemodialysis only).

Assessment

1. Check the client's medical history for hypersensitivity to particular types of anticonvulsant drugs. Note the derivatives of that particular type as they should also be avoided.
2. Note the client's orientation as to time and place, affect, reflexes, and vital signs and record as baseline data.
3. Check intervals of EEG for regions of abnormal spike or line flat patterns. Also examine EEG for temporal lobe foci, and for spike and dome patterns before instituting therapy.
4. Determine the frequency and severity of client's seizures noting location, duration, consciousness, and any other reportable characteristics.
5. Assess the condition of the client's skin and mucous membranes.
6. If the client is female and of childbearing age, determine the likelihood of pregnancy. Some of these drugs have been linked to fetal abnormalities.
7. Obtain a CBC, blood glucose level, liver and renal function studies as well as urinalysis prior to initiating therapy.

Interventions

1. Monitor blood pressure, pulse, and respirations. Observe for signs and symptoms of impending seizures.
2. Note any evidence of CNS side effects, such as complaints of blurred vision, dimmed vision, slurred speech, nystagmus, or confusion.

3. Observe for muscle twitching, loss of muscle tone, episodes of bizarre behavior, and/or subsequent amnesia and document.

4. Check if the physician wishes the client to receive folic acid supplements to prevent megaloblastic anemia.

5. Check if the physician wishes the client to receive vitamin D supplementation to prevent hypocalcemia. The usual dose is 4,000 units of vitamin D weekly.

6. Clients who are to be on prolonged therapy need to have a diet rich in vitamin D.

7. Frequently check for decreased levels of serum calcium since phenytoin can contribute to demineralization of bone. This can result in osteomalacia in adults and rickets in children. The risk is particularly great in clients who are inactive.

8. Anticipate that the physician will order vitamin K to be administered to pregnant women 1 month before delivery. This is to prevent postpartum hemorrhage and bleeding in the newborn and the mother.

9. For clients who require IV administration of anticonvulsant drugs, monitor closely for respiratory depression and cardiovascular collapse.

Client/Family Teaching

1. Gastrointestinal distress may be lessened by taking the drugs with large amounts of fluid or with food.

2. During the initiation of therapy the anticonvulsant drugs may cause a decrease in mental alertness, drowsiness, headache, vertigo, and ataxia. CNS symptoms are often dose-related and may disappear with a change of dosage or continued therapy. Therefore, the client should be warned to avoid hazardous tasks until the drug therapy has been regulated and the symptoms disappear.

3. Take the prescribed amount of drug ordered. The doses of anticonvulsant drugs are not to be increased, decreased, or discontinued without the physician's approval. There is a danger that convulsions may result.

4. Avoid the use of alcohol and any other CNS depressants because they may interfere with the action of anticonvulsants.

5. For complaints of altered sleep patterns, explain the nature of the disturbance and suggest ways to counteract the problem.

6. For alteration in bowel habits, suggest increased fluid intake and include fruit and other foods with roughage in the diet.

7. For clients who develop gingival hyperplasia, advocate the use of intensified oral hygiene, the use of a soft tooth brush, massage of the gums, and daily use of dental floss. It is also important to have routine dental visits.

8. If slurred speech develops, advocate slowing speech patterns to avoid the problem.

9. If rash, fever, severe headaches, stomatitis, rhinitis, urethritis, or balanitis (inflammation of the glans penis) occur, instruct clients to report immediately to the physician. These are early

symptoms of hypersensitivity and may require a change in medication.

10. Review the importance of avoiding fever, low glucose levels, and low sodium conditions. These conditions lower the seizure threshold.

11. Report sore throat, easy bruising, petechiae, or nosebleeds, all of which are signs of hematologic toxicity.

12. Instruct client to report jaundice, dark urine, anorexia, and abdominal pain. These may be signs of hepatotoxicity.

13. Stress the importance of monthly liver function studies so as to detect early signs of hepatitis, hepatocellular degeneration, and fatal hepatocellular necrosis.

14. If the client is female and likely to become pregnant, discuss the possible effects of the medication on pregnancy.

15. If the client is a lactating mother, observe and report signs of toxicity in the nursing infant.

16. Provide a list of drug and food interactions as well as side effects associated with drug therapy. Explain what to do should these occur and when to contact the physician.

17. Remind the client of the importance of reporting for all scheduled laboratory studies including CBC, renal and liver function studies as well as drug levels on a regular basis.

18. Instruct clients to report any unusual incidents in their life to the physician. There may be a need to alter the dosage of drug, especially if the client is undergoing physical trauma or emotional distress.

19. Individuals on anticonvulsant therapy should carry identification indicating the form of epilepsy and the drug therapy being taken.

Evaluation: Evaluate client for:

- Compliance with the prescribed medication regimen
- A decrease in the frequency of seizures and an improved level of seizure control
- Evidence of freedom from complications of drug therapy
- Laboratory confirmation that serum drug levels are within desired therapeutic range

ANTIDIABETIC AGENTS, ORAL

See also the following individual entries:

Acetohexamide
Chlorpropamide
Glipizide
Glyburide
Tolazamide
Tolbutamide
Tolbutamide Sodium

General Statement: Several oral antidiabetic agents are available for clients with non-insulin–dependent diabetes. These agents are sulfonylureas, which are related chemically to sulfonamides; however, they are devoid of antibacterial activity. Oral hypoglycemic drugs are classified as either first- or second-generation. *Generation* refers to structural changes in the basic molecule. Second-generation oral hypoglycemic drugs are more lipophilic and, as such, have greater hypoglycemic potency. Also, second-generation drugs are bound to plasma protein by covalent bonds, whereas first-generation drugs are bound to plasma protein by ionic bonds. The implication is that the second-generation drugs are potentially less susceptible to displacement from plasma protein by drugs such as salicylates and oral anticoagulants.

These agents are used chiefly for clients with maturity-onset, mild, nonketotic diabetes, usually associated with obesity, when the condition cannot be controlled by diet alone but the client does not require insulin. The oral antidiabetics should not be used in unstable or brittle diabetes, whatever the client's age.

Action/Kinetics: These drugs are believed to act by one or more of the following mechanisms: (1) the sensitivity of pancreatic islet cells is increased; (2) the pancreatic beta cell membrane is directly depolarized, leading to insulin secretion; or (3) the peripheral tissues become more sensitive to insulin due to an increase in the number of insulin receptors or an increased ability of circulating insulin to combine with receptors. The drugs are ineffective in the complete absence of functioning beta islet cells. All of the oral hypoglycemic drugs are significantly bound (90%) to plasma protein.

Clients whose condition is to be controlled by oral antidiabetics should undergo a 7-day therapeutic trial. A drop in blood sugar level, a decrease in glucosuria, and disappearance of pruritus, polyuria, polydipsia, and polyphagia indicate that the patient can probably be managed on oral antidiabetic agents. These drugs should not be used in patients with ketosis. If the patient is transferred from insulin to an oral antidiabetic drug, the hormone should be discontinued gradually over a period of several days. The sulfonylureas have similar pharmacologic actions but differ in their pharmacokinetic properties (see individual agents).

Uses: Non-insulin–dependent diabetes mellitus (type II) that does not respond to diet management alone. As an adjunct to stabilize insulin-dependent maturity-onset diabetes.

Contraindications: Stress before and during surgery, severe trauma, fever, infections, pregnancy, diabetes complicated by recurrent episodes of ketoacidosis or coma; juvenile, growth-onset, insulin-dependent, or brittle diabetes; impaired endocrine, renal, or liver function. Not indicated for clients whose diabetes can be controlled by diet alone. Relapse may occur with the sulfonylureas in undernourished clients. Long-acting products in geriatric clients.

Special Concerns: Use with caution during lactation since hypoglycemia may occur in the infant. Safety and effectiveness in children have not been established. Geriatric clients may be more sensitive to oral hypoglycemics and hypoglycemia may be more difficult to recognize in these clients. Use with caution in debilitated and malnourished clients.

Side Effects: Hypoglycemia is the most common side effect. *CV:* Chronic use of oral hypoglycemic drugs has been associated with an increased risk of cardiovascular mortality. *GI:* Nausea, heartburn, diarrhea, full feeling. *CNS:* Fatigue, dizziness, fever, headache, weak-

...lepatic: Cholestatic ...vation of hepatic ...*ermatologic:* Skin ...ia, erythema, pruri- ...hotophobia. *Hemato-* ...bocytopenia, leukope- ..., and eosinophilia are ...ommon. Also, agranulo- ...molytic anemia, pancyto- ...astic anemia.

...nce to drug action de- ...a in a small percentage of ...ents.

Symptoms of Overdose: Hypo-glycemia. The following symptoms of hypoglycemia are listed in their general order of appearance: tingling of lips and tongue, hunger, nausea, decreased cerebral function (lethargy, yawning, confusion, agitation, nervousness), increased sympathetic activity (tachycardia, sweating, tremor), seizures, stupor, coma.

Drug Interactions

Acetazolamide / ↑ Blood sugar in prediabetics and diabetics on oral hypoglycemics

Alcohol / Possible Antabuse-like syndrome, especially flushing of face and shortness of breath. Also, ↓ effect of oral hypoglycemic due to ↑ breakdown by liver

Anabolic steroids / ↑ Hypoglycemic effect of oral antidiabetics

Anticoagulants, oral / ↑ Effect of oral hypoglycemics by ↓ breakdown by liver and ↓ plasma protein binding

Beta-adrenergic blocking agents / ↓ Hypoglycemic effect of oral hypoglycemics; also, symptoms of hypoglycemia may be masked

Calcium channel blockers / ↑ Requirements for sulfonylureas

Chloramphenicol / ↑ Effect of oral hypoglycemics by ↓ breakdown by liver and ↓ renal excretion

Cimetidine / ↑ Effect of oral hypoglycemics due to ↓ breakdown by liver

Clofibrate / ↑ Hypoglycemic effect of oral antidiabetics due to ↓ plasma protein binding

Corticosteroids / ↑ Requirements for sulfonylureas

Diazoxide / Effects of both drugs decreased

Digitoxin / ↓ Effect of digitoxin by ↑ breakdown by liver

Fenfluramine / Additive hypoglycemia

Guanethidine / ↑ Effect of oral hypoglycemics

Isoniazid / ↑ Requirements for sulfonylureas

MAO inhibitors / ↑ Hypoglycemic effect of oral antidiabetics due to ↓ breakdown by liver

Methyldopa / ↑ Effect of sulfonylureas due to ↓ breakdown by liver

Miconazole / ↑ Effect of oral hypoglycemics

Nicotinic acid / ↓ Effect of oral hypoglycemics

Nonsteroidal anti-inflammatory drugs / ↑ Hypoglycemic effect of oral antidiabetics

Oral contraceptives / ↓ Hypoglycemic effect of oral antidiabetics

Phenobarbital / ↓ Effect of oral hypoglycemics due to ↑ breakdown by liver

Phenothiazines / ↑ Requirements for sulfonylureas due to ↓ release of insulin

Phenylbutazone / ↑ Effect of oral hypoglycemics due to ↓ breakdown by liver, ↓ plasma protein binding, and ↓ renal excretion

Phenytoin / ↓ Effect of sulfonylureas due to ↓ insulin release

Probenecid / ↑ Effect of oral hypoglycemics

Ranitidine / ↑ Effect of oral hypoglycemics

Rifampin / ↓ Effect of sulfonylureas due to ↑ breakdown by liver

Salicylates / ↑ Effect of oral hypoglycemics by ↓ plasma protein binding

Sulfonamides / ↑ Effect of oral hypoglycemics by ↓ plasma protein binding and ↓ breakdown by liver

Sympathomimetics / ↑ Requirements for sulfonylureas

Thiazides / ↑ Requirements for sulfonylureas

Thyroid hormone / ↑ Requirements for sulfonylureas

Laboratory Test Interference:
↑ BUN and serum creatinine.

Dosage: PO. See individual preparations. Adjust dosage according to needs of client. Exercise and diet are of primary importance in the control of diabetes.

NURSING CONSIDERATIONS

See also *Nursing Considerations* for *Insulins (applicable to all clients with diabetes controlled by medication whether insulin or an oral hypoglycemic),* p. 160.

Administration/Storage

1. Oral drugs may be taken with food to decrease the incidence of gastric upset.
2. If ketonuria, acidosis, increased glycosuria, or serious side effects occur, withdraw the medication.

3. *Treatment of Ove* hypoglycemia is tr oral glucose and adju. dose of the drug o patterns. Severe hypogly requires hospitalization. centrated (50%) dextrose given by rapid IV and is f lowed by continuous infusio of 10% dextrose at a rate that will maintain blood glucose above 100 mg/dl. Client should be monitored for at least 24–48 hr as hypoglycemia may recur (clients with chlorpropamide toxicity should be monitored for 3–5 days due to the long duration of action of this drug).

TRANSFER FROM INSULIN

1. If the client has been receiving 20 units or less of insulin daily, maintenance dosage of oral hypoglycemic agents may be instituted, and the insulin discontinued abruptly.
2. For clients receiving 20–40 units of insulin daily, institute a maintenance dosage of oral hypoglycemic agent and reduce insulin dose by 25%–30%. Insulin should be discontinued gradually, using the absence of glucose in the urine as a guide.
3. For clients receiving more than 40 units of insulin daily, institute a maintenance dosage and reduce insulin by 20%. Discontinue insulin gradually, using glucose in the urine as a guide. It may be advisable to hospitalize clients on such high doses of insulin while they are being transferred to oral hypoglycemic agents.
4. Be prepared to begin treatment with IV dextrose solution if the

client develops severe hypoglycemia.
5. Review the drugs with which
oral hypoglycemic agents interact and determine if the
client is taking any of them.

TRANSFER FROM ONE ORAL ANTIDIABETIC AGENT TO ANOTHER

1. Except for chlorpropamide, no
conversion period is necessary. When transferring clients
from chlorpropamide, caution
should be exercised for 1–2
weeks due to the long half-life
of chlorpropamide.
2. Mild symptoms of hyperglycemia may appear during the
transfer period. Clients should
perform finger sticks or test
their urine for glucose and
ketone bodies regularly (1–3
times daily) during the transfer
period. Positive results must be
reported to the physician.
3. No transition period is needed
when a client is transferred
from one sulfonylurea to
another. However, if a client is
to be transferred from chlorpropamide, caution should be
exercised due to the pro-
longed duration of action of
this drug.

THERAPEUTIC FAILURE OF HYPO-
GLYCEMIC AGENTS: Diabetic clients who do not respond to the
sulfonylureas are said to be *primary
failures*. Clients may respond to the
sulfonylureas during the initial
months of therapy, yet fail to respond thereafter. These clients are
referred to as *secondary failures*.

Assessment

1. Document any stress the client
may be experiencing. Clients

about to undergo surgical procedures, who have suffered
severe trauma, who have a
fever and infection, or who are
pregnant should not be placed
on oral hypoglycemic agents.
2. Note the potential of the client
to understand the complexities
of the transfer process.
3. Assess clients as to their ability
to adhere to the established
protocol.
4. If the client is female, sexually
active, and of childbearing age,
note if she is taking oral contraceptives. The effectiveness of
oral contraceptive agents is
lessened by oral hypoglycemic
agents.

Interventions

1. Assess clients taking a sulfonylurea closely during the first
7 days of treatment to determine their therapeutic response.
2. Closely supervise and observe
the client during the 3–5 days
after the transfer.

Client/Family Teaching

1. Instruct the client in testing
blood or urine at home for
glucose and maintaining a written record of glucose levels for
review by the health care provider.
2. Review the symptoms of hypoglycemia and hyperglycemia.
Advise that juice with sugar,
honey, or corn syrup may help
with hypoglycemic episodes.
3. Instruct that the medication
helps to control hyperglycemia
but does not cure diabetes.
Stress that the therapy is usually long term.
4. Explain the need to adhere to
the prescribed diet if sulfonyl-

urea is to be effective. Remind clients that most secondary failures are due to poor dietary compliance. Also, stress the importance of regular exercise.

5. Advise that self-administering insulin may be necessary if complications occur. Instruct the client in self-administration of insulin and how to maintain a record of site rotations.

6. Explain the importance of not changing brands of insulin or syringes. Review equipment, methods of storage, and proper method for safely discarding used syringes.

7. Advise clients to report to the physician when not feeling as well as usual, or if they develop pruritus, skin rash, jaundice, dark urine, fever, sore throat, nausea or vomiting, or diarrhea.

8. If the client is scheduled for a thyroid test, report to the laboratory the fact that the client is taking a sulfonylurea. The drug interferes with the uptake of radioactive iodine.

9. Avoid alcohol when taking oral hypoglycemic agents as a disulfuram-like reaction may occur.

10. Stress the need for close medical supervision for the first 6 weeks of therapy.

11. Stress the need for periodic laboratory tests as ordered by the physician. Oral hypoglycemic agents can cause blood dyscrasias.

12. Remind the client to carry sugar or candy and identification at all times, listing the medications currently prescribed.

Evaluation: Evaluate client for:
• Evidence of an understanding of illness and assess for compliance with prescribed treatment and dietary regime
• Reports of a decrease in the frequency of hypo- or hyperglycemic episodes
• Freedom from complications with prescribed drug therapy
• Laboratory confirmation that serum glucose levels are within desired range

ANTIEMETICS

See also the following individual entries:

Buclizine Hydrochloride
Cyclizine Hydrochloride
Dimenhydrinate
Diphenhydramine Hydrochloride
Dronabinol
Hydroxyzine Hydrochloride
Hydroxyzine Pamoate
Meclizine Hydrochloride
Nabilone
Ondansetron Hydrochloride
Phosphorated Carbohydrate Solution
Prochlorperazine
Prochlorperazine Edisylate
Prochlorperazine Maleate
Scopolamine Hydrobromide
Trimethobenzamide Hydrochloride

General Statement: Nausea and vomiting can be caused by a variety of conditions, such as infections, drugs, radiation, motion, organic disease, or psychological factors. The underlying cause of the symptoms must be elicited before emesis is corrected.

The act of vomiting is complex. The vomiting center in the medulla responds to stimulation from many peripheral areas, as well as to stimuli from the CNS itself, the chemoreceptor trigger zone in the medulla, the vestibular apparatus of the ear, and the cerebral cortex.

The selection of an antiemetic depends on the cause of the symptoms, as well as on the manner in which the vomiting is triggered.

Many drugs used for other conditions, such as the antihistamines, phenothiazines, barbiturates, and scopolamine, have antiemetic properties and can be so used. (For details see appropriate sections.) These agents often have serious side effects (mostly CNS depression) that make their routine use undesirable.

Drug Interaction: Because of their antiemetic and antinauseant activity, the antiemetics may mask overdosage caused by other drugs.

NURSING CONSIDERATIONS

Assessment

1. Take a complete client history, determining if nausea is an unusual occurrence or if it is a recurring phenomenon.
2. Determine the extent of the nausea and what event seems to have triggered it.
3. Note the number of times the client has had to take an antiemetic in the past and under what conditions.

Interventions

1. Assess for other side effects, such as increased intracranial pressure or intestinal obstruction. Antiemetic drugs may mask signs of underlying pathology or overdosage of other drugs.
2. Monitor fluid status and observe for symptoms of dehydration.

Client/Family Teaching

1. Caution the client that the drug tends to cause drowsiness and dizziness. Advise the client to avoid driving or performing other hazardous tasks until individual response to the drug has been evaluated.
2. Review measures to decrease nausea such as ice chips, sips of water, non-greasy foods, removal of noxious stimuli from the environment (odors or materials), and frequent oral hygiene.
3. Advise client to dangle legs before standing and to rise slowly to prevent symptoms of orthostatic hypotension.

Evaluation: Evaluate client for:
- Reports of effective control of nausea and vomiting
- Evidence of dehydration, R/T, nausea, and vomiting
- Improved nutritional status once nausea and vomiting have been controlled as evidenced by weight gain and/or increase in caloric intake

ANTIHISTAMINES (H$_1$–BLOCKERS)

See also the following individual entries:

Astemizole
Brompheniramine Maleate
Buclizine Hydrochloride
Chlorpheniramine Maleate
Cyclizine Hydrochloride
Cyclizine Lactate
Cyproheptadine Hydrochloride
Dexchlorpheniramine Maleate
Dimenhydrinate
Diphenhydramine
    Hydrochloride

Meclizine Hydrochloride
Promethazine Hydrochloride
Terfenadine
Tripelennamine Hydrochloride
Triprolidine Hydrochloride

Action/Kinetics: The effects of histamine may be reversed either by drugs that block histamine receptors (antihistamines) or by drugs that have effects opposite to those of histamine (e.g., epinephrine). Antihistamines used for the treatment of allergic conditions are referred to as *H₁-receptor blockers* while antihistamines used for the treatment of GI disorders (e.g., peptic ulcer) are referred to as *H₂-receptor blockers* (see *Cimetidine, Famotidine, Nizatidine,* and *Ranitidine*).

Antihistamines do not prevent the release of histamine; rather, they compete with histamine for histamine receptors (competitive inhibition), thus preventing or reversing the effects of histamine. Antihistamines prevent or reduce increased capillary permeability (i.e., decrease edema, itching) and bronchospasms. Allergic reactions unrelated to histamine release are not affected by antihistamines.

The H_1-blockers manifest varying degrees of CNS depression, as well as anticholinergic, antiemetic, and antiserotonin effects.

From a chemical point of view, the antihistamines can be divided into the following classes.

1. **Ethylenediamine Derivatives.** This group manifests low to moderate sedative effects and almost no anticholinergic or antiemetic activity. They frequently cause GI distress. Available agents: pyrilamine, tripelennamine.
2. **Ethanolamine Derivatives.** This group is most likely to cause CNS depression (drowsiness). There is a low incidence of GI side effects. There are significant anticholinergic and antiemetic effects. Available agents: carbinoxamine, clemastine, diphenhydramine.
3. **Alkylamines.** Members of this group are among the most potent antihistamines. They are effective at relatively low dosage and are most suitable agents for daytime use. This group manifests minimal sedation, moderate anticholinergic effects, and no antiemetic effects. Paradoxical excitation may also occur. Individual response to agents is variable. Available agents: brompheniramine, chlorpheniramine, dexchlorpheniramine, triprolidine.
4. **Phenothiazines.** These agents possess significant antihistaminic action, varying degrees of sedation, and a high degree of both anticholinergic and antiemetic effects. Available agents: methdilazine, promethazine, trimeprazine.
5. **Piperidines.** Members of this group have prolonged antihistaminic activity, with a comparatively low incidence of drowsiness, moderate anticholinergic activity, and no antiemetic effects. Available agents: azatadine, cyproheptadine, diphenylpyraline, phenindamine.
6. **Miscellaneous.** The two drugs in this group are specific in that they bind to peripheral rather than central H_1-histamine receptors. They have no sedative, anticholinergic, or antiemetic effects. Available agents: astemizole, terfenadine.

The kinetics of most antihistamines are similar. **Onset:** 15–30 min; **peak:** 1–2 hr; **duration:** 4–6 hr (piperidines have a longer duration). Many antihistamines are available as timed-release preparations. Most antihistamines are metabolized by the liver and excreted in the urine.

Uses: Treatment of vasomotor, perennial, or seasonal allergic rhinitis and allergic conjunctivitis. Treatment of angioedema, urticarial transfusion reactions, urticaria, pruritus. Atopic dermatitis, contact dermatitis, pruritus ani, pruritus vulvae, insect bites. Sneezing and rhinorrhea due to the common cold. Treatment of anaphylaxis, parkinsonism, drug-induced extrapyramidal reactions, vertigo. Prophylaxis and treatment of motion sickness, including nausea and vomiting. Nighttime sleep aid.

Contraindications: Hypersensitivity to the drug, narrow-angle glaucoma, prostatic hypertrophy, stenosing peptic ulcer, and pyloroduodenal or bladder neck obstruction. Pregnancy or possibility thereof (some agents), lactation, premature and newborn infants. The phenothiazine-type antihistamines are contraindicated in CNS depression from any cause, bone marrow depression, jaundice, dehydrated or acutely ill children, and in comatose patients.

Special Concerns: Administer with caution to clients with convulsive disorders, to geriatric clients, in respiratory disease, and to infants and children (may cause hallucinations, convulsions, and death).

Side Effects: *CNS:* Sedation ranging from mild drowsiness to deep sleep. Dizziness, lassitude, headache, confusion, disturbed coordination, muscular weakness. Paradoxical excitation (especially in children and the elderly) including restlessness, irritability, insomnia, hysteria, tremors, euphoria, nervousness, delirium, palpitations, and even convulsions. Also, hallucinations, disorientation, disturbing dreams or nightmares, catatonia, pseudoschizophrenia, extrapyramidal reactions. Antihistamines can precipitate epileptiform seizures in clients with focal lesions. *GI:* Epigastric distress, dryness of mouth, anorexia or increased appetite, weight gain, nausea, vomiting, and diarrhea or constipation. *CV:* Palpitations, increased heart rate, postural hypotension, extrasystoles, bradycardia, reflex tachycardia, ECG changes, cardiac arrest. *GU:* Urinary frequency, retention, or difficulty. Impotence, decreased libido, menstrual irregularities, induced lactation, gynecomastia, inhibition of ejaculation. *Respiratory:* Dryness of nose, mouth, throat; nasal stuffiness, respiratory depression, wheezing and tightness of chest. *Hematologic:* Anemias (hemolytic, hypoplastic, aplastic), leukopenia, pancytopenia, thrombocytopenic purpura, agranulocytosis, thrombocytopenia. *Allergic:* Edema (peripheral, angioneurotic, laryngeal), anaphylaxis, rash, photosensitivity, urticaria, dermatitis, lupus-like syndrome, asthma. *Miscellaneous:* Hands become heavy and weak, tingling, excess sweating, chills, erythema, stomatitis, glycosuria, double vision, vertigo, tinnitus, acute labyrinthitis, neuritis, blurred vision, oculogyric crisis, torticollis.

Topical use: Prolonged use may result in local irritation and allergic contact dermatitis.

Symptoms of Acute Toxicity:

Antihistamines have a wide therapeutic range. Overdosage can nevertheless be fatal. Children are particularly susceptible. Overdosage can cause both CNS overstimulation and depression. The overstimulation is characterized by hallucinations, incoordination, and tonic-clonic convulsions. Fixed, dilated pupils, flushing, and fever are common in children. Cerebral edema, deepening coma, and respiratory collapse occur usually within 2–18 hr.

Overdosage in adults usually starts with severe CNS depression.

Drug Interactions

Alcohol, ethyl / See *CNS depressants*

Anticoagulants / Antihistamines may ↓ the anticoagulant effects

Antidepressants, tricyclic / Additive anticholinergic side effects

CNS depressants, antianxiety agents, barbiturates, narcotics, phenothiazines, procarbazine, sedative-hypnotics / Potentiation or addition of CNS depressant effects. Concomitant use may lead to drowsiness, lethargy, stupor, respiratory depression, coma, and possibly death

Heparin / Antihistamines may ↓ the anticoagulant effects

MAO inhibitors / Intensification and prolongation of anticholinergic side effects

Note: Also see *Drug Interactions* for *Phenothiazines,* p. 204.

Laboratory Test Interference: Discontinue antihistamines 4 days before skin testing to avoid false (−).

Dosage: Usually PO. Parenteral administration is seldom used because of irritating nature of drugs. Topical usage is also limited because antihistamines often cause hypersensitivity reactions. When given for motion sickness, antihistamines are usually given 30–60 min before anticipated travel. See individual drugs.

NURSING CONSIDERATIONS

Administration/Storage

1. Inject IM preparations deep into the muscle. Preparations tend to be irritating to the tissues.
2. Sustained-release preparations should be swallowed whole. Scored tablets may be broken before swallowing. If the client has difficulty swallowing capsules, they can be opened and the contents put into soft food for ingestion.
3. Topical preparations should not be applied to raw, blistered, or oozing areas of the skin.
4. Do not apply to the eyes, around the genitalia, or to mucous membranes.
5. Oral preparations may cause gastric irritation. Therefore, administer the medication with meals, milk, or a snack.
6. Have syrup of ipecac available to induce vomiting in the event of overdosage.
7. *Treatment of Overdose:*
   - Treat symptoms and provide supportive care.
   - Vomiting is induced with syrup of ipecac (do not use for phenothiazine overdosage) followed by activated charcoal and a cathartic. If vomiting has not been induced within 3 hr of ingestion,

gastric lavage can be undertaken.

- Hypotension can be treated with a vasopressor such as norepinephrine, dopamine, or phenylephrine (do not use epinephrine).
- For convulsions, use only short-acting depressants (e.g., diazepam). IV physostigmine can be used to treat centrally mediated convulsions.
- Ice packs and a cool sponge bath are effective in reducing fever in children.
- Severe cases of overdose can be treated by hemoperfusion.

Assessment

1. Note any history of drug sensitivity to antihistamines and record.
2. Note if the client has any medical history of ulcers or glaucoma or if the client is pregnant. Antihistamines are contraindicated under these circumstances.
3. Assess the extent of the allergic response for which the antihistamine is being ordered.
4. Review the medications the client is currently taking, noting those with which there may be an interaction.
5. Determine if the client is to have skin testing conducted. Antihistamines should be *discontinued* 4 days prior to testing to avoid false (−) results.
6. Obtain baseline blood pressure, pulse, and respirations and document.
7. Assess lung sounds and note characteristics of secretions produced.

Interventions

1. Note client complaints of severe CNS depression. This is a symptom of overdosage and may require the administration of syrup of ipecac. See Treatment of Overdose under Administration/Storage.
2. Monitor the blood pressure, pulse, and respirations. If the client develops hypotension or palpitations, document and report to the physician.
3. Monitor I & O. If the clients experience difficulty in voiding, have them void prior to receiving the medication.
4. If the client complains of constipation, encourage the client to take at least 3,000 ml of fluids per day, unless the client's condition requires restriction of fluids. Instruct client to increase the amount of exercise performed and increase the intake of fruits, fruit juices, and fiber. A stool softener may also be indicated if these measures are not successful.
5. Monitor lung sounds and secretion production. If bronchial secretions are thick, increase fluid intake to decrease the viscosity of secretions and avoid milk temporarily.
6. If the client is hospitalized and sedated with antihistamines, put up the side rails, ambulate with assistance, and incorporate safety precautions.
7. If the client complains of dizziness, weakness, or lassitude, assist with ambulation and report these symptoms.
8. If clients complain of local irritation, they may have developed an adverse reaction to the drug. Document and report to the physician.

Client/Family Teaching

1. Report all side effects to the physician immediately. Include onset of the side effects and duration, describing exactly what occurred. The physician may order a drug with fewer side effects. However, the client should not discontinue taking the medication without first consulting the physician.
2. Caution the client not to drive a car or operate other machinery until response to the medication (drowsiness) has worn off. Sedative effect may disappear spontaneously after several days of therapy.
3. Provide a printed list of drugs to avoid. Advise the client to consult with the physician concerning any depressants that may be ordered since antihistamines tend to potentiate the effects of other CNS depressants.
4. Report the development of sore throat, fever, unexplained bruising, bleeding, or petechiae. A CBC and platelets may be indicated to rule out a blood dyscrasia.
5. Advise clients that there is potential for developing a sensitivity to sun or ultraviolet light. Avoid any undue exposure to the sun, use a sunscreen, and wear a hat and long sleeves when in the sun.
6. If the drug is being used for motion sickness, it should be taken 30 min before it is time to use the vehicle or board a plane.
7. Avoid alcohol, any other CNS depressants, or OTC products unless cleared by the physician.
8. Advise that symptoms of dry mouth may be reduced by frequent rinsing with water, good oral hygiene, and the use of sugarless gum or candies.

Evaluation: Evaluate client for:
- Reports of a reduction in the frequency and intensity of allergic manifestations
- Control of itching and associated swelling
- Prevention of motion sickness
- Effective nighttime sedation
- A reduction in the original complaints for which the drug was prescribed

ANTIHYPERTENSIVE AGENTS

See also the following drug classes and individual drugs:

Agents Acting Directly on Vascular Smooth Muscle

Diazoxide
Hydralazine Hydrochloride
Nitroprusside Sodium

Angiotensin-Converting Enzyme Inhibitors

Benazepril
Captopril
Enalapril
Fosinopril
Lisinopril
Quinapril
Ramipril

Beta-Adrenergic Blocking Agents
See p. 113.

Centrally Acting Agents

Clonidine Hydrochlordie
Guanabenz Acetate
Guanfacine Hydrochloride
Methyldopa
Methyldopate Hydrochloride

Combination Drugs Used for Hypertension

Amiloride and
Hydrochlorothiazide
Lisinopril and
Hydrochlorothiazide
Methyldopa and
Hydrochlorothiazide
Propranolol and
Hydrochlorothiazide
Reserpine and Chlorothiazide
Reserpine, Hydralazine, and
Hydrochlorothiazide
Triamterene and
Hydrochlorothiazide

Miscellaneous Agents

Labetalol
Minoxidil, Oral

Peripherally Acting Agents

Doxazosin
Guanadrel Sulfate
Guanethidine Sulfate
Phenoxybenzamine
Hydrochloride
Phentolamine Mesylate
Prazosin Hydrochloride
Terazosin

General Statement: Hypertension is a condition in which the mean arterial blood pressure is elevated. It is one of the most widespread chronic conditions for which medication is prescribed and taken on a regular basis. Most cases of hypertension are of unknown etiology and result from a generalized increase in resistance to flow in the peripheral vessels (arterioles). Such cases are known as primary or essential hypertension. Treatment of essential hypertension is aimed at reducing blood pressure to normal or near-normal levels, because this is believed to prevent or halt the slow, albeit permanent, damage caused by constant excess pressure.

Essential hypertension is commonly classified according to its severity as mild, moderate, or severe. Most early cases of hypertension are mild. Moderate or severe (malignant) hypertension can result in degenerative changes in the brain, heart, and kidneys and can be fatal.

Other types of hypertension (secondary hypertension) have a known etiology and can result from a complication of pregnancy (toxemic hypertension) or certain other diseases that cause impairment of kidney function. It can also be caused by a tumor of the adrenal gland (pheochromocytoma) or by blockage of certain arteries leading into the kidney (renal hypertension). The latter two cases can be corrected by surgery.

Most pharmacologic agents used to treat hypertension lower blood pressure by relaxing the constricted arterioles leading to a decrease in the resistance to peripheral blood flow. These drugs exert this effect by decreasing the influence of the sympathetic nervous system on smooth muscle of arterioles, by directly relaxing arteriolar smooth muscle, or by acting on the centers in the brain that control blood pressure.

Antihypertensive drug therapy is usually initiated when the diastolic blood pressure is greater than 90 mm Hg. Initial approaches of antihypertensive treatment include weight reduction, sodium restriction, alcohol restriction, stopping smoking, exercise, and behavior modification. Antihypertensive drug therapy is undertaken in a stepped care fashion. A single drug from one of the following classes should be considered as initial therapy: diuretic, beta-adrenergic blocking agent, calcium channel blocker, or an angiotensin-converting enzyme (ACE) inhibitor. This therapy should be continued for 1–3 months. If the response to the drug is inadequate and if the client is adhering to the dosage regimen and is not experiencing significant side effects, one of the following three options should be considered: (1) add a drug from a different drug class; (2) increase the dose of the first drug, provided it is less than the recommended maximum dose; or (3) discontinue the initial drug and begin therapy with a drug from another drug class. When additional drugs (up to three or four different drugs may be required to control blood pressure) are added to the regimen, they should act by different mechanisms than the drugs already being used. A diuretic should be considered as either the initial or the second drug for antihypertensive drug therapy. The goal of drug therapy is to control the hypertension with the fewest number of drugs at the lowest effective dose. Importantly, the physician should attempt to decrease the dosage or number of antihypertensive drugs at regular intervals along with insisting that the client adhere to the regimen established (i.e., weight control, sodium restriction).

The following drugs are used for stepped care: thiazide diuretics, beta-adrenergic blocking agents, calcium channel blocking drugs, ACE inhibitors, centrally acting alpha-blockers (step II), peripherally acting drugs (step II), vasodilators (step III), and miscellaneous agents. Certain drugs, such as guanethidine (step IV) and captopril are reserved for later use due to their potential side effects.

Other drugs used to treat hypertension include: sedatives and antianxiety agents, rauwolfia alkaloids, ganglionic blocking agents, and one of the monoamine oxidase inhibitors.

NURSING CONSIDERATIONS

Assessment

1. Determine baseline blood pressure before starting any antihypertensive therapy. To ensure accuracy of baseline readings, take blood pressure at least three times during one visit and record.
2. Evaluate the extent of client's understanding of the disease of hypertension and the therapy as prescribed.
3. Ascertain life-style changes clients may have to make to achieve the goal of lowered blood pressure.
4. Assess the probability of the client's willingness to adhere to prescribed therapy.
5. Determine client's ability to take own blood pressure measurements.

Interventions

1. Periodically reassess blood pressure measurements as determined by the client's condition. Monitor I&O and weights.
2. Record significant changes in blood pressure readings or lack of response to medication on the client's record and report to the physician.

Client/Family Teaching

1. Discuss goals of drug therapy in the management of hypertension.
2. Adhere to a low-sodium, low-fat diet; utilize dietitian assist-

ance in meal planning as needed.

3. Explain the importance of adhering to the treatment plan prescribed by the physician. Review the importance of exercise, proper diet, and rest, and of complying with the prescribed drug therapy.

4. Instruct that medication controls but does not cure hypertension. Remind client to take medication despite feeling better and not to stop abruptly as rebound hypertension may occur.

5. Teach clients and a family member how and when to take blood pressure recordings. Assist them to develop a method and explain the importance of keeping a written record to share with the health care provider so that prescribed therapy may be evaluated at each visit.

6. Teach the client and family how to accurately monitor fluid intake and output and weights. Advise to keep a record for physician review and to report any overt changes.

7. Discuss the expected drug responses and the toxic side effects of prescribed drugs. Report these symptoms immediately to the physician.

8. Explain that weakness, dizziness, and fainting may occur with rapid changes of position from supine to standing. Advise to rise slowly from a lying or sitting position and to dangle legs for several minutes before standing to minimize the occurrence of orthostatic hypotension.

9. If clients accidentally miss a dose of medication and if it is remembered at the time of the next dose of drug, they should not double up or take two doses close together.

10. Stress the importance of routine eye exams to detect early retinal changes.

11. Avoid the concomitant use of other medications that could lower blood pressure (e.g., alcohol, barbiturates, CNS depressants) or that could elevate blood pressure (e.g., OTC cold remedies).

12. Avoid any OTC medications, especially cold remedies, without first consulting the physician or pharmacist. Sympathomimetic amines in products used to treat asthma, colds, and allergies are to be used with extreme caution.

13. Advise that exercising in hot weather may enhance the occurrence of hypotensive effects.

14. Avoid excessive amounts of caffeine (tea, coffee, chocolate, or colas).

15. Emphasize the importance and review additional interventions for BP control, some of which may include dietary restrictions of sodium, weight reduction, decreased use of alcohol, discontinuation of tobacco products, exercise programs (and assist to identify one which the client may feel comfortable with) and methods to reduce and deal with stress.

Evaluation: Evaluate client for:
- Evidence of knowledge and understanding of illness, and assess response to therapy and to teaching and level of compliance
- Evidence of a consistent re-

duction in BP as documented in client log
- Evidence of weight loss if on
a reducing diet
- Freedom from complica-
tions/side effects of drug
therapy

Special Concerns

1. Remind clients to always keep
all medications out of the reach
of children.
2. Monitor elderly clients closely.
They tend to have greater sensitivity to drugs and may develop untoward side effects
more quickly than younger
clients.

ANTI-INFECTIVES

*See also the following individual
drugs and drug classes:*

Amebicides and
  Trichomonacides
Aminoglycosides
Anthelmintics
Antimalarials
Antiviral Drugs
Azithromycin
Aztreonam for Injection
Bacitracin
Cephalosporins
Chloramphenicol
Ciprofloxacin Hydrochloride
Clarithromycin
Clindamycin
Eflornithine Hydrochloride
Erythromycins
Fluoroquinolones
Imipenem-Cilastatin Sodium
Lincomycin
Mupirocin
Ofloxacin
Penicillins
Pentamidine Isethionate
Polymyxin B Sulfate
Spectinomycin Hydrochloride

Sulfonamides
Tetracyclines
Vancomycin

General Statement: The beginning of modern medicine is generally related to two events: the proof
by Pasteur that many diseases are
caused by microorganisms and the
discovery of effective anti-infective
drugs. The first of these drugs were
the sulfonamides (1938), followed
by penicillin during the early 1940s.
Since then, dozens of anti-infectives
have been added to the list. More-
over, significant progress has been
made in the development of antiviral drugs.

Unfortunately, the advent of the
anti-infectives has not been a pure
panacea. Some of the bacteria and
other microorganisms have adapted to the anti-infectives, and there
has been a gradual emergence of
bacteria resistant to certain anti-
infectives, especially the antibiotics.
Fortunately, most resistant strains
can be eradicated by new and/or
different antibiotics, antibiotic combinations, or higher dosages.
Nevertheless, awareness of the
problem has prompted somewhat
greater scrutiny by the physician as
to when and how to prescribe
antibiotics.

The following general guidelines
apply to the use of most anti-infective drugs:

1. Anti-infective drugs can be divided into those that are *bacteriostatic;* that is, arrest the
multiplication and further development of the infectious
agent, or *bactericidal;* that is,
eradicate all living microorganisms. Both time of administration and length of therapy may
be affected by this difference.
2. Some anti-infectives halt the

growth of or eradicate many different microorganisms and are termed *broad-spectrum antibiotics*. Others affect only certain specific organisms and are termed *narrow-spectrum antibiotics*.

3. Some of the anti-infectives elicit a hypersensitivity reaction in some persons. Penicillins cause more severe and more frequent hypersensitivity reactions than any other drug.

4. Because of differences in susceptibility of infectious agents to anti-infectives, the sensitivity of the microorganism to the drug ordered should be determined before treatment is initiated. Several sensitivity tests are commonly used for this purpose. The most widely used test—the Kirby-Bauer or disk-diffusion test—gives qualitative results; there are also various quantitative tests aimed at determining the minimal inhibitory concentration (MIC).

5. Certain anti-infective agents have marked side effects, some of the more serious of which are neurotoxicity, including ototoxicity, and nephrotoxicity. Care must be taken not to administer two anti-infectives with similar side effects concomitantly, or to administer these drugs to clients in whom the side effects might be damaging (e.g., a nephrotoxic drug to a client suffering from kidney disease). The choice of anti-infective also depends on its distribution in the body (i.e., whether it passes the blood-brain barrier).

6. Another difficulty associated with anti-infective therapy is that these drugs can eradicate the normal intestinal flora necessary for proper digestion, synthesis of vitamin K, and control of fungi that may gain access to the GI tract (superinfection).

Action/Kinetics: The mechanism of action of the anti-infectives varies. The following modes of action have been identified.[*] Note the considerable overlap among these mechanisms:

1. Inhibition of synthesis of or activation of enzymes that disrupt bacterial cell walls leading to loss of viability and possibly cell lysis (e.g., penicillins, cephalosporins, cycloserine, bacitracin, vancomycin, miconazole, ketoconazole, clotrimazole).

2. Direct effect on the microbial cell membrane to affect permeability and leading to leakage of intracellular components (e.g., polymyxin, colistimethate, nystatin, amphotericin).

3. Effect on the function of bacterial ribosomes to cause a reversible inhibition of protein synthesis (e.g., chloramphenicol, tetracyclines, erythromycin, clindamycin).

4. Bind to the 30S ribosomal subunit that alters protein synthesis and leads to cell death (e.g., aminoglycosides).

5. Effect on nucleic acid metabo-

[*]Sande, M.A., Kapusnik-Uner, J.E., Mandel, G.L.: Antimicrobial agents. In *Goodman and Gilman's The Pharmacological Basis of Therapeutics*, 8th ed. Edited by Gilman, A.G., Rall, T.W., Nies, A.S., Taylor, P. New York, Pergamon Press, 1990, p. 1019.

lism, inhibits DNA-dependent RNA polymerase (e.g., rifampin), or inhibition of DNA supercoiling and DNA synthesis (e.g., quinolones).

6. Antimetabolites that block specific metabolic steps essential to the life of the microorganism (e.g., trimethoprim, sulfonamides).

7. Bind to viral enzymes that are essential for DNA synthesis leading to a halt of viral replication (e.g., acyclovir, ganciclovir, vidarabine, zidovudine).

Uses: Antibiotics as a group are effective against most bacterial pathogens, as well as against some of the rickettsias and a few of the larger viruses. They are ineffective against viruses that cause influenza, hepatitis, and the common cold. Other anti-infectives are effective against a number of parasites including helminths, the malarial parasite, fungi, trichomonas, and others.

The choice of the anti-infective depends on the nature of the illness to be treated, the sensitivity of the infecting agent, and the client's previous experience with the drug. Hypersensitivity and allergic reactions may preclude the use of the agent of choice.

In addition to their use in acute infections, anti-infectives may be given prophylactically in the following instances:

1. To protect persons exposed to a known specific organism

2. To prevent secondary bacterial infections in acutely ill clients suffering from infections unresponsive to antibiotics

3. To reduce risk of infection in clients suffering from various chronic illnesses

4. To inhibit spread of infection from a clearly defined focus, as after accidents or surgery

5. To "sterilize" the bowel or other areas of the body in preparation for extensive surgery

Instead of using a single agent, the physician may sometimes prefer to prescribe a combination of anti-infective agents.

Contraindications: Hypersensitivity or allergic reaction to certain anti-infectives is common and may preclude the use of a particular agent.

Side Effects: The antibiotics and anti-infective agents have few direct toxic effects. Kidney and liver damage, deafness, and blood dyscrasias are occasionally observed.

The following undesirable manifestations, however, occur frequently:

1. Antibiotic therapy often suppresses the normal flora of the body, which in turn keeps certain pathogenic microorganisms, such as *Candida albicans, Proteus,* or *Pseudomonas,* from causing infections. If the flora is altered, *superinfections* (monilial vaginitis, enteritis, urinary tract infections), which necessitate the discontinuation of therapy or the use of other antibiotics, can result.

2. Incomplete eradication of an infectious organism. Casual use of anti-infectives favors the emergence of *resistant* strains insensitive to a particular drug.

Resistant strains often are either mutants of the original infectious agents that have developed a slightly different metabolic pathway and can exist despite the antibiotic, or are variants that have developed the ability to release a chemical substance—for instance, the enzyme penicillinase—which can destroy the antibiotic.

To minimize the chances for the development of resistant strains, anti-infectives are usually given for a prescribed length of time after acute symptoms have subsided. Casual use of antibiotics is discouraged for the same reasons.

Laboratory Tests: The bacteriologic sensitivity of the infectious organism to the anti-infective (especially the antibiotic) should be tested by the laboratory before initiation of therapy and during treatment.

NURSING CONSIDERATIONS

Administration/Storage

1. Check expiration date on container.
2. Check for recommended method of storage for the drug and store accordingly.
3. Clearly mark the date and time of reconstitution, your initials, and the strength of solutions of all drugs. Note the length of time that the drug may be stored after dilution and store under appropriate conditions.
4. Complete the administration of anti-infective agents by IVPB (or as ordered) before the drug loses potency.
5. *Treatment of Overdose:* Discontinue the drug and treat

symptomatically. Supportive measures should be instituted as needed. Hemodialysis may be used although its effectiveness is questionable, depending on the drug and the status of the client (i.e., more effective in impaired renal function).

Assessment

1. Determine if client has experienced any unusual reaction or problems associated with penicillin or related drug therapy.
2. Ensure that diagnostic cultures and sensitivity tests have been done before administering the first dose of anti-infective. Use correct procedure for obtaining, storing, and transporting specimen to the laboratory.

Interventions

1. Report to the physician any history of allergic responses to any anti-infective agents.
2. Conspicuously mark in red, on the client's chart, medication record, care plan, and bed the fact that the client has an allergy and to what. Inform client not to take that drug again unless the physician gives approval after reviewing the history of past allergic reactions to this medication.
3. Ensure that epinephrine, oxygen, antihistamines, and corticosteroids are immediately available to treat an acute allergic response.
4. Once drug therapy is initiated, ask the client about any unusual reactions or problems with the medication. Review with the client possible side effects

such as hives, rashes, difficulty breathing, etc. If any of these occur, they may indicate a hypersensitivity or allergic response and the drug should be discontinued and the physician notified immediately.

5. If the anti-infective is mainly excreted by the kidneys, anticipate reduced dosage in clients with renal dysfunction. Nephrotoxic drugs are usually contraindicated in persons with renal dysfunction because toxic levels of the drugs are rapidly attained when renal function is impaired.

6. Notify physician when two or more anti-infectives are ordered for the same client, especially if the drugs have similar side effects, such as nephrotoxicity and/or neurotoxicity.

7. Assess client for therapeutic response, such as reduction of fever, increased appetite, and increased sense of well-being.

8. Assess client for superinfections, particularly of fungal origin, characterized by black furred tongue, nausea, and diarrhea.

9. *Prevent superinfections by*
   - Limiting client's exposure to persons suffering from an active infectious process
   - Rotating the site of IV administration and by changing IV tubing every 24–48 hr
   - Providing and emphasizing need for good hygiene
   - Instructing care provider to wash own hands carefully before and after contact with the client

10. Have the order for an anti-infective (administered in the hospital) evaluated at least every 5–7 days for renewal, revision, or cancellation.

11. Schedule drug administration throughout 24-hr period to maintain appropriate drug levels. A drug administration schedule is determined by the half-life ($t\frac{1}{2}$) of the drug, the severity of the infection, and the client's need for sleep.

12. Obtain and monitor serum drug levels throughout therapy to ensure that client is receiving the appropriate dose.

Client/Family Teaching

1. Use anti-infectives only under medical supervision.

2. Do not share medications with friends or family members.

3. Teach the proper method for taking medication and time intervals at which to take the prescribed anti-infective.

4. Provide a printed list of adverse side effects. Report signs and symptoms of allergic reactions and superinfections.

5. Prevent recurrence by completing recommended course of therapy, even though client may feel well.

6. Discard any drug remaining after course of therapy is completed.

7. Advise clients with diabetes to perform finger sticks as opposed to urine testing for the most reliable sugar levels.

Evaluation: Evaluate client for a positive clinical response as evidenced by:
   - A reduction of fever
   - A decrease in WBCs
   - An increased appetite
   - Reports of symptomatic improvement
   - Laboratory evidence of therapeutic serum drug levels
   - Freedom from complications of drug therapy

ANTINEOPLASTIC AGENTS

See also the following individual entries:

Altretamine
Asparaginase
Bleomycin Sulfate
Busulfan
Carboplatin for Injection
Carmustine
Chlorambucil
Cisplatin
Cyclophosphamide
Cytarabine
Dacarbazine
Dactinomycin
Daunorubicin
Diethylstilbestrol Diphosphate
Doxorubicin
Estramustine Phosphate Sodium
Etoposide
Floxuridine
Fludarabine Phosphate
Fluorouracil
Flutamide
Goserelin Acetate
Hydroxyurea
Idrarubicin Hydrochloride
Ifosfamide
Interferon Alfa-n3
Interferon Alfa-2a
Interferon Alfa-2b
Leuprolide
Levamisole Hydrochloride
Lomustine
Mechlorethamine
    Hydrochloride
Medroxyprogesterone Acetate
Megestrol Acetate
Melphalan
Mercaptopurine
Mesna
Methotrexate
Methotrexate Sodium
Mitomycin
Mitotane
Mitoxantrone Hydrochloride
Pentostatin
Pipobroman
Plicamycin
Polyestradiol Phosphate
Procarbazine Hydrochloride
Streptozocin
Tamoxifen
Testolactone
Thioguanine
Thiotepa
Vinblastine Sulfate
Vincristine Sulfate

General Statement: Significant progress continues to be made in the drug therapy of neoplastic diseases. Some types of cancer can now be considered "curable" by chemotherapy alone. In many other forms of cancer, especially in cases of suspected metastatic disease, chemotherapy is an important adjunct in treatment. Progress can be attributed, in part, to the more judicious use of an increasing number of combination regimens of antineoplastic agents, the composition and time of administration of which are based on a better understanding of the characteristics of a specified neoplastic disease, on the kinetics of the cell cycle (see *Action/Kinetics*), and on the mechanism of action of the drugs used. Some of the principles underlying successful cancer chemotherapy are reviewed below. Extensive nursing implications to increase the comfort of the client during cancer therapy are provided.

General Impact of Antineoplastic Agents: Many antineoplastic agents slow down the disease process and induce a remission. All antineoplastic agents are cytotoxic (i.e., cell poisons) and therefore interfere with normal as well as neoplastic cells. However, neoplastic cells are much more active and multiply more rapidly than normal cells, and are thus more affected by the antineoplastic agents. Normal tissue cells, such as those of the bone marrow, the GI mucosal epithelium, and hair follicles are naturally active and particularly susceptible to antineoplastic agents. The margin between the dose of antineoplastic drug needed to destroy the neoplastic cells and that needed to cause bone marrow damage, for example, is narrow. Thus, clients who receive antineoplastic agents are closely watched for signs of bone marrow depression, which is characterized by low blood counts (leukocytes, erythrocytes, platelets). Since white blood cells (WBCs) or platelets show the effect of an overdose more rapidly than do erythrocytes, the platelet and WBC counts are often used as a guide to dosage. If a blood or marrow test indicates a precipitous fall in the WBC or platelet count, the antineoplastic agent may have to be discontinued or the dosage modified significantly. Drugs are usually withheld when the WBC count falls below 2,000/mm^3 and the platelet count falls below 100,000/mm^3. Sometimes the effect of the antineoplastic drugs on the bone marrow is cumulative, with the depression of WBCs and platelets occurring weeks or months after initiation of therapy. Thus, clients must be followed carefully. Antineoplastic agents should be administered only by people knowledgeable in their management. Facilities must be available for frequent laboratory evaluations, especially total blood counts and bone marrow tests. The toxicity of the antineoplastic agents is manifested in the lining of the GI tract by development of oral ulcers, intestinal bleeding, and diarrhea. Finally, since hair follicles are also rapidly proliferating tissue, alopecia often accompanies the drug treatment of antineoplastic disease. Antineoplastic agents fall into several broad categories: Alkylating Agents, Antimetabolites, Antibiotics, Natural Products and Miscellaneous Agents, Hormonal and Antihormonal Agents, and Radioactive Isotopes. The choice of the chemotherapeutic agent(s) depends both on the type of the tumor and on its site of growth. Although it has been said that cancer is not one disease but many, a simpler major subdivision involves separation into solid tumors and hematologic malignancies. The former are confined to a specific tissue or organ site initially and usually involve surgery and/or irradiation. Chemotherapy is used to eradicate remaining cells or metastases, or when primary treatment is insufficient or impossible. Chemotherapy is usually the major form of therapy in hematologic malignancies (i.e., leukemias, lymphomas); some cures have been achieved, notably in Hodgkin's disease and the leukemias of childhood. General information applying to all antineoplastic agents (*Action, Uses, Contraindications, Side Effects, Administration,* and extensive *Nursing Considerations*) is presented below.

Action: During division, cells go through a definite number of stages during which they are more or less susceptible to various chemotherapeutic agents (see *Action/Kinetics* of various agents). Some agents, notably the alkylating agents, are effective during all stages of the cycle, while others, the antimetabolites, for example, are effective only during stages of DNA synthesis. The various cell stages are described in Figure 1.

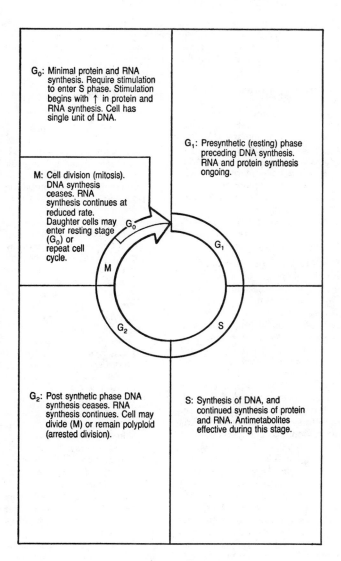

Figure 1 Cell stages.

Uses: Most of the drugs discussed in this section are used exclusively for neoplastic disease. A few are used on an experimental basis for some of the rheumatic diseases.

Contraindications: Hypersensitivity to drug. Most antineoplastic agents are contraindicated for a period of 4 weeks after radiation therapy or chemotherapy with similar drugs. Use with caution, and at reduced dosages, in clients with preexisting bone marrow depression, malignant infiltration of bone marrow or kidney, or liver dysfunction. The safe use of these drugs during pregnancy has not been established; they are contraindicated during the first trimester.

Side Effects: *Bone marrow depression* (leukopenia, thrombocytopenia, agranulocytosis, anemia) *is the major danger of antineoplastic therapy. Bone marrow depression can sometimes be irreversible. It is mandatory that the client have frequent total blood counts and bone marrow examinations. Precipitous falls must be reported to a physician.* Other side effects include: *GI:* Nausea, vomiting (may be severe), anorexia, diarrhea (may be hemorrhagic), stomatitis, enteritis, abdominal cramps, intestinal ulcers. *Hepatic:* Hepatic toxicity including jaundice and changes in liver enzymes. *Dermatologic:* Dermatitis, erythema, various dermatoses including maculopapular rash, alopecia (reversible), pruritus, urticaria, cheilosis. *Immunologic:* Immunosuppression with increased susceptibility to viral, bacterial, or fungal infections. *CNS:* Depression, lethargy, confusion, dizziness, headache, fatigue, malaise, fever, weakness. *GU:* Acute renal failure, reproductive abnormalities including amenorrhea and azoospermia. **Note:** Alkylating agents, in particular, may be both carcinogenic and mutagenic.

GENERAL NURSING CONSIDERATIONS FOR ANTINEOPLASTIC AGENTS

Administration/Storage

1. Antineoplastic drugs should be prepared only by trained personnel; preparation is generally contraindicated by pregnant women.
2. Antineoplastic drugs should be prepared under a laminar flow (biologic) hood.
   - If a laminar flow hood is not available, preparation should be done in a work area away from cooling or heating vents and away from other people. The work area should be covered with a disposable plastic liner.
   - Use latex gloves to protect the skin when reconstituting antineoplastic drugs. Do not use gloves made of polyvinyl chloride since these are permeable to some cytotoxic drugs. Use caution in preparation, particularly to prevent skin reactions. Prevent contact of the drugs with skin or mucous membranes. If this occurs, wash the area immediately with copious amounts of water and document accordingly.
   - Wash the hands well both before and after removing the gloves used for drug preparation.
   - Before beginning preparation the nurse should put on a disposable, nonpermeable surgical gown with a closed front and knit cuffs that completely cover the wrists.

- Wear goggles. Should material accidentally enter the eyes, wash eyes out well with isotonic saline eyewash (or water if isotonic saline is unavailable) and immediately see an ophthalmologist for further care.

3. Use piggyback setup with an electronic infusion pump.

4. Start infusion with a solution not containing the vesicant drug.

5. If possible, do not use the dorsum of the hand, wrist, or antecubital fossa as the site of infusion.

6. Avoid administering medication through a previously used site.

7. After IV has been started and unmedicated solution is being infused, check for blood return and for pain, redness, or edema before starting solution containing medication.

8. Luer-Lok fittings should be a part of all syringes and IV equipment used. Equipment should be disposable.
   - If the drug is to be reconstituted from a vial, vent the vial at the beginning of the procedure. This lowers the internal pressure and reduces the risk of spilling or spraying solution when the needle is withdrawn from the diaphragm.
   - Use a sterile alcohol wipe around the needle and vial top when withdrawing the drug.
   - Place a sterile alcohol wipe around the needle when expelling air from the syringe.

9. Once the drug has been prepared the external surfaces of syringes and bottles should be wiped with an alcohol sponge. All disposable equipment should be placed in a separate disposable plastic bag and marked for incineration.

10. Instruct client to report pain, redness, or edema near the injection site during or after treatment.

11. Due to effects on the reproductive system, client should be advised to practice some form of reliable contraception.

12. Nurses should wear latex gloves when disposing of vomitus, urine, or feces from clients receiving cytotoxic drug therapy.

13. Maintain a record of all exposure during preparation, administration, cleanup, and spills. Follow appropriate institutional guidelines governing exposures allowed extravasation and periodic laboratory evaluations.

Interventions

1. Establish a team involving the client, family, nurse, physician, pharmacist, social worker, and other health care workers to develop a holistic, therapeutic plan for the client's physical, emotional, social, and spiritual concerns.

2. Initially, identify one family member through which the health care team can direct and receive information and have that person function as a liaison for all family members. This should be someone in whom the client has complete confidence.

3. Whenever possible, assure that the members of the health team are people who are com-

mitted to a long-term relationship with the client. This assures that there will be consistency in follow-through of care and provides the client with the emotional support that will be necessary for treatment in the long months and possibly years ahead.

4. Utilize the nursing process format while working with the client and family. Learn from the client and family what they understand from what the physician has explained to them and clarify any misconceptions they may have.

5. Work closely with the client and family as they experience the effects and problems of chemotherapy associated with cure, remission, or palliation.

NURSING CONSIDERATIONS DURING INITIATION OF CHEMOTHERAPY

Assessment

1. Conduct a complete physical assessment of the client. Determine the client's emotional status, and note any history of hypersensitivity to drugs or foods.

2. Examine the client's mouth for any abnormalities or problems. If possible or indicated, contact the client's dentist to clarify any findings.

3. Determine what experience the client has had concerning surgery, prior radiation therapy, or with chemotherapy.

4. If dealing with someone who has just moved to the area or who is visiting and has experienced problems concerning the illness, contact the health professional with whom the client has been working to learn of any potential problems.

5. Ensure that the necessary blood work has been completed. This provides important baseline data against which to measure client progress.

6. Review the client's current pain control regimen. Make sure that pain medication is made available and in quantities necessary to relieve pain.

Interventions

1. Place client on careful intake and output and record.

2. Instruct client to report any pain, redness, or edema that occurs near the site of injection during or after treatment.

3. Report extravasation to the physician and follow the institutional protocol for minimizing the effects.

4. Chart administration of antineoplastic drugs on the medication record and according to the established protocol for the institution.
   - Record client's drug protocol on medication administration record.
   - Day 1 is the first day of the first dose.
   - Number each day after that in sequence, even though client may not receive drug daily.
   - Indicate when the nadir (the time of most severe physiologic depression) is likely to occur so that possible complications, such as infection

and bleeding, can be anticipated and treated early.

- When the drug regimen is repeated, the first day of therapy is charted as day 1.

5. Establish appropriate principles to promote client compliance.

6. Assist the client and family in locating an appropriate support group in their community to assist them in coping with the client's illness, associated therapy, and emotional turmoil in the family unit.

Client/Family Teaching

1. Stress the importance of complying with all aspects of the therapeutic regimen.

2. Supply information and literature appropriate to the particular type of cancer or illness the client has.

3. Outline the types of side effects the client may be expected to experience and identify a means for coping with these problems.

4. Explain that local cancer support groups in their community may assist them to understand and perhaps begin to cope with their illness.

5. Appropriate literature, such as *Chemotherapy and You,* published by the U.S. Department of Health and Human Services, NIH Publication 81–1136, may be useful as a guide during treatment. The American Cancer Association provides free, many booklets related to the various types of cancers, chemotherapy, and how to deal with the side effects of treatments. Encourage clients to go

to their library and physician with unanswered questions.

6. Identify how and where to contact their health care providers to report any side effects, ask questions, or to request clarification of instructions.

7. Review the drugs to be used and the anticipated results.

8. In the event that antineoplastic agents are prepared and administered in the home, families need to be advised as to the proper disposal of urine, feces, and vomitus.

9. If solutions are prepared in the home and accidents of spilling the drug occur, medical attention must be sought immediately. The health department should be notified. The name of the drug and the type and duration of exposure must be recorded and reported.

10. When the clients are at home, instruct them to maintain accurate intake and output records. Provide them with appropriate conversion charts as necessary.

Evaluation: Evaluate client for:

- Evidence of knowledge and understanding of illness, drug side effects, and goals of therapy
- Complaints of nausea and vomiting, anorexia, or diarrhea and determine the effectiveness of the currently prescribed agents
- Evidence of hepatic toxicity or changes in liver enzymes
- The presence of and extent of psychologic depression, lethargy or other signs of

possible changes in mental status.

- Any evidence of acute renal failure.
- Reports that pain is controlled

NURSING CONSIDERATIONS FOR BONE MARROW DEPRESSION

LEUKOPENIA

Assessment

1. Check WBC count (normal values: 5,000–10,000/mm^3).
2. Review differential (normal values: neutrophils 60%–70%, lymphocytes 25%–30%, monocytes 2%–6%, eosinophils 1%–3%, basophils 0.25%–0.5%).
3. Note any sudden sharp drop in WBC count or a reduction below 2,000/mm^3, because these findings might necessitate reduction in dosage or withdrawal of the drug. Withhold drug and report.
4. Check temperature q 4 hr and recheck in 1 hr if there is a slight elevation. Report fever above 38°C (100°F) because client has limited resistance to infection resulting from leukopenia and immunosuppression.
5. Assess skin and orifices of body for signs of infection. Early identification is extremely important, since due to the absence of granulocytes, local abscesses do not form with pus, but infection becomes systemic as a septicemia.
6. Be aware of any signs of infection. Check the oral cavity for sores or the presence of ulcerated areas. Check urine for odor or particulate matter.

7. Be alert to any client report of increased weakness or fatigue. These symptoms may indicate anemia or electrolyte imbalance.
8. Continually assess for any changes in client morale.

Interventions

1. *Prevent infection by* using strict medical asepsis.
2. Provide frequent good physical care.
3. Maintain a clean environment.
4. Use pHisoHex or an antiseptic to wash client who has a tendency to have skin eruptions.
5. Provide mouth care q 4–6 hr, with either normal saline or hydrogen peroxide diluted to half strength with water. Follow with a substrate of milk of magnesia. (Make substrate of milk of magnesia by discarding the clear liquid in the top of the bottle and using the thick white liquid that remains to coat the oral mucosa.) Do not use lemon or glycerin, because they tend to reduce the production of saliva and change the pH of the mouth. Mucosal deterioration occurs if mouth care is not provided at least q 6 hr.
6. Cleanse and dry the rectal area after each bowel movement. Apply A&D ointment if there is irritation.
7. Be prepared to initiate reverse isolation if WBC count falls below 1,500–2,000/mm^3 by:
   - Maintaining client in private room and explaining reasons for this procedure
   - Practicing universal precautions; use gloves, masks, and gowns as ordered

- Limiting articles brought into room
- Providing private bathroom or bedside commode
- Minimizing unnecessary traffic into and out of room
- Screening visitors for infection before they enter room and limiting visitations

8. Prevent nosocomial infections from invasive procedures by:
   - Cleansing skin with an antiseptic before procedure
   - Changing tubing of IV infusion q 24 hr
   - Changing site of IV infusion q 48 hr, if client does not have an implanted venous access device

THROMBOCYTOPENIA

Assessment

1. Obtain platelet count (normal values: 200,000–300,000/mm^3). Client with a platelet count below 150,000/mm^3 should be monitored closely.
2. Check urine for blood cells.
3. Check stool for occult blood.
4. Inspect skin for petechiae or bruising.
5. Assess all orifices for bleeding.
6. Assess blood pressure of hospitalized client q.d. and prn.

Interventions

1. Prevent bleeding by minimizing SC or IM injections. When injections are necessary, apply pressure for 3–5 min to prevent leakage or hematoma.
2. Report and document any unusual bleeding after injection.
3. Do not apply a blood pressure cuff or other tourniquet for excessive periods of time.
4. Advise the client to use safety

measures to *prevent bleeding* from cuts or bruises by:
- Not picking at their nose, as bleeding may result
- Using an electric razor for shaving rather than a blade
- Providing a soft-bristled toothbrush or having client massage gums with fingers to limit irritation
- Rearranging furniture so that area for ambulation is unimpeded and also, to prevent bumping into furniture at night when getting out of bed to go to the bathroom
- Having a night light to permit visualization in the event client must get up during the night

5. *Assist with the treatment of bleeding*
   - Due to epistaxis by pinching nose for 10 min and applying pressure to upper lip to stop nosebleed
   - With transfusion (usually ordered if platelet count falls below 150,000/mm^3). Take baseline vital signs before start of transfusion and then q 15 min after transfusion is started. Monitor vital signs for at least 2 hr after transfusion is completed. Assess for histoincompatibility, indicated by chills, fever, and urticaria. Stop transfusion, provide supportive care, and follow appropriate institutional protocol.

ANEMIA

Assessment

1. Check hemoglobin (normal values: 14–16 g/100 ml blood) and hematocrit (normal values:

men, 40%–54%; women, 37%–47%).

2. Assess client for pallor, lethargy, or unusual fatigue.

Interventions

1. *Minimize anemia by:*
   - Providing a nutritious diet that client can tolerate
   - Administering or instructing client to take vitamins and iron supplements as ordered
2. *Assist with treatment of anemia by:*
   - Administering diet high in iron that client can tolerate
   - Administering vitamins and iron supplements as ordered
   - Assisting with transfusion, as noted above, for treatment of thrombocytopenia

NURSING CONSIDERATIONS FOR GI TOXICITY

NAUSEA/VOMITING

Assessment

1. Determine if the client is refusing food or fluids or just experiencing anorexia.
2. Compare client's nutritional status and weight with the baseline established at the start of therapy and monitor on subsequent visits.
3. Include the family in discussions on nutrition problems as they often supply information the client either forgets to mention or is afraid to talk about.
4. Examine the frequency, character, and amount of vomitus. If the client has been vomiting at home be sure the family member in attendance has been taught to follow this procedure and document accordingly.
5. List antiemetics prescribed and their results.

Interventions

1. *Prevent nausea and vomiting by:*
   - Premedicating with antiemetic as ordered, before administering antineoplastic drug. Usually the antiemetic is ordered to be administered 30 min before or just after administration of antineoplastic agent.
   - Administering antineoplastic on an empty stomach, with meals, or at bedtime, to minimize nausea and vomiting and to produce the most therapeutic effect for the client
   - Teaching client and/or family how to insert an antiemetic suppository
   - Providing ice chips at onset of nausea
   - Providing carbonated beverages to counteract nausea
   - Encouraging ingestion of dry carbohydrates such as toast and dry crackers before initiating activity
   - Waiting for nausea and vomiting to pass before serving food
   - Providing small, nutritious snacks and planning meal schedules to coincide with client's best tolerance time
   - Providing nourishing foods that the client likes
   - Encouraging intake of a high-protein diet
   - Freezing dietary supplements and serving them like ice cream to make them more palatable
   - Avoiding foods with overpowering aroma
   - Encouraging client to chew foods well

- Providing good oral hygiene both before and after meals
- Encourage the client to eat favorite foods where possible. Such encouragement tends to ensure some nutrition will be provided even though the client feels ill.
- Where possible, encourage clients to eat their meals with others, preferably at a table. Sharing with other clients has been shown to encourage some clients to eat.

2. *Assist with the treatment of nausea and vomiting by:*
- Administering antiemetic, as ordered, or contacting physician if antiemetic has not been ordered. All vomiting should be reported to physician, because a change in chemotherapeutic regimen or correction of electrolyte balance may be required.
- Providing supportive care to keep client as comfortable, clean, and free from odor as possible
- Explaining to client that GI discomfort is generally a sign that the drug is also affecting tumor cells
- Try other antiemetic agents if one prescribed is ineffective.
- Attending to correction of electrolyte balance and providing hyperalimentation as necessary
- Screening visitors and calls until client feels able to resume these interactions

DIARRHEA/ABDOMINAL CRAMPING

Assessment

1. Note frequency and severity of cramping caused by hypermotility.

2. Document frequency, color, consistency, and amount of diarrhea, all of which indicate amount of tissue destruction occurring.
3. Assess for signs of dehydration and acidosis indicating electrolyte imbalance, and maintain careful intake and output records.

Interventions

1. *Prevent diarrhea/abdominal cramping by:*
- Providing a bland low-roughage diet
- Increasing the use of constipating foods, such as hard cheeses, in the diet

2. *Assist with the treatment of diarrhea by:*
- Administering antidiarrheal, if ordered, or contacting physician if antidiarrheal has not been ordered. Diarrhea or abdominal cramping should be reported, because a change in chemotherapeutic regimen or correction of electrolyte balance may be required.
- Increasing fluids, unless contraindicated
- Assisting with correction of electrolyte imbalance
- Providing good skin care, especially to the perianal area to prevent skin breakdown. Apply A&D ointment for perianal tenderness. Change client's gown and bed linens frequently; use room deodorizers as needed.

STOMATITIS (MUCOSAL ULCERATION)

Assessment: Assess for dryness of the mouth, erythema, and white patchy areas of the oral mucous membranes that indicate developing stomatitis. Assessment should be done each time the drug/drugs are administered.

Interventions

1. *Prevent stomatitis by:*
   - Assessing oral cavity t.i.d. and reporting bleeding gums or burning sensation especially when acid liquids such as fruit juice are ingested
   - Setting up a regular schedule for oral care
   - Providing good mouth care
   - Applying Vaseline to lips at least t.i.d.
2. *Assist with treatment of stomatitis by:*
   - Continuing to provide good oral care
   - Applying topical viscous anesthetic, such as lidocaine (Xylocaine), before meals, or providing a swish of lidocaine to anesthetize oral mucosa. Client may swallow lidocaine after swishing it around oral cavity but should be encouraged to expectorate it. A physician's order is required for the use of lidocaine.
   - Providing bland foods at medium temperatures
   - Administering nystatin solution or clotrimazole troches for fungal infections

NURSING CONSIDERATIONS FOR NEUROTOXICITY

Assessment

1. Assess for symptoms of minor neuropathies, such as tingling in hands and feet and loss of deep tendon reflexes.

2. Assess for symptoms of serious neuropathies, such as weakness of hands, ataxia, loss of coordination, foot drop, wrist drop, or paralytic ileus.
3. Note what kind of activities the clients liked to do that required using their hands. This could be an important clue when asking clients about changes in sensation or weakness involving the hands.

Interventions

1. *Prevent functional loss due to neurotoxicity by:*
   - Reporting symptoms of neuropathies to the physician early and discussing findings. The physician may decide to change the medication regimen
   - Practicing and teaching seizure precautions
2. *Assist with treatment of neuropathies by:*
   - Using appropriate safety measures in caring for client with a functional loss
   - Maintaining good body alignment by frequent and anatomically correct repositioning. Determine the need for range-of-motion exercises.
   - Obtaining medical orders for stool softeners and laxatives as needed

NURSING CONSIDERATIONS FOR OTOTOXICITY

Assessment: Assess for hearing difficulties before initiating therapy.

Interventions

1. Instruct client to report tinnitus or alteration in hearing.

2. Perform audiometry testing, if indicated, throughout therapy.

NURSING CONSIDERATIONS FOR HEPATOTOXICITY

Assessment

1. Obtain and assess the following liver function tests:
   - Serum bilirubin (normal values: 0.3–1.0 mg/dl). An elevation may indicate liver disease or an increased rate of RBC hemolysis is present.
   - AST (normal values: 5–40 units/ml). Elevation is indicative of changes in the liver, skeletal muscles, lungs, pancreas, and heart. Hepatitis produces striking elevations in the AST.
   - ALT (normal values: 5–35 units/ml). Elevation may be indicative of conditions leading to hepatic necrosis.
   - LDH (normal values: 100–225 units/ml). Elevation may be indicative of hepatitis, pulmonary infarction, and congestive heart failure.
2. Observe for signs of liver involvement, such as abdominal pain, high fever, diarrhea, and yellowing of skin and sclera.

Interventions

1. Prevent further hepatotoxicity by reporting elevations in liver function tests and signs of liver involvement to physician, as these are indications for changing medication regimen.
2. Assist with the treatment for hepatotoxicity by providing supportive nursing care to relieve symptoms, such as pain, fever, diarrhea, and symptoms associated with jaundice.

NURSING CONSIDERATIONS FOR RENAL TOXICITY

Assessment

1. Obtain and assess the following renal function tests:
   - BUN (normal values: 10–20 mg/dl)
   - Serum uric acid (normal values: 2.0–7.8 mg/dl)
   - Creatinine clearance (normal values: women, 0.8–1.7 g/24 hr; men, 1.0–1.9 g/24 hr)
   - Quantitative uric acid (normal values: 250–750 mg/day)
2. Observe and document any stomach pain, swelling of feet or lower legs, shakiness, unusual body movement, and stomatitis.

Interventions

1. Record intake and output.
2. Limit hyperuricemia by encouraging extra fluid intake to speed excretion of uric acid and to decrease hazard of crystal and urate stone formation.
3. Test pH and assist with alkalinization of urine as ordered.

NURSING CONSIDERATIONS FOR IMMUNOSUPPRESSION

Assessment

1. Assess for the presence of fever, chills, or sore throat.
2. Note any changes in WBC count and differential.

Interventions

1. Assist with treatment of client with immunosuppression by:
   - Preventing infection as noted under bone marrow depression for leukopenia

- Advising delay of active immunization for several months after therapy is completed because there may be either a hypo- or hyperactive response

NURSING CONSIDERATIONS FOR GU ALTERATIONS

Assessment

1. Assess for altered GU function.
2. Determine client understanding that most symptoms, such as amenorrhea, cease after medication is discontinued.
3. Ascertain client's comprehension of risks before initiation of therapy, by asking whether physician has informed client that sterility may be a permanent result of therapy.

Intervention: Prevent teratogenesis by teaching client and partner of childbearing age to use contraceptive measures to avoid pregnancy, both during and for several months after therapy. Drug could have a teratogenic effect on the fetus if the woman were to conceive during this period.

NURSING CONSIDERATIONS FOR ALOPECIA

Assessment: Assess client understanding that body hair might fall out during therapy, but that it will grow back. Reinforce that hair may be of a different texture or color, but will start to grow in again about 8 weeks after therapy is completed.

Interventions

1. Minimize alopecia by:
   - Assisting with the application of scalp tourniquet 10–15 min before, during, and for 10–15 min after medication is administered
   - Applying ice packs to scalp 10–15 min before, during, and for 10–15 min after administration of medication
2. Alternatives for managing alopecia include:
   - Encouraging client to shop for a wig before hair loss begins
   - Shaving head, if hair starts to fall out in large clumps, and using a wig or scarf until scalp hair has grown in again
   - Using a wig or scarf while hair is falling out and growing in again
   - Wearing a night cap at bedtime. This assures that hair that falls out during the night will be collected in one place and will not be all over the bed in the morning.
   - Encouraging expression of feelings related to changes in self-image

NURSING CONSIDERATIONS FOR ALTERATIONS IN SKIN

Assessment

1. Assess skin turgor and integrity. Document baseline data for comparison.
2. Anticipate and explain to family that some clients have slight changes in skin color during therapy.

Interventions

1. Maintain cleanliness of skin through bathing and frequent linen changes.
2. Prevent dryness and replenish moisture of skin with emollient lotions.
3. Prevent excessive exposure to sun or artificial ultraviolet light.
4. Use a special mattress or bed to redistribute weight on bony

prominences and to minimize pressure and friction on pressure points.

5. Ensure adequate nutritional intake.

6. Refer for assistance with makeup application as needed.

Evaluation: Evaluate client for:

- Evidence of a reduction in the size and spread of tumor or malignant process
- Clinical evidence of successful administration of chemotherapy with a minimum of adverse side effects

---

ANTIPARKINSON AGENTS

See also the following individual entries:

Amantadine Hydrochloride
Benztropine Mesylate
Biperiden Hydrochloride
Biperiden Lactate
Bromocriptine Mesylate
Carbidopa
Carbidopa/Levodopa
Levodopa
Pergolide
Procyclidine Hydrochloride
Selegiline
Trihexyphenidyl Hydrochloride

General Statement: Parkinson's disease is a progressive disorder of the nervous system, affecting mostly people over the age of 50. The symptoms include slowness of motor movements (bradykinesia and akinesia), stiffness or resistance to passive movements (rigidity), muscle weakness, tremors, speech impairment, sialorrhea (salivation), and postural instability. Parkinsonism is a frequent side effect of certain antipsychotic drugs, including prochlorperazine, chlorpro-

mazine, and reserpine. Drug-induced symptoms usually disappear when the responsible agent is discontinued. Extrapyramidal Parkinson-like symptoms can accompany brain injuries (strokes, tumors) or other diseases of the nervous system. The cause of Parkinson's disease is unknown; however, it is associated with a depletion of the neurotransmitter dopamine in the nervous system. Administration of levodopa—the precursor of dopamine—relieves symptoms in 75%–80% of the clients. Anticholinergic agents also have a beneficial effect by reducing tremors and rigidity and improving mobility, muscular coordination, and motor performance. They are often administered together with levodopa. Certain antihistamines, notably diphenhydramine (Benadryl), are also useful in the treatment of parkinsonism. Clients suffering from Parkinson's disease need emotional support and encouragement because the debilitating nature of the disorder often causes depression. Comprehensive treatment also includes physical therapy.

NURSING CONSIDERATIONS

See *Nursing Considerations* for individual drugs.

ANTITHYROID DRUGS

See also the following individual entries:

Methimazole
Propylthiouracil

Action/Kinetics: Antithyroid drugs include thiouracil derivatives and large doses of iodide. These drugs inhibit (partially or completely) the production of thyroid hormones by the thyroid gland. The drugs act by preventing the incorporation of iodide into tyrosine and coupling of iodotyrosines. Since these agents do not affect release or activity of preformed hormone, it may take several weeks for the therapeutic effect to become established.

Uses: Hyperthyroidism; prior to surgery or radiotherapy. Adjunct in treatment of thyrotoxicosis or thyroid storm. Propylthiouracil is also used to reduce mortality due to alcoholic liver disease.

Contraindications: Lactation (may cause hypothyroidism in the infant).

Special Concerns: Pregnancy category: D. Use with caution in the presence of cardiovascular disease. Prothrombin time should be monitored during therapy as propylthiouracil may cause hypoprothrombinemia and bleeding.

Side Effects: *Hematologic:* Agranulocytosis, thrombocytopenia, granulocytopenia, hypoprothrombinemia, aplastic anemia, leukopenia. *GI:* Nausea, vomiting, taste loss, epigastric pain, sialadenopathy. *CNS:* Headache, paresthesia, drowsiness, vertigo, depression, CNS stimulation. *Dermatologic:* Skin rash, urticaria, alopecia, skin pigmentation, pruritus, exfoliative dermatitis, erythema nodosum. *Miscellaneous:* Jaundice, arthralgia, myalgia, neuritis, edema, lymphadenopathy, vasculitis, lupus-like syndrome, drug fever, periarteritis, hepatitis, nephritis, interstitial pneumonitis, insulin autoimmune syndrome resulting in hypoglycemic coma. *Symptoms of Overdose:* Nausea, vomiting, headache, fever, pruritus, epigastric distress, arthralgia, pancytopenia, agranulocytosis (most serious). Rarely, exfoliative dermatitis, hepatitis, neuropathies, CNS stimulation or depression.

NURSING CONSIDERATIONS

Administration/Storage

1. The medication should be taken every 8 hr around the clock.
2. *Treatment of Overdose:* Maintain a patent airway and support ventilation and perfusion. Very carefully monitor and maintain vital signs, blood gases, and serum electrolytes. Monitor bone marrow function.

Assessment

1. Note if the client is taking any medications that may interact unfavorably with the antithyroid drug and document.
2. If the client is female and of childbearing age, determine if pregnant.
3. Determine that baseline prothrombin times, CBC, and thyroid function studies have been performed.

Interventions

1. Note any client complaint of unusual bleeding, nausea, loss of taste, or epigastric pain. These symptoms should be reported to the physician.
2. Observe for the presence of skin rashes, urticaria, alopecia, changes in skin pigmentation or pruritus. Document and report to the physician.

Client/Family Teaching

1. Advise that it takes up to 12 weeks for the drug to produce

the full effect. Stress that the drug must be taken regularly and exactly as directed. Hyperthyroidism may recur if the drug is not taken properly.

2. Review the symptoms of hyperthyroidism or thyrotoxicosis (palpitations, increased heart rate, nervousness, sleeplessness, sweating, diarrhea, weight loss, fever) and advise client to report if persistent.

3. Review the symptoms of hypothyroidism (weak, listless, tired, headache, dry skin, cold intolerance, constipation) and advise client to report as dosage may require adjustment.

4. Report any sore throat, enlargement of the cervical lymph nodes, GI disturbances, fever, rash, or jaundice. These symptoms may necessitate either a reduction of the dosage of drug or withdrawal of the drug by the physician.

5. Discuss the potential loss of taste perception. If this occurs, advise clients to increase the use of herbs and nonsodium seasonings.

6. Review symptoms of iodism (cold symptoms, skin lesions, stomatitis, GI upset, metallic taste) and advise client to report.

7. Identify the dietary sources of iodine (iodized salt, shellfish, turnips, cabbage, kale) that may need to be omitted from the diet.

8. Explain that if the drug is taken as ordered for 1 or more years, more than half the clients achieve a permanent remission.

9. Stress the importance of reporting for follow-up lab studies and medical evaluations to determine the response to drug therapy.

10. Advise client to carry identification at all times listing problems and medications currently prescribed.

Evaluation: Evaluate client for:
- Laboratory confirmation that thyroid function studies are within desired range
- Clinical evidence of the control of symptoms associated with hyperthyroidism
- A decrease in the vascularity and friability of the thyroid gland in preparation for surgery
- A reduction in mortality in alcoholic liver disease

BARBITURATES

See also the following individual entries:

Pentobarbital
Pentobarbital Sodium
Phenobarbital
Phenobarbital Sodium
Secobarbital
Secobarbital Sodium

General Statement: The barbiturates, especially their sodium salts, are readily absorbed after oral, rectal, or parenteral administration. They are distributed throughout all tissues, cross the placental barrier, and appear in breast milk. Toxic doses depress the activity of tissues in addition to the CNS, including the cardiovascular system. In some patients, barbiturates manifest an unusual action, including an excitatory response.

Action/Kinetics: Barbiturates produce all levels of CNS depression, ranging from mild depression (sedation) following low doses to hypnotic (sleep-inducing) effects, and even coma and death, as dosage is increased. Certain barbiturates are also effective anticonvulsants. The depressant and anticonvulsant effects may be related to their ability to increase and/or mimic the inhibitory activity of the neurotransmitter gamma-aminobutyric acid (GABA) on nerve synapses. For example, the sedative-hypnotic effects of barbiturates may be due to an effect in the thalamus to inhibit ascending conduction in the reticular activating system, thus interfering with the transmission of impulses to the cerebral cortex. The anticonvulsant effects are believed to result from depression of monosynaptic and polysynaptic impulses in the CNS; barbiturates may also increase the threshold for electrical stimulation in the motor cortex. Importantly, barbiturates are not analgesics and therefore should not be given to patients for the purpose of ameliorating pain. The main difference between the various barbiturates is in the onset of action. *Ultrashort-acting:* **Onset: IV,** immediate; **duration:** up to 30 min. *Short-acting:* **Onset: PO,** 10–15 min; **peak effect:** 3–4 hr. *Intermediate-acting:* **Onset: PO,** 45–60 min; **peak effect:** 6–8 hr. *Long-acting:* **Onset: PO,** 60 or more min; **peak effect:** 10–12 hr. **Rectal administration:** Onset times are similar to PO. **IV Administration:** From immediate for short-acting drugs up to 5 min for long-acting drugs. **Duration of sedation:** 3–6 hr after **IV;** 6–8 hr, for all other routes. **Note:** It is currently believed that there is little difference in the duration of hypnosis after the use of any barbiturate; however, there is a difference in the time of onset. Thus, although widely used, the classification by duration of action may be outdated. Barbiturates are metabolized almost completely in the liver (except for barbital and phenobarbital) and are excreted in the urine.

Uses: Preanesthetic medication, anesthesia (thiobarbiturates), sedation, hypnotic, and for the control of acute convulsive conditions (only phenobarbital, mephobarbital, metharbital), as in epilepsy, tetanus, and eclampsia. The benzodiazepines have replaced barbiturates for the treatment of many conditions. See also information on individual drugs.

Contraindications: Hypersensitivity to barbiturates, severe trauma, pulmonary disease, edema, uncontrolled diabetes, history of porphyria, and for clients in whom they produce an excitatory response.

Special Concerns: Barbiturates should be used with caution during pregnancy (category: D) and lactation and in clients with CNS depression, hypotension, marked asthenia (characteristic of Addison's disease, hypoadrenalism, and severe myxedema), porphyria, fever, anemia, hemorrhagic shock, cardiac, hepatic or renal damage, history of alcoholism in suicidal clients. Geriatric clients usually manifest increased sensitivity to barbiturates, as evidenced by confusion, excitement, mental depression, and hypothermia.

Side Effects: *CNS:* Depression of CNS (sleepiness, drowsiness), ataxia, vertigo, nightmares, lethargy, hangover, agitation, confusion, hyperkinesia, paradoxical excitement, nervousness, hallucinations, psychiatric disturbances, insomnia, dizziness, anxiety, delirium, stupor. *CV:* Bradycardia, hypotension, syncope, circulatory collapse. *Respiratory:* Respiratory depression, bronchospasm, hypoventilation, apnea, laryngospasm. *GI:* Nausea, vomiting, diarrhea, constipation, epigastric pain. *Allergic:* Skin rashes, angioneurotic edema, serum sickness, urticaria, morbilliform rash. Rarely, exfoliative dermatitis, Stevens-Johnson syndrome. *Miscellaneous:* Pain syndrome (myalgia, neuralgia, arthritic pain). *After SC use:* Tissue necrosis, pain, tenderness, redness, permanent neurologic damage if injected near peripheral nerves. *After IV use:* Thrombophlebitis. *After IM use:* Pain at injection site. Barbiturates can induce physical and psychologic dependence if high doses are used regularly for long periods of time. Withdrawal symptoms usually begin after 12–16 hr of abstinence. Manifestations of withdrawal include anxiety, weakness, nausea, vomiting, muscle cramps, delirium, and even tonic-clonic seizures. *Symptoms of Acute Toxicity:* Characterized by cortical and respiratory depression; anoxia; peripheral vascular collapse; feeble, rapid pulse; pulmonary edema; decreased body temperature; clammy, cyanotic skin; depressed reflexes; stupor; and coma. After initial constriction the pupils become dilated. Death results from respiratory failure or arrest followed by cardiac arrest. *Symptoms of Chronic Toxicity:* Prolonged use of barbiturates at high doses may lead to physical and psychologic dependence, as well as tolerance. Doses of 600–800 mg daily for 8 weeks may lead to physical dependence. The addict usually ingests 1.5 g/day. Addicts prefer short-acting barbiturates. Symptoms of dependence are similar to those associated with chronic alcoholism, and withdrawal symptoms are equally severe. Withdrawal symptoms usually last for 5–10 days and are terminated by a long sleep.

Drug Interactions

GENERAL CONSIDERATIONS

1. Barbiturates stimulate the activity of enzymes responsible for the metabolism of a large number of other drugs by a process known as *enzyme induction.* As a result, when barbiturates are given to patients receiving such drugs, their therapeutic effectiveness is markedly reduced or even abolished.
2. The CNS depressant effect of the barbiturates is potentiated by many drugs. Concomitant administration may result in coma or fatal CNS depression. Barbiturate dosage should either be reduced or eliminated when other CNS drugs are given.
3. Barbiturates also potentiate the toxic effects of many other agents.

Alcohol / Potentiation or addition of CNS depressant effects. Concomitant use may lead to drowsiness, lethargy, stupor, respiratory collapse, coma, or death
Anesthetics, general / See *Alcohol*
Anorexiants / ↓ Effect of anorexiants due to opposite activities
Antianxiety drugs / See *Alcohol*
Anticoagulants, oral / ↓ Effect of anticoagulants due to ↓ absorption from GI tract and ↑ breakdown by liver

Antidepressants, tricyclic / ↓ Effect of antidepressants due to ↑ breakdown by liver

Antidiabetic agents / Prolong the effects of barbiturates

Antihistamines / See *Alcohol*

Beta-adrenergic agents / ↓ Beta blockade due to ↑ breakdown by the liver

Chloramphenicol / ↑ Effect of barbiturates by ↓ breakdown by the liver and ↓ effect of chloramphenicol by ↑ breakdown by liver

CNS depressants / See *Alcohol*

Corticosteroids / ↓ Effect of corticosteroids due to ↑ breakdown by liver

Digitoxin / ↓ Effect of digitoxin due to ↑ breakdown by liver

Doxorubicin / ↓ Effect of doxorubicin

Doxycycline / ↓ Effect of doxycycline due to ↑ breakdown by liver

Estrogens / ↓ Effect of estrogen due to ↑ breakdown by liver

Furosemide / ↑ Risk or intensity of orthostatic hypotension

Griseofulvin / ↓ Effect of griseofulvin due to ↓ absorption from GI tract

Haloperidol / ↓ Effect of haloperidol due to ↑ breakdown by liver

MAO Inhibitors / ↑ Effect of barbiturates due to ↓ breakdown by liver

Methoxyflurane / ↑ Kidney toxicity due to ↑ breakdown of methoxyflurane by liver to toxic metabolites

Narcotic analgesics / See *Alcohol*

Oral contraceptives / ↓ Effect of contraceptives due to ↑ breakdown by liver

Phenothiazines / ↓ Effect of phenothiazines due to ↑ breakdown by liver; also see *Alcohol*

Phenytoin / ↓ Effect variable; monitor carefully

Procarbazine / ↑ Effect of barbiturates

Quinidine / ↓ Effect of quinidine due to ↑ breakdown by liver

Rifampin / ↓ Effect of barbiturates due to ↑ breakdown by liver

Sedative-hypnotics, nonbarbiturate / See *Alcohol*

Theophyllines / ↓ Effect of theophyllines due to ↑ breakdown by liver

Valproic acid / ↑ Effect of barbiturates due to ↓ breakdown by liver

Laboratory Test Interferences

1. **Interference with test method:** ↑ 17-Hydroxycortico-steroids.
2. **Caused by pharmacologic effects:** ↑ Creatinine phospho-kinase, alkaline phosphatase, serum transaminase, serum testosterone (in certain women), urinary estriol, porphobilino-gen, coproporphyrin, uropor-phyrin. ↓ Prothrombin time in patients on coumarin. ↑ or ↓ Bilirubin. False + lupus erythe-matosus test.

Dosage: See individual drugs. Aim for minimum effective dosage. As hypnotics, barbiturates should be administered intermittently because tolerance develops. Elderly clients should receive one-half of the adult dose, and children should receive one-quarter to one-half the adult dose.

NURSING CONSIDERATIONS

Administration/ Storage

1. When used as hypnotics, barbiturates should not be given for more than 14–28 days.

2. Aqueous solutions of sodium salts are unstable and must be used within 30 min after preparation.
3. Discard parenteral solutions that contain precipitate.
4. During IV administration:
   - Closely monitor the IV administration for the correct rate of flow. A too rapid injection may produce respiratory depression, dyspnea, and shock.
   - Monitor the site of the IV injection closely for extravasation, which may cause pain, nerve damage, and necrosis.
   - Note any redness or swelling along the site of the vein. This is evidence of thrombophlebitis.
5. Maintain an accurate record of the barbiturates on hand and the amounts dispensed following appropriate institutional and DEA guidelines.
6. *Treatment of Acute Toxicity:*
   - Maintenance of an adequate airway, oxygen intake, and carbon dioxide removal are essential.
   - After oral ingestion, gastric lavage or gastric aspiration may delay absorption. Emesis should not be induced once the symptoms of overdosage are manifested, as the client may aspirate the vomitus into the lungs. Also, if the dose of barbiturate is high enough, the vomiting center in the brain may be depressed.
   - Absorption following SC or IM administration of the drug may be delayed by the use of ice packs or tourniquets.

- Maintain renal function.
- Removal of the drug by peritoneal dialysis or an artificial kidney should be carried out.
- Supportive physiologic methods have proven superior to use of analeptics.

7. *Treatment of Chronic Toxicity:* Cautious withdrawal of the hospitalized addict over a 2–4-week period. A stabilizing dose of 200–300 mg of a short-acting barbiturate is administered q 6 hr. The dose is then reduced by 100 mg daily until the stabilizing dose is reduced by one-half. The client is then maintained on this dose for 2–3 days before further reduction. The same procedure is repeated when the initial stabilizing dose has been reduced by three-quarters. If a mixed spike and slow activity appear on the EEG, or if insomnia, anxiety, tremor, or weakness is observed, the dosage is maintained at a constant level or increased slightly until symptoms disappear.

Assessment

1. Note any history of adverse side effects to any of the barbiturate family of drugs.
2. Discuss the client's sleeping pattern with the client and family. This information is important in the physician's decision concerning the type of barbiturate to prescribe.
3. Determine the client's usual bedtime and the usual wakening hours.
4. If the client is of childbearing age determine if pregnancy is likely. Other measures should

be found to encourage sleep if pregnancy is a probability.

5. Determine the cause of the client's inability to sleep. A person in pain who gains relief of the pain may not need sleeping medication. Note evidence of fear and anxiety that may interfere with sleep.

6. Assess the client's environmental preferences for sleep, such as room temperature, lights, and sounds.

7. Note presence of sensory alterations that could cause sleeplessness or disruptions in sleep time.

Interventions

1. Prior to administering the drug, discuss the goals of the medication therapy with the client.

2. Review the treatment for chronic and acute toxicity associated with barbiturates.

3. Do not awaken a client to administer a sleeping medication.

4. Assist the client during ambulation and use side rails once the client is in bed. Clients who receive hypnotic medications may become confused and unsteady. This is a particular problem among the elderly.

5. Use supportive measures such as a back rub, warm drinks, a quiet atmosphere and a calm attitude to encourage relaxation.

6. When the drug is administered PO, remain with the client to determine that the drug has been swallowed. If the client is disoriented and/or wearing dentures, check the buccal cavity, under the tongue, and under denture plates. Routinely check the bedside area to ensure that the client is not hoarding medication.

7. Anticipate that some clients may experience a period of transitory elation, confusion, or euphoria before sedation, and provide appropriate nursing measures to calm the client and prevent injury.

8. If clients become confused after taking the barbiturate, do not apply cuffs or other restraints. Rather remain with them and try to soothe and orient them by turning on a light and talking quietly and calmly until they are relaxed.

9. If the client asks for a second sleeping medication during the night, try to determine the cause of the sleeplessness. Institute comfort measures. If the client has pain, relieve the pain first. Wait approximately 20–30 min and then give the second dose of sleeping medication if the client has not yet fallen asleep.

10. Keep a careful check of the length of time the client has been receiving barbiturates. Therapy that requires sedative doses of medication over an 8-week period of time will cause physical dependence. Remind the medical staff of the amount of time the client has been taking the medication. If the client is not responding as anticipated, review the need to alter the dose and explore other related factors, such as the environment, the existence of psychologic stress, or possibly drug dependence.

11. Assess the client for evidence of physical and/or psychologic dependence and tolerance.

Note any changes in the vital signs and condition of the client's skin. Document and report these findings to the physician.

12. Be alert to signs and symptoms of porphyria, characterized by nausea, vomiting, abdominal pain, and muscle spasms. Document and report the incidence and anticipate that the drug will be discontinued.

13. If the client receiving barbiturates is a child, supervise the child's play activity, especially if child is riding a bicycle or engaging in other potentially dangerous forms of play.

14. At each visit, review the goals of therapy with the client and the effectiveness of the medication regimen. Investigate any problems noted by the client. When clients are receiving barbiturates on an outpatient basis, be alert to the number of times they return for prescription refills. Frequency of refills may indicate the client has developed a dependency or that the client may be selling the drug for profit.

15. Monitor the client's CBC, differential, and platelet count. Some clients may develop hematologic disorders such as agranulocytosis, megaloblastic anemia, and/or thrombocytopenia.

16. If the barbiturate is administered IV to counteract acute convulsions or for anesthesia anticipate that the therapy will be of limited duration.

Client/Family Teaching

1. Avoid the use of alcoholic beverages. These potentiate the effects of barbiturates.

2. Do not drive a car or operate other hazardous machinery after taking the medication.

3. Take the medication only as prescribed.

4. Avoid the use of OTC drugs or other medications unless the physician has first been consulted.

5. If the client is taking barbiturates for insomnia, suggest that the drug be taken a half hour before bedtime.

6. To avoid an accidental overdose, keep the medication in a medicine closet or in a drawer *away from* the bedside.

7. Keep all medications out of the reach of children. Large doses may be fatal and the potential for abuse exists.

8. If taking a barbiturate for 8 or more weeks, client should not discontinue the drug suddenly. To do so may result in withdrawal symptoms such as weakness, anxiety, delirium, and tonic-clonic seizures.

9. Dosages of drug should not be reduced without first checking with the physician.

10. Report to the physician immediately, any signs of hematologic toxicity such as signs of infection (sore throat or fever) or increased bleeding tendencies (nosebleeds or easy bruising).

11. Identify alternative methods to promote relaxation and sleep (such as progressive muscle relaxation, guided imagery or soft music); support the client in exploring these methods.

Evaluation: Evaluate client for any of the following:

• Reports of a reduction in muscle spasms, tremulousness, and level of anxiety in preparation for anesthesia

- Evidence of effective sedation
- Reports of improved sleeping patterns with less frequent awakenings
- Evidence of effective control of seizures

BENZODIAZEPINES

See also the following individual entries:

Alprazolam
Chlordiazepoxide
Clorazepate Dipotassium
Diazepam
Estazolam
Flurazepam
Halazepam
Lorazepam
Oxazepam
Prazepam
Quazepam
Temazepam
Triazolam

General Statement: The benzodiazepines exhibit a wide margin of safety between therapeutic and toxic doses. For example, ataxia and sedation are observed at doses higher than those required to achieve antianxiety effects. The major difference among benzodiazepines appears to be a function of duration of action and other pharmacokinetic properties. All antianxiety agents have the ability to cause psychologic and physical dependence. Withdrawal symptoms usually start within 12–48 hr after stopping the drug and last for 12–48 hr. When the client has received large doses of these drugs for weeks or months, dosage should be reduced gradually over a period of 1–2

weeks. Alternatively, a short-acting barbiturate may be substituted and then withdrawn gradually. Abrupt withdrawal of high dosage of the drug may be accompanied by coma, convulsions, and even death.

Action/Kinetics: The major antianxiety agents include the benzodiazepines and meprobamate. The benzodiazepines are thought to affect the limbic system and reticular formation to reduce anxiety. This effect is believed to be mediated through the action of the benzodiazepines to increase or facilitate the inhibitory neurotransmitter activity of GABA which is one of the inhibitory CNS neurotransmitters. Two benzodiazepine receptor subtypes have been identified in the brain–BZ_1 and BZ_2. Receptor subtype BZ_1 is believed to be associated with sleep mechanisms, whereas receptor subtype BZ_2 is associated with memory, motor, sensory, and cognitive function. When used for 3–4 weeks for sleep, certain benzodiazepines may cause REM rebound when discontinued. Meprobamate and the benzodiazepines also possess varying degrees of anticonvulsant activity, skeletal muscle relaxation, and the ability to alleviate tension. The rate of absorption from the GI tract will determine the onset and intensity of action of the various benzodiazepines. The benzodiazepines generally have long half-lives (1–8 days); thus cumulative effects can occur. Also, several of the benzodiazepines are metabolized to active metabolites in the liver, which prolongs their duration of action. Benzodiazepines are widely distributed throughout the body. Approximately 70%–99% of an administered dose is bound to plasma protein. Metabolites of benzodiazepines are excreted through the kidneys.

Uses: Management of anxiety and tension occurring alone or as a side effect of other conditions, including menopausal syndrome, premenstrual tension, asthma, and angina pectoris. Neurologic conditions involving muscle spasm and tetanus. Insomnia (recurring or due to poor sleeping habits) characterized by difficulty in falling asleep, frequent awakenings during the night, or early morning awakening. Adjunct in treatment of rheumatoid arthritis, osteoarthritis, trauma, low back pain, torticollis, and selected convulsive disorders including status epilepticus. Premedication for surgery or electric cardioversion. Rehabilitation of chronic alcoholics, delirium tremens, nocturnal enuresis in childhood. *Investigational:* Irritable bowel syndrome.

Contraindications: Hypersensitivity, acute narrow-angle glaucoma, psychoses. Use of flurazepam for insomnia in children less than 15 years of age and use of estazolam, quazepam, temazepam, or triazolam for insomnia in children less than 18 years of age.

Special Concerns: Pregnancy category: X (estazolam, quazepam, temazepam, triazolam). Use with caution in impaired hepatic or renal function and in the geriatric or debilitated client. Use during lactation may cause sedation, weight loss, and possibly feeding difficulties in the infant. Geriatric clients may be more sensitive to the effects of benzodiazepines; symptoms may include oversedation, dizziness, confusion, or ataxia. When used for insomnia, rebound sleep disorders may occur following abrupt withdrawal of certain benzodiazepines.

Side Effects: *CNS:* Drowsiness, fatigue, confusion, ataxia, sedation, dizziness, vertigo, depression, apathy, lightheadedness, delirium, headache, lethargy, disorientation, hypoactivity, crying, anterograde amnesia, slurred speech, stupor, coma, fainting, difficulty in concentration, euphoria, nervousness, irritability, akathisia, hypotenia, vivid dreams, "glassy-eyed," hysteria, suicide attempt, psychosis. Paradoxical excitement manifested by anxiety, acute hyperexcitability, increased muscle spasticity, insomnia, hallucinations, sleep disturbances, rage, and stimulation. *GI:* Increased appetite, constipation, diarrhea, anorexia, nausea, vomiting, weight gain or loss, dry mouth, bitter or metallic taste, increased salivation, coated tongue, sore gums, difficulty in swallowing, gastritis, fecal incontinence. *Respiratory:* Respiratory depression and sleep apnea, especially in clients with compromised respiratory function. *Dermatologic:* Urticaria, rash, pruritus, alopecia, hirsutism, dermatitis, edema of ankles and face. *Endocrine:* Increased or decreased libido, gynecomastia, menstrual irregularities. *GU:* Difficulty in urination, urinary retention, incontinence, dysuria, enuresis. *CV:* Hypertension, hypotension, bradycardia, tachycardia, palpitations, edema, cardiovascular collapse. *Hematologic:* Anemia, agranulocytosis, leukopenia, eosinophilia, thrombocytopenia. *Ophthalmologic:* Diplopia, conjunctivitis, nystagmus, blurred vision. *Miscellaneous:* Joint pain, lymphadenopathy, muscle cramps, paresthesia, dehydration, lupus-like symptoms, sweating, shortness of breath, flushing, hiccoughs, fever, hepatic dysfunction. *Following IM use:* Redness, pain, burning. *Following IV use:* Thrombosis and phlebitis at site. *Symptoms of Overdose:* Severe drowsiness, confusion with reduced or absent reflexes, tremors, slurred speech, staggering, hypotension, shortness of breath, labored breathing, respiratory depression, impaired coordination, seizures, weakness, slow heart rate, coma. **Note:** Geriatric clients, debilitated clients, young children, and clients with liver disease are more sensitive to the CNS effects of benzodiazepines.

Drug Interactions

Alcohol / Potentiation or addition of CNS depressant effects. Concomitant use may lead to drowsiness, lethargy, stupor, respiratory collapse, coma, or death

Anesthetics, general / See *Alcohol*

Antacids / ↓ Rate of absorption of benzodiazepines

Antidepressants, tricyclic / Concomitant use with benzodiazepines may cause additive sedative effect and/or atropine-like side effects

Antihistamines / See *Alcohol*

Barbiturates / See *Alcohol*

Cimetidine / ↑ Effect of benzodiazepines by ↓ breakdown in liver

CNS depressants / See *Alcohol*

Digoxin / Benzodiazepines ↑ effect of digoxin by ↑ serum levels

Disulfiram / ↑ Effect of benzodiazepines by ↓ breakdown in liver

Erythromycin / ↑ Effect of benzodiazepines by ↓ breakdown in liver

Fluoxetine / ↑ Effect of benzodiazepines due to ↓ breakdown in liver

Isoniazid / ↑ Effect of benzodiazepines due to ↓ breakdown in liver

Ketoconazole / ↑ Effect of benzodiazepines due to ↓ breakdown in liver

Levodopa / Effect may be ↓ by benzodiazepines

Metoprolol / ↑ Effect of benzodiazepines due to ↓ breakdown in liver

Narcotics / See *Alcohol*

Neuromuscular blocking agents / Benzodiazepines may ↑, ↓, or have no effect on the action of neuromuscular blocking agents

Oral contraceptives / ↑ Effect of benzodiazepines due to ↓ breakdown in liver; or, ↑ rate of clearance of benzodiazepines that undergo glucuronidation (e.g., lorazepam, oxazepam)

Phenothiazines / See *Alcohol*

Phenytoin / Concomitant use with benzodiazepines may cause ↑ effect of phenytoin due to ↓ breakdown by liver

Probenecid / ↑ Effect of selected benzodiazepines due to ↓ breakdown by liver

Propoxyphene / ↑ Effect of benzodiazepines due to ↓ breakdown by liver

Propranolol / ↑ Effect of benzodiazepines due to ↓ breakdown by liver

Ranitidine / May ↓ absorption of benzodiazepines from the GI tract

Rifampin / ↓ Effect of benzodiazepines due to ↑ breakdown by liver

Sedative-hypnotics, nonbarbiturate / See *Alcohol*

Theophyllines / ↓ Sedative effect of benzodiazepines

Valproic acid / ↑ Effect of benzodiazepines due to ↓ breakdown by liver

Laboratory Test Interference:
↑ AST, ALT, LDH, alkaline phosphatase.

Dosage: See individual drugs.

NURSING CONSIDERATIONS

Administration/Storage

1. Persistent drowsiness, ataxia, or visual disturbances may require dosage adjustment.
2. Lower dosage is usually indicated for older clients.
3. GI effects are decreased when drugs are given with meals or shortly afterward.
4. Withdraw drugs gradually.
5. Review the list of drug interactions prior to taking the client's history and beginning drug therapy.
6. In case of overdose, a benzodiazepine antagonist (flumazenil) should be readily available.
7. *Treatment of Overdose:* Supportive therapy. Gastric lavage, provided that an endotracheal tube with an inflated cuff is used to prevent aspiration of vomitus. Emesis only if drug ingestion was recent and client is fully conscious. Activated charcoal and saline cathartic may be given after emesis or lavage. Adequate respiratory function must be maintained. Hypotension may be reversed by IV fluids, norepinephrine, or metaraminol. Excitation should **not** be treated with barbiturates.

Assessment

1. Note any history of adverse reactions to this class of drugs.
2. Assess the client's life-style and general level of health.
3. Note the manner in which the client responds to questions and discusses the problem.
4. Determine if the client has had any prior treatment for the same problems and the outcome.
5. Obtain baseline CBC, liver and renal function studies to determine potential problems or impaired function.
6. Review the client's physical history for any contraindications to drug therapy.
7. List drugs client currently taking to prevent any unfavorable interactions.

Interventions

1. Document any symptoms consistent with overdosage.
2. Determine the presence of any blood dyscrasias that could preclude administering the drug.
3. If the client complains of a sore throat, fever, or weakness, assess for blood dyscrasias. Obtain CBC with differential, notify the physician, and anticipate that the drug may be withheld until appropriate data can be evaluated.
4. Monitor the blood pressure before and after the client receives an IV dose of antianxiety medication. Keep the client in a recumbent position for 2–3 hr after IV administration. Determine the presence and degree of hypotension and document.
5. Anticipate that the dosage of drug will be the lowest possible effective one, especially when administering the drug to the elderly or debilitated client.
6. When the drug is administered

to a hospitalized client, remain with client until the drug is swallowed.

7. If the client exhibits ataxia, or complains of weakness or lack of coordination when ambulating, provide assistance. Use side rails once the client is back in bed.

8. Note any early symptoms of cholestatic jaundice, such as client complaint of nausea, diarrhea, upper abdominal pain, or the presence of high fever or rash. Check liver functions studies and report to the physician.

9. If there is any yellowing of the client's sclera, skin, or mucous membranes, the client is exhibiting a late sign of cholestatic jaundice and biliary tract obstruction. Withhold the medication, document and report to the physician.

10. If the client appears overly sleepy, confused, or becomes comatose, withhold the drug, document, and report to the physician.

11. If the client has suicidal tendencies, anticipate that the drug will be prescribed in small doses. Be alert to signs of increased depression and report immediately.

12. If the prescription is for a client who has a history of alcoholism or of taking excessive quantities of drug, carefully supervise the amount of drug prescribed and dispensed.

13. Note any other evidences of client physical or psychologic dependence.

14. Assess for manifestations of ataxia, slurred speech, and vertigo. Such symptoms are characteristic of chronic intoxica-

tion and are usually indications that the client is taking more than the recommended dose of drug.

15. For clients receiving the medication on an outpatient basis, determine the frequency of the requests for medication. Count the number of pills or capsules left at the time of the request for refills or renewal of the prescription if the frequency seems out of the ordinary. The client may be taking larger doses than are recommended.

Client/Family Teaching

1. Stress that these drugs may reduce the ability to handle potentially dangerous equipment, such as automobiles and other machinery.

2. Avoid alcohol while taking anti-anxiety agents. Alcohol potentiates the depressant effects of both the alcohol and the medication.

3. Do not take any unprescribed or OTC medications without first consulting with the physician.

4. Arise slowly from a supine position and dangle the legs over the side of the bed for a few minutes before standing up.

5. If feeling faint client should sit or lie down immediately and lower the head.

6. Encourage working clients to allow extra time to prepare for their daily activities to enable them to take the necessary precautions before arising, thereby reducing one source of anxiety and stress.

7. Do not stop taking the drug suddenly. Any sudden with-

drawal of the drug after a prolonged period of therapy or after excessive use may cause a recurrence of the preexisting symptoms of anxiety. It may also cause a withdrawal syndrome, manifested by increased anxiety, anorexia, insomnia, vomiting, ataxia, muscle twitching, confusion, and hallucinations. Some clients may develop seizures and convulsions.

8. Instruct the client and family in several relaxation techniques that may assist in lowering their anxiety levels.

Evaluation: Evaluate client for:
- Reports of symptomatic improvement noting a decreased frequency in the occurrence of anxiety and tension episodes as well as evidence of new coping strategies
- Evidence of a reduction in the frequency and intensity of muscle spasms and tremulousness
- Reports of improved sleeping patterns with less frequent awakenings, especially early morning
- Reports of effective control of seizures

BETA-ADRENERGIC BLOCKING AGENTS

See also the following individual agents:

Acebutolol Hydrochloride
Atenolol
Betaxolol Hydrochloride
Carteolol Hydrochloride
Esmolol Hydrochloride

Levobunolol Hydrochloride
Metipranolol Hydrochloride
Metoprolol Tartrate
Nadolol
Penbutolol Sulfate
Pindolol
Propranolol Hydrochloride
Timolol Maleate

Action/Kinetics: Beta-adrenergic blocking agents combine reversibly with beta-adrenergic receptors to block the response to sympathetic nerve impulses, circulating catecholamines, or adrenergic drugs. Beta-adrenergic receptors have been classified as beta-1 (predominantly in the cardiac muscle) and beta-2 (mainly in the bronchi and vascular musculature). Blockade of beta-1 receptors decreases heart rate, myocardial contractility, and cardiac output; in addition, AV conduction is slowed. These effects lead to a decrease in blood pressure, as well as a reversal of cardiac arrhythmias. Blockade of beta-2 receptors increases airway resistance in the bronchioles and inhibits the vasodilating effects of catecholamines on peripheral blood vessels. The various beta-blocking agents differ in their ability to block beta-1 and beta-2 receptors (see individual drugs); also, certain of these agents have intrinsic sympathomimetic action.

Uses: Depending on the drug, these agents may be used to treat one or more of the following conditions: hypertension, angina pectoris, cardiac arrhythmias, myocardial infarction, prophylaxis of migraine, tremors (essential, lithium-induced, parkinsonism), situational anxiety, aggressive behavior, antipsychotic-induced akathisia, esophageal varices rebleeding, and alcohol withdrawal syndrome. Propranolol is indicated for a number of other conditions (see information on propranolol).

Contraindications: Sinus bradycardia, greater than first degree heart block, cardiogenic shock, congestive heart failure unless secondary to tachyarrhythmia treatable with beta-blockers, overt cardiac failure. Most are contraindicated in chronic bronchitis, asthma, bronchospasm, emphysema.

Special Concerns: Use with caution in diabetes, thyrotoxicosis, and impaired hepatic and renal function. Safe use during pregnancy and lactation and in children has not been established. Also, see individual agents.

Side Effects: *CV:* Bradycardia, hypotension (especially following IV use), congestive heart failure, cold extremities, claudication, worsening of angina, strokes, edema, syncope, arrhythmias, chest pain, peripheral ischemia, flushing, shortness of breath, sinoatrial block, pulmonary edema, vasodilation, increased heart rate, palpitations, conduction disturbances, first and third degree heart block, worsening of AV block, thrombosis of renal or mesenteric arteries, precipitation or worsening of Raynaud's phenomenon. Sudden withdrawal of large doses may cause angina, ventricular tachycardia, fatal myocardial infarction, or sudden death. *GI:* Nausea, vomiting, diarrhea, flatulence, dry mouth, constipation, anorexia, cramps, bloating, gastric pain, dyspepsia, distortion of taste, weight gain or loss, retroperitoneal fibrosis, ischemic colitis. *Hepatic:* Hepatomegaly, acute pancreatitis, elevated liver enzymes. *Respiratory:* Asthma-like symptoms, bronchospasms, bronchial obstruction, wheeziness, laryngospasm with respiratory distress, worsening of chronic obstructive lung disease, dyspnea, cough, nasal stuffiness, rhinitis, pharyngitis, rales. *CNS:* Dizziness, fatigue, lethargy, vivid dreams, depression, hallucinations, delirium, psychoses, paresthesias, insomnia, nervousness, nightmares, headache, vertigo, disorientation of time and place, hypoesthesia or hyperesthesia, decreased concentration, short-term memory loss, change in behavior, emotional lability, slurred speech, lightheadedness. In the elderly, paranoia, disorientation, and combativeness have occurred. *Hematologic:* Agranulocytosis, thrombocytopenia. *Allergic:* Fever, sore throat, respiratory distress, rash, laryngospasm, pharyngitis, anaphylaxis. *Skin:* Pruritus, rashes, increased skin pigmentation, sweating, dry skin, alopecia, skin irritation, psoriasis (reversible). *Musculoskeletal:* Joint and muscle pain, arthritis, arthralgia, back pain, muscle cramps. *GU:* Impotence, decreased libido, dysuria, urinary tract infection, nocturia, urinary retention or frequency, pollakiuria. *Ophthalmic:* Visual disturbances, eye irritation, dry or burning eyes, blurred vision, conjunctivitis. *Other:* Hyperglycemia or hypoglycemia, lupus-like syndrome, Peyronie's disease, tinnitus, increase in symptoms of myasthenia gravis, facial swelling, decreased exercise tolerance, rigors, speech disorders. *Symptoms of Overdose:* Cardiovascular symptoms include bradycardia, hypotension, congestive heart failure, cardiogenic shock, intraventricular conduction disturbances, AV block, pulmonary edema, asystole, and tachycardia. Also, overdosage of pindolol may cause hypertension and overdosage of propranolol may result in systemic vascular resistance. CNS symptoms include respiratory depression, decreased consciousness, coma, and seizures. Miscellaneous symptoms include bronchospasm (especially in clients with obstructive pulmonary disease), hyperkalemia, and hypoglycemia.

Drug Interactions

Anesthetics, general / Additive depression of myocardium

Anticholinergic agents / Counteract bradycardia produced by beta-adrenergic blockers

Antihypertensives / Additive hypotensive effect

Chlorpromazine / Additive beta-adrenergic blocking action

Cimetidine / ↑ Effect of beta blockers due to ↓ breakdown by liver

Clonidine / Paradoxical hypertension; also, ↑ severity of rebound hypertension

Disopyramide / ↑ Effect of both drugs

Epinephrine / Beta blockers prevent beta-adrenergic action of epinephrine but not alpha-adrenergic action → ↑ systolic and diastolic blood pressure and ↓ heart rate

Furosemide / ↑ Beta-adrenergic blockade

Hydralazine / ↑ Beta-adrenergic blockade

Indomethacin / ↓ Effect of beta blockers possibly due to inhibition of prostaglandin synthesis

Insulin / Beta blockers ↑ hypoglycemic effect of insulin

Lidocaine / ↑ Effect of lidocaine due to ↓ breakdown by liver

Methyldopa / Possible ↑ blood pressure to alpha-adrenergic effect

Nonsteroidal anti-inflammatory drugs / ↓ Effect of beta blockers, possibly due to inhibition of prostaglandin synthesis

Oral contraceptives / ↑ Effect of beta blockers due to ↓ breakdown by liver

Phenformin / ↑ Hypoglycemia

Phenobarbital / ↓ Effect of beta blockers due to ↑ breakdown by liver

Phenothiazines / ↑ Effect of both drugs

Phenytoin / Additive depression of myocardium; also phenytoin ↓ effect of beta blockers due to ↑ breakdown by liver

Prazosin / ↑ First-dose effect of prazosin (acute postural hypotension)

Reserpine / Additive hypotensive effect

Rifampin / ↓ Effect of beta blockers due to ↑ breakdown by liver

Ritodrine / Beta blockers ↓ effect of ritodrine

Salicylates / ↓ Effect of beta blockers, possibly due to inhibition of prostaglandin synthesis

Succinylcholine / Beta blockers ↑ effects of succinylcholine

Sympathomimetics / Reverse effects of beta blockers

Theophylline / Beta blockers reverse the effect of theophylline; also, beta blockers ↓ renal clearance of theophylline

Tubocurarine / Beta blockers ↑ effects of tubocurarine

Verapamil / Possible side effects

since both drugs ↓ myocardial contractility or AV conduction.

Laboratory Test Interference: ↓ Serum glucose.

Dosage: See individual drugs.

NURSING CONSIDERATIONS

Administration/Storage

1. Sudden cessation of beta blockers may precipitate or worsen angina.
2. *Treatment of Overdosage:*
   - To improve blood supply to the brain, place client in a supine position and raise the legs.
   - Measure blood glucose and serum potassium. Monitor blood pressure and ECG continuously.
   - Provide general supportive treatment such as inducing emesis or gastric lavage and artificial respiration.
   - *Seizures:* Give IV diazepam or phenytoin.
   - *Excessive bradycardia:* If hypotensive, give atropine, 0.6 mg; if no response, give q 3 min for a total of 2–3 mg. Cautious administration of isoproterenol may be tried. Also, glucagon, 5–10 mg rapidly over 30 seconds, followed by continuous IV infusion of 5 mg/hr may reverse bradycardia. Transvenous cardiac pacing may be needed for refractory cases.
   - *Cardiac failure:* Digitalis, diuretic, and oxygen; if failure is refractory, IV aminophylline or glucagon may be helpful.
   - *Hypotension:* Place client in Trendelenburg position. IV fluids unless pulmonary edema is present; also vaso-

pressors such as norepinephrine (may be drug of choice), dobutamine, dopamine with monitoring of blood pressure. If refractory, glucagon may be helpful. In intractable cardiogenic shock, intra-aortic balloon insertion may be required.
   - *Premature ventricular contractions:* Lidocaine or phenytoin. Disopyramide, quinidine, and procainamide should be avoided as they depress myocardial function further.
   - *Bronchospasms:* Give a beta-2 adrenergic agonist, epinephrine, or theophylline.
   - *Heart block, second or third degree:* Isoproterenol or transvenous cardiac pacing.

Assessment

1. Take the client's pulse and blood pressure prior to beginning therapy.
2. Obtain serum glucose level, liver and renal function studies as a baseline against which to measure results after medication regimen begins.
3. Note any history of diabetes or impaired renal function.

Interventions

1. Take pulse rate and BP, at least once a day to assure that the client has not developed tachycardia or bradycardia.
2. When assessing the client's respirations note the rate and quality. Drugs in this category may cause dyspnea and bronchospasm.
3. Monitor I&O and daily weights. Observe for increasing dyspnea, coughing, client complaint

of difficulty breathing or fatigue, or the presence of edema. These are symptoms of congestive heart failure and indicate that the client may require digitalization, diuretics, and/or discontinuation of drug therapy.

4. Assess any client complaints of "having a cold, easy fatigue, or feeling of lightheadedness." These side effects may indicate a need to have the medication changed.

5. If working with a client with diabetes be especially cognizant of symptoms of hypoglycemia, such as hypotension or tachycardia. Most beta-adrenergic blocking agents mask these signs.

Client/Family Teaching

1. Instruct in taking blood pressures and pulse rates. Assess client/family knowledge and understanding of illness, and level of compliance as based on response to therapy and teaching.

2. Develop a method to maintain accurate written records of blood pressures and pulse rates. Instruct client to maintain a written record for review by the health care provider so that medication can be adjusted as needed.

3. Provide written instructions as to when to call the physician, for example if the pulse rate goes below 50 beats/min or the blood pressure is less than 90 mm Hg systolic.

4. Once dose is established, take and record BP at least twice a week and take pulse rate immediately prior to first dose each day unless otherwise directed.

5. Reinforce that when prescribed for BP control, medication controls hypertension but does not cure it. Stress the importance of continuing to take the medication despite feeling better and not to stop abruptly as rebound hypertension may occur.

6. Advise client to always consult a physician before interrupting therapy because abrupt withdrawal of most beta-adrenergic blocking agents may precipitate angina, myocardial infarction, or rebound hypertension.

7. Some drugs may cause blurred vision, dizziness or drowsiness; do not engage in activities that require mental alertness until drug effects become apparent.

8. Advise client to rise from a sitting or lying position slowly and to dangle legs before standing to avoid symptoms of orthostatic hypotension.

9. Dress warmly during cold weather because diminished blood supply to extremities may cause client to be more sensitive to the cold. Advise to check extremities for warmth.

10. Avoid excessive intake of coffee, tea, or cola. Consult with physician before taking any OTC preparations.

11. Clients with diabetes should be attentive to symptoms of hypoglycemia and should perform finger sticks more often while on drug therapy. Document and report any overt changes.

12. Report any asthma-like symptoms, cough, or nasal stuffiness to the physician as these may be symptoms of congestive heart failure and require further evaluation.

13. Report any bothersome side effects to the physician, especially new-onset depression.
14. Always keep all medications out of the reach of children.

Evaluation: Evaluate client for:
- Evidence of a decrease in blood pressure
- Reports of a reduction in the frequency and severity of anginal attacks
- Reports of a reduction in anxiety levels
- Clinical evidence of a decrease in tremors
- Reports of effective migraine prophylaxis
- ECG confirmation of control of cardiac arrhythmias
- Any evidence of intolerance to drug therapy

CALCIUM CHANNEL BLOCKING AGENTS

See also the following individual entries:

Bepridil Hydrochloride
Diltiazem Hydrochloride
Felodipine
Isradipine
Nicardipine Hydrochloride
Nifedipine
Nimodipine
Verapamil Hydrochloride

Action/Kinetics: Calcium ions are important for generation of action potentials and for excitation/contraction of muscles. For contraction of cardiac and smooth muscle to occur, extracellular calcium must move into the cell through openings called *calcium channels*. The calcium channel blocking agents (also called *slow channel blockers* or *calcium antagonists*) inhibit the influx of calcium through the cell membrane, resulting in a depression of automaticity and conduction velocity in both smooth and cardiac muscle. This leads to a depression of contraction in these tissues. Although all drugs in this class act similarly, they have different degrees of selectivity on vascular smooth muscle, myocardium, and conduction and pacemaker tissues. In the myocardium, these drugs dilate coronary vessels and inhibit spasms of coronary arteries. They also decrease total peripheral resistance, thus reducing energy and oxygen requirements of the heart. These effects benefit various types of angina. These agents also are effective against certain cardiac arrhythmias by slowing AV conduction and prolonging repolarization. In addition, they depress the amplitude, rate of depolarization, and conduction in atria.

Uses: See individual drugs. Depending on the drug, calcium channel blockers are used for angina pectoris (chronic stable, unstable, or vasospastic) and essential hypertension. Selected drugs are used for arrhythmias (verapamil) or subarachnoid hemorrhage (nimodipine).

Contraindications: Sick sinus syndrome, second or third degree AV block (except with a functioning pacemaker). Use of bepridil, diltiazem, or verapamil for hypotension (less than 90 mm Hg). Lactation.

Special Concerns: Pregnancy category: C. Abrupt withdrawal of calcium channel blockers may result in increased frequency and duration of chest pain. Safety and effectiveness of bepridil, diltiazem, felodipine, and isradipine have not been established in children.

Side Effects: Side effects vary from one calcium channel blocker to another; refer to individual drugs. *Symptoms of Overdose:* Nausea, weakness, drowsiness, dizziness, slurred speech, confusion, marked and prolonged hypotension, bradycardia, junctional rhythms, second or third degree block.

Drug Interactions

Beta-adrenergic blocking agents / Beta blockers may cause depression of myocardial contractility and AV conduction
Cimetidine / ↑ Effect of calcium channel blockers due to ↓ first-pass metabolism
Fentanyl / Severe hypotension or increased fluid volume requirements
Ranitidine / ↑ Effect of calcium channel blockers due to ↓ first-pass metabolism

NURSING CONSIDERATIONS

Administration/Storage: *Treatment of Overdosage:*
- Treatment is supportive. Monitor cardiac and respiratory function.
- If client is seen soon after ingestion, emetics or gastric lavage should be considered followed by cathartics.
- *Hypotension:* IV calcium, dopamine, isoproterenol, metaraminol, norepinephrine. Also, provide IV fluids. Place client in Trendelenburg position.
- *Ventricular tachycardia:* IV procainamide or lidocaine; also, cardioversion may be necessary. Also, provide slow-drip IV fluids.
- *Bradycardia, asystole, AV*

block: IV atropine sulfate (0.6–1 mg), calcium gluconate (10% solution), isoproterenol, norepinephrine; also, cardiac pacing may be indicated. Provide slow-drip IV fluids.

Assessment

1. Note if the client has had any experience with calcium channel blocking drugs in the past and, if so, the response of the client to the drugs.
2. Determine that baseline weight, vital signs, and ECG have been performed.

Interventions

1. These drugs cause peripheral vasodilation. Therefore, clients should have their blood pressure and pulse monitored during the initial administration of the drug. Any excessive hypotensive response and increased heart rate may precipitate angina.
2. Monitor I&O and daily weights. Assess for symptoms of CHF (weight gain, peripheral edema, dyspnea, rales, jugular vein distention).

Client/Family Teaching

1. Discuss the goals of therapy (e.g., to decrease the diastolic BP by 10 mm Hg, to decrease the heart rate by 20 beats/min etc).
2. Teach how to take pulse and BP at home. This should be done at the same time of day and at least twice a week.
3. Develop a method to maintain a written record of BP and pulse and to note any response after taking the drug. This re-

cord should be brought for the physician to review at each visit.

4. Evaluate client understanding and adherence to prescribed drug regimen. Correct any misunderstandings the client may have.

5. Review benefits of the drug and any possible side effects. Encourage the client to report any new signs or symptoms to the health care provider.

6. Advise not to perform activities that require mental alertness until drug effects are realized.

7. Report any side effects such as dizziness, vertigo, unusual flushing, facial warmth, or headaches.

8. If postural hypotension occurs, advise the client to change positions slowly, especially when standing up from a reclining position. Sit down immediately if faintness occurs. Move slowly from lying down to a sitting or standing position.

9. Explain that long periods of standing, excessive heat, hot showers or baths, and ingestion of alcohol may exacerbate postural hypotension.

10. Avoid alcohol and any OTC preparations without physician approval.

11. Stress that if the client notices any swelling of the hands or feet, pronounced dizziness, or chest pain accompanied by diaphoresis, or shortness of breath, or if severe headaches occur, the physician should be notified immediately.

12. Take calcium channel blocking agents with meals to reduce GI irritation.

Evaluation: Evaluate client for:

- Clinical evidence of a decrease in blood pressure and/or a decrease in pulse rate depending on the goals of therapy. Review the client's BP and pulse record and progress in attaining these goals
- Reports of a reduction in the frequency and intensity of anginal attacks
- ECG evidence of control of cardiac arrhythmias

CALCIUM SALTS

See also the following individual entries:

Calcium Carbonate
Calcium Chloride
Calcium Citrate
Calcium Glubionate
Calcium Gluceptate
Calcium Gluconate
Calcium Lactate
Dibasic Calcium Phosphate Dihydrate

Classification: Electrolyte, mineral.

Action/Kinetics: Calcium is essential for maintaining normal function of nerves, muscles, the skeletal system, and permeability of cell membranes and capillaries. For example, calcium is necessary for activation of many enzyme reactions and is required for nerve impulses; contraction of cardiac, smooth, and skeletal muscle, renal function, respiration, and blood coagulation. It has a role in the release of neurotransmitters and hormones; in the uptake and binding of amino acids, in vitamin B_{12}

absorption, and in gastrin secretion. The normal serum calcium concentration is 9–10.4 mg/dl (4.5–5.2 mEq/L). When the calcium level of the extracellular fluid falls below this level, calcium is first mobilized from bone. However, eventually blood calcium depletion may be significant. Hypocalcemia is characterized by muscular fibrillation, twitching, skeletal muscle spasms, leg cramps, tetanic spasms, cardiac arrhythmias, smooth muscle hyperexcitability, mental depression, and anxiety states. Excessive, chronic hypocalcemia is characterized by brittle, defective nails, poor dentition, and brittle hair. The daily RDA for elemental calcium is 0.8 g/day for adults over 25 years of age and children 1–10 years of age, 1.2 g for pregnant or lactating women and both males and females 11–24 years of age, 0.6 g for children 6–12 months of age, and 0.4 g for infants less than 6 months of age. Calcium deficiency can be corrected by the administration of various calcium salts. Calcium is well absorbed from the upper GI tract. However, severe low-calcium tetany is best treated by IV administration of calcium gluconate. The presence of vitamin D is necessary for maximum calcium utilization. The hormone of the parathyroid gland is necessary for the regulation of the calcium level.

Uses: IV: Acute hypocalcemic tetany secondary to renal failure, hypoparathyroidism, premature delivery, maternal diabetes mellitus in infants, and poisoning due to magnesium, oxalic acid, radiophosphorus, carbon tetrachloride, fluoride, phosphate, strontium, and radium. To treat depletion of electrolytes. Also during cardiac resuscitation when epinephrine or isoproterenol has not improved myocardial contraction (may also be given into the ventricular cavity for this purpose). To reverse cardiotoxicity or hyperkalemia. **IM or IV:** Reduce spasms in renal, biliary, intestinal, or lead colic. To relieve muscle cramps due to insect bites and to decrease capillary permeability in various sensitivity reactions. **PO:** Osteoporosis, osteomalacia, chronic hypoparathyroidism, rickets, latent tetany, hypocalcemia secondary to use of anticonvulsant drugs. Myasthenia gravis, Eaton-Lambert syndrome, supplement for pregnant, postmenopausal, or nursing women. Also, prophylactically for primary osteoporosis. *Investigational:* As an infusion to diagnose Zollinger-Ellison syndrome and medullary thyroid carcinoma. To antagonize neuromuscular blockade due to aminoglycosides.

Contraindications: Digitalized clients, sarcoidosis, renal or cardiac disease. Cancer clients with bone metastases. Renal calculi, hypophosphatemia, hypercalcemia.

Special Concerns: Calcium requirements decrease in geriatric clients; thus, dose may have to be adjusted. Also, low levels of active vitamin D metabolites may impair calcium absorption in older clients. Use with caution in cor pulmonale, respiratory acidosis, renal disease or failure, ventricular fibrillation, hypercalcemia.

Side Effects: Following PO use: GI irritation, constipation. **Following IV use:** Venous irritation, tingling sensation, feeling of oppression or heat, chalky taste. Rapid IV administration may result in vasodilation, decreased blood pressure and heart rate, cardiac arrhythmias, syncope, or cardiac arrest. **Following IM use:** Burning feeling, necrosis, tissue sloughing, cellulitis, soft tissue calcification. **Note:** If calcium is injected into the myocardium rather than into the ventricle, laceration of coronary arteries, cardiac tamponade, pneumothorax, and ventricular fibrillation may occur. *Symptoms due to excess calcium (hypercalcemia):* Lassitude, fatigue, GI symptoms (anorexia, nausea, vomiting, abdominal pain, dry mouth, thirst), polyuria, depression of nervous and neuromuscular function (emotional disturbances, confusion, skeletal muscle weakness, and constipation), confusion, delirium, stupor, coma, impairment of renal function (polyuria, polydipsia, and azotemia), renal calculi, arrhythmias, and bradycardia.

Drug Interactions

Atenolol / ↓ Effect of atenolol due to ↓ bioavailability and plasma levels

Cephalocin / Incompatible with calcium salts

Corticosteroids / Interfere with absorption of calcium from GI tract

Digitalis / Increased digitalis arrhythmias and toxicity. Death has resulted from combination of digitalis and IV calcium salts

Iron salts / ↓ Absorption of iron from the GI tract

Milk / Excess of either may cause hypercalcemia, renal insufficiency with azotemia, alkalosis, and ocular lesions

Norfloxacin / ↓ Bioavailability of norfloxacin

Sodium polystyrene sulfonate / Metabolic alkalosis and ↓ binding of resin to potassium in clients with renal impairment

Tetracyclines / ↓ Effect of tetracyclines due to ↓ absorption from GI tract

Thiazide diuretics / Hypercalcemia due to thiazide-induced renal tubular reabsorption of calcium and bone release of calcium

Verapamil / Calcium antagonizes the effect of verapamil

Vitamin D / Enhances intestinal absorption of dietary calcium

Dosage: See individual agents: calcium carbonate, calcium glubionate, calcium gluceptate, calcium gluconate, calcium lactate, dibasic calcium phosphate dihydrate.

NURSING CONSIDERATIONS

Administration/Storage

ORAL

1. Administer 1–1.5 hr after meals. Alkalis and large amounts of fat decrease the absorption of calcium.
2. If the client has difficulty swallowing large tablets, obtain a calcium in water suspension. Because calcium goes into suspension six times more readily in hot water than in cold water, the solution can be prepared by diluting the medication with *hot* water. Solution may then be cooled before administering to the client.

IV

1. Administer slowly, observing vital signs closely for evidence of bradycardia and hypotension.
2. Prevent leakage of medication into the tissues. These salts are extremely irritating.

IM

1. Rotate the injection sites because this medication may cause sloughing of tissue.
2. Do not administer IM calcium gluconate to children.

Treatment of Overdose: Discontinue therapy; consider hemodialysis.

Assessment

1. Note if the client is receiving digitalis products. Document and report to the physician because the drug is contraindicated.
2. Obtain baseline renal function studies to determine if renal disease is present.

Interventions

1. Monitor serum calcium levels.
2. If the client goes into hypocalcemic tetany, provide appropriate safety precautions to protect the client from injury.
3. Observe for symptoms of hypercalcemia, such as fatigue and CNS depression.

Client/Family Teaching

1. Explain that calcium requirements are best met by dietary sources (including milk in the diet).
2. Stress that multivitamin and mineral preparations are expensive and do not contain sufficient calcium to meet the daily calcium requirements.
3. Provide printed instructions concerning prescribed diet. Have a dietitian work with client to assist with proper selection of foods and meal planning.

Evaluation: Evaluate client for:
- Evidence of resolution of clinical symptoms of hypocalcemia
- Reports of relief of muscle cramps
- Laboratory confirmation that serum calcium level is within desired range (8.8-10.4 mg/dl)

CARDIAC GLYCOSIDES

See also the following individual entries:

Deslanoside
Digitoxin
Digoxin

General Statement: Cardiac glycosides, such as digitoxin, are plant alkaloids. They are probably the oldest, yet still the most effective, drugs for treating congestive heart failure (CHF). By improving myocardial contraction, they improve blood supply to all organs, including the kidney, thereby improving function. This action results in diuresis, thereby correcting the edema often associated with cardiac insufficiency. Digitalis glycosides are also used for the treatment of cardiac arrhythmias, since they decrease pulse rate as well. The cardiac glycosides are cumulative in action. This effect is partially responsible for the difficulties associated with their use.

Action/Kinetics: Cardiac glycosides increase the force of myocardial contraction (positive inotropic effect). This effect is due to inhibition of movement of sodium and potassium ions across myocardial cell membranes due to complexing with adenosine triphosphatase. This results in an increase of calcium influx and an increased release of free calcium ions within the myocardial cells, which then potentiate the contractility of cardiac muscle fibers. The digitalis glycosides also decrease the rate of conduction and increase the refractory period of the AV node. This effect is due to an increase in parasympathetic tone and a decrease in sympathetic tone. The cardiac glycosides are absorbed from the GI tract. Absorption varies from 40% to 90%, depending on the preparation and *brand*. With most preparations, peak plasma concentrations are reached within 2–3 hr. Half-life ranges from 1.7 days for digoxin to 7 days for digitoxin. The drugs are primarily excreted through the kidneys, either unchanged (digoxin) or metabolized (digitoxin). The initial dose of digitalis glycosides is larger (loading dose) and is traditionally referred to as the *digitalizing dose (DD);* subsequent doses are referred to as *maintenance doses (MD).*

Uses: CHF, especially secondary to hypertension, coronary artery or atherosclerotic heart disease, valvular heart disease. Control of rapid ventricular contraction rate in clients with atrial fibrillation or flutter. Slow heart rate in sinus tachycardia due to CHF. Supraventricular tachycardia. Prophylaxis and treatment of recurrent paroxysmal atrial tachycardia with paroxysmal AV junctional rhythm. In conjunction with propranolol for angina. Cardiogenic shock (value not established).

Contraindications: Coronary occlusion or angina pectoris in the absence of CHF or hypersensitivity to cardiogenic glycosides.

Special Concerns: Use with caution in clients with ischemic heart disease, acute myocarditis, ventricular tachycardia, hypertrophic subaortic stenosis, hypoxic or myxedemic states, Adams-Stokes or carotid sinus syndromes, cardiac amyloidosis, or cyanotic heart and lung disease, including emphysema and partial heart block. Electric pacemakers may sensitize the myocardium to cardiac glycosides. The cardiac glycosides should also be given cautiously and at reduced dosage to elderly, debilitated clients, pregnant women and nursing mothers, and to newborn, term, or premature infants who have immature renal and hepatic function. Similar precautions also should be observed for clients with reduced renal and/or hepatic function, since such impairment retards excretion of cardiac glycosides.

Side Effects: Cardiac glycosides are extremely toxic and have caused death even in clients who have received the drugs for long periods of time. There is a narrow margin of safety between an effective therapeutic dose and a toxic dose. Overdosage caused by the cumulative effects of the drug is a constant danger in therapy with cardiac glycosides. Digitalis toxicity is characterized by a wide variety of symptoms, which are hard to differentiate from those of the cardiac disease itself. *CV:* Changes in the rate, rhythm, and irritability of the heart and the mechanism of the heartbeat. Extrasystoles, bigeminal pulse, coupled rhythm, ectopic beat, and other forms of arrhythmias have been noted. Death most often results from ventricular fibrillation. Cardiac glycosides should be discontinued in adults when pulse rate falls below 60 beats/min. All cardiac changes are best detected by the electrocardiogram (ECG), which is also most useful in clients suffering from intoxication. Acute hemorrhage. *GI:* Anorexia, nausea, vomiting, excessive salivation, epigastric distress, abdominal pain, diarrhea, bowel necrosis. Clients on digitalis therapy may experience two vomiting stages. The first is an early sign of toxicity and is a direct effect of digitalis on the GI tract. Late vomiting indicates stimulation of the vomiting center of the brain, which occurs after the heart muscle has been saturated with digitalis. *CNS:* Headaches, fatigue, lassitude, irritability, malaise, muscle weakness, insomnia, stupor. Psychotomimetic effects (especially in elderly or arteriosclerotic clients or neonates) including disorientation, confusion, depression, aphasia, delirium, hallucinations, and, rarely, convulsions. *Neuromuscular:* Neurologic pain involving the lower third of the face and lumbar areas, paresthesia. *Visual disturbances:* Blurred vision, flickering dots, white halos, borders around dark objects, diplopia, amblyopia, color perception changes. *Hypersensitivity (5–7 days after starting therapy):* Skin reactions (urticaria, fever, pruritus, facial and angioneurotic edema). *Other:* Chest pain, coldness of extremities. *Symptoms of Overdose (Toxicity):* GI symptoms include anorexia, nausea, vomiting, diarrhea, abdominal discomfort. CNS symptoms include blurred, yellow, or green vision and halo effect; headache, weakness, drowsiness, mental depression, apathy, restlessness, disorientation, confusion, seizures, EEG abnormalities, delirium, hallucinations, psychosis.

Cardiac effects include ventricular tachycardia, unifocal or multiform premature ventricular contractions, paroxysmal and nonparoxysmal nodal rhythms, AV dissociation, accelerated junctional rhythm, excessive slowing of the pulse, AV block (may proceed to complete block), atrial fibrillation, ventricular fibrillation (most common cause of death). *Children:* Atrial arrhythmias and atrial tachycardia with AV block are the most common signs of toxicity; in neonates excessive slowing of sinus rate, sinoatrial (SA) arrest, and prolongation of PR interval occur.

Drug Interactions: One of the most serious side effects of digitalis-type drugs is hypokalemia (lowering of serum potassium levels). This may lead to cardiac arrhythmias, muscle weakness, hypotension, and respiratory distress. Other agents causing hypokalemia reinforce this effect and increase the chance of digitalis toxicity. Such reactions may occur in clients who have been on digitalis maintenance for a long time.

Aminoglycosides / ↓ Effect of digitalis glycosides due to ↓ absorption from GI tract
Aminosalicylic acid / ↓ Effect of digitalis glycosides due to ↓ absorption from GI tract
Amphotericin B / ↑ K depletion caused by digitalis; ↑ incidence of digitalis toxicity
Antacids / ↓ Effect of digitalis glycosides due to ↓ absorption from GI tract
Calcium preparations / Cardiac arrhythmias if parenteral calcium given with digitalis
Chlorthalidone / ↑ K and Mg loss with ↑ chance of digitalis toxicity
Cholestyramine / Cholestyramine

binds digitoxin in the intestine and ↓ its absorption

Colestipol / Colestipol binds digitoxin in the intestine and ↓ its absorption

Ephedrine / ↑ Chance of cardiac arrhythmias

Epinephrine / ↑ Chance of cardiac arrhythmias

Ethacrynic acid / ↑ K and Mg loss with ↑ chance of digitalis toxicity

Furosemide / ↑ K and Mg loss with ↑ chance of digitalis toxicity

Glucose infusions / Large infusions of glucose may cause ↓ in serum K and ↑ chance of digitalis toxicity

Hypoglycemic drugs / ↓ Effect of digitalis glycosides due to ↑ breakdown by liver

Methimazole / ↑ Chance of toxic effects of digitalis

Metoclopramide / ↓ Effect of digitalis glycosides by ↓ absorption from GI tract

Muscle relaxants, nondepolarizing / ↑ Risk of cardiac arrhythmias

Propranolol / Propranolol potentiates digitalis-induced bradycardia

Reserpine / ↑ Chance of cardiac arrhythmias

Spironolactone / Either ↑ or ↓ toxic effects of digitalis glycosides

Succinylcholine / ↑ Chance of cardiac arrhythmias

Sulfasalazine / ↓ Effect of digitalis glycosides by ↓ absorption from GI tract

Sympathomimetics / ↑ Chance of cardiac arrhythmias

Thiazides / ↑ K and Mg loss with ↑ chance of digitalis toxicity

Thyroid hormones / ↑ Effectiveness of digitalis glycosides

Laboratory Test Interferences: May ↓ prothrombin time. Alters tests for 17-ketosteroids and 17-hydroxycorticosteroids.

Dosage: PO, IM, or IV. *Highly individualized.* See individual drugs: digitoxin, digoxin. Initially, the drugs are usually given at higher ("digitalizing" or loading) doses. These are reduced as soon as the desired therapeutic effect is achieved or undesirable toxic reactions develop. The client's response to cardiac glycosides is gauged by clinical and ECG observations. The rates at which clients become digitalized vary considerably. Clients with mild signs of congestion can often be digitalized gradually over a period of several days. Clients suffering from more serious congestion, for example, those showing signs of acute left ventricular failure, dyspnea, or lung edema, can be digitalized more rapidly by parenteral administration of a fast-acting cardiac glycoside. Once digitalization has been attained (pulse 68–80 beats/min) and symptoms of CHF have subsided, the client is put on maintenance dosage. Depending on the drug and the age of the client, the daily maintenance dose is often approximately 10% of the digitalizing dose.

NURSING CONSIDERATIONS

Administration/Storage

1. Many cardiac glycosides have similar names. However, their dosage and duration of their effect differ markedly. Therefore, check the doctor's order, the medication administration record/card and the bottle label of the medication to be administered. If a client questions the drug (size, color, etc.)

recheck the drug order, bottle label, and the name of the client to whom the drug is to be given.

2. Measure all PO liquid cardiac medications precisely, using a calibrated dropper or a syringe.

3. The half-life of cardiac glycosides is prolonged in the elderly. When working with elderly clients, anticipate the doses of drug will be smaller than for those in other age groups.

4. Obtain written guidelines orders indicating the pulse rates, both high and low, at which cardiac glycosides are to be withheld. Any change in rate or rhythm may indicate digitalis toxicity.

5. *Treatment of Overdose in Adults:*
   - Discontinue drug and admit to the intensive care area for continuous monitoring of ECG.
   - If serum potassium is below normal, potassium chloride should be administered in divided oral doses totaling 3–6 g (40–80 mEq). Potassium should not be used when severe or complete heart block is due to digitalis and not related to tachycardia.
   - *Atropine:* A dose of 0.01 mg/kg IV to treat severe sinus bradycardia or slow ventricular rate due to second-ary AV block.
   - *Cholestyramine, colestipol, activated charcoal:* To bind digitalis in the intestine thus preventing enterohepatic recirculation.
   - *Digoxin immune FAB:* See

drug entry. Given in approximate equimolar quantities as digoxin, it reverses signs and symptoms of toxicity.
   - *Lidocaine:* A dose of 1 mg/kg given over 5 min followed by an infusion of 15–50 mcg/kg/min to maintain normal cardiac rhythm.
   - *Phenytoin:* For cases unresponsive to potassium, can give a dose of 0.5 mg/kg at a rate not exceeding 50 mg/min (given at 1–2 hr intervals). The maximum dose should not exceed 10 mg/kg/day.
   - *Countershock:* A direct-current countershock can be used **only as a last resort.**

6. *Treatment of Overdose in Children:* Give potassium in divided doses totaling 1–1.5 mEq/kg (if correction of arrhythmia is urgent, a dose of 0.5 mEq/kg/hr can be used) with careful monitoring of the ECG. The potassium IV solution should be dilute to avoid local irritation although IV fluid overload must be avoided. Digoxin immune FAB may also be used.

FOR CLIENTS STARTING ON A DIGITALIZING DOSE

Assessment

1. Note any drugs the client may be taking that would adversely interact with digitalis glycosides.

2. Obtain and review the following laboratory tests before administering the medication: hemoglobin, hematocrit, serum electrolytes, calcium, magnesium, and liver and renal function tests.

3. Ascertain that an ECG has been completed and reviewed before administration.

FOR CLIENTS BEING DIGITALIZED AND FOR CLIENTS ON A MAINTENANCE DOSE OF A CARDIAC GLYCOSIDE

Interventions

1. Observe cardiac monitor for evidence of bradycardia and/or arrhythmias, or count the apical pulse rate for at least 1 min before administering the drug.
   - If the adult pulse rate is below 60 beats/min or if an arrhythmia not previously noted occurs, withhold the drug, notify the physician, and document these findings.
   - If a child's pulse rate is 90–110 beats/min or if an arrhythmia is present, withhold the drug and notify the physician.
2. With another nurse simultaneously take the client's apical/radial pulse for 1 min. If there is a pulse deficit, withhold the drug, and report to the physician. A pulse deficit may indicate that the client is having an adverse reaction to the drug.
3. Weigh the client prior to initiating therapy and daily after beginning therapy. Weight gain may indicate the presence of edema.
4. Place the client on intake and output. Determine that the client is adequately hydrated and that elimination is in line with the intake. Adequate intake will help prevent cumulative toxic effects of the drug.
5. Provide the client with foods, such as orange juice and bananas, which are high in potassium.
6. Anticipate that clients taking nonpotassium-sparing diuretics as well as a cardiac glycoside will require potassium supplements.
7. If a potassium supplement is needed, ask the pharmacist to provide the client with the most palatable preparation available. (Potassium preparations are usually bitter.)
8. If the client complains of gastric distress, an antacid preparation may be ordered.
   - Antacids containing aluminum or magnesium and kaolin/pectin mixtures should be given 6 hr before or 6 hr after dose of cardiac glycoside to prevent decreased therapeutic effect of glycoside.
9. When the drug is given to newborns, use a cardiac monitor to identify early evidence of toxicity. Any excessive slowing of sinus rate, sinoatrial arrest, or prolonged PR interval should be reported immediately and the drug withheld.
10. Be especially alert to cardiac arrhythmias in children. This sign of toxicity occurs more frequently in children than in adults.
11. Monitor serum digoxin levels (therapeutic range 0.5–2.0 ng/ml) and become familiar with medications that enhance the effects of digoxin.
12. Elderly clients must be observed for early signs and symptoms of toxicity, because their rate of drug elimination is slower than with other clients. Nausea, vomiting, anorexia,

and/or confusion may be signs of toxicity and should be reported immediately.

13. During digitalization the client should be in a closely monitored environment where emergency equipment is readily available.

14. Have digoxin antidote available (Digoxin immune FAB) for management of clients with severe toxicity.

Client/Family Teaching

1. Stress the need for close medical and nursing supervision and the importance of reporting any signs of change however minor they may seem.

2. Review how to count the pulse accurately before taking the medication. Review all written instructions several times in the days prior to discharge.

3. Maintain a written record of pulse rates and medication administration for review by health care provider.

4. Emphasize guidelines for withholding medication and reporting abnormal pulse rate to physician.

5. Use the same brand of cardiac glycoside administered in the hospital. Different preparations have varying degrees of potency and pharmacokinetics and should not be used unless designated by the physician.

6. Follow directions carefully for taking the medication. If one dose of drug is accidentally missed, do not double up on the next dose. Call the physician and report the incident.

7. Develop a checklist to be marked after taking medications. This is particularly important when working with elderly clients who may tend to have memory loss.

8. Take medication after meals to lessen gastric irritation.

9. Discard any previously prescribed cardiac glycoside, to avoid taking medications by mistake.

10. Review the toxic symptoms of prescribed drugs. Provide a printed list of the toxic symptoms, stressing early recognition and prompt reporting to the physician. Anorexia is often the earliest symptom.

11. Weigh in every morning at the same time before breakfast, and in similar clothing. Report any rapid weight gain and bring written record of weight to physician at time of appointment.

12. Review and explain any dietary and activity restrictions.

13. Maintain a sodium-restricted diet. Provide a printed list of foods low in sodium.

14. Follow a potassium-rich diet and provide a list of potassium-rich foods. This is particularly important when working with clients on a limited income because it enables them to make choices they can afford. Utilize dietitian as needed to assist with shopping and meal planning.

15. Consult with the physician before taking any other medications, whether prescribed or OTC, because drug interactions occur frequently with cardiac glycosides.

16. Report any persistent cough, difficulty breathing, or edema to the physician. These are all signs of CHF and demand immediate medical attention.

17. Help clients contact community health agencies designed to assist them in maintaining health.
18. Stress the importance of returning for scheduled follow-up visits and laboratory tests.

Evaluation: Evaluate client for:
- A positive response to digitalization, as evidenced by improved cardiac rate and rhythm, improvement in breathing patterns, decrease in severity of CHF, improved cardiac output, reduction in weight, and/or improved diuresis
- Laboratory confirmation that serum levels of drug are within therapeutic range (e.g., digoxin 0.5–2.0 ng/ml).

CENTRALLY ACTING SKELETAL MUSCLE RELAXANTS

See also the following individual entries:

Baclofen
Carisoprodol
Chlorzoxazone
Cyclobenzaprine
Dantrolene Sodium
Diazepam
Methocarbamol
Orphenadrine Citrate

Action/Kinetics: The centrally acting skeletal muscle relaxants decrease muscle tone and involuntary movement. Many relieve anxiety and tension as well. Although the precise mechanism of action is unknown, most of these agents depress spinal polysynaptic reflexes. Their beneficial effects may also

be attributable to their antianxiety activity. Several of the drugs in this group also manifest analgesic properties.

Uses: Musculoskeletal and neurologic disorders associated with muscle spasms, hyperreflexia, and hypertonia, including parkinsonism, tetanus, tension headaches, acute muscle spasms caused by trauma, and inflammation (e.g., low back syndrome, sprains, arthritis, bursitis). They also may be useful in the management of cerebral palsy and multiple sclerosis.

Side Effects: Side effects often involve the CNS, GI system, and urinary system. Symptoms of allergy may also be manifested. For specific side effects, see individual drugs.

Symptoms of Overdose: Often extensions of the side effects. Stupor, coma, shock-like syndrome, respiratory depression, loss of muscle tone, and impaired deep tendon reflexes may also occur.

Drug Interactions: Centrally acting muscle relaxants may increase the sedative and respiratory depressant effects of CNS depressants (e.g., alcohol, barbiturates, sedatives and hypnotics, and antianxiety agents).

Dosage: For dosage, see individual agents.

NURSING CONSIDERATIONS

Administration

1. Crush tablets or empty capsules into a small amount of fruit juice if the client is unable to swallow.
2. If the skeletal muscle relaxant is to be discontinued after long-term use, the dose of drug should be tapered to prevent

rebound spasticity, hallucinations, or other withdrawal symptoms.
3. Review list of drug interactions.
4. The lowest possible dosage of drug should be determined and used to treat the client's symptoms.
5. Have emergency drugs, gastric lavage, oxygen, pressor agents, and IV fluids available in the event of a drug overdose.
6. *Treatment of Overdose:* Symptomatic. Emesis or gastric lavage (followed by activated charcoal). If necessary, artificial respiration, oxygen administration, pressor agents, and IV fluids may be used. It may be possible to increase the rate of excretion of selected drugs by diuretics (including mannitol), peritoneal dialysis, or hemodialysis.

Assessment

1. Obtain a complete drug history.
2. Note any history of prior seizures. Some drugs in this category may cause deterioration of seizure control.
3. Assess the extent of the client's musculoskeletal and neurologic disorders associated with muscle spasm. Note muscle stiffness, pain, and extent of ROM.
4. Conduct a thorough baseline mental status examination against which to measure subsequent examinations.

Interventions

1. Monitor blood pressure every 4 hr when therapy is initiated in a hospital setting.
2. Supervise ambulation and transfers and ensure a safe client environment. With these drugs, sedentary or immobilized clients are more prone to hypotension upon ambulation.
3. Note client complaints of nausea, anorexia, or changes in taste perception. Notify physician if these symptoms persist as nutritional state may become impaired.
4. Monitor the client's urinary output. Anticipate the need to use drugs to increase the rate of excretion if the output is too low.
5. Check the client's muscle responses and deep tendon reflexes for symptoms of drug overdosage.

Client/Family Teaching

1. Review the goals of the medication therapy with the client and family and determine to what extent they have been met.
2. Do not operate dangerous machinery or drive a car when taking these drugs because they may impair mental alertness.
3. Review additional therapies that may be prescribed for muscle spasm (heat, rest, physical therapy).
4. If the urine becomes dark, the skin or sclera appears yellow, or if the client develops pruritus, notify the physician and discontinue using the medication.
5. Avoid using antihistamines because these drugs may produce an additive depressant effect.
6. Avoid the use of alcohol and any other CNS depressants.
7. Stress the importance of re-

porting for all scheduled lab and medical follow-up visits so that therapy can be evaluated and drug dosage adjusted as needed.

Evaluation: Evaluate client for:
- Reports of symptomatic improvement in extent and intensity of muscle spasm and pain
- Clinical evidence of increased ROM with measurable improvement in muscle tone and involuntary movements
- Reports of effective control of tension headaches

CEPHALOSPORINS

See also the following individual entries:

Cefaclor
Cefadroxil Monohydrate
Cefamandole Nafate
Cefazolin Sodium
Cefixime
Cefmetazole Sodium
Cefonicid Sodium
Cefoperazone Sodium
Ceforanide
Cefotaxime Sodium
Cefotetan Disodium
Cefoxitin Sodium
Ceftazidime
Ceftizoxime Sodium
Ceftriaxone Sodium
Cefuroxime Axetil
Cefuroxime Sodium
Cephalexin
Cephalothin Sodium
Cephapirin Sodium
Cephradine
Moxalactam Disodium

General Statement: The cephalosporins are semisynthetic antibiotics resembling the penicillins both chemically and pharmacologically. Some cephalosporins are rapidly absorbed from the GI tract and quickly reach effective concentrations in the urinary, GI, and respiratory tracts except in clients with pernicious anemia or obstructive jaundice. The drugs are eliminated rapidly in clients with normal renal function.

The cephalosporins are broad-spectrum antibiotics classified as first-, second-, and third-generation drugs. The difference among generations is based on antibacterial spectra; third-generation cephalosporins have more activity against gram-negative organisms and resistant organisms and less activity against gram-positive organisms than first-generation drugs. Third-generation cephalosporins are also stable against beta-lactamases. Cephalosporins can be destroyed by cephalosporinase. Also, the cost increases from first- to third-generation cephalosporins.

Action/Kinetics: The cephalosporins interfere with a final step in the formation of the bacterial cell wall (inhibition of mucopeptide biosynthesis), resulting in unstable cell membranes that undergo lysis (same mechanism of actions as penicillins). Also, cell division and growth are inhibited. The cephalosporins are most effective against young, rapidly dividing organisms. The $t^{1/2}$ ranges from 69 to 132 min, and serum protein binding ranges from 5% to 86%. Cephalosporins are widely distributed to most tissues and fluids. First- and second-generation drugs do not enter the CSF well but third-generation drugs enter inflamed meninges readily. The cephalosporins are rapidly excreted by the kidneys.

Uses: Cephalosporins are effective against infections of the biliary tract, GI tract, GU system, bones, joints, upper and lower respiratory tract, skin, and skin structures. Also, gynecologic infections, meningitis, osteomyelitis, endocarditis, intra-abdominal infections, peritonitis, otitis media, gonorrhea, septicemia, and prophylaxis prior to surgery. A listing of the organisms against which cephalosporins are effective follows.

First-Generation Cephalosporins. Gram-positive cocci including *Staphylococcus aureus, S. epidermidis, S. pyogenes, Streptococcus pneumoniae, S. viridans,* group A and B streptococci, and anaerobic streptococci. Activity against gram-negative bacteria includes *Escherichia coli, Hemophilus influenzae, Klebsiella,* and *Proteus mirabilis.*

Second-Generation Cephalosporins. Spectrum similar to that of first-generation cephalosporins. Also active against certain gram-negative bacteria and anaerobes including *Providencia rettgeri, Bacteroides* species, *Peptococcus,* and *Peptostreptococcus* species. Selected second-generation cephalosporins are effective against the following genera: *Citrobacter, Enterobacter, Providencia, Clostridium,* and *Fusobacterium,* as well as *Morganella morganii, Neisseria gonorrhoeae,* and *Proteus vulgaris.*

Third-Generation Cephalosporins. Less active against gram-positive cocci. Spectrum similar to first- and second-generation cephalosporins. Most are also active against the following gram-negative and anaerobic species: *Acinetobacter, Citrobacter, Enterobacter, Providencia, Salmonella, Serratia, Shigella, Bacteroides, Clostridium,* *Fusobacterium, Peptococcus,* and *Peptostreptococcus.* Most are effective against *Morganella morganii, Neisseria gonorrhoeae, Neisseria meningitidis, Proteus vulgaris, Pseudomonas aeruginosa,* and *Bacteroides fragilis.* Selected third-generation cephalosporins are effective against *Hemophilus parainfluenzae, Moraxella catarrhalis, Salmonella thypi, Clostridium difficile,* and *Eubacterium* species.

Contraindications: Hypersensitivity to cephalosporins. Clients hypersensitive to penicillin may occasionally cross-react to cephalosporins.

Special Concerns: Safe use in pregnancy and lactation has not been established. Use with caution in the presence of impaired renal or hepatic function or together with other nephrotoxic drugs. Creatinine clearances should be performed on all clients with impaired renal function who receive cephalosporins. Use with caution in clients over 50 years of age.

Side Effects: *GI:* Nausea, vomiting, diarrhea, abdominal cramps or pain, dyspepsia, glossitis, heartburn, sore mouth or tongue, dysgeusia, anorexia, flatulence, cholestasis. Pseudomembranous colitis. *Allergic:* Urticaria, rashes (maculopapular, morbilliform, or erythematous), pruritus (including anal and genital areas), fever, chills, erythema, angioedema, serum sickness, joint pain, exfoliative dermatitis, chest tightness, myalgia, erythema multiforme, edema, itching, numbness, chills, Stevens-Johnson syndrome, anaphylaxis. **Note:** Cross-allergy may be manifested between cephalosporins and penicillins. *Hematologic:* Leukopenia, leukocytosis, lymphocytosis, neutropenia (transient), eosinophilia, thrombocytopenia, thrombocythemia, agranulocytosis, granulocytopenia, bone marrow depression, hemolytic anemia, pancytopenia, decreased platelet function, aplastic anemia, hypoprothrombinemia (may lead to bleeding), thrombocytosis (transient). *CNS:* Headache, malaise, fatigue, vertigo, dizziness, lethargy, confusion, paresthesia. *Hepatic:* Hepatomegaly, hepatitis. Intrathecal use may result in hallucinations, nystagmus, or seizures. *Miscellaneous:* Superinfection including oral candidiasis and enterococcal infections, hypotension, sweating, flushing, dyspnea, interstitial pneumonitis.

IV or IM use may result in local swelling, inflammation, cellulitis, paresthesia, burning, phlebitis, thrombophlebitis. IM use may also cause pain and induration, tenderness, increased temperature. Sterile abscesses have been observed following SC use. Nephrotoxicity (↑ BUN with and without ↑ serum creatinine) may occur in clients over 50 and in young children.

Symptoms of Overdose: Parenteral use of large doses of cephalosporins may cause seizures, especially in clients with impaired renal function.

Drug Interactions

Aminoglycosides / ↑ Risk of renal toxicity with certain cephalosporins
Anticoagulants / Certain cephalosporins ↑ prothrombin time
Bacteriostatic agents / ↓ Effect of cephalosporins
Bumetanide / ↑ Risk of renal toxicity

Colistimethate / ↑ Risk of renal toxicity
Colistin / ↑ Risk of renal toxicity
Ethacrynic acid / ↑ Risk of renal toxicity
Furosemide / ↑ Risk of renal toxicity
Polymyxin B / ↑ Risk of renal toxicity
Probenecid / ↑ Effect of cephalosporins by ↓ excretion by kidneys
Vancomycin / ↑ Risk of renal toxicity

Laboratory Test Interferences: False + for urinary glucose with Benedict's solution, Fehling's solution, or Clinitest tablets. Enzyme tests (Clinistix, Tes-Tape) are unaffected. False + Coombs' test and urinary 17-ketosteroids.

↑ AST, ALT, total bilirubin, GGTP, LDH, alkaline phosphatase.

Dosage: See individual drugs.

NURSING CONSIDERATIONS

See also *General Nursing Considerations For All Anti-Infectives,* p. 83

Administration/Storage

1. Parenteral solutions infused too rapidly may cause pain and irritation; infuse over 30 min unless otherwise indicated.
2. Therapy should be continued for at least 2–3 days after symptoms of infection have disappeared.
3. For group A beta-hemolytic streptococcal infections, therapy should be continued for at least 10 days to prevent the development of glomerulonephritis or rheumatic fever.
4. *Treatment of Overdose:* If seizures occur, discontinue the drug immediately and give

anticonvulsant drugs. Hemodialysis may also be effective.

Assessment

1. Assess client with a history of hypersensitivity reaction to penicillin for cross-sensitivity to cephalosporins. Have epinephrine readily available.
2. Assess client's financial status. Many in this group of antibiotics are quite expensive and clients on fixed incomes with limited health benefits may be unable to afford the prescription expense.
3. Document symptoms of infection and ensure that appropriate cultures have been performed prior to initiating drug therapy.

Interventions

1. The cephalosporins all have similar sounding and similarly spelled names. Use care when transcribing physician's orders for administration of these drugs and request clarification as needed.
2. Pseudomembranous colitis may occur in clients receiving cephalosporins. If diarrhea develops, report to physician immediately and continue to monitor for signs and laboratory evidence of electrolyte imbalance.
3. Obtain liver and renal function studies and anticipate lower doses for clients with renal impairment. For dialysis clients, administer after treatment.
4. If GI upset occurs, the drug may be administered with meals.

5. Drug may cause a false + Coomb's test. Document appropriately and instruct client.

Client/Family Teaching

1. Emphasize that oral medications should be taken on an empty stomach, unless otherwise directed.
2. Report any symptoms that may necessitate drug withdrawal such as vaginal itching or drainage, fever, or diarrhea.
3. Explain that yogurt or buttermilk may be prescribed for diarrhea related to intestinal superinfections.
4. Advise to report signs of superinfection (black furry tongue, vaginal itching or discharge, and loose, foul-smelling stools). Nystatin may be ordered for secondary infections.
5. Stress the importance of taking medication as ordered and of reporting side effects so that appropriate therapy may be initiated.
6. Explain that medication may cause a false + Coombs' test. This would be of concern if client is being cross-matched for blood transfusions or in newborns whose mothers have taken cephalosporins during pregnancy.

Evaluation: Evaluate client for:
- Evidence (presence/absence) of pretreatment symptoms and C&S results to determine effectiveness of treatment
- Clinical evidence of resolution of infection and reports of improvement in presenting symptoms

CHOLINERGIC BLOCKING AGENTS

Atropine Sulfate
Benztropine Mesylate
Biperiden Hydrochloride
Biperiden Lactate
Dicyclomine Hydrochloride
Glycopyrrolate
Methantheline Bromide
Procyclidine Hydrochloride
Propantheline Bromide
Scopolamine Hydrobromide
Scopolamine Transdermal
   Therapeutic System
Trihexyphenidyl Hydrochloride

Action/Kinetics: The cholinergic blocking agents prevent the neurotransmitter acetylcholine from combining with receptors on the postganglionic parasympathetic nerve terminal (muscarinic site). In therapeutic doses, these drugs have little effect on transmission of nerve impulses across ganglia (nicotinic sites) or at the neuromuscular junction.

The main effects of cholinergic blocking agents are:

1. To reduce spasms of smooth muscles like those controlling the urinary bladder or spasms of bronchial and intestinal smooth muscle.
2. To block vagal impulses to the heart, resulting in an increase in the rate and speed of impulse conduction through the atrioventricular conducting system.
3. To suppress or decrease gastric secretions, perspiration, salivation, and secretion of bronchial mucus.
4. To relax the sphincter muscles of the iris and cause pupillary dilation (mydriasis) and loss of

accommodation for near vision (cycloplegia).
5. To act in diverse ways on the CNS, producing such reactions as depression (scopolamine) or stimulation (toxic doses of atropine). Many of the anticholinergic drugs also have antiparkinsonism effects. They abolish or reduce the signs and symptoms of Parkinson's disease, such as tremors and rigidity, and result in some improvement in mobility, muscular coordination, and motor performance. These effects may be due to blockade of the effects of acetylcholine in the CNS. This section also discusses miscellaneous synthetic antispasmodics related to anticholinergic drugs.

The anticholinergics that are related to atropine are quickly absorbed following oral ingestion. These agents cross the blood-brain barrier and may exert significant CNS effects. Examples of these drugs are scopolamine, l-hyoscyamine, and belladonna alkaloids. The drugs classified as quaternary ammonium anticholinergic drugs are erratically absorbed from the GI tract and exert minimal CNS effects, since they do not cross the blood-brain barrier. Examples of these drugs are glycopyrrolate, methantheline, propantheline, tridihexethyl chloride, clidinium bromide, isopropamide, and others.

Uses: See individual drugs.

Contraindications: Glaucoma, adhesions between iris and lens of the eye, tachycardia, myocardial ischemia, unstable cardiovascular state in acute hemorrhage, partial obstruction of the GI and biliary tracts, prostatic hypertrophy, renal disease, myasthenia gravis, hepatic disease, paralytic ileus, pyloroduodenal stenosis, pyloric obstruction, intestinal atony, ulcerative colitis, obstructive uropathy. Cardiac clients, especially when there is danger of tachycardia; older persons suffering from atherosclerosis or mental impairment. Lactation.

Special Concerns: Use with caution in pregnancy. Infants and young children are more susceptible to the toxic side effects of anticholinergic drugs. Of particular importance is use of such drugs in children when the ambient temperature is high; due to suppression of sweat glands, the body temperature may increase rapidly. Geriatric clients are particularly likely to manifest anticholinergic side effects such as dry mouth, constipation, and urinary retention (especially in males). Geriatric clients are also more likely to experience agitation, confusion, drowsiness, excitement, glaucoma, and impaired memory. Use with caution in hyperthyroidism, congestive heart failure, cardiac arrhythmias, hypertension, Down syndrome, asthma, spastic paralysis, blonde individuals, allergies, and chronic lung disease.

Side Effects: These are desirable in some conditions and undesirable in others. Thus, the anticholinergics have an antisalivary effect that is useful in parkinsonism. This same effect is unpleasant when the drug is used for spastic conditions of the GI tract.

Most side effects are dose-related and decrease when dosage decreases. Sometimes it helps to discontinue the medication for several days. With this in mind, anticholinergic drugs have the following side effects. *GI:* Nausea, vomiting, dry mouth, dysphagia, constipation, heartburn, change in taste perception, bloated feeling, paralytic ileus. *CNS:* Dizziness, drowsiness, nervousness, disorientation, headache, weakness, insomnia, fever (especially in children). Large doses may produce CNS stimulation including tremor and restlessness. Anticholinergic psychoses: ataxia, euphoria, confusion, disorientation, loss of short-term memory, decreased anxiety, fatigue, insomnia, hallucinations, dysarthria, agitation. *CV:* Palpitations. *GU:* Urinary retention or hesitancy, impotence. *Ophthalmologic:* Blurred vision, dilated pupils, photophobia, cycloplegia, precipitation of acute glaucoma. *Allergic:* Urticaria, skin rashes, anaphylaxis. *Other:* Flushing, decreased sweating, nasal congestion, suppression of glandular secretions including lactation. Heat prostration (fever and heat stroke) in presence of high environmental temperatures due to decreased sweating.

Symptoms of Overdose (Belladonna poisoning):

Infants and children are especially susceptible to the toxic effects of atropine and scopolamine. Poisoning (dose-dependent) is characterized by the following symptoms: dry mouth, burning sensation of the mouth, difficulty in swallowing and speaking, blurred vision, photophobia, rash, tachycardia, increased respiration, increased body temperature (up to 109°F, 42.7°C), restlessness, irritability, confusion, muscle incoordination, dilated pupils, hot dry skin, respiratory depression and paralysis, tremors, seizures, hallucinations, and death.

Drug Interactions

Amantadine / Additive anticholinergic side effects

Antacids / ↓ Absorption of anticholinergics from GI tract

Antidepressants, tricyclic / Additive anticholinergic side effects

Antihistamines / Additive anticholinergic side effects

Atenolol / Anticholinergics ↑ effects of atenolol

Benzodiazepines / Additive anticholinergic side effects

Corticosteroids / Additive increase in intraocular pressure

Cyclopropane / ↑ Chance of ventricular arrhythmias

Digoxin / ↑ Effect of digoxin due to ↑ absorption from GI tract

Disopyramide / Potentiation of anticholinergic side effects

Guanethidine / Reversal of inhibition of gastric acid secretion caused by anticholinergics

Haloperidol / Additive increase in intraocular pressure

Histamine / Reversal of inhibition of gastric acid secretion caused by anticholinergics

Levodopa / Possible ↓ effect of levodopa due to ↑ breakdown of levodopa in stomach (due to delayed gastric emptying time)

MAO inhibitors / ↑ Effect of anticholinergics due to ↓ breakdown by liver

Meperidine / Additive anticholinergic side effects

Methylphenidate / Potentiation of anticholinergic side effects

Metoclopramide / Anticholinergics block action of metoclopramide

Nitrates, nitrites / Potentiation of anticholinergic side effects

Nitrofurantoin / ↑ Bioavailability of nitrofurantoin

Orphenadrine / Additive anticholinergic side effects

Phenothiazines / Additive anticholinergic side effects; also, effects of phenothiazines may be ↓

Primidone / Potentiation of anticholinergic side effects

Procainamide / Additive anticholinergic side effects

Quinidine / Additive anticholinergic side effects

Reserpine / Reversal of inhibition of gastric acid secretion caused by anticholinergics

Sympathomimetics / ↑ Bronchial relaxation

Thiazide diuretics / ↑ Bioavailability of thiazide diuretics

Thioxanthines / Potentiation of anticholinergic side effects

Dosage: See individual drugs.

NURSING CONSIDERATIONS

Administration / Storage

1. Check dosage and measure the drug exactly. Some drugs in this category are given in small amounts. As a consequence, overdosage is quickly achieved and can lead to toxicity.

2. Review the list of drugs with which drugs in this category interact.

3. *Treatment of Overdose (Belladonna poisoning):*
   - Gastric lavage or induction of vomiting followed by activated charcoal. General supportive measures.
   - Anticholinergic effects can be reversed by physostigmine (Eserine), 1–3 mg IV (effectiveness uncertain; thus use other agents if possible). Neostigmine methylsulfate, 0.5–2 mg IV, repeated as necessary.
   - If there is excitation, diazepam, a short-acting barbiturate, IV sodium thiopental

(2% solution), or chloral hydrate (100–200 ml of a 2% solution by rectal infusion) may be given.

- For fever, cool baths may be used. Keep client in a darkened room if photophobia is manifested.
- Artificial respiration should be instituted if there is paralysis of respiratory muscles.

Assessment

1. Assess for a history of asthma, glaucoma, or duodenal ulcer, all of which contraindicate the use of these drugs.
2. Note client history of renal disease, cardiac problems, or hepatic disease.
3. Determine the age of the client. Elderly clients, especially those with mental impairment or atherosclerosis, should not receive these drugs.

Interventions

1. If the client complains of a dry mouth, provide frequent mouth care and cold drinks, especially postoperatively. Sugarless hard candies and chewing gum may also be of some benefit.
2. Observe the client for evidence of drug interactions that may occur. A reduction in dosage of one of the medications may be necessary.

Client/Family Teaching

1. Explain that certain side effects are to be expected and describe these. Report these to the physician, who may alleviate symptoms by reducing the dose of drug or by temporarily stopping the drug. Sometimes the client may be expected to tolerate certain side effects such as dry mouth or blurred vision because of the overall beneficial effects of drug therapy.
2. Stress the importance of maintaining the dietary regimen prescribed by the physician. Assist the client to understand and plan diet. Consult with the dietitian as necessary for assistance in meal planning.
3. Remind the client that antiparkinsonism drugs are not to be withdrawn abruptly. If the medication is changed, one drug should be withdrawn slowly and the other started in small doses.

ADDITIONAL NURSING CONSIDERATIONS RELATED TO PATHOLOGIC CONDITIONS FOR WHICH THE DRUG IS ADMINISTERED

CARDIOVASCULAR

Interventions

1. Monitor heart rate, BP, and respiratory rate. Assess client for any changes and report.
2. Note any client complaints of palpitations, document, and report to the physician.

OCULAR

Assessment: Document intraocular pressures and assess visual fields.

Interventions: Note any client complaint of dizziness or blurred vision. Provide assistance with ambulation and institute safety measures.

Client/Family Teaching

1. Explain how long vision will be affected by the medication and

assist the client in planning activities for safety.

2. Advise that temporary stinging and blurred vision will occur.

3. Caution that night vision may be impaired.

4. Explain that photophobia, which may occur, can be relieved by wearing dark glasses.

5. Report any marked changes in vision, eye irritation. or persistent headaches immediately.

6. Review the appropriate methods for instillation of drops or ointment and observe client administration technique.

GASTROINTESTINAL

Client/Family Teaching

1. Advise clients receiving medication for treatment of GI pathology to take the medication early enough before a meal (at least 20 min) so that the medication will be effective when needed.

2. Clients with GI pathology should be instructed on how to maintain the prescribed diet. Provide printed information related to the diet and refer to the dietitian as needed.

3. Instruct the client to continue taking the medication as ordered and to notify the physician of any adverse side effects.

GENITOURINARY

Interventions

1. Assess middle-aged male clients in particular for infrequent voiding. This is evidence of urinary retention and should be documented and reported to the physician.

2. Monitor I&O. Palpate abdomen for evidence of bladder disten-

tion and determine the need for catheterization.

3. If impotence occurs, it may be drug-related. The client should be encouraged to consult with the physician.

Evaluation: Evaluate client for:

• Reports of a reduction in muscle spasms

• Evidence of an increased heart rate

• Evidence of a decrease in the production of secretions

• Reports of a reduction in muscle tremors, rigidity, and spasticity

DIURETICS

See also the following individual entries:

Acetazolamide
Acetazolamide Sodium
Aldactazide
Amiloride Hydrochloride
Bumetanide
Chlorothiazide
Chlorothiazide Sodium
Chlorthalidone
Dyazide
Ethacrynate Sodium
Ethacrynic Acid
Furosemide
Hydrochlorothiazide
Indapamide
Spironolactone
Triamterene

General Statement: The kidney is a complex organ with three main functions:

1. Elimination of waste materials and return of useful metabolites to the blood.

2. Maintenance of the acid-base balance.

3. Maintenance of an adequate electrolyte balance, which in turn governs the amount of fluid retained in the body.

Malfunction of one or more of these regulatory processes may result in the retention of excessive fluid by various tissues (edema). The latter can be an important manifestation of many conditions (e.g., congestive heart failure, pregnancy, and premenstrual tension).

Action: Diuretic drugs increase the urinary output of water and sodium (prevention or correction of edema), mostly through one of the following mechanisms:

1. Increasing the glomerular filtration rate.
2. Decreasing the rate at which sodium is reabsorbed from the glomerular filtrate by the renal tubules; therefore, water is excreted along with sodium.
3. Promoting the excretion of sodium, and therefore water, by the kidney.

Some of the commonly used diuretics, especially the thiazides, also have an antihypertensive effect. Diuretic drugs can enhance the normal function of the kidney but cannot stimulate a failing kidney into functioning. According to their mode of action and chemical structure, the diuretics fall into the following classes: thiazides (benzothiadiazides); carbonic anhydrase inhibitors (used mainly for glaucoma); osmotic diuretics; loop diuretics; and potassium-sparing drugs.

Uses: Edema, congestive heart failure, hypertension, pregnancy, and premenstrual tension. See also individual agents.

NURSING CONSIDERATIONS
Administration

1. If a diuretic is to be taken daily, administer it in the morning so that the major diuretic effect will occur before bedtime.
2. Liquid potassium preparations are bitter. Therefore, when they are to be used, administer with fruit juice or milk to make them more palatable.

Assessment

1. Obtain baseline serum electrolyte levels as well as client weight, intake and output and record.
2. Determine the extent of the client's edema and assess skin turgor, mucous membranes, and lung fields.
3. Review drugs the client has been taking to identify those with which diuretics interact.
4. Conduct baseline studies of renal and hepatic function.

Interventions

1. Weigh the client each morning after the client has voided and before the client has eaten or taken fluids. Record the weight and report any sudden increase in weight to the physician.
2. Monitor the client's intake and output. Report any absence of or decrease in diuresis and note any changes in lung sounds.
3. Check ambulatory clients for edema in the extremities. Check clients on bed rest for edema in the sacral area. Measure daily, document the extent of edema or ascites, and report to the physician.
4. Monitor for serum electrolyte

levels and the following *signs of electrolyte imbalance:*

- *Hyponatremia* (low-salt syndrome)—characterized by muscle weakness, leg cramps, dryness of mouth, dizziness, and GI disturbances.
- *Hypernatremia* (excessive sodium retention in relation to body water)—characterized by CNS disturbances such as confusion, loss of sensorium, stupor, and coma. Poor skin turgor or postural hypotension are not as prominent as when there are combined deficits of sodium and water.
- *Water intoxication* (caused by defective water diuresis)—characterized by lethargy, confusion, stupor, and coma. Neuromuscular hyperexcitability with increased reflexes, muscular twitching, and convulsions if water intoxication is acute.
- *Metabolic acidosis*—characterized by weakness, headache, malaise, abdominal pain, nausea, and vomiting. Hyperpnea occurs in severe metabolic acidosis. Signs of volume depletion, such as poor skin turgor, soft eyeballs, and a dry tongue may also be observed.
- *Metabolic alkalosis*—characterized by irritability, neuromuscular hyperexcitability, and, in severe cases, tetany.
- *Hypokalemia* (deficiency of potassium in the blood)—characterized by muscular weakness, failure of peristalsis, postural hypotension, respiratory embarrassment, and cardiac arrhythmias.

- *Hyperkalemia* (excess of potassium in the blood)—characterized by early signs of irritability, nausea, intestinal colic, and diarrhea; and by later signs of weakness, flaccid paralysis, dyspnea, difficulty in speaking, and arrhythmias.

5. All signs of electrolyte imbalance should be reported to the physician and documented in the chart. Electrolyte levels should be monitored and the physical safety of the client should be safeguarded.

6. If the client is receiving enteric-coated potassium tablets, monitor for the presence of abdominal pain, distention, or GI bleeding. These tablets can cause small bowel ulceration. If these symptoms occur, discontinue the tablets. Also, monitor the client's stool to ensure that the tablets have not passed through intact.

7. If the client is also receiving antihypertensive drugs, monitor for excessively low blood pressure. Diuretics potentiate the effects of antihypertensive agents.

8. Diuretics may precipitate symptoms of diabetes mellitus in clients with latent or mild diabetes. Therefore, test the urine or perform finger sticks routinely in clients with diabetes and observe for signs of hyperglycemia.

9. If the client is taking digitalis, check the apical pulse. Hyper- or hypokalemia associated with diuretic therapy may potentiate the toxic effects of digitalis and precipitate cardiac arrhythmias.

10. Assess the client for complaints of sore throat, the presence of a

skin rash, and yellowing of the skin or sclera, and report. These may be signs of blood dyscrasias due to drug hypersensitivity.

11. If the client has a history of liver disease, be alert for electrolyte imbalances, which could cause stupor, coma, and death.

12. If the client has a history of gout, note any increase in the frequency of acute attacks that may be precipitated by diuretics. Document and report to the physician.

Client/Family Teaching

1. Instruct clients in taking their blood pressure and pulse, in recording the measurements and how to determine if adverse effects have occurred that need to be reported to the physician. These measurements may assist the physician to determine if symptoms are drug related and if the dosage of drug is appropriate.

2. Maintain a written record of weight. Explain that there may be some weight loss from the diuresis related to the drug therapy.

3. Advise that the drug may cause frequent, copious voiding and to take in the morning to prevent disruption of sleep. Assist the client in planning activities to accommodate this occurrence. Assure the client that there is no need to be alarmed by the diuresis.

4. Advise clients who need additional potassium intake to include foods in the diet that are high in potassium. Eating such foods is preferable to taking potassium chloride supplements. Provide the client with a list of foods high in potassium such as citrus, grape, cranberry, apple, pear, and apricot juices; bananas; meat, fish, or fowl; cereals; and tea and cola beverages. Refer the client to a dietitian as needed, for assistance in shopping and planning appropriate menus.

5. Unless the client has a preexisting condition such as gastric ulcer or diabetes, clients who are taking diuretics and who require potassium supplements should be encouraged to drink a large glass of orange juice daily.

6. Use caution in driving a car or operating other hazardous machinery until drug effects become apparent. Weakness and/ or dizziness may occur with diuresis.

7. Rise slowly from bed and sit down or lie down if feeling faint or dizzy.

8. Advise that the use of alcohol, standing for prolonged periods, and exercise in hot weather may enhance effects of orthostatic hypotension.

9. Instruct clients to notify physician immediately if they experience dizziness, nausea, muscle weakness, cramps, or tingling of the extremities.

10. Advise client to wear protective clothing, sunscreens, and sunglasses in the sun to prevent photosensitivity reactions.

11. Do not take any OTC preparations without first consulting with the physician or pharmacist.

Evaluation: Evaluate client for:
- Evidence of a reduction in blood pressure

- Reports of an increase in urine output
- Evidence of a reduction in edema with resultant weight loss
- Adequate tissue perfusion as evidenced by warm dry skin and good pulses
- Freedom from complications of drug therapy
- Laboratory confirmation of normal electrolyte levels and fluid balance

ERYTHROMYCINS

See also the following individual entries:

Erythromycin Base
Erythromycin Estolate
Erythromycin Ethylsuccinate
Erythromycin Gluceptate
Erythromycin Lactobionate
Erythromycin Stearate

Action/Kinetics: The erythromycins are produced by strains of *Streptomyces erythraeus* and have bacteriostatic and bactericidal activity (at high concentrations or if microorganism is particularly susceptible).

The erythromycins inhibit protein synthesis of microorganisms by binding reversibly to a ribosomal subunit (50S), thus interfering with the transmission of genetic information and inhibiting protein synthesis. The drugs are effective only against rapidly multiplying organisms. The erythromycins are absorbed from the upper part of the small intestine. Erythromycins for oral use are manufactured in enteric-coated or film-coated forms to prevent destruction by gastric acid. Erythromycin is approximately 70% bound to plasma proteins and achieves concentrations in body tissues about 40% of those in the plasma. Erythromycin diffuses into body tissues; peritoneal, pleural, ascitic, and amniotic fluids; saliva; through the placental circulation; and across the mucous membrane of the tracheobronchial tree. It diffuses poorly into spinal fluid, although penetration is increased in meningitis. Alkalinization of the urine (to pH 8.5) increases the gram-negative antibacterial action. **Peak serum levels: PO,** 1–4 hr. **t½:** 1.5–2 hr, *but prolonged in clients with renal impairment.* The drug is partially metabolized by the liver and primarily excreted in bile. Erythromycins are also excreted in breast milk.

Uses

1. Upper respiratory tract infections due to *Streptococcus pyogenes* (group a beta-hemolytic streptococci), *S. pneumoniae,* and *Hemophilus influenzae* (combined with sulfonamides).
2. Mild to moderate lower respiratory tract infections due to *S. pyogenes* and *S. pneumoniae.* Respiratory tract infections due to *Mycoplasma pneumoniae.*
3. Pertussis (whooping cough) caused by *Bordetella pertussis;* may also be used as prophylaxis of pertussis in exposed individuals.
4. Mild to moderate skin and skin structure infections due to *S. pyogenes* and *Staphylococcus aureus.*
5. As an adjunct to antitoxin in diphtheria (caused by *Corynebacterium diphtheriae*), to prevent carriers, and to eradicate the organism in carriers.

6. Intestinal amebiasis due to *Entamoeba histolytica*.
7. Acute pelvic inflammatory disease due to *Neisseria gonorrhoeae*.
8. Erythrasma due to *C. minutissimum*.
9. *Chlamydia trachomatis* infections causing urogenital infections during pregnancy, conjunctivitis in the newborn, or pneumonia during infancy. Also, uncomplicated chlamydial infections of the urethra, endocervix, or rectum in adults (when tetracyclines are contraindicated or not tolerated).
10. Nongonococcal urethritis caused by *Ureaplasma urealyticum* when tetracyclines are contraindicated or not tolerated.
11. Legionnaire's disease due to *Legionella pneumophilia*.
12. As an alternative to penicillin (in penicillin-sensitive clients) to treat primary syphilis caused by *Treponema pallidum*.
13. Prophylaxis of initial or recurrent attacks of rheumatic fever in clients allergic to penicillin or sulfonamides.
14. Infections due to *Listeria monocytogenes*.
15. Bacterial endocarditis due to alpha-hemolytic streptococci, Viridans group, in clients allergic to penicillins.

Investigational: Infections due to *N. gonorrhoeae,* including uncomplicated urethral, rectal, or endocervical infections and disseminated gonococcal infections; severe or prolonged diarrhea due to *Campylobacter jejuni;* genital, inguinal, or anorectal infections due to *Lymphogranuloma venereum;* chancroid due to *Haemophilus ducreyi.*
Many erythromycins are available in ointments and solutions for ophthalmic, otic, and dermatologic use.

Contraindications: Hypersensitivity to erythromycin; in utero syphilis.

Special Concerns: Most erythromycins are pregnancy category B. Use with caution in liver disease and during lactation.

Side Effects: Erythromycins have a low incidence of side effects (except for the estolate salt). *GI* (most common): Nausea, vomiting, diarrhea, cramping, abdominal pain, stomatitis, anorexia, melena, heartburn, pruritus ani, pseudomembranous colitis. *Allergic:* Skin rashes with or without pruritus, bullous fixed eruptions, urticaria, eczema, anaphylaxis (rare). *CNS:* Fear, confusion, altered thinking, uncontrollable crying or hysterical laughter, feeling of impending loss of consciousness. *CV:* Rarely, ventricular arrhythmias. *Miscellaneous:* Superinfection, hepatotoxicity, ototoxicity. *Following topical use:* Itching, burning, irritation, or stinging of skin. Dry, scaly skin.

IV use may result in venous irritation and thrombophlebitis; IM use produces pain at the injection site, with development of necrosis or sterile abscesses.

Symptoms of Overdose: Nausea, vomiting, diarrhea, epigastric distress, acute pancreatitis (mild), hearing loss (with or without tinnitus and vertigo).

Drug Interactions

Alfentanil / ↓ Excretion of alfentanil → ↑ effect
Anticoagulants / ↑ Anticoagulant effect → hemorrhage
Bromocriptine / ↑ Serum levels

of bromocriptine → ↑ pharmacologic and toxic effects

Carbamazepine / ↑ Effect of carbamazepine due to ↓ breakdown by liver

Cyclosporine / ↑ Effect of cyclosporine due to ↓ excretion

Digoxin / Erythromycin ↑ bioavailability of digoxin

Disopyramide / ↑ Plasma levels of disopyramide → arrhythmias and ↑ QTc intervals

Ergot alkaloids / Acute ergotism manifested by peripheral ischemia

Methylprednisolone / ↑ Effect of methylprednisolone due to ↓ breakdown by liver

Penicillin / Erythromycins either ↓ or ↑ effect of penicillins

Sodium bicarbonate / ↑ Effect of erythromycin in urine due to alkalinization

Theophylline / ↑ Effect of theophylline due to ↓ breakdown in liver

Triazolam / ↑ Bioavailability of triazolam → ↑ CNS depression

Laboratory Test Interferences: False + or ↑ values of urinary catecholamines, urinary steroids, and AST and ALT.

Dosage: PO and **IM** (painful); some preparations can be given **IV.** See individual drugs.

NURSING CONSIDERATIONS

See also *General Nursing Considerations For All Anti-Infectives,* p. 83

Administration/Storage

1. Inject deep into muscle mass. Injections are painful and irritating.
2. *Treatment of Overdose:* Induce vomiting. General supportive measures. Allergic reactions

should be controlled with conventional therapy.

Assessment

1. Note if client is allergic to any other antibiotic drugs.
2. Document symptoms of infection and ensure that appropriate cultures have been performed prior to initiating therapy.
3. Assess for skin reactions when using erythromycin ointment. Discontinue use and report to physician.
4. When using ophthalmic solutions, assess for mild reaction which, although usually transient, should be reported to the physician.

Interventions

1. Do not administer with or immediately prior to ingestion of fruit juice or other acidic drinks because acidity may decrease activity of drug. However, adequate water (up to 8 oz) should be consumed with each dose.
2. Do not routinely administer PO medication with meals because food decreases the absorption of most erythromycins. However, physician may order medication to be given with food to reduce GI irritation.
3. Instill otic solutions at room temperature. Gently pull pinna of ear down and back for children under 3 years of age; pull pinna of ear up and back for clients over 3 years of age.
4. Observe for evidence of impaired liver function, especially among the elderly. Review appropriate lab data.

5. Monitor for indications of superinfection, such as furry tongue, vaginal itching, rectal itching, or diarrhea.
6. Note evidence of rash or any complaints of irritation of the mouth or tongue.
7. Note any evidence of hearing loss, which is usually temporary.

Client/Family Teaching

1. Question clients to ensure they are eating a balanced diet and that fluid intake is adequate.
2. Doses of erythromycins should be evenly spaced throughout a 24-hr period.
3. If clients have difficulty with nausea, have them notify the physician so the prescription can be changed to coated tablets that can be taken with meals.
4. If tablets are not coated, advise client to take them 2 hr after meals.
5. Do not take erythromycins with juices.
6. Remind client to clean affected area before applying ointment.
7. Instill otic solutions at room temperature. Demonstrate the appropriate method for administration and have client/family return demonstrate.

Evaluation: Evaluate client for:
- Evidence of knowledge and understanding of illness, level of compliance, and assess response to prescribed therapy as well as to teaching
- Clinical evidence of resolution of infection (negative laboratory culture reports, ↓

temperature, improved appetite)
- Reports of symptomatic improvement

ESTROGENS

See also the following individual entries:

Chlorotrianisene
Diethylstilbestrol Diphosphate
Esterified Estrogens
Estradiol Transdermal System
Estrogenic Substances, Aqueous
Estrogens Conjugated, Oral
Estrogens Conjugated, Parenteral
Oral Contraceptives
Polyestradiol Phosphate

General Statement: Estrogens are first produced in large quantities during puberty and are responsible for the development of primary and secondary female sex characteristics. From puberty on, estrogens are secreted primarily by the ovarian follicles during the early phase of the menstrual cycle. Their production decreases sharply at menopause, but small quantities continue to be produced. Men also produce some estrogens. During each menstrual cycle, estrogens trigger the proliferative phase of the endometrium, affect the vaginal tract mucosa and breast tissue, and increase uterine tone. During adolescence, estrogens cause closure of the epiphyseal junction. Large doses inhibit the development of the long bones by causing premature closure and inhibiting endochondral bone formation. In adult women, estrogens participate in bone maintenance by aiding the deposition of calcium in the protein matrix of bones. They increase elastic elements in the skin, tend to cause sodium and fluid retention, and produce an anabolic effect by enhancing the turnover of dietary nitrogen and other elements into protein. Furthermore, they tend to keep plasma cholesterol at relatively low levels. All natural estrogens, including estradiol, estrone, and estriol, are steroids. These compounds are either obtained from the urine of pregnant mares or prepared synthetically. Nonsteroidal estrogens, including diethylstilbestrol and chlorotrianisene, are prepared synthetically.

Action/Kinetics: Estrogens combine with receptors in the cytoplasm of the cell, resulting in an increase in protein synthesis. For example, estrogens are required for development of secondary sex characteristics, development and maintenance of the female genital system and breasts. They also produce effects in the pituitary and hypothalamus. Natural estrogens are generally administered parenterally because they are either destroyed in the GI tract or have a significant first-pass effect; hence, adequate plasma levels are never reached. Synthetic derivatives can be given PO and are rapidly absorbed, distributed, and excreted. Estrogens are metabolized in the liver and excreted in urine (major portion) and feces.

Uses: Systemic. Primary ovarian failure, female hypogonadism or castration, menopausal symptoms (especially flushing, sweating, chills), atrophic vaginitis, kraurosis vulvae, abnormal uterine bleeding (progestins are preferred), postpartum breast engorgement. Adjunct to diet and calcium for prophylaxis of osteoporosis. Palliative treatment in advanced, inoperable, metastatic breast carcinoma in postmenopausal women and in men. Advanced inoperable carcinoma of the prostate. Certain estrogens are used as postcoital contraceptives. Mestranol or ethinyl estradiol in combination with a progestin are components of oral contraceptives. **Vaginal.** Atrophic vaginitis, atrophic dystrophy of the vulva due to menopause or ovariectomy.

Contraindications: Cancerous or precancerous lesions of the breast (until 5 years after menopause) and of the genital tract. Administer with caution, if at all, to clients with a history of thrombophlebitis, thromboembolism, asthma, epilepsy, migraine, cardiac failure, renal insufficiency, diseases involving calcium or phosphorus metabolism, or a family history of mammary or genital tract cancer. Estrogen therapy may be contraindicated in clients with blood dyscrasias, hepatic disease, or thyroid dysfunction. Prolonged therapy is inadvisable in women who plan to become pregnant. Undiagnosed abnormal genital bleeding. Estrogens are also contraindicated in clients who have not yet completed bone growth. Estrogens should not be used during pregnancy because they may damage the fetus (pregnancy category: X). Use during lactation.

Special Concerns: Safety and effectiveness have not been determined in children and should be used with caution in adolescents in whom bone growth is incomplete.

Side Effects: Systemic use. Side effects to estrogens are dose dependent. *CV:* Potentially, the most serious side effects involve the cardiovascular system. Thromboembolism, thrombophlebitis, myocardial infarction, pulmonary embolism, retinal thrombosis, mesenteric thrombosis, subarachnoid hemorrhage, postsurgical thromboembolism. Hypertension, edema, stroke. *GI:* Nausea, vomiting, abdominal cramps, bloating, diarrhea, changes in appetite. *Dermatologic:* Most common are chloasma or melasma. Also, erythema multiforme, erythema nodosum, hirsutism, alopecia, hemorrhagic eruptions. *Hepatic:* Cholestatic jaundice, aggravation of porphyria, benign (most common) or malignant liver tumors. *GU:* Breakthrough bleeding, spotting, changes in amount and/or duration of menstrual flow, amenorrhea (following use), dysmenorrhea, premenstrual-like syndrome. Increased incidence of *Candida* vaginitis. *CNS:* Mental depression, dizziness, changes in libido, chorea, headache, aggravation of migraine headaches, fatigue, nervousness. *Ocular:* Steepening of corneal curvature resulting in intolerance of contact lenses. Optic neuritis or retinal thrombosis, resulting in sudden or gradual, partial or complete loss of vision, double vision, papilledema. *Hematologic:* Increase in prothrombin and blood coagulation factors VII, VIII, IX, and X. Decrease in antithrombin III. *Miscellaneous:* Breast tenderness, enlargement, or secretions. Increased risk of gallbladder disease. Premature closure of epiphyses in children. Increased frequency of benign or malignant tumors of the cervix, uterus, vagina, and other organs. Weight gain. Increased risk of congenital abnormalities. Hypercalcemia in clients with metastatic breast carcinoma. In males, estrogens may cause gynecomastia, loss of libido, decreased spermatogenesis, testicular atrophy, and feminization. Prolonged use of high doses may inhibit the function of the anterior pituitary. Estrogen therapy affects many laboratory tests. **Vaginal use.** *GU:* Vaginal bleeding, vaginal discharge, endometrial withdrawal bleeding, serious bleeding in ovariectomized women with endometriosis. *Miscellaneous:* Breast tenderness.

Drug Interactions

Anticoagulants, oral /
   ↓ Anticoagulant response by ↑ activity of certain clotting factors

Anticonvulsants / Estrogen-induced fluid retention may precipitate seizures. Also, contraceptive steroids ↑ effect of anticonvulsants by ↓ breakdown in liver and ↓ plasma protein binding

Antidiabetic agents / Estrogens may impair glucose tolerance and thus change requirements for antidiabetic agent

Barbiturates / ↓ Effect of estrogen by ↑ breakdown by liver

Phenytoin / See *Anticonvulsants*

Rifampin / ↓ Effect of estrogen due to ↑ breakdown by liver

Succinylcholine / Estrogens may ↑ effects of succinylcholine

Tricyclic antidepressants / Possible increased effects of tricyclic antidepressants

Laboratory Test Interferences: Alter liver function tests and thyroid function tests. False + urine glucose test. ↓ Serum cholesterol, total serum lipids, pregnanediol excretion, serum folate. ↑ Serum triglyceride levels, thyroxine-binding globulin, sulfobromophthalein retention, prothrombin; factors VII, VIII, IX, X. Impaired glucose tolerance, reduced response to metyrapone.

Dosage: PO, IM, SC, vaginal, topical, or by implantation. The dosage of estrogens is highly individualized and is aimed at the minimal effective amount.

NURSING CONSIDERATIONS

Administration/Storage

1. Estrogens may be administered orally, parenterally, topically, intravaginally, or by implanting pellets.
2. The dose is highly individualized and is aimed at the minimal amount that will be effective.
3. Most orally administered estrogens are metabolized rapidly and, with the exception of chlorotrianisene, must be administered daily.
4. Parenterally administered estrogens are released more slowly from their aqueous suspensions or oily solutions. When administered by injection, the drug should be administered slowly and deeply.
5. To avoid continuous stimulation of reproductive tissue, cyclic therapy consisting of 3 weeks on and 1 week off is usually recommended.
6. To reduce postpartum breast engorgement, doses are administered during the first few days after delivery.

Assessment

1. Obtain a health history of the client, noting any history of thromboembolic problems before administering the drug.
2. Note if the client has diabetes.
3. Obtain baseline serum glucose level if client is diabetic and liver function studies if long-term therapy is anticipated.
4. List any history of depression, migraine headaches, or attempted suicide, document, and report to the physician.

Interventions

1. Observe the client for alterations in mental attitude. Signs of depression, withdrawal, complaints of insomnia or anorexia, or a lack of attention to personal appearance should be documented and called to the attention of the physician.
2. Monitor BP and liver function studies.
3. If the client has diabetes, monitor serum glucose and triglyceride levels and report any elevations to the physician.
4. If the client has a history of problems with blood coagulation factors, monitor these and the prothrombin time routinely and report any increase to the physician.

Client/Family Teaching

1. Medical supervision is essential during prolonged estrogen therapy. Advise physician if any new changes occur during drug therapy.
2. Advise the client who is receiving cyclical therapy to take the medication for 3 weeks and then to omit it for 1 week. Menstruation may then occur, but pregnancy will not occur because ovulation is suppressed. Instruct the client to keep a record of menstruation and any problem encountered such as missed menses, spotting, or irregularity, and report these to the physician.
3. Notify the physician immediately if pregnancy is suspected.

4. Explain to the client that breast tenderness may occur. Also, there may be enlargement or breast secretion. Instruct the client in breast self-examination and encourage client to perform this exam monthly. Any continued problems or changes in the breasts should be reported to the physician.

5. If the client has a history of thromboembolic problems, instruct her in how to take blood pressure and pulse, and how to keep an accurate written record to share with the physician at the next visit.

6. Report immediately to the physician if there are leg pains, sudden onset of chest pain, dizziness, shortness of breath, weakness of the arms or legs or any evidence of numbness.

7. Report any unusual vaginal bleeding. This may be caused by excessive amounts of estrogen and the dosage may need to be reduced.

8. Warn that nausea, bloating, abdominal cramping, changes in appetite, and vomiting may occur. These usually disappear with the continuation of therapy. Taking medication with meals or a light snack will prevent gastric irritation and usually eliminate the nausea. If the medication is to be taken once a day, taking it at bedtime may eliminate the problem.

9. Some clients may develop changes in the curvature of the cornea, making it difficult to wear contact lenses. The client who wears contact lenses needs to be made aware of this potential problem and advised to consult an ophthalmologist if evidenced.

10. Report any skin changes such as alopecia or melasma. The dose of drug may need to be changed or the physician may elect to use a different drug.

11. If the client has diabetes, estrogen can alter glucose tolerance. Advise particularly close monitoring of blood and urine to detect hyperglycemia and glycosuria, and to report any increase immediately to the physician. The dose of antidiabetic medication may need to be changed.

12. Discuss with male clients who are receiving estrogen therapy the fact that they may develop feminine characteristics or suffer from impotence. These symptoms usually disappear once the course of therapy has been completed.

13. If the treatment demands the use of vaginal suppositories, teach the client how to correctly insert the suppository. Advise the client to wear a perineal pad if there is an increase in vaginal discharge during the treatment. Remind the client to store the suppositories in the refrigerator.

14. If the client is to apply a vaginal preparation, it is best done at bedtime. Advise the client to wear a sanitary napkin when vaginal preparations are being used. Remind her to avoid the use of tampons.

15. Sometimes estrogen ointments may cause systemic reactions. Explain this to clients using the ointment and tell them to notify the physician.

16. If the client is pregnant and is planning to breast-feed her baby, she should notify her physician. A woman who is

planning to breast-feed should not take estrogens and should consult with her physician for alternative forms of contraception.

17. If the client smokes, explain the added dangers in combination with this drug therapy and assist client in efforts to stop smoking.

18. Explain that some potential risks have been associated with estrogen therapy, related to endometrial cancer. Check with the physician to ensure that the client is aware of these.

Evaluation: Evaluate client for any of the following:

- Control of symptoms of estrogen imbalance
- Effective as an adjunct in slowing postmenopausal osteoporosis
- Reports of symptomatic relief of postmenopausal symptoms
- Evidence of control of tumor size and spread in metastatic breast and prostate cancers
- Effective contraception

FLUOROQUINOLONES

See also the following individual entries:

Ciprofloxacin
Norfloxacin
Ofloxacin

Action/Kinetics: These antibiotics are synthetic, broad-spectrum antibacterial agents. The fluorine molecule confers increased activity against gram-negative organisms as well as broadens the spectrum against gram-positive organisms. These drugs act as bactericidal agents by interfering with DNA gyrase, an enzyme needed for the synthesis of bacterial DNA. Ciprofloxacin and ofloxacin achieve therapeutic levels in most parts of the body; however, norfloxacin does not achieve sufficient blood levels and is thus approved only for urinary tract infections. Food may delay the absorption of ciprofloxacin and norfloxacin.

Uses: See individual drugs. Generally ciprofloxacin and ofloxacin are used for lower respiratory tract infections, skin and skin structure infections, bone and joint infections, urinary tract infections, infectious diarrhea. In addition ofloxacin is used for sexually transmitted diseases. Norfloxacin is approved only for complicated and uncomplicated urinary tract infections and experimentally for urethral gonorrhea or endocervical gonococcal infections caused by penicillinase- or nonpenicillinase-producing *Neisseria gonorrhoeae*.

Contraindications: Hypersensitivity to the quinolone group of antibiotics, including cinoxacin and nalidixic acid. Lactation. Use in children less than 18 years of age.

Special Concerns: Pregnancy category: C.

Side Effects: See individual drugs. The following side effects are common to each of the fluoroquinolone antibiotics. *GI:* Nausea, vomiting, diarrhea, abdominal pain or discomfort, dry or painful mouth, heartburn, dyspepsia, flatulence, constipation, pseudomembranous colitis (except for ofloxacin). *CNS:* Headache, dizziness, malaise, lethargy, fatigue, drowsiness, somnolence, depression, insomnia, seizures, paresthesia, hallucinations.

Dermatologic: Rash, pruritus. *Hypersensitivity reactions:* Pharyngeal or facial edema, dyspnea, urticaria, itching, tingling, loss of consciousness, cardiovascular collapse. *Other:* Visual disturbances, hearing loss, superinfection, phototoxicity, eosinophilia.

Drug Interactions

Antacids / ↓ Serum levels of fluoroquinolones due to ↓ absorption from the GI tract

Anticoagulants / ↑ Effect of anticoagulant

Antineoplastic agents / ↓ Serum levels of fluoroquinolones

Cyclosporine / ↑ Risk of nephrotoxicity

Iron salts / ↓ Serum levels of fluoroquinolones due to ↓ absorption from the GI tract

Probenecid / ↑ Serum levels of fluoroquinolones due to ↓ renal clearance

Sucralfate / ↓ Serum levels of fluoroquinolones due to ↓ absorption from the GI tract

Theophylline / ↑ Plasma levels and ↑ toxicity of theophylline due to ↓ clearance

Zinc salts / ↓ Serum levels of fluoroquinolones due to ↓ absorption from the GI tract

Laboratory Test Interferences: ↑ ALT, AST.

Dosage: See individual drugs.

NURSING CONSIDERATIONS

See also *General Nursing Considerations* for *All Anti-Infectives,* p. 83.

Administration/Storage

1. Clients should drink liberal amounts of fluids.
2. Products containing iron or zinc and antacids containing magnesium or aluminum should not be taken simultaneously or within 2 hr before or after dosing with fluoroquinolones.
3. *Treatment of Overdose:* For acute overdose, vomiting should be induced or gastric lavage performed. The client should be carefully observed and, if necessary, symptomatic and supportive treatment given. Hydration should be maintained.

Assessment

1. Note any previous experiences with antibiotics in this class and document results.
2. Determine that baseline CBC, liver, and renal function studies as well as laboratory cultures have been performed.
3. List medications client currently prescribed noting any that may interact unfavorably.

Interventions

1. Monitor VS, I&O, and encourage increased intake of fluids.
2. Observe client closely for any evidence of adverse effects as hypersensitivity reactions may be observed even following the first dose. The drug should be discontinued at the first sign of skin rash or other allergic reactions.
3. During prolonged or chronic administration of fluoroquinolones, periodic assessment of renal, hepatic, and hematopoietic function should be performed.

Client/Family Teaching

1. Take only as directed and preferably not with meals as food may delay the absorption of ciprofloxacin and norfloxacin.

2. Review list of drug side effects noting those that require immediate reporting and also advise client to report any other persistent, bothersome symptoms.
3. Describe symptoms of a hypersensitivity reaction and stress the importance of immediate reporting; instruct client to discontinue drug therapy in this event.
4. Advise client not to take any mineral supplements or antacids containing magnesium or aluminum concomitantly or within 2 hr of drug therapy.

Evaluation: Evaluate client for:

- Reports of symptomatic improvement
- Clinical evidence of resolution of infection
- Laboratory evidence of negative culture reports

HISTAMINE H$_2$ ANTAGONISTS

See also the following individual entries:

Cimetidine
Famotidine
Nizatidine
Ranitidine

Action/Kinetics: Histamine H$_2$ antagonists are competitive blockers of histamine. As such they inhibit all phases of gastric acid secretion including that caused by histamine, gastrin, and muscarinic agents. Both fasting and nocturnal acid secretion are inhibited. In addition, the volume and hydrogen ion concentration of gastric juice are decreased. Cimetidine, famotidine, and ranitidine have no effect on gastric emptying; cimetidine and famitidine have no effect on lower esophageal pressure. Fasting or postprandial serum gastrin is not affected by famotidine, nizatidine, or ranitidine. Cimetidine is known to affect the cytochrome P-450 drug metabolizing system for other drugs. Ranitidine also affects the P-450 enzyme system, but its effect on elimination of other drugs is not significant. Neither famotidine nor nizatidine affects the P-450 enzyme system.

Uses: See individual drugs. Treatment of duodenal ulcer and maintenance therapy after healing of the active ulcer. Benign gastric ulcer. Pathologic hypersecretory conditions (except nizatidine) including Zollinger-Ellison syndrome, systemic mastocytosis, and multiple endocrine adenomas. Cimetidine and ranitidine are approved for use in gastroesophageal reflex disease. *Investigational:* All drugs except nizatidine are used experimentally for prevention of aspiration pneumonitis, prophylaxis of stress ulcers, and acute upper GI bleeding.

Contraindications: Hypersensitivity to H$_2$-receptor antagonists.

Special Concerns: Pregnancy category: B (cimetidine, famotidine, ranitidine); pregnancy category: C (nizatidine). Use with caution in impaired hepatic and renal function. Safety and effectiveness have not been established for use in children.

Side Effects: The following side effects are common to all or most of the H$_2$-histamine antagonists. See individual drugs for complete listing.

GI: Nausea, vomiting, abdominal discomfort, diarrhea, constipation, hepatocellular effects. *CNS:* Headache, fatigue, somnolence, dizziness, confusion, hallucinations. *Dermatologic:* Rash, urticaria, pruritus, alopecia (rare), erythema multiforme (rare). *Other:* Thrombocytopenia, gynecomastia, impotence, loss of libido, cardiac arrhythmias following rapid IV use (rare), arthralgia (rare), anaphylaxis (rare).

Symptoms of Overdose: No experience is available for deliberate overdose.

Dosage: See individual drugs.

NURSING CONSIDERATIONS

Administration/Storage

1. These drugs may be taken without regard for meals.
2. Doses of antacids should be staggered if used with cimetidine or ranitidine.
3. *Treatment of Overdose:* Induce vomiting or perform gastric lavage to remove any unabsorbed drug. Monitor the client and undertake supportive therapy.

Assessment

1. Assess client symptoms of epigastric or abdominal pain noting onset, duration, intensity, and any previous treatment and the results.
2. Obtain baseline CBC, liver and renal function studies.
3. Perform baseline CNS assessment noting level of orientation.

Client/Family Teaching

1. Advise client to take medication as prescribed and not to stop if pain subsides or if "feeling better" as drug is necessary to inhibit gastric acid secretion.
2. Any evidence of confusion or disorientation should be reported immediately to the physician. This has been noted more often in the elderly and severely ill.
3. Avoid alcohol, aspirin-containing products, and foods that may cause GI irritation.
4. Instruct client to inform physician of drug therapy when undergoing skin testing. These drugs generally should be discontinued 24 hr before testing begins as a false negative response may be evident in tests with allergen extracts.
5. Smoking may interfere with drug's action. Advise client to stop smoking and most especially not to smoke following the last prescribed dose of the day. Offer referrals and assistance in accessing formal smoking cessation programs.
6. Advise that any new evidence of bleeding, such as blood-tinged emesis or dark tarry stools as well as dizziness or rash, require immediate reporting.
7. Stress the importance of reporting for all scheduled follow-up studies and advise that a response to these agents does not preclude gastric malignancy.

Evaluation: Evaluate client for:
- Radiographic or endoscopic evidence of duodenal ulcer healing
- Clinical evidence of reduced gastric irritation and bleeding with reports of a reduction in abdominal pain

INSULINS

See also the following individual entries:

Human Insulin
Insulin Injection
Insulin Injection Concentrated
Insulin Zinc Suspension
Insulin Zinc Suspension, Extended
Insulin Zinc Suspension, Prompt
Isophane Insulin Suspension
Isophane Insulin Suspension and Insulin Injection

General Statement: Diabetes mellitus is a disease in which the islets of Langerhans in the pancreas produce either no insulin or insufficient quantities of insulin. Diabetes mellitus is classified as insulin-dependent (type I; formerly referred to as *juvenile-onset*) and non-insulin–dependent (type II; formerly referred to as *maturity-onset*). Diabetes mellitus can be treated successfully by the administration of insulin isolated from the pancreas of cattle or hogs or of human insulin made either semisynthetically or derived from recombinant DNA technology.

The structure of insulin from pork sources more closely resembles human insulin than that from beef sources.

Proinsulin still remains the major impurity in insulin products. Such impurities may lead to local or systemic allergic reactions as well as antibody-mediated insulin resistance. In recent years, however, technology has improved so that insulin preparations currently marketed in the United States do not contain more than 25 parts per million (ppm) of proinsulin. Insulin products that contain less than 20 ppm of proinsulin are referred to as *improved single peak* insulins; those products that contain 10 ppm or less of proinsulin are referred to as *purified insulins*. In reality, purified pork insulins have approximately 1 ppm of proinsulin and human insulins made semisynthetically or from recombinant DNA have 1 and 0 ppm, respectively.

Insulin preparations with different times of onset, peak activity, and duration of action have been developed. Such products are prepared by precipitating insulin in the presence of zinc chloride to form zinc insulin crystals and/or by combining insulin with a protein such as protamine. Based on these modifications, insulin products are classified as fast-acting, intermediate-acting, and long-acting. These preparations permit the physician to select the preparation best suited to the life-style of the client.

RAPID-ACTING INSULIN

1. Insulin injection (Regular Insulin, Crystalline Zinc Insulin, Unmodified Insulin)
2. Prompt insulin zinc suspension (Semilente)

INTERMEDIATE-ACTING INSULIN

1. Isophane insulin suspension (NPH)
2. Insulin zinc suspension (Lente)

LONG-ACTING INSULIN

Extended insulin zinc suspension (Ultralente)

Note: Insulin preparations with various times of onset and duration of action are often mixed to obtain optimum control in diabetic clients.

Action/Kinetics: Insulin, following combination with insulin receptors on cell plasma membranes, facilitates the transport of glucose into cardiac and skeletal muscle and adipose tissue. It also increases synthesis of glycogen in the liver. Insulin stimulates protein synthesis and lipogenesis and inhibits lipolysis and release of free fatty acids from fat cells.

This latter effect prevents or reverses the ketoacidosis sometimes observed in the diabetic. Insulin also causes intracellular shifts in magnesium and potassium. Since insulin is a protein, it is destroyed in the GI tract. Thus, it must be administered subcutaneously so that it is readily absorbed into the bloodstream and distributed throughout the extracellular fluid. Insulin is metabolized mainly by the liver.

Uses: Replacement therapy in type I diabetes. Diabetic ketoacidosis or diabetic coma (use regular insulin). Insulin is also indicated in type II diabetes when other measures have failed (e.g., diet, exercise, weight reduction) or with surgery, trauma, infection, fever, endocrine dysfunction, pregnancy, gangrene, Raynaud's disease, or kidney or liver dysfunction.

Purified or human insulins are used for local insulin allergy, lipodystrophy at the injection site, immunologic insulin resistance, temporary insulin use (e.g., surgery, acute stress, gestational diabetes), and newly diagnosed diabetes.

Regular insulin is used in IV hyperalimentation solutions, in IV dextrose to treat severe hyperkalemia, and IV as a provocative test for growth hormone secretion.

Insulin and oral hypoglycemic drugs have been used in type II diabetics who are difficult to control with diet and oral therapy alone.

Diet: The dietary control of diabetes is as important as medication with appropriate drugs. The role of the nurse and dietitian in teaching the client how to eat properly cannot be underestimated.

As a first step, the physician must determine the individual client's dietary requirements. Since there is a close relationship between carbohydrate (CHO), fat (F), and protein (P), intake of each of these nutrients must be regulated. The prescribed amount of CHO, P, and F eaten at each meal must remain constant.

The nurse and/or dietitian must teach the client how to calculate exchange values of various foods. Food lists and food-exchange values published by the American Diabetes Association and the American Dietetic Association are valuable teaching aids.

Diabetic clients should adhere to a regular meal schedule. Clients taking large amounts of insulin will frequently be better controlled when they have four to six small meals daily rather than three large ones. The frequency of meals and the overall caloric intake vary with the type of drug taken. Diabetic children may be on a less restricted diet, adjusting the insulin dosage according to blood and urine glucose readings. Children with negative urine glucose tend to become hypoglycemic rapidly with exercise or decrease in appetite, and many physicians allow for glucose spilling.

Contraindications: Hypersensitivity to insulin.

Special Concerns: Pregnant diabetic clients often manifest decreased insulin requirements during the first half of pregnancy and increased requirements during the latter half. Lactation may decrease insulin requirements.

Side Effects: *Hypoglycemia:* Due to insulin overdose, delayed or decreased food intake, too much exercise in relationship to insulin dose, or when transferring from one preparation to another. Even carefully controlled clients occasionally develop signs of insulin overdosage characterized by hunger, weakness, fatigue, nervousness, pallor or flushing, profuse sweating, headache, palpitations, numbness of mouth, tingling in the fingers, tremors, blurred and double vision, hypothermia, excess yawning, mental confusion, incoordination, tachycardia, and loss of consciousness.

Symptoms of hypoglycemia may mimic those of psychic disturbances. Severe prolonged hypoglycemia may cause brain damage, and in the elderly, may mimic stroke.

Allergic: Urticaria, angioedema, lymphadenopathy, bullae, anaphylaxis. Occurs mostly following intermittent insulin therapy or IV administration of large doses to insulin-resistant patients. Antihistamines or corticosteroids may be used to treat these symptoms. Clients who are highly allergic to insulin and cannot be treated with oral hypoglycemics may respond to human insulin products.

At site of injection: Swelling, stinging, redness, itching, warmth. These symptoms often disappear with continued use. Lipoatrophy or hypertrophy of subcutaneous fat tissue (minimize by rotating site of injection).

Insulin resistance: Usual cause is obesity. Acute resistance may occur following infections, trauma, surgery, emotional disturbances, or other endocrine disorders.

Ophthalmologic: Blurred vision, transient presbyopia. Occurs mainly during initiation of therapy or in clients who have been uncontrolled for a long period of time.

Hyperglycemic rebound (Somogyi effect): Usually in clients who receive chronic overdosage.

DIFFERENTIATION BETWEEN DIABETIC COMA AND HYPOGLYCEMIC REACTION (INSULIN SHOCK): Coma in diabetes may be caused by uncontrolled diabetes (high sugar content in blood or urine, ketoacidosis) or by too much insulin (insulin shock, hypoglycemia).

Diabetic coma and insulin shock can be differentiated in the following manner:

Hyperglycemia (Diabetic Coma)

Onset / Gradual (days)
Medication / Insufficient insulin
Food intake / Normal or excess
Overall appearance / Extremely ill
Skin / Dry and flushed
Infection / Frequent
Fever / Frequent
Mouth / Dry
Thirst / Intense
Hunger / Absent
Vomiting / Common
Abdominal pain / Frequent
Respiration / Increased, air hunger
Breath / Acetone odor
Blood pressure / Low
Pulse / Weak and rapid

Vision / Dim
Tremor / Absent
Convulsions / None
Urine sugar / High
Ketone bodies / High
Blood sugar / High

Hypoglycemia (Insulin Shock)

Onset / Sudden (24–48 hr)
Medication / Excess insulin
Food intake / Probably too little
Overall appearance / Very weak
Skin / Moist and pale
Infection / Absent
Fever / Absent
Mouth / Drooling
Thirst / Absent
Hunger / Occasional
Vomiting / Absent
Abdominal pain / Rare
Respiration / Normal
Breath / Normal
Blood pressure / Normal
Pulse / Full and bounding
Vision / Diplopia
Tremor / Frequent
Convulsions / In late stages
Urine sugar / Absent in second specimen
Ketone bodies / Absent in second specimen
Blood sugar / Less than 60 mg/ 100 ml

Source: Adapted with permission from *The Merck Manual,* 11th ed.

Diabetic coma is usually precipitated by the client's failure to take insulin. Hypoglycemia is often precipitated by the client's unpredictable response, excess exertion, stress due to illness or surgery, errors in calculating dosage, or failure to eat.

TREATMENT OF DIABETIC COMA OR SEVERE ACIDOSIS: Administer 30–60 units regular insulin. This is followed by doses of 20 units or more every 30 min. To avoid a hypoglycemic state, 1 g dextrose is administered for each unit of insulin given. Treatment is often supplemented by electrolytes and fluids. Urine samples are collected for analysis, and vital signs are monitored as ordered.

TREATMENT OF HYPOGLYCEMIA (INSULIN SHOCK): Mild hypoglycemia can be relieved by oral administration of CHOs such as orange juice, candy, or a lump of sugar. If the patient is comatose, adults may be given 10–30 ml of 50% dextrose solution IV; children should receive 0.5–1 ml/kg of 50% dextrose solution. Epinephrine, hydrocortisone, or glucagon may be used in severe cases to cause an increase in blood glucose.

Drug Interactions

Alcohol, ethyl / ↑ Hypoglycemia → low blood sugar and shock
Anabolic steroids / ↑ Hypoglycemic effect of insulin
Beta-adrenergic blocking agents / ↑ Hypoglycemic effect of insulin
Chlorthalidone / ↓ Hypoglycemic effect of antidiabetics
Clofibrate / ↑ Hypoglycemic effects of insulin
Contraceptives, oral / ↑ Dosage of antidiabetic due to impairment of glucose tolerance
Corticosteroids / ↓ Effect of insulin due to corticosteroid-induced hyperglycemia
Dextrothyroxine / ↓ Effect of insulin due to dextrothyroxine-induced hyperglycemia
Diazoxide / Diazoxide-induced hyperglycemia ↓ diabetic control
Digitalis glycosides / Use with caution, as insulin affects serum potassium levels
Diltiazen / ↓ Effect of insulin
Dobutamine / ↓ Effect of insulin
Epinephrine / ↓ Effect of insulin due to epinephrine-induced hyperglycemia

Estrogens / ↓ Effect of insulin due to impairment of glucose tolerance

Ethacrynic acid / ↓ Hypoglycemic effect of antidiabetics

Fenfluramine / Additive hypoglycemic effects

Furosemide / ↓ Hypoglycemic effect of antidiabetics

Glucagon / Glucagon-induced hyperglycemia ↓ effect of antidiabetics

Guanethidine / ↑ Hypoglycemic effect of insulin

MAO inhibitors / MAO inhibitors ↑ and prolong hypoglycemic effect of antidiabetics

Oxytetracycline / ↑ Effect of insulin

Phenothiazines / ↑ Dosage of antidiabetic due to phenothiazine-induced hyperglycemia

Phenytoin / Phenytoin-induced hyperglycemia ↓ diabetic control

Propranolol / Propranolol inhibits rebound of blood glucose after insulin-induced hypoglycemia

Salicylates / ↑ Effect of hypoglycemic effect of insulin

Sulfinpyrazone / ↑ Hypoglycemic effect of insulin

Tetracyclines / May ↑ hypoglycemic effect of insulin

Thiazide diuretics / ↓ Hypoglycemic effect of antidiabetics

Thyroid preparations / ↓ Effect of antidiabetic due to thyroid-induced hyperglycemia

Triamterene / ↓ Hypoglycemic effect of antidiabetic

Laboratory Test Interferences: Alters liver function tests and thyroid function tests. False + Coombs' test, ↑ serum protein, ↓ serum amino acids, calcium, cholesterol, potassium, and urine amino acids.

Dosage: Insulin is usually administered SC. Insulin injection (regular insulin) is the **only** preparation that may be administered IV. This route should be used only for clients with severe ketoacidosis or diabetic coma.

Dosage for insulin is always expressed in USP units.

Dosage is established and monitored by blood glucose (often using glucose monitoring machines in the home), urine glucose, and acetone tests. Dosage is highly individualized. Furthermore, since the requirements of clients may change with time, dosage must be checked at regular intervals. It is usually advisable to hospitalize clients while their daily insulin and caloric requirements are being established.

In pregnancy, insulin requirements may increase suddenly during the last trimester. After delivery, requirements may suddenly drop to prepregnancy levels. To prevent the development of hypoglycemia, insulin is often discontinued on the day of delivery and glucose is administered IV.

The various insulin preparations can be mixed to obtain the combination best suited for the individual client. However, mixing must be done according to the directions received from the physician and/or pharmacist.

NURSING CONSIDERATIONS

Also includes general applications for all clients with diabetes controlled by medication (whether it be insulin or an oral hypoglycemic agent).

Administration/Storage

1. Read the product information brochure and any important notes inserted into the package of prescribed insulin.
2. Discard open vials that have not been used for several weeks or any whose expiration date has passed.
3. Refrigerate stock supply of insulin but avoid freezing. Freezing destroys the manner in which insulin is suspended in the formulation.
4. Store insulin vial in a cool place, avoiding extremes of temperature or exposure to sunlight.
5. The following guidelines should be followed with respect to mixing the various insulins.
   - Regular insulin may be mixed with NPH or Lente insulins. However, to avoid transfer of the longer-acting insulin into the regular insulin vial, regular insulin should be drawn into the syringe first.
   - A mixture of regular insulin with NPH or Lente insulin should be administered within 15 min of mixing due to binding of regular insulin by excess protamine and/or zinc in the longer-acting preparations.
   - Lente, Semilente, or Ultralente insulins may be mixed with each other in any proportion; however, these insulins should not be mixed with NPH insulins.
   - When used in an insulin infusion pump, insulin may be mixed in any proportion with either 0.9% sodium chloride injection or water for injection. Due to stability changes, such mixtures should be used within 24 hr of their preparation.
6. Store compatible mixtures of insulin for no longer than 1 month at room temperature or 3 months at 2°C–8°C (36°F–46°F). However, bacterial contamination may occur.
7. To ensure a constant amount of precipitate in each dose, invert the vial several times to mix before the material is withdrawn. Avoid vigorous shaking and frothing of the material. (Regular and globin insulin are the only two insulins that do not have a precipitate.)
8. Discard any vial in which the precipitate is clumped or granular in appearance or which has formed a solid deposit of particles on the side of the vial.
9. To prevent dosage error, do not alter the order of mixing insulins or change the model or brand of syringe or needle.
10. Administer at a 90° angle when using a 1/2-inch needle and at a 45° angle when using a 5/8-inch needle for injection.
11. Provide an automatic injector for clients who are fearful of injecting themselves.
12. Assist the visually impaired client with diabetes to obtain information and devices for self-administration of insulin by consulting their local diabetes association or by writing to the American Diabetes Association, 149 Madison Avenue, New York, NY 10016 (telephone: 212-725-4925), for their buyer's guide, which lists numerous available products for diabetics. Clients may also contact

The Lighthouse, Inc., 800 Second Avenue, New York, NY 10017 (telephone: 212-808-0077) for additional information on visual impairments.

13. Lipoatrophy may occur. This may appear as mild dimpling of the skin or as deep pits in young girls and women, and lipodystrophy, appearing as well-developed muscle on the anterior and lateral thighs of young boys and men. To prevent this problem, rotate the sites of SC injections of insulin.

- Make a chart indicating the injection sites (see Figure 2).
- Allow 3–4 cm between injection sites.
- Do not inject in the same site for at least 1 month.
- Avoid injecting within 1 cm around the umbilicus because of the high vascularity in this area.
- Avoid injections around the waistline because of the sensitive nerve supply to this area.
- Use insulin at room temperature to prevent lipodystrophy.

14. Note that rotation of injection sites may lead to differences in blood levels of insulin.

15. If the insulin has been refrigerated, allow it to remain at room temperature for at least 1 hr before using.

16. Apply pressure for a minute after injection, but do not massage since this may interfere with the rate of absorption.

17. If breakfast must be delayed because of laboratory tests, delay administering the morning dose of insulin.

18. Care of reusable syringes and needles.

- Do not use heavily chlorinated water or water with a high chemical content for sterilizing syringes. To sterilize, boil the syringe and needle for 5 min.
- Needle and syringe can be sterilized by soaking in isopropyl alcohol for at least 5 min. The alcohol must evaporate from the equipment before use to prevent reduction in the strength (dilution) of the insulin.
- Clean syringes covered by a

Figure 2 Pattern for varying insulin injection sites. If you follow the sketch, you will see that the right arm is marked A, the right side of the abdomen is B, and the right thigh is C. Crossing to the left side of the body, the left thigh is marked D, the abdomen E, and the left arm F. Each of these areas can be thought of as a rectangle which may be divided, as shown, into eight different squares more than one inch on each side. These squares are numbered, starting from the upper and outside corner, which is number one, to the lowest corner, which is number eight, with all even numbers toward the middle of the body. If you select square number one and inject into it at each of the six areas A through F, it will take you six days to return again to A. Then selecting square number two and injecting into it at each of the six areas again rotates you around your body, returning in six days to area A. Follow with square number three, and so forth. It is easy to see that this procedure provides 48 different places in which to make your injections. If you make one injection daily, it will be that many days before you return to the A-1 square . . . . almost seven weeks. (Figure and legend courtesy of Becton Dickinson and Company.)

Setting Up An Easy Rotation Cycle

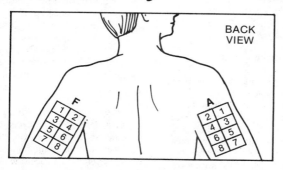

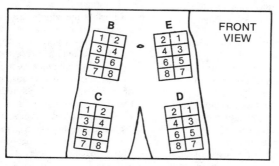

Injection Log

SITE		1	2	3	4	5	6	7	8
right arm	A								
right abdomen	B								
right thigh	C								
left thigh	D								
left abdomen	E								
left arm	F								

precipitate with a cotton-tip-ped swab soaked in vinegar; then thoroughly rinse syringe in water and sterilize it. Clean needles with a wire and sharpen with a pumice stone.

Assessment

1. Obtain a thorough nursing history from the client and/or family.
2. Assess the client for symptoms of hyperglycemia: thirst, polydypsia, polyuria, drowsiness, loss of appetite, fruity odor to the breath, and flushed dry skin. Note state of consciousness.
3. Assess the client for symptoms of hypoglycemia: drowsiness, chills, confusion, anxiety, cold sweats and cool pale skin, excessive hunger, nausea, headache, irritability, shakiness, rapid pulse, and unusual weakness or tiredness.
4. Determine when clients first noticed changes in their physical condition and what these changes were.
5. Note if the client and/or family has noticed any psychological changes and list what they consisted of.
6. Identify and list other medications the client may be taking.
7. Weigh the client. This is especially important when working with elderly clients because the amount of hypoglycemic agent prescribed is determined by their weight.
8. Perform baseline serum electrolytes, blood sugar, phosphate, magnesium, and glycosolated hemoglobin levels as indicated.

Interventions

1. If the client has symptoms of a *hyperglycemic reaction,* obtain medical supervision as rapidly as possible.
   - Have regular insulin available for administration.
   - Immediately obtain a blood sample for glucose or perform a finger stick before administering medication.
   - After administering the insulin, monitor the client closely.
   - Observe the client for further signs of hyperglycemia such as shortness of breath, facial flushing, air hunger, soft eyeballs, and acetone on the breath.
   - Check urine glucose, urine acetone, blood glucose, and other related laboratory data.
2. Check the client for early symptoms of *hypoglycemia,* such as easy fatigue, hunger, headache, drowsiness, nausea, lassitude, and tremulousness.
   - More marked symptoms such as weakness, sweating, tremors, and/or nervousness may occur later.
   - Observe the client at night for excessive restlessness and profuse sweating.
   - Obtain a blood sugar level and/or finger stick and promptly administer a carbohydrate (orange juice, candy, or a lump of sugar, if the client is conscious) and notify the physician.
   - If the client is conscious and has been taking long-acting insulin, also administer a slowly digestible carbohydrate, such as bread with corn syrup or honey. Provide

additional carbohydrates such as crackers and milk for the next 2 hr.

- If the client is in the hospital, have available 10%–20% dextrose solution for IV fluid therapy and D 50% bristojets for IV push.
- If the client is unconscious, apply honey or Karo syrup to the buccal membrane or administer glucagon if available.

3. Some clients experience a Somogyi effect and are often mistaken for clients who do not follow the prescribed methods of therapy. The Somogyi effect occurs when hypoglycemia triggers the release of epinephrine, glucocorticoids, and growth hormone, which stimulates glycogenesis and results in a higher blood glucose level. Reduction in the dosage of insulin is necessary to stabilize the client. This should be anticipated in the client who has originally been treated for hypoglycemia.

4. Juveniles with diabetes demand closer attention and observation for hypoglycemia. They are more susceptible to insulin shock than clients with diabetes in other age groups and have a more limited response to glucagon.

5. Assess juvenile diabetics more closely for infection or emotional disturbances that may increase their insulin requirements.

6. For the elderly client who has been newly diagnosed as having diabetes, the initial doses of insulin should be low, gradually increasing the dose until the desired effects have been achieved.

- Be alert for signs of hypoglycemia, such as slurred speech and mental confusion.
- If the client is to be on NPO status for whatever reason, consult the physician about the dosage adjustment that will be required.

7. Review the client's entire medication regimen for drugs that may enhance or antagonize antidiabetic agents being used. A dosage adjustment of antidiabetic agents may be necessary.

Client/Family Teaching

1. Review with the client and family the nature of diabetes mellitus and its signs and symptoms. Advise that medications assist to control diabetes but do not cure it.

2. Explain the necessity for close, regular medical supervision.

3. If the client is testing urine, explain how to test the urine for sugar and acetone and demonstrate how this test should be conducted. When testing the urine for glycosuria with Clinitest Tablets, Tes-Tape, Diastix, or Clinistix, as recommended by the physician, provide the client with printed instructions.

- Test a fresh second-voided specimen.
- Empty the bladder by voiding about 1 hr before mealtime.
- As soon as the client can void again, obtain the specimen and test.
- If the client is taking other medications, note what they are and determine if they may interfere with the test.

Notify the lab and use appropriate tests if interference may be a problem.

4. If the client is performing finger sticks to monitor glucose levels, demonstrate how this test should be conducted. If using a glucose monitoring machine, have clients perform a return demonstration to assure they know the proper technique, proper calibration, method of operation, and maintenance for the device. Some general principles may be followed.
   - Rotate sites.
   - Cleanse area with soap and water or alcohol prior to stabbing.
   - Stab finger and let a bead of blood form.
   - Wipe off with a cotton ball.
   - Then, let the bead of blood reform and apply to the test strip.
   - Follow specific guidelines for the individual device in use.

5. Discuss the fact that regimens are specific to the individual client, based on age, the severity of the diabetes, weight, any other medical problems the client may have, as well as the philosophy of the health care team.

6. Instruct clients in administering insulin and have them perform a return demonstration.

7. Provide a chart and instruct clients in how to chart the injection sites and how to avoid either lipoatrophy or lipodystrophy of injection sites.
   - For self injection, instruct the client to brace the arm against a hard surface such as the wall or a chair.
   - Cleanse the area thoroughly, allow the area to dry, then, depending on the condition of the skin, either pinch the skin between the thumb and forefingers of one hand, or spread the skin using the thumb and fingers of one hand.
   - Insert the needle at a 45° angle into the subcutaneous tissue and aspirate to be sure that the needle is not in a blood vessel.
   - Inject the insulin and withdraw the needle.

8. Explain the use and care of equipment, as well as the provision and storage of medication.

9. Advise to always have an extra vial of insulin and extra equipment on hand for administration when traveling, at home, or when hospitalized.

10. Have regular insulin available for emergency use.

11. Explain the importance of exercise and the effect of exercise on the utilization of carbohydrates and increasing carbohydrate needs.

12. Stress the importance of adhering to the prescribed diet. Emphasize weight control and ingestion of food relative to the peak action of the insulin being used. Record weekly weights and report any major variations.

13. Provide a food exchange list, explain it, and refer the client to a dietitian for assistance in meal planning.

14. Explain the importance of carrying candy or sugar at all times to counteract hypoglycemia should it occur.

15. Discuss the possibility of allergic responses. Itching, redness,

swelling, stinging, or warmth may occur at the injection site. These will usually disappear after a few weeks of therapy. However, they should be reported to the physician because the type of insulin may need to be changed. Purified or human insulins are used for local insulin allergy and lipodystrophy at the injection site.

16. Provide a printed chart explaining symptoms of hypoglycemia and hyperglycemia (see Interventions) and instructions concerning what to do for each. Also, instruct the client to notify the physician when either event occurs, explaining as specifically as possible what happened and what activity the client was engaged in. The dosage of insulin may need to be adjusted.

17. The client may have blurred vision at the beginning of insulin therapy. Advise the client that the condition should subside in 6–8 weeks. The effect is caused by the fluctuation of blood glucose levels, which produce osmotic changes in the lens of the eye and within the ocular fluids. If the condition does not clear up in 8 weeks, the client should be advised to have an eye examination and evaluation.

18. If the client feels ill and omits a meal because of fever, nausea, or vomiting, the next dose of insulin should be omitted unless the urine or finger stick test indicates an increase in sugar levels. Report this problem to the physician immediately for guidance in regulating

insulin and test glucose levels every 4 hr or as directed.

19. If client becomes ill, the physician should be notified immediately. Explain that to prevent coma, the client should maintain adequate hydration by drinking 1 cup or more of noncaloric fluids such as coffee, tea, water, or broth every hour. The client or family member should conduct urine testing or finger sticks more frequently under these circumstances.

20. If foods have been omitted, replace them by a similar amount of carbohydrate such as orange juice or some other easily absorbed form of carbohydrate.

21. If the supply of insulin is exhausted or the equipment to administer is not available, decrease the food intake by one-third and drink plenty of fluids. Omit the insulin and obtain the necessary supplies as soon as possible in order to return to the prescribed diet and insulin dosage.

22. Explain the importance of good hygienic practices to prevent infection.

23. Advise the client to wear a Medic Alert bracelet or carry a card identifying the client as having diabetes, currently prescribed medications, who to notify and what to do in the event the client is unable to respond.

24. Avoid alcoholic beverages because alcohol can cause hypoglycemia. Excessive intake of alcohol may require a reduction in the dosage of insulin because alcohol potentiates the hypoglycemic effect of insulin.

It also causes a disulfiram-type reaction with oral hypoglycemic agents.

25. Caution clients to use only the insulin prescribed and to check carefully each time they purchase insulin to be certain it is the correct form, brand, and strength they have been taking. If there is any change in insulin purity, strength, type, source of the insulin, or manufacturer, there may be a need to adjust the dosage of insulin.

26. Check vials of insulin carefully before each dose is taken. Regular insulin should be clear, whereas other forms may be cloudy.

27. Two kinds of insulin can be mixed in the same syringe if the following guidelines are followed:
   - Regular insulin can be mixed with any other insulin.
   - Lente forms can be mixed with other Lente insulins but cannot be mixed with other insulins with the exception of regular insulin.
   - A single form of insulin in a syringe can be stable for weeks or a month.
   - Except for the commercially prepared mixtures, mixtures of insulin are not stable and should be administered within 5 min of preparation.
   - When insulins are mixed, regular (unmodified) insulin should always be drawn up in the syringe first. Instruct the client to use the same procedure at all times when drawing up two insulins to avoid contamination of the two vials of insulin.

28. Refer the client and family to the American Diabetes Association and local support groups for additional information and support and to a dietitian for assistance with dietary modification. Support groups may assist clients and families to understand and learn to cope with this disease.

29. Stress the importance of follow-up visits and laboratory studies to evaluate the effectiveness of therapy.

Evaluation: Evaluate client for:
- Evidence of an understanding and effective management of their diabetes; note the development of positive coping strategies
- Laboratory confirmation that serum glucose and acetone levels are within desired range
- Evidence of healthy and intact skin at injection sites

INTRAVENOUS NUTRITIONAL THERAPY

See also the following individual entries:

Amino Acid Formulation for Hepatic Failure or Hepatic Encephalopathy
Amino Acid Formulation for High Metabolic Stress
Amino Acid Formulation for Renal Failure
Crystalline Amino Acid Infusion
IV Fat Emulsion

Action/Kinetics: Intravenous nutrition is an important treatment regimen for clients in whom oral feeding is not possible or is inadequate. A large number of products provide one or more of the following nutrients: dextrose, electrolytes, amino acids, fat emulsion, vitamins, minerals, and fluids. These preparations are administered IV either peripherally or via a central venous catheter. Such regimens are often referred to as total parenteral nutrition (TPN). The success of TPN is gauged by weight gain and positive nitrogen balance.

The proper administration of TPN products requires a thorough knowledge of the nutritional needs of the clients, as well as of their fluid and electrolyte balance. Central administration, via a central venous catheter, is used in clients requiring long-term parenteral nutrition or in those clients who are severely debilitated. Peripheral parenteral administration is used for short-term parenteral nutrition (up to 12 days), in situations where the caloric requirements are not excessive, or as a supplement to oral feeding. Clients receiving TPN must be frequently evaluated by means of complete laboratory tests.

Uses: In situations where GI absorption of nutrients is impaired due to disease, obstruction, or other drug therapy (e.g., cancer chemotherapy). Following GI surgery or in situations where nutrient requirements are increased as in trauma, burns, or severe infections.

Special preparations are available for use in renal failure, hepatic failure or encephalopathy, or in acute metabolic stress.

Contraindications: Hypersensitivity to specific proteins or inborn errors of amino acid metabolism. Products for general nutritional purposes (e.g., crystalline amino acid infusions) should not be used in severe kidney or liver disease, hyperammonemia, hepatic coma, or encephalopathy. Also, severe uncorrected acid-base imbalance.

Special Concerns: Use with caution in pregnancy. Sodium-containing products should be used with caution in clients with congestive heart failure, renal insufficiency, or edema. Potassium-containing products should be used cautiously in clients with severe renal failure or hyperkalemia. Products containing acetate should be used with care in alkalosis and hepatic insufficiency.

Side Effects: *Metabolic:* Metabolic acidosis or alkalosis, hyperammonemia, ketosis, dehydration, hypo- or hypervitaminosis, elevated hepatic enzymes, electrolyte imbalances, hypophosphatemia, hypocalcemia, osteoporosis, glycosuria, hypervolemia, osmotic diuresis. Rapid withdrawal of concentrated dextrose solutions may result in hypoglycemia. Essential fatty acid deficiency following long-term use of fat-free products (symptoms include dry, scaly skin, rash resembling eczema, alopecia, slow wound healing, and fatty infiltration of the liver). *Dermatologic:* Skin rashes, flushing, sweating. *Other:* Nausea, vertigo, fever, headache, dizziness. *At site of catheter:* Venous thrombosis, phlebitis.

Drug Interactions

Folic acid / Precipitation of calcium as calcium folate
Sodium bicarbonate / Precipitation of calcium and magnesium carbonate; ↓ effect of insulin and vitamin B complex with C
Tetracyclines / ↓ Effect of amino acids to conserve protein

Dosage: The dose, route of administration, and content of the infusion are determined individually for each client depending on the nutritional need, physical state, and length of therapy anticipated.

NURSING CONSIDERATIONS

Administration/Storage

1. Appropriate laboratory monitoring with baseline values and evaluation are required before and during administration.
2. Dextrose, 12.5% or greater, should not be used in peripheral venous infusions.
3. Blood should not be administered through the same infusion site. An exception would be a multilumen catheter in the subclavian (or large central) vein.
4. Solutions must be prepared aseptically under a laminar flow hood in the pharmacy.
5. Solutions should be used as soon as possible after preparation. No more than 24 hr should elapse for administration of a single bottle.
6. The IV administration set should be replaced daily.
7. Appropriate guidelines must be followed for clients in whom indwelling catheters will be in place for a long period of time.
8. Administer TPN solutions using an electronic infusion device whenever possible.
9. If the infusion must be discontinued, do not stop the infusion abruptly. Infuse dextrose 10% at the TPN rate until the next bag/bottle is available.

Assessment

1. Obtain a thorough nursing history.
2. Determine that a full nutritional assessment has been per-

formed by the dietitian (including height, weight, anthropometric measurements, caloric needs, lab values, and evaluation of nitrogen balance, as well as GI tract function) prior to initiating therapy.
3. Obtain baseline laboratory data including hepatic and renal function studies, blood glucose level, electrolyte levels, pH, protein level, and albumin level prior to initiating therapy.
4. Consult the nutritional support team for a more thorough evaluation of client needs.
5. Determine if the client has a history of allergic responses to protein hydrolysate. This is characterized by pruritus, urticaria, and wheals. Report positive responses and observations to the physician and nutritional support team.

Interventions

1. Monitor blood glucose levels at least every 6 hr initially; use urine, finger sticks, or serum determinations. Generally blood glucose levels over 200 mg/100 ml or fractional urine determinations of $3^+ - 4^+$ indicate the need for insulin to be added to the TPN solution.
2. Obtain written parameters and guidelines from the physician for controlling hyperglycemia.
3. If the blood glucose level exceeds 1,000 mg/100 ml, immediately discontinue TPN and substitute a hypo-osmolar solution to prevent neurologic dysfunction and coma.
4. Monitor and record vital signs, intake and output, and weights throughout TPN therapy.
5. Auscultate chest and observe

for evidence of peripheral edema as a symptom of fluid overload and report.

6. Report chills, fever, and diaphoresis and follow nutritional support team guidelines for managing infections.

Client/Family Teaching

1. For clients receiving intravenous nutritional therapy at home, review the appropriate procedure for site care, accessing the site, spiking and hanging the fluids, inserting the tubing, and operating the infusion pump, as well as removing and capping the site. Observe client performing procedure on several occasions and offer support and encouragement as needed. Provide printed, easy to follow guidelines and stress the importance of using aseptic technique.

2. List symptoms that require immediate reporting: fever, chills, sweating, pain, bleeding, blockage, drainage, and leaking at infusion site.

3. Advise that most therapy may be administered during the night so as not to interfere with client's daily routine.

4. Coordinate discharge with home health care agency to facilitate adjustment of client and provide appropriately prescribed equipment and support to client and family. Provide a number to call if client has questions or needs help.

Evaluation: Evaluate client for:

• Appropriate nutrient replacement as evidenced by weight gain, proper healing, and improved parameters as compared to baseline nutritional assessment

• Freedom from complication of intravenous nutritional therapy

LAXATIVES

See also the following individual entries:

Bisacodyl
Bisacodyl Tannex Enema
Cascara Sagrada
Castor Oil
Castor Oil, Emulsified
Docusate Calcium
Docusate Potassium
Docusate Sodium
Glycerin Suppositories
Lactulose
Magnesium Hydroxide
Magnesium Sulfate
Methylcellulose
Mineral Oil
Phenolphthalein
Psyllium Hydrophilic Muciloid
Senna
Sennosides A and B, Calcium Salts
Sodium Phosphate and Sodium Biphosphate

General Statement: Difficult or infrequent passage of stools (constipation) is a symptom of many conditions ranging from purely organic causes (obstruction, megacolon) to common functional disorders. Clients confined to bed may often develop constipation. Constipation may also be of psychologic origin. The underlying cause of constipation should be elucidated by a physician, especially since a marked change in bowel habits may be a symptom of a pathologic condition.

Laxatives are effective because they act locally, either by specifically stimulating the smooth muscles of the bowel or by changing the bulk or consistency of the stools. Laxatives can be divided into four categories.

1. *Stimulant laxatives:* Substances that chemically stimulate the smooth muscles of the bowel to increase contractions. Drugs include bisacodyl, cascara, danthron, phenolphthalein, and senna.
2. *Saline laxatives:* Substances that increase the bulk of the stools by retaining water. Includes magnesium salts and sodium phosphate.
3. *Bulk-forming laxatives:* Nondigestible substances that pass through the stomach and then increase the bulk of the stools. Examples are methylcellulose, psyllium, and polycarbophil.
4. *Emollient and lubricant laxatives:* Agents that soften hardened feces and facilitate their passage through the lower intestine. Examples include docusate and mineral oil.

Many laxative products contain two or more drugs with laxative properties. Today laxatives are prescribed less frequently for chronic constipation than in the past. In fact, continued use of laxatives has been held responsible for some cases of chronic constipation and other intestinal disorders because the client may start to depend on the psychologic effect and physical stimulus of the drug rather than on the body's own natural reflexes. Prevention of constipation should include adequate fluid intake and diet, as well as daily exercise.

Uses: Laxatives are indicated for the following conditions: anorectal lesions like hemorrhoids; for diagnostic procedures and in conjunction with surgery or anthelmintic therapy; and in cases of chemical poisoning. Short-term treatment of constipation.

Contraindications: Severe abdominal pain that *might* be caused by appendicitis, enteritis, ulcerative colitis, diverticulitis, intestinal obstruction. The administration of laxatives in such cases might cause rupture of the abdomen or intestinal hemorrhage. Children under the age of 2.

Side Effects: Excess activity of the colon resulting in nausea, diarrhea, or vomiting. Dehydration, disturbance of the electrolyte balance. Dependency occurs if used chronically.
    Bulk laxatives: Obstruction in the esophagus, stomach, small intestine, or rectum. *Stimulant laxatives:* Chronic abuse may lead to malfunctioning colon.

Drug Interactions

Anticoagulants, oral /
    ↓ Absorption of vitamin K from GI tract induced by laxatives may ↑ effects of anticoagulants and result in bleeding
Digitalis / Cathartics may ↓ absorption of digitalis
Tetracyclines / ↓ Effect of tetracyclines due to ↓ absorption from GI tract

NURSING CONSIDERATIONS

Administration

1. When administering a laxative, note the length of time it takes for the laxative to take effect and give it so that the result of the laxative will not interfere with the client's rest.
2. Administer laxatives at a temperature that makes them more agreeable to the client.

3. If the laxative is to be administered in a liquid, try to select one that the client finds palatable.

4. Administer laxatives at a time that will not interfere with the client's digestion and absorption of nutrients.

5. If the laxative is ordered to prepare the client for a diagnostic study, check the directions carefully to ensure accurate administration in preparation for the study.

Assessment

1. Determine the extent of the client's problem with constipation. Note how long the client has had to rely on laxatives.

2. Note if the client has abdominal pain and discomfort, its exact location, and the type of discomfort the client is experiencing. The symptoms may indicate appendicitis or some other intestinal disorder and laxatives would be contraindicated.

3. Note the age of the client, state of health, and nutritional status.

4. Identify any special restriction or limitation due to illness. This may include fluid restriction as well as a sodium-restricted diet.

5. List other medications the client is taking that may contribute to a constipation problem.

6. Identify if the client has had any recent changes in life-style that may contribute to the current problem.

7. Determine the character of the client's stool and the frequency of bowel movements expected by the client. The client's definition of constipation may determine if, in fact, constipation exists.

8. Note the type of laxative the client has been taking and the relative effectiveness associated with this laxative.

Interventions

1. If the client is in a hospital or is ill at home, provide a commode at the bedside. This will promote better bowel function by encouraging the client to move about and ensure privacy.

2. Encourage the client to alter dietary habits to include bulk foods and sufficient fluid in the daily diet to enhance elimination.

3. Discuss with clients the need for regular exercise, as well as a need for a reduction of their dependence on laxatives.

Client/Family Teaching

1. Discuss the need to have a regular schedule for defecation.

2. Instruct the client to keep a record of bowel function and response to all laxatives taken.

3. If the laxative is to be taken in preparation for a diagnostic study, review the directions with the client and provide a printed set of instructions to follow. If the client is unable to read, try to ensure that someone in the family or a friend can review the directions with the client so that an accurate result of the test can be obtained.

4. Instruct the client in techniques that facilitate elimination. Sitting with the legs slightly elevated and leaning forward

to increase abdominal pressure often encourages elimination.

5. Discuss the dangers of relying on laxatives for bowel movements and stress the use of diet to achieve the same purpose. Two or three prunes a day are preferable to laxatives.

6. Consult the physician if constipation persists because there could be a physiologic problem that requires attention.

7. If the client is pregnant, advise her to consult with the physician before taking any laxatives to treat constipation.

8. Advise nursing mothers to avoid using laxatives unless approved by the physician. Many are excreted in breast milk and can cause the infant to develop diarrhea.

Evaluation: Evaluate client for:
- Relief of constipation as evidenced by evacuation of a soft formed stool
- Reports that bowel movements occur regularly with a minimum of difficulty and without having to resort to the chronic use of laxatives, enemas, or suppositories
- Evidence of effective colon prep for diagnostic procedures

NARCOTIC ANALGESICS

See also the following individual entries:

Alfentanil Hydrochloride
Buprenorphine Hydrochloride
Butorphanol Tartrate
Codeine Phosphate
Codeine Sulfate
Dezocine
Empirin with Codeine
Fentanyl Citrate
Fentanyl Transdermal System
Fiorinal
Fiorinal with Codeine
Hydromorphone Hydrochloride
Meperidine Hydrochloride
Methadone Hydrochloride
Morphine Sulfate
Nalbuphine Hydrochloride
Oxycodone Hydrochloride
Oxycodone Terephthalate
Paregoric
Pentazocine Hydrochloride with Naloxone
Pentazocine Lactate
Percocet
Percodan
Phenaphen with Codeine
Propoxyphene Hydrochloride
Propoxyphene Napsylate
Sufentanil
Synalgos-DC
Talwin Nx
Tylenol with Codeine
Tylox
Vicodin

General Statement: The narcotic analgesics include opium, morphine, codeine, various opium derivatives, and totally synthetic substances with similar pharmacologic properties. Of these, meperidine (Demerol) is the best known. The relative activity of all narcotic analgesics is measured against morphine.

Opium itself is a mixture of alkaloids obtained since ancient times from the poppy plant. Morphine and codeine are two of the pure chemical substances isolated from opium. Certain drugs (pentazocine, butorphanol, nalbuphine) have both narcotic agonist and antagonist properties. Such drugs may precipitate a withdrawal syndrome if given to clients dependent on narcotics.

Action/Kinetics: The most important effect of the narcotic analgesics is on the CNS. In addition to an alteration of pain perception (analgesia), the drugs, especially at higher doses, induce euphoria, drowsiness, changes in mood, mental clouding, and deep sleep.

The narcotic analgesics also depress respiration. The effect is noticeable with small doses. Death by overdosage is almost always the result of respiratory arrest.

The narcotic analgesics have a nauseant and emetic effect (direct stimulation of the chemoreceptor trigger zone). They depress the cough reflex, and small doses of narcotic analgesics (codeine) are part of several antitussive preparations.

The narcotic analgesics have little effect on blood pressure when the client is in a supine position. However, most narcotics decrease the capacity of the client to respond to stress. Morphine and other narcotic analgesics induce peripheral vasodilation, which may result in hypotension.

Many narcotic analgesics constrict the pupil. With such drugs, pupillary constriction is the most obvious sign of dependence.

The narcotic analgesics also decrease peristaltic motility. The constipating effects of these agents (Paregoric) are sometimes used therapeutically in severe diarrhea. The narcotic analgesics also increase the pressure within the biliary tract.

The narcotic analgesics attach to specific receptors located in the CNS (cortex, brain stem, and spinal cord), resulting in analgesia. Although the details are unknown, the mechanism is believed to involve decreased permeability of the cell membrane to sodium, which results in diminished transmission of pain impulses. Five categories of opioid receptors have been identified: mu, kappa, sigma, delta, and epsilon. Narcotic analgesics are believed to exert their activity at mu, kappa, and sigma receptors. Mu receptors are thought to mediate supraspinal analgesia, euphoria, and respiratory depression. Pentazocine-like spinal analgesia, miosis, and sedation are mediated by kappa receptors while sigma receptors mediate dysphoria, hallucinations, as well as respiratory and vasomotor stimulation (caused by drugs with antagonist activity). For kinetics, see individual agents.

Uses: Severe pain, especially of coronary, pulmonary, or peripheral origin. Hepatic and renal colic. Preanesthetic medication and adjuncts to anesthesia. Postsurgical pain. Acute vascular occlusion, especially of coronary, pulmonary, and peripheral origin. Diarrhea and dysentery. Pain from myocardial infarction, carcinoma, burns. Postpartum pain. Some members of this group are primarily used as antitussives. Methadone is used for heroin withdrawal and maintenance.

Contraindications: Asthmatic conditions, emphysema, kyphoscoliosis, severe obesity, convulsive states as in epilepsy, delirium tremens, tetanus and strychnine poisoning, diabetic acidosis, myxedema, Addison's disease, hepatic cirrhosis, and children under 6 months.

Special Concerns: Use cautiously in clients with head injury or after head surgery because of morphine's capacity to elevate intracranial pressure and mask the pupillary response.

Use with caution in the elderly, the debilitated, in young children, in individuals with increased intracranial pressure, in obstetrics, and with clients in shock or during acute alcoholic intoxication.

Morphine should be used with extreme caution in clients with pulmonary heart disease (cor pulmonale). Deaths following ordinary therapeutic doses have been reported. Use cautiously in clients with prostatic hypertrophy, because it may precipitate acute urinary retention.

Use cautiously in clients with reduced blood volume, such as in hemorrhaging clients who are more susceptible to the hypotensive effects of morphine.

Since the drugs depress the respiratory center, they should be given early in labor, at least 2 hr before delivery, to reduce the danger of respiratory depression in the newborn. When given before surgery, the narcotic analgesics should be given at least 1-2 hr preoperatively so that the danger of maximum depression of respiratory function will have passed before anesthesia is initiated.

These drugs should sometimes be withheld prior to diagnostic procedures so that the physician can use pain to locate dysfunction.

Side Effects: *Respiratory:* Respiratory depression, apnea. *CNS:* Dizziness, lightheadedness, sedation, lethargy, headache, euphoria, mental clouding, fainting. Idiosyncratic effects including excitement, restlessness, tremors, delirium, insomnia. *GI:* Nausea, vomiting, constipation, increased pressure in biliary tract, dry mouth, anorexia. *CV:* Flushing, changes in heart rate and blood pressure, circulatory collapse. *Allergic:* Skin rashes including pruritus and urticaria. Sweating, laryngospasm, edema. *Miscellaneous:* Urinary retention, oliguria, reduced libido, changes in body temperature. Narcotics cross the placental barrier and depress respiration of the fetus or newborn.

DEPENDENCE AND TOLERANCE: It is important to remember that all drugs of this group are addictive. Psychologic and physical dependence and tolerance develop even when clients use clinical doses. Tolerance is characterized by the fact that the client requires shorter periods of time between doses or larger doses for relief of pain. Tolerance usually develops faster when the narcotic analgesic is administered regularly and when the dose is large.

Symptoms of Acute Toxicity:

Severe toxicity is characterized by profound respiratory depression, apnea, deep sleep, stupor or coma, circulatory collapse, seizures, cardiopulmonary arrest, and death. Less severe toxicity results in symptoms including CNS depression, miosis, respiratory depression, deep sleep, flaccidity of skeletal muscles, hypotension, bradycardia, hypothermia, pulmonary edema, pneumonia, shock. The respiratory rate may be as low as 2-4 breaths/min. The client may be cyanotic. Urine output is decreased, the skin feels clammy, and body temperature decreases. If death occurs, it almost always results from respiratory depression.

Symptoms of Chronic Toxicity:

The problem of chronic dependence on narcotics occurs not only as a result of "street" use but is also found often among those who have easy access to narcotics (physicians, nurses, pharmacists). All the principal narcotic analgesics (morphine, opium, heroin, codeine, meperidine, and others) have, at times, been used for nontherapeutic purposes.

The nurse must be aware of the problem and be able to recognize signs of chronic dependence. These are constricted pupils, GI effects (constipation), skin infections, needle scars, abscesses, and itching, especially on the anterior surfaces of the body, where the client may inject the drug.

Withdrawal signs appear after drug is withheld for 4–12 hr. They are characterized by intense craving for the drug, insomnia, yawning, sneezing, vomiting, diarrhea, tremors, sweating, mental depression, muscular aches and pains, chills, and anxiety. Although the symptoms of narcotic withdrawal are uncomfortable, they are rarely life-threatening. This is in contrast to the withdrawal syndrome from depressants, where the life of the individual may be endangered because of the possibility of tonic-clonic seizures.

Drug Interactions

Alcohol, ethyl / Potentiation or addition of CNS depressant effects; concomitant use may lead to drowsiness, lethargy, stupor, respiratory collapse, coma, or death
Anesthetics, general / See *Alcohol*
Antianxiety drugs / See *Alcohol*
Antidepressants, tricyclic / ↑ Narcotic-induced respiratory depression
Antihistamines / See *Alcohol*
Barbiturates / See *Alcohol*
Cimetidine / ↑ CNS toxicity (e.g., disorientation, confusion, respiratory depression, apnea, seizures) with narcotics

CNS depressants / See *Alcohol*
MAO inhibitors / Possible potentiation of either MAO inhibitor (excitation, hypertension) or narcotic (hypotension, coma) effects; death has resulted
Methotrimeprazine / Potentiation of CNS depression
Phenothiazines / See *Alcohol*
Sedative-hypnotics, nonbarbiturate / See *Alcohol*
Skeletal muscle relaxants (surgical) / ↑ Respiratory depression and ↑ muscle relaxation

Laboratory Test Interferences: Altered liver function tests. False + or ↑ urinary glucose test (Benedict's). ↑ Plasma amylase or lipase.

Dosage: See individual drugs.

The dosage of narcotics and the reaction of a client to the dosage depend on the amount of pain. Two to four times the usual dose may be tolerated for relief of excruciating pain. However, the nurse should be aware that if, for some reason, the pain disappears, severe respiratory depression may result. This respiratory depression is not apparent while the pain is still present.

NURSING CONSIDERATIONS

Administration/Storage

1. Review the list of drugs with which narcotics interact and their associated effects.
2. Request that the physician rewrite the orders at timed intervals as required for continued administration.
3. Record the amount of narcotic used on the narcotic inventory sheet, indicating what was administered, the date, the time, the dose, and to whom, or if the drug was wasted and in-

clude an appropriate witness as necessary.

4. *Treatment of Acute Overdose:* Initial treatment is aimed at combating progressive respiratory depression by maintaining a patent airway and by artificial respiration. Gastric lavage and induced emesis are indicated in case of oral poisoning. The narcotic antagonist naloxone (Narcan), 0.4 mg IV, is effective in the treatment of acute overdosage. Respiratory stimulants (e.g., caffeine) should not be used to treat depression from the narcotic overdosage.

Assessment

1. Note if the client has had any prior experience with narcotic analgesics such as an adverse reaction with the drug or category of drugs prescribed.
2. Determine the amount of pain or discomfort, its location, intensity, and duration, frequency of occurrence, and what drug has been effective in the past. The amount and type of narcotic ordered should be individualized according to the client's response.
3. Use a pain rating scale so that clients can calculate or describe their level of pain. This may be used as a baseline against which to measure the effectiveness of drug therapy.
4. Obtain baseline vital signs prior to administering the drug. Generally, if the respiratory rate is less than 12/min or the systolic BP is less than 90 mm Hg, a narcotic should not be administered unless there is ventilatory support or specific physician-written guidelines, with parameters for administration.

5. Note the client's weight, age, and general body size. Too large a dosage of medication for the client's weight and age can result in serious side effects. For the elderly client, the blood levels may be higher, resulting in longer periods of pain relief.
6. Document the amount of time that has elapsed between the doses for the client to have relief from recurring pain.
7. Note precipitating factors as well as the impact of the pain on the client's ability to function.
8. Document any history of asthma or other conditions that tend to compromise respirations.
9. If the client is of childbearing age, discuss the possibility of pregnancy. Narcotics cross the placental barrier and depress the respirations of the fetus. The drugs may be contraindicated under certain circumstances.
10. Baseline CBC, liver and renal functions studies as well as electrolytes should be considered.

Interventions

1. Use supportive nursing measures such as relaxation techniques, repositioning the client, and reassurance to assist in relieving pain.
2. Explore the problem and source of the client's pain. Use nonnarcotic analgesic medications when possible. Coadministration may increase analgesic effects and permit lower doses of the narcotic analgesic.

3. Administer the medication when it is needed. *Prolonging the medication until the client experiences the maximum amount of pain reduces the effectiveness of the medication.*
4. Monitor vital signs and mental status.
   - Monitor the respiratory rate for signs of respiratory depression. Obtain written parameters for administration of narcotic analgesics, as necessary.
   - Narcotic analgesics depress the cough reflex. Therefore, turn clients every 2 hr, have them cough and take deep breaths to prevent atelectasis. Consider incentive spirometry.
   - Monitor BP. Hypotension is more apt to occur in the elderly and in those who are receiving other medications with hypotension as a side effect.
   - Monitor the heart rate. If the pulse drops below 60 beats/min in the adult or 110 beats/min in an infant, withhold the drug and notify the physician.
   - Observe the client for any decrease in blood pressure, deep sleep, or constricted pupils. Withhold the drug if any of these symptoms occur. Document and report to the physician.
   - Note the effects of the drug on the client's mental status. A client who has experienced pain, fear, or anxiety may become euphoric and excited. Record this and report.
5. Report if the client develops nausea and vomiting. If this occurs, the physician may order an antiemetic or change the medication therapy.
6. If the client is taking a narcotic medication by mouth, a snack or milk may decrease gastric irritation and lessen nausea.
7. Monitor bowel function. Narcotics, especially morphine, can have a depressant effect on the GI tract. Clients may become constipated as a consequence. If their condition permits, increase the fluid intake to 2,500–3,000 ml/day and increase their intake of fruit juices, fruits, and fiber as well as level and frequency of exercise as tolerated.
8. Narcotic drugs may cause urinary retention. Monitor the client's intake and urinary output and palpate the abdomen to detect for evidence of bladder distention. Encourage the client to attempt to empty the bladder every 3–4 hr. Question clients about difficulty voiding, pain in the bladder area, sensation of not emptying the bladder, or any unusual odors.
9. Note client complaint of difficulty with vision. Examine the client's pupillary response to light. If the client's pupils remain constricted, notify the physician and note this on the client's record.
10. If the client is bedridden, put up side rails and provide other protective safety measures. Assist with ambulation, BR, and transfers.
11. When administering medication, reassure client that flushing and a feeling of warmth sometimes may occur with therapeutic doses of drug.
12. Because clients may perspire

profusely when receiving a narcotic, be prepared to bathe them and change their clothes and linens frequently.

13. If a client is to be receiving a narcotic preparation over a period of time, monitor renal and liver function studies.

14. Assess hospitalized clients receiving around-the-clock therapy for evidence of tolerance and addiction.

15. In clients with terminal disease states, dependence on drug therapy is not considered a problem, whereas *adequate pain control is of the utmost concern*.

Client/Family Teaching

1. Inform the client and family that the drug may become habit-forming and include them in exploring alternative methods for pain control.

2. Review the side effects of the drug and discuss the goals of therapy.

3. Provide a printed card listing the possible side effects of drug therapy. Review these with the client on discharge and again when the client returns for a visit to the office or clinic.

4. Avoid consuming alcohol in any form.

5. Do not take OTC drugs without first consulting the physician. Many have small amounts of alcohol. Also, they may interact unfavorably with the prescribed medication.

6. For fecal impaction, describe preventive actions, such as increased fluid intake, increased use of fruit and fruit juices, and the possible need for a stool softener.

7. If the client is to go home on a narcotic medication, explain that the drug can cause drowsiness and dizziness. Therefore, client should use caution when operating a motor vehicle or performing other tasks that require mental alertness.

8. Advise to rise slowly from a lying to sitting position and to dangle legs before standing, to minimize orthostatic effects.

9. If the client is to be treated by a physician other than the one prescribing the medication, tell the physician about the drug being used and the reason for the prescribed therapy.

10. Stress the importance of storing all drugs in a safe place, out of the reach of children. Always store away from the bedside to prevent accidental overdosage.

11. During prolonged usage, advise client not to stop medications abruptly as withdrawal symptoms may occur.

12. Stress the importance of follow-up care and review the anticipated goals of the therapy with the client and family and determine whether or not these have been achieved.

13. Determine the extent of the pain relief achieved with each dosage of medication (e.g., pain level decreased from a level 5 to a level 2, 20 min after administration of medication).

14. If the goals have not been achieved, determine the source of the problem and modify the next plan of action.

Evaluation: Evaluate client for:
- Reports of effective control of severe pain without altered hemodynamics or impaired level of consciousness

- The absence of symptoms of acute toxicity, tolerance, or addiction, during short-term therapy

NARCOTIC ANTAGONISTS

See also the following individual entries:

Naloxone
Naltrexone

General Statement: The narcotic antagonists are able to prevent or reverse many of the pharmacologic actions of morphine-type analgesics and meperidine. For example, respiratory depression induced by these drugs is reversed within minutes. Naloxone is considered a pure antagonist in that it does not produce morphine-like effects.

The narcotic antagonists are not effective in reversing the respiratory depression induced by barbiturates, anesthetics, or other nonnarcotic agents. Narcotic antagonists almost immediately induce withdrawal symptoms in narcotic addicts and are sometimes used to unmask dependence.

Action/Kinetics: Narcotic antagonists block the action of narcotic analgesics by displacing previously given narcotics from their receptor sites or by preventing narcotics from attaching to the opiate receptors, thereby preventing access by the analgesic. This type of antagonism is competitive.

NURSING CONSIDERATIONS

Assessment

1. Determine the etiology of respiratory depression. Narcotic antagonists do not relieve the toxicity of nonnarcotic CNS depressants.
2. Assess and obtain baseline vital signs before administering any narcotic antagonist.

Interventions

1. Monitor respirations closely after the duration of action of the narcotic antagonist. Additional doses of drug may be necessary.
2. Observe for the appearance of withdrawal symptoms after administration of the narcotic antagonist. Withdrawal symptoms are characterized by restlessness, lacrimation, rhinorrhea, yawning, perspiration, vomiting, diarrhea, sweating, anxiety, pain, chills, and an intense craving for the drug.
3. Have emergency drugs and equipment readily available.
4. If the client is comatose, turn frequently and position on the side to prevent aspiration.
5. Maintain a safe, protective environment. Use side rails and soft supports as needed.
6. Assess vital signs after drug administration to determine the effectiveness of the drug.
7. Note the appearance of narcotic withdrawal symptoms after the antagonist has been administered.
8. If the narcotic antagonist is being used to diagnose narcotic use or dependence, observe the initial dilation of the client's pupils, followed by constriction.

Evaluation: Evaluate client for effective reversal of toxic effects of narcotic analgesic as evidenced by increased level of consciousness and improved respiratory rate and pattern.

NASAL DECONGESTANTS

See also the following individual entries:

Ephedrine Hydrochloride
Ephedrine Sulfate
Epinephrine Hydrochloride
Naphazoline Hydrochloride
Oxymetazoline Hydrochloride
Phenylephrine Hydrochloride
Xylometazoline Hydrochloride

Action/Kinetics: The most commonly used agents for relief of nasal congestion are the adrenergic drugs. They act by stimulating alpha-adrenergic receptors, thereby constricting the arterioles in the nasal mucosa; this reduces blood flow to the area, decreasing congestion. Both topical (sprays, drops) and oral agents may be used.

Uses: PO. Nasal congestion due to hay fever, common cold, allergies, or sinusitis. To help sinus or nasal drainage. To relieve congestion of eustachian tubes. **Topical.** Nasal and nasopharyngeal mucosal congestion due to hay fever, common cold, allergies, or sinusitis. With other therapy to decrease congestion around the eustachian tubes. Relieve ear block and pressure pain during air travel.

Contraindications: Severe hypertension, coronary artery disease.

Special Concerns: Use with caution in hyperthyroidism, arteriosclerosis, increased intraocular pressure, prostatic hypertrophy, angina, diabetes, ischemic heart disease, hypertension. Also, clients receiving MAO inhibitors may manifest hypertensive crisis following the use of oral nasal decongestants. Use with caution in geriatric clients and during pregnancy and lactation.

Side Effects: *Topical use:* Stinging and burning, mucosal dryness, sneezing, local irritation, rebound congestion (rhinitis medicamentosa). Systemic use may produce the following symptoms. *CV:* Cardiovascular collapse with hypotension, arrhythmias, palpitations, precordial pain, tachycardia, transient hypertension, bradycardia. *CNS:* Anxiety, dizziness, headache, fear, restlessness, tremors, insomnia, tenseness, lightheadedness, drowsiness, psychologic disturbances, weakness, psychoses, hallucinations, seizures, depression. *GI:* Nausea, vomiting, anorexia. *Ophthalmologic:* Irritation, photophobia, tearing, blurred vision, blepharospasm. *Other:* Dysuria, sweating, pallor, breathing difficulties, orofacial dystonia.

  Note: Ephedrine may also produce anorexia and urinary retention in men with prostatic hypertrophy.

Dosage: See individual drugs.

NURSING CONSIDERATIONS

Administration/Storage

1. Most nasal decongestants are used topically in the form of sprays, drops, or solutions.
2. Solutions of topical nasal decongestants may become contaminated with use. This may result in the growth of bacteria and fungi. Thus, the dropper or spray tip should be rinsed in hot water after each use and covered.
3. During administration, have facial tissues and a receptacle available for used tissues.

Interventions

1. Use separate equipment for each client to prevent the

spread of infection. If only one container of medication is available, use an individual dropper for each client.

2. Instruct the client to blow the nose gently before administering therapy. If the client is unable to blow the nose, clear the nasal passages with a bulb-type aspirator.

3. After completing the treatment, rinse the dropper or tip of spray container. Dry with a tissue and cover, using care not to introduce water into the spray container. Wipe the tip of the nasal jelly tube with a damp tissue and replace the cap.

Client/Family Teaching

1. Instruct in the appropriate technique for preparing the nasal passages.

2. Review the method of administration of the prescribed medication, whether drops, spray, or jelly.

3. Discuss and demonstrate the proper use and care of equipment.

Evaluation: Evaluate client for:

- Reports of decreased nasal congestion, relief of symptoms of eustachian tube congestion, and a reduction in allergic manifestations
- Freedom from complications of drug therapy as well as equipment contaminations

NEUROMUSCULAR BLOCKING AGENTS

See also the following individual entries:

Atracurium Besylate
Doxacurium Chloride
Pancuronium Bromide
Pipecuronium Bromide
Succinylcholine Chloride
Tubocurarine Chloride
Vecuronium Bromide

General Statement: The drugs considered in this section interfere with nerve impulse transmission between the motor end plate and the receptors of skeletal muscle (i.e., peripheral action). Upon stimulation, these muscles normally contract when acetylcholine is released from storage sites embedded in the motor end plate.

The drugs fall into two groups: competitive (nondepolarizing) agents and depolarizing agents. Competitive agents—atracurium, doxacurium, gallamine, metocurine, pancuronium, tubocurarine, vecuronium—compete with acetylcholine for the receptor site in the muscle cells. These agents are also called *curariform* because their mode of action is similar to that of the poison curare. The depolarizing agent—succinylcholine—initially excites skeletal muscle and then prevents the muscle from contracting by prolonging the time during which the receptors at the end plate cannot respond to acetylcholine (depolarization during refractory time).

The muscle paralysis caused by the neuromuscular blocking agents is sequential. Therapeutic doses produce muscle depression in the following order: heaviness of eyelids, difficulty in swallowing and talking, diplopia, progressive weakening of the extremities and neck, followed by relaxation of the trunk and spine. The diaphragm (respiratory paralysis) is affected last. The drugs do not affect consciousness, and their use, in the absence of adequate levels of general anesthesia, may be frightening to the patient.

There is a narrow margin of safety between a therapeutically effective dose causing muscle relaxation and a toxic dose causing respiratory paralysis. **The neuromuscular blocking agents are always administered by a physician.** However, the nurse must be prepared to maintain and monitor respiration until the effect of the drug subsides.

Uses: See individual agents.

Special Concerns: The neuromuscular blocking agents should be used with caution in clients with myasthenia gravis; renal, hepatic, or pulmonary impairment; respiratory depression; and in elderly or debilitated clients.

Depolarizing agents should be used with caution for clients with electrolyte imbalance, especially hyperkalemia, and in those taking digitalis.

Side Effects: Respiratory paralysis. Severe and prolonged muscle relaxation. *CV:* Cardiac arrhythmias, bradycardia, hypotension, cardiac arrest. *GI:* Excessive salivation during light anesthesia. *Miscellaneous:* Bronchospasms, hyperthermia, hypersensitivity (rare). See also individual agents.

Symptoms of Overdose: Decreased respiratory reserve, extended skeletal muscle weakness, prolonged apnea, low tidal volume, sudden release of histamine, cardiovascular collapse.

Drug Interactions: The following drug interactions are for non-depolarizing skeletal muscle relaxants. For Succinylcholine, see p. 1165.

Aminoglycoside antibiotics / Additive muscle relaxation
Amphotericin B / ↑ Muscle relaxation
Anesthetics, inhalation / Additive muscle relaxation
Clindamycin / Additive muscle relaxation
Colistin / ↑ Muscle relaxation
Furosemide / ↑ Effect of skeletal muscle relaxants
Lincomycin / ↑ Muscle relaxation
Magnesium salts / ↑ Muscle relaxation
Methotrimeprazine / ↑ Muscle relaxation
Narcotic analgesics / ↑ Respiratory depression and ↑ muscle relaxation
Phenothiazines / ↑ Muscle relaxation
Polymyxin B / ↑ Muscle relaxation
Procainamide / ↑ Muscle relaxation
Procaine / ↑ Muscle relaxation by ↓ plasma protein binding
Quinidine / ↑ Muscle relaxation
Thiazide diuretics / ↑ Muscle relaxation due to hypokalemia

NURSING CONSIDERATIONS

Administration/Storage

1. When the drug is to be administered by a constant infusion, use a microdrip tubing administration set and/or an infusion control device.
2. During drug administration, have a suction machine, oxygen, and resuscitation equipment immediately available for emergency use.
3. *Treatment of Overdose:* There are no known antidotes.

- Use a peripheral nerve stimulator to monitor and assess the client's response to the neuromuscular blocking medication.
- Have anticholinesterase drugs, such as edrophonium, pyridostigmine, or neostigmine available to counteract respiratory depression due to paralysis of skeletal muscles. These drugs increase the body's production of acetylcholine. To minimize the muscarinic cholinergic side effects, atropine should also be given.
- Correct blood pressure, electrolyte imbalance, or circulating blood volume by fluid and electrolyte therapy. Vasopressors can be used to correct hypotension due to ganglionic blockade.

Assessment

1. Note age and condition of the client. Elderly and debilitated clients should not receive drugs in this category.
2. If the client has any history of renal disease, obtain renal function studies prior to beginning therapy.
3. Note all other drugs the client is receiving. Often clients requiring neuromuscular blocking agents are also receiving other drugs that may have the effect of prolonging client response to the neuromuscular blocking agent being used.
4. Question the client concerning changes in vision, ability to chew or to move the fingers, and document findings.
5. Note initial selective paralysis followed by paralysis in the

following sequence: levator muscles of the eyelids, mastication muscles, limb muscles, abdominal muscles, glottis muscles, intercostal muscles, and the diaphragm muscles. Of note is that neuromuscular recovery occurs in the reverse order.

Interventions

1. Drugs should only be administered in a closely monitored environment and used only for intubated clients.
2. Monitor the client's blood pressure and pulse frequently. Respirations and pulmonary status should be monitored continuously. Ensure that cardiac and ventilator alarms are set appropriately and checked at frequent intervals.
3. Observe for excessive bronchial secretions or respiratory wheezing. Report if evident and suction to maintain patent endotracheal tube.
4. Perform frequent neurovascular assessments.
5. Observe the client closely for drug interactions. These can potentiate muscular relaxation and prove fatal. If interactions occur, consult the physician immediately to obtain orders for the appropriate medication to counteract the observed effects.
6. Consciousness and pain thresholds are not affected by neuromuscular blocking agents. Most clients can still hear, feel, and see while they are receiving blocking agents. Therefore, inappropriate talking should be avoided and adequate anesthesia should be administered

when painful procedures are necessary.

7. Clients requiring prolonged ventilatory therapy should be adequately sedated with analgesics and/or benzodiazepines.

8. Administer eye drops and eye patches to protect corneas during prolonged therapy as needed.

Evaluation: Evaluate client for:

• Evidence of desired level of muscle paralysis

• Adequate suppression of twitch response upon peripheral nerve stimulation tests

---

NONSTEROIDAL ANTI-INFLAMMATORY DRUGS

See also the following individual entries:

Carprofen
Diclofenac Sodium
Etodolac
Fenoprofen Calcium
Flurbiprofen Sodium
Ibuprofen
Indomethacin
Indomethacin Sodium
    Trihydrate
Ketoprofen
Ketorolac Tromethamine
Meclofenamate Sodium
Naproxen
Naproxen Sodium
Piroxicam
Sulindac
Suprofen
Tolmetin Sodium

General Statement: Arthritis, which means inflammation of the joints, refers to approximately 80 different conditions also called rheumatic, collagen, or connective tissue diseases. The most prominent symptoms of these conditions are painful, inflamed joints, but the cause for this joint inflammation varies from disease to disease. The joint pain of gout, for example, results from sodium urate crystals formed as a consequence of the overproduction or underelimination of uric acid. Osteoarthritis is caused by the degeneration of the joint; rheumatoid arthritis and systemic lupus erythematosus (SLE) are autoimmune diseases. Immune factors trigger the release of corrosive enzymes in the joints in a complex manner. Infectious arthritis is the result of rapid joint destruction by microorganisms like gonococci that invade the joint cavity. Treatment must be aimed at the cause of the particular form of arthritis, and a thorough diagnostic evaluation must therefore precede the initiation of therapy. Gout is treated with uricosuric agents, which alter uric acid metabolism; infectious arthritis responds to antibiotics; osteoarthritis, rheumatoid arthritis, ankylosing spondylitis, and SLE respond to anti-inflammatory drugs. Rheumatoid arthritis may also be treated with two remitting agents (gold and penicillamine) or to hydroxychloroquine sulfate. Aspirin is an important agent in the treatment of all rheumatic diseases. Corticosteroids are used, preferably for short-term therapy only, for some of the more resistant cases of rheumatoid arthritis and SLE or for situations of exacerbation of these diseases. Corticosteroids also are used for intra-articular injection. Drug therapy of the arthritides must be supplemented by a physical therapy program, as well as proper rest and diet. Total joint replacement is also an important mode of therapy to correct the ravages of arthritis.

Action/Kinetics: Over the past decade, a growing number of nonsteroidal anti-inflammatory drugs (NSAIDs) have been developed, with anti-inflammatory, analgesic, and antipyretic effects. Chemically, these drugs are related to indene, indole, or propionic acid. As in the case of aspirin, the therapeutic actions of these agents are believed to result from the inhibition of the enzyme cyclooxygenase, resulting in decreased prostaglandin synthesis. The agents are effective in reducing joint swelling, pain, and morning stiffness, as well as in increasing mobility in individuals with arthritis. They do not alter the course of the disease, however. Their anti-inflammatory activity is comparable to that of aspirin.

The analgesic activity is due, in part, to relief of inflammation. Also, the drugs may inhibit lipoxygenase, inhibit synthesis of leukotrienes, inhibit release of lysosomal enzymes, and inhibit neutrophil aggregation. Rheumatoid factor production may also be inhibited. The antipyretic action is believed to occur by decreasing prostaglandin synthesis in the hypothalamus, resulting in an increase in peripheral blood flow and heat loss as well as promoting sweating.

The NSAIDs have an irritating effect on the GI tract. They differ from one another slightly with respect to their rate of absorption, length of action, anti-inflammatory activity, and effect on the GI mucosa. Most are rapidly and completely absorbed from the GI tract; food delays the rate, but not the total amount, of drug absorbed. These drugs are metabolized in the kidney and are excreted through the urine, mainly as metabolites.

Uses: Rheumatoid arthritis (acute flares and long-term management in adults and children), osteoarthritis, ankylosing spondylitis, gout, and other musculoskeletal diseases. Treatment of nonrheumatic inflammatory conditions including bursitis, acute painful shoulder, synovitis, tendinitis, or tenosynovitis. Mild to moderate pain including primary dysmenorrhea, episiotomy pain, strains and sprains, postextraction dental pain. Dysmenorrhea. *Investigational:* Depending on the drug, can be used for sunburn, to abort an acute migraine attack, prophylaxis of migraine, premenstrual syndrome.

Contraindications: Most for children under 14 years of age. Lactation. Hypersensitivity to any of these agents or to aspirin. Individuals in whom aspirin, NSAIDs, or iodides have caused acute asthma, rhinitis, urticaria, nasal polyps, bronchospasm, angioedema or other symptoms of allergy or anaphylaxis.

Special Concerns: Pregnancy category: B (diclofenac, flurbiprofen, ketoprofen, ketorolac, naproxen) or C (etodolac, mefenamic acid, tolmetin). Clients intolerant to one of the NSAIDs may be intolerant to others in this group. Use with caution in clients with a history of GI disease, reduced renal function, in geriatric clients, in clients with intrinsic coagulation defects or those on anticoagulant therapy, in compromised cardiac function, in hypertension, in conditions predisposing to fluid retention, and in the presence of existing controlled infection. The safety and efficacy of most NSAIDs have not been determined in children. Safety and efficacy have not been determined in functional class IV rheumatoid arthritis (i.e., clients incapacitated, bedridden, or confined to a wheelchair).

Side Effects: *GI (most common):* Peptic or duodenal ulceration and GI bleeding, intestinal ulceration with obstruction and stenosis, reactivation of preexisting ulcers. Heartburn, dyspepsia, nausea, vomiting, anorexia, diarrhea, constipation, increased or decreased appetite, indigestion, stomatitis, epigastric pain, abdominal cramps or pain, gastroenteritis, paralytic ileus, salivation, dry mouth, glossitis, pyrosis, icterus, rectal irritation, gingival ulcer, occult blood in stool, hematemesis, gastritis, proctitis, eructation, sore or dry mucous membranes, ulcerative colitis, rectal bleeding, melena, perforation and hemorrhage of esophagus, stomach, duodenum, small or large intestine. *CNS:* Dizziness, drowsiness, vertigo, headaches, nervousness, migraine, anxiety, mental confusion, aggravation of parkinsonism and epilepsy, lightheadedness, paresthesia, peripheral neuropathy, akathisia, excitation, tremor, seizures, myalgia, asthenia, malaise, insomnia, fatigue, drowsiness, confusion, emotional lability, depression, inability to concentrate, psychoses, hallucinations, depersonalization, amnesia, coma, syncope. *CV:* Congestive heart failure, hypotension, hypertension, arrhythmias, peripheral edema and fluid retention, vasodilation, exacerbation of angiitis, palpitations, tachycardia, chest pain, sinus bradycardia, peripheral vascular disease, peripheral edema. *Respiratory:* Bronchospasm, laryngeal edema, rhinitis, dyspnea, pharyngitis, hemoptysis, shortness of breath, eosinophilic pneumonitis. *Hematologic:* Bone marrow depression, neutropenia, leukopenia, pancytopenia, eosinophila, thrombocytopenia, granulocytopenia, agranulocytosis, aplastic anemia, hemolytic anemia, decreased hemoglobin and hematocrit, hypocoagulability, epistaxis. *Ophthalmologic:* Amblyopia, visual disturbances, corneal deposits, retinal hemorrhage, scotomata, retinal pigmentation changes or degeneration, blurred vision, photophobia, diplopia, iritis, loss of color vision (reversible), optic neuritis, cataracts, swollen, dry, or irritated eyes. *Dermatologic:* Pruritus, skin eruptions, sweating, erythema, eczema, hyperpigmentation, ecchymoses, petechiae, rashes, urticaria, purpura, onycholysis, vesiculobullous eruptions, cutaneous vasculitis, toxic epidermal necrolysis, angioneurotic edema, erythema nodosum, Stevens-Johnson syndrome, exfoliative dermatitis, photosensitivity, alopecia, skin irritation, peeling, erythema multiforme, desquamation, skin discoloration. *GU:* Menometrorrhagia, menorrhagia, impotence, menstrual disorders, hematuria, cystitis, azotemia, nocturia, proteinuria, urinary tract infections, polyuria, dysuria, urinary frequency, oliguria, pyuria, anuria, renal insufficiency, nephrosis, nephrotic syndrome, glomerular and interstitial nephritis, urinary casts, acute renal failure in clients with impaired renal function, renal papillary necrosis *Metabolic:* Hyperglycemia, hypoglycemia, glycosuria, hyperkalemia, hyponatremia, diabetes mellitus. *Other:* Tinnitus, hearing loss or disturbances, ear pain, deafness, metallic or bitter taste in mouth, thirst, chills, fever, flushing, jaundice, sweating, breast changes, gynecomastia, muscle cramps, dyspnea, involuntary muscle movements, muscle weakness, facial edema, pain, serum sickness, aseptic meningitis, hypersensitivity reactions including asthma, acute respiratory distress, shock-like syndrome, angioedema, angiitis, dyspnea, anaphylaxis.

Symptoms of Overdose: CNS symptoms include dizziness, drowsiness, mental confusion, lethargy, disorientation, intense headache, paresthesia, and seizures. GI symptoms include nausea, vomiting, gastric irritation, and abdominal pain. Miscellaneous symptoms include tinnitus, sweating, blurred vision, increased serum creatinine and BUN, and acute renal failure.

Drug Interactions

Anticoagulants / Concomitant use results in ↑ prothrombin time

Aspirin / ↓ Effect of NSAIDs due to ↓ blood levels; also, ↑ risk of adverse GI effects

Beta-adrenergic blocking agents / ↓ Antihypertensive effect of blocking agents

Cimetidine / ↑ or ↓ Plasma levels of NSAIDs

Cyclosporine / ↑ Risk of nephrotoxicity

Lithium / ↑ Serum lithium levels

Loop diuretics / ↓ Effect of loop diuretics

Methotrexate / ↑ Risk of methotrexate toxicity

Phenobarbital / ↓ Effect of NSAIDs due to ↑ breakdown by liver

Phenytoin / ↑ Effect of phenytoin due to ↓ plasma protein binding

Probenecid / ↑ Effect of NSAIDs due to ↑ plasma levels

Sulfonamides / ↑ Effect of sulfonamides due to ↓ plasma protein binding

Sulfonylureas / ↑ Effect of sulfonylureas due to ↓ plasma protein binding

Dosage: See individual drugs.

NURSING CONSIDERATIONS

Administration/Storage

1. Alcohol and aspirin should not be taken together with NSAIDs.
2. Can be taken with food, milk, or antacids should GI upset occur.
3. NSAIDS may have an additive analgesic effect when administered with narcotic analgesics thus permitting lower narcotic dosages.
4. Clients who do not respond clinically to one NSAID may respond to another.
5. *Treatment of Overdose:* There are no antidotes; treatment includes general supportive measures. Since the drugs are acidic, it may be beneficial to alkalinize the urine and induce diuresis to hasten excretion.

Assessment

1. Note any history of allergic responses to aspirin or other anti-inflammatory agents. These drugs are contraindicated in this event.
2. Determine if the client has asthma or nasal polyps. This condition may be exacerbated by the use of NSAIDs.
3. Note the age of the client. Children under 14 years of age should not receive drugs in this category.
4. Determine if the client is taking oral hypoglycemic agents or insulin and document this information.
5. Interview clients concerning other medications they are currently taking. Determine if

any of these drugs are on the drug interaction list and report.

6. Document location, intensity, and type of pain experienced. Assess joint mobility and ROM.

Client/Family Teaching

1. Take NSAIDs with a full glass of water or milk, with meals, or with an antacid prescribed by the physician and remain upright 30 min following administration to reduce gastric irritation.

2. Report to the physician symptoms of GI irritation not relieved by adhering to the prescribed protocol.

3. Comply with the drug regimen because regular intake of drug is necessary to sustain anti-inflammatory effects.

4. Discuss the need for regular medical supervision so that dosages of drug can be adjusted based on the client's condition, age, changes in disease activity, and overall drug response.

5. Report any episodes of bleeding, blurred vision or other eye symptoms, tinnitus, skin rashes, purpura, weight gain or edema.

6. Use caution in operating machinery or in driving a car because medication may cause dizziness or drowsiness.

7. Avoid alcohol, aspirin, acetaminophen, and any other OTC preparations without first consulting the physician or pharmacist.

8. If the client has diabetes mellitus, explain the possible increase in hypoglycemic effect of the drugs on hypoglycemic agents. Advise clients to pay particular attention to urine and blood testing and report any symptoms of hypoglycemic effects to the physician. The dosage of agent and NSAID may need to be adjusted.

9. Remind clients to tell other physicians and health care providers of the medication being taken to avoid having prescriptions written for drugs that would interact unfavorably with NSAIDs.

Evaluation: Evaluate client for:
- Evidence of improved joint mobility and increased ROM
- Reports of symptomatic improvement in level of experienced discomfort and pain

---

OPHTHALMIC CHOLINERGIC (MIOTIC) AGENTS

See also the following individual entries:

Physostigmine Salicylate
Physostigmine Sulfate
Pilocarpine Hydrochloride
Pilocarpine Nitrate
Pilocarpine Ocular Therapeutic System
Pilocarpine and Epinephrine
Pilocarpine and Physostigmine
Timolol Maleate

General Statement: Cholinergic agents are commonly used for the treatment of glaucoma and less frequently for the correction of accommodative esotropia.

Action/Kinetics: The ophthalmic cholinergic drugs fall into two classes: direct-acting (carbachol, pilocarpine) and indirect-acting (demecarium, echothiophate, isoflurophate, neostigmine, physostigmine), which inhibit the enzyme acetylcholinesterase. In the treatment of glaucoma, the drugs lead to an accumulation of acetylcholine, which stimulates the ciliary muscles and increases contraction of the iris sphincter muscle. This opens the angle of the eye and results in increased outflow of aqueous humor and consequently in a decrease of intraocular pressure. This effect is of particular importance in narrow-angle glaucoma. Hourly tonometric measurements are recommended during initiation of therapy. The drugs also cause spasms of accommodation.

Uses: *Glaucoma:* Primary acute narrow-angle glaucoma (acute therapy) and primary chronic wide-angle glaucoma (chronic therapy). Selected cases of secondary glaucoma. Diagnosis and treatment of accommodative esotropia. Antidote against harmful effects of atropine-like drugs in clients with glaucoma. Alternately with a mydriatic drug to break adhesions between lens and iris. See also individual drugs.

Contraindications: *Direct-acting drugs:* Inflammatory eye disease (iritis), asthma, hypertension. *Indirect-acting drugs:* Same as for *direct-acting drugs,* as well as acute-angle glaucoma, history of retinal detachment, ocular hypotension accompanied by intraocular inflammatory processes, intestinal or urinary obstruction, peptic ulcer, epilepsy, parkinsonism, spastic GI conditions, vasomotor instability, severe bradycardia or hypotension, and recent myocardial infarctions. During lactation.

Special Concerns: Pregnancy category: X for demecarium, echothio-

phate, and isoflurophate. Geriatric clients must be carefully monitored.

Side Effects: *Local:* Painful contraction of ciliary muscle, pain in eye, blurred vision, spasms of accommodation, darkened vision, failure to accommodate to darkness, twitching, headaches, painful brow. Most of these symptoms lessen with prolonged usage. Iris cysts and retinal detachment (indirect-acting drugs only).

Systemic: Systemic absorption of drug may cause nausea, GI discomfort, diarrhea, hypotension, bronchial constriction, and increased salivation.

Dosage: See individual drugs.

NURSING CONSIDERATIONS
Administration

1. To prevent the overflow of solution into the nasopharynx after topical instillation of drops, exert pressure on the nasolacrimal duct for 1–2 min before the client closes the eyelids.
2. Have epinephrine and atropine available for emergency treatment of increased intraocular pressure.

Interventions

1. Report redness around the cornea. Epinephrine or phenylephrine hydrochloride (10%) may be ordered with demecarium bromide, echothiophate iodide, or isoflurophate to minimize this kind of reaction.
2. Report any changes in vision, eye irritation, or evidence of severe headaches.

Client/Family Teaching

1. Review and demonstrate the appropriate method for instilling eye drops or ointment. Observe client self-administering prescribed medications.
2. Stress the importance of taking the eye drops exactly as prescribed.
3. Side effects can be minimized by taking at least one dose of medication at bedtime.
4. Advise the client not to drive for 1–2 hr after instilling cholinergic agents. Caution that night vision may be impaired.
5. Pain and blurred vision may occur. This problem usually diminishes with prolonged use of the drug. However, if these symptoms persist, call the physician.
6. If bothersome side effects persist, notify the physician. The dosage of medication may need to be changed.
7. Explain that painful eye spasms may be relieved by applying cold compresses.
8. Provide the client with a schedule for eye examinations. Stress the importance of adhering to the schedule and refilling the prescriptions as needed.

Evaluation: Evaluate client for:

- A positive clinical response based on ophthalmic examinations that show improved visual fields and tonometric measurements that show evidence of a decrease in intraocular pressures
- Evidence of compliance with prescribed therapy and any reports of side effects that may require a change in the dosage or agent.

ORAL CONTRACEPTIVES: ESTROGEN-PROGESTERONE COMBINATIONS

See also the following individual entries:

Brevicon
Demulen
Genora
Levlen
Loestrin
Lo-Ovral
Modicon
Nelova
Norcept
Nordette
Norethin
Norinyl
Norlestrin
Ortho-Novum
Ovcon
Ovral
Tri-Norinyl
Triphasil

General Statement: The majority of oral contraceptives contain both an estrogen and a progestin in each tablet; such products are referred to as *combination oral contraceptives*. There are three types of combination products: (1) monophasic—contain the same amount of estrogen and progestin in each tablet; (2) biphasic—contain the same amount of estrogen in each tablet but the progestin content is lower for the first 10 days of the cycle and higher for the last 11 days; (3) triphasic—the estrogen content may be the same or may vary throughout the medication cycle; the progestin content varies. The purpose of the biphasic and triphasic products is to provide hormones in a manner similar to that occurring physiologically. This is said to decrease breakthrough bleeding during the medication cycle.

The other type of oral contraceptive is the progestin-only ("mini-pill") product, which contains small amounts of a progestin in each tablet.

Action/Kinetics: The combination oral contraceptives are thought to act by inhibiting ovulation due to an inhibition (through negative feedback mechanism) of luteinizing hormone (LH) and follicle-stimulating hormone (FSH), which are required for development of ova. These products also alter the cervical mucus so that it is not conducive to sperm penetration, and render the endometrium less suitable for implantation of the blastocyst should fertilization occur.

Although oral contraceptives may be associated with serious side effects, a number of noncontraceptive health benefits have been confirmed. These include increased regularity of the menstrual cycle, decreased incidence of dysmenorrhea, decreased blood loss, decreased incidence of functional ovarian cysts and ectopic pregnancies, and decreased incidence of diseases such as fibroadenomas, fibrocystic disease, acute pelvic inflammatory disease, endometrial cancer, and ovarian cancer.

The progestin-only products do not consistently inhibit ovulation. However, these products also alter the cervical mucus, render the endometrium unsuitable for implantation, and may alter tubal transport of the ovum. This method of contraception is less reliable than combination therapy.

Uses: Contraception, menstrual irregularities, menopausal symptoms. High doses are used for endometriosis and hypermenorrhea.

Contraindications: History of cerebrovascular disease (e.g., coronary artery disease, myocardial infarction, angina pectoris, cerebral vascular disease), thrombophlebitis, and/or pulmonary embolism, hypertension, ocular proptosis, partial or complete loss of vision, defects in the visual field, diplopia, carcinoma of the breast or genital tract, adolescents with incomplete epiphyseal closure, impaired hepatic function, undiagnosed genital bleeding. Smoking.

Special Concerns: Pregnancy category: X. Use with caution in clients with asthma, epilepsy, migraine, diabetes, metabolic bone disease, renal or cardiac disease, and a history of mental depression. Use with caution in clients taking ampicillin, antiepileptic drugs, phenylbutazone, and rifampin, since intermittent bleeding (spotting) and unwanted pregnancy may result.

Side Effects: The oral contraceptives have wide-ranging effects. These are particularly important, since the drugs may be given for several years to healthy women. Many authorities have voiced concern about the long-term safety of these agents. Some advise discontinuing therapy after 18–24 months of continuous use. The majority of side effects of oral contraceptives are due to the estrogen component. These are listed under *Estrogens*.

Other side effects include auditory disturbances, Raynaud's syndrome, pancreatitis, rhinitis, hemolytic uremic syndrome, and a possible association with systemic lupus erythematosus. Also, there is an increased risk of congenital abnormalities if oral contraceptives are given to pregnant women. Oral contraceptives decrease the quantity and quality of breast milk. Selected studies have concluded that the risk of breast cancer may be increased in women who started long-term use of oral contraceptives before age 25 and in long-term users of oral contraceptives before their first pregnancy.

Drug Interactions

Acetaminophen /   ↓ Hepatotoxicity of acetaminophen due to ↑ breakdown by liver; this effect ↓ therapeutic effect

Anticoagulants, oral /   ↓ Effect of anticoagulants by increasing levels of certain clotting factors

Ascorbic acid /   ↑ Effect of oral contraceptives due to ↓ breakdown by liver

Barbiturates /   ↓ Effect of oral contraceptives due to ↑ breakdown by liver

Benzodiazepines /   ↑ or ↓ Effect of benzodiazepines due to changes in breakdown by liver

Caffeine /   ↑ Effect of caffeine due to ↓ breakdown by liver

Carbamazepine /   ↓ Effect of oral contraceptives due to ↑ breakdown by liver

Clofibrate /   ↑ Excretion of the active form of clofibrate (clofibric acid)

Corticosteroids /   ↑ Effect of corticosteroids due to ↓ breakdown by liver

Griseofulvin /   May ↓ effect of oral contraceptives

Guanethidine /   ↓ Effect of guanethidine

Hypoglycemics /   Oral contraceptives ↓ effect of hypoglycemics

Insulin /   Oral contraceptives may ↑ insulin requirements

Isoniazid /   ↓ Effect of oral contraceptives due to ↑ breakdown by liver

Lorazepam /   ↑ Clearance of lorazepam due to ↑ breakdown by liver

Metoprolol /   ↑ Effect of metoprolol due to ↓ breakdown by liver

Neomycin /   ↓ Effect of oral contraceptive due to ↑ breakdown by liver

Oxazepam /   ↑ Clearance of oxazepam due to ↑ breakdown by liver

Penicillins /   May ↓ effect of oral contraceptives

Phenylbutazone /   ↓ Effect of contraceptives due to ↑ breakdown by liver

Phenytoin /   ↓ Effect of oral contraceptives due to ↑ breakdown by liver

Rifampin /   ↓ Effect of contraceptives due to ↑ breakdown by liver

Temazepam /   ↑ Clearance of temazepam due to ↑ breakdown by liver

Tetracyclines /   ↓ Effect of contraceptives due to tetracycline-induced inhibition of gut bacteria that hydrolyze steroid conjugates

Theophyllines /   Oral contraceptives ↑ effect of theophyllines due to ↓ breakdown by liver

Tricyclic antidepressants /   Oral contraceptives ↑ effect of antidepressants due to ↓ breakdown by liver

Troleandomycin /   ↑ Chance of jaundice

Laboratory Test Interferences: Altered liver and thyroid function tests. ↓ Prothrombin time, 17-hydroxycorticosteroids, 17-ketosteroids, and 17-ketogenic steroids. (Therapy with ovarian hormones should be discontinued 60 days before performance of laboratory tests.) ↑ Gamma globulins.

Dosage: See *Administration/Storage*.

NURSING CONSIDERATIONS

See also *Nursing Considerations* for *Estrogens,* p. 150, and *Progesterone and Progestins,* p. 210.

Administration/Storage

1. Tablets should be taken at approximately the same time each day (e.g., with a meal or at bedtime).
2. Spotting or breakthrough bleeding may occur for the first 1–2 cycles; if it continues past this time, consult the physician.
3. For the initial cycle, an **additional** form of contraception should be used for the first week.
4. The type of oral contraceptive preparation will determine the precise manner in which the drug is taken:
   • For the 21-day regimen, one tablet is taken daily beginning on day 5 of menses (day 1 is the first day of menstrual flow). No tablets are taken for 7 days.
   • For a 28-day regimen, hormone-containing tablets are taken for the first 21 days, followed by 7 days of inert or iron-containing tablets.
   • Certain products, including the biphasic and selected triphasic oral contraceptives, are termed *Sunday start.* The first tablet should be taken

the Sunday following the beginning of menses (if menses begins on Sunday, the first tablet should be taken that day). **Note:** The biphasic and triphasic products have varying amounts of estrogen and/or progestin, depending on the stage of the cycle; the client should understand fully how these preparations are to be taken and which tablets are to be taken at various times during the medication cycle.
   • For progestin-only products, the first tablet is taken on the first day of menses; thereafter, one tablet is taken every day of the year.
5. It is recommended that for a women beginning combination oral contraceptive therapy, a product be chosen that contains the least amount of estrogen for that particular client.
6. If a woman fails to take one or more tablets, the following recommendations should be followed:
   • If one tablet is missed, it should be taken as soon as it is remembered. Alternatively, two tablets can be taken the following day.
   • If two tablets are missed, two tablets can be taken each day for two days; alternatively, two tablets can be taken on the day the missed tablets are remembered, with the second missed tablet being discarded.
   • If three tablets are missed, a new medication cycle should be initiated 7 days after the last tablet was taken, and an additional form of contraception should be used until

the start of the next menstrual period.

Note: With each succeeding tablet missed, the possibility increases that ovulation will occur.

Assessment

1. Note any previous experience with these medications and results or problems experienced.
2. Determine the client's beliefs and needs concerning contraception and instruct accordingly.

Client/Family Teaching

1. Advise the client to take the tablets exactly as prescribed to prevent pregnancy.
2. Remind the client if she misses taking 1 tablet she should take the tablet as soon as the oversight has been detected.
3. If 2 consecutive tablets have been missed, the dosage must be doubled for the next 2 consecutive days. The regular schedule may then be resumed. However, the client or her partner should use additional contraceptive measures for the remainder of the cycle.
4. If 3 tablets are missed, discontinue the therapy and start a new course as indicated by the type of medication. Alternative contraceptive measures should be used when the tablets are not taken and should be continued for 7 days after a new course has been started.
5. If client develops pain in the legs or chest, respiratory distress, an unexplained cough, severe headaches, dizziness, or blurred vision, discontinue the

therapy and notify the physician immediately.
6. Oral contraceptives decrease the viscosity of cervical mucus, increasing the susceptibility to vaginal infections. These are difficult to treat successfully; therefore, good hygienic practice is essential.
7. If the client has persistent nausea, edema, and skin eruptions beyond the four cycles, she should consult with the physician for a possible adjustment of drug dosage or for a different combination.
8. Report any symptoms of eye pathology, such as headaches, dizziness, blurred vision, or partial loss of sight immediately.
9. Alterations in thought processes, depression, or fatigue should be reported to the physician because a medication preparation with less progesterone activity may be indicated.
10. Androgenic effects, such as weight gain, increased oiliness of the skin, acne, or hirsutism, should be reported because a change in medication or dosage may be in order.
11. Report any missed menstrual periods. If two consecutive periods are missed, discontinue the therapy until pregnancy has been ruled out.
12. Advise the client not to take the tablets longer than 18 months without consulting her physician.
13. Explain the need to practice another form of contraception if receiving ampicillin, anticonvulsants, phenylbutazone, rifampin, or tetracycline. These drugs may cause intermittent

bleeding and the drug interactions could result in an unwanted pregnancy.

14. Contraceptives interfere with the elimination of caffeine. Therefore, advise clients to limit their caffeine consumption to prevent insomnia, irritability, tremors, and cardiac irregularities.

15. If the woman is breast-feeding her infant, another form of contraception should be used until lactation is well established.

16. **Do not smoke.** Offer encouragement and assist the client to quit. Suggest participation in smoking cessation programs that have proven effective.

17. Be certain that the client is made aware of all potential inherent risks related to this therapy prior to initiating drug therapy.

18. Stress the importance for the client to report for a yearly Pap smear and physical examination.

Evaluation: Evaluate client for:
- Effective contraception
- Menstrual regularity
- Decreased menstrual blood loss resulting from hormone imbalances

PENICILLINS

See also the following individual entries:

Amoxicillin
Amoxicillin and Potassium Clavulanate
Ampicillin
Ampicillin Oral
Ampicillin Sodium Parenteral
Ampicillin Sodium/Sulbactam Sodium
Ampicillin Trihydrate with Probenecid
Bacampicillin Hydrochloride
Carbenicillin Indanyl Sodium
Cloxacillin Sodium Monohydrate
Dicloxacillin Sodium Monohydrate
Methicillin Sodium
Mezlocillin Sodium
Nafcillin Sodium
Oxacillin Sodium
Penicillin G Benzathine, Parenteral
Penicillin G, Benzathine and Procaine Combined
Penicillin G Potassium for Injection
Penicillin G Potassium, Oral
Penicillin G, Procaine, Aqueous
Penicillin G Sodium for Injection
Penicillin V Potassium
Piperacillin Sodium
Ticarcillin Disodium
Ticarcillin Disodium and Clavulanate Potassium

Classification: Anti-infective.

Action/Kinetics: The bactericidal action of penicillins depends on their ability to bind penicillin-binding proteins (PBP-1 and PBP-3) in the cytoplasmic membranes of bacteria, thus inhibiting cell wall synthesis. Some penicillins act by acylation of membrane-bound transpeptidase enzymes, thereby preventing cross-linkage of peptidoglycan chains, which are necessary for bacterial cell wall strength and rigidity. Cell division and growth are inhibited and often lysis and elongation of susceptible bacteria occur. Penicillin is most effective against young, rapidly dividing organisms and has little effect on mature resting cells. Depending on the concentration of the drug at the site of infection and the susceptibility of the infectious microorganism, penicillin is either bacteriostatic or bactericidal. Penicillins are distributed throughout most of the body and pass the placental barrier. They also pass into synovial, pleural, pericardial, peritoneal, ascitic, and spinal fluids. Although normal meninges and the eyes are relatively impermeable to penicillins, they are better absorbed by inflamed meninges and eyes. **Peak serum levels, after PO:** 1 hr. **t¹/₂:** 30–110 min; protein binding: 20%–98% (see individual agents). The renal, cardiac, and hematopoietic functions, as well as the electrolyte balance, of clients receiving penicillin should be monitored at regular intervals. Excreted largely unchanged by the urine as a result of glomerular filtration and active tubular secretion.

Uses: See individual drugs. Depending on the penicillin, these drugs are effective against one or more of the following organisms. **Gram-positive organisms:** *Bacillus anthracis,* beta-hemolytic streptococci, *Corynebacterium diphtheriae, Listeria monocytogenes,* staphylococci, *Staphylococcus aureus,* streptococci, *Streptococcus faecalis, Streptococcus pneumoniae,* and *Streptococcus viridans.* **Gram-negative organisms:** Acinetobacter species, Citrobacter species, Enterobacter species, *Escherichia coli, Hemophilus influenzae,* Klebsiella species, *Moraxella catarrhalis, Morganella morganii, Neisseria gonorrhoeae, Neisseria meningitidis, Proteus mirabilis, Proteus vulgaris,* Providencia species, *Pro-*

videnica rettgeri, Providencia stuartii, Pseudomonas aeruginosa, Salmonella species, Serratia species, Shigella species, and *Streptobacillus moniliformis.* **Anaerobic organisms:** *Actinomyces bovis,* Bacteroides species, Clostridium species, Eubacterium species, Fusobacterium species, Peptococcus species, Peptostreptococcus species, *Treponema pallidum,* Veillonella species.

Contraindications: Hypersensitivity to penicillins, imipenem, and cephalosporins. Oral use of penicillins during the acute stages of empyema, bacteremia, pneumonia, meningitis, pericarditis, and purulent or septic arthritis.

Special Concerns: Most penicillins are pregnancy category B. Use of penicillins during lactation may lead to sensitization, diarrhea, candidiasis, and skin rash in the infant. Use with caution in clients with a history of asthma, hay fever, or urticaria. Clients with cystic fibrosis have a higher incidence of side effects with broad spectrum penicillins. Safety and effectiveness of carbenicillin, piperacillin, and the beta-lactamase inhibitor/penicillin combinations (e.g., amoxicillin/potassium clavulanate, ticarcillin/ potassium clavulanate) have not been determined in children less than 12 years of age. The incidence of resistant strains of staphylococci to penicillinase-resistant penicillins is increasing. Use of prolonged therapy may lead to superinfection (i.e., bacterial or fungal overgrowth of nonsusceptible organisms).

Side Effects: Penicillins are potent sensitizing agents; it is estimated that up to 10% of the US population is allergic to the antibiotic. Hypersensitivity reactions are reported to be on the increase in pediatric populations. Sensitivity reactions may be immediate (within 20 min) or delayed (as long as several days or weeks after initiation of therapy). *Allergic:* Skin rashes (including maculopapular and exanthematous), exfoliative dermatitis, erythema multiforme (rarely, Stevens-Johnson syndrome), hives, pruritus, wheezing, anaphylaxis, fever, eosinophilia, angioedema, serum sickness, laryngeal edema, laryngospasm, prostration, angioneurotic edema, bronchospasm, hypotension, vascular collapse, death. *GI:* Diarrhea (may be severe), abdominal cramps or pain, nausea, vomiting, bloating, flatulence, increased thirst, bitter/unpleasant taste, glossitis, gastritis, stomatitis, dry mouth, sore mouth or tongue, furry tongue, black "hairy" tongue, bloody diarrhea, rectal bleeding, enterocolitis, pseudomembranous colitis. *CNS:* Dizziness, insomnia, hyperactivity, fatigue, prolonged muscle relaxation. Neurotoxicity including lethargy, neuromuscular irritability, seizures, hallucinations following large IV doses (especially in clients with renal failure). *Hematologic:* Thrombocytopenia, leukopenia, agranulocytosis, anemia, thrombocytopenic purpura, hemolytic anemia, granulocytopenia, neutropenia, bone marrow depression. *Renal:* Oliguria, hematuria, hyaline casts, proteinuria, pyuria (all symptoms of interstitial nephritis), nephropathy. Electrolyte imbalance following IV use. *Miscellaneous:* Hepatotoxicity (cholestatic jaundice), superinfection, swelling of face and ankles, anorexia, hyperthermia, transient hepatitis, vaginitis, itchy eyes. IM injection may cause pain and induration at the injection site, ecchymosis, and hematomas. IV use may cause vein irritation, deep vein thrombosis, and thrombophlebitis. For **emergency treatment** of severe allergic or anaphylactic reactions, administer epinephrine (0.3–0.5 ml of a 1:1,000 solution SC or IM, or 0.2–0.3 ml diluted in 10 ml saline, given slowly by IV). Corticosteroids should be on hand. In those instances where penicillin is the drug of choice, the physician may decide to use it even though the client is allergic, adding a medication to the regimen to control the allergic response. *Symptoms of Overdose:* Neuromuscular hyperexcitability, convulsive seizures. Massive IV doses may cause agitation, asterixis, hallucinations, confusion, stupor, multifocal myoclonus, seizures, coma, hyperkalemia, and encephalopathy.

Drug Interactions

Aminoglycosides / Penicillins ↓ effect of aminoglycosides

Antacids / ↓ Effect of penicillins due to ↓ absorption from GI tract

Antibiotics, Chloramphenicol, Erythromycins, Tetracyclines / ↓ Effect of penicillins

Anticoagulants / Penicillins may potentiate pharmacologic effect

Aspirin / ↑ Effect of penicillins by ↓ plasma protein binding

Chloramphenicol / Either ↑ or ↓ effects

Erythromycins / Either ↑ or ↓ effects

Heparin / ↑ Risk of bleeding following parenteral penicillins

Oral contraceptives / ↓ Effect of oral contraceptives

Phenylbutazone / ↑ Effect of penicillins by ↓ plasma protein binding

Probenecid / ↑ Effect of penicillins by ↓ excretion

Tetracyclines / ↓ Effect of penicillins

Laboratory Test Interferences:
↓ Hematocrit, hemoglobin, WBC lymphocytes, serum potassium, albumin, total proteins, uric acid. ↑ Basophils, lymphocytes, monocytes, platelets, serum alkaline phosphatase, serum sodium. ↑ AST, ALT, bilirubin, LDH following semisynthetic penicillins.

Dosage: Penicillins are available in a variety of dosage forms for oral, parenteral, inhalation, and intrathecal administration. Dosages for individual drugs are given in drug entries. Long-acting preparations are frequently used. Oral doses must be higher than IM or SC doses because a large fraction of penicillin given orally may be destroyed in the stomach.

NURSING CONSIDERATIONS

See also *General Nursing Considerations for All Anti-Infectives,* p. 83

Administration/Storage

1. IM and IV administration of penicillin causes a great deal of local irritation. These antibiotics should thus be injected slowly.
2. IM injections are made deeply into the gluteal muscle. IV injections are usually made through the tubing of an IV infusion.

Assessment

1. Assess rigorously for allergic reactions because the incidence is higher with penicillin therapy than with other antibiotics. If a reaction occurs, the drug must be discontinued immediately. Epinephrine,

oxygen, antihistamines, and corticosteroids must be immediately available.
2. Anticipate that allergic reactions are more likely to occur in clients with a history of asthma, hay fever, urticaria, or allergy to cephalosporins.

Interventions

1. Detain client in an ambulatory care site for at least 20 min after administering a penicillin injection to assess for the onset of anaphylaxis. Be prepared for prompt treatment of anaphylactic reaction.
2. Do not administer long-acting types of penicillin IV, because these types are only for IM use. They may cause emboli or CNS or cardiac pathology if administered IV.
3. Do not massage repository (long-acting) penicillin products after injection, because rate of absorption should not be increased.
4. Prevent rapid administration of IV penicillin because this method may cause local irritation and may precipitate convulsions.
5. The elderly may be more sensitive to the effects of penicillin than are younger people. Therefore, care should be exerted when calculating the dose based on client weight and height.
6. Most penicillins are excreted in breast milk and should be prescribed cautiously to nursing mothers.

Client/Family Teaching

1. Review the drugs prescribed, their side effects, and the expected outcome of therapy.

2. Review the signs and symptoms of allergic reaction, instructing the client to stop the medication when noted and to check with medical supervision as soon as possible.
3. Take oral penicillin with a glass of water 1 hr before or 2–3 hr after meals.
4. Explain when to return for repository penicillin injections to complete treatment, as ordered.
5. Complete entire prescribed course of therapy, even though client may feel well. A person with alpha-hemolytic streptococcus infection must continue with penicillin therapy for a minimum of 10 days, and preferably 14 days, to prevent development of rheumatic fever or glomerulonephritis.
6. Review signs and symptoms of superinfections and instruct client to report these to the physician.

Evaluation: Evaluate client for:
- Evidence of knowledge and understanding of illness and compliance with prescribed therapy
- Status (presence/absence) of pretreatment symptoms and C&S results to determine effectiveness of treatment, reviewing appropriate lab data
- Reports of symptomatic improvement

PHENOTHIAZINES

See also the following individual entries:

Acetophenazine Maleate
Chlorpromazine
Chlorpromazine Hydrochloride

Fluphenazine Decanoate
Fluphenazine Enanthate
Fluphenazine Hydrochloride
Mesoridazine Besylate
Perphenazine
Prochlorperazine
Prochlorperazine Edisylate
Prochlorperazine Maleate
Promazine Hydrochloride
Thioridazine Hydrochloride
Trifluoperazine
Triflupromazine Hydrochloride

General Statement: The advent of antipsychotic drugs was responsible for a major change in the treatment of the mentally ill. Reserpine, an alkaloid derived from *Rauwolfia serpentina,* and chlorpromazine, both of which appeared during the early 1950s, almost singlehandedly revolutionized the care of the mentally ill both inside and outside the hospital. Clients who had not been helped for decades with electroshock, insulin therapy, and/or other forms of treatment could now often be discharged from the hospital. Antipsychotic drugs do not cure mental illness, but they calm the intractable client, relieve the despondency of the severely depressed, activate the immobile and withdrawn, and make some clients more accessible to psychotherapy.

Most phenothiazines induce some sedation, especially during the initial phase of the treatment. Medicated clients can, however, be easily roused. In this manner, the phenothiazines differ markedly from the narcotic analgesics and sedative hypnotics. However, phenothiazines potentiate the analgesic properties of opiates and prolong the action of CNS depressant drugs.

The drugs also decrease spontaneous motor activity, as in parkinsonism, and many lower blood pressure.

According to their detailed chemical structure, the phenothiazines belong to three subgroups:

1. Dimethylaminopropyl compounds
2. Piperazine compounds
3. Piperidine compounds

Drugs belonging to the *dimethylaminopropyl subgroup,* which includes chlorpromazine, are often the first choice for clients in acute excitatory states. Drugs belonging to this subgroup cause more sedation than other phenothiazines and are especially indicated for clients exhausted by lack of sleep.

Members of the *piperazine subgroup* act most selectively on the subcortical sites. This accounts for the fact that they can be administered in relatively small doses. This, in turn, results in minimal drowsiness and undesirable motor effects. The piperazines also have the greatest antiemetic effects because they specifically depress the chemoreceptor trigger zone (CTZ) of the vomiting center. Members of the *piperidyl subgroup* are less toxic in terms of extrapyramidal effects. Mellaril, a member of this group, has little effectiveness as an antiemetic drug.

Action/Kinetics: It has been postulated that excess amounts of dopamine in certain areas of the CNS cause psychoses. Phenothiazines are thought to act by blocking postsynaptic mesolimbic dopamine receptors, leading to a reduction in psychotic symptoms. Phenothiazines block both D_1 and D_2 dopamine receptors. The antiemetic effects are thought to be due to inhibition or blockade of dopamine

(D_2) receptors in the chemoreceptor trigger zone in the medulla as well as by peripheral blockade of the vagus nerve in the GI tract. Relief of anxiety is manifested as a result of an indirect decrease in arousal and increased filtering of internal stimuli to the brain stem reticular system. Alpha-blockade produces sedation. Phenothiazines also raise pain threshold and produce amnesia due to suppression of sensory impulses. In addition, these drugs produce anticholinergic and antihistaminic effects and depress the release of hypothalamic and hypophyseal hormones. Peripheral effects include anticholinergic and alpha-adrenergic blocking properties. Kinetic information on the phenothiazines is scarce and often unreliable.

Generally, peak plasma levels occur 2–4 hr after oral administration. Phenothiazines are widely distributed throughout the body. They have an average half-life of 10–20 hr. Most are metabolized in the liver and excreted by the kidney. Studies have shown that both oral dosage forms and suppositories from different manufacturers differ in their bioavailability. It is recommended that brands not be interchanged unless data indicating bioequivalance are available.

Uses: Psychoses, especially if excessive psychomotor activity manifested. Involutional, toxic, or senile psychoses. Used in combination with MAO inhibitors in depressed clients manifesting anxiety, agitation, or panic (use with caution). With lithium in acute manic phase of manic-depressive illness. As an adjunct in alcohol withdrawal to reduce anxiety, tension, depression, nausea, and/or vomiting. For severe behavioral problems in children, manifested by hyperexcitable and/or combative behavior; also, for short-term use in hyperactive children who exhibit excess motor activity and conduct disorders.

Prophylaxis and control of severe nausea and vomiting due to cancer chemotherapy, radiation therapy, postoperatively. Intractable hiccoughs, intermittent porphyria, tetanus (as adjunct). As preoperative and/or postoperative medications. Some phenothiazines are antipruritics. See also individual drugs.

Contraindications: Severe CNS depression, coma, clients with subcortical brain damage, bone marrow depression, lactation. In clients with a history of seizures and in those on anticonvulsant drugs. Geriatric or debilitated clients, hepatic or renal disease, cardiovascular disorders, glaucoma, prostatic hypertrophy. Contraindicated in children with chickenpox, CNS infections, measles, gastroenteritis, dehydration due to increased risk of extrapyramidal symptoms.

Special Concerns: Phenothiazines should be used with caution in clients exposed to extreme heat or cold and in those with asthma, emphysema, or acute respiratory tract infections. Safe use during pregnancy not established; thus use only when benefits outweigh risks. Children may be more sensitive to the neuromuscular or extrapyramidal effects (especially dystonias); those especially at risk include children with chickenpox, CNS infections, measles, dehydration, or gastroenteritis. Thus, generally, phenothiazines are not recommended for use in children less than 12 years of age. Geriatric clients often manifest higher plasma levels due to decreases in lean body mass, total body water, and albumin and an increase in total body fat. Also, geriatric clients may be more likely to manifest orthostatic hypotension, anticholinergic effects, sedative effects, and extrapyramidal side effects.

Side Effects: *CNS:* Depression, drowsiness, dizziness, lethargy, fatigue. Extrapyramidal effects, Parkinson-like symptoms including shuffling gait or tic-like movements of head and face, tardive dyskinesia (see below), akathisia, dystonia. Seizures, especially in clients with a history thereof. Neuroleptic malignant syndrome (rare). *CV:* Orthostatic hypotension, increase or decrease in blood pressure, tachycardia, fainting. *GI:* Dry mouth, anorexia, constipation, paralytic ileus, diarrhea. *Endocrine:* Breast engorgement, galactorrhea, gynecomastia, increased appetite, weight gain, hyper- or hypoglycemia, glycosuria. Delayed ejaculation, increased or decreased libido. *GU:* Menstrual irregularities, loss of bladder control, urinary difficulty. *Dermatologic:* Photosensitivity, pruritus, erythema, eczema, exfoliative dermatitis, pigment changes in skin (long-term use of high doses). *Hematologic:* Aplastic anemia, leukopenia, agranulocytosis, eosinophilia, thrombocytopenia. *Ophthalmologic:* Deposition of fine particulate matter in lens and cornea leading to blurred vision, changes in vision. *Respiratory:* Laryngospasm, bronchospasm, laryngeal edema, breathing difficulties. *Miscellaneous:* Fever, muscle stiffness, decreased sweating, muscle spasm of face, neck, or back, obstructive jaundice, nasal congestion, pale skin, mydriasis, systemic lupus-like syndrome.

Tardive dyskinesia has been observed with all classes of antipsychotic drugs, although the precise cause is not known. The syndrome is most commonly seen in older clients, especially women, and in individuals with organic brain syndrome. It is often aggravated or precipitated by the sudden discontinuance of antipsychotic drugs and may persist indefinitely after the drug is discontinued. Early signs of tardive dyskinesia include fine vermicular movements of the tongue and grimacing or tic-like movements of the head and neck. Although there is no known cure for the syndrome, it may not progress if the dosage of the drug is slowly reduced. Also, a few drug-free days may unmask the symptoms of tardive dyskinesia and help in early diagnosis.

Symptoms of Overdose: CNS depression including deep sleep and coma, hypotension, extrapyramidal symptoms, agitation, restlessness, seizures, hypothermia, hyperthermia, autonomic symptoms, cardiac arrhythmias, ECG changes.

Drug Interactions

Alcohol, ethyl / Potentiation or addition of CNS depressant effects. Concomitant use may lead to drowsiness, lethargy, stupor, respiratory collapse, coma, or death

Aluminum salts (antacids) / ↓ Absorption from GI tract

Amphetamine / ↓ Effect of amphetamine by ↓ uptake of drug to the site of action

Anesthetics, general / See *Alcohol*

Antacids, oral / ↓ Effect of phenothiazines due to ↓ absorption from GI tract

Antianxiety drugs / See *Alcohol*

Anticholinergic drugs / Additive anticholinergic side effects and/or ↓ antipsychotic effect

Antidepressants, tricyclic / Additive anticholinergic side effects

Antidiabetic agents / ↓ Effect of antidiabetic agents, since phenothiazines ↑ blood sugar

Bacitracin / Additive respiratory depression

Barbiturate anesthetics / ↑ Chance of tremor, involuntary muscle activity, and hypotension

Barbiturates / See *Alcohol;* also, barbiturates may ↓ effect due to ↑ breakdown by liver

Bromocriptine / Phenothiazines ↓ effect

Capreomycin / Additive respiratory depression

Charcoal / ↓ Effect of phenothiazines due to ↓ absorption from GI tract

CNS depressants / See *Alcohol;* also, ↓ effect of phenothiazines due to ↑ breakdown by liver

Colistimethate / Additive respiratory depression

Diazoxide / Additive hyperglycemic effect

Guanethidine / ↓ Effect of guanethidine by ↓ uptake of drug at the site of action

Hydantoins / ↑ Risk of hydantoin toxicity

Lithium carbonate / ↑ Risk of extrapyramidal symptoms, disorientation, or unconsciousness

MAO inhibitors / ↑ Effect of phenothiazines due to ↓ breakdown by liver

Meperidine / ↑ Risk of hypotension and sedation

Metoprolol / Additive hypotensive effects

Narcotics / See *Alcohol*

Phenytoin / ↑ Effect of phenytoin
due to ↓ breakdown by liver
Polymyxin B / Additive
respiratory depression
Propranolol / Additive
hypotensive effects
Quinidine / Additive cardiac
depressant effect
Sedative-hypnotics,
nonbarbiturate / See *Alcohol*
Succinylcholine / ↑ Muscle
relaxation
Tricyclic antidepressants /
↑ Serum levels of tricyclic
antidepressant

Laboratory Test Interferences:
False + : Bile (urine dipstick), ferric
chloride, pregnancy tests, urinary
porphobilinogen, urinary steroids,
urobilinogen (urine dipstick). False
(−): Inorganic phosphorus, urinary
steroids. *Caused by pharmacologic
effects:* ↑ Alkaline phosphatase, bilirubin, serum transaminases, serum
cholesterol, urinary catecholamines. ↓ Glucose tolerance, serum
uric acid, 5-hydroxyindoleacetic
acid (5-HIAA), FSH, growth hormone, LH, vanillylmandelic acid.

Dosage: See individual drugs.
The phenothiazines are effective
over a wide dosage range. Dosage
is usually increased gradually to
minimize side effects over 7 days
until the minimal effective dose is
attained. Dosage is increased more
gradually in elderly or debilitated
clients because they are more susceptible to the effects and side
effects of drugs. After symptoms are
controlled, dosage is gradually reduced to maintenance levels. It is
usually desirable to keep chronically ill clients on maintenance levels
indefinitely.
Medication, especially in clients
on high dosages, should not be
discontinued abruptly.

NURSING CONSIDERATIONS
Administration/Storage
1. Do not interchange brands of
   oral form of drug or suppositories. They may differ in bioavailability.
2. Do not use pink or markedly
   discolored solutions.
3. When preparing or administering parenteral solutions, both
   nurse and client should avoid
   contact of drug with skin, eyes,
   and clothing to prevent contact
   dermatitis.
4. Do not mix antipsychotic drugs
   with other drugs in the same
   syringe.
5. A specific rate of flow of drug
   should be ordered when administering parenteral solutions.
6. To lessen the pain of the injection, dilute commercially available injectable solutions in
   saline or local anesthetic.
7. When administering the drug
   IM, inject the drug deeply into
   the muscle.
8. Massage the area of the injection site after IM administration
   to reduce the pain.
9. Prevent extravasation of the IV
   solution.
10. Store solutions in a cool dry
    place in amber-colored con-
    tainers.
11. *Treatment of Overdose:* Emet-
    ics are not to be used as they
    are of little value and may
    cause a dystonic reaction of the
    head or neck that may result in
    aspiration of vomitus.
    • Hypotension: Volume re-
      placement; norepinephrine
      or phenylephrine may be
      used (do not use epineph-
      rine).
    • Ventricular arrhythmias: phe-
      nytoin, 1 mg/kg IV, not to

exceed 50 mg/min; may be repeated q 5 min up to 10 mg/kg.

- Seizures or hyperactivity: Diazepam or pentobarbital.
- Extrapyramidal symptoms: Antiparkinson drugs, diphenyhydramine, barbiturates.

Note: These *Nursing Considerations* apply to all antipsychotic agents except lithium.

Assessment

1. Take a complete drug history noting any past incidence of drug hypersensitivity.
2. When performing the nursing history, determine if there is any history of seizures. The drugs in this class may lower the seizure threshold.
3. Document baseline mental status noting mood, behavior, and any evidence of depression.
4. When working with elderly clients, assess their baseline level of mental acuity and document.
5. If administering the drug to children, note the extent of the client's hyperexcitability.
6. If the client is a child, assess the possibility of the child having chickenpox or measles.
7. Note any history of asthma or emphysema.
8. Obtain baseline readings of blood pressure and pulse before administering any antipsychotic drug. Assess the BP when the client is in a reclining position, standing position, and sitting position.
9. Ensure that the client has baseline CBC with differential, liver function studies, urinalysis, an EEG, and ocular examination prior to initiating therapy.
10. Note all medications the client may be taking to determine if any may interact unfavorably with the antipsychotic agent being considered.

Interventions

1. If drug is administered IV, the rate of flow should be monitored carefully and the blood pressure taken at frequent intervals.
2. Note client complaints of undue distress when in a hot or cold room. The client's heat regulating mechanism may be affected by the drug.
   - If the client complains of feeling cold, provide extra blankets.
   - If the client complains of feeling too warm, suggest bathing in tepid water.
   - Clients should *NOT* use heating pads or hot water bottles if they feel cold.
3. If the client becomes excessively active or depressed, document and report to the physician. The medication may need to be changed.
4. Note the presence of spasms of the client's face, neck, back, or tongue. The physician may determine that the condition can be treated with antihistamines, or the decision may be to discontinue the drug.
5. When working with elderly clients be particularly observant for symptoms of tardive dyskinesia. Clients may exhibit puffing of the cheeks or tongue, develop chewing movements, and involuntary movements of the extremities

and trunk. Such symptoms should be reported immediately to the physician and the drug discontinued.

6. If the client develops a sore throat, persistent fever, malaise, and weakness, document and report. These may be signs associated with agranulocytosis. The drug should be withheld until the appropriate blood work has been performed and the tests are evaluated by the physician.

7. Measure intake and output and observe for abdominal distention. Report any urinary retention. The dosage of medication may need to be reduced, antispasmodics may be indicated, or the drug may need to be changed.

8. Question clients concerning constipation. Encourage them to maintain an adequate fluid intake and to eat a diet high in roughage. Laxatives may be required.

9. Conduct periodic ocular examinations to detect any early visual disturbances.

10. Note any changes in carbohydrate metabolism (e.g., glycosuria, weight loss, polyphagia, increased appetite, or excessive weight gain). These signs may require a change in diet or medication therapy. These symptoms can be particularly significant if the client has diabetes.

11. Premenopausal women need to know that the menstrual cycle may become irregular. They may develop engorged breasts and begin lactating. The client needs to be reassured that this condition may be altered by a change in the medication therapy.

12. Some clients may develop a hypersensitivity reaction such as fever, asthma, laryngeal edema, angioneurotic edema, and anaphylactic reaction. **Stop** medication, notify physician, and treat symptomatically.

13. Be aware that clients on long-term therapy may develop a yellow-brown skin reaction that may turn grayish purple.

14. Note evidence of early cholestatic jaundice, such as high fever, client complaint of upper abdominal pain, nausea, diarrhea, and rash. Obtain liver function studies and compare with the baseline measurements.

15. If the client develops yellowing of the sclera, skin, or mucous membranes, withhold the drug. Record these observations and report to the physician because these signs may indicate that the client has a biliary obstruction.

16. The antiemetic effects of phenothiazines may mask other pathology such as toxicity to other drugs, intestinal obstruction, or brain lesions. Careful observations of the client are therefore essential.

17. If the client is receiving barbiturates to relieve anxiety during phenothiazine therapy, anticipate the dose of the barbiturate will be reduced.

18. If barbiturates are being administered as an anticonvulsant, the dosage of barbiturates will not be reduced.

19. If administering phenothiazines to a child, note neuromuscular reactions, especially if the child is dehydrated or has an acute infection. These children are more susceptible to side effects.

20. If the medication is to be administered IV, keep the client recumbent for at least 1 hr after the IV is completed.
    - Monitor the blood pressure for hypotension, compare to the baseline measurements.
    - After 1 hr, slowly elevate the head of the bed, and observe for tachycardia, faintness, or complaint of dizziness.
    - Keep side rails up.
21. If the drug is to be discontinued, it should be done gradually to minimize the possible onset of severe GI disturbances or symptoms of tardive dyskinesia.
22. If clients are in a hospital setting, remain with them to assure that the medication has been swallowed. It may be advisable to give a liquid preparation of the drug to permit better control over drug taking and improve compliance.
23. If clients develop respiratory symptoms, instruct them to take slow, deep breaths. The drug may depress the cough reflex.
24. When clients are being seen on an outpatient basis, check on the number of times they request prescription refills. They may be hoarding medication, especially if they are depressed.

Client/Family Teaching

1. May take with food or milk to minimize GI upset.
2. Advise young women that the drug may cause menstrual irregularity and can cause false + pregnancy tests. If the client suspects she may be pregnant, she should notify her physician.
3. Encourage female clients to keep an accurate record of their menstrual periods.
4. Male clients should be told they may experience decreased libido and develop breast enlargement. Reassure client and instruct him to report these symptoms to the physician so that the medication can be adjusted.
5. Many clients develop photosensitivity reactions. Advise them to wear protective clothing and sunglasses when in the sun and to avoid sunbathing. They should also use large quantities of sun screens for added protection.
6. Drug may discolor the urine pink or reddish brown.
7. To prevent a dry mouth, rinse the mouth frequently, increase fluid intake, chew sugarless gum, and/or suck on hard candies.
8. Increase fluids and bulk in the diet to minimize the constipating effects of these drugs.
9. Avoid driving a car or operating heavy machinery or engaging in any activities that require mental alertness for at least 2 weeks after the therapy has started. Consult with physician for evaluation of client's response to treatment before resuming any of these activities.
10. If the client develops blurred vision, avoid driving the car and notify physician.
11. Remind clients that long-term therapy may affect their vision. Therefore, they should schedule regular ophthalmic examinations.
12. Rise slowly from a lying or sitting position and dangle legs

before standing to avoid orthostatic symptoms.

13. Report any elevation of body temperature, feeling of weakness, or sore throat. These may be indications of blood dyscrasias and require immediate attention.

14. Do not stop taking the drug abruptly. An abrupt cessation of high doses of phenothiazines can cause nausea, vomiting, tremors, sensations of warmth and cold, sweating, tachycardia, headache, and insomnia.

15. Review the goals of therapy with client and family and assess degree to which they have been attained. Remind the client and family that it may be weeks or months before the full effects of the medication will be noticed.

16. Stress the importance of taking the drug as prescribed after discharge and remind client to advise all health care providers of the medications currently prescribed.

17. Avoid alcohol and any other CNS depressants without physician approval.

18. Stress the importance of reporting for periodic laboratory studies and follow-up care for evaluation and adjustment of drug dosage.

Evaluation: Evaluate client for:
- Evidence of a decrease in excitable, withdrawn, or paranoid behaviors, comparing baseline evaluations of behavior with present level
- Orientation as to time, place, and understanding of the illness
- Evidence of adherence to the prescribed drug regimen

and assess for any evidence of extrapyramidal effects of drug therapy
- Reports of relief of nausea and vomiting

PROGESTERONE AND PROGESTINS

See also the following individual entries:

Levonorgestrel Implants
Medroxyprogesterone Acetate
Megestrol Acetate
Oral Contraceptives

General Statement: Progesterone is a natural female ovarian steroid hormone produced in large amounts during pregnancy. It is chiefly secreted by the corpus luteum during the second half of the menstrual cycle and is produced by the placenta during pregnancy.

The hormone acts on the thick muscles of the uterus (myometrium) and on its lining (endometrium). It prepares the lining for the implantation of the fertilized ovum. Under the influence of progesterone, the estrogen-primed endometrium enters its "secretory phase" during which it thickens and secretes large quantities of mucus and glycogen. The myometrium relaxes under the effect of progesterone. During puberty, progesterone participates in the maturation of the female body, acting on the breasts and the vaginal mucosa.

Progesterone interacts, by a feedback mechanism, with follicle-stimulating hormone (FSH) and luteinizing hormone (LH), produced by the anterior pituitary. When progesterone and estrogen are high, there is a decrease in the production of FSH and LH. This inhibits ovulation and accounts for the fact that progesterone is an effective contraceptive. Natural progesterone has to be injected, but a whole series of compounds with progesterone-type activity (collectively called *progestins*) can be taken orally. These substances are now routinely substituted for natural progesterone. Progesterone is essential for the maintenance of pregnancy.

Although progesterone stimulates the development of alveolar mammary tissue during pregnancy, it does not initiate lactation. On the contrary, it suppresses the lactogenic hormone; lactation starts postpartum only when progesterone and estrogen levels have decreased.

Action/Kinetics: Physiologic doses are used for replacement therapy and to suppress gonadotropin production, which inhibits ovulation. Pharmacologic doses have several uses (see below). Progesterone must be administered parenterally because of major inactivation in the liver (first-pass effect). The hormones are metabolized in the liver and a major portion is excreted in the urine (urinalysis is used to monitor progesterone levels).

Uses: Abnormal uterine bleeding, primary or secondary amenorrhea (used with an estrogen), endometriosis, premenstrual tension. Alone or with an estrogen for contraception. May also be used in combination with an estrogen for endometriosis and hypermenorrhea. Certain types of cancer. **Note:** Not to be used to prevent habitual abortion or to treat threatened abortion.

Contraindications: Genital malignancies, thromboembolic disease, vaginal bleeding of unknown origin, impaired liver function. Pregnancy, especially during the first four months. Cancer of the breast, missed abortion, as a diagnostic test for pregnancy. Lactation.

Special Concerns: Use with caution in case of asthma, epilepsy, depression, and migraine.

Side Effects: Occasionally noted with short-term dosage, frequently observed with prolonged high dosage. *GU:* Spotting, irregular periods, amenorrhea, changes in amount and/or duration of menstrual flow, changes in cervical secretions and cervical erosion, breast tenderness or secretions. *Dermatologic:* Allergic rashes, pruritus, acne, melasma, chloasma, alopecia, hirsutism. *CNS:* Depression, pyrexia, insomnia. *Miscellaneous:* Weight gain or loss, cholestatic jaundice, masculinization of the female fetus, nausea, edema, precipitation of acute intermittent porphyria, photosensitivity.

Drug Interactions: Rifampin and possibly phenobarbital ↓ the effect of progesterone by ↑ breakdown by the liver.

Dosage: Progesterone must be administered parenterally. Other progestins can be administered PO and parenterally. The usual schedule of administration for *functional uterine bleeding, amenorrhea, infertility, dysmenorrhea, premenstrual tension, and contraception* is days 5 through 25 of the menstrual cycle, with day 1 being the first day of menstrual flow.

NURSING CONSIDERATIONS

Assessment

1. Assess the client's history for evidence of thrombophlebitis,

pulmonary embolism, or cerebrovascular accidents.
2. Obtain a baseline blood pressure, pulse, and weight and document.
3. Determine if the client has any history of psychic depression.
4. Note if the client has diabetes mellitus.
5. Determine that baseline laboratory studies have been performed.

Interventions

1. Monitor the blood pressure and pulse and report any changes from the baseline findings.
2. Observe the client's extremities for evidence of edema, document, and report to the physician.
3. Check the client for any physical changes such as yellowing of the sclera and report if evident.

Client/Family Teaching

1. Describe the symptoms of thrombic disorders such as pains in the legs, sudden onset of chest pain, shortness of breath, and coughing for no apparent reason. Instruct the client to report these symptoms to the physician immediately.
2. Advise clients to weigh themselves at least twice a week and to report any unusual weight gain. Rapid weight gain may indicate the presence of edema.
3. Discuss the need to report any yellowing of the skin or sclera. This indicates jaundice and may necessitate the discontinuation of the medication or a change in the dosage.

4. To avoid gastric irritation and nausea, advise the client to take the medication with a light snack, in the evening.
5. Explain that gastric distress usually subsides after the first few cycles of the drug. However, if these symptoms persist, they should be reported to the physician.
6. If any episodes of bleeding occur, they should also be reported.
7. Discuss the fact that progestins may reactivate or worsen a psychic depression. Advise family to take particular note of any psychic changes the client may undergo, the circumstance of the depression, and to report this to the physician.
8. Advise clients with diabetes that progesterone may alter glucose tolerance. Instruct them to report positive urine tests for glucose and abnormal finger stick results promptly because the dosage of antidiabetic medication may need to be adjusted.
9. Early symptoms of ophthalmic pathology, such as headaches, dizziness, blurred vision, or partial loss of vision, should be reported when noted.
10. Advise clients to stop smoking. If they express difficulty, offer assistance and suggest an anti-smoking program.
11. Emphasize the need to report to the physician regularly for medical follow-up.

Evaluation: Evaluate client for:
- Control of abnormal bleeding
- Effective hormone replacement therapy

- Establishment of menstrual regularity
- Effective contraceptive agent

SUCCINIMIDES

See also the following individual entries:

Ethosuximide
Methsuximide
Phensuximide

General Statement: Three succinimide derivatives are currently used primarily for the treatment of absence seizures (petit mal): ethosuximide, methsuximide, and phensuximide. Ethosuximide is currently the drug of choice. Methsuximide should be used only when the client is refractory to other drugs. These drugs may be given concomitantly with other anticonvulsants if other types of epilepsy are manifested with absence seizures.

Action/Kinetics: The succinimide derivatives suppress the paroxysmal three cycle per second spike and wave activity that is associated with lapses of consciousness seen in absence seizures. They apparently do so by depressing the motor cortex and by raising the threshold of the CNS to convulsive stimuli. The drugs are rapidly absorbed from the GI tract.

Uses: Primarily absence seizures (petit mal).

Contraindications: Hypersensitivity to succinimides.

Special Concerns: Safe use during pregnancy has not been established. Must be used with caution in clients with abnormal liver and kidney function.

Side Effects: *CNS:* Drowsiness, ataxia, dizziness, headaches, euphoria, lethargy, fatigue, insomnia, irritability, nervousness, dream-like state, hyperactivity. Psychiatric or psychologic aberrations such as mental slowing, hypochondriasis, sleep disturbances, inability to concentrate, depression, night terrors, instability, confusion, aggressiveness. Rarely, auditory hallucinations, paranoid psychosis, increased libido, suicidal behavior. *GI:* Nausea, vomiting, hiccoughs, anorexia, diarrhea, gastric distress, weight loss, abdominal and epigastric pain, cramps, constipation. *Hematologic:* Leukopenia, granulocytopenia, eosinophilia, agranulocytosis, pancytopenia with or without bone marrow suppression, monocytosis. *Dermatologic:* Pruritus, urticaria, erythema multiforme, lupus erythematosus, Stevens-Johnson syndrome, pruritic erythematous rashes, skin eruptions, alopecia, hirsutism, photophobia. *GU:* Urinary frequency, vaginal bleeding, renal damage, microscopic hematuria. *Miscellaneous:* Blurred vision, muscle weakness, hyperemia, hypertrophy of gums, swollen tongue, myopia, periorbital edema.

Symptoms of Acute Overdose: Confusion, sleepiness, slow shallow respiration, nausea, vomiting, CNS depression with coma and respiratory depression, hypotension, cyanosis, hyper- or hypothermia, absence of reflexes, unsteadiness, flaccid muscles.

Symptoms of Chronic Overdose: Ataxia, dizziness, drowsiness, confusion, depression, proteinuria, skin rashes, hangover, irritability, poor judgment, nausea, vomiting, muscle weakness, periorbital edema, hepatic dysfunction, fatal bone marrow aplasia, delayed onset of coma, nephrosis, hematuria, casts.

Drug Interactions: Succinimides may increase the effects of hydantoins by decreasing breakdown by the liver.

Dosage: *Individualized.* See individual agents. Succinimides may be given in combination with other anticonvulsants if two or more types of seizures are present.

NURSING CONSIDERATIONS

See also *Nursing Considerations* for *Anticonvulsants*, p. 63.

Administration/Storage: *Treatment of Overdose:* General supportive measures. Charcoal hemoperfusion may be helpful.

Client/Family Teaching

1. Report any increase in frequency of tonic-clonic (grand mal) seizures immediately.
2. Alert the family to the possibility of transient personality changes, hypochondriacal behavior, and aggressiveness. Stress the need to report these personality changes immediately to the physician.
3. Report any persistent fever, swollen glands, and bleeding gums. These may be symptoms of a blood dyscrasia.
4. Report for CBCs and liver and renal function studies on a scheduled basis.
5. Caution should be exercised while driving or performing other tasks requiring alertness and coordination as the drugs may cause, dizziness, blurred vision, and drowsiness.

Evaluation: Evaluate client for:
- Evidence of a decrease in the frequency of petit mal seizures
- Freedom from side effects of drug therapy.

SULFONAMIDES

See also the following individual entries:

Mafenide Acetate
Pediazole
Sulfacetamide Sodium
Sulfacytine
Sulfadiazine
Sulfadiazine Sodium
Sulfamethizole
Sulfamethoxazole
Sulfamethoxazole and
    Phenazopyridine
Sulfamethoxazole and
    Trimethoprim
Sulfasalazine
Sulfisoxazole
Sulfisoxazole Acetyl
Sulfisoxazole Diolamine
Sulfisoxazole and
    Phenazopyridine

Action/Kinetics: Sulfonamides are structurally related to para-aminobenzoic acid and, as such, competitively inhibit the enzyme dihydropteroate synthetase, which is responsible for incorporating para-aminobenzoic acid into dihydrofolic acid. Thus, the synthesis of dihydrofolic acid is inhibited, resulting in a decrease in tetrahydrofolic acid, which is required for synthesis of DNA, purines, and thymidine. Thus, sulfonamides halt multiplication of bacteria (bacteriostatic) but do not kill fully formed microorganisms. Resistance to sulfonamides has occurred with increasing frequency.

The various sulfonamides are absorbed and excreted at widely differing rates. This has an important bearing on their therapeutic use. For instance, agents that are poorly absorbed from the GI tract are particularly indicated for intestinal infections because they remain localized in the intestine for a long time.

Sulfonamides are absorbed into the bloodstream and distributed throughout all tissues, including the CSF, where concentrations attain 50%–80% of those found in the blood. The sulfonamides are metabolized in the liver and primarily excreted by the kidneys. Small amounts are found in the feces, bile, breast milk, and other secretions.

It is always desirable to determine the susceptibility of the pathogen before, or soon after, initiation of therapy.

Sulfonamides have the advantage of being relatively inexpensive.

Uses: The range of usefulness of the sulfonamides has been greatly reduced by the emergence of resistant strains of bacteria and the development of more effective antibiotics.

Acute, nonobstructive urinary tract infections caused by *Escherichia coli, Klebsiella, Enterobacter, Staphylococcus aureus, Proteus mirabilis, P. vulgaris*. Drug of choice for nocardiosis. Elimination of meningococci from the nasopharynx in asymptomatic *Neisseria meningitidis* carriers when organism is sulfonamide-sensitive group A strain. As an alternative to penicillin for prophylaxis of rheumatic fever. As an alternative to tetracyclines for chlamydial infections or for trachoma and inclusion conjunctivitis or lymphogranuloma venereum. In conjunction with pyrimethamine for toxoplasmosis. In combination with quinine sulfate and pyrimethamine for chloroquine-resistant *Plasmodium falciparum*. In combination with penicillin or erythromycin for otitis media. Chancroid. In conjunction with streptomycin for meningitis caused by *H. influenzae*.

Contraindications: Except for hypersensitivity reactions to sulfonamides and chemically related drugs (e.g., thiazides, sulfonylureas, loop diuretics, carbonic anhydrase inhibitors, local anesthetics, PABA-containing sunscreens), there are few absolute contraindications. Sulfonamides, however, are potentially dangerous drugs and cause a 5% overall incidence of major and minor side effects.

Sulfonamides may cause mental retardation and never should be administered during the third term of pregnancy, to nursing mothers, or to infants under 2 months of age, except for the treatment of congenital toxoplasmosis (a serious parasitic disease that can cause brain inflammation) or in life-threatening situations. Porphyria. Group A beta-hemolytic streptococcal infections.

Special Concerns: Sulfonamides should be used with caution, and in reduced dosage, in clients with impaired liver or renal function, intestinal or urinary tract obstructions, blood dyscrasias, allergies, asthma, and hereditary glucose-6-phosphate dehydrogenase deficiency. Use with caution if exposed to sunlight or ultraviolet light as photosensitivity may occur.

Side Effects: *GI:* Nausea, vomiting, diarrhea, abdominal pain, glossitis, stomatitis, anorexia, pseudomembranous enterocolitis, pancreatitis. *Allergic:* Rash, pruritus, photosensitivity, erythema nodosum or multiforme, generalized skin eruptions, Stevens-Johnson syndrome, conjunctivitis, rhinitis, balanitis. Serum sickness, urticaria, pruritus, exfoliative dermatitis, anaphylaxis, epidermal necrolysis with or without corneal damage, periorbital edema, conjunctival and scleral injection, allergic myocarditis, decreased pulmonary function, disseminated lupus erythematosus, periarteritis nodosa, arteritis. *CNS:* Headaches, dizziness, mental depression, seizures, hallucinations, vertigo, insomnia, apathy, ataxia, confusion, psychoses, drowsiness, restlessness. *Renal:* Renal damage due to precipitation of sulfonamide or its acetyl derivative in the tubules (manifested by crystalluria, hematuria, oliguria); nephrotic syndrome. *Hematologic:* Acute hemolytic anemia especially in glucose-6-phosphate dehydrogenase deficiency, aplastic anemia, leukopenia, agranulocytosis, thrombocytopenia, methemoglobinemia, purpura megaloblastic anemia, hypoprothrombinemia, Heinz body anemia. *Miscellaneous:* Jaundice, hepatitis, hepatocellular necrosis, tinnitus, hypoglycemia, arthralgia, acidosis, superinfection, hearing loss, transverse myelitis, drug fever, pyrexia, alopecia, arthralgia, myalgia, periarteritis nodosum.

By killing the intestinal flora, the sulfonamides also reduce the bacterial synthesis of vitamin K. This may result in hemorrhage. Administration of vitamin K to patients on long-term sulfonamide therapy is recommended.

Symptoms of Overdose: Nausea, vomiting, anorexia, colic, dizziness, drowsiness, headache, unconsciousness, toxic fever. More serious manifestations include acute hemolytic anemia, agranulocytosis, acidosis, maculopapular dermatitis, hepatic jaundice, sensitivity reactions, toxic neuritis, death (several days after the first dose).

Drug Interactions

Anesthetics, local / ↓ Effect of sulfonamides

Antacids / ↓ Effect of sulfonamides due to ↓ absorption from GI tract

Anticoagulants, oral / ↑ Effect of anticoagulants due to ↓ in plasma protein binding

Antidiabetics, oral / ↑ Hypoglycemic effect due to ↓ in plasma protein binding

Cyclosporine / ↓ Effect of cyclosporine and ↑ nephrotoxicity

Methenamine / ↑ Chance of sulfonamide crystalluria due to acid urine

Methotrexate / ↑ Effect of methotrexate due to ↓ plasma protein binding and ↓ renal tubular excretion → bone marrow suppression

Oxacillin / ↓ Effect of oxacillin due to ↓ absorption from GI tract

Paraldehyde / ↑ Chance of sulfonamide crystalluria

Phenylbutazone / ↑ Effect of sulfonamides by ↑ blood levels

Phenytoin / ↑ Effect of phenytoin due to ↓ breakdown in liver

Probenecid / ↑ Effect of sulfonamides by ↓ in plasma protein binding

Salicylates / ↑ Effect of sulfonamides by ↑ blood levels

Laboratory Test Interferences: False + or ↑ liver function tests (amino acids, bilirubin, BSP), renal function (BUN, nonprotein nitrogen, creatinine clearance), blood counts, prothrombin time, Coombs'

test. False + or ↑ urine glucose (copper reduction methods, such as Benedict's solution or Clinitest), protein, urobilinogen.

Dosage: See individual drugs.

Sulfonamides are usually given PO. Dosage is adjusted individually. An initial loading dose is usually recommended. Short-acting compounds must be given q 4–6 hr.

Topical application of sulfonamides is rarely ordered today, except for mafenide acetate, which is used as a 10% ointment to treat burn infections.

Creams of triple sulfa or sulfisoxazole are used for vaginitis.

When sulfonamides are given as adjuncts to GI surgery, medication is usually started 3–5 days before surgery and is given for 1–2 weeks postoperatively after peristalsis has resumed.

NURSING CONSIDERATIONS

See also *General Nursing Considerations For All Anti-Infectives,* p. 83

Administration/Storage: *Treatment of Overdose:* Immediately discontinue the drug.
- Induce emesis or perform gastric lavage, especially if large doses were taken.
- To hasten excretion, alkalinize the urine and force fluids (if kidney function is normal). If there is renal blockage due to sulfonamide crystals, catheterization of the ureters may be needed.
- In the event of agranulocytosis, antibiotic therapy is needed to combat infection.
- To treat severe anemia or thrombocytopenia, blood or platelet transfusions are required.

Assessment

1. Obtain a thorough nursing and drug history.
2. Note if the client has ever received sulfonamide therapy and the response.
3. Question clients concerning any possible intestinal problems, urinary tract obstructions, or allergies.
4. If the client is pregnant, the physician should be told so that another type of medication not harmful to a developing fetus may be used.
5. Document symptoms of infection. Ensure that appropriate liver and renal function studies as well as C&S data have been performed prior to initiating therapy.
6. Obtain baseline CBC, blood sugar levels, and bleeding times, and monitor throughout drug therapy.

Interventions

1. During drug therapy, assess clients for any of the following reactions that may require withdrawal of the drug:
   - Skin rashes, abdominal pain, reports of anorexia, irritation of the mouth or tingling of the extremities
   - Blood dyscrasias (characterized by sore throat, fever, pallor, purpura, jaundice, or weakness)
   - Serum sickness (characterized by eruptions of purpuric spots and pain in limbs and joints). Serum sickness may develop 7–10 days after initiation of therapy.
   - Early symptoms of Stevens-Johnson syndrome (characterized by high fever, severe

headaches, stomatitis, conjunctivitis, rhinitis, urethritis, and balanitis [inflammation of the tip of the penis])
- Jaundice, which may indicate hepatic involvement, with onset 3–5 days after initiation of therapy
- Renal involvement (characterized by renal colic, oliguria, anuria, hematuria, and proteinuria)
- Ecchymosis and hemorrhage (caused by decreased synthesis of vitamin K by intestinal bacteria)
- Hemolytic anemia especially in the elderly
- Behavioral changes or acute mental disturbances

2. Monitor intake and output and record. Encourage adequate fluid intake to prevent crystalluria. Observe urinalysis for evidence of crystals. Minimum output of urine should be 1,500 ml daily. Test pH level of urine to determine excess acidity. Administration of a particularly insoluble sulfonamide may require alkalinization of urine. The drug of choice for this purpose is sodium bicarbonate.

3. If administering long-acting sulfonamides, adequate fluid intake must be maintained for 24–48 hr after the drug has been discontinued.

Client/Family Teaching

1. Provide a printed list of drug side effects and advise which to report immediately.

2. Take drug on time and as prescribed and remain under medical supervision during course of therapy despite feeling better.

3. Certain sulfonamides may color urine orange-red or brown. This should not be cause for alarm but should be reported to the physician.

4. Take medication with 6–8 oz (180–240 ml) of water and maintain adequate fluid intake for 24–48 hr after discontinuing drug.

5. Explain how to monitor intake and output and instruct client to maintain a record during the course of therapy. Unless contraindicated, encourage client to consume at least 3 L of fluid/day.

6. Demonstrate how to test urine pH daily and advise when to report changes in acidity because additional drug therapy may need to be instituted.

7. Discourage the use of vitamin C while on therapy since it may make the urine more acidic and contribute to crystal formation.

8. If clients are also taking anticoagulants, instruct them to be particularly alert to evidence of an increase in bleeding tendencies (bruising, cuts that bleed for a longer time than usual, etc.) and to report.

9. Avoid prolonged exposure to sunlight because drug may cause a photosensitivity reaction. Wear protective clothing, sunglasses, and sunscreen when exposure is necessary.

10. Report any changes in vision or hearing to the physician.

11. Do not perform activities that require mental alertness until drug effects realized.

Evaluation: Evaluate client for:
- Evidence of knowledge and understanding of illness and level of compliance

- Negative laboratory C&S results and note any evidence of organism resistance to sulfonamide
- Clinical evidence of resolution of infection and reports of symptomatic improvement

SYMPATHOMIMETIC DRUGS

See also the following individual entries:

Albuterol
Bitolterol Mesylate
Dobutamine Hydrochloride
Dopamine Hydrochloride
Ephedrine
Ephedrine Hydrochloride
Ephedrine Sulfate
Epinephrine
Epinephrine Bitartrate
Epinephrine Borate
Epinephrine Hydrochloride
Ethylnorepinephrine
  Hydrochloride
Isoetharine Hydrochloride
Isoetharine Mesylate
Isoproterenol Hydrochloride
Isoproterenol Sulfate
Levarterenol Bitartrate
Mephentermine Sulfate
Metaproterenol Sulfate
Metaraminol Bitartrate
Naphazoline Hydrochloride
Oxymetazolone Hydrochloride
Phenylephrine Hydrochloride
Phenylpropanolamine
  Hydrochloride
Pirbuterol Acetate
Pseudoephedrine
  Hydrochloride
Pseudoephedrine Sulfate
Terbutaline Sulfate
Xylometazoline Sulfate

General Statement: The adrenergic drugs supplement, mimic, and reinforce the messages transmitted by the natural neurohormones—norepinephrine and epinephrine. These hormones are responsible for transmitting nerve impulses at the postganglionic neurojunctions of the sympathetic nervous system. The adrenergic drugs work in two ways: (1) by mimicking the action of norepinephrine or epinephrine (directly acting sympathomimetics) or (2) by causing or regulating the release of the natural neurohormones from their storage sites at the nerve terminals (indirectly acting sympathomimetics). Some drugs exhibit a combination of effects 1 and 2.

The myoneural junction is equipped with special receptors for the neurohormones. These receptors have been classified into two types: alpha (α) and beta (β), according to whether they respond to norepinephrine, epinephrine, or isoproterenol and to certain blocking agents. Alpha-adrenergic receptors are blocked by phenoxybenzamine and phentolamine, whereas beta-adrenergic receptors are blocked by propranolol and similar drugs.

Both alpha and beta receptors have been divided into subtypes. Thus adrenergic stimulation of receptors will manifest the following general effects:

Alpha-1-adrenergic: /
  Vasoconstriction, decongestion, constriction of the pupil of the eye, contraction of splenic capsule, contraction of the trigone-sphincter muscle of the urinary bladder.
Alpha-2-adrenergic: / Presynaptic to regulate amount of transmitter released; decrease tone, motility, and secretory

activity of the GI tract (possibly involved in hypersecretory response also); decrease insulin secretion.

Beta-1-adrenergic: / Myocardial contraction (inotropic), regulation of heartbeat (chronotropic), improved impulse conduction, increase lipolysis.

Beta-2-adrenergic: / Peripheral vasodilation, bronchial dilation; decrease tone, motility, and secretory activity of the GI tract; increase renin secretion.

In addition, adrenergic agents affect the exocrine glands, the salivary glands, and the CNS. The adrenergic stimulants discussed in this section act preferentially on one or more of the above receptor subtypes; their pharmacologic effect must be carefully monitored and balanced.

Uses: Sympathomimetic agents are mainly used for the treatment of shock induced by sudden cardiac arrest, decompensation, myocardial infarction, trauma, bronchodilation, acute renal failure, drug reactions, anaphylaxis. Adrenergic drugs are also used to reverse bronchospasm caused by bronchial asthma, emphysema, chronic bronchitis, and other respiratory disorders. Sympathomimetic drugs having predominantly alpha-receptor activity are used for the relief of nasal and nasopharyngeal congestion due to rhinitis, sinusitis, head colds. See individual drugs.

Contraindications: Tachycardia due to arrhythmias or digitalis toxicity.

Special Concerns: Use with caution in hyperthyroidism, diabetes, prostatic hypertrophy, seizures, de-generative heart disease, especially in geriatric clients or those with asthma, emphysema, or psychoneuroses. Also, use with caution in clients with coronary insufficiency, coronary artery disease, hypertension, or history of stroke.

Side Effects: *CV:* Tachycardia, arrhythmias, palpitations, blood pressure changes, anginal pain, precordial pain, pallor, cerebral hemorrhage. *GI:* Nausea, vomiting, heartburn, anorexia, altered taste. *CNS:* Restlessness, anxiety, tension, insomnia, hyperkinesis, drowsiness, vertigo, irritability, dizziness, headache, tremors. *Other:* Pulmonary edema, respiratory difficulties, muscle cramps, coughing, bronchospasms, irritation of oropharynx.

Drug Interactions

Beta-adrenergic blocking agents / Inhibit adrenergic stimulation of the heart and bronchial tree; cause bronchial constriction; hypertension, asthma, not relieved by adrenergic agents

Ammonium chloride / ↓ Effect of sympathomimetics due to ↑ excretion by kidney

Anesthetics / Halogenated anesthetics sensitize heart to adrenergics—causes cardiac arrhythmias

Anticholinergics / Concomitant use aggravates glaucoma

Antidiabetics / Hyperglycemic effect of epinephrine may necessitate ↑ in dosage of insulin or oral hypoglycemic agents

Corticosteroids / Chronic use with sympathomimetics may result in or aggravate glaucoma; aerosols containing sympathomimetics and corticosteroids may be lethal in asthmatic children

Digitalis glycosides / Combination may cause cardiac arrhythmias

Furazolidone / Furazolidone ↑ alpha-adrenergic effects of sympathomimetics

Guanethidine / Direct-acting sympathomimetics ↑ effects of guanethidine, while indirect-acting sympathomimetics ↓ effects of guanethidine

MAO inhibitors / All effects of sympathomimetics are potentiated; symptoms include hypertensive crisis with possible intracranial hemorrhage, hyperthermia, convulsions, coma; death may occur

Methyldopa / ↑ Effects of sympathomimetics

Methylphenidate / Potentiates pressor effect of sympathomimetics; combination hazardous in glaucoma

Oxytocics / ↑ Chance of severe hypertension

Phenothiazines / ↑ Risk of cardiac arrhythmias

Reserpine / ↑ Risk of hypertension following use of direct-acting sympathomimetics and ↓ effect of indirect-acting sympathomimetics

Sodium bicarbonate / ↑ Effect of sympathomimetics due to ↓ excretion by kidney

Thyroxine / Potentiation of pressor response of sympathomimetics

Tricyclic antidepressants / ↑ Effect of direct-acting sympathomimetics and ↓ effect of indirect-acting sympathomimetics

NURSING CONSIDERATIONS

Administration/Storage

1. Review the list of drugs with which adrenergic agents interact.

2. Discard colored solutions.

3. When administering IV infusions of adrenergic drugs, use an electronic infusion device and administer in a monitored environment.

Assessment

1. Determine if the client has any history of sensitivity to adrenergic drugs.

2. In taking the nursing history, note especially if the client has a history of tachycardia, endocrine disturbances, or respiratory tract problems and document.

3. Obtain baseline data regarding the client's general physical condition and hemodynamic status including ECG, VS, and appropriate laboratory data.

Interventions

1. During the period of dosage adjustment, closely monitor and record blood pressure and pulse.

2. Monitor intake and output and vital signs throughout therapy.

3. Assess IV site frequently to ensure patency.

Client/Family Teaching

1. Discuss prescribed drug and provide printed material regarding potential side effects of this drug therapy.

2. Explain the adverse side effects of the drugs and the importance of reporting all side effects to the physician.

3. Instruct the client not to increase the dosage of medication and not to take the medication more frequently than prescribed while on maintenance doses. If symptoms be-

come more severe, client should consult the physician.

4. Advise the client to take the medication early in the day because these drugs may cause insomnia.

SPECIAL NURSING CONSIDERATIONS FOR ADRENERGIC BRONCHODILATORS

Assessment

1. Obtain a full baseline client history prior to starting the drug therapy.
2. Review the contraindications for adrenergic bronchodilators.
3. Note any previous experience client may have had with this class of drugs.
4. Assess and record the client's vital signs prior to administering the medication.
5. Obtain arterial blood gases as a baseline against which to measure the influence of medication once therapy begins.

Interventions

1. Monitor BP and pulse after therapy begins to assess client's cardiovascular response.
2. Observe the effects of the drug on the client's CNS and if pronounced, adjust the dosage of medication and the frequency of administration.
3. If the client has status asthmaticus and abnormal arterial blood gases, continue to provide oxygen mixture and ventilating assistance even though the symptoms appear to be relieved by the bronchodilator.
4. To prevent depression of respiratory effort, administer oxygen on the basis of the evaluation of the client's clinical symptoms and the arterial blood gases.
5. If 3–5 aerosol treatments of the same agent have been administered within the last 6–12 hr, with only minimal relief, further treatment is not advised.
6. If the client's dyspnea worsens after repeated excessive use of the inhaler, paradoxical airway resistance may occur. Be prepared to assist with alternative therapy.

Client/Family Teaching

1. To improve lung ventilation and reduce fatigue during eating, start inhalation therapy upon arising in the morning and before meals.
2. A single aerosol treatment is usually enough to control an asthma attack. Overuse of adrenergic bronchodilators may result in reduced effectiveness, possible paradoxical reaction, and cardiac arrest.
3. Increased fluid intake aids in liquefying secretions.
4. If more than 3 aerosol treatments in a 24-hr period are required for relief, contact the physician.
5. If dizziness or chest pain occurs, or if there is no relief when the usual dose of medication is used, consult the physician.
6. Avoid OTC preparations and any other adrenergic medications unless expressly ordered by the physician.
7. Regular, consistent use of the medication is essential for maximum benefit, but overuse can be life-threatening.
8. Demonstrate how to accom-

plish postural drainage. Explain how to cough productively and show family how to clap and vibrate the chest to promote good respiratory hygiene.

9. Explain the appropriate technique for use and care of prescribed inhalers and respiratory equipment.

10. For clients using inhalable medications and bronchodilators, advise to use the bronchodilator first and to wait 5 min before administering the other medication unless otherwise ordered by the physician.

11. Advise client to avoid crowds during "flu seasons", to dress warmly in cold weather, and to stay in air conditioning during hot, humid days to prevent exacerbations of illness.

Evaluation: Evaluate client for:

- Evidence of knowledge and understanding of the illness and determine compliance with prescribed medication regimen
- A positive clinical response as evidenced by a reduction in the symptoms for which the therapy was originally prescribed

TETRACYCLINES

See also the following individual entries:

Doxycycline Calcium
Doxycycline Hyclate
Doxycycline Monohydrate
Oxytetracycline
Oxytetracycline Hydrochloride
Tetracycline
Tetracycline Hydrochloride

Action/Kinetics: The tetracyclines inhibit protein synthesis by microorganisms by binding to a crucial ribosomal subunit (50S), thereby interfering with protein synthesis. The drugs block the binding of aminoacyl transfer RNA to the messenger RNA complex. Cell wall synthesis is not inhibited. The drugs are mostly bacteriostatic and are effective only against multiplying bacteria. Tetracyclines are well absorbed from the stomach and upper small intestine. They are well distributed throughout all tissues and fluids and diffuse through noninflamed meninges and the placental barrier. They become deposited in the fetal skeleton and calcifying teeth. **t½:** 7–18.6 hr (see individual agents) and is increased in the presence of renal impairment. The drugs bind to serum protein (range: 20%–93%; see individual agents). The drugs are concentrated in the liver in the bile and are excreted mostly unchanged in the urine and feces.

Uses: Used mainly for infections caused by *Rickettsia, Chlamydia,* and *Mycoplasma.* Due to development of resistance, tetracyclines are usually not used for infections by common gram-negative or gram-positive organisms.

Tetracyclines are the drugs of choice for rickettsial infections such as Rocky Mountain spotted fever, endemic typhus, and others. They are also the drugs of choice for psittacosis, lymphogranuloma venereum, and urethritis due to *Mycoplasma hominis* and *Ureaplasma urealyticum.* Epididymo-orchitis due to *Chlamydia trachomatis* and/or *Neisseria gonorrhoeae.* Atypical pneumonia caused by *Mycoplasma pneumoniae.* Adjunct in the treatment of trachoma.

Tetracyclines are the drugs of choice for gram-negative bacteria causing bartonellosis, brucellosis, granuloma inguinale, cholera. They are used as alternatives for the treatment of plague, tularemia, chancroid, or *Campylobacter fetus* infections. Prophylaxis of plague after exposure. Infections caused by *Acinetobacter, Bacteroides, Enterobacter aerogenes, Escherichia coli, Shigella.* Respiratory and/or urinary tract infections caused by *Hemophilus influenzae* or *Klebsiella pneumoniae.*

As an alternative to penicillin for uncomplicated gonorrhea or disseminated gonococcal infections, especially with penicillin allergy. Acute pelvic inflammatory disease. Tetracyclines are also useful as an alternative to penicillin for early syphilis.

Although not generally used for gram-positive infections, tetracyclines may be beneficial in anthrax, *Listeria* infections, and actinomycosis. They have also been used in conjunction with quinine sulfate for chloroquine-resistant *Plasmodium falciparum* malaria and as an intracavitary injection to control pleural or pericardial effusions caused by metastatic carcinoma. As an adjunct to amebicides in acute intestinal amebiasis. Used orally to treat uncomplicated endocervical, rectal, or urethral *Chlamydia* infections.

Topical uses include skin granulomas caused by *Mycobacterium marinum;* ophthalmic bacterial infections causing blepharitis, conjunctivitis, or keratitis; and as an adjunct in the treatment of ophthalmic chlamydial infections such as trachoma or inclusion conjunctivitis. Tetracyclines are used as an alternative to silver nitrate for prophylaxis of neonatal gonococcal ophthalmia. Vaginitis. Severe acne.

Contraindications: Hypersensitivity; avoid drug during tooth development stage (last trimester of pregnancy, neonatal period, during breast-feeding, and during childhood up to 8 years) because tetracyclines interfere with enamel formation and dental pigmentation. Never administer intrathecally.

Special Concerns: Use with caution and at reduced dosage in clients with impaired kidney function.

Side Effects: *GI* (most common): Nausea, vomiting, thirst, diarrhea, anorexia, sore throat, flatulence, epigastric distress, bulky loose stools. Less commonly, stomatitis, dysphagia, black hairy tongue, glossitis, or inflammatory lesions of the anogenital area. Rarely, pseudomembranous colitis. Oral dosage forms may cause esophageal ulcers, especially in clients with esophageal obstructive element or hiatal hernia. *Allergic* (rare): Urticaria, pericarditis, polyarthralgia, fever, rash, pulmonary infiltrates with eosinophilia, angioneurotic edema, worsening of systemic lupus erythematosus, anaphylaxis, purpura. *Skin:* Photosensitivity, maculopapular and erythematous rashes, exfoliative dermatitis (rare), onycholysis, discoloration of nails. *CNS:* Dizziness, lightheadedness, unsteadiness, paresthesias. *Hematologic:* Eosinophilia, hemolytic anemia, neutropenia, thrombocytopenia, thrombocytopenic purpura. *Hepatic:* Fatty liver, increases in liver enzymes; rarely, hepatotoxicity, hepatitis, hepatic cholestasis. *Miscellaneous:* Candidal superinfections including oral and vaginal candidiasis, discoloration of infants' and children's teeth, bone lesions, delayed bone growth, abnormal pigmentation of the conjunctiva, pseudotumor cerebri in adults and bulging fontanels in infants.

IV administration may cause thrombophlebitis; IM injections are painful and may cause induration at the injection site.

The administration of deteriorated tetracyclines may result in Fanconi-like syndrome characterized by nausea, vomiting, acidosis, proteinuria, glycosuria, aminoaciduria, polydipsia, polyuria, hypokalemia.

Drug Interactions

Aluminum salts / ↓ Effect of tetracyclines due to ↓ absorption from GI tract

Antacids, oral / ↓ Effect of tetracyclines due to ↓ absorption from GI tract

Anticoagulants, oral / IV tetracyclines ↑ hypoprothrombinemia

Bismuth salts / ↓ Effect of tetracyclines due to ↓ absorption from GI tract

Bumetanide / ↑ Risk of kidney toxicity

Calcium salts / ↓ Effect of tetracyclines due to ↓ absorption from GI tract

Cimetidine / ↓ Effect of tetracyclines due to ↓ absorption from GI tract

Contraceptives, oral / ↓ Effect of oral contraceptives

Digoxin / Tetracyclines ↑ bioavailability of digoxin

Diuretics, thiazide / ↑ Risk of kidney toxicity

Ethacrynic acid / ↑ Risk of kidney toxicity

Furosemide / ↑ Risk of kidney toxicity

Insulin / Tetracyclines may ↓ insulin requirement

Iron preparations / ↓ Effect of tetracyclines due to ↓ absorption from GI tract

Lithium / Either ↑ or ↓ levels of lithium

Magnesium salts / ↓ Effect of tetracyclines due to ↓ absorption from GI tract

Methoxyflurane / ↑ Risk of kidney toxicity

Penicillins / Tetracyclines may mask bactericidal effect of penicillins

Sodium bicarbonate / ↓ Effect of tetracyclines due to ↓ absorption from GI tract

Zinc salts / ↓ Effect of tetracyclines due to ↓ absorption from GI tract

Laboratory Test Interferences: False + or ↑ urinary catecholamines and urinary protein (degraded); ↑ coagulation time. False (−) or ↓ urinary urobilinogen, glucose tests (see *Nursing Considerations*). Prolonged use or high doses may change liver function tests and WBC counts.

Dosage: See individual drugs.

NURSING CONSIDERATIONS

See also *General Nursing Considerations For All Anti-Infectives*, p. 83

Administration/Storage

1. Do not use outdated or deteriorated drugs because a Fanconi-like syndrome may occur (see *Side Effects*).
2. Discard unused capsules to prevent use of deteriorated medication.
3. Administer IM into large muscle mass to avoid extravasation into subcutaneous or fatty tissue.
4. Administer on an empty stomach at least 1 hr before or 2 hr after meals. Withhold antacids, iron salts, dairy foods, and

other foods high in calcium for at least 2 hr after PO administration. Do not administer milk with tetracyclines.

Assessment

1. Note any evidence of impaired kidney function.
2. Determine if client has any history of colitis or other bowel problems.
3. If the client is female and pregnant, determine what trimester she is in.
4. Note symptoms of infection and ensure that baseline laboratory studies have been performed including BUN, creatinine, C&S etc.

Interventions

1. If client experiences gastric distress following administration of medication, report to physician. Suggest that the client be permitted to have a light meal with the medication to reduce distress. An alternative would be to reduce the individual dose of the medication but increase the frequency of administration.
2. Monitor VS and I&O. Maintain adequate intake and output because renal dysfunction may result in drug accumulation, leading to toxicity. Assess client with impaired kidney function for increased BUN, acidosis, anorexia, nausea, vomiting, weight loss, and dehydration. Continue assessment after cessation of therapy because symptoms may appear latently.
3. Prevent or treat pruritus ani by cleansing the anal area with water several times a day and/or after each bowel movement. Observe for symptoms of enterocolitis, such as diarrhea, pyrexia, abdominal distention, and scanty urine. These symptoms may necessitate discontinuing drug and substituting another antibiotic.
4. If GI disturbances occur, avoid antacids that contain calcium, magnesium, or aluminum.
5. Assess client on IV therapy for nausea, vomiting, chills, fever, and hypertension resulting from too rapid administration or an excessively high dose. Slow rate of IV infusion and report if symptoms occur.
6. Observe infant for bulging fontanelle, which may be caused by a too rapid rate of IV infusion. Slow IV infusion rate and report.
7. Indications of side effects such as sore throat, dysphagia, fever, dizziness, hoarseness, and inflammation of mucous membranes of the body. Candidal superinfections should be documented and reported.
8. Assess client with impaired hepatic or renal function for altered level of consciousness or other CNS disturbances and report.
9. Observe for onycholysis (loosening or detachment of the nail from the nail bed) or discoloration and take appropriate precautions.

Client/Family Teaching

1. Avoid direct or artificial sunlight, which can cause a severe sunburn-like reaction, and report erythema if it occurs. Wear protective clothing, sunglasses, and a sunscreen if exposure is necessary.
2. Zinc tablets or vitamin prep-

arations containing zinc may interfere with absorption of tetracyclines. Identify food sources high in zinc that should be avoided (oysters, fresh and raw; cooked lobster, dry oat flakes, steamed crabs, veal, liver, etc.)

3. Do not take tetracyclines with milk, cheese, ice cream, yogurt, or other foods containing calcium. If dose is taken with meals, avoid these foods for 2 hr after the meal.

4. Tetracyclines interfere with formation of tooth enamel and dental pigmentation from pregnancy through age 8.

5. Explain how to prevent or treat pruritus ani by cleansing the anal area with water several times a day and/or after each bowel movement.

Evaluation: Evaluate client for:
- Evidence of knowledge and understanding of illness and level of compliance as based on response to therapy and teaching
- Laboratory C&S reports to evaluate response to therapy and for any evidence of organism resistance to drug therapy
- Clinical evidence of resolution of infection and reports of symptomatic improvement

THEOPHYLLINE DERIVATIVES

See also the following individual entries:

Aminophylline
Oxtriphylline
Theophylline

General Statement: Asthma is a disease characterized by difficulty in breathing, resulting from smooth muscle contraction of the bronchi and bronchioles, edema of the mucosa of the respiratory tract, or mucus secretions that adhere to the walls of the bronchi and bronchioles. The cause of asthma is not known with certainty but, in some clients, allergy is the underlying reason.

The overall objectives of drug therapy for asthma are to open blocked airways and to alter the characteristics of respiratory tract fluid. The drugs and drug classes used to treat asthma are bronchodilators, such as theophyllines and sympathomimetic amines, mucolytics, corticosteroids, and cromolyn sodium.

Action/Kinetics: The theophylline derivatives are plant alkaloids, which, like caffeine, belong to the xanthine family. They stimulate the CNS, directly relax the smooth muscles of the bronchi and pulmonary blood vessels (relieve bronchospasms), produce diuresis, inhibit uterine contractions, stimulate gastric acid secretion, and increase the rate and force of contraction of the heart. The bronchodilator activity of theophyllines is due to direct relaxation of the bronchiolar smooth muscle and pulmonary blood vessels, which relieves bronchospasm. Theophylline was thought to act by inhibiting phosphodiesterase, which resulted in an increase in cyclic adenosine monophosphate (cAMP). cAMP increased the release of endogenous epinephrine resulting in bronchodilation. However, this effect is negligible at doses used clinically. Although the exact mechanism is not known, theophyllines may act by altering the calcium levels of smooth muscle, blocking adenosine receptors, inhibiting the effect of prostaglandins on smooth muscle, and inhibiting the release of slow-reacting substance of anaphylaxis (SRS-A) and histamine. Aminophylline, oxtriphylline, and theophylline sodium glycinate release free theophylline in vivo. Response to the drugs is highly individualized. Theophylline is well absorbed from uncoated plain tablets and oral liquids. *Theophylline salts:* **Onset:** 1–5 hr, depending on route and formulation. **Therapeutic plasma levels:** 10–20 mcg/ml. $t^{1/2}$: 3–15 hr in nonsmoking adults, 4–5 hr in adult heavy smokers, 1–9 hr in children, and 20–30 hr for premature neonates. An increased $t^{1/2}$ may be seen in individuals with CHF, alcoholism, liver dysfunction, or respiratory infections. Because of great variations in the rate of absorption (due to dosage form, food, dose level) as well as its extremely narrow therapeutic range, theophylline therapy is best monitored by determination of the serum levels. If these determinations cannot be obtained, saliva (contains 60% of corresponding theophylline serum levels) determinations can be used. 85%–90% metabolized in the liver and various metabolites, including the active 3-methylxanthine. Theophylline is metabolized partially to caffeine in the neonate. The premature neonate excretes 50% unchanged theophylline and may accumulate the caffeine metabolite. Excretion is through the kidneys (about 10% unchanged in adults).

Uses: Prophylaxis and treatment of bronchial asthma. Reversible bronchospasms associated with chronic bronchitis, emphysema, and chronic obstructive pulmonary disease. *Investigational:* Treatment of neonatal apnea and Cheyne-Stokes respiration.

Contraindications: Hypersensitivity to any xanthine, peptic ulcer, seizure disorders (unless on medication), hypotension, coronary artery disease, angina pectoris.

Special Concerns: Safe use during pregnancy (category: C) has not been established. Use during lactation may result in irritability, insomnia, and fretfulness in the infant. Use with caution in premature infants due to the possible accumulation of caffeine. Xanthines are not usually tolerated by small children because of excessive CNS stimulation. Geriatric clients may manifest an increased risk of toxicity. Use with caution in the presence of gastritis, alcoholism, acute cardiac diseases, hypoxemia, severe renal and hepatic disease, severe hypertension, severe myocardial damage, hyperthyroidism, glaucoma.

Side Effects: Side effects are uncommon at serum theophylline levels less than 20 mcg/ml. At levels greater than 20 mcg/ml, 75% of individuals experience side effects including nausea, vomiting, diarrhea, irritability, insomnia, and headache. At levels of 35 mcg/ml or greater, individuals may manifest cardiac arrhythmias, hypotension, tachycardia, hyperglycemia, seizures, brain damage, or death. *GI:* Nausea, vomiting, diarrhea, anorexia, epigastric pain, hematemesis, dyspepsia, rectal irritation (following use of suppositories), rectal bleeding, gastroesophageal reflux during sleep or while recumbent (theophylline). *CNS:* Headache, insomnia, irritability, fever, dizziness, lightheadedness, vertigo, reflex hyperexcitability, seizures, depression, speech abnormalities, alternating periods of mutism and hyperactivity, brain damage, death. *CV:* Hypotension, life-threatening ventricular arrhythmias, palpitations, tachycardia, peripheral vascular collapse, extrasystoles. *Renal:* Proteinuria, excretion of erythrocytes and renal tubular cells, dehydration due to diuresis, urinary retention (men with prostatic hypertrophy). *Other:* Tachypnea, respiratory arrest, fever, flushing, hyperglycemia, antidiuretic hormone syndrome, leukocytosis, rash, alopecia. **Note:** Aminophylline given by rapid IV may produce hypotension, flushing, palpitations, precordial pain, headache, dizziness, or hyperventilation. Also, the ethylenediamine in aminophylline may cause allergic reactions, including urticaria and skin rashes.

Symptoms of Overdose: Agitation, headache, nervousness, insomnia, tachycardia, extrasystoles, anorexia, nausea, vomiting, fasciculations, tachypnea, tonic/clonic seizures. The first signs of toxicity may be seizures or ventricular arrhythmias. Toxicity is usually associated with parenteral administration but can be observed after oral administration, especially in children.

Drug Interactions

Allopurinol / ↑ Theophylline levels

Aminogluthethimide / ↓ Theophylline levels

Barbiturates / ↓ Theophylline levels

Benzodiazepines / Sedative effect may be antagonized by theophylline

Beta-adrenergic agonists / Additive effects

Beta-adrenergic blocking agents / ↑ Theophylline levels

Calcium channel blocking drugs / ↑ Theophylline levels

Carbamazepine / Either ↑ or ↓ theophylline levels

Charcoal / ↓ Theophylline levels

Cimetidine / ↑ Theophylline levels

Ciprofloxacin / ↑ Plasma levels of theophylline with ↑ possibility of side effects

Corticosteroids / ↑ Theophylline levels

Digitalis / Theophylline ↑ toxicity of digitalis

Disulfram / ↑ Theophylline levels

Ephedrine and other sympathomimetics / ↑ Theophylline levels

Erythromycin / ↑ Effect of theophylline due to ↓ breakdown by liver

Ethacrynic acid / Either ↑ or ↓ theophylline levels

Furosemide / Either ↑ or ↓ theophylline levels

Halothane / ↑ Risk of cardiac arrhythmias

Interferon / ↑ Theophylline levels

Isoniazid / Either ↑ or ↓ theophylline levels

Ketamine / Seizures of the extensor-type

Ketoconazole / ↓ Theophylline levels

Lithium / ↓ Effect of lithium due to ↑ rate of excretion

Loop diuretics / ↓ Theophylline levels

Mexiletine / ↑ Theophylline levels

Muscle relaxants, nondepolarizing / Theophylline ↓ effect of these drugs

Oral contraceptives / ↑ Effect of theophyllines due to ↓ breakdown by liver

Phenytoin / ↓ Theophylline levels

Propofol / Theophyllines ↓ sedative effect of propofol

Quinolones / ↑ Theophylline levels

Reserpine / ↑ Risk of tachycardia

Rifampin / ↓ Theophylline levels

Sulfinpyrazone / ↓ Theophylline levels

Sympathomimetics / ↓ Theophylline levels

Tetracyclines / ↑ Risk of theophylline toxicity

Thiabendazole / ↑ Theophylline levels

Thyroid hormones / ↓ Theophylline levels in hypothyroid clients

Tobacco smoking / ↓ Effect of theophylline due to ↑ breakdown by liver

Troleandomycin / ↑ Effect of theophylline due to ↓ breakdown by liver

Verapamil / ↑ Effect of theophyllines

Laboratory Test Interferences: ↑ Plasma free fatty acids, bilirubin, urinary catecholamines, erythrocyte sedimentation rate. Interference with uric acid tests and tests for furosemide, probenecid, theobromine, and phenylbutazone.

Dosage: Individualized. Initially, dosage should be adjusted according to plasma level of drug. Usual: 10–20 mcg theophylline/ml plasma. The dose of the various salts should be equivalent based on the content of anhydrous theophylline. See individual agents.

NURSING CONSIDERATIONS

Administration/Storage

1. Review the list of agents with which theophylline derivatives interact.

2. Dilute drugs and maintain proper infusion rates to minimize problems of overdosage. Use an infusion pump to regulate infusion of IV solutions.

3. Wait to initiate oral therapy for at least 4–6 hr after switching from IV therapy.

4. *Treatment of Overdose:*
   - Have ipecac syrup, gastric lavage equipment, and cathartics available to treat overdose if the client is conscious and not having seizures. Otherwise a mechanical ventilator, oxygen, diazepam, and IV fluids may be necessary for the treatment of overdosage.
   - For postseizure coma, an airway must be maintained and the client oxygenated. To remove the drug, perform only gastric lavage and give the cathartic and activated charcoal by a large bore gastric lavage tube. Charcoal hemoperfusion may be necessary.
   - Atrial arrhythmias may be treated with verapamil and ventricular arrhythmias may be treated with lidocaine or procainamide.
   - IV fluids are used to treat acid-base imbalance, hypotension, and dehydration. Hypotension may also be treated with vasopressors.
   - Tepid water sponge baths or a hypothermic blanket are used to treat hyperpyrexia.
   - Apnea is treated with artificial respiration.
   - Serum levels of theophylline must be monitored until they fall below 20 mcg/ml as secondary rises of theophylline may occur, especially with sustained-release products.

Assessment

1. Assess the client for any history of hypersensitivity to xanthine compounds.
2. Note if the client has a history of hypotension, coronary artery disease, angina, peptic ulcer disease, or seizure disorders. These drugs generally should not be used in clients with these problems.
3. Determine if the client smokes cigarettes or has a history of smoking marijuana. These habits induce hepatic metabolism of the drug. Smokers require an increase in the dosage of drug from 50%–100%.
4. Assess diet habits because these can influence the excretion of theophylline. A client eating a high-protein and/or low-carbohydrate diet will have an increased excretion of the drug. Clients eating a low-protein and/or high-carbohydrate diet will have a decrease in the excretion of theophylline. Therefore, dietary intake is an important part of the premedication assessment.
5. Document onset of symptoms and obtain a description of what client experienced that required medication therapy. Obtain baseline blood pressure and pulse prior to starting drug therapy.

Interventions

1. Monitor BP and pulse closely during therapy. Report any wide variations from normal to the physician.
2. Observe closely for signs of toxicity such as nausea, anorexia, insomnia, irritability, hyperexcitability, or cardiac arrhythmias. Document and report to the physician.
3. Observe small children in particular for excessive CNS stimulation; children often are unable to report side effects.
4. To avoid epigastric pain when the drug is administered orally, give the medication with a snack or with meals.
5. Monitor for therapeutic serum levels of theophylline in the 10–20 mcg/ml range. Levels above 20 mcg/ml require an adjustment in the dosage of drug.

Client/Family Teaching

1. Notify the physician if nausea, vomiting, GI pain, or restlessness occurs.
2. Take the medication around the clock and only as prescribed, because more is *not* better.
3. Do not smoke because smoking may aggravate underlying medical conditions as well as interfere with drug absorption.
4. Explain to clients how to protect themselves from acute exacerbations of illness by avoiding crowds, dressing warmly in cold weather, covering their mouth and nose so that cold air is not directly inhaled, staying in air conditioning during excessively hot and humid weather, maintaining proper diet and nutrition and adequate fluid intake.
5. Provide printed material listing the early signs and symptoms of infections, adverse side effects of drug therapy, and when to call the physician.
6. When secretions become thick

and tacky, increase intake of fluids. This thins secretions and assists in their removal.

7. Avoid overexertion at all times.
8. Hold medication and report immediately any side effects or CNS depression in children and infants receiving drug therapy.
9. Review dietary restrictions and advise to limit intake of xanthine-containing products such as coffee, colas, and chocolate.

Evaluation: Evaluate client for:
- Evidence of a positive clinical response characterized by improved airway exchange, a decrease in wheezing, and reports of improved breathing patterns
- Evidence of knowledge and understanding of illness and assess compliance with prescribed regimen
- Laboratory confirmation that serum drug levels are within therapeutic range (10–20 mcg/ml)

THIAZIDES AND RELATED DIURETICS

See also the following individual entries:

Aldactazide
Chlorothiazide
Chlorothiazide Sodium
Chlorthalidone
Dyazide
Hydrochlorothiazide
Indapamide

Action/Kinetics: The thiazide diuretics are related chemically to the sulfonamides. They are devoid of anti-infective activity but can cause the same hypersensitivity reactions as the sulfonamides.

The thiazides and related diuretics promote diuresis by decreasing the rate at which sodium and chloride are reabsorbed by the distal renal tubules of the kidney. By increasing the excretion of sodium and chloride, they force excretion of additional water. They also increase the excretion of potassium and, to a lesser extent, bicarbonate, as well as decrease the excretion of calcium and uric acid. Sodium and chloride are excreted in approximately equal amounts. The thiazides do not affect the glomerular filtration rate.

The antihypertensive mechanism of action of the thiazides is attributed to direct dilation of the arterioles, as well as to a reduction in the total fluid volume of the body and altered sodium balance. *Diuretic effect:* Usual, **Onset:** 1–2 hr. **Peak:** 4–6 hr. **Duration:** 6–24 hr. *Antihypertensive effect:* **Onset:** several days. *Optimal therapeutic effect:* 3–4 weeks.

Most thiazides are absorbed from the GI tract; a large fraction is excreted unchanged in urine.

Uses: Edema due to congestive heart failure, nephrosis, nephritis, renal failure, premenstrual syndrome, hepatic cirrhosis, corticosteroid or estrogen therapy. Hypertension. *Investigational:* Alone or in combination with allopurinol (or amiloride) for prophylaxis of calcium nephrolithiasis. Nephrogenic diabetes insipidus.

Contraindications: Hypersensitivity to drug, anuria, renal decompensation. Impaired renal function and advanced hepatic cirrhosis.

Drugs should not be used indiscriminately in clients with edema and toxemia of pregnancy, even though they may be therapeutically useful, because the thiazides may have adverse effects on the newborn (thrombocytopenia and jaundice).

Thiazides and related diuretics may precipitate myocardial infarctions in elderly clients with advanced arteriosclerosis, especially if the client is also receiving therapy with other antihypertensive agents.

Clients with advanced heart failure, renal disease, or hepatic cirrhosis are most likely to develop hypokalemia.

Thiazides may activate or worsen systemic lupus erythematosus.

Special Concerns: Geriatric clients may manifest an increased risk of hypotension and changes in electrolyte levels. Administer with caution to debilitated clients or to those with a history of hepatic coma or precoma, gout, diabetes mellitus, or during pregnancy and lactation. Particular care must be exercised when thiazides are administered concomitantly with drugs that also cause potassium loss, such as digitalis, corticosteroids, and some estrogens.

Side Effects: *Electrolyte imbalance:* Hypokalemia (most frequent) characterized by cardiac arrhythmias. Hyponatremia characterized by weakness, lethargy, epigastric distress, nausea, vomiting. Hypokalemic alkalosis. *GI:* Dry mouth, thirst, stomach pain or upset, sore throat, diarrhea, bitter taste, anorexia. *CNS:* Mood changes, vertigo, paresthesias, weakness, restlessness, anxiety, depression, nervousness, neuropathy, tiredness, fever, syncope, dizziness. *CV:* Irregular heart rate, orthostatic hypotension, venous thrombosis, excessive volume depletion, palpitations, cold extremities, allergic myocarditis. *Allergic:* Skin rashes, urticaria, photosensitivity, purpura, vasculitis, necrotizing angiitis, anaphylaxis, pruritus, hives, dry skin, pneumonitis, pulmonary edema. *Hematologic:* Agranulocytosis, thrombocytopenia, aplastic anemia, leukopenia, neutropenia, hemolytic anemia. *Endocrine:* Hyperglycemia, aggravation of preexisting diabetes mellitus, hyperuricemia, electrolyte imbalance. *GU:* Frequent urination, polyuria, nocturia, impotence, reduced libido, crystalluria. *Respiratory:* Respiratory distress, dyspnea, pneumonitis, sinus congestion, epistaxis, cough, sore throat. *Miscellaneous:* Muscle cramps, joint pain and swelling, impaired liver function, pancreatitis, jaundice, hepatic coma, acute attacks of gout, blurred vision, rhinorrhea, flushing, chills, weight loss.

Symptoms of Overdose: Electrolyte imbalance including potassium deficiency (manifested by confusion, dizziness, GI disturbances, and muscle weakness), nausea, and vomiting. More severe toxicity causes hypotension, GI irritation and hypermotility, depressed respiration, and coma.

Drug Interactions

Anticholinergic agents / ↑ Effect of thiazides due to ↑ amount absorbed from GI tract

Anticoagulants, oral / ↑ Effect of anticoagulants by concentrating circulating clotting factors and ↑ clotting factor synthesis in liver

Antidiabetic agents / Thiazides antagonize hypoglycemic effect of antidiabetic agents

Antihypertensive agents / Thiazides potentiate the effect of antihypertensive agents

Cholestyramine / ↓ Effect of thiazides due to ↓ absorption from GI tract

Colestipol / ↓ Effect of thiazides due to ↓ absorption from GI tract

Corticosteroids / Enhanced potassium loss due to potassium-losing properties of both drugs

Diazoxide / Enhanced hypotensive effect. Also, ↑ hyperglycemic response

Digitalis glycosides / Thiazides produce ↑ potassium and magnesium loss with ↑ chance of digitalis toxicity

Ethanol / Additive orthostatic hypotension

Fenfluramine / ↑ Antihypertensive effect of thiazides

Furosemide / Profound diuresis and electrolyte loss

Guanethidine / Additive hypotensive effect

Indomethacin / ↓ Effect of thiazides, possibly by inhibition of prostaglandins

Lithium / Increased risk of lithium toxicity due to ↓ renal excretion

Muscle relaxants, nondepolarizing / ↑ Effect of muscle relaxants due to hypokalemia

Norepinephrine / Thiazides ↓ arterial response to norepinephrine

Quinidine / ↑ Effect of quinidine due to ↑ renal tubular reabsorption

Reserpine / Additive hypotensive effect

Sulfonamides / ↑ Effect of thiazides due to ↓ plasma protein binding

Tetracyclines / ↑ Risk of azotemia

Tubocurarine / ↑ Muscle relaxation and ↑ hypokalemia

Vasopressors (sympathomimetics) / Thiazides ↓ responsiveness of arterioles to vasopressors

Laboratory Test Interferences: Hypokalemia, hypercalcemia, hyponatremia, hypomagnesemia, hypochloremia, hypophosphatemia, hyperuricemia. ↑ BUN, creatinine, glucose in blood and urine. ↓ Serum protein-bound iodine levels (no signs of thyroid disturbance). Initial ↑ in total cholesterol, LDL cholesterol, and triglycerides.

Dosage: Drugs are preferentially given **PO,** but some preparations can be given parenterally. They are usually given in the morning, so the peak effect occurs during the day.

NURSING CONSIDERATIONS

See also *Nursing Considerations* for *Diuretics,* p. 141.

Administration/Storage

1. May be taken with food or milk if GI upset occurs.
2. Clients resistant to one type of thiazide may respond to another.
3. Thiazides should not be taken with any other medication (including OTC drugs for asthma, cough and colds, hay fever, weight control) unless approved by the physician.
4. To minimize electrolyte imbalance, thiazides may be taken every other day or on a 3–5 day basis for treatment of edema.
5. To prevent excess hypotension, the dose of other antihypertensive agents should be reduced when beginning thiazide therapy.
6. *Treatment of Overdose:*
   - Induce emesis or perform gastric lavage followed by activated charcoal. Undertake measures to prevent aspiration.
   - Electrolyte balance, hydra-

tion, respiration, cardiovascular, and renal function must be maintained.

- Although GI effects are usually of short duration, treatment may be required.

Assessment

1. Note if the client has any history of hypersensitivity to the drug.
2. Obtain baseline electrolytes, renal and liver function tests prior to initiating therapy.
3. Note any history of heart disease, an indication that the client will require close monitoring once the drug has been administered.
4. Determine if client has a history of gout and check baseline uric acid level.

Interventions

1. If the client is to undergo surgery, anticipate that the drug will be stopped at least 48 hr before the procedure. Thiazide inhibits the pressor effects of epinephrine.
2. Evaluate dietary potassium intake. Potassium chloride supplements should be given only when dietary measures are inadequate.
3. If potassium supplements are required, use liquid preparations to avoid ulcerations that may be produced by potassium salts in the solid dosage form. Exceptions include slow-K (potassium salt imbedded in a wax matrix) and micro-K (microencapsulated potassium salt).
4. If the client has diabetes, monitor blood glucose levels more frequently after beginning thiazide therapy. It may be necessary to change the dose of insulin or oral hypoglycemic agent.

Client/Family Teaching

1. Avoid alcoholic beverages because alcohol, in combination with thiazides, causes severe hypotension.
2. Avoid eating licorice; it may precipitate severe hypokalemia.
3. Eat a diet high in potassium. Encourage clients to include orange juice, bananas, citrus fruits, broccoli, spinach, tomato juice, cucumbers, beets, dried fruits, or apricots.
4. Take thiazide diuretic in the morning to avoid interrupting sleep with the frequent need to void.
5. If clients have a history of gout, advise them to reduce their intake of purines. Provide a printed list of foods to avoid.
6. Advise the client to maintain a written record of weight. Explain that there may be some weight loss from the diuresis related to the drug therapy.
7. Caution client to rise slowly and to dangle legs before standing to minimize orthostatic effects. Sit or lie down if feeling faint or dizzy.
8. If the client has diabetes, discuss the importance of more careful monitoring of urine and finger sticks for glucose determinations. Advise the client how to adjust the hypoglycemic agent in accordance with the physician's prescribed orders and to keep the physician informed of any changes in blood glucose levels or the effectiveness of the hypoglycemic agent being used.

9. Explain the importance of taking thiazides as directed and stress the importance of reporting for scheduled follow-up visits to evaluate the effectiveness of drug therapy. Provide the client with a list of side effects that should be reported to the physician should they occur.

Evaluation: Evaluate client for:

- Evidence of a positive clinical response to the symptoms for which the therapy was prescribed (e.g., ↓ edema, ↓ BP, and ↑ urinary output)
- Evidence of knowledge and understanding of illness and assess compliance with prescribed therapy

THYROID DRUGS

See also the following individual entries:

Levothyroxin Sodium
Liothyronine Sodium
Liotrix
Thyrogolublin
Thyroid Desiccated
Thyrotropin

General Statement: The thyroid manufactures two active hormones: thyroxine and triiodothyronine, both of which contain iodine. These thyroid hormones are released into the bloodstream, where they are bound to protein.

Diseases involving the thyroid fall into two groups:

1. Hypothyroidism or diseases in which little or no hormone is produced. These can be subdivided into cretinism, resulting from a deficiency of thyroid hormone during fetal and early life, and myxedema, a deficiency of thyroid hormone in the adult. Cretinism is characterized by arrested physical and mental development, with dystrophy of the bones and soft parts and lowered basal metabolism. Myxedema is characterized by a dry, waxy swelling, with abnormal deposits of mucin in the skin. The edema is nonpitting and the facial changes are distinctive, with swollen lips and a thickened nose. Primary myxedema results from atrophy of the thyroid gland. Secondary myxedema may result from hypofunction of the pituitary gland or prolonged administration of antithyroid drugs.

2. Hyperthyroidism or conditions associated with an overproduction of hormones, as in Graves' or Basedow's disease (diffuse enlargement of the thyroid gland; often characterized by protruding eyes) and Plummer's disease, in which extra thyroid hormone is produced by a single "hot" thyroid nodule. These conditions are usually characterized by hypertrophy and hyperplasia of the thyroid and a state of extreme nervousness.

EUTHYROID OR SIMPLE, NONTOXIC GOITER (ENDEMIC GOITER): In these states, a normal or near-normal amount of hormone is produced by an enlarged thyroid gland. This condition can occur when the dietary intake of iodine is below normal. Today the disease is much rarer because iodine is added as a matter of routine to cooking salt.

In these individuals, the thyroid tends to become enlarged, especially during adolescent growth and pregnancy. Surgery may be necessary to alleviate the pressure on the trachea caused by the enlarged thyroid and to prevent the oxygen supply from being diminished.

Drugs used in the treatment of thyroid disease fall into two groups: (1) thyroid preparations used to correct thyroid deficiency diseases and (2) antithyroid drugs that reduce production of hormones by an overactive gland.

The external supply of thyroid hormones usually results in a reduction in the amount of natural hormone produced by the thyroid gland.

The accurate determination of thyroid function is crucial for the treatment of thyroid disease. Thyroid function can be evaluated by (1) total levothyroxine (T_4), (2) free levothyroxine, (3) serum liothyronine (T_3), (4) liothyronine resin uptake (RT_3U), (5) free thyroxine index, and (6) thyroid-stimulating hormone (TSH). The results of some of the tests are at times skewed by medications the client is taking, so that the effect of these drugs must be considered when evaluating the test.

Thyroid conditions are often treated by fixed combinations of levothyroxine sodium and liothyronine sodium in a ratio of 4:1. Such a preparation is liotrix (Euthroid, Thyrolar). For all information regarding these drugs, see drug entries for levothyroxine sodium and liothyronine sodium.

Action/Kinetics: The thyroid hormones regulate growth by controlling protein synthesis and regulating energy metabolism by increasing the resting or basal metabolic rate (BMR). Other metabolic effects include increased conversion of cholesterol to bile acids, increase in protein-bound iodine (PBI), increased carbohydrate utilization, and participation in the calcification of long bones.

The hormones also have a cardiostimulatory effect and can increase renal blood flow as well as the glomerular filtration rate (GFR) (diuresis). The thyroid gland is under the control of the hypothalamus and the pituitary gland, which produce TSH-releasing factor and thyrotropin (TSH), respectively. Like other hormone systems, the thyroid, pituitary, and hypothalamus work together in a feedback mechanism. Excess thyroid hormone causes a decrease in TSH, and a lack of thyroid hormone causes an increase in the production and secretion of TSH.

Uses: Replacement therapy in primary and secondary myxedema, myxedemic coma, nontoxic goiter, hypothyroidism, some thyroid tumors, chronic thyroiditis, sporadic cretinism, and thyrotropin-dependent tumors. With antithyroid drugs for thyrotoxicosis (to prevent goiter or hypothyroidism).

Contraindications: Uncorrected adrenal insufficiency, myocardial infarction, hyperthyroidism, and thyrotoxicosis. Adrenal insufficiency unless treatment with adrenocortical steroids is initiated first. Not to be used to treat obesity or infertility.

Special Concerns: Pregnancy category: A. Geriatric clients may be more sensitive to the usual adult dosage of these hormones. Use with extreme caution in the presence of angina pectoris, hypertension, and other cardiovascular diseases, renal insufficiency, and ischemic states.

Side Effects: Thyroid preparations have cumulative effects, and overdosage (e.g., symptoms of hyperthyroidism) may occur. *CV:* Arrhythmias, palpitations, angina, increased heart rate and pulse pressure, cardiac arrest, aggravation of congestive heart failure. *GI:* Cramps, diarrhea, nausea, appetite changes. *CNS:* Headache, nervousness, mental agitation, irritability, insomnia, tremors. *Miscellaneous:* Weight loss, hyperhidrosis, excessive warmth, irregular menses, heat intolerance, fever, dyspnea.

Drug Interactions

Anticoagulants / ↑ Effect of anticoagulants by ↑ hypoprothrombinemia

Antidepressants, tricyclic / ↑ Effect of antidepressants and ↑ effect of thyroid

Antidiabetic agents / Hyperglycemic effect of thyroid preparations may necessitate ↑ in dose of antidiabetic agent

Cholestyramine / ↓ Effect of thyroid hormone due to ↓ absorption from GI tract

Corticosteroids / Thyroid preparations increase tissue demands for corticosteroids. Adrenal insufficiency must be corrected with corticosteroids before administering thyroid hormones. In clients already treated for adrenal insufficiency, dosage of corticosteroids must be increased when initiating therapy with thyroid drug

Digitalis compounds / ↓ Effect of digitalis, with worsening of arrhythmias or congestive heart failure

Epinephrine / Cardiovascular effects ↑ by thyroid preparations

Estrogens / Estrogens may ↑ requirements for thyroid hormone

Ketamine / Concomitant use may result in severe hypertension and tachycardia

Levarterenol / Cardiovascular effects ↑ by thyroid preparations

Phenytoin / ↑ Effect of thyroid hormone by ↓ plasma protein binding

Salicylates / Salicylates compete for thyroid-binding sites on protein

Laboratory Test Interferences: Alter thyroid function tests. ↑ Prothrombin time. ↓ Serum cholesterol.

Dosage: Thyroid drugs are started with a low dose that is gradually increased until a satisfactory response is achieved within safe dose limits. When necessary, a decrease in dosage and a more gradual upward adjustment relieve severe side effects.

NURSING CONSIDERATIONS

Administration/Storage

1. The treatment is initiated with small doses that are gradually increased.
2. The dose of medication for a child may be the same as the dosage for an adult.
3. When changing from one thyroid drug to another, follow the specific instructions to prevent overdosage or relapse.
4. Store thyroid preparations in a cool, dark place away from moisture and light.

Assessment

1. Take a complete nursing history.
2. Review all medications the client is currently receiving to be

sure none interacts unfavorably with the antithyroid medication.
3. Note if the client is taking antidiabetic agents or is on anticoagulant therapy and document.
4. Assess the client's general physical condition and note whether the client has a history of angina, cardiac problems or any other health problems.
5. Take a baseline ECG against which to compare subsequent ECG tracings once therapy has been instituted.
6. Ensure that all laboratory studies and levels have been performed before initiating therapy.

Interventions

1. Monitor the client's thyroid function studies closely.
2. Observe the client for side effects of the drug. Complaints of headache, insomnia, and tremors should be documented and reported to the physician.
3. Observe the client on anticoagulant therapy for bleeding from any orifice or for purpura. Monitor PT/PTT closely because the action of anticoagulants is potentiated by thyroid preparations.
4. Clients with a history of angina or other cardiovascular disorders need to have their blood pressure and pulse monitored closely. If the pulse increases to more than 100 beats/min, withhold the drug and notify the physician, unless otherwise directed.
5. Take an ECG at regular intervals during the drug therapy

and compare with the baseline tracing.
6. Note the client's general response to the therapy. Complaints of abdominal cramps, weight gain, dyspnea, palpitations, angina, fatigue, or observing increased pallor or edema may indicate that the client is experiencing cardiac problems and further assessment by the physician is indicated.
7. Monitor weights. Observe for evidence of heat intolerance and client weight loss. Document and report to the physician.

Client/Family Teaching

1. Stress that the drug must be taken only while the client is under medical supervision and that it must be taken for life.
2. Side effects of the medication may not appear for 4–6 weeks after the start of therapy. Therefore, explain to clients that they should notify the physician of any new signs or symptoms. The same is true if the dosage of drug is increased.
3. Report immediately to the physician any excessive weight loss, palpitations, leg cramps, nervousness, or insomnia. Provide a printed list of the symptoms that require immediate medical attention and a number to call to report these events.
4. If the client has diabetes, explain that thyroid preparations may require adjustment of the dosage of insulin. Therefore, it is important to monitor the urine and/or blood sugar levels closely and to report any changes to the physician.

5. Note that certain foods, such as cabbage, turnips, pears, and peaches, are goitrogenic and may alter the requirements for thyroid hormone. Provide a list of such foods and have the dietitian discuss diet and assist with meal planning.

6. Thyroid hormones increase the client's toxicity to iodine. Therefore explain the need to avoid foods high in iodine (dried kelp, iodized salt, saltwater fish/shellfish), multivitamins, dentifrices, and other nonprescription medications containing iodine.

7. Have the dietitian counsel clients regarding diet so they will select foods according to the increased energy demands resulting from the medication therapy.

8. Thyroid preparations potentiate the action of anticoagulants; therefore, if the client is also receiving anticoagulant therapy, explain the importance of reporting any excessive bruising or bleeding.

9. Female clients should keep a record of their menstrual periods and report any changes.

10. Take the thyroid medication in a single morning dose to reduce the likelihood of nighttime insomnia.

11. Do not change brands of medication unless clients have first consulted with the physician.

12. Keep all scheduled follow-up visits and scheduled laboratory tests.

Evaluation: Evaluate client for:
- Evidence that appropriate weight and normal sleep patterns are maintained
- Laboratory confirmation that thyroid function studies are within desired range
- Evidence of increased mental alertness and improvement in hair and skin condition

TRICYCLIC ANTIDEPRESSANTS

See also the following individual entries:

Amitriptyline Hydrochloride
Amoxapine
Clomipramine
Desipramine Hydrochloride
Doxepin Hydrochloride
Imipramine Hydrochloride
Imipramine Pamoate
Maprotiline Hydrochloride
Nortriptyline Hydrochloride
Protriptyline Hydrochloride
Triavil
Trimipramine Maleate

General Statement: The tricyclic antidepressants are chemically related to the phenothiazines and, as such, they exhibit many of the same pharmacologic effects (e.g., anticholinergic, antiserotonin, sedative, antihistaminic, and hypotensive). The tricyclic antidepressants are less effective for depressed clients in the presence of organic brain damage or schizophrenia. Also, they can induce mania; this possibility should be kept in mind when given to clients with manic-depressive psychoses.

Action/Kinetics: Tricyclic antidepressants prevent the reuptake of norepinephrine or serotonin, or both, into the storage granules of the presynaptic nerves. This results in increased concentrations of these neurotransmitters in the synapses, which alleviates depression. (**Note:** Endogenous depression is thought to be caused by low concentrations of norepinephrine and/or serotonin.) The tricyclic antidepressants are well absorbed from the GI tract. All these drugs have a long serum half-life. Up to 4–6 days may be required to reach steady plasma levels, and maximum therapeutic effects may not be noted for 2–4 weeks. Because of the long half-life, single daily dosage may suffice. The tricyclic antidepressants are more than 90% bound to plasma protein. They are partially metabolized in the liver and excreted primarily in the urine.

Uses: Endogenous and reactive depressions. Preferred over MAO inhibitors because they are less toxic. See individual drugs for special uses, such as use in depression associated with anxiety and disturbances in sleep.

Contraindications: Severely impaired liver function. Use during acute recovery phase from myocardial infarction. Concomitant use with MAO inhibitors.

Special Concerns: Use with caution in clients with epilepsy, cardiovascular diseases, glaucoma, benign prostatic hypertrophy, suicidal tendencies, a history of urinary retention, and the elderly. Concomitant use with MAO inhibitors should be undertaken with caution. Use during pregnancy only when benefits clearly outweigh risks. Use with caution during lactation. Generally not recommended for children less than 12 years of age. Geriatric clients may be more sensitive to the anticholinergic and sedative side effects.

Side Effects: Most frequent side effects are sedation and atropine-like reactions. *CNS:* Confusion, anxiety, restlessness, insomnia, nightmares, hallucinations, delusions, mania or hypomania, headache, dizziness, inability to concentrate, panic reaction, worsening of psychoses, fatigue, weakness. *Anticholinergic:* Dry mouth, blurred vision, mydriasis, constipation, paralytic ileus, urinary retention or difficulty in urination. *GI:* Nausea, vomiting, anorexia, gastric distress, unpleasant taste, stomatitis, glossitis, cramps, increased salivation, black tongue. *CV:* Fainting, tachycardia, hypo- or hypertension, arrhythmias, heart block, possibility of palpitations, myocardial infarction, stroke. *Neurologic:* Paresthesias, numbness, incoordination, neuropathies, extrapyramidal symptoms including tardive dyskinesia, dysarthria, seizures. *Dermatologic:* Skin rashes, urticaria, flushing, pruritus, petechiae, photosensitivity, edema. *Endocrine:* Testicular swelling and gynecomastia in males, increase or decrease in libido, impotence, menstrual irregularities and galactorrhea in females, hypo- or hyperglycemia, changes in secretion of antidiuretic hormone. *Miscellaneous:* Sweating, alopecia, nasal congestion, lacrimation, increase in body temperature, chills, urinary frequency including nocturia. Bone marrow depression including thrombocytopenia, leukopenia, agranulocytosis, eosinophilia.

High dosage increases the frequency of seizures in epileptic clients and may cause epileptiform attacks in normal subjects.

Symptoms of Overdose: CNS symptoms include agitation, confusion, hallucinations, hyperactive reflexes, choreoathetosis, seizures, coma. Anticholinergic symptoms include dilated pupils, dry mouth, flushing, and hyperpyrexia. Cardiovascular toxicity includes depressed myocardial contractility, decreased heart rate, decreased coronary blood flow, tachycardia, intraventricular block, complete AV block, re-entry ventricular arrhythmias, premature ventricular contractions, ventricular tachycardia or fibrillation, sudden cardiac arrest, hypotension, pulmonary edema.

Drug Interactions

Acetazolamide / ↑ Effect of tricyclics by ↑ renal tubular reabsorption of the drug

Alcohol, ethyl / Concomitant use may lead to ↑ GI complications and ↓ performance on motor skill tests—death has been reported

Ammonium chloride / ↓ Effect of tricyclics by ↓ renal tubular reabsorption of the drug

Anticholinergic drugs / Additive anticholinergic side effects

Anticoagulants, oral / ↑ Hypoprothrombinemia due to ↓ breakdown by liver

Anticonvulsants / Tricyclics may ↑ incidence of epileptic seizures

Antihistamines / Additive anticholinergic side effects

Ascorbic acid / ↓ Effect of tricyclics by ↓ renal tubular reabsorption of the drug

Barbiturates / Additive depressant effects; also, barbiturates may ↑ breakdown of antidepressants by liver

Benzodiazepines / Tricyclic antidepressants ↑ effect of benzodiazepines

Beta-adrenergic blocking agents / Tricyclic antidepressants ↓ effect of the blocking agents

Charcoal / ↓ Absorption of tricyclic antidepressants → decreased effectiveness (or toxicity)

Chlordiazepoxide / Concomitant use may cause additive sedative effects and/or additive atropine-like side effects

Cimetidine / ↑ Effect of tricyclics (especially serious anticholinergic symptoms) due to ↓ breakdown by liver

Clonidine / Dangerous ↑ in blood pressure and hypertensive crisis

Diazepam / Concomitant use may cause additive sedative effects and/or additive atropine-like side effects

Dicumarol / Tricyclic antidepressants may ↑ the t½ of dicumarol → increased anticoagulation effects

Disulfiram / ↑ Levels of tricyclic antidepressant; also, possibility of acute organic brain syndrome

Ephedrine / Tricyclics ↓ effects of ephedrine by preventing uptake at its site of action

Estrogens / Depending on the dose, estrogens may ↑ or ↓ the effects of tricyclics

Ethchlorvynol / Combination may result in transient delirium

Fluoxetine / Fluoxetine ↑ pharmacologic and toxic effects of tricyclic antidepressants (effect may persist for several weeks after fluoxetine is discontinued)

Furazolidone / Toxic psychoses possible

Glutethimide / Additive anticholinergic side effects

Guanethidine / Tricyclics ↓ the antihypertensive effect of guanethidine by preventing uptake at its site of action

Haloperidol / ↑ Effect of tricyclics due to ↓ breakdown by liver

Levodopa / ↓ Effect of levodopa due to ↓ absorption

MAO inhibitors / Concomitant use may result in excitation, increase in body temperature, delirium, tremors, and convulsions although combinations have been used successfully

Meperidine / Tricyclics enhance narcotic-induced respiratory depression; also, additive anticholinergic side effects

Methyldopa / Tricyclics may block hypotensive effects of methyldopa

Methylphenidate / ↑ Effect of tricyclics due to ↓ breakdown by liver

Narcotic analgesics / Tricyclics enhance narcotic-induced respiratory depression; also, additive anticholinergic effects

Oral contraceptives / ↑ Plasma levels of tricyclic antidepressants due to ↓ breakdown by liver

Oxazepam / Concomitant use may cause additive sedative effects and/or atropine-like side effects

Phenothiazines / Additive anticholinergic side effects; also, phenothiazines ↑ effects of tricyclics due to ↓ breakdown by liver

Procainamide / Additive cardiac effects

Quinidine / Additive cardiac effects

Reserpine / Tricyclics ↓ hypotensive effect of reserpine

Sodium bicarbonate / ↑ Effect of tricyclics by ↑ renal tubular reabsorption of the drug

Sympathomimetics / Potentiation of sympathomimetic effects → hypertension or cardiac arrhythmias

Tobacco (smoking) / ↓ Serum levels of tricyclic antidepressants due to ↑ breakdown by liver

Thyroid preparations / Mutually potentiating effects observed

Vasodilators / Additive hypotensive effect

Laboratory Test Interferences: ↑ Alkaline phosphatase, bilirubin; ↑ or ↓ blood glucose. False + or ↑ urinary catecholamines.

Dosage: See individual drugs.

Dosage levels vary greatly in effectiveness from one client to another; therefore, dosage regimens must be carefully individualized.

NURSING CONSIDERATIONS

Administration/Storage

1. In adolescents and elderly clients, initial dosage should be lower than in adults; the dose may then be gradually increased as required.

2. The dosage of drug should be highly individualized according to the client's age, weight, physical and mental condition, and response to the therapy.

3. For maintenance therapy, a single daily dose may suffice.

4. The dose is usually administered at bedtime, so any anticholinergic and/or sedative effects will not be bothersome.

5. To reduce incidence of sedation and anticholinergic effects, small dosages of the drug should be used first and then gradually increased to the desired dosage levels.

6. *Treatment of Overdose:*
   - Admit client to hospital and monitor ECG closely for 3–5 days.
   - Empty stomach in alert clients by inducing vomiting followed by gastric lavage and charcoal administration **after insertion of cuffed**

endotracheal tube. Maintain respiration and avoid the use of respiratory stimulants.

- Normal or half-normal saline is used to prevent water intoxication.
- To reverse the cardiovascular effects (e.g., hypotension and cardiac dysrhythmias), hypertonic sodium bicarbonate, IM, is given by IV infusion. The usual dose is 0.5–2 mEq/kg by IV bolus followed by IV infusion to maintain the blood at pH 7.5. If hypotension is not reversed by bicarbonate, vasopressors (e.g., dopamine) and fluid expansion may be needed. If the cardiac dysrhythmias do not respond to bicarbonate, lidocaine or phenytoin may be used.
- Isoproterenol may be effective in controlling bradyarrhythmias and torsade de pointes ventricular tachycardia. Propranolol, 0.1 mg/kg IV (up to 0.25 mg by IV bolus) is used to treat life-threatening ventricular arrhythmias in children.
- Shock and metabolic acidosis are treated with IV fluids, oxygen, bicarbonate, and corticosteroids.
- Control hyperpyrexia by external means (ice pack, cool baths, spongings).
- To reduce possibility of convulsions, minimize external stimulation. If necessary, use diazepam or phenytoin to control convulsions. Avoid barbiturates if MAO inhibitors have been used recently.

Assessment

1. Assess extent of dysphoric mood, appetite, and any reports of weight changes.
2. Note client report of sleep disturbances, lethargy, apathy, impaired thought processes, or lack of responses.
3. Assess for evidence of suicide ideations.
4. Obtain baseline CBC and liver function studies before initiating therapy.
5. Record ECG, heart sounds, and evaluate neurologic functioning as baseline data.
6. Obtain baseline ophthalmic exam and note any reports of visual disturbances and the presence of glaucoma.
7. Note any evidence of urinary retention, especially among the elderly.

Interventions

1. Monitor clients for any changes in vision, such as client complaint of headaches, halos, or eye pain.
2. Assess clients closely if they also develop dilated pupils or complain of nausea. These symptoms may be serious, especially if the client has angle-closure glaucoma and may require a change in medication.
3. Note any signs of an allergic response to the drug, such as skin rash, alopecia, and eosinophilia.
4. Note client complaints of constipation. Provide a diet high in fiber, an increased fluid intake, and a stool softener as needed.
5. Routinely check client's CBC for eosinophil count, thrombocytes, and leukocytes. Check for evidence of agranulocyto-

sis, especially common among elderly women and during the second month of drug therapy. Document and report to the physician because the drug may need to be withheld.

6. Obtain ECGs periodically throughout drug therapy and compare to the baseline ECG. If the client has a history of cardiovascular disorders, assess for tachycardia and any increase in attacks of angina because these may lead to a myocardial infarction or stroke.

7. Note complaints of sore throat, fever, easy bruising, unusual bleeding, presence of petechiae or purpura. These are symptoms of blood dyscrasias. Withhold drug and notify the physician. Place client in protective isolation and practice universal precautions until the CBC with leukocyte counts has been evaluated.

8. Assess GI complaints of anorexia, nausea, vomiting, epigastric distress, diarrhea, a blackened tongue, and a peculiar taste in the mouth. Document and notify the physician because these symptoms require an adjustment of dosage. Administering the medication with or immediately following meals may reduce gastric irritation.

9. Query client concerning adverse endocrine disturbances such as increased or decreased libido, gynecomastia, testicular swelling, and impotence. Discuss these with the client's physician and the client and mutually devise a plan to assist client to deal with the problem.

10. Monitor clients with diabetes mellitus, especially when tricyclic therapy is initiated or discontinued. These drugs may alter blood sugar levels in either direction and require an adjustment in the dose of hypoglycemic agent.

11. In clients with a history of hyperthyroidism, be alert for cardiac arrhythmias that may be precipitated by tricyclic drugs.

12. Assess clients for changes in baseline behavior, indicating further psychological disturbances such as mood swings, increases in agitation, and anxiety. Document and report because a change in medication may be indicated.

13. Monitor intake and output. Check for abdominal distention, urinary retention, and for the absence of bowel sounds (as in paralytic ileus) because these conditions may require immediate attention and a reduction in drug dose.

14. Note symptoms of cholestatic jaundice and biliary tract obstruction such as high fever, yellowing of the skin, mucous membranes and sclera, pruritus as well as upper abdominal pain. Document and report because a change in therapy may be indicated.

15. If the client has been receiving electroshock therapy, check with the physician before administering tricyclic drugs. The combination may be hazardous.

16. Ascertain if the drug is to be discontinued several days prior to surgery. The tricyclic compounds may adversely affect blood pressure during surgery.

17. If withdrawal of the drug is required for any reason, expect

the procedure to occur slowly in order to avoid any withdrawal symptoms.

18. MAO inhibitors are usually contraindicated with tricyclic antidepressants. If used in conjunction with tricyclic drugs, the dosages should be small and the client should be under close medical supervision.

19. Note if any epileptiform seizures are precipitated by the drug. Incorporate seizure precautions when evident.

Client/Family Teaching

1. Stress the importance of maintaining an environment conducive to regular sleep patterns during the initiation of tricyclic therapy.

2. Advise to take medications that may cause sedation at bedtime to minimize excess daytime sedation and to take medications that cause insomnia in the morning or upon arising.

3. Do not ingest any other drugs or alcohol while taking tricyclic antidepressants without the express consent of the physician. This rule should also be followed for 2 weeks after completing tricyclic drug therapy.

4. It may require 2–4 weeks for the client to realize a maximum clinical response. Apprise clients of the delay in response and encourage them to stay on the treatment regimen.

5. Use caution when performing hazardous tasks requiring mental alertness or physical coordination because the drug may cause drowsiness or ataxia.

6. Rise gradually from a supine position and do not remain standing in one place for any length of time. If the client feels faint, advise to lie down to minimize orthostatic hypotension. Review appropriate safety measures.

7. Provide nutritional guidance to avoid or counteract problems associated with drug therapy such as anorexia, nausea, or nervous eating. Take medication with meals to decrease GI upset.

8. Increase oral hygiene and take frequent sips of water, suck on hard candy, or chew sugarless gum to maintain a moist mouth.

9. Discuss changes in libido or reproductive function. Encourage involvement in marital and family therapy.

10. Advise clients with diabetes to monitor blood glucose levels carefully because drug may affect carbohydrate metabolism, and adjustment of hypoglycemic drugs and diet may be indicated.

11. If the client becomes photosensitive, stay out of the sun. Wear protective clothing, sunglasses, and a sunscreen if exposure is necessary.

12. Report any alterations in perceptions, such as the development of hallucinations, blurred vision, or excessive stimulations. Especially evaluate clients recovering from depression for suicidal tendencies.

13. Instruct the family on methods to help clients alter their behavior. Encourage participation in prescribed psychotherapy programs.

Evaluation

1. Evaluate client for evidence of a reduction in level of depres-

sion such as improved appetite, renewed interest in outside activities, socialization, client reports of improved sleeping patterns, more energy, and a general sense of well being.

2. Assess level of compliance and attempt to determine if the client is hoarding drugs.

3. Review goals of therapy and results to date and determine the client's need for continued drug therapy.

VITAMIN K

See also the following individual entries:

Menadiol Sodium Diphosphate
Phytonadione

Classification: Fat-soluble vitamin, blood clotting factor.

Action/Kinetics: Vitamin K is essential for the hepatic synthesis of factors II, VII, IX, and X, all of which are essential for blood clotting. The chief manifestation of vitamin K deficiency is an increase in bleeding tendency, demonstrated by ecchymoses, epistaxis, hematuria, GI bleeding, postoperative and intracranial hemorrhage.

Vitamin K is available as phytonadione (vitamin K_1), a synthetic lipid-soluble analog and menadiol sodium diphosphate (vitamin K_4), a water-soluble synthetic analog.

Uses: Primary and drug-induced hypoprothrombinemia, especially that caused by anticoagulants of the coumarin and phenindione type. Vitamin K cannot reverse the anticoagulant activity of heparin.

Parenteral use for vitamin K malabsorption syndromes. Adjunct during whole blood transfusions.

Preoperatively to prevent the danger of hemorrhages in surgical clients who may require anticoagulant therapy.

Certain forms of liver disease. Hemorrhagic states associated with obstructive jaundice, celiac disease, ulcerative colitis, sprue, biliary fistula, cystic fibrosis of the pancreas, regional enteritis, resection of intestine.

Contraindications: Severe liver disease.

Special Concerns: Use in infants. Use with caution during lactation. Use with caution in clients with sulfite sensitivity.

Side Effects: *Allergic:* Rash, urticaria, anaphylaxis. *After PO use:* Nausea, vomiting, stomach upset, headache. *After parenteral use:* Flushing, alteration of taste, sweating, hypotension, dizziness, rapid and weak pulse, dyspnea, cyanosis, delayed skin reactions. Pain, swelling, and tenderness at injection site. *Newborns:* Hyperbilirubinemia and fatal kernicterus.

Drug Interactions

Antibiotics / Antibiotics may inhibit the body's production of vitamin K and may lead to bleeding. Vitamin K supplements should be given

Anticoagulants, oral / Vitamin K antagonizes anticoagulant effect

Cholestyramine / ↓ Effect of phytonadione and menadione due to ↓ absorption from GI tract

Colestipol / ↓ Effect of phytonadione and menadione due to ↓ absorption from GI tract

Hemolytics / ↑ Potential for toxicity (especially with menadione)

Mineral oil / ↓ Effect of phytonadione and menadione due to ↓ absorption from GI tract

Quinidine, Quinine / ↑ Requirement for vitamin K

Salicylates / High doses of salicylates → ↑ requirements for vitamin K

Sulfonamides / ↑ Requirements for vitamin K

Sucralfate / ↓ Effect of phytonadione and menadione due to ↓ absorption from GI tract

Dosage: See individual drugs.

NURSING CONSIDERATIONS

Assessment

1. Determine if client has any sensitivity to sulfites and document.
2. Note drugs the client is taking to determine how they may interact with vitamin K
3. Obtain baseline PT/PTT, liver and hematologic values prior to initiating therapy.
4. Determine if client has any history or laboratory evidence of advanced liver disease.
5. Note indications for drug therapy.

Interventions

1. Monitor liver function studies and hematologic values during drug therapy.
2. Note any evidence of frank bleeding. Test stools, urine, and GI drainage for occult blood.

Client/Family Teaching

1. Advise client to take only as directed.
2. Review dietary sources high in vitamin K (dairy products, meats, and green leafy vegetables).
3. Report any evidence of unusual bruising or bleeding immediately.
4. Avoid alcohol and aspirin as well as any other OTC preparations without physician consent.

Evaluation: Evaluate client for evidence of a positive clinical response to drug therapy based on physical findings and laboratory data and determine the need for continued drug therapy.

CHAPTER THREE
A–Z Listing of Drugs

A

Acebutolol hydrochloride
(ays-**BYOU**-toe-lohl)
Monitan✹, Sectral (Rx)

See also *Beta-Adrenergic Blocking Agents,* p. 113.

Classification: Beta-adrenergic blocking agent.

Action/Kinetics: Predominantly beta-1 blocking activity but will inhibit beta-2 receptors at higher doses. Acebutolol also has some intrinsic sympathomimetic activity. **t½:** 3–4 hr. Low lipid solubility. Metabolized in liver and excreted in urine and bile.

Uses: Hypertension (either alone or with other antihypertensive agents such as thiazide diuretics). Premature ventricular contractions.

Additional Contraindication: Severe, persistent bradycardia.

Special Concerns: Pregnancy category: B. Dosage has not been established in children.

Dosage: Capsules. *Hypertension:* **initial,** 400 mg once daily (although 200 mg b.i.d. may be needed for optimum control; **then,** 400–800 mg daily (range: 200–1,200 mg daily). *Premature ventricular contractions:* **Initial,** 200 mg b.i.d.; **then,** increase dose gradually to reach 600–1,200 mg/day. Dosage should be decreased in geriatric patients (should not exceed 800 mg daily) and in those with impaired kidney or liver function (decrease dose by 50% when creatinine clearance is 50 ml/min/1.73 m² and by 75% when it is less than 25 ml/min/1.73 m²).

NURSING CONSIDERATIONS

See also *Nursing Considerations for Antihypertensive Agents,* p. 78.

Administration/Storage

1. When treatment is discontinued, the drug should be withdrawn gradually over a 2-week period.
2. The bioavailability increases in elderly clients; thus, such clients may require lower maintenance doses (no more than 800 mg daily).
3. Acebutolol may be combined with another antihypertensive agent.

Client/Family Teaching

1. Advise that drug may cause drowsiness and not to perform tasks that require mental alertness until drug effects realized.
2. Drug may cause an increased sensitivity to cold.

A

Evaluation: Evaluate client for:
- Decrease in blood pressure
- Reduction of ventricular irritability with a ↓ in PVCs

Acetaminophen (Apap, Paracetamol)

(ah-SEAT-ah-MIN-oh-fen)

Capsules: Anacin-3✻, Anacin-3 Extra Strength✻, Panadol, Apacet Extra Strength, Meda Cap, Ty-Tab. Granules: Snaplets-FR Granules. Oral Solution/Elixir: Aceta, Actamin, Actamin Extra, Alba-Temp 300, Apacet Oral Solution, Atasol✻, Children's Anacin-3 Elixir, Children's Genapap Elixir, Children's Panadol, Children's Tylenol Elixir, Dolanex, Dorcal Children's Fever and Pain Reducer, Genapap, Halenol Elixir, Infants' Anacin-3, Infants' Genapap, Infants' Tylenol, Liquiprin Children's Elixir, Myapap, Myapap Elixir, Oraphen-PD, Panadol, Pedric, PMS Acetaminophen✻, Robigesic✻, St. Joseph Aspirin-Free Fever Reducer for Children, Tempra, Tenol, Tylenol, Tylenol Extra Strength, Valdol Liquid. Oral Suspension: Liquiprin Infants' Drops. Tablets: 222 AF✻, Aceta, Actamin, Actamin Extra, Aminofen, Aminofen Max, Anacin-3, Anacin-3 Extra Strength, Anacin-3 Maximum Strength Caplets, Apacet, Apacet Extra Strength, Apacet Extra Strength Caplets, Apo-Acetaminophen✻, Atasol✻, Atasol Caplets✻, Atasol Forte✻, Atasol Forte Caplets✻, Banesin, Conacetol, Dapa, Datril Extra-Strength, Datril Extra-Strength Caplets, Genapap, Genapap Extra Strength, Genapap Extra Strength Caplets, Genebs, Genebs Extra Strength, Genebs Extra Strength Caplets, Halenol, Halenol Extra Strength, Halenol Extra Strength Caplets, Meda Tab, Neo-Dol✻, Panadol, Panadol Caplets, Panadol Junior Strength Caplets, Panex, Panex-500, Phenaphen Caplets, PMS-Acetaminophen✻, Robigesic✻, Rounox✻, Tapanol, Tapanol Extra Strength, Tapanol Extra Strength Caplets, Tapar, Tenol, Tylenol, Tylenol Caplets, Tylenol Extra Strength, Tylenol Extra Strength Caplets, Tylenol Extra Strength Gelcaps, Tylenol Junior Strength Caplets, Ty-Tab, Ty-Tab Caplets, Ty-Tab Extra Strength, Valadol, Valorin, Valorin Extra. Tablets, Chewable: Children's Anacin-3, Children's Genapap, Children's Panadol, Children's Tylenol, Children's Ty-Tab, Panadol✻, St. Joseph Aspirin-Free Fever Reducer for Children, Tempra, Tempra Double Strength. Suppositories: Abenol✻, Acephen, Children's Feverall, Junior Strength Feverall, Neopap, Suppap-120, Suppap-325, Suppap-650. Wafers: Pedric. (OTC)

Acetaminophen, buffered

(ah-SEAT-ah-MIN-oh-fen)

Bromo Seltzer (OTC)

Classification: Nonnarcotic analgesic, para-aminophenol type.

Action/Kinetics: The only para-aminophenol derivative currently used is acetaminophen. It decreases fever by an effect on the hypothalamus leading to sweating and vasodilation. Acetaminophen also inhibits the effect of pyrogens on the hypothalamic heat-regulating centers. It may cause analgesia by inhibiting CNS prostaglandin synthesis; however, due to minimal effects on peripheral prostaglandin synthesis, acetaminophen has no anti-inflammatory or uricosuric effects. It does not manifest any anticoagulant effect and does not produce ulceration of the GI tract. The magnitude of its antipyretic and analgesic effects is comparable to that of aspirin.

Peak plasma levels: 30–120 min. **t½:** 45 min–3 hr. **Therapeutic serum levels** (analgesia): 5–20 mcg/ml. **Plasma protein binding:** Approximately 25%. Acetaminophen is metabolized in the liver and is excreted in the urine as glucuronide and sulfate conjugates. However, an intermediate hydroxylated metabolite is hepatotoxic following large doses of acetaminophen.

Acetaminophen is often combined with other drugs, as in Darvocet-N, Parafon Forte, Phenaphen with Codeine, and Tylenol with Codeine.

The buffered product is a mixture of acetaminophen, sodium bicarbonate, and citric acid that effervesces when placed in water. This product has a high sodium content (0.76 g/¾ capful).

Uses: Control of pain due to headache, dysmenorrhea, arthralgia, myalgia, musculoskeletal pain, immunizations, teething, tonsillectomy. To reduce fever in bacterial or viral infections. As a substitute for aspirin in upper GI disease, aspirin allergy, bleeding disorders, patients on anticoagulant therapy, and gouty arthritis. *Investigational:* In children receiving DPT vaccination to decrease incidence of fever and pain at injection site.

Contraindications: Renal insufficiency, anemia. Clients with cardiac or pulmonary disease are more susceptible to toxic effects of acetaminophen.

Special Concerns: Evidence indicates that acetaminophen may have to be used with caution in pregnancy.

Side Effects: Few when taken in usual therapeutic doses. Chronic and even acute toxicity can develop after long symptom-free usage. *Hematologic:* Methemoglobinemia, hemolytic anemia, neutropenia, thrombocytopenia, pancytopenia, leukopenia. *Allergic:* Skin rashes, fever. *Miscellaneous:* CNS stimulation, hypoglycemia, jaundice, drowsiness, glossitis.

Symptoms of Overdose: There may be few initial symptoms. *Hepatic toxicity. CNS:* CNS stimulation, general malaise, delirium followed by depression, seizures, coma, death. *GI:* Nausea, vomiting, diarrhea, gastric upset. *Miscellaneous:* Sweating, chills, fever, vascular collapse.

Drug Interactions

Alcohol, ethyl / Chronic use of alcohol ↑ toxicity of larger therapeutic doses of acetaminophen

Anticoagulants, oral / Acetaminophen may ↑ hypoprothrombinemic effect

Barbiturates / ↑ Potential of hepatotoxicity due to ↑ breakdown of acetaminophen by liver

Carbamazepine / ↓ Potential of hepatotoxicity due to ↑ breakdown of acetaminophen by liver

Diflunisal / ↑ Plasma levels of acetaminophen

Caffeine / ↑ Analgesic effect of acetaminophen

Chloramphenicol / Acetaminophen ↑ serum chloramphenicol levels

Hydantoins / ↑ Potential of hepatotoxicity due to ↑ breakdown of acetaminophen by liver

Oral contraceptives / ↑ Breakdown of acetaminophen by liver

Phenobarbital / ↑ Potential of hepatotoxicity due to ↑ breakdown of acetaminophen by liver

Phenytoin / ↑ Potential of hepatotoxicity due to ↑ breakdown of acetaminophen by liver

Sulfinpyrazone / ↑ Potential of hepatotoxicity due to ↑ breakdown of acetaminophen by liver

Dosage: Capsules, Granules, Elixir, Oral Solution, Oral Suspension, Tablets, Suppositories, Wafers. Adults: 325–650 mg q 4 hr; doses up to 1 g q.i.d. may be used. Daily dosage should not exceed 4 g. **Pediatric:** Doses given 4–5 times/day. **Up to 3 months:** 40 mg/dose; **4–12 months:** 80 mg/dose; **1–2 years:** 120 mg/dose; **2–3 years:** 160 mg/dose; **4–5 years:** 240 mg/dose; **6–8 years:** 320 mg/dose; **9–10 years:** 400 mg/dose; **11–12 years:** 480 mg/dose. *Alternative pediatric dose:* 10 mg/kg/dose.

Suppositories. Adults, 650 mg q 4–6, hr not to exceed 6 suppositories per day. **Pediatric, less than 3 years:** Physician should be consulted; **3–6 years:** 120 mg q 4–6 hr, not to exceed 2.6 g/day; **6–12 years:** 325 mg q 4–6 hr not to exceed 720 mg/day.

Buffered. Adult, usual: 1 or 2 three-quarter capfuls are placed into an empty glass; add half a glass of cool water. May be taken while fizzing or after settling. Can be repeated every 4 hr as required or directed by physician.

NURSING CONSIDERATIONS

Administration/Storage

1. Suppositories should be stored below 80°F (27°C).
2. *Treatment of Overdose:* Initially, induction of emesis, gastric lavage, activated charcoal. Oral *N*-acetylcysteine (see p. 258) is said to reduce or prevent hepatic damage by inactivating acetaminophen metabolites, which cause liver effects. CNS stimulation, excitement, and delirium are symptoms of toxicity. Have acetylcysteine available for treatment of overdosage.

Assessment

1. If the client is to receive long-term therapy, liver function studies should be conducted prior to initiating drug therapy.
2. Document presence of fever. Question client concerning pain, noting type, location, duration, and intensity.

Interventions

1. Note the presence of bluish color of the mucosa and fingernails or client complaints of dyspnea, weakness, headache, or vertigo. These symptoms of methemoglobinemia are caused by anoxia and require immediate attention.
2. Observe for pallor, weakness, and complaints of heart palpitations. Document and report as these symptoms may signal

the presence of hemolytic anemia.

3. To assess for evidence of nephritis, check the client's urine for occult blood and the presence of albumin on a routine basis, especially when client is receiving long-term drug therapy.

4. Clients complaining of dyspnea, rapid weak pulse, cold extremities, clammy sweat, or subnormal temperatures are displaying symptoms of chronic poisoning and may collapse with confusion. All complaints and symptoms observed during drug therapy should be reported to the physician immediately .

Client/Family Teaching

1. Teach symptoms of acute toxicity such as nausea, vomiting, and abdominal pain. Instruct clients to notify the physician immediately.

2. Provide printed information to familiarize clients with the signs and symptoms of severe poisoning. Instruct them to report all such signs and symptoms immediately.

3. Review signs that may indicate possible chronic overdose of medication, such as unexplained bleeding, bruising, sore throat, malaise, and fever.

4. Phenacetin, the major active metabolite of acetaminophen, may cause the urine to become dark brown or wine in color.

5. Teach clients to read the labels on all OTC preparations that they take. Many contain acetaminophen and, as a result, can produce toxic reactions if taken over a period of time with the prescribed drug.

6. Explain that so-called headache and minor pain relievers containing combinations of salicylates, acetaminophen, and caffeine may be no more beneficial than aspirin alone and that such combinations may be more dangerous. When in doubt consult pharmacist or physician.

7. Any pain or fever that persists for 3–5 days requires medical attention.

Evaluation: Evaluate for a positive clinical response as demonstrated by a reduction in fever and/or subjective reports of control of pain.

Acetazolamide
(ah-set-ah-**ZOE**-la-myd)
AK-Zol, Apo-Acetazolamide ✽, Daranide, Dazamide, Diamox, Diamox Sequels, Neptazane, Novo-Zolamide ✽ (Rx)

Acetazolamide sodium
(ah-set-ah-**ZOE**-la-myd)
Diamox (Rx)

See also *Anticonvulsants,* p. 61.

Classification: Anticonvulsant (miscellaneous), diuretic (carbonic anhydrase inhibitor).

Action/Kinetics: Acetazolamide is a sulfonamide derivative possessing carbonic anhydrase inhibitor activity. As an anticonvulsant, beneficial effects may be due to inhibition of carbonic anhydrase in the CNS, which increases carbon dioxide tension resulting in a decrease in neuronal conduction. Systemic acidosis may also be involved. As a diuretic, the drug inhibits carbonic anhydrase in the kidney, which decreases formation of bicarbonate and hydrogen ions from carbon dioxide, thus reducing the availability of these ions for active transport. Use as a diuretic is limited because the drug promotes metabolic acidosis, which inhibits diuretic activity. This may be partially circumvented by giving acetazolamide on alternate days. Acetazolamide also reduces intraocular pressure.

Absorbed from the GI tract and widely distributed throughout the body, including the CNS. Excreted unchanged in the urine. **Tablets: Onset,** 60–90 min; **peak:** 2–4 hr; **duration:** 8–12 hr. **Sustained-release capsules: Onset,** 2 hr; **peak:** 8–12 hr; **duration:** 18–24 hr. **Injection (IV): Onset,** 2 min; **peak:** 15 min; **duration:** 4–5 hr. The drug is eliminated mainly unchanged through the kidneys.

Uses: Adjunct in clonic-tonic, myoclonic seizures, absence seizures (petit mal), mixed seizures, simple partial seizure patterns. Open-angle, secondary, angle-closure, or malignant glaucoma. Prophylaxis or treatment of acute mountain sickness. *Investigational:* Hypokalemic and hyperkalemic forms of familial periodic paralysis; to induce forced alkaline diuresis; to increase excretion of certain weakly acidic drugs; prophylaxis of uric acid or cystine renal calculi.

Contraindications: Low serum sodium and potassium levels. Renal and hepatic dysfunction. Hyperchloremic acidosis, adrenal insufficiency, hypersensitivity to thiazide diuretics. Not to be used chronically in presence of noncongestive angle-closure glaucoma.

Special Concerns: Use with caution in the presence of mild acidosis, advanced pulmonary disease, and pregnancy.

Side Effects: *Short-term therapy* (minimal adverse reactions): Anorexia, polyuria, drowsiness, confusion, paresthesia. *Long-term therapy:* Acidosis, transient myopia. *Rarely:* Urticaria, glycosuria, hepatic insufficiency, melena, flaccid paralysis, convulsions. Also, side effects similar to those produced by sulfonamides.

Drug Interactions: Also see *Diuretics,* p. 140.

Amphetamine / ↑ Effect of amphetamine by ↑ renal tubular reabsorption
Ephedrine / ↑ Effect of ephedrine by ↑ renal tubular reabsorption
Lithium carbonate / ↓ Effect of lithium by ↑ renal excretion
Methotrexate / ↓ Effect of methotrexate due to ↑ renal excretion
Primidone / ↓ Effect of primidone due to ↓ GI absorption
Pseudoephedrine / ↑ Effect of pseudoephedrine by ↑ renal tubular reabsorption
Quinidine / ↑ Effect of quinidine by ↑ renal tubular reabsorption
Salicylates / ↓ Effect of salicylates by ↑ renal excretion

Dosage: Extended-release Capsules, Tablets. *Seizures.* **Adults/children:** 4–30 mg/kg/day in divided doses. Optimum daily dosage: 375–1,000 mg (doses higher than 1,000 mg do not increase therapeutic effect). *If used as adjunct to other anticonvulsants:* **Initial,** 250 mg once daily; dose can be increased up to 1,000 mg/day if necessary.

Glaucoma, simple open-angle: 0.25–1 g daily in divided doses. *Glaucoma, closed-angle prior to surgery or secondary:* 0.25 g q 4 hr, 0.25 g b.i.d., or 0.5 g followed by 0.125–0.25 g q 4 hr. **Extended-release capsules:** 500 mg b.i.d. in the morning and evening. **Pediatric:** 8–30 mg/kg (usual: 10–15 mg/kg or 300–900 mg/m²) daily in divided doses.

Acute mountain sickness: 250 mg b.i.d.–q.i.d. (500 mg 1–2 times daily of extended-release capsules). During rapid ascent, 1 g daily is recommended.

NURSING CONSIDERATIONS

See also *Nursing Considerations* for *Diuretics,* p. 141, *Sulfonamides,* p. 216, and *Anticonvulsants,* p. 63.

Administration/Storage

1. Change over from other anticonvulsant therapy to acetazolamide should be gradual.
2. Use parenteral solutions within 24 hr after reconstitution.
3. IV administration is preferred; IM administration is painful due to alkalinity of solution.
4. Reconstitute with at least 5 ml of sterile water for injection.
5. Tolerance after prolonged use may necessitate dosage increase.
6. Do not administer the sustained-release dosage form as an anticonvulsant.
7. When used for prophylaxis of mountain sickness, dosage should be initiated 1–2 days before ascent and should be continued for at least 2 days while at high altitudes.
8. Due to possible differences in bioavailability, brands should not be interchanged.

Assessment

1. Obtain a complete nursing history, noting indications for drug use.
2. Evaluate laboratory findings for levels of electrolytes, uric acid and glucose. Document any evidence of liver and renal dysfunction prior to administering the medication.
3. Obtain a complete client drug history to ensure that the client is not receiving any drug therapy that interacts with the medication.
4. When administered for glaucoma, record baseline intra-ocular pressure readings.

Client/Family Teaching

1. Taking the drug with food may decrease gastric irritation and GI upset.
2. The drug increases the frequency of voiding. Therefore, take the medication early in the day to avoid interrupting sleep.
3. Clients with diabetes should be warned that the drug may increase blood glucose levels. Therefore, they should monitor serum glucose levels carefully and report increases because the dose of hypoglycemic agent may require adjustment.
4. If nausea, dizziness, muscle weakness, or cramps occur, report these to the physician.
5. Note any changes in the color of stools and report.
6. Emphasize importance of reporting for scheduled laboratory studies.
7. Evaluate drug effects before undertaking tasks that require mental alertness.

A

Evaluation: Evaluate for a positive clinical response based on pretreatment symptoms as evidenced by:
- ↓ in seizure activity
- ↓ in intraocular pressure recordings
- Prevention of mountain sickness

Acetohexamide
(ah-seat-oh-**HEX**-ah-myd)
Dimelor✲, Dymelor (Rx)

See also *Antidiabetic Agents, Oral,* p. 65.

Classification: First-generation sulfonylurea.

Action/Kinetics: Onset: 1 hr. **t½:** 1.3 hr for acetohexamide and 6–8 hr for active metabolite. **Duration:** 12–24 hr. Metabolized in the liver to a potent active metabolite. Excreted through the kidney (80%) and feces (10%).

Special Concerns: Pregnancy category: C.

Additional Side Effects: Hair loss.

Dosage: PO. Adults, initial: 250 mg daily; **maintenance:** 500 mg daily, adjusting dosage thereafter until optimum control is achieved. Doses in excess of 1.5 g daily are not recommended. **Geriatric clients, initial:** 125–250 mg daily; **then,** adjust dosage gradually until desired effect is achieved.

NURSING CONSIDERATIONS

See *Nursing Considerations* for *Antidiabetic Agents, Oral,* p. 68.

Administration/Storage: Doses of 1 g or over should be divided, usually before the morning and evening meals.

Acetohydroxamic acid (AHA)
(ah-**SEAT**-oh-hy-drox-**AM**-ick **AH**-sid)
Lithostat (Rx)

Classification: Antiurolithic, adjunct to treat urinary tract infections.

Action/Kinetics: This drug inhibits the enzyme urease, which decreases the hydrolysis of urea to ammonia. Thus, there is a decrease in both urine alkalinity and ammonia concentration. It is especially useful in urinary tract infections of urea-splitting organisms. Following administration of acetohydroxamic acid, urinary pH decreases, leading to increased efficacy of antibiotics. The drug is not antibacterial itself. Well absorbed from the GI tract and distributed throughout the body. **Peak blood levels:** 15–60 min. **t½:** 5–10 hr. To be effective the drug must be excreted unchanged in the urine (approximately 35%–65%).

Uses: Adjunct in urinary tract infections due to urea-splitting organisms. Prophylaxis of struvite calculi formation produced by urease-producing bacteria such as *Proteus.*

Contraindications: Should not be used instead of surgery or antibiotic therapy. Renal dysfunction. In females not using contraception. Pregnancy, lactation.

Special Concerns: Pregnancy category: X.

Side Effects: The incidence of adverse effects is high (30%). *GI:* Nausea, vomiting, anorexia. *CNS:* Headaches (common), malaise, depression, tremors, nervousness, anxiety. *Hematologic:* Hemolytic anemia, reticulocytosis without anemia. *Other:* Phlebitis in the legs; nonpruritic, macular skin rash; alopecia. *Symptoms of Overdose:* Hemolysis in reduced renal function, nausea, vomiting, anorexia, malaise, lethargy, tremulousness, decreased sense of well-being.

Drug Interactions

Alcohol / Nonpruritic, macular skin rash within 30–60 min
Iron / ↓ Absorption of iron due to chelation by acetohydroxamic acid

Dosage: Tablets. Adults: 250 mg t.i.d.–q.i.d. up to a maximum of 1.5 g daily. **Pediatric: initially,** 10 mg/kg/day; **then,** adjust dose depending on response and hematologic picture. **Serum creatinine greater than 1.8 mg/dl:** maximum of 1 g/day in divided doses at 12-hr intervals.

NURSING CONSIDERATIONS

Administration/Storage: *Treatment of Overdose:* Discontinue the medication. Monitor hematology profile. Blood transfusions may be required.

Client/Family Teaching

1. Complaints of headaches, especially during the first 2–3 days of therapy, are common and respond well to aspirin.
2. Assure that nausea, vomiting, anorexia, and malaise are usually transient. Drug therapy is rarely terminated because of these symptoms.
3. Demonstrate how to inspect lower legs for redness, tenderness, and pain, which are signs of superficial phlebitis and should be reported to the physician.
4. If loss of body hair is severe, wigs and eye makeup may be used.
5. Warn client to forego ingestion of alcohol while on this drug, because a rash may develop.
6. Because drug chelates iron, iron-deficiency anemia may result. Supplemental iron tablets may be recommended.
7. Instruct females of childbearing age to practice some form of birth control.

Evaluation: Evaluate client for:
- ↓ in urinary pH
- Subjective reports of symptomatic improvement

Acetophenazine maleate

(ah-**SEAT**-oh-**FEN**-ah-zeen)
Tindal (Rx)

See also *Phenothiazines,* p. 201.

Classification: Antipsychotic, piperazine-type phenothiazine.

Action/Kinetics: Acetophenazine manifests a low incidence of orthostatic hypotension, moderate sedation and anticholinergic effects but a high incidence of extrapyramidal effects.

Uses: Psychoses.

Special Concerns: Dosage has not been established in children less than 12 years of age.

Dosage: Tablets. Adults and children over 12 years, usual: 20 mg t.i.d. (range: 40–80 mg daily in divided doses); 80–120 mg daily in divided doses for hospitalized schizophrenic clients (doses as high as 400–600 mg/day may be needed in severe schizophrenia).

Emaciated, geriatric, and debilitated clients require a lower initial dose.

NURSING CONSIDERATIONS

See also *Nursing Considerations* for *Phenothiazines,* p. 205.

Assessment

1. Note the age of the client since elderly clients usually require lower drug dosage.
2. Identify if the client is taking lithium. Acetophenazine potentiates CNS toxicity.

Client/Family Teaching

1. Administer 1 hr before bedtime if client has difficulty sleeping.
2. Provide clients with a list of potential drug reactions that they should report to the physician.
3. Remind client to call the physician if any side effects occur and *not* to stop taking the medication abruptly.

Acetylcysteine
(ah-see-till-**SIS**-tay-een)
Airbron ✹, Mucomyst, Mucosol, Parvolex (Rx)

Classification: Mucolytic.

Action/Kinetics: Acetylcysteine reduces the viscosity of purulent and nonpurulent pulmonary secretions and facilitates their removal by splitting disulfide bonds. Action increases with increasing pH (peak: pH 7–9). **Onset, inhalation:** Within 1 min; **by direct instillation:** immediate. **Time to peak effect:** 5–10 min.

Uses: Adjunct in the treatment of acute and chronic bronchitis, em-

physema, tuberculosis, pneumonia, bronchiectasis, atelectasis. Routine care of clients with tracheostomy, pulmonary complications after thoracic or cardiovascular surgery, or in posttraumatic chest conditions. Pulmonary complications of cystic fibrosis. Diagnostic bronchial asthma. Antidote in acetaminophen poisoning to reduce hepatotoxicity. *Investigational:* As an ophthalmic solution for dry eye.

Contraindications: Sensitivity to drug.

Special Concerns: Pregnancy category: B. Use with caution during lactation, in the elderly, and in clients with asthma.

Side Effects: *Respiratory:* Acetylcysteine increases the incidence of bronchospasm in clients with asthma. The drug may also increase the amount of liquefied bronchial secretions, which must be removed by suction if cough is inadequate. Bronchial and tracheal irritation, tightness in chest, bronchoconstriction. *GI:* Nausea, vomiting, stomatitis. *Other:* Rashes, fever, drowsiness, rhinorrhea.

Drug Interactions: Acetylcysteine is incompatible with antibiotics and should be administered separately.

Dosage: Nebulization, direct application, or direct intratracheal instillation using 10% or 20% solution. *Nebulization into face mask, tracheostomy, mouth piece:* 1–10 ml of 20% solution or 2–10 ml of 10% solution 3–4 times daily. *Closed tent or croupette:* 300 ml of 10% or 20% solution/treatment. *Direct instillation into tracheostomy:* 1–2 ml of 10%–20% solution q 1–4 hr. *Percutaneous intratracheal catheter:* 1–2 ml of

20% solution or 2–4 ml of 10% solution q 1–4 hr by syringe attached to catheter. *Instillation to particular portion of bronchopulmonary tree using small plastic catheter into the trachea:* 2–5 ml of 20% solution instilled into the trachea by means of a syringe connected to a catheter. *Diagnostic procedures:* 2–3 doses of 1–2 ml of 20% or 2–4 ml of 10% solution by nebulization or intratracheal instillation before the procedure. *Acetaminophen overdosage:* **PO, initial:** 140 mg/kg; **then,** 70 mg/kg q 4 hr for a total of 17 doses.

NURSING CONSIDERATIONS

Administration/ Storage

1. Use nonreactive plastic, glass, or stainless steel equipment for administration.
2. The 10% solution may be used undiluted.
3. Use either water for injection or saline to dilute the 20% solution.
4. Administer the medication via face mask, face tent, oxygen tent, head tent, or by positive-pressure breathing apparatus as indicated.
5. Administer with compressed air for nebulization. Hand nebulizers are contraindicated.
6. After prolonged nebulization, dilute the last fourth of the medication with sterile water for injection to prevent concentration of the medication.
7. The solution may develop a light purple color. This does not affect the action of the medication.
8. Closed bottles of solution remain stable for 2 years when stored at 20°C. Open bottles should be stored at 2°C–8°C and should be used within 96

hr. Once a bottle has been opened, record the time and date of opening so that the drug will not be used beyond the 96-hr period.
9. Acetylcysteine is incompatible with antibiotics and must be administered separately.
10. Have an endotracheal tube available and a suction machine at the bedside for removal of increased bronchial secretions.

Assessment

1. Determine from the client and history when bronchial spasms occur.
2. Discuss conditions likely to cause congestion and wheezing and document.
3. Identify the previous approaches (successful and unsuccessful) used in treating their conditions.
4. Determine if the client is currently taking any antibiotic medications.

Interventions

1. If bronchospasm occurs, have a bronchodilator, such as isoproterenol for aerosol inhalation, readily available.
2. Position the client to facilitate the removal of secretions.
3. If the client is unable to cough up secretions, provide mechanical suction for their removal.
4. Monitor vital signs, intake and output.
5. Wash the client's face following nebulization treatment. The medication may cause the face to become sticky.
6. Advise the client that the nauseous odor present when the treatment begins will likely become less noticeable.

Evaluation: Evaluate client for:

- Improved airway exchange when used as a mucolytic
- Reduction in acetaminophen levels and associated liver toxicity when used as an antidote

---

Acetylsalicylic acid

(ah-**SEE**-till-sal-ih-**SILL**-ick **AH**-sid)

Apo-Asa ✹, Arthrisin ✹, Artria S.R., A.S.A., A.S.A. Enseals, Astrin ✹, Aspergum, Aspirin, Bayer Aspirin, Bayer Timed-Release Arthritic Pain Formula ✹, Corphyen ✹, Easprin, Ecotrin, Empirin, Entrophen ✹, 8-Hour Bayer Timed-Release, Measurin, Norwich Aspirin, Novasen ✹, PMS-ASA ✹, Riphen ✹, Sal-Adult ✹, Sal-Infant ✹, Supasa ✹, ZOR-prin (OTC) (Easprin and ZORprin are Rx)

Acetylsalicylic acid, buffered

(ah-**SEE**-till-sal-ih-**SILL**-ick **AH**-sid)

Alka-Seltzer Effervescent Pain Reliever and Antacid, APF Arthritic Pain Formula ✹, Arthritis Pain Formula, Ascriptin, Ascriptin A/D, Buffaprin, Bufferin, Buffinol, Cama Arthritis Pain Formula, Magnaprin, Magnaprin Arthritis Strength, Maprin, Maprin I-B (OTC)

Classification: Nonnarcotic analgesic, antipyretic, anti-inflammatory agent.

Action/Kinetics: Aspirin manifests antipyretic, anti-inflammatory, and analgesic effects. The antipyretic effect is due to an action on the hypothalamus, resulting in heat loss by vasodilation of peripheral blood vessels and promoting sweating. The anti-inflammatory effects are probably mediated through inhibition of cyclo-oxygenase, which results in a decrease in prostaglandin synthesis and other mediators of the pain response. Prostaglandins have been implicated in the inflammatory process, as well as in mediation of pain. Thus, if levels are decreased, the inflammatory reaction may subside. The mechanism of action for the analgesic effects of aspirin is not known fully but is partly attributable to improvement of the inflammatory condition. Aspirin also produces inhibition of platelet aggregation by decreasing the synthesis of endoperoxides and thromboxanes—substances that mediate platelet aggregation.

Large doses of aspirin (5 g/day or more) increase uric acid secretion, while low doses (2 g/day or less) decrease uric acid secretion. However, aspirin antagonizes drugs used to treat gout.

Aspirin is rapidly absorbed after PO administration. Aspirin is hydrolyzed to the active salicylic acid, which is 70%–90% protein bound. For arthritis and rheumatic disease, blood levels of 150–300 mcg/ml should be maintained. For analgesic and antipyretic, blood levels of 25–50 mcg/ml should be achieved. For acute rheumatic fever, blood levels of 150–300 mcg/ml should be achieved. **Therapeutic salicylic acid serum levels:** 150–300 mcg/ml, although tinnitus occurs at serum levels above 200 mcg/ml and serious toxicity above 400 mcg/ml. $t^{1/2}$: aspirin, 15–20 min; salicylic acid, 2–20 hr, depending on the dose. Salicylic acid and metabolites are excreted by the kidney. The bioavailability of enteric-coated salicylate products may be poor.

Aspirin is found in many combination products including Darvon Compound, Empirin Compound Plain and with Codeine, Equagesic, Fiorinal Plain and with Codeine, Norgesic and Norgesic Forte, and Synalgos DC.

Uses: Pain arising from integumental structures, myalgias, neuralgias, arthralgias, headache, dysmenorrhea, and similar types of pain. Antipyretic.   Anti-inflammatory agent in conditions such as arthritis, osteoarthritis, systemic lupus erythematosus, acute rheumatic fever, gout, and many other conditions. Aspirin is also used to reduce the risk of recurrent transient ischemic attacks and strokes in men. Decrease risk of death from nonfatal myocardial infarction in clients who have a history of infarction or who manifest unstable angina; aortocoronary bypass surgery. Gout. May be effective in less severe postoperative and postpartum pain; pain secondary to trauma and cancer. *Investigational:* Chronic use to prevent cataract formation; low doses to prevent toxemia of pregnancy; in pregnant women with inadequate uteroplacental blood flow. Reduce colon cancer mortality (low doses).

Contraindications: Hypersensitivity to salicylates. Clients with asthma, hay fever, or nasal polyps have a higher incidence of hypersensitivity reactions. Severe anemia, history of blood coagulation defects, in conjunction with anticoagulant therapy. Salicylates can cause congestive failure when taken in the large doses used for rheumatic diseases. Vitamin K deficiency; one week before and after surgery. In pregnancy, especially the last trimester as the drug may cause problems in the newborn child or complications during delivery. In children or teenagers with chickenpox or flu due to possibility of development of Reye's syndrome.

Controlled-release aspirin is not recommended for use as an antipyretic or short-term analgesic because adequate blood levels may not be reached. Also, controlled-release products are not recommended for children less than 12 years of age and in children with fever accompanied by dehydration.

Special Concerns: Pregnancy category: C. Use with caution during lactation. Salicylates are to be used with caution in the presence of gastric or peptic ulcers, in mild diabetes, erosive gastritis or bleeding tendencies, and in clients with cardiac disease. Use with caution in liver or kidney disease. Aspirin products now carry the following labeling: "It is especially important not to use aspirin during the last three months of pregnancy unless specifically directed to do so by a doctor because it may cause problems in the newborn child or complications during delivery."

Side Effects: The toxic effects of the salicylates are dose-related. *GI:* Dyspepsia, heartburn, anorexia, nausea, occult blood loss, epigastric discomfort, massive GI bleeding, potentiation of peptic ulcer. *Allergic:* Bronchospasm, asthma-like symptoms, anaphylaxis, skin rashes, angioedema, urticaria, rhinitis, nasal polyps. *Hematologic:* Prolongation of bleeding time, thrombocytopenia, leukopenia, purpura, shortened erythrocyte survival time, decreased plasma iron levels. *Miscellaneous:* Thirst, fever, dimness of vision.

Note: Use of aspirin in children

and teenagers with flu or chicken-pox may result in the development of Reye's syndrome. Also, dehydrated, febrile children are more prone to salicylate intoxication.

Salicylism—mild toxicity. Seen at serum levels between 150–200 mcg/ml. *GI:* Nausea, vomiting, diarrhea, thirst. *CNS:* Tinnitus (most common), dizziness, difficulty in hearing, mental confusion, lassitude. *Miscellaneous:* Flushing, sweating, tachycardia. Symptoms of salicylism may be observed with doses used for inflammatory disease or rheumatic fever.

Severe salicylate poisoning. Seen at serum levels over 400 mcg/ml. *CNS:* Excitement, confusion, disorientation, irritability, hallucinations, lethargy, stupor, coma, respiratory failure, seizures. *Metabolic:* Respiratory alkalosis (initially), respiratory acidosis and metabolic acidosis, dehydration. *GI:* Nausea, vomiting. *Hematologic:* Platelet dysfunction, hypoprothrombinemia, increased capillary fragility. *Miscellaneous:* Hyperthermia, hyperventilation, hemorrhage, pulmonary edema, cardiovascular collapse, renal failure, tetany, hypoglycemia (late).

For treatment, see *Nursing Considerations,* p. 264.

Drug Interactions

Acetazolamide / ↑ CNS toxicity of salicylates; also, ↑ excretion of salicylic acid if urine kept alkaline

Alcohol, ethyl / ↑ Chance of GI bleeding caused by salicylates

Alteplase, recombinant / ↑ Risk of bleeding

Aminosalicylic acid (PAS) / Possible ↑ effect of PAS due to ↓ excretion by kidney or ↓ plasma protein binding

Ammonium chloride / ↑ Effect of salicylates by ↑ renal tubular reabsorption

Angiotensin-converting enzyme (ACE) inhibitors / ↓ Effect of ACE inhibitors possibly due to prostaglandin inhibition

Antacids / ↓ Salicylate levels in plasma due to ↑ rate of renal excretion

Anticoagulants, oral / ↑ Effect of anticoagulant by ↓ plasma protein binding and plasma prothrombin

Antirheumatics / Both are ulcerogenic and may cause ↑ GI bleeding

Ascorbic acid / ↑ Effect of salicylates by ↑ renal tubular reabsorption

Beta-adrenergic blocking agents / Salicylates ↓ action of beta-blockers, possibly due to prostaglandin inhibition

Charcoal, activated / ↓ Absorption of salicylates from GI tract

Corticosteroids / Both are ulcerogenic; also, corticosteroids may ↓ blood salicylate levels by ↑ breakdown by liver and ↑ excretion

Dipyridamole / Additive anticoagulant effects

Furosemide / ↑ Chance of salicylate toxicity due to ↓ renal excretion; also, salicylates may ↓ effect of furosemide in clients with impaired renal function or cirrhosis with ascites

Heparin / Inhibition of platelet adhesiveness by aspirin may result in bleeding tendencies

Hypoglycemics, oral / ↑ Hypoglycemia due to ↓ plasma protein binding and ↓ excretion

A

Indomethacin / Both are ulcerogenic and may cause ↑ GI bleeding

Insulin / Salicyaltes ↑ hypoglycemic effect of insulin

Methionine / ↑ Effect of salicylates by ↑ renal tubular reabsorption

Methotrexate / ↑ Effect of methotrexate by ↓ plasma protein binding; also, salicylates block renal excretion of methotrexate

Nitroglycerin / Combination may result in unexpected hypotension

Nizatidine / ↑ Serum levels of salicylates

Nonsteroidal anti-inflammatory drugs / Additive ulcerogenic effects; also, aspirin may ↓ serum levels of NSAIDs

Phenylbutazone / Combination may produce hyperuricemia

Phenytoin / ↑ Effect of phenytoin by ↓ plasma protein binding

Probenecid / Salicylates inhibit uricosuric activity of probenecid

Sodium bicarbonate / ↓ Effect of salicylates by ↑ rate of excretion

Spironolactone / Aspirin ↓ diuretic effect of spironolactone

Sulfinpyrazone / Salicylates inhibit uricosuric activity of sulfinpyrazone

Sulfonamides / ↑ Effect of sulfonamides by ↑ blood levels of salicylates

Valproic acid / ↑ Effect of valproic acid due to ↓ plasma protein binding

Laboratory Test Interferences: False + or ↑ : Amylase, AST, ALT, uric acid, PBI, urinary VMA (most tests), catecholamines, urinary glucose (Benedict's, Clinitest), and urinary uric acid (at high doses) values. False (−) or ↓ : CO_2 content, glucose (fasting), potassium, urinary VMA (Pisano method), and thrombocyte values.

Dosage: Capsules, Tablets, Chewable Tablets, Chewing Gum, Tablets, Delayed-Release Tablets, Extended-Release Tablets. Adults: *Analgesic/antipyretic:* 325–500 mg q 3 hr, 325–600 mg q 4 hr, or 650–1,000 mg q 6 hr. *Arthritis/rheumatic diseases:* 3.6–5.4 g/day in divided doses. *Juvenile rheumatoid arthritis:* 80–100 mg/kg/day (alternate dose: 3 g/m²) in divided doses q 4–6 hr.

Pediatric: *Analgesic, antipyretic:* 65 mg/kg/day (alternate dose: 1.5 g/m²/day) in divided doses q 4–6 hr, not to exceed 3.6 g/day. Alternatively, the following dosage regimen can be used: **Pediatric, 2–4 years:** 160 mg q 4 hr as needed; **4–6 years:** 240 mg q 4 hr as needed; **6–9 years:** 320–325 mg q 4 hr as needed; **9–11 years:** 320–400 mg q 4 hr as needed; **11–12 years:** 320–480 mg q 4 hr as needed.

Acute rheumatic fever: **Adults, initial,** 5–8 g daily. **Pediatric, initial,** 100 mg/kg/day (3 g/m²/day); **then,** decrease to 75 mg/kg daily for 4–6 weeks. *Inhibitor of platelet aggregation:* 325 mg daily with the following exceptions: *Recurrent cerebral thromboembolism:* 1 g daily. *Transient ischemic attacks associated with mitral valve prolapse:* 325–1,000 mg daily. *Prophylaxis of thrombosis or occlusion of coronary bypass graft:* 325 mg 7 hr postoperatively via a nasogastric tube; **then,** 325 mg t.i.d. with 75 mg dipyridamole daily.

Note: Doses as low as 80–100 mg daily are being studied for use in unstable angina, myocardial infarction, and aortocoronary bypass surgery.

Suppositories. *Analgesic/antipyretic:* **Adults:** 325–650 mg q 4 hr as needed. **Pediatric:** See above. *Antirheumatic:* **Adults:** 3.6–5.4 g/day in divided doses. **Pediatric:** 80–100 mg/kg daily in divided doses.

NURSING CONSIDERATIONS

Administration/Storage

1. To reduce gastric irritation, administer with meals, milk, or crackers.
2. If ordered by the physician, sodium bicarbonate may be given concurrently to lessen gastric irritation.
3. Enteric-coated tablets or buffered tablets are better tolerated by some clients.
4. Aspirin should be taken with a full glass of water to prevent lodging of the drug in the esophagus.
5. Individuals allergic to tartrazine should not take aspirin.
6. Have epinephrine available to counteract hypersensitivity reactions should they occur. Asthma caused by hypersensitive reaction to salicylates may be refractory to epinephrine, so antihistamines should also be available for parenteral and oral use.
7. *Treatment of Overdose:* Initially induce vomiting or perform gastric lavage followed by activated charcoal (most effective if given within 2 hr of ingestion). Monitor salicylate levels, acid-base and fluid and electrolyte balance. For seizures, give diazepam. Treat hyperthermia if present. Alkaline diuresis will enhance renal excretion. Hemodialysis is effective but should be reserved for severe poisonings.

Interventions for Salicylate Toxicity

1. If the client has had repeated administration of large doses of salicylates, note evidence of hyperventilation or client complaints of auditory or visual disturbances (symptoms of salicylism). Report these to the physician and record on the client's chart.
2. Severe salicylate poisoning, whether due to overdose or accumulation, will have an exaggerated effect on the CNS and the metabolic system.
   - Clients may develop a salicylate jag characterized by garrulous behavior. They may act as if they were inebriated.
   - Convulsions and coma may follow.
3. When working with febrile children or the elderly who have been treated with aspirin, maintain adequate fluid intake. These two categories of clients are more susceptible to salicylate intoxication if they are dehydrated.
4. Have the following emergency supplies available for treatment of *acute salicylate toxicity:*
   - Apomorphine
   - Emetics and equipment for gastric lavage
   - IV equipment and solutions of dextrose, saline, potassium, and sodium bicarbonate; vitamin K
   - Short-acting barbiturates such as pentobarbital or secobarbital to treat convulsions

- Oxygen and a ventilator

Assessment

1. Take a complete drug history and note any evidence of hypersensitivity. Clients who have tolerated salicylates well in the past may suddenly have an allergic or anaphylactoid reaction.
2. If aspirin is being administered for pain, determine the type and pattern of pain, if the pain is unusual, or if it is recurring. Use a rating scale to assess the level of pain. Note the effectiveness of aspirin if used in the past for pain control.
3. Determine the precipitating factors related to the problem.
4. Note if the client has asthma, hay fever, or nasal polyps.
5. If the client is a child, determine if it is possible for the child to have chickenpox or the flu.
6. Note any client history of peptic ulcers or other conditions that could suggest potential problems with the use of salicylates.
7. Determine if the client is to have diagnostic tests. Many of these can be affected by the use of salicylates.
8. Determine if the client has a history of any bleeding tendencies.
9. Review the drugs the client is taking to determine the possibility of drug interactions.

Interventions

1. If client is hospitalized, administer salicylates only on an order from the physician and at the time scheduled.
2. Minimize distress by assisting the client to preserve energy.

3. Provide a comforting, relaxing environment.
4. When administering salicylates for antipyretic effect, assure that the physician has indicated the temperature at which the drug should be administered.
   - Monitor the client's temperature at least 1 hr after administering the medication.
   - Check for marked diaphoresis, and if present, dry the client, change the linens, provide fluids, and prevent chilling.
5. Note if blood is present in the stool or urine. Document and report to the physician.
6. Observe client receiving anticoagulant therapy for bruises or bleeding of the mucous membranes. Large doses of salicylates may increase the prothrombin time.
7. Assess for gastric irritation and pain.

Client/Family Teaching

1. Do not take salicylates if product is off-color or has a strange odor.
2. Explain that if sodium bicarbonate is to be used it should be taken only with physician's consent. Sodium bicarbonate may decrease the serum level of aspirin more rapidly than normal, thus reducing the effectiveness of the aspirin.
3. Discuss the toxic symptoms to be reported: ringing in the ears, difficulty hearing, dizziness or fainting spells, unusual increase in sweating, severe abdominal pain, or mental confusion. Instruct client to call the physician if any of these symptoms occur.

4. If the client has diabetes mellitus, discuss the possibility of hypoglycemia occurring because salicylates potentiate the effects of the antidiabetic drugs. Clients should monitor their blood glucose levels carefully and contact the physician for possible adjustment in drug dosage should hypoglycemia occur.

5. In cardiac clients on large doses of drug, advise that they should be alert to symptoms of CHF and to report to the physician.

6. Remind clients to tell their dentist and other health providers that they are taking salicylates and the reasons for this therapy.

7. Before purchasing other OTC preparations, tell the physician, pharmacist or nurse that you are taking salicylates and the quantity used per day.

8. Salicylates should be administered to children only upon the recommendation of their physician.

9. If a child refuses to take the medication or vomits it, discuss with the physician the possibility of using aspirin suppositories or acetaminophen.

10. If a client is to undergo surgery, consult the physician about whether to continue salicylates. Aspirin and NSAID's that may interfere with blood clotting mechanisms are usually discontinued a week before surgery to prevent the possibility of postoperative bleeding.

11. Warn clients to avoid indiscriminate use of salicylate drugs.

12. Parents should be advised not to give aspirin routinely to children under 12 years of age without first consulting the physician.

13. Children who are dehydrated and who have a fever are especially susceptible to aspirin intoxication from even small amounts of aspirin.

14. Report to the physician any gastric irritation and pain experienced by the child. These may be symptoms of hypersensitivity or toxicity.

Evaluation: Evaluate client for:
- Subjective reports of relief of discomfort
- Fever reduction; signs of infection where a fever may be masked by salicylates
- Improved joint mobility
- Freedom from complications of drug therapy

———— COMBINATION DRUG ————
Actifed Capsules, Syrup, Tablets, Actifed 12-Hour Capsules
(**AK**-tih-fed)
(OTC)

Classification/Content: Each capsule or tablet contains: *Antihistamine:* Triprolidine HCl, 2.5 mg. *Decongestant:* Pseudoephedrine HCl, 60 mg. Each 5 ml of the syrup contains one-half the amount of the above drugs, while the 12-hour capsule contains twice the amount of the above drugs. Also see information on individual components.

Uses: Treatment of nasal congestion, runny nose, itching of nose or throat, itchy or watery eyes due to the common cold, allergic rhinitis (i.e., hay fever), or other upper respiratory problems.

Dosage: Capsules. Adults and children over 12 years: One q 4–6 hr, not to exceed four capsules daily. Consult physician if capsules are indicated for children under 12 years of age. **Tablets: Adults and children over 12 years of age:** One q 4–6 hr; **pediatric, 6–12 years of age:** ½ tablet q 4–6 hr. Consult physician if tablets are indicated for children under 6 years of age. No more than four doses of the tablets should be given daily. **Syrup: Adults and children over 12 years of age:** 10 ml q 4–6 hr; **pediatric, 6–12 years of age:** 5 ml q 4–6 hr. Consult physician if syrup is indicated for children under 6 years of age. No more than four doses of the syrup should be given daily. **12-Hour Capsules: Adults and children over 12 years of age:** One q 12 hr, not to exceed two capsules daily.

NURSING CONSIDERATIONS

See *Nursing Considerations* for *Antihistamines,* p. 74.

Acyclovir (Acycloguanosine)

(ay-**SYE**-kloh-veer, ay-**SYE**-kloh-**GWON**-oh-seen)

Zovirax (Rx)

Classification: Antiviral anti-infective.

Action/Kinetics: Acyclovir is converted by herpes simplex virus (HSV)-infected cells to acyclovir triphosphate, which interferes with herpes simplex virus DNA polymerase, thereby inhibiting DNA replication. Systemic absorption is minimal from the GI tract (although therapeutic levels are reached) and following topical administration.

Peak levels after PO: 1.5–2 hr. **t½, PO:** 3.3 hr. Metabolites and unchanged drug (up to 85%) are excreted through the kidney. Dosage should be reduced in clients with impaired renal function.

Uses: PO. Initial and recurrent genital herpes in immunocompromised and nonimmunocompromised clients. Prophylaxis of frequently recurrent genital herpes infections in nonimmunocompromised clients. Treatment of chickenpox in children ranging from 2 to 18 years of age. **Parenteral.** Initial therapy for severe genital herpes in clients who are not immunocompromised; initial and recurrent mucosal and cutaneous HSV-1 and HSV-2 infections in immunocompromised individuals. Varicella zoster infections (shingles) in immunocompromised clients. Herpes simplex encephalitis (HSE) in clients over 6 months of age. **Topical.** Acyclovir decreases healing time and duration of viral shedding in initial herpes genitalis. Also used for limited non–life-threatening mucocutaneous herpes simplex virus infections in immunocompromised clients. The drug does not seem to be beneficial in recurrent herpes genitalis or in herpes labialis in nonimmunocompromised clients. *Investigational:* Cytomegalovirus and HSV infection following bone marrow or renal transplantation; herpes simplex ocular infections; herpes simplex proctitis; herpes simplex whitlow; herpes zoster encephalitis; disseminated primary eczema herpeticum; herpes simplex-associated erythema multiform; infectious mononucleosis, varicella pneumonia, varicella zoster in immunocompromised clients.

A

Contraindications: Hypersensitivity to formulation. Use in the eye. Use to prevent recurrent HSV infections.

Special Concerns: Pregnancy category: C. Use with caution during lactation. Use with caution with concomitant intrathecal methotrexate or interferon. Safety and efficacy of oral form not established in children.

Side Effects: PO. *Short-term treatment. GI:* Nausea, vomiting, diarrhea, anorexia, sore throat, taste of drug. *CNS:* Headache, dizziness, fatigue. *Miscellaneous:* Edema, skin rashes, leg pain, inguinal adenopathy. *Long-term treatment. GI:* Nausea, vomiting, diarrhea, sore throat. *CNS:* Headache, vertigo, insomnia, fatigue, fever, depression, irritability. *Other:* Arthralgia, rashes, palpitations, superficial thrombophlebitis, muscle cramps, menstrual abnormalities, acne, lymphadenopathy, alopecia. **Parenteral.** *At injection site:* Phlebitis, inflammation. *CNS:* Encephalopathic changes, jitters, headache. *Miscellaneous:* Skin rashes, urticaria, sweating, hypotension, nausea, thrombocytosis. **Topical.** Transient burning, stinging, pain. Pruritus, rash, vulvitis. **Note:** All of these effects have also been reported with the use of a placebo preparation. *Symptoms of Overdose:* Increased BUN and serum creatinine, renal failure following parenteral overdose.

Dosage: Capsules, Suspension, Tablets. *Initial genital herpes:* 200 mg q 4 hr (while awake) for a total of 5 capsules/day for 10 days. *Chronic genital herpes:* 200 mg t.i.d. for up to 12 months. Up to five 200-mg capsules/day may be required. *Intermittent therapy:* 200 mg q 4 hr (while awake) for a total of 5 capsules/day for 5 days. *Herpes zoster, acute treatment:* 800 mg q 4 hr 5 times/day for 7–10 days. *Chickenpox:* 20 mg/kg (of the suspension) q.i.d. for 5 days. **IV infusion.** *Mucosal and cutaneous herpes simplex in immunocompromised clients:* **Adults,** 5 mg/kg infused at a constant rate over 1 hr, q 8 hr (15 mg/kg/day) for 7 days. **Children less than 12 years of age:** 250 mg/m² infused at a constant rate over 1 hr, q 8 hr for 7 days. *Varicella-zoster infections (shingles):* **Adults,** 10 mg/kg infused over a constant rate over 1 hr, q 8 hr for 7 days. **Children less than 12 years of age:** 500 mg/m² infused at a constant rate over at least 1 hr, q 8 hr for 7 days. *Herpes simplex encephalitis:* **Adults:** 10 mg/kg infused at a constant rate over at least 1 hr, q 8 hr for 10 days. **Children less than 12 years of age:** 500 mg/m² infused at a constant rate over at least 1 hr, q 8 hr for 10 days. **Topical (5% ointment), Adults and children:** Lesion should be covered with sufficient amount of ointment (0.5-in. ribbon/4 sq in. of surface area) q 3 hr, 6 times/day for 7 days.

NURSING CONSIDERATIONS

See also *General Nursing Considerations For All Anti-Infectives,* p. 83.

Administration/Storage

1. Reconstituted solution should be used within 12 hr.
2. If refrigerated, reconstituted solution may show a precipitate, which dissolves at room temperature.
3. Store ointment in a dry place at room temperature.
4. To prevent spread of infection to other body sites, use a finger cot or rubber glove when applying the cream.

5. Do not exceed recommended dose.
6. Medication should not be shared with others.
7. Both the oral and parenteral dose and/or dosing interval should be adjusted in acute or chronic renal impairment.
8. The suspension may be used to treat varicella zoster infections.
9. *Treatment of Overdose:* Hemodialysis (peritoneal dialysis is less effective).

Client/Family Teaching

1. Cover all lesions with acyclovir as ordered, but do not exceed the frequency or length of time of recommended treatment.
2. Apply acyclovir ointment in the amount directed with a finger cot or rubber glove to prevent transmission of infection.
3. Report any burning, stinging, itching, and rash if they occur due to application of acyclovir.
4. Complete the examination and tests to rule out possible presence of other sexually transmitted diseases.
5. Return for medical supervision if herpes simplex virus recurs because acyclovir is ineffective for treatment of reinfection.
6. Acyclovir will not prevent transmission of disease to others or prevent reinfection.
7. The total dose and dosage schedule differ depending on whether the infection is initial or chronic and whether intermittent therapy regimen is being used. Therefore, following prescribed dosage and duration of treatment is extremely important.
8. Use condoms for sexual intercourse to prevent reinfections while undergoing treatment.
9. Abstain from intercourse during acute outbreaks.

Evaluation: Evaluate client for a positive clinical response as evidenced by:
- Subjective reports of less severe and less frequent recurrences of genital herpes
- Crusting and healing of herpes lesions

Adenosine
(ah-**DEN**-oh-seen)
Adenocard (Rx)

Classification: Antiarrhythmic.

Action/Kinetics: Adenosine is found naturally in all cells of the body. The substance slows conduction time through the AV node, interrupts the reentry pathways through the AV node, and restores normal sinus rhythm in paroxysmal supraventricular tachycardia (including Wolff-Parkinson-White syndrome). **t½:** Less than 10 sec (taken up by erythrocytes and vascular endothelial cells). Exogenous adenosine becomes part of the body pool and is metabolized mainly to inosine and adenosine monophosphate (AMP).

Uses: Conversion of sinus rhythm of paroxysmal supraventricular tachycardia. Symptomatic relief of varicose vein complications with stasis dermatitis.

Contraindications: Second- or third-degree AV block or sick sinus syndrome (except in clients with a functioning artificial pacemaker). Also, atrial flutter, atrial fibrillation, ventricular tachycardia.

Special Concerns: Use during pregnancy only when clearly needed (pregnancy category: C). Use with caution in clients with asthma.

A

Side Effects: *CV:* Facial flushing (common), headache, chest pain, sweating, palpitations, hypotension. *CNS:* Lightheadedness, dizziness, numbness, tingling in arms, heaviness in arms, blurred vision, apprehension. *GI:* Nausea, metallic taste, tightness in throat. *Respiratory:* Shortness of breath or dyspnea (common), chest pressure, hyperventilation. *Miscellaneous:* Pressure in head, burning sensation, neck and back pain, pressure in groin.

Drug Interactions

Carbamazepine / ↑ Degree of heart block
Caffeine / Competitively antagonizes effect of adenosine
Dipyridamole / ↑ Effect of adenosine
Theophylline / Competitively antagonizes effect of adenosine

Dosage: Rapid IV bolus only, initial: 6 mg over 1–2 sec. If the first dose does not reverse the supraventricular tachycardia within 1–2 min, 12 mg should be given as a rapid IV bolus. The 12-mg dose may be repeated a second time, if necessary. Doses greater than 12 mg are not recommended.

NURSING CONSIDERATIONS

See also *Nursing Considerations* for *Antiarrhythmic Drugs,* p. 52.

Administration/Storage

1. Store at room temperature. Do not refrigerate as crystallization may occur.
2. The solution should be clear at the time of use.
3. Discard any unused portion because the product contains no preservatives.
4. The drug should be administered directly into a vein. If it is to be given into an IV line,

introduce the drug in the most proximal line and follow with a rapid saline flush.

Interventions

1. Document client complaints of chest pressure, shortness of breath, heaviness of the arms, palpitations, or dyspnea.
2. Note any facial flushing and reassure the client. This is a common side effect of therapy and the physician should be informed.
3. If client complains of numbness, tingling in the arms, blurred vision, or appears apprehensive, check BP and pulse. Then notify the physician as this may be an indication to discontinue the drug therapy.

Evaluation: Evaluate client for:
- Conversion of paroxysmal SVT to NSR
- Subjective reports of symptomatic relief when used as therapy for stasis dermatitis

---

Albumin, Normal Human Serum, 5%
(al-**BYOU**-min)
Albuminar-5, Albutein 5%, Buminate 5%, Normal Serum Albumin (Human) 5% Solution, Plasbumin-5 (Rx)

Albumin, Normal Human Serum, 25%
(al-**BYOU**-min)
Albuminar-25, Albutein 25%, Buminate 25%, Normal Serum Albumin (Human) 25% Solution, Plasbumin-25 (Rx)

Classification: Blood volume expander.

Action/Kinetics: Prepared from whole blood, serum, plasma, or placentas from healthy human donors. It is supplied as a 5% (isotonic and isosmotic with normal human plasma) and 25% (salt-poor solution of which each 50 ml is osmotically equivalent to 250 ml of citrated plasma) strength. It contains sodium, 130–160 mEq/L.

Uses: Blood volume expander in shock, following surgery, hemorrhage, burns, or other trauma. Hypoproteinemia due to toxemia of pregnancy, anuria, acute hepatic cirrhosis or coma, acute nephrotic syndrome, tuberculosis, and premature infants. As an adjunct to exchange transfusions in hyperbilirubinemia and erythroblastosis fetalis. Adult respiratory distress syndrome, cardiopulmonary bypass (presurgically to dilute blood), acute liver failure (with or without coma), renal dialysis, acute nephrosis. Sequestration of protein-rich fluids as in extensive cellulitis, mediastinitis, pancreatitis, and acute peritonitis. To avoid excessive hypoproteinemia in exchange transfusions or where large volumes of washed or previously frozen red blood cells have been used.

Contraindications: Severe anemia, cardiac failure, allergy to albumin, renal insufficiency, presence of increased intravascular volume, chronic nephrosis, clients on cardiopulmonary bypass.

Special Concerns: Pregnancy category: C. This product is not a substitute for whole blood.

Side Effects: *Allergic:* Chills, fever, headache, rash, nausea, vomiting, flushing, urticaria, tachycardia, hypotension, respiratory and blood pressure changes, increased salivation. *CV:* Hypotension in clients on

cardiopulmonary bypass. Rapid administration may cause pulmonary edema, dyspnea, and vascular overload.

Laboratory Test Interference: ↑ Serum alkaline phosphatase.

Dosage: 5%, IV infusion, individualized. *Hypoproteinemia:* Rate not to exceed 5–10 ml/min. *Burns:* Sufficient solution to establish and maintain a plasma albumin level of 2–3 g/100 ml (total serum protein of approximately 5.2 g/100 ml). *Shock:* **Adults and children, initial,** 500 ml as rapidly as tolerated; repeat after 30 min if response inadequate. **Infants and neonates:** 10–20 ml/kg. **25%.** *Hypoproteinemia with or without edema:* **Adults:** 50–75 g/day; **pediatric:** 25 g/day. Rate should not exceed 2 ml/min. *Nephrosis:* 100 ml daily for 7–10 days, given with a loop diuretic. *Burns:* Determined by extent; dose must be sufficient to maintain plasma albumin levels of 2–3 g/100 ml with a plasma oncotic pressure of 20 mm Hg. *Shock:* Dose determined by client's condition. For significantly reduced blood volume, give as rapidly as desired; for normal or slightly low blood volume, give 1 ml/min. *Hyperbilirubinemia and erythroblastosis fetalis:* 4 ml/kg (1 g/kg) 1–2 hr before transfusion of blood. *Erythrocyte resuspension:* Usually, 25 g/L of erythrocytes. *Renal dialysis:* 100 ml (avoid fluid overload).

NURSING CONSIDERATIONS
Administration/Storage
1. Do not use turbid or sedimented solution.
2. Preparation does not contain preservatives. Use each opened bottle at once.
3. Use the accompanying vented

A

IV administration sets when administering commercial vials of blood volume expanders.

4. May be given as rapidly as needed initially. However, as plasma volume approaches normal, the 5% solution should not be given faster than 2–4 ml/min and the 25% solution should not be given faster than 1 ml/min.

5. In hypoproteinemia, the 5% solution should not be given faster than 5–10 ml/min and the 25% solution should not be given faster than 2–3 ml/min to minimize the possibility of circulatory overload and pulmonary edema.

6. Albumin should not be considered as a nutrient.

7. These products should be stored at room temperature, not to exceed 30°C (86°F).

Assessment

1. Note laboratory reports that may indicate the presence of any contraindications to therapy (e.g., anemia, renal insufficiency).

2. Obtain and record client blood pressure, pulse, and respirations as a baseline against which to measure subsequent readings.

3. Weigh client, if possible, before the start of therapy.

Interventions

1. Note symptoms of pulmonary edema, demonstrated by cough, dyspnea, rales, and cyanosis. **Stop** the administration of albumin and notify the physician immediately if any of these symptoms occur. Obtain chest X ray.

2. Record intake and output and client weight.

3. Observe client for diuresis and reduction of edema if present.

4. Check client for evidence of dehydration such as dry, cracked lips, flushed, dry skin, reduced urinary output, usually dark colored urine, or loss of skin turgor. This necessitates further administration of IV fluids.

5. Take blood pressure and pulse frequently (usually q 15 min initially).

6. Note evidence of hemorrhage or shock, which may occur following surgery or trauma. A rapid increase in blood pressure causes bleeding in severed blood vessels that had not been noted previously.

Evaluation: Evaluate client for:
- ↑ blood pressure and circulating blood volume
- Prevention or reversal of hypoproteinemia

Albuterol (Salbutamol)
(al-**BYOU**-ter-ohl)
Novo-Salmol ✹, Proventil, Ventodisk ✹, Ventolin, Ventolin Rotacaps, Volmax ✹ (Rx)

See also *Sympathomimetic Drugs*, p. 218.

Classification: Direct-acting adrenergic (sympathomimetic) agent.

Action/Kinetics: Albuterol stimulates beta-2 receptors of the bronchi, leading to bronchodilation. Causes less tachycardia and is longer-acting than isoproterenol. Has minimal beta-1 activity. **Onset, PO:** 15–30 min; **inhalation,** 5–15 min. **Peak effect, PO:** 2–3 hr; **inhalation,** 60–90 min (after two inhalations). **Duration, PO:** 8 hr (up to 12 hr for extended-release); **inhalation,** 3–6 hr. Metabolites and unchanged drug excreted in urine and feces. **Tablets not to be used in children less than 12 years of age.**

Use: Bronchial asthma; bronchospasm due to bronchitis or emphysema; bronchitis; reversible obstructive pulmonary disease in those 4 years of age and older; exercise-induced bronchospasm. Prophylaxis of bronchial asthma or bronchospasms. Parenteral for treatment of status asthmaticus.

Special Concerns: Pregnancy category: C. Dosage has not been established for the syrup in children less than 2 years of age, for tablets in children less than 6 years of age, and for extended-release tablets in children less than 12 years of age. Aerosol for prevention of exercise-induced bronchospasm is not recommended for children less than 12 years of age.

Dosage: Aerosol for Inhalation. Adults and children over 12 years of age: *Bronchodilation:* 0.18–0.2 mg (2 inhalations) q 4–6 hr (Ventolin aerosol may be used in children over 4 years of age). *Prophylaxis of exercise-induced bronchospasm:* 0.18–0.2 mg (2 inhalations) 15 min before exercise. **Solution for Inhalation. Adults and children over 12 years of age:** *Bronchodilation:* 1.25–5 mg (of the base) in 2–5 ml of sterile 0.9% sodium chloride or sterile water for inhalation administered by intermittent positive-pressure breathing (IPPB) or nebulization. **Capsule for Inhalation. Adults and children over 4 years of age:** *Bronchodilation:* 0.2–0.4 mg q 4–6 hr (for prophylaxis of exer-

cise-induced bronchospasm, give 15 min before exercise). **Syrup. Adults and children over 14 years of age:** 2–4 mg t.i.d.–q.i.d., up to a maximum of 8 mg q.i.d. **Children, 6–14 years, initial:** 2 mg (base) t.i.d.–q.i.d.; **then,** as necessary to a maximum of 24 mg daily in divided doses. **Children, 2–6 years, initial:** 0.1 mg/kg t.i.d.; **then,** increase as necessary up to 0.2 mg/kg, not to exceed 4 mg t.i.d. **Tablets.** *Bronchodilation:* **Adults and children over 12 years of age, initial:** 2–4 mg (of the base) t.i.d.–q.i.d.; **then,** increase dose as needed up to a maximum of 8 mg t.i.d.–q.i.d. In geriatric patients or those sensitive to beta-agonists, start with 2 mg t.i.d.–q.i.d. and then increase dose gradually, if needed. **Extended-release Tablets. Adults:** *Bronchodilation,* 4 or 8 mg (of the base) q 12 hr up to a maximum of 32 mg daily.

NURSING CONSIDERATIONS

See also *Nursing Considerations* for *Sympathomimetic Drugs,* p. 220.

Administration/Storage

1. Do not exceed the recommended dose.
2. If the dose of drug used previously does not provide relief, contact the physician immediately.
3. When using albuterol inhalers, do not use other inhalation medication unless prescribed by the physician.
4. The contents of the container are under pressure. Therefore, do not store near heat or open flames and do not puncture the container.
5. When given by nebulization, either a face mask or mouthpiece may be used. Compressed air or oxygen with a gas

A

flow of 6–10 L/min should be used, with a single treatment lasting from 5–15 min.

6. When given by IPPB, the inspiratory pressure should be from 10–20 cm water with the duration of treatment ranging from 5–20 min depending on the client and instrument control.

7. The MDI (metered-dose inhaler) may be administered on a mechanical ventilator through an adapter.

Assessment

1. Obtain a baseline history and assess client's CNS before initiating therapy.

2. Assess lung sounds. Note evidence of client anxiety because this may contribute to air hunger.

3. Determine if the client is able to self-administer the medication.

Interventions

1. Maintain a calm, reassuring attitude. If the client is acutely ill, do not leave unattended.

2. Monitor the client's CNS for effects of the therapy, adjusting the dose or frequency of medication, if needed.

3. Observe for evidence of allergic responses.

Evaluation: Evaluate for improved breathing patterns and airway exchange.

––––––– COMBINATION DRUG –––––––
Aldactazide
(al-DAK-tah-zyd)
(Rx)

Content/Classification: This drug is a combination of a thiazide and potassium-sparing diuretic. *Diuretic:* Spironolactone, 25 or 50 mg. *Diuretic/antihypertensive:* Hydrochlorothiazide, 25 or 50 mg. Also see information on individual components, p. 1155 and p. 718.

Contraindications: Use in pregnancy only if benefits outweigh risks.

Uses: Congestive heart failure, essential hypertension, nephrotic syndrome. Edema and/or ascites in cirrhosis of the liver.

Dosage: Tablets. *Edema:* **Adults, usual:** 100 mg of each drug daily (range: 25–200 mg), given as single or divided doses. **Pediatric, usual:** equivalent to 1.65–3.3 mg/kg spironolactone. *Essential hypertension:* **Adults, usual:** 50–100 mg of each drug daily in single or divided doses.

NURSING CONSIDERATIONS

See *Nursing Considerations* for *Diuretics,* p. 141, and *Antihypertensive Agents,* p. 78.

Alfentanil hydrochloride
(al-FEN-tah-nil)
Alfenta (C-II, Rx)

See also *Narcotic Analgesics,* p. 174.

Classification: Narcotic analgesic.

Action/Kinetics: Onset: Immediate. **t½:** 1–2 hr (after IV use).

Uses: *Continuous infusion:* With nitrous oxide/oxygen to maintain general anesthesia. *Incremental doses:* Adjunct with barbiturate/nitrous oxide/oxygen to maintain general anesthesia. *Anesthetic induction:* As primary agent when endotracheal intubation and mechanical ventilation are necessary.

Contraindications: Use during labor.

Special Concerns: Pregnancy category: C. Use in children less than 12 years of age is not recommended. Use with caution during lactation.

Additional Side Effects: Bradycardia, postoperative confusion, blurred vision, hypercapnia, shivering, and asystole hypercapnia. Neonates with respiratory distress syndrome have manifested hypotension with doses of 20 mcg/kg.

Dosage: *Continuous infusion, duration 45 min or more:* **Initial for induction:** 50–75 mcg/kg; **maintenance, with nitrous oxide/oxygen:** 0.5–3 mcg/kg/min. Following the induction dose, the infusion rate requirement should be reduced by 30%–50% for the first hour of maintenance. *Induction of anesthesia, duration 45 min or more:* **Initial for induction:** 130–245 mcg/kg; **maintenance:** 0.5–1.5 mcg/kg/min. If a general anesthetic is used for maintenance, the concentration of inhalation agents should be reduced by 30%–50% for the first hour. *Anesthetic adjunct, 30–60 min duration:* **Initial for induction:** 20–50 mcg/kg; **maintenance:** 5–15 mcg/kg, up to a total dose of 75 mcg/kg. *Anesthetic adjunct, less than 30 min duration:* **Initial for induction:** 8–20 mcg/kg; **maintenance:** 3–5 mcg/kg (or 0.5–1 mcg/kg/min, up to a total dose of 8–40 mcg/kg). If there is a lightening of general anesthesia or the client manifests signs of surgical stress, the rate of administration of alfentanil may be increased to 4 mcg/kg/min or a bolus dose of 7 mcg/kg may be used. If the situation is not controlled following three bolus doses over 5 min, an inhalation anesthetic, a barbiturate, or a vasodilator should be used. It signs of lightening anesthesia are noted within the last 15 min of surgery, a bolus dose of 7 mcg/kg should be given rather than increasing the infusion rate. A potent inhalation anesthetic may be used as an alternative.

NURSING CONSIDERATIONS

See also *Nursing Considerations* for *Narcotic Analgesics,* p. 177.

Administration/Storage

1. The dosage of drug must be individualized for each client and for each use.
   - For elderly or debilitated clients the dosage of drug should be reduced.
   - For obese clients who are more than 20% above their ideal body weight, the dosage should be based on lean body weight.
2. The injectable form may be reconstituted with either normal saline, 5% dextrose in normal saline, lactated Ringer's solution, or 5% dextrose in water.
3. The infusion should be discontinued 10–15 min prior to the end of surgery.

Assessment

1. Note if the client has a history of drug sensitivity. The drug should be avoided if this is evident.
2. Determine if the client's pain is the result of a head injury. The drug is contraindicated in this instance.

A

3. Obtain baseline vital signs prior to administering the medication. Assisted or controlled ventilation may be required.

Client/Family Teaching

1. Some clients may develop muscular rigidity. If this occurs, report it to the physician before proceeding with the next dose of medication.
2. Advise to avoid alcohol or CNS depressants for at least 24 hr following drug administration.

Evaluation: Evaluate client for evidence of:
- Desired level of analgesia
- Reduction of motor activity

Alglucerase
(al-**GLOO**-sir-ace)
Ceredase (Rx)

Classification: Treatment of Gaucher's disease.

Action/Kinetics: Gaucher's disease is a rare congenital disorder of lipid metabolism where there is a deficiency in beta-glucocerebrosidase leading to an accumulation of lipid glucocerebroside in the liver, spleen, and bone marrow. Symptoms of the disease include an enlarged spleen, increased skin pigmentation, bone lesions, severe anemia, and thrombocytopenia. Alglucerase, which is a modified form of beta-glucocerebrosidase, is derived from human placental tissue; it catalyzes the hydrolysis of the glycolipid glucocerebroside to glucose and ceramide, which is part of the normal degradation pathway for membrane lipids. Following IV infusion, steady state enzyme levels

were observed in 60 min. $t^{1/2}$: 3.6–10.4 min.

Uses: Chronic enzyme replacement in clients with confirmed diagnosis of type I Gaucher's disease who meet the following criteria: moderate-to-severe anemia, thrombocytopenia with bleeding tendency, significant hepatomegaly or splenomegaly, and bone disease.

Special Concerns: Pregnancy category: C. Use with caution during lactation. Since alglucerase is derived from human placental tissue, there is always the risk of some viral contamination; however, the drug product has been found to be free from hepatitis B surface antigen and for antigens of the human immunodeficiency virus (HIV-1).

Side Effects: Nausea, vomiting, chills, abdominal discomfort, slight fever.

Dosage: IV infusion. Initial: Up to 60 U/kg/infusion with infusions usually given q 2 weeks. Dose is then adjusted downward for maintenance therapy; dosage can be lowered q 3–6 months with some clients responding to doses as low as 1 U/kg.

NURSING CONSIDERATIONS
Administration/Storage

1. Although the dose is usually given every 2 weeks, the severity of the disease (and client convenience) may require administration as frequently as every other day or as infrequently as every 4 weeks.
2. Response parameters should be closely monitored as the dose is progressively lowered.
3. Prior to administration, the drug is diluted with normal

saline to a final volume not to exceed 100 ml. An in-line particulate filter is recommended for the infusion apparatus.

4. The product should not be shaken as shaking may denature the glycoprotein, making it inactive.

5. The product should be stored at 4°C (39°F). If the bottle shows any discoloration or particulate matter, it should not be used.

6. Since the product does not contain any preservative, it should not be stored for subsequent use after being opened.

7. Small dosage adjustments (either increased or decreased) may be made to avoid discarding partially used bottles provided that the monthly administered dosage is not altered.

Assessment

1. Note onset and list symptoms of disease requiring treatment.
2. Obtain baseline CBC and determine laboratory confirmation of type I Gaucher's disease noting the presence of anemia, thrombocytopenia with bleeding tendency, enlarged liver and spleen, and any evidence of bone disease (potential for pathologic fractures due to demineralization).
3. Perform a baseline assessment to use as data to determine the effectiveness of drug therapy.

Client/Family Teaching

1. Explain that the client may experience "flu-like" symptoms (nausea, vomiting, fever, chills, and abdominal discomfort) but that this is usually only temporary.
2. Advise client that the drug has been derived from pooled human placental tissue and review the potential risks.
3. Stress the importance of reporting for scheduled visits as the dose is progressively lowered based on response parameters.

Evaluataion: Evaluate client for:

- Evidence of a reduction in splenomegaly and hepatomegaly within 6 months of continued alglucerase therapy
- Laboratory evidence of improved hematologic parameters (e.g., ↑ Hb, Hct, erythrocyte, and platelet counts)

Allopurinol
(al-oh-**PYOUR**-ih-nohl)
Alloprin✶, Apo-Allopurinol✶, Novopurol✶, Purinol✶, Zyloprim (Rx)

Classification: Antigout agent.

Action/Kinetics: Allopurinol and its major metabolite, oxipurinol, are potent inhibitors of xanthine oxidase, an enzyme involved in the synthesis of uric acid, without disrupting the biosynthesis of essential purine. This results in decreased levels of uric acid. The drug also increases reutilization of xanthine and hypoxanthine for synthesis of nucleotide and nucleic acid synthesis by acting on the enzyme hypoxanthine-guanine phosphoribosyltransferase. The resultant increases in nucleotides cause a negative feedback to inhibit synthesis of purines and a decrease in uric acid levels. **Peak plasma levels:** 1.5 hr for allopurinol and 4.5 hr for oxipurinol. **Onset:** 2–3 days. **t½** (allopurinol); 1–3 hr; **t½** (oxipurinol): 12–30 hr. **Peak serum levels, allopurinol:** 2–3 mcg/ml; **oxipurinol:** 5–6.5 mcg/ml (up to 50 mcg/ml in clients with impaired renal function). **Maximum therapeutic effect:** 1–3 weeks. Well absorbed from GI tract, metabolized in liver, excreted in urine and feces (20%).

Uses: Primary or secondary gout (acute attacks, tophi, joint destruction, nephropathy, uric acid lithiasis). Clients with leukemia, lymphoma, or other malignancies in whom drug therapy causes elevations of serum and urinary uric acid. Recurrent calcium oxalate calculi. *Investigational:* Mixed with methylcellulose as a mouthwash to prevent stomatitis following fluorouracil administration.

Contraindications: Hypersensitivity to drug. Clients with idiopathic hemochromatosis or relatives of clients suffering from this condition. Children except as an adjunct in treatment of neoplastic disease. Severe skin reactions on previous exposure.

Special Concerns: Pregnancy category: C. Use with caution during lactation. Use with caution in clients with liver or renal disease. In children use has been limited to rare inborn errors of purine metabolism or hyperuricemia as a result of malignancy or cancer therapy.

Side Effects: *Dermatologic* (most frequent): Pruritic maculopapular skin rash (may be accompanied by fever and malaise). Exfoliative urticarial, purpura-type dermatitis and alopecia. Stevens-Johnson syndrome. Skin rash has been accompanied by hypertension and cataract development. *Allergy:* Fever, chills, leukopenia, eosinophilia, arthralgia, skin rash, pruritus, nausea, vomiting, nephritis. *GI:* Nausea, vomiting, diarrhea, gastritis, dyspepsia, abdominal pain (intermittent). *Hematologic:* Leukopenia, eosinophilia, thrombocytopenia, leukocytosis. *Hepatic:* Hepatomegaly, cholestatic jaundice, hepatic necrosis, granulomatous hepatitis. *Neurologic:* Headache, peripheral neuropathy, paresthesia, somnolence, neuritis. *CV:* Necrotizing angiitis, hypersensitivity vasculitis. *Miscellaneous:* Ecchymosis, epistaxis, taste loss, arthralgia, acute attacks of gout, fever, myopathy, renal failure, uremia, alopecia.

Drug Interactions

ACE inhibitors / ↑ Risk of hypersensitivity reactions

Aluminum salts / ↓ Effect of allopurinol

Ampicillin / ↑ Risk of ampicillin-induced skin rashes

Anticoagulants, oral / ↑ Effect of anticoagulant due to ↓ breakdown by liver

Azathioprine / ↑ Effect of azathioprine due to ↓ breakdown by liver

Cyclophosphamide / ↑ Risk of bleeding or infection due to ↑ myelosuppressive effects of cyclophosphamide

Iron preparations / Allopurinol ↑ hepatic iron concentrations

Mercaptopurine / ↑ Effect of mercaptopurine due to ↓ breakdown by liver

Theophylline / Allopurinol ↑ plasma theophylline levels → to possible toxicity

Thiazide diuretics / ↑ Risk of hypersensitivity reactions to allopurinol

Uricosuric agents / ↓ Effect of oxipurinol due to ↑ rate of excretion

Laboratory Test Interferences: ↑ ALT, AST, alkaline phosphatase. ↑ Serum cholesterol. ↓ Serum glucose levels.

Dosage: Tablets. *Gout/hyperuricemia:* **Adults,** 200–600 mg/day, depending on severity (minimum effective dose: 100–200 mg/day). Maximum daily dose should not exceed 800 mg. *Prevention of uric acid nephropathy during treatment of neoplasms:* 600–800 mg/day for 2–3 days (with high fluid intake). *Prophylaxis of acute gout:* **Initial,** 100 mg/day; increase by 100 mg at weekly intervals until serum uric acid level of 6 mg/100 ml or less is reached. **Pediatric,** *Hyperuricemia associated with malignancy,* **6–10 years of age:** 300 mg/day either as a single dose of 100 mg t.i.d.; **under 6 years of age:** 150 mg/day in 3 divided doses. *Recurrent calcium oxalate calculi:* 200–300 mg daily in one or more doses (dose may be adjusted according to urinary levels of uric acid). Transfer from colchicine, uricosuric agents, and/or anti-inflammatory agents to allopurinol should be made gradually by decreasing the dosage of the above agents and increasing the dosage of allopurinol until a normal serum uric acid level is achieved.

NURSING CONSIDERATIONS

Administration/Storage

1. Administer with food or immediately after meals to lessen potential gastric irritation.
2. At least 10–12 eight ounce glasses of fluid should be taken each day.
3. To prevent the formation of uric acid stones, the urine should be kept slightly alkaline.

Assessment

1. Take a complete drug history, noting any medications that might interact with allopurinol.
2. Review client orders, determine if the client is scheduled for diagnostic tests with which allopurinol would interact.
3. If the client is female and of childbearing age and sexually active, or if the woman is nursing, allopurinol is contraindicated.

Interventions

1. If the client has been taking a uricosuric agent and is to be placed on allopurinol, anticipate that the dosage of the uricosuric agent will be gradually decreased as the dosage of allopurinol is gradually increased.
2. Assess for changes in vision. If changes occur, advise the client to have an ophthalmologic exam.
3. Monitor the CBC with differential, platelet count, liver and renal function studies, and serum uric acid on a routine basis during therapy.
4. Dosage should be decreased with renal impairment.

Client/Family Teaching

1. Take medication at or following meal time to decrease GI upset.
2. Advise clients to monitor their weight if they are experiencing nausea and vomiting or other signs of gastric irritation. If the condition persists and the client notes weight loss, report to the physician.

3. If a skin rash occurs, report to the physician. Skin rashes may start after months of drug therapy. If they are caused by allopurinol, the drug needs to be discontinued.
4. Unless otherwise indicated, advise clients to maintain a fluid intake that will result in a minimum excretion of 2 L of urine daily. This will assist to prevent kidney damage.
5. Advise clients not to take iron salts while they are taking allopurinol. High concentrations of iron may occur in the liver.
6. Avoid excessive intake of vitamin C, which may lead to increased potential for the formation of kidney stones.
7. Avoid alcoholic beverages. These decrease the effect of allopurinol.
8. Provide the client with a printed list of foods high in purine to avoid. These may include sardines, row, scallops, anchovies, organ meat, and mincemeat.

Evaluation: Evaluate client for:
- Decrease in serum and urinary uric acid levels
- Reports of symptomatic improvement

Alpha₁-Proteinase Inhibitor (Human) (Alpha₁-PI)

(**AL**-fah-1-**PROH**-tee-in-ayz)

Prolastin (Rx)

Classification: Alpha$_1$-proteinase inhibitor.

Action/Kinetics: Alpha$_1$-PI is the enzyme that is deficient in alpha$_1$-antitrypsin disease. This disease causes a progressive breakdown of elastin tissues in the alveoli, resulting in emphysema. Often fatal, alpha$_1$-antitrypsin disease is usually manifested in the third and fourth decades of life. Prolastin is a sterile, lyophilized product obtained from pooled human plasma that is nonreactive for the human immunodeficiency virus (HIV) antibody and the hepatitis B surface antigen. **t$^{1/2}$:** 4.5 days. **Therapeutic serum levels:** Approximately 80 mg/dl, although such levels may not reflect actual functional alpha$_1$-PI levels.

Use: Panacinar emphysema due to congenital alpha$_1$-proteinase deficiency.

Contraindications: Clients with PiMZ or PiMS phenotypes of alpha$_1$-antitrypsin deficiency.

Special Concerns: Use during pregnancy (category: C) only if benefits clearly outweigh risks. Safety and efficacy for use in children not determined. Use with caution in clients at risk for circulatory overload.

Side Effects: Although precautions are taken during the manufacture of this product, it is possible that hepatitis and other infectious viruses may be present. *Miscellaneous:* Delayed fever up to 12 hr following treatment, dizziness, lightheadedness, mild transient leukocytosis.

Dosage: IV only. Adults: 60 mg/kg each week at a rate of 0.08 ml/kg/min (or greater).

NURSING CONSIDERATIONS
Administration/Storage
1. Administer within 3 hr after reconstitution.
2. Administer only via IV. Follow

recommended procedures for reconstitution.

3. Prolastin should be stored at 2°C–8°C and should not be frozen.

4. When reconstituted, Prolastin is equal to or greater than 20 mg/ml and has a pH of 6.6–7.4.

5. The reconstituted drug should not be mixed with other diluents except for normal saline.

6. Clients should be immunized against hepatitis B prior to using Prolastin. If time does not permit adequate immunization, a single dose of Hepatitis B Immune Globulin (Human), 0.06 ml/kg IM, should be given at the time of the initial dose of Prolastin.

7. Equipment used and any unused reconstituted alpha$_1$-proteinase inhibitor (human) should be appropriately discarded.

Assessment

1. Obtain a complete nursing history and lung assessment.

2. Obtain a hepatitis profile. If the client has not received hepatitis B immunization, document and provide predrug therapy.

Interventions

1. Observe the client for delayed fever, which may occur within 12 hr. This is usually resolved in 24 hr.

2. Note any complaints of light-headedness or dizziness and report to the physician.

Client/Family Teaching

1. Advise that cigarette smoking may accelerate and aggravate condition by causing an increase of elastin secretion.

2. Discuss familial tendency to alpha$_1$-antitrypsin deficiency, and explain the need for all relatives to be screened and provided appropriate counseling.

3. Stress the importance of reporting weekly for medication to maintain an adequate anti-elastase barrier.

4. Explain that therapy must continue throughout the client's lifetime.

5. Discuss that the product is prepared from human plasma and explain the potential associated risks.

Evaluation

1. Prolastin levels should be within therapeutic range (80 mg/dl).

2. ABGs are within acceptable range and client experiences less difficulty and effort with breathing.

3. Appropriate family members are identified, screened, and counseled.

Alprazolam

(al-**PRAYZ**-oh-lam)

Apo-Alpraz✢, Xanax (C-IV, Rx)

See also *Benzodiazepines*, p. 108.

Classification: Antianxiety agent.

Action/Kinetics: Peak plasma levels: PO, 8–37 ng/ml after 1–2 hr. **t½:** 12–15 hr. 80% plasma protein bound. Metabolized to alpha-hydroxyalprazolam, an active metabolite. **t½:** 12–15 hr. Excreted in urine.

Uses: Anxiety. Anxiety associated with depression with or without agoraphobia. *Investigational:*

Agorophobia with social phobia, depression, premenstrual syndrome.

Special Concerns: Pregnancy category: D.

Dosage: Tablets. *Anxiety disorder:* **Adults, initial:** 0.25–0.5 mg t.i.d.; **then,** titrate to needs of client, with total daily dosage not to exceed 4 mg. **In elderly or debilitated: initial,** 0.25 mg b.i.d.–t.i.d.; **then,** adjust dosage to needs of client. *Antipanic agent:* 0.5 mg t.i.d.; increase dose as needed up to a maximum of 10 mg daily. *Agoraphobia with social phobia:* 2–8 mg daily. *Premenstrual syndrome:* 0.25 mg t.i.d.

NURSING CONSIDERATIONS

See also *Nursing Considerations* for *Benzodiazepines,* p. 111.

Administration/Storage: The daily dose should not be decreased more than 0.5 mg q 3 days if therapy is terminated or the dose decreased.

Interventions

1. Use side rails and support devices as needed, especially at night because elderly clients tend to become somewhat confused
2. Anticipate reduced dosage in the elderly and debilitated client.

Evaluation: Evaluate for:
- Evidence of positive behaviors in clients being treated for phobias
- Subjective reports of a reduction in the levels of anxiety as well as evidence of new coping strategies
- Improvement of PMS symptoms with a minimum of unwanted drug side effects

---

Alprostadil (PGE₁)

(al-PROSS-tah-dill)
Prostin VR✱, Prostin VR Pediatric (Rx)

Classification: Prostaglandin.

Action/Kinetics: Alprostadil is one of the prostaglandins that is a naturally occurring acidic lipid. Alprostadil relaxes smooth muscle of the ductus arteriosus leading to increased pulmonary blood flow with increased blood oxygenation and lower body perfusion. Clients with low pO_2 values respond best. The drug may also cause vasodilation, inhibit platelet aggregation, and stimulate both intestinal and uterine smooth muscle. When injected intracavernosally, alprostadil relaxes the trabecular cavernous smooth muscles and causes dilation of penile arteries. This results in increased arterial blood flow to the corpus cavernosa and thus swelling and elongation of the penis. **Onset, systemic:** 1.5–3 hr for acyanotic congenital heart disease and 15–30 min for cyanotic congenital heart disease. **Time to peak effect:** 3 hr for coarctation of the aorta and 1.5 hr for interruption of aortic arch. **Duration:** Closure of the ductus arteriosus usually begins 1–2 hr after infusion discontinued. Alprostadil is rapidly metabolized (80% in one pass) by oxidation in the lung, and metabolites are excreted by the kidney.

Uses: For temporary maintenance of patency of the ductus arteriosus (until surgery can be performed) in neonates with congenital heart defects. *Investigational:* Diagnosis and treatment of impotence.

Contraindications: Respiratory distress syndrome (hyaline membrane disease). Use with caution in neonates with bleeding tendencies. History of priapism, sickle cell disease.

Side Effects: *Respiratory:* Apnea (in 10%–12% of neonates), especially in neonates less than 2 kg at birth; bronchial wheezing, bradypnea, hypercapnia, respiratory depression. *CNS:* Fever, seizures, hypothermia, jitteriness, lethargy, cerebral bleeding, stiffness, hyperextension of the neck, irritability. *CV:* Flushing, especially after intra-arterial dosage, bradycardia, hypotension, tachycardia, cardiac arrest, edema, congestive heart failure, shock, arrhythmias. *GI:* Diarrhea, hyperbilirubinemia, gastric regurgitation. *Renal:* Hematuria, anuria. *Skeletal:* Cortical proliferation of long bones. *Hematologic:* Disseminated intravascular coagulation, thrombocytopenia, anemia, bleeding. *Miscellaneous:* Sepsis, peritonitis, hypoglycemia, hypokalemia or hyperkalemia. *Symptoms of Overdose:* Apnea, bradycardia, flushing, hypotension, pyrexia.

Laboratory Test Interferences: ↑ Bilirubin. ↓ Glucose, serum calcium. ↑ or ↓ Potassium.

Dosage: Continuous IV infusion or umbilical artery: Initial, 0.05–0.1 mcg/kg/min; **then,** after response achieved, decrease infusion rate to lowest dose that will maintain response (e.g., 0.1–0.05 to 0.025–0.01 mcg/kg/min). **Note:** If 0.1 mcg/kg/min is insufficient, dosage can be increased up to 0.4 mcg/kg/min. **Intracavernosal:** 2.5–20 mcg (up to 40 mcg) with dose adjusted according to response; should not be given more than 3 times a week or for 2 days in succession.

NURSING CONSIDERATIONS

Administration/Storage

1. Administer only in pediatric intensive care facilities.
2. Dilute 500 mcg with either sodium chloride injection or dextrose injection in volumes appropriate for the infant's fluid intake and suitable for the type of infusion pump available.
3. Use a Y set-up.
4. Discard any unused solutions and prepare a fresh infusion solution every 24 hr.
5. Sterile solutions should be infused for the shortest time and at the lowest dose that will produce the desired effect.
6. Have a respirator available at the cribside.
7. Store ampules at 2°C–8°C (36°F–46°F).
8. *Treatment of Overdose:* Reduce rate of infusion if symptoms of hypotension or pyrexia occur; discontinue infusion if symptoms of apnea or bradycardia occur.

Assessment

1. Assess the client's cardiac function, blood pressure, and respiratory function and document prior to administering the medication.
2. Determine if the neonate has restricted pulmonary blood flow.
3. Note evidence of bleeding tendencies and sickle cell anemia as these are contraindications to drug therapy.

A

Interventions

1. Monitor arterial pressure intermittently by umbilical artery catheter, auscultation, Dinemapp or with a Doppler transducer. If the arterial pressure falls significantly, decrease the rate of flow immediately. Obtain written guidelines for arterial pressures from the physician.
2. Observe the infant for apnea, bradycardia, pyrexia, flushing, and hypotension. These are symptoms of *overdosage*. The following guidelines are appropriate.
   - If the infant develops apnea or bradycardia, stop the administration of drug, change to the unmedicated solution, start resuscitation, and report to the physician.
   - If the infant develops pyrexia or hypotension, reduce the rate of IV flow and report to the physician. The rate of IV flow will likely be reduced until the temperature and blood pressure return to baseline values.
   - If flushing occurs, report to the physician. This symptom indicates an incorrect intra-arterial placement of the catheter. The catheter requires repositioning.
3. If the infant has restricted pulmonary blood flow, monitor the blood gases. A positive response to alprostadil is indicated by at least a 10 mm Hg increase in blood pO_2.
4. If the infant has restricted systemic blood flow, monitor the systemic blood pressure and serum pH. If the infant has acidosis, a positive response to alprostadil would be indicated by an increased pH, an increase in blood pressure, and a decreased ratio of pulmonary artery pressure to aortic pressure.

Evaluation: Evaluate client for:

- Improved pulmonary blood flow with a resultant increased blood oxygenation level
- Freedom from complications of drug therapy

Alteplase, recombinant

(**AL**-teh-playz)

Activase, Activase rt-PA✱ (Rx)

Classification: Thrombolytic agent (tissue plasminogen activator).

Action/Kinetics: Alteplase, a tissue plasminogen activator, is synthesized by a human melanoma cell line using recombinant DNA technology. This enzyme binds to fibrin in a thrombus, causing a conversion of plasminogen to plasmin. This conversion results in local fibrinolysis and a decrease in circulating fibrinogen. Within 10 min following termination of an infusion, 80% of the alteplase has been cleared from the plasma by the liver. The enzyme activity of alteplase is 580,000 IU/mg. **t½, initial:** 4 min; **final:** 35 min (elimination phase).

Uses: Lysis of coronary thrombi following acute myocardial infarction. The drug thus reduces the incidence of congestive heart failure and improves ventricular function. Acute pulmonary thromboembolism. *Investigational:* Unstable angina pectoris.

Contraindications: Severe (uncontrolled) hypertension. Clients with a risk of internal bleeding and history of cerebrovascular accident, intracranial or intraspinal surgery or trauma (within 2 months), aneurysm, bleeding diathesis, intracranial neoplasm, arteriovenous (AV) malformation or aneurysm, severe uncontrolled hypertension, and active internal bleeding.

Special Concerns: Use with caution in the presence of recent GI or GU bleeding (within 10 days), subacute bacterial endocarditis, acute pericarditis, significant liver dysfunction, concomitant use of oral anticoagulants, diabetic hemorrhagic retinopathy, septic thrombophlebitis or occluded AV cannula (at infected site), pregnancy (category: C) and lactation, mitral stenosis with atrial fibrillation. Since fibrin will be lysed during therapy, careful attention should be given to potential bleeding sites such as sites of catheter insertion and needle puncture sites. Use with caution within 10 days of major surgery (e.g., obstetrics, coronary artery bypass) and in clients over 75 years of age. Safety and efficacy have not been established in children. **Note:** Doses greater than 150 mg have been associated with an increase in intracranial bleeding.

Side Effects: *Bleeding tendencies:* Internal bleeding (including the GI and GU tracts and intracranial or retroperitoneal sites). Superficial bleeding (e.g., gums, sites of recent surgery, venous cutdowns, arterial punctures). Ecchymosis, epistaxis. *GI:* Nausea, vomiting. *Miscellaneous:* Fever, urticaria, hypotension.

Drug Interactions

Acetylsalicylic acid / ↑ Risk of bleeding
Dipyridamole / ↑ Risk of bleeding

Heparin / ↑ Risk of bleeding, especially at arterial puncture sites

Dosage: IV infusion only. *Acute myocardial infarction:* 100 mg total dose subdivided as follows: 60 mg (34.8 million IU) the first hour with 6–10 mg given in a bolus over the first 1–2 min and the remaining 50–54 mg given over the hour; 20 mg (11.6 million IU) over the second hour and 20 mg given over the third hour. **Clients less than 65 kg:** 1.25 mg/kg given over 3 hr, with 60% given the first hour with 6%–10% given by direct IV injection within the first 1–2 min; 20% is given the second hour and 20% during the third hour. Doses of 150 mg have caused an increase in intracranial bleeding. *Pulmonary embolism:* 100 mg over 2 hr; heparin therapy should be instituted near the end of or right after the alteplase infusion when the partial thromboplastin or thrombin time returns to twice that of normal or less.

NURSING CONSIDERATIONS

Administration/Storage

1. Alteplase therapy should be initiated as soon as possible after onset of symptoms.
2. Nearly 90% of clients also receive heparin concomitantly with alteplase and either aspirin or dipyridamole during or after heparin therapy.
3. The product must be reconstituted with only sterile water for injection without preservatives immediately prior to use. The reconstituted preparation contains 1 mg/ml and is a colorless to pale yellow transparent solution.
4. Using an 18-gauge needle, the

stream of sterile water for injection should be directed into the lyophilized cake. The product should be left undisturbed for several minutes to allow dissipation of any large bubbles.

5. If necessary, the reconstituted solution may be further diluted immediately prior to use in an equal volume of 0.9% sodium chloride injection or 5% dextrose injection to yield a concentration of 0.5 mg/ml. Dilution should be accomplished by gentle swirling or slow inversion.

6. Either glass bottles or polyvinyl chloride bags may be used for administration.

7. Alteplase is stable for up to 8 hr following reconstitution or dilution. Stability will not be affected by light.

8. Use an electronic infusion device for medication administration. Do not add any other medications to the line.

9. Lyophilized alteplase should be stored at room temperatures not to exceed 30°C or under refrigeration between 2°C–8°C.

10. *Treatment of Overdose:* Discontinue therapy immediately as well as any concomitant heparin therapy.

Assessment

1. Ensure that bleeding times have been completed before initiating therapy. These serve as baseline data against which to determine client response to therapy and any associated changes that may need to occur.

2. Note any client history of hypertension or internal bleeding.

3. Record client age and determine whether or not client has had recent surgery.

4. Assess client's overall physical condition and document.

5. Obtain a drug history and determine if client is currently taking any oral anticoagulant drugs.

Interventions

1. Carefully review and follow instructions for drug reconstitution.

2. Review the contraindications carefully before initiating therapy.

3. Anticipate concurrent heparin administration by infusion.

4. Have available emergency drugs and resuscitative equipment.

5. Clients receiving therapy should be observed in a closely monitored environment.

6. Anticipate and assess for reperfusion reactions such as:
   • reperfusion arrhythmias usually of short duration. These may include accelerated idioventricular rhythm and sinus bradycardia.
   • a reduction of chest pain.
   • a return of the elevated ST segment to near baseline levels.

7. Check all access sites for any evidence of bleeding.

8. During IV therapy, arterial sticks require 30 min of manual pressure followed by application of a pressure dressing.

9. In the event of any uncontrolled bleeding, terminate the

alteplase and heparin infusions and notify the physician immediately.

10. During treatment for pulmonary embolism, ensure that the partial thromboplastin time or prothrombin time is no more than twice that of normal before heparin therapy is added.

Client/Family Teaching

1. Review the inherent risks of drug therapy during acute coronary artery occlusion.
2. Stress that to be effective, the therapy should be instituted within 4–6 hr of onset of symptoms of acute myocardial infarction.

Evaluation

1. Evaluate for restoration of coronary perfusion as evidenced by improved circulation and/or improved parameters indicative or left ventricular function.
2. Evaluate for evidence of adverse side effects such as rust colored urine, GI bleeding, CHF, or signs of intracranial bleeding (increased intracranial pressure) that would necessitate termination of therapy.

Altretamine

(all-**TRET**-ah-meen)

Hexalen, Hexastat✹ (Rx)

See also *Antineoplastic Agents,* p. 85.

Classification: Antineoplastic, miscellaneous.

Action/Kinetics: The mechanism of action of altretamine is unknown although metabolism of the drug is required for cytotoxicity. Altretamine is well absorbed following oral ingestion and undergoes rapid demethylation in the liver, yielding the principal metabolites–pentamethylmelamine and tetramethylmelamine. **Peak plasma levels:** 0.5–3 hr. **t½:** 4.7–10.2 hr. Metabolites of the drug are excreted mainly through the kidney.

Uses: Used alone in the palliative treatment of persistent or recurrent ovarian cancer after first-line cisplatin- or alkylating agent-based combination therapy.

Contraindications: Preexisting bone marrow depression or severe neurologic toxicity, although the drug has been used safely in clients with preexisting cisplatin neuropathies. Use during lactation.

Special Concerns: Pregnancy category: D. Safety and effectiveness have not been determined in children. High daily doses may result in gradual onset of nausea and vomiting.

Side Effects: *GI:* Nausea and vomiting (most common). *Neurologic:* Peripheral sensory neuropathy, fatigue, anorexia, seizures. *Hematologic:* Leukopenia, thrombocytopenia, anemia. *Miscellaneous:* Hepatic toxicity, skin rash, pruritus, alopecia.

Drug Interactions: Use with MAO inhibitors may cause severe orthostatic hypotension, especially in clients over the age of 60 years.

Laboratory Test Interferences: ↑ Serum creatinine, BUN, alkaline phosphatase.

Dosage: Capsules: 260 mg/m²/day given either for 14 or 21 consecutive days in a 28-day cycle. The total daily dose is given as four divided oral doses after meals and at bedtime.

NURSING CONSIDERATIONS

See also *Nursing Considerations* for *Antineoplastic Agents,* p. 88.

Assessment

1. Determine that a baseline neurologic examination has been performed and document.
2. Obtain hematologic studies prior to initiating drug therapy.

Interventions

1. Anticipate neurotoxicity as a side effect of drug therapy. A neurologic exam should be performed prior to each course of altretamine.
2. If prescribed, administer pyridoxine with altretamine. This may reduce the severity of the neurotoxic effects.

Client/Family Teaching

1. Report any adverse symptoms, such as tingling, decreased sensation, dizziness, nausea, and vomiting. Drug dose may need to be decreased or therapy discontinued.
2. Practice barrier contraception as drug may cause fetal damage.
3. Emphasize the importance of reporting for monthly hematologic studies.

Aluminum hydroxide gel

(ah-**LOO**-mih-num)

Alternagel, Amphojel, Concentrated Aluminum Hydroxide, Gaviscon✿, Nephrox (OTC)

Aluminum hydroxide gel, dried

(ah-**LOO**-mih-num)

Alu-Cap, Alu-Tab, Amphojel Tablets, Basaljel✿, Dialume (OTC)

See also *Antacids,* p. 37.

Classification: Antacid.

Action/Kinetics: Aluminum hydroxide is nonsystemic, has demulcent activity, and is constipating. Aluminum hydroxide and phosphorus form insoluble phosphates that are eliminated in the feces. This yields a relatively phosphorus-free urine and prevents phosphate stone formation in susceptible clients. Acid-neutralizing capacity: 6.5–18 mEq/tablet, capsule, or 5 ml. Aluminum-containing antacids are believed to have a cytoprotective effect on the gastric mucosa (perhaps by stimulating prostaglandin synthesis), which protects against mucosal damage by aspirin and ethanol. Small amounts are absorbed from the intestine.

Additional Uses: Hyperphosphatemia, chronic renal failure.

Contraindications: Sensitivity to aluminum. Peptic ulcer associated with pancreatic deficiency, diarrhea, or low-phosphorus diet. Aluminum hydroxide preparations contain sodium and thus should not be administered to clients on a low-sodium diet.

Side Effects: Chronic use may lead to bone pain, muscle weakness, or malaise due to chronic phosphate deficiency and osteomalacia. Constipation, intestinal obstruction. Decreased absorption of fluoride. Accumulation of aluminum in bone, CNS, and serum, which may be neurotoxic (e.g., encephalopathy has been reported).

Additional Drug Interactions: Aluminum hydroxide gel inhibits the absorption of barbiturates, digoxin, phenytoin, corticosteroids, quinidine, warfarin, and isoniazid, thereby decreasing their effect.

Dosage: Capsules, Suspension, Tablets. *Antacid:* **Adults, usual:** 500–1,800 mg 3–6 times/day after meals, between meals, and at bedtime. *Hyperphosphatemia:* **Children:** 50–150 mg/kg/day in divided doses q 4–6 hr; adjust dosage until normal serum phosphate levels achieved.

NURSING CONSIDERATIONS

See also *Nursing Considerations* for *Antacids*, p. 38.

Administration/Storage

1. Administer the gel in a half glass of water.
2. If administering the medication via stomach tube, dilute commercial solution 2 or 3 times with water. Administer this solution at a rate of 15–20 ml/min. The total daily dose should be approximately 1.5 L of the diluted suspension.

Assessment

1. Note any client history of hypersensitivity to aluminum products.
2. Determine if the client is, for any reason, on a prescribed low-sodium diet. Aluminum preparations may then be contraindicated.
3. Discuss with the client the kind of epigastric discomfort being experienced. Determine if the pain is localized, burning, and gnawing, if it occurs 2–3 hr after a meal, and/or if it occurs during the early morning.
4. Obtain baseline data concerning the presence of occult blood in the stools.
5. Obtain laboratory tests such as CBC, liver and renal function studies.
6. Assess the client's bowel sounds, skin integrity, and neurologic status and document findings.
7. List any other drugs the client may be taking, either prescribed or OTC preparations.

Interventions

1. Monitor for relief of epigastric pain and report any incidence of continued distress.
2. Monitor for additive effects the drug may have on GI motility. Palpate the abdomen and listen to bowel sounds for evidence of any problems.
3. Observe for acid rebound effects, evidenced by client complaint of nocturnal pain. Document and report to the physician.
4. Determine the urinary phosphate level monthly when the drug is used in the management of phosphatic urinary calculi.
5. If clients are being treated for phosphatic urinary calculi, refer them to a dietitian for a low-phosphate diet. The diet generally should consist of 1.3 g phosphorus, 700 mg calcium, 13 g nitrogen, and 2,500 cal/day for the duration of the therapy.

Client/Family Teaching

1. If clients are given tablets, instruct them to chew the tab-

lets before swallowing and to take them with a glass of milk or water.

2. Report any changes in bowel elimination to the physician.

3. Remind the client that these products are not indicated for prolonged, continual use except under the supervision of a physician. If the symptoms persist, report them to the physician so that further evaluation and therapy may be prescribed.

Evaluation: Evaluate client for:
- Reduction in epigastric discomfort
- Decrease in serum phosphate levels

Amantadine hydrochloride
(ah-**MAN**-tah-deen)
Symadine, Symmetrel (Rx)

Classification: Antiviral and antiparkinson agent.

Action/Kinetics: As an antiviral agent, amantadine is believed to prevent penetration of the virus into cells, possibly by inhibiting uncoating of the RNA virus. Amantadine may also prevent the release of infectious viral nucleic acid into the host cell. The drug reduces symptoms of viral infections if given within 24–48 hr after onset of illness. For the treatment of parkinsonism, amantadine may increase the release of dopamine from synaptosomes or block the reuptake of dopamine into presynaptic neurons. Either of these mechanisms results in an increase in the levels of dopamine in dopaminergic synapses in the corpus striatum. Well absorbed from GI tract. **Onset:** 48

hrs. **Peak serum concentration:** 0.2 mcg/ml after 1–4 hr. **t½:** range of 9–37 hr, longer in presence of renal impairment. Ninety percent excreted unchanged in urine.

Use: Influenza A viral infections of the respiratory tract (prophylaxis and treatment of high-risk clients with immunodeficiency, cardiovascular, metabolic, neuromuscular, or pulmonary disease). Symptomatic treatment of idiopathic parkinsonism and parkinsonism syndrome resulting from encephalitis, carbon monoxide intoxication, drugs, or cerebral arteriosclerosis. The drug decreases extrapyramidal symptoms, including akinesia, rigidity, tremors, excessive salivation, gait disturbances, and total functional disability. Favorable results have been obtained in about 50% of the clients. Improvements can last for up to 30 months, although some clients report that the effect of the drug wears off in 1–3 months. A rest period or an increased dosage may reestablish effectiveness. For parkinsonism, amantadine hydrochloride is usually used concomitantly with other agents, such as levodopa and anticholinergic agents.

Contraindications: Hypersensitivity to drug.

Special Concerns: Administer with caution to clients with liver and renal disease, history of epilepsy, CHF, peripheral edema, orthostatic hypotension, recurrent eczematoid dermatitis, or severe psychosis, in clients taking CNS stimulant drugs, to those exposed to rubella, and to nursing mothers. Safe use for those who may become pregnant (category: C), for lactating mothers, and in children less than one year have not been established.

Side Effects: *GI:* Nausea, vomiting, constipation, anorexia, xerostomia. *CNS:* Depression, psychosis, convulsions, hallucinations, lightheadedness, confusion, ataxia, irritability, anxiety, headache, dizziness, fatigue, insomnia. *CV:* Congestive heart failure, orthostatic hypotension, peripheral edema. *Miscellaneous:* Urinary retention, leukopenia, neutropenia, mottling of skin of the extremities due to poor peripheral circulation (livedo reticularis), skin rashes, visual problems, slurred speech, oculogyric episodes, dyspnea, weakness, eczematoid dermatitis. *Symptoms of Overdose:* Anorexia, nausea, vomiting, CNS effects.

Drug Interactions

Anticholinergics / Additive anticholinergic effects (including hallucinations, confusion), especially with trihexyphenidyl and benztropine
CNS stimulants / May ↑ CNS and psychic effects of amantadine; use cautiously together
Hydrochlorothiazide/triamterene combination / ↓ Urinary excretion of amantadine → ↑ plasma levels
Levodopa / Potentiated by amantadine

Dosage: Capsules, Syrup. *Antiviral.* **Adults:** 200 mg daily as a single or divided dose. **Children, 1–9 years:** 4.4–8.8 mg/kg/day up to a maximum of 150 mg/day in 1 or 2 divided doses (use syrup); **9–12 years:** 100 mg b.i.d. *Prophylactic treatment:* Institute before or immediately after exposure and continue for 10–21 days if used concurrently with vaccine or for 90 days without vaccine. *Symptomatic*

management: Initiate as soon as possible and continue for 24–48 hr after disappearance of symptoms. Dose should be decreased in renal impairment (see package insert). Dose should be reduced to 100 mg daily for persons with active seizure disorders due to the increased risk of seizure frequency using daily doses of 200 mg. *Parkinsonism:* When used as sole agent, usual dose is 100 mg b.i.d.; may be necessary to increase up to 400 mg/day in divided doses. When used with other antiparkinson drugs: 100 mg 1–2 times/day. *Drug-induced extrapyramidal symptoms:* 100 mg b.i.d. (up to 300 mg/day may be required in some). Dosage should be reduced in clients with impaired renal function.

NURSING CONSIDERATIONS

See also *General Nursing Considerations For All Anti-Infectives,* p. 83.

Administration/Storage:

1. Protect capsules from moisture.
2. Therapy should be started for viral illness as soon as possible after symptoms begin and for 24–48 hr after symptoms disappear.
3. *Treatment of Overdose:* Gastric lavage or induction of emesis followed by supportive measures. Ensure that client is well hydrated; give IV fluids if necessary. To treat CNS toxicity, IV physostigmine, 1–2 mg given q 1–2 hr in adults or 0.5 mg at 5–10 min intervals (maximum of 2 mg/hr) in children. Sedatives and anticonvulsants may be given if needed; antiarrhythmics and vasopressors may also be required.

A

Assessment

1. Obtain a thorough nursing history and note any evidence of seizures, CHF, and renal insufficiency.
2. Determine if client has a history of active seizure disorder as drug must be reduced to prevent breakthrough seizures.
3. Anticipate that following loss of effectiveness of the drug, benefits may be regained by increasing the dosage or discontinuing the drug for several weeks and then reinstituting it.

Interventions

1. Observe clients with a history of epilepsy or other seizures for an increase in seizure activity and take appropriate precautions.
2. Assess clients with a history of CHF or peripheral edema for increased edema and/or respiratory distress and report promptly.
3. Monitor intake and output. Observe clients with renal impairment for crystalluria, oliguria, and increased BUN or creatinine levels and report promptly.
4. Monitor CNS and immediately report any mental status changes.

Client/Family Teaching

1. Do not drive a car or work in a situation where alertness is important because medication can affect vision, concentration, and coordination.
2. Rise slowly from a prone position because orthostatic hypotension may occur.
3. Lie down if dizzy or weak to relieve symptoms of orthostatic hypotension.
4. Report diffuse patchy discoloration or mottling of the skin. Discoloration lessens when legs are elevated and usually fades completely within weeks after discontinuing drug.
5. Report any exposure to rubella because drug may increase susceptibility to disease.
6. Susceptible individuals should avoid crowds during "flu" season.
7. Psychological changes such as confusion, nervousness, or depression should be reported.
8. Notify physician of any persistent or bothersome side effects.
9. Administer last daily dose several hours before retiring to prevent insomnia.
10. Clients with seizure disorders should be advised to report any early signs or symptoms of seizure activity as dosage may require adjustment.

Evaluation

1. Client/family will demonstrate an understanding of the disease process and its progression.
2. Evaluate for evidence of decreased extrapyramidal symptoms in clients with parkinsonism.
3. Note subjective reports of improvement in symptoms of influenza A viral infections.

Amikacin sulfate

(am-ih-**KAY**-sin)

Amikin (Rx)

See also *Anti-Infectives,* p. 80, and *Aminoglycosides,* p. 23.

Classification: Antibiotic, aminoglycoside.

Action/Kinetics: Amikacin is derived from kanamycin. Its spectrum is somewhat broader than that of other aminoglycosides, including *Serratia* and *Acinetobacter* species, as well as certain staphylococci and streptococci. Amikacin is effective against both penicillinase- and nonpenicillinase-producing organisms. **Therapeutic serum levels: IM,** 8–16 mcg/ml after 45–120 min. **t½:** 2–3 hr.

Special Concerns: Pregnancy category: D. Use with caution in premature infants and neonates.

Dosage: IM (preferred) and **IV, adults, children, and older infants:** 15 mg/kg/day in 2–3 equally divided doses q 8–12 hr for 7–10 days; **maximum daily dose:** 15 mg/kg. *Uncomplicated urinary tract infections:* 250 mg b.i.d.; **newborns:** loading dose of 10 mg/kg followed by 7.5 mg/kg q 12 hr. *Impaired renal function:* Normal loading dose of 7.5 mg/kg; **then** administration should be monitored by serum level of amikacin (35 mcg/ml maximum) or creatinine clearance rates. Duration of treatment: **Usual:** 7–10 days.

NURSING CONSIDERATIONS

See also *Nursing Considerations* for *Aminoglycosides,* p. 25.

Administration/Storage (for IV Administration)

1. Add 500-mg vial to 200 ml of sterile diluent, such as normal saline or D₅W.
2. Administer over a 30- to 60-min period for children and adults.
3. Administer to infants in the amount of fluid ordered by the physician. The IV administration to infants should be over 1–2 hr.
4. Store colorless liquid at room temperature for no longer than 2 years.
5. Potency is not affected if the solution turns a light yellow.

Amiloride hydrochloride
(ah-**MILL**-oh-ryd)
Midamor (Rx)

Classification: Diuretic, potassium-sparing.

Action/Kinetics: Amiloride acts on the distal tubule to inhibit sodium exchange for potassium which results in increased secretion of sodium and water and conservation of potassium. The drug also has weak diuretic and antihypertensive activity. **Onset:** 2 hr. **Peak effect:** 6–10 hr. **Peak plasma levels:** 3–4 hr. **Duration:** 24 hr. **t½:** 6–9 hr. 23% is bound to plasma protein. Approximately 50% is excreted unchanged by kidney and 40% by the feces unchanged.

Uses: Adjunct with thiazides or other kaliuretic diuretics in the treatment of hypertension or edema due to congestive heart failure, hepatic cirrhosis, and nephrotic syndrome to help restore normal serum potassium or prevent hypokalemia. *Investigational:* Prophylaxis and treatment of hypokalemia in clients for whom other treatments are inappropriate.

Contraindications: Hyperkalemia (greater than 5.5 mEq potassium/L). In clients receiving other potassium-sparing diuretics or potassium supplements. Impaired renal function. Diabetes mellitus.

Special Concerns: Pregnancy category: B. Use with caution in metabolic or respiratory acidosis; during lactation. Geriatric clients may have a greater risk of developing hyperkalemia.

Side Effects: *Electrolyte:* Hyperkalemia, hyponatremia, and hypochloremia if used with other diuretics. *CNS:* Headache, dizziness, encephalopathy, tremors, paresthesias, mental confusion, insomnia, decreased libido, depression, sleepiness, vertigo, nervousness. *GI:* Nausea, anorexia, vomiting, diarrhea, changes in appetite, gas and abdominal pain, dry mouth, flatulence, abdominal fullness, GI bleeding, thirst, dyspepsia, heartburn. *Respiratory:* Dyspnea, cough, shortness of breath. *Musculoskeletal:* Weakness, muscle cramps, fatigue; joint, neck and back pain; pain in extremities. *GU:* Impotence, polyuria, dysuria, bladder spasms, urinary frequency. *CV:* Angina, palpitations, arrhythmias, orthostatic hypotension. *Miscellaneous:* Aplastic anemia, neutropenia, visual disturbances, nasal congestion, tinnitus, increased intraocular pressure, skin rash, itching, pruritus, alopecia.

Symptoms of Overdose: Electrolyte imbalance, dehydration.

Drug Interactions

Angiotensin-converting enzyme inhibitors / ↑ Risk of significant hyperkalemia
Lithium / ↓ Renal excretion of lithium → ↑ chance of toxicity
Potassium products / Hyperkalemia with possibility of cardiac arrhythmias or cardiac arrest
Spironolactone, Triamterene / Hyperkalemia, hyponatremia, hypochloremia

Dosage: Tablets. *As single agent or with other diuretics:* **Adults, initial,** 5 mg/day; 10 mg/day may be necessary in some clients. Doses as high as 20 mg/day may be used, if needed, with careful monitoring of electrolytes.

NURSING CONSIDERATIONS

See also *Nursing Considerations* for *Diuretics,* p. 141.

Administration/Storage

1. Administer with food to reduce chance of GI upset.
2. *Treatment of Overdose:* Induce emesis or gastric lavage. Treat hyperkalemia by IV sodium bicarbonate or oral or parenteral glucose with a rapid-acting insulin. Sodium polystyrene sulfonate, orally or by enema, may also be used.

Interventions

1. Monitor renal function studies, intake and output, and weights.
2. Monitor serum electrolytes. Assess for hyperkalemia and for indications to withdraw the drug. Cardiac irregularities may be precipitated.
3. Do not encourage potassium supplementation or foods rich in potassium because drug does not promote potassium excretion.
4. Do not administer with other potassium-sparing diuretics.

Evaluation: Evaluate for a positive clinical response as evidenced by:
- ↓ blood pressure

- ↑ diuresis
- Normal serum potassium level

——— COMBINATION DRUG ———
Amiloride and Hydrochlorothiazide
(ah-**MILL**-oh-ryd, hy-droh-klor-oh-**THIGH**-ah-zyd)
Apo-Amilzide, Moduretic, Moduret✿, Nu-Amilzide (Rx)

See also *Amiloride,* p. 293, and *Hydrochlorothiazide,* p. 718.

Classification/Content: *Diuretic, potassium-sparing:* Amiloride HCl, 5 mg. *Antihypertensive/diuretic:* Hydrochlorothiazide, 50 mg.

Uses: Hypertension or congestive heart failure, especially when hypokalemia occurs. May be used alone or with other antihypertensive drugs, such as beta-adrenergic blocking drugs and methyldopa.

Special Concerns: Pregnancy category: C. Use with caution during lactation. Geriatric clients may be more sensitive to the hypotensive and electrolyte effects of this combination; also, age-related decreases in renal function may require a decrease in dosage.

Dosage: Tablets. Initial: 1 tablet daily; **then,** dosage may be increased to 2 tablets daily.

NURSING CONSIDERATIONS

See *Nursing Considerations* for individual agents.

Administration/Storage
1. This drug should be taken with food.
2. The daily dose may be given as a single dose or in divided doses.

3. More than two tablets daily are not usually necessary.
4. Maintenance therapy may be intermittent.

Amino Acid Formulation for Hepatic Failure or Hepatic Encephalopathy
(ah-**ME**-no **AH**-sid)
HepatAmine (Rx)

Classification: Nutritional agent.

Action/Kinetics: This product contains both essential and nonessential amino acids with high levels of branched chain amino acids as leucine, isoleucine, and valine. The branched chain amino acids improve mental status and EEG patterns. Fat emulsion, dextrose, electrolytes, and vitamins may be added if required.

Use: To normalize amino acid levels and improve nitrogen balance in clients with cirrhosis and hepatitis who manifest hepatic encephalopathy.

Additional Contraindication: Anuria.

Special Concerns: Pregnancy category: C.

Dosage: IV: 80–120 g amino acids (equivalent to 12–18 g nitrogen) daily.

NURSING CONSIDERATIONS

See also *Nursing Considerations* for *Intravenous Nutritional Therapy,* p. 170.

Administration/Storage
1. The total daily fluid (500 ml HepatAmine mixed with 500

ml 50% dextrose supplemented with electrolytes and vitamins) intake is usually 2–3 L given over a period of 8–12 hr. Clients with restrictions on fluid intake may only tolerate 1–2 L.

2. Infusion rates should be slow to start and gradually increased from 60–125 ml/hr.

3. The product may be given either peripherally or by central venous indwelling catheter.

Amino Acid Formulation for High Metabolic Stress
(ah-ME-noh AH-sid)
Aminosyn-HBC 7%, 4% BranchAmin, FreAmine HBC 6.9% (Rx)

Classification: Nutritional agent.

Action/Kinetics: The products contain mixtures of essential and nonessential amino acids with high amounts of branched chain amino acids, isoleucine, leucine, and valine. The products reverse negative nitrogen balance or prevent nitrogen losses.

Use: Prophylaxis of nitrogen loss or treatment of negative nitrogen balance in individuals if adequate protein intake is not possible by the oral, gastronomy, or jejunostomy routes when GI protein absorption is impaired or there is impairment of nitrogen homeostasis due to sepsis or severe trauma.

Additional Contraindications: Anuria, electrolyte imbalance, acid-base imbalance, hepatic coma.

Special Concerns: Pregnancy category: C.

Dosage: IV. *Adults with adequate calories:* 1.5 g/kg (approximate).

NURSING CONSIDERATIONS

See also *Nursing Considerations* for *Intravenous Nutritional Therapy,* p. 170.

Administration/Storage: This product may be administered either peripherally or by central venous indwelling catheter.

Amino Acid Formulations for Renal Failure
(ah-ME-noh AH-sid)
Aminess 5.2%, Aminosyn-RF 5.2%, 5.4% NephrAmine, RenAmin (Rx)

Classification: Nutritional agent.

Action/Kinetics: The nutritional requirements for clients with renal disease are different from those for clients with normal renal function. Administration of minimal amounts of essential amino acids enhances utilization of urea. Administration of nonessential amino acids should be restricted. These products promote protein synthesis and improve cellular metabolic balance.

Use: Treatment of uremia when oral nutrition is not practical or feasible.

Additional Contraindications: Acid-base imbalance, electrolyte imbalance, hyperammonemia.

Special Concerns: Pregnancy category: C. Use with caution in children with acute renal failure and in infants with low birth weight. The risk of hyperammonemia may be increased in infants due to the absence of arginine in Aminess and NephrAmine (Aminosyn-RF and RenAmin contain arginine).

Dosage: IV. Adults: *Aminess 5.2%,* 400 ml mixed with 500 ml of 70% dextrose (solution contains 2.3% essential amino acids and 30% dextrose). *Aminosyn-RF 5.2%,* 300 ml (up to 600 ml may be used) mixed with 500 ml of 70% dextrose (solution contains 1.96% essential amino acids and 44% dextrose). *5.4% NephrAmine,* 250 ml (up to 500 ml may be used) mixed with 500 ml of 70% dextrose (solution contains 1.8% essential amino acids and 47% dextrose). *RenAmin,* 250–500 ml.

Pediatric: *Individualized,* **usual,** 0.5–1 g/kg/day (initial doses should be lower and then slowly increased).

NURSING CONSIDERATIONS

See also *Nursing Considerations* for *Intravenous Nutritional Therapy,* p. 170.

Administration/Storage

1. These products should be given through a central venous catheter at an initial rate not to exceed 20–30 ml/hr for the first 6–8 hr. Then the rate can be increased by 10 ml/hr each 24 hr to a maximum of 60–100 ml/hr.
2. Use of Aminess or NephrAmine in infants may increase the chance of hyperammonemia because these products do not contain arginine.
3. If the hypertonic dextrose solution is discontinued, rebound hypoglycemia may be prevented by giving 5% or 10% dextrose solutions.

Aminocaproic acid   A

(ah-ME-noh-kah-**PROH**-ick **AH**-sid)

Amicar (Rx)

Classification: Hemostatic, systemic.

Action/Kinetics: Inhibits action of plasminogen (clotting factor), thereby preventing fibrinolysis (clot dissolution). Rapidly absorbed from the GI tract. **Peak plasma levels:** 2 hr. **Effective plasma levels:** 0.13 mg/ml. **Duration (after IV):** 3 hr or less. Rapidly excreted through the kidney, mostly unchanged.

Uses: Excessive bleeding associated with systemic hyperfibrinolysis and urinary fibrinolysis. Surgical complications following heart surgery and portacaval shunt in cancer of the lung, prostate, cervix, stomach, and other types of surgery associated with heavy postoperative bleeding. Aplastic anemia. *Investigational:* Prevention of recurrence of subarachnoid hemorrhage, megakaryocytic thrombocytopenia, prophylaxis and treatment of hereditary angioneurotic edema, acute promyelocytic leukemia with accompanying coagulopathy.

Contraindications: Clients with active, intravascular clotting possibly associated with fibrinolysis and bleeding.

Special Concerns: Use with caution, or not at all, in clients with uremia or cardiac, renal, or hepatic disease. Use during pregnancy only if benefits clearly outweigh risks.

Side Effects: *GI:* Nausea, cramping, diarrhea. *CNS:* Dizziness, malaise, headache, delirium; auditory, visual, and kinesthetic hallucina-

tions. *CV:* Hypotension, thrombophlebitis. *Other:* Tinnitus, conjunctival suffusion, myopathies, nasal
stuffiness, skin rash, prolongation
of menses, reversible acute renal
failure.

Drug Interactions

Anticoagulants, oral / ↓ Anticoagulant effects
Contraceptives, oral (Estrogen) /
Combination with aminocaproic
acid may lead to hyper-
coagulable condition

Laboratory Test Interferences:
↑ Serum aldolase, AST, creatinine
phosphokinase, and potassium.

Dosage: Syrup, Tablets. *Acute
bleeding:* **Initial priming dose,** 5
g during first hour; **then,** 1–1.25 g
q hr for 8 hr or until bleeding is
controlled. **Maximum daily dose:**
30 g. *After prostatic surgery:* 6 g
over the first 24 hr may be sufficient. *Prevention of hemorrhage after
dental surgery:* 6 g immediately
after surgery followed by 6 g q 6 hr
for 9–19 days.
   IV infusion. *Acute bleeding:*
Initial priming dose: 4–5 g during first hour; **then,** 1 g q hr for 8
hr (or until desired response is
obtained). *Subarachnoid hemorrhage, recurrent:* 36 g daily (18 g in
400 ml 5% dextrose solution infused over 12 hr) for 10 days.
Switch to oral therapy after this
time.

NURSING CONSIDERATIONS

Administration/Storage

1. For IV use, may be mixed with
   saline, 5% dextrose, sterile
   water, or Ringer's solution. It
   should *never* be injected undiluted.
2. For IV, priming dose is dissolved in 250 ml of solution;

continuous infusion is at the
rate of 1–1.25 g/hr for 8 hr in
50 ml of diluent.

Assessment

1. Obtain CBC, platelet count,
   bleeding parameters, liver and
   renal function studies prior to
   instituting therapy.
2. Determine baseline BP and
   pulse before starting IV.
3. Note any history of prior incidence of uremia, cardiac, renal,
   or hepatic disease.
4. Determine if client is taking
   any oral contraceptives (estrogen). Interaction with aminocaproic acid can lead to hypercoagulable condition.
5. Note presence of menses.

Interventions

1. Infusions should be administered utilizing an electronic
   infusion device.
2. Assess client frequently for
   hypotension, bradycardia, and
   arrhythmias, symptoms indicating that the rate of IV administration is too fast. Slow rate of
   IV infusion and report if such
   symptoms occur.
3. With all systemic hemostatics,
   observe carefully for signs and
   symptoms of thrombosis, such
   as leg pain, chest pain, or
   respiratory distress.
4. Have available vitamin K or
   protamine sulfate for emergency use.
5. Keep tablets and raspberry-fla-
   vored syrup out of the reach of
   children.

Evaluation

1. Assess client for control of
   bleeding and appropriate lab
   data to evaluate response to
   therapy.

2. Note presence of adverse side effects such as nausea, cramping, or diarrhea.
3. If client is experiencing menses, observe for excessive bleeding.

Aminophylline

(am-in-**OFF**-ih-lin)

Aminophyllin, Palaron✲, Phyllocontin, Phyllocontin-350✲, Truphyllin (Rx)

See also *Theophylline Derivatives,* p. 226.

Action/Kinetics: Aminophylline contains 79% theophylline.

Additional Uses: Neonatal apnea, respiratory stimulant in Cheyne-Stokes respiration. Parenteral form has been used for biliary colic, as a cardiac stimulant, diuretic, and an adjunct in treating congestive heart failure, although such uses have been replaced by more effective drugs.

Special Concerns: Pregnancy category: C. Use with caution when aminophylline and sodium chloride are used with adrenocorticosteroids or in clients with edema.

Additional Side Effects: The ethylenediamine in the product may cause exfoliative dermatitis or urticaria.

Dosage: Oral Solution, Tablets. *Bronchodilator, acute attacks, in clients not currently on theophylline therapy:* **Adults and children up to 16 years of age, loading dose:** Equivalent of 5–6 mg of anhydrous theophylline/kg. *Bronchodilator, acute attacks, in clients currently receiving theophylline:* **Adults and children up to 16 years of age:** If possible, a serum theophylline level should be obtained first. Then, base loading dose on the premise that each 0.5 mg theophylline/kg of lean body weight will result in a 0.5–1.6 mcg/ml increase in serum theophylline levels. If immediate therapy is needed and a serum level cannot be obtained, a single dose of the equivalent of 2.5 mg/kg of anhydrous theophylline can be given. *Maintenance in acute attack, based on equivalent of anhydrous theophylline:* **Young adult smokers,** 4 mg/kg q 6 hr; **healthy, nonsmoking adults,** 3 mg/kg q 8 hr; **geriatric clients or clients with cor pulmonale,** 2 mg/kg q 8 hr; **clients with congestive heart failure or liver failure,** 2 mg/kg q 8–12 hr. **Pediatric, 12–16 years,** 3 mg/kg q 6 hr; **9–12 years:** 4 mg/kg q 6 hr; **1–9 years:** 5 mg/kg q 6 hr; **6–12 months,** Use the formula: dose (mg/kg q 8 hr) = (0.05) (age in weeks) + 1.25; **Up to 6 months,** Use the formula: dose (mg/kg q 8 hr) = (0.07) (age in weeks) + 1.7. *Chronic therapy, based on equivalent of anhydrous theophylline:* **Adults, initial,** 6–8 mg/kg up to a maximum of 400 mg daily in 3–4 divided doses at 6–8 hr intervals; **then,** dose can be increased in 25% increments at 2–3 day intervals up to a maximum of 13 mg/kg or 900 mg daily, whichever is less. **Pediatric, initial,** 16 mg/kg up to a maximum of 400 mg daily in 3–4 divided doses at 6–8 hr intervals; **then,** dose may be increased in 25% increments at 2–3 day intervals up to the following maximum doses (without measuring serum theophylline): **16 years and older,** 13 mg/kg or 900 mg daily, whichever is less; **12–16 years:** 18 mg/kg daily; **9–12 years:** 20 mg/kg daily; **1–9 years:** 24 mg/kg daily; **Up to 12 months,**

A

Use the following formula: dose (mg/kg daily) = (0.3) (age in weeks) + 8.0.

Enteric-coated Tablets. *Bronchodilator, chronic therapy, based on equivalent of anhydrous theophylline:* **Adults, initial,** 6–8 mg/kg up to a maximum of 400 mg daily in 3–4 divided doses q 6–8 hr; **then,** dose may be increased, if needed and tolerated, by increments of 25% at 2–3 day intervals up to a maximum of 13 mg/kg/day or 900 mg/day, whichever is less, without measuring serum theophylline. **Pediatric, over 12 years of age, initial,** 4 mg/kg q 8–12 hr; **then,** dose may be increased by 2–3 mg/kg/day at 3-day intervals up to the following maximum doses (without measuring serum levels): **16 years and older:** 13 mg/kg/day or 900 mg/day, whichever is less; **12–16 years:** 18 mg/kg daily.

Extended-release Tablets. *Bronchodilator, chronic therapy, based on equivalent of anhydrous theophylline:* **Adults, initial,** 4 mg/kg q 8–12 hr; **then,** dose may be increased by 2–3 mg/kg/day at 3-day intervals to a maximum of 13 mg/kg or 900 mg/day, whichever is less. **Pediatric, initial,** Same as adults; **then,** dose may be increased by 2–3 mg/kg/day at 3-day intervals up to the following maximum doses: **16 years and older:** 13 mg/kg/day or 900 mg/day, whichever is less. **12–16 years:** 18 mg/kg/day.

Enema. For use as a bronchodilator for loading doses and for maintenance in acute attacks, see doses for oral solution and tablets.

IV infusion. *Bronchodilator, acute attacks, for clients not currently on theophylline:* **Adults and children up to 16 years, loading dose based on anhydrous theophylline,** 5 mg/kg given over a period of 20 min. *Bronchodilator, acute attack, for clients currently on theophylline:* **Adults and children up to 16 years, loading dose based on anhydrous theophylline,** If possible, a serum theophylline level should be obtained first. Then, base loading dose on the premise that each 0.5 mg theophylline/kg of lean body weight will result in a 0.5–1.6 mcg/ml increase in serum theophylline levels. If immediate therapy is needed and a serum level cannot be obtained, a single dose of the equivalent of 2.5 mg/kg of anhydrous theophylline can be given. *Maintenance for acute attacks, based on equivalent of anhydrous theophylline:* **Young adult smokers,** 0.7 mg/kg/hr; **nonsmoking, healthy adults,** 0.43 mg/kg/hr; **geriatric clients or clients with cor pulmonale:** 0.26 mg/kg/hr; **clients with congestive heart failure or liver failure:** 0.2 mg/kg/hr. **Pediatric, 12–16 years, nonsmokers,** 0.5 mg/kg/hr; **9–12 years,** 0.7 mg/kg/hr; **1–9 years,** 0.8 mg/kg/hr; **up to 1 year,** Based on the following formula: dose (mg/kg/hr) = (0.008) (age in weeks) + 0.21.

NURSING CONSIDERATIONS

See also *Nursing Considerations* for *Theophylline Derivatives,* p. 229.

Administration/Storage

1. To avoid hypotension, administer IV doses of medication at a rate not to exceed 25 mg/min.
2. Only the 25 mg/ml injection (which should be further diluted) should be used for IV administration. Use an infusion pump to regulate infusion rates of IV solutions.

3. IM injection is not recommended due to severe, persistent pain at the site of injection.
4. A minimum of 4–6 hr should elapse when switching from IV infusion to the first dose of PO therapy.
5. Enteric-coated tablets may be incompletely and slowly absorbed.
6. Enteric-coated and extended-release tablets are not recommended for children less than 12 years of age.
7. Use of aminophylline suppositories is not recommended due to the possibility of slow and unreliable absorption.

Interventions

1. Monitor pulse and BP closely during IV administration. Aminophylline may cause a transitory lowering of the blood pressure. If this occurs, the dosage of drug and rate of flow should be adjusted immediately.
2. Report serum levels greater than 20 mcg/ml.
3. Observe for symptoms of toxicity, i.e., nausea, vomiting, restlessness, convulsions, and arrhythmias, and report.

Evaluation: Evaluate client for:
• Improved airway exchange on auscultation
• ABGs within desired range

Amiodarone hydrochloride
(am-ee-**OH**-dah-rohn)
Cordarone (Rx)

See also *Antiarrhythmic Drugs,* p. 51.

Classification: Antiarrhythmic, type III.

Action/Kinetics: The antiarrhythmic activity is due to an increase in the duration of the myocardial cell action potential as well as alpha- and beta-adrenergic blockade. **Onset:** Several days up to 1–3 weeks. Drug may accumulate in the liver, lung, spleen, and adipose tissue. **Therapeutic serum levels:** 0.5–2.5 mcg/ml. **t½:** Biphasic: initial t½: 2.5–10 days; final t½: 40–55 days (usual). Effects may persist for several weeks or months after therapy is terminated. Effective plasma concentrations are difficult to predict although concentrations below 1 mg/L are usually ineffective, whereas those above 2.5 mg/L are not necessary. Neither amiodarone nor its metabolite, desethylamiodarone, is dialyzable.

Uses: This drug should be reserved for life-threatening ventricular arrhythmias unresponsive to other therapy. Amiodarone has been used for recurrent ventricular fibrillation and recurrent, hemodynamically unstable ventricular tachycardia.

Contraindications: Marked sinus bradycardia due to severe sinus node dysfunction, second- or third-degree AV block, syncope caused by bradycardia (except when used with a pacemaker). Lactation.

Special Concerns: Should be used in pregnancy only when benefits outweigh the potential risks (pregnancy category: C). Safety and efficacy in children have not been determined. The drug may be more sensitive in geriatric clients, especially on thyroid function.

Side Effects: Adverse reactions, some potentially fatal, are common

A

with doses greater than 400 mg/day. *Pulmonary:* Interstitial pneumonitis, alveolitis, pulmonary inflammation or fibrosis. *CV:* Worsening of arrhythmias, symptomatic bradycardia, sinus arrest, sinoatrial (SA) node dysfunction, congestive heart failure, edema, hypotension, cardiac conduction abnormalities, coagulation abnormalities. *Hepatic:* Increases in AST and ALT, abnormal liver function tests. *CNS:* Malaise, tremor, lack of coordination, fatigue, ataxia, paresthesias, peripheral neuropathy, dizziness, insomnia, headache, decreased libido. *Ophthalmologic:* Corneal microdeposits (asymptomatic) in clients on therapy for 6 months or more, photophobia, dry eyes, blurred vision, halos. *GI:* Nausea, vomiting, constipation, anorexia, abdominal pain, abnormal smell and taste, abnormal salivation. *Dermatologic:* Photosensitivity, solar dermatitis, blue-gray pigmentation after prolonged exposure, rash, alopecia, spontaneous ecchymosis, flushing. *Miscellaneous:* Hypothyroidism or hyperthyroidism. *Symptoms of Overdose:* Bradycardia, hypotension, disorders of cardiac rhythm.

Drug Interactions

Anticoagulants / ↑ Effect → bleeding disorders
Beta-adrenergic blocking agents / ↑ Chance of bradycardia, sinus arrest, or AV block
Digoxin, digitoxin / ↑ Serum digoxin, digitoxin levels → toxicity
Quinidine / ↑ Serum quinidine → toxicity
Procainamide / ↑ Serum procainamide → toxicity
Phenytoin / ↑ Serum phenytoin levels → toxicity

Dosage: Tablets. Due to the drug's side effects, unusual pharmacokinetic properties, and difficult dosing schedule, amiodarone should be administered in a hospital only by physicians trained in treating life-threatening arrhythmias. Loading doses are required to ensure a reasonable onset of action. *Life-threatening arrhythmias:* **PO, loading dose:** 800–1,600 mg/day for 1–3 weeks (or until initial response occurs); **then,** reduce dose to 600–800 mg/day for one month. **Maintenance dose:** 200–400 mg/day.

NURSING CONSIDERATIONS

See also *Nursing Considerations* for *Antiarrhythmic Drugs,* p. 52.

Administration/Storage

1. Daily doses of 1,000 mg or more should be administered in divided doses with meals.
2. To minimize side effects, the lowest effective dose should be determined. If side effects occur, the dose should be reduced.
3. If dosage adjustments are required, the client should be monitored for an extended period of time due to the long and variable half-life of the drug and the difficulty in predicting the time needed to achieve a new steady-state plasma drug level.
4. When initiating amiodarone therapy, other antiarrhythmic drugs should be gradually discontinued.
5. *Treatment of Overdose:* Use supportive treatment. A beta-adrenergic agonist or a pacemaker is used to treat bradycardia; hypotension due to insufficient tissue perfusion is treat-

ed with a vasopressor or positive inotropic agents.

Assessment

1. Determine if the client is taking any other antiarrhythmic medications.
2. Assess quality of respirations and breath sounds.
3. Note the client's baseline vital signs and perfusion (skin temperature, color). Record client pulse rate several times in similar circumstances, where possible, to establish a baseline against which to measure responses after initiating therapy.
4. Obtain baseline data concerning the client's vision before starting therapy.

Interventions

1. During administration, observe ECG for increased arrhythmias and heart rates less than 60 beats/min and report if evident.
2. Monitor BP and assess for evidence of hypotension.
3. Note client complaints of shortness of breath, painful breathing, or cough. Assess pulmonary status and document.
4. Observe for CNS symptoms such as tremor, lack of coordination, paresthesias, and dizziness.
5. Anticipate reduced dosages of digoxin, warfarin, quinidine, procainamide, and phenytoin if administered concomitantly with amiodarone hydrochloride.
6. Monitor thyroid studies because drug inhibits conversion of T_4 to T_3.
7. Note client complaints of headaches, depression, or insomnia. Also observe for any change in client behavior such as decreased interest in personal appearance or apparent hallucinations. These findings may indicate a need for a change in drug therapy.
8. Clients should have periodic ophthalmic examinations because small yellow-brown granular corneal deposits may develop during prolonged therapy.

Client/Family Teaching

1. Some clients may develop crystals on the skin, producing a bluish color. In this event, avoid exposure to the sun because the crystals create photosensitivity. Notify physician so dosage of drug can be adjusted.
2. Report all side effects and avoid direct exposure to sunlight. Wear protective clothing and a sunscreen if exposure is necessary.
3. Report any bleeding or bruising promptly, to enable the physician to avoid the development of coagulation disorders.
4. Wheezing, fever, coughing, or dyspnea are all symptoms of pulmonary problems and require prompt attention.
5. Stress the importance of reporting for laboratory studies as scheduled.
6. Carry a Medic Alert card at all times.

Evaluation: Evaluate for a positive clinical response as evidenced by termination and control of life-threatening ventricular arrhythmias.

A

Amitriptyline hydrochloride

(ah-me-**TRIP**-tih-leen)

Amitril, Apo-Amitriptyline ✦, Elavil, Endep, Enovil, Levate ✦, Novo-Triptyn ✦, PMS Amitriptyline (Rx)

See also *Tricyclic Antidepressants*, p. 239.

Classification: Tricyclic antidepressant.

Action/Kinetics: Amitriptyline is metabolized to an active metabolite, nortriptyline. Has significant anticholinergic and sedative effects with moderate activity to cause orthostatic hypotension. **Effective plasma levels of amitriptyline and nortriptyline:** Approximately 110–250 ng/ml. **t½:** 31–46 hr. Up to one month may be required for beneficial effects to be manifested.

Amitriptyline is also found in Limbitrol and Triavil.

Uses: Relief of symptoms of depression including depression accompanied by anxiety and insomnia. Chronic pain due to cancer or other pain syndromes. Prophylaxis of cluster and migraine headaches. *Investigational:* Pathologic laughing and crying secondary to forebrain disease, bulimia nervosa, antiulcer agent, enuresis.

Special Concerns: Pregnancy category: C.

Dosage: Syrup, Tablets. *Antidepressant:* **Adults (outpatients):** 75 mg/day in divided doses; may be increased to 150 mg/day. *Alternate dosage:* **Initial,** 50–100 mg at bedtime; **then,** increase by 25–50 mg, if necessary, up to 150 mg daily. **Hospitalized clients: initial,** 100 mg/day; may be increased to 200–300 mg/day. **Maintenance: usual,** 40–100 mg/day (may be given as a single dose at bedtime). **Adolescent and geriatric:** 10 mg t.i.d. and 20 mg at bedtime up to a maximum of 100 mg daily. **Pediatric, 6–12 years:** 10–30 mg (1–5 mg/kg) daily in 2 divided doses. *Chronic pain:* 50–100 mg daily. *Enuresis:* **Pediatric, over 6 years:** 10 mg daily as a single dose at bedtime; dose may be increased up to a maximum of 25 mg. **Less than 6 years:** 10 mg daily as a single dose at bedtime.

IM only. *Antidepressant:* **Adults,** 20–30 mg q.i.d.; switch to **PO** therapy as soon as possible.

NURSING CONSIDERATIONS

See also *Nursing Considerations* for *Tricyclic Antidepressants*, p. 242.

Administration/Storage

1. Increases in dosage should be made in late afternoon or at bedtime.
2. Beneficial antidepressant effects may not be noted for 30 days.
3. Sedative effects may be manifested prior to antidepressant effects.

Client/Family Teaching

1. Take with food to minimize gastric upset.
2. Warn clients not to drive a car or operate hazardous machinery because drug causes a high degree of sedation.
3. Urine may appear blue-green in color.
4. Client may take entire dose at bedtime if sedation is manifested during waking hours.

—— *COMBINATION DRUG* ——
Amitriptyline and Perphenazine
(ah-me-**TRIP**-tih-leen, per-**FEN**-ah-zeen)

Elavil Plus✹, Etrafon 2-10✹, Etrafon-A✹, Etrafon-D✹, Etrafon-F✹, PMS-Levazine 2/25✹, PMS-Levazine 4/25✹, Triavil 2-10, 2-25, 4-10, 4-25, and 4-50 (Rx)

Classification/Content: See also information on individual components.

Antidepressant: Amitriptyline HCl, 10, 25, or 50 mg. *Antipsychotic:* Perphenazine, 2 or 4 mg.

There are five different strengths of Triavil: Triavil 2–10, Triavil 2–25, Triavil 4–10, Triavil 4–25, and Triavil 4–50. **Note:** The first number refers to the number of milligrams of perphenazine and the second number refers to the number of milligrams of amitriptyline.

Uses: Depression with moderate to severe anxiety and/or agitation. Depression and anxiety in clients with chronic physical disease. Also schizophrenic clients with symptoms of depression.

Contraindications: Use during pregnancy is not recommended. CNS depression due to drugs. In presence of bone marrow depression. Concomitant use with monoamine oxidase inhibitors. During acute recovery phase from myocardial infarction. Use in children.

Dosage: PO. Adults, initial: One tablet of Triavil 2–25 or 4–25 t.i.d.–q.i.d. or one tablet of Triavil 4–50 b.i.d. Schizophrenic clients should receive an initial dose of two tablets of Triavil 4–50 t.i.d., with a fourth dose at bedtime, if necessary. Initial dosage for geriatric or adolescent clients in whom anxiety dominates is Triavil 4–10 t.i.d.–q.i.d., with dosage adjusted as required. **Maintenance:** One tablet Triavil 2–25 or 4–25 b.i.d.–q.i.d. or one tablet Triavil 4–50 b.i.d.

NURSING CONSIDERATIONS

See *Nursing Considerations* for *Tricyclic Antidepressants,* p. 242, and *Amitriptyline hydrochloride,* p. 304.

Administration/Storage

1. Triavil is not recommended for children.
2. Total daily dosage of Triavil should not exceed four of the 4–50 tablets or eight tablets of all other dosage strengths.
3. The therapeutic effect may take up to several weeks to be manifested.
4. Once a satisfactory response has been observed, the dose should be reduced to the smallest amount required for relief of symptoms.

Amoxapine
(ah-**MOX**-ah-peen)
Asendin (Rx)

See also *Tricyclic Antidepressants,* p. 239.

Classification: Tricyclic antidepressant.

Action/Kinetics: In addition to its effect on monoamines, this drug also blocks dopamine receptors. Is metabolized to the active metabolites 7-hydroxy- and 8-hydroxy-amoxapine. **Peak blood levels:** 90 min. **Effective plasma levels:** 200–500 ng/ml. **t½:** 8 hr; t½ of

A

major metabolite: 30 hr. Excreted in urine.

Uses: Endogenous and reactive depression. Antianxiety agent.

Contraindications: Avoid high dose levels in clients with a history of convulsive seizures. Not to be used during acute recovery period after myocardial infarction.

Special Concerns: Pregnancy category: C. Safe use in children under 16 years of age and during lactation not established.

Additional Side Effects: Tardive dyskinesia. Overdosage may cause seizures (common), neuroleptic malignant syndrome, testicular swelling, impairment of sexual function, and breast enlargement in males and females. Also, renal failure may be seen 2–5 days after overdosage.

Dosage: Tablets. Adults: *individualized,* **initial,** 50 mg t.i.d. Can be increased to 100 mg t.i.d. during first week. Doses greater than 300 mg daily should not be used unless this dose has been ineffective for at least 14 days. **Maintenance:** 300 mg as a single dose at bedtime. **Hospitalized clients:** Up to 150 mg q.i.d. **Geriatric, initial,** 25 mg b.i.d.–t.i.d. If necessary, increase to 50 mg b.i.d.–t.i.d. after first week. **Maintenance:** Up to 300 mg once daily at bedtime.

NURSING CONSIDERATIONS

See also *Nursing Considerations* for *Tricyclic Antidepressants,* p. 242.

Interventions

1. Observe client for early CNS manifestations of tardive dyskinesia.

2. Assess closely for any evidence of toxic effects and report to physician.

Client/Family Teaching

1. Take with food to minimize gastric upset.
2. Administer entire dose at bedtime if sedation is persistent.

Amoxicillin (amoxycillin)

(ah-mox-ih-**SILL**-in)

Amoxil, Amoxil Pediatric Drops, APO-Amoxi✤, Biomox, Novamoxin✤, Nu-Amoxi✤, Polymox, Polymox Drops, Trimox 125, 250, and 500, Wymox (Rx)

See also *Anti-Infectives,* p. 80, and *Penicillins,* p. 197.

Classification: Antibiotic, penicillin.

Action/Kinetics: Semisynthetic broad-spectrum penicillin closely related to ampicillin. Destroyed by penicillinase, acid stable, and better absorbed than ampicillin. From 50% to 80% of an oral dose is absorbed from the GI tract. **Peak serum levels: PO:** 4–11 mcg/ml after 1–2 hr. **t½:** 60 min. Mostly excreted unchanged in urine.

Uses: Gram-positive streptococcal infections including *Streptococcus faecalis, S. pneumoniae,* and non-penicillinase-producing staphylococci. Gram-negative infections due to *Hemophilus influenzae, Proteus mirabilis, Escherichia coli,* and *Neisseria gonorrhoeae.*

Dosage: Capsules, Oral Suspension, Chewable Tablets. *Susceptible infections of ear, nose, throat, GU tract, skin and soft tissues, lower* respiratory tract: **Adults,** 250–500 mg q 8 hr; **pediatric under 20 kg:** 20–40 (or more) mg/kg daily in three equal doses. The pediatric dose should not exceed the maximum adult dose. *Prophylaxis of bacterial endocarditis:* 3 g 60 min prior to procedure (dental, oral, or upper respiratory tract) and 1.5 g 6 hr later. Alternatively, ampicillin, 1–2 g (50 mg/kg for children) plus gentamicin, 1.5 mg/kg (2 mg/kg for children) not to exceed 80 mg, both either IM or IV 30 min before procedure followed by amoxicillin, 1.5 g (25 mg/kg for children) 6 hr after initial dose. Amoxicillin may be given as an alternate procedure for GU or GI procedures at a dose of 3 g 1 hr before procedure followed by 1.5 g 6 hr after the initial dose.

Gonococcal infections: 3 g with probenecid, 1 g, given as a single dose. In addition, tetracycline, 0.5 mg, q.i.d. for 7 days. *Gonococcal infection in pregnancy:* 3 g with probenecid, 1 g, given as a single dose. In addition, erythromycin base, 0.5 g q.i.d. for 7 days. *Disseminated gonococcal infections:* 3 g with probenecid, 1 g, given as a single dose; **then,** 0.5 g q.i.d. for 7 days. *Acute pelvic inflammatory disease:* 3 g with probenecid, 1 g, given as a single dose. In addition, doxycycline, 100 mg b.i.d. for 10–14 days. *Sexually transmitted epididymo-orchitis:* 3 g with probenecid, 1 g, given as a single dose. In addition, tetracycline, 0.5 g q.i.d. for 10 days. *Bacterial vaginosis:* 0.5 g q.i.d. for 7 days. *Chlamydia trachomatis during pregnancy (as an alternative to erythromycin):* 0.5 g t.i.d. for 7 days.

NURSING CONSIDERATIONS

See also *Nursing Considerations* for *Penicillins,* p. 200.

Administration/Storage

1. Dry powder is stable at room temperature for 18–30 months. Reconstituted suspension is stable for 1 week at room temperature and for 2 weeks at 2°C–8°C.
2. Chewable tablets are available for pediatric use. These may be administered with food.

—— *COMBINATION DRUG* ——
Amoxicillin and Potassium clavulanate
(ah-mox-ih-**SILL**-in, poh-**TASS**-ee-um klav-you-**LAN**-ayt)
Augmentin '125,' '250,' and '500' Clavulin✿ (Rx)

See also *Anti-Infectives,* p. 80, and *Penicillins,* p. 197.

Classification: Antibiotic, penicillin.

Action/Kinetics: *For details, see amoxicillin.* Potassium clavulanate inactivates lactamase enzymes, which are responsible for resistance to penicillins. Thus, this preparation is effective against microorganisms that have manifested resistance to amoxicillin. For potassium clavulanate: **Peak serum levels:** 1–2 hr. **t½:** 1 hr. **Note:** Both the "250" and "500" tablets contain 125 mg potassium clavulanate.

Uses: For beta-lactamase–producing strains of the following organisms: *Hemophilus influenzae* causing lower respiratory tract infections, otitis media, and sinusitis; *Staphylococcus aureus, Escherichia coli,* and *Klebsiella,* causing skin and skin structure infections; *E. coli, Klebsiella,* and *Enterobacter,* causing urinary tract infections.

A

Dosage: Oral Suspension, Chewable Tablets, Tablets. Adults, usual: One "250" tablet q 8 hr; **children less than 40 kg,** 20 mg/kg daily in divided doses q 8 hr. *Respiratory tract and severe infections:* **Adults,** one "500" tablet q 8 hr; **children, less than 40 kg,** 40 mg/kg daily in divided doses q 8 hr (this dose is also used in children for otitis media, lower respiratory tract infections, or sinusitis). *Chancroid:* One "500" tablet t.i.d. for 7 days (alternative to erythromycin). *Disseminated gonococcal infections:* Following therapy with an appropriate cephalosporin, uncomplicated disease therapy may be completed with 1 "500" mg tablet t.i.d. for 1 week.

NURSING CONSIDERATIONS

See also *Nursing Considerations* for *Penicillins,* p. 200.

Administration/Storage

1. Both the "250" and "500" tablets contain 125 mg clavulanic acid; therefore, two "250" tablets are not the same as one "500" tablet.
2. The reconstituted suspension should be refrigerated and discarded after 10 days.

Amphetamine sulfate

(am-**FET**-ah-meen)
(C-II) (Rx)

See also *Amphetamines and Derivatives,* p. 29.

Classification: CNS stimulant.

Action/Kinetics: After PO administration, completely absorbed in 3 hr. **Duration: PO,** 4–24 hr; **t½:** 10–30 hr, depending on urinary pH. Excreted in urine. Acidification will increase excretion, whereas alkalinization will decrease it. For every one unit increase in pH, the plasma half-life will increase by 7 hr.

Uses: Attention deficit disorders in children, narcolepsy.

Special Concerns: Pregnancy category: C. Use is not recommended in children less than 3 years of age for attention deficit disorders and in children less than 6 years of age for narcolepsy. Use is no longer recommended as an appetite suppressant.

Dosage: Tablets. *Narcolepsy:* **Adults,** 5–20 mg 1–3 times daily. **Children over 12 years, initial:** 5 mg b.i.d.; increase in increments of 10 mg/day at weekly intervals until optimum dose is reached. **Children, 6–12 years, initial:** 2.5 mg b.i.d.; increase in increments of 5 mg at weekly intervals until optimum dose is reached (maximum is 60 mg daily). *Attention deficit disorders in children:* **3–6 years, initial:** 2.5 mg/day; increase by 2.5 mg/day at weekly intervals until optimum dose is achieved (usual range 0.1–0.5 mg/kg/dose each morning). **6 years and older, initial:** 5 mg 1–2 times/day; increase in increments of 5 mg weekly until optimum dose is achieved (rarely over 40 mg/day).

NURSING CONSIDERATIONS

See also *Nursing Considerations* for *Amphetamines and Derivatives,* p. 31.

Administration/Storage

1. When used as an anorexiant, the drug should be used only for short-term therapy.
2. When used for attention deficit

disorders or narcolepsy, the first dose should be given on awakening with an additional one or two doses given at intervals of 4–6 hr.

3. The last dose of medication should be given 6 hr before bedtime.

4. The peak effects of the drug are observed 2–3 hr after administration. The effects last from 4–24 hr.

Assessment

1. Perform a baseline CNS assessment prior to initiating therapy.

2. Obtain a baseline ECG before starting therapy.

3. Note the client's age. If the client is of childbearing age and is sexually active, determine the possibility of pregnancy because amphetamines are contraindicated.

Interventions

1. Note any symptoms of impaired mental processes or emotional liability. Document and report to the physician.

2. If children are receiving amphetamines, assess the child's growth. Children may have their growth retarded as a result of the medication. Children should periodically have the drug discontinued to allow growth to proceed normally and to determine if the drug therapy needs to be continued.

Client/Family Teaching

1. Report any noted changes in mood or affect to the physician.

2. Do not use caffeine or caffeine-containing beverages. Provide a printed list of such products.

3. Avoid taking OTC preparations that contain caffeine, phenyl-propanolamine, and other drugs that can affect the cardiovascular system.

4. Avoid using heavy machinery or driving a car until the effects of the medication can be evaluated.

5. Monitor weight and maintain a written record to share with the health care provider at each client visit.

6. To prevent constipation, drink at least 2,500 ml of fluid daily and increase the amount of high-fiber foods, including fruits, in the daily diet.

7. Advise clients who have a dry mouth to chew sugarless gum or candies and to rinse the mouth frequently with nonalcoholic mouth rinses.

Evaluation

1. Review with the client and family the goals of therapy and assess any reported changes in behavior.

2. Assess child for improved attention span and/or a decreased incidence of falling asleep during the day (narcolepsy).

3. Document weight reduction.

Amphotericin B

(am-foe-**TER**-ih-sin)
Fungizone Intravenous (Rx)

See also *Anti-Infectives*, p. 80.

Classification: Antibiotic, antifungal.

Action/Kinetics: This antibiotic is produced by *Streptomyces nodosus;* it is fungistatic or fungicidal depending on the concentration of the drug in body fluids and the susceptibility of the fungus. Amphotericin B binds to specific chemical structures—sterols—of the fungal cellular membrane, increasing cellular permeability and promoting loss of potassium and other substances. Amphotericin B is used either IV or topically. It is highly bound to serum protein (90%) **Peak plasma levels:** 0.5–2 mcg/ml. **t½, initial:** 24 hr; **second phase:** 15 days. Slowly excreted by kidneys.

Uses: The drug is toxic and should be used only for clients under close medical supervision with progressive or potentially fatal fungal infections. *IV:* Disseminated North American blastomycosis, cryptococcosis, and other systemic fungal infections, including coccidioidomycosis, histoplasmosis, mucomycosis, sporotrichosis, aspergillosis, disseminated candidiasis, and monilial overgrowth resulting from oral antibiotic therapy. Secondary therapy to treat American mucocutaneous leishmaniasis. *Topical:* Cutaneous and mucocutaneous infections of *Candida (Monilia)* infections.

Contraindications: Hypersensitivity to drug. Use to treat common forms of fungal diseases showing only positive skin or serologic tests.

Special Concerns: Pregnancy category: B. The bone marrow depressant effects may result in increased incidence of microbial infection, delayed healing, and gingival bleeding. Although used in children, safety and efficacy have not been determined.

Side Effects: After topical use. Irritation, pruritus, dry skin. **After IV use.** *GI:* Nausea, vomiting, diarrhea, dyspepsia, anorexia, abdominal cramps, epigastric pain, melena, hemorrhagic gastroenteritis. *CNS:* Fever, chills, headache, malaise, vertigo; rarely, seizures, peripheral neuropathy, and other neurologic symptoms. *CV:* Thrombophlebitis, phlebitis. Rarely, arrhythmias, hyper- or hypotension, ventricular fibrillation, cardiac arrest. *Renal:* Anuria, oliguria, azotemia, hypokalemia, renal tubular acidosis, nephrocalcinosis, hyposthenuria. *Hematologic:* Normochromic, normocytic anemia. Rarely, coagulation defects, thrombocytopenia, leukopenia, agranulocytosis, eosinophilia, leukocytosis. *Dermatologic:* Maculopapular rash, pruritus. *Miscellaneous:* Muscle and joint pain, generalized pain, weight loss, tinnitus, blurred or double vision, hearing loss, hepatic failure, dyspnea, flushing, anaphylaxis.

Drug Interactions

Aminoglycosides / Additive nephrotoxicity and/or ototoxicity

Corticosteroids, Corticotropin / ↑ K depletion caused by amphotericin B

Cyclosporine / ↑ Nephrotoxic effects of cyclosporine

Digitalis glycosides / ↑ K depletion caused by amphotericin B; ↑ Incidence of digitalis toxicity

Flucytosine / Synergistic antifungal effect

Miconazole / Amphotericin B ↓ effect of miconazole

Rifampin / Synergistic antifungal effect

Skeletal muscle relaxants, surgical (e.g., succinylcholine, *d*-tubocurarine*) / ↑ Muscle relaxation

Tetracyclines / Synergistic antifungal effect

Laboratory Test Interferences: ↑ AST, ALT, alkaline phosphatase, creatinine, BUN, NPN, BSP retention values.

Dosage: Slow IV infusion, initial: 0.25 mg/kg/day. May be increased gradually by 0.1–0.2 mg/kg/day, up to a maximum dose of 1.5 mg/kg/day to 1.5 mg/kg every other day. A test dose (1 mg) should be given first to assess client tolerance. Depending on use, treatment may be required for several months. **Topical (lotion, cream, ointment—each 3%):** Apply liberally to affected areas b.i.d.–q.i.d. Depending on the type of lesion, up to 4 weeks of therapy may be necessary.

NURSING CONSIDERATIONS

See also *General Nursing Considerations For All Anti-Infectives,* p. 83.

Administration/Storage

1. Follow directions on vial for dilution. Use only distilled water without a bacteriostatic agent or 5% dextrose as diluent to avoid precipitation of drug.
2. Strict aseptic technique must be used in preparation because there is no bacteriostatic agent in the medication.
3. Use a sterile 20-gauge needle every time entrance is made into the vial.
4. Do not use saline solution or distilled water with bacteriostatic agent as a diluent because a precipitate may result.
5. Do not use the initial concentrate if any precipitate is present.
6. An in-line membrane filter with a pore diameter of 1 micron may be used.
7. Protect from light during administration and storage.
8. Minimize local inflammation and danger of thrombophlebitis by administering the solution below the recommended dilution of 0.1 mg.
9. Initiate therapy in the most distal veins.
10. Have on hand 200–400 units of heparin sodium, since it may be ordered for the infusion to prevent thrombophlebitis.
11. Administer IV infusion for 6 hr.
12. After reconstitution, amphotericin may be stored for 24 hr in a dark room or in a refrigerator for 1 week without significant loss of potency.
13. Use dilutions of 0.1 mg/ml immediately after preparation.
14. Rub creams and lotions into lesion.

Assessment

1. Assess for any history of adverse effects and hypersensitivity to any anti-infectives or drugs in the antifungal category.
2. During the nursing and drug history, assess mental status and note client age.

Interventions

1. Ascertain if the physician wants the client to receive antipyretics, antihistamines, and/or antiemetic drugs during therapy to reduce side effects.
2. Determine if a 1-mg test dose has been administered to assess client's tolerance to amphotericin.
3. Infuse IV slowly and interrupt if client develops any adverse effects and notify physician.

A

4. Monitor vital signs frequently during IV administration.
5. Monitor intake and output. Report a reduction in output and blood sediment or cloudiness in the urine.
6. Weigh client twice weekly as a means of determining signs of possible malnutrition or dehydration.
7. Anticipate hypokalemia in clients concomitantly taking digoxin. Observe for toxicity, muscle weakness and monitor serum digoxin levels.

Client/Family Teaching

1. Report any incidents of anorexia, nausea, vomiting, headache, or chills.
2. Stress the importance of reporting any decrease in intake and output.
3. Amphotericin therapy usually requires 6–10 weeks to ensure an adequate response to therapy and to prevent any relapse.
4. If diarrhea develops, try small frequent meals. GI effects may be reduced by administering an antihistamine or antiemetic before drug therapy and by administering the drug before mealtime.
5. Neurologic symptoms such as tinnitus, blurred vision, or vertigo should be reported immediately.
6. Review guidelines for therapy with creams and lotions:
   • Drug does not stain skin when it is rubbed into lesion.
   • Any discoloration of fabric caused by cream or lotion may be removed by washing with soap and water.
   • Any discoloration of clothing

caused by ointment may be removed with a standard cleaning fluid.
   • Report any increased itching, burning, or rash at site of local application.

Evaluation

1. Assess client/family knowledge and understanding of illness, response to therapy and teaching.
2. Note any alteration in renal function as well as cloudiness or bloody sediment in the urine.
3. Intrathecal administration of amphotericin may cause inflammation of the spinal roots; assess for sensory loss or foot drop in these clients.
4. Note clinical evidence of resolution of fungal infection.

Ampicillin oral
(am-pih-**SILL**-in)
APO-Ampi✣, D-Amp, Novo-Ampicillin✣, Nu-Ampi✣, Omnipen, Penbritin✣, Polycillin, Polycillin Pediatric Drops, Principen, Totacillin (Rx)

——— COMBINATION DRUG ———
Ampicillin with Probenecid
(am-pih-**SILL**-in, proh-**BEN**-ih-sid)
Ampicin-PRB✣, Polycillin-PRB, Probampacin (Rx)

Ampicillin sodium, parenteral
(am-pih-**SILL**-in)
Ampicin✣, Omnipen-N, Penbritin✣, Polycillin-N, Totacillin-N (Rx)

See also *Anti-Infectives,* p. 80, and *Penicillins,* p. 197.

Classification: Antibiotic, penicillin.

Action/Kinetics: Synthetic, broad-spectrum antibiotic suitable for gram-negative bacteria. Acid resistant, destroyed by penicillinase. Absorbed more slowly than other penicillins. From 30%–60% of oral dose absorbed from GI tract. **Peak serum levels: PO:** 1.8–2.9 mcg/ml after 2 hr; **IM,** 4.5–7 mcg/ml. **t½:** 80 min—range 50–110 min. Partially inactivated in liver; 25%–85% excreted unchanged in urine.

Uses: Infections of respiratory, GI, and GU tracts caused by *Shigella, Salmonella, Escherichia coli, Hemophilus influenzae, Proteus* strains, *Neisseria gonorrhoeae, N. meningitidis,* and *Enterococcus.* Also, otitis media in children, bronchitis, rat-bite fever, and whooping cough. Penicillin G-sensitive staphylococci, streptococci, pneumococci.

Additional Drug Interactions

Allopurinol / ↑ Incidence of skin rashes
Ampicillin / ↓ Effect of oral contraceptives

Dosage: Ampicillin: Capsules, Oral Suspension; Ampicillin sodium: IV, IM. *Respiratory tract and soft tissue infections:* **PO, 20 kg or more:** 250 mg q 6 hr; **less than 20 kg:** 50 mg/kg/day in equally divided doses q 6–8 hr. **IV, IM, 40 kg or more:** 250–500 mg q 6 hr; **less than 40 kg:** 25–50 mg/kg/day in equally divided doses q 6–8 hr.
Disseminated gonococcal infections: **PO,** 1 g q 6 hr.
Bacterial meningitis: **Adults,** A total of 8–12 g daily given in divided doses q 3–4 hr. **Pediatric:** 100–200 mg/kg daily in divided

doses q 3–4 hr. *Bacterial endocarditis prophylaxis* (dental, oral, or upper respiratory tract procedures; GI or GU tract surgery or instrumentation): **Adult, IM, IV:** 1–2 g (use 2 g for GI or GU tract surgery) plus gentamicin, 1.5 mg/kg (not to exceed 80 mg) IM or IV, given 30 min before procedure followed by amoxicillin, 1.5 g, 6 hr after initial dose; or, repeat parenteral dose 8 hr after initial dose. **Pediatric:** Ampicillin, 50 mg/kg with gentamicin, 2 mg/kg 30 min prior to procedure followed by amoxicillin, 25 mg/kg, after 6 hr or a parenteral dose of ampicillin is given after 8 hr. *Septicemia:* **Adults/children:** 150–200 mg/kg, IV for first 3 days, then IM q 3–4 hr.
Ampicillin with Probenecid: Oral Suspension. *Urethral, endocervical, or rectal infections due to Neisseria gonorrhoeae:* 3.5 g ampicillin and 1 g probenecid as a single dose. *Prophylaxis of infection in rape victims:* 3.5 g with 1 g probenecid.

NURSING CONSIDERATIONS

See also *Nursing Considerations* for *Penicillins,* p. 200.

Administration/Storage

1. After reconstitution for IM or direct IV administration, the solution of sodium ampicillin must be used within the hour.
2. For IM use, dilute only with sterile water for injection or bacteriostatic water for injection.
3. For IV "piggyback," ampicillin may be reconstituted with sodium chloride injection.
4. IV injections of reconstituted sodium ampicillin should be given slowly; 2 ml should be

given over a period of at least 3–5 min.

5. For administration by IV drip, check compatibility and length of time that drug retains potency in a particular solution.

6. If the creatinine clearance is less than 10 ml/min, the dosing interval should be increased to 12 hr.

Interventions

1. Obtain and monitor liver and renal function studies. If creatinine clearance is less than 10 ml/min, the dosing interval should be increased to 12 hr.

2. When administering IM, tell the client that it will be painful.

3. Rotate and document injection sites.

4. Monitor urinary output and serum potassium in the elderly.

Client/Family Teaching

1. Teach the person administering the drug the appropriate method for administration and storage.

2. Take the drug for the prescribed number of days even if the symptoms subside.

3. If side effects occur, call the physician and refrain from taking the drug until medically cleared.

4. Take the medication 1 hr before or 2 hr after meals.

5. Ampicillin chewable tablets should not be swallowed whole.

6. Do not save any of the drug for future use or share with family members or friends who may seem to have the same type of infection.

7. Drug may decrease effectiveness of oral contraceptives.

Advise client to practice alternative method of contraception during this period.

Evaluation

1. Assess client/family knowledge and understanding of illness, response to therapy and teaching.

2. Observe skin closely for rashes because they occur more often with this drug than with other penicillins.

3. If clients develop a skin rash, have them tested for mononucleosis because this may be the cause of the rash.

4. Review lab data. Note any evidence of resistance to anti-infective drug therapy.

———— COMBINATION DRUG ————

Ampicillin sodium/Sulbactam sodium

(am-pih-**SILL**-in/sull-**BACK**-tam)

Unasyn (Rx)

See also *Anti-Infectives,* p. 80, and *Penicillins,* p. 197.

Classification: Antibiotic, penicillin.

Action/Kinetics: For details, see *Ampicillin oral.* Sulbactam is present in this product because it irreversibly inhibits beta-lactamases, thus ensuring activity of ampicillin against beta-lactamase–producing microorganisms. Thus, sulbactam broadens the antibiotic spectrum of ampicillin to those bacteria normally resistant to it. **Peak serum levels, after IV infusion:** 15 min. **$t^{1/2}$, both drugs:** about 1 hr. From 75%–85% of both drugs are excreted unchanged in the urine within 8 hr after administration.

Uses: To treat infections caused by beta-lactamase–producing strains of the following: (a) skin and skin structure infections caused by *Staphylococcus aureus, Escherichia coli, Klebsiella* species (including *K. pneumoniae*), *Proteus mirabilis, Bacteroides fragilis, Enterobacter* species, and *Acinetobacter calcoaceticus;* (b) intra-abdominal infections caused by *E. coli, Klebsiella* species (including *E. pneumoniae*), *Bacteroides* (including *B. fragilis* and *Enterobacter*) (c) gynecologic infections caused by *E. coli* and *Bacteroides* (including *B. fragilis*). **Note:** Mixed infections caused by ampicillin-susceptible organisms and beta-lactamase–producing organisms are susceptible to this product; thus, additional antibiotics do not have to be used.

Special Concerns: Safety and efficacy in children less than 12 years of age have not been established.

Side Effects: *At site of injection:* Pain and thrombophlebitis. *GI:* Diarrhea, nausea, vomiting, flatulence, abdominal distention, glossitis. *CNS:* Fatigue, malaise, headache. *GU:* Dysuria, urinary retention. *Miscellaneous:* Itching, chest pain, edema, facial swelling, erythema, chills, tightness in throat, epistaxis, substernal pain, mucosal bleeding, candidiasis.

  Symptoms of Overdose: Neurologic symptoms, including convulsions.

Laboratory Test Interferences: ↑ AST, ALT, alkaline phosphatase, lactic dehydrogenase, creatinine, BUN; also, ↑ basophils, eosinophils, lymphocytes, monocytes, platelets. ↓ Serum albumin and total proteins, hemoglobin, hematocrit, red blood cells, white blood cells, and platelets. Presence of red blood cells and hyaline casts in urine.

Dosage: IV, IM: 1 g ampicillin/0.5 g sulbactam to 2 g ampicillin/1 g sulbactam q 6 hr, not to exceed 4 g sulbactam daily. Doses must be decreased in renal impairment.

NURSING CONSIDERATIONS

See also *Nursing Considerations* for *Penicillins,* p. 200, and *Ampicillin,* p. 313.

Administration/Storage

1. For IV use, drug can be given by slow injection over 10–15 min or, if mixed with 50–100 ml of diluent, can be given over 15–30 min.
2. For IV use, the drug can be reconstituted with any of the following: 5% dextrose injection, 5% dextrose injection in 0.45% saline, 10% invert sugar, lactated Ringer's injection, 0.9% sodium chloride injection, M/6 sodium lactate injection, or sterile water for injection.
3. For IM use, the drug can be reconstituted with sterile water for injection or 0.5% or 2% lidocaine HCl injection.
4. After reconstitution, solutions should stand so that any foaming will dissipate and the vial can be inspected visually to ensure dissolution.
5. Solutions for IM administration must be used within 1 hr after preparation.
6. If aminoglycosides are prescribed concomitantly, administer each separately, because ampicillin will inactivate aminoglycosides.
7. *Treatment of Overdose:* Both ampicillin and sulbactam may be removed by hemodialysis.

Assessment: Determine if client has mononucleosis because drug, in this event, may cause skin rash.

Interventions

1. Anticipate reduced doses in clients with impaired renal function.
2. IM injections are extremely painful; follow manufacturer's recommendations for IM reconstitution and tell the client to expect some discomfort.

Evaluation: Assess lab culture and sensitivity reports to determine effectiveness of drug therapy.

Amrinone lactate
(AM-rih-nohn)
Inocor (Rx)

Classification: Cardiac inotropic agent.

Action/Kinetics: Amrinone causes an increase in cardiac output by increasing the force of contraction of the heart, probably by inhibiting phosphodiesterase. It reduces afterload and preload by directly relaxing vascular smooth muscle. **Time to peak effect:** 10 min. **t½, after rapid IV:** 3.6 hr; **after IV infusion:** 5.8 hr. **Plasma levels:** 3.0 mcg/ml. **Duration:** 30 min–2 hr, depending on the dose. The drug is excreted primarily in the urine both unchanged and as metabolites.

Uses: Congestive heart failure (short-term therapy in clients unresponsive to digitalis, diuretics, and/or vasodilators). Can be used in digitalized clients.

Contraindications: Hypersensitivity to bisulfites. Severe aortic or pulmonary valvular disease in lieu of surgery. Acute myocardial infarction.

Special Concerns: Safety and efficacy in pregnancy (category: C), lactation, and in children not established.

Side Effects: *GI:* Nausea, vomiting, abdominal pain, anorexia. *CV:* Hypotension, arrhythmias. *Allergic:* Pericarditis, pleuritis, ascites. *Other:* Thrombocytopenia, hepatotoxicity, fever, chest pain, burning at site of injection. *Symptom of Overdose:* Hypotension.

Drug Interactions: Excessive hypotension when used with disopyramide.

Dosage: **IV. Initial:** 0.75 mg/kg as bolus slowly over 2–3 min; may be repeated after 30 min if necessary. **Maintenance, IV infusion:** 5–10 mcg/kg/min. Daily dose should not exceed 10 mg/kg although up to 18 mg/kg/day has been used in some clients for short periods.

NURSING CONSIDERATIONS

Administration/Storage

1. Amrinone may be administered undiluted or diluted in 0.9% or 0.45% saline to a concentration of 1–3 mg/ml. Diluted solutions should be used within 24 hr.
2. Amrinone should not be diluted with solutions containing dextrose (glucose) prior to injection. However, the drug may be injected into running dextrose (glucose) infusions through a Y connector or directly into the tubing.
3. Administer solution with an electronic infusion device.
4. Amrinone should not be administered in an IV line con-

taining furosemide because a precipitate will form.

5. Protect from light and store at room temperature.

6. *Treatment of Overdose:* Reduce or discontinue drug administration and begin general supportive measures.

Assessment

1. Determine that baseline vital signs and ECG have been performed.
2. Obtain baseline electrolytes, CBC, and platelet count.

Interventions

1. Clients should be on a cardiac monitor while receiving amrinone lactate.
2. Monitor serum potassium levels, CBC, and platelets; report any bruises or bleeding.
3. Monitor BP frequently, note any drop in blood pressure because drug can cause hypotension.

Evaluation

1. Evaluate for unusual hypersensitivity reactions, including pericarditis, pleuritis, and ascites.
2. Assess for a positive response to therapy such as improvement in cardiac output, decrease in preload and afterload, and improvement in symptoms of congestive heart failure.

Amyl nitrite

(AM-ill)

Amyl Nitrite Aspirols, Amyl Nitrite Vaporole (Rx)

See also *Antianginal Drugs—Nitrates/Nitrites,* p. 47.

Classification: Coronary vasodilator, antidote for cyanide poisoning.

Action/Kinetics: Amyl nitrite is believed to act by reducing systemic and pulmonary arterial pressure (afterload) and by decreasing cardiac output due to peripheral vasodilation as opposed to causing coronary artery dilation. Vascular relaxation occurs due to stimulation of intracellular cyclic guanosine monophosphate. As an antidote to cyanide poisoning, amyl nitrite promotes formation of methemoglobin which combines with cyanide to form the nontoxic cyanmethemoglobin. **Onset (inhalation):** 30 sec. **Duration:** 3–5 min. About 33% is excreted through the kidneys.

Uses: Prophylaxis or relief of acute attacks of angina pectoris; acute cyanide poisoning. *Investigational:* Diagnostic aid to assess reserve cardiac function.

Special Concerns: Pregnancy category: X. Use of amyl nitrite in children has not been studied. Hypotensive effects are more likely to occur in geriatric clients.

Dosage: Inhalation. *Angina pectoris:* 0.18–0.3 ml (1 container crushed). Usually, 1–6 inhalations from one container produces relief. Dosage may be repeated after 3–5 min. *Antidote for cyanide poisoning:* Administer for 30–60 sec q 5 min until client is conscious; is then repeated at longer intervals for up to 24 hr.

NURSING CONSIDERATIONS

See also *Nursing Considerations* for *Antianginal Drugs—Nitrates/Nitrites,* p. 49.

Administration/Storage

1. Administer only by inhalation.
2. Containers should be protec-

A

ted from light and stored at a temperature of 46°F (8°C)–59°F (15°C).

3. *Amyl nitrite vapors are highly flammable. Do not use near flame or intense heat.*

Assessment

1. Take a history of common precipitating incidents that immediately precede the onset of chest pain.
2. Determine and document the degree, location, type, and duration of chest pain, and the direction in which it radiates.
3. Note the presence of risk factors and list.
4. Determine and document source of cyanide poisoning and presenting symptoms.

Client/Family Teaching

1. Discuss and mutually set the goals of therapy with client and family.
2. Assist client to identify changes in life-style that may reduce the need for amyl nitrite.
3. Enclose fabric-covered ampule in a handkerchief or piece of cloth and crush by hand.
4. Sit down during inhalation to avoid hypotension.
5. Drug has a pungent odor, but several deep breaths must nevertheless be taken to attain drug effects.
6. Always store medication out of reach of children.
7. The medication has the potential for abuse and must be stored appropriately.

Evaluation: Evaluate for a positive clinical response as evidenced by:

- Termination of angina attack
- Resolution of symptoms of cyanide toxicity

Anistreplase
(an-ih-**STREP**-layz)
Eminase (Rx)

Classification: Thrombolytic enzyme.

Action/Kinetics: Anistreplase is prepared by acylating human plasma derived from lys-plasminogen and purified streptokinase derived from group C beta-hemolytic streptococci. When prepared, anistreplase is an inactive derivative of a fibrinolytic enzyme although the compound can still bind to fibrin. Anistreplase is activated by deacylation and subsequent release of the anisoyl group in the blood stream. The production of plasmin from plasminogen occurs in both the blood stream and the thrombus leading to thrombolysis. The drug will lyse thrombi obstructing coronary arteries and reduce the size of infarcts. **t½:** 70–120 min.

Uses: Management of acute myocardial infarction in adults, resulting in improvement of ventricular function and reduction of mortality. Treatment should be initiated as soon as possible after the onset of symptoms of acute myocardial infarction.

Contraindications: Use in active internal bleeding; within 2 months of intracranial or intraspinal surgery or trauma; history of cerebrovascular accident; intracranial neoplasm, arteriovenous (AV) malformation, or aneurysm; known bleeding diathesis; severe, uncontrolled hypertension; severe allergic reactions to streptokinase.

Special Concerns: Pregnancy category: C. Use with caution in nursing mothers. Safety and effectiveness have not been determined in children.

Note: The risks of anistreplase therapy may be increased in the following conditions; thus, benefit versus risk must be assessed prior to use. Within 10 days of major surgery (e.g., coronary artery bypass graft, obstetric delivery, organ biopsy, previous puncture of noncompressible vessels); cerebrovascular disease; within 10 days of GI or GU bleeding; within 10 days of trauma including cardiopulmonary resuscitation; systolic blood pressure greater than 180 mm Hg or diastolic blood pressure greater than 110 mm Hg; likelihood of left heart thrombus (e.g., mitral stenosis with atrial fibrillation); subacute bacterial endocarditis; acute pericarditis; hemostatic defects including those secondary to severe hepatic or renal disease; pregnancy; clients older than 75 years of age; diabetic hemorrhagic retinopathy or other hemorrhagic ophthalmic conditions; septic thrombophlebitis or occluded AV cannula at seriously infected site; clients on oral anticoagulant therapy; any condition in which bleeding constitutes a significant hazard or would be difficult to manage due to its location.

Side Effects: *Bleeding:* Including at the puncture site (most common), nonpuncture site hematoma, hematuria, hemoptysis, GI hemorrhage, intracranial bleeding, gum/mouth hemorrhage, epistaxis, anemia, eye hemorrhage. *CV:* Arrhythmias, conduction disorders, hypotension; cardiac rupture, chest pain, emboli (causal relationship to use of anistreplase unknown). *Allergic:* Anaphylaxis, bronchospasm, angioedema, urticaria, itching, flushing, rashes, eosinophilia, delayed purpuric rash which may be associated with arthralgia, ankle edema, mild hematuria, GI symptoms, and proteinuria. *GI:* Nausea, vomiting. *Hematologic:* Thrombocytopenia. *CNS:* Agitation, dizziness, paresthesia, tremor, vertigo. *Respiratory:* Dyspnea, lung edema. *Miscellaneous:* Chills, fever, headache, shock.

Drug Interactions: Increased risk of bleeding or hemorrhage if used with heparin, oral anticoagulants, vitamin K antagonists, aspirin, or dipyridamole.

Laboratory Test Interferences: ↑ Transaminase levels, thrombin time, activated partial thromboplastin time, and prothrombin time. ↓ Plasminogen and fibrinogen.

Dosage: IV only: 30 units over 2–5 min into an IV line or vein as soon as possible after onset of symptoms.

NURSING CONSIDERATIONS

See also *Nursing Considerations* for *Alteplase, Recombinant,* p. 285.

Administration/Storage

1. The drug is reconstituted by slowly adding 5 ml of sterile water for injection. To minimize foaming, gently roll the vial after directing the stream of sterile water against the side of the vial. The vial should not be shaken.
2. The reconstituted solution should be colorless to pale yellow without any particulate matter or discoloration.
3. The reconstituted solution should not be further diluted before administration.
4. The reconstituted solution should not be added to any infusion fluids and no other medications should be added

to the vial or syringe containing anistreplase.

5. The solution should be discarded if not administered within 30 min of reconstitution.

Assessment

1. Note any history and any evidence of bleeding.
2. Obtain client blood pressure and pulse readings as baseline data, before initiating therapy.
3. Take a full drug history. Note especially if client has been taking aspirin, anticoagulants, or vitamin K antagonists.
4. Determine that appropriate laboratory studies have been completed prior to starting drug therapy.

Interventions

1. Invasive procedures should be avoided to minimize bleeding tendencies. Incorporate bleeding precautions.
2. If an arterial puncture is necessary following use of anistreplase, an upper extremity vessel accessible to manual compression should be used. Apply 30 min of manual pressure followed by application of a pressure dressing. Puncture site should be checked frequently for any evidence of bleeding.
3. Monitor closely and document reperfusion arrhythmias.

Evaluation

1. Note resistance to the effects of anistreplase, which may be observed if the drug is given more than 5 days after a previous dose, after streptokinase therapy, or after a streptococcal infection.
2. Increased antistreptokinase antibody levels between 5 days and 6 months after anistreplase or streptokinase administration may increase the risk of allergic reactions.
3. Assess for a reduction in infarct size and improved ventricular function.

Antithrombin III (Human)
(an-tee-THROM-bin)
ATnativ (Rx)

Classification: Antithrombin.

Action/Kinetics: Antithrombin III (human) is derived from pooled human plasma obtained from healthy donors. It is identical with heparin cofactor I, which is a component of plasma necessary for heparin to exert its anticoagulant effect. Plasma used for antithrombin III (human) has been found to be nonreactive for hepatitis B surface antigen and negative for antibody to human immunodeficiency virus (HIV). The drug also undergoes heat treatment for 10 hr to prevent transmittal of viral infections. One unit is the amount of antithrombin III (AT-III) in 1 ml of normal pooled human plasma. Antithrombin III inactivates all coagulation enzymes except factor VIIa and factor XIII.

Uses: Hereditary AT-III deficiency in pregnant clients, in clients requiring surgery, and in individuals with thromboembolism.

Special Concerns: Pregnancy category: C. Safety and effectiveness have not been determined in children. Even though special precautions are taken, individuals may develop signs or symptoms of viral infections, including non-A, non-B hepatitis.

Side Effects: No side effects have been reported to date.

Drug Interactions: The anticoagulant effect of heparin is increased when used concomitantly with AT-III; the dose of heparin should be decreased during AT-III therapy.

Dosage: IV. The dose must be individualized depending on the status of the client. Assuming a plasma volume of 40 ml/kg, an initial loading dose may be calculated as follows:

Dosage units = [desired AT-III level (%)−baseline AT-III (%)] × body weight (kg)/1% (IU/kg)

Administration of 1 IU/kg raises the level of AT-III by 1%–2.1%. The drug may be infused slowly over 5–10 min at a rate of 50 IU (1 ml)/min, not to exceed 100 IU (2 ml)/min.

NURSING CONSIDERATIONS

Administration/Storage

1. To reconstitute, the powder should be dissolved by gently swirling in 10 ml sterile water for injection, 0.9% sodium chloride injection, or 5% dextrose injection. The product should not be shaken.
2. After reconstitution, the drug should be brought to room temperature and administered within 3 hr.
3. After the initial dose (which may increase AT-III levels to 120% of normal), the dose should be adjusted to maintain AT-III levels greater than 80% of normal.
4. AT-III levels should be measured at least twice daily initially

and until the client is stabilized and then once daily, immediately before the next infusion.
5. Anticipate a loading dose followed by once daily dosing, based on frequent plasma AT-III levels. Dosing recommendations are only guidelines; the exact loading and maintenance doses must be individualized depending on the status of the client, response to therapy, and actual plasma AT-III levels achieved.

Assessment

1. Perform a complete nursing history on clients with hereditary AT-III deficiency, noting any positive family history of venous thrombosis.
2. Determine that AT-III levels have been obtained prior to drug therapy and before each subsequent infusion.
3. Document pretreatment weight.

Interventions

1. Observe for elevated BP and dyspnea during IV administration; slow infusion rate and notify physician if evident.
2. Monitor vital signs closely throughout drug therapy.
3. Note early signs and symptoms of acute thrombosis. Perform routine vascular checks and monitor AT-III levels.
4. Observe for any evidence of bleeding. Anticipate a reduced dose of heparin when administered concomitantly with AT-III.
5. Anticipate that when AT-III is given for clients with heredity deficiency to control an acute thrombosis or to prevent

thrombosis due to surgery or in obstetrics, that levels should be maintained for 2–8 days, depending on the status of the client.

Client/Family Teaching

1. Explain the high risk of thrombosis during pregnancy and surgery in clients with hereditary deficiencies because their AT-III levels are generally 50% of the level of normal.
2. Stress that the disease is inherited and refer for appropriate medical follow-up, counseling and family planning.
3. Discuss the associated risks of drug therapy because product is derived from pooled human plasma.

Evaluation

1. Serum AT-III levels greater than 80% of normal during therapy for high-risk procedures.
2. Freedom from complications of disease deficiency and replacement drug therapy.

Asparaginase
(ah-**SPAIR**-ah-jin-ays)
**Colaspase, Elspar, Kidrolase ✿
(Abbreviation: Lcf-ASP) (Rx)**

Classification: Antineoplastic, miscellaneous.

Action/Kinetics: Drug isolated from *Escherichia coli*. Cell cycle specific (G_1 phase). Neoplastic cells are unable to synthesize sufficient asparagine, an amino acid, to meet their metabolic needs. The supply of asparagine is further decreased by the enzyme asparaginase, which breaks down asparagine to aspartic acid and ammonia. Asparaginase

interferes with synthesis of DNA, RNA, and protein and is cell-cycle specific for the G_1 phase of cell division. **Time to peak plasma levels, after IM:** 14–24 hr. **$t^{1/2}$, after IV:** 8–30 hr; **after IM:** 39–49 hr. The drug accumulates in plasma and tissue, and a small amount (1%) appears in CSF. Excretion is unknown. More toxic in adults than in children.

Use: Acute lymphocytic leukemia in children; mostly used in combination with other drugs. Not to be used for maintenance therapy. *Investigational:* Acute myelocytic and myelomonocytic leukemia, chronic lymphocytic leukemia, Hodgkin's and non-Hodgkin's lymphomas, melanosarcoma.

Contraindications: Anaphylactic reactions to asparaginase, acute hemorrhagic pancreatitis. Lactation. Institute retreatment with great care.

Special Concerns: Pregnancy category: C. Use with caution in presence of liver dysfunction.

Additional Side Effects: Hypersensitivity reaction including those with negative skin tests. Hyperglycemia, uricemia, azotemia, acute hemorrhagic pancreatitis, fatal hyperthermia. Hallucinations, Parkinson-like syndrome (rare).

Drug Interactions

Methotrexate / Asparaginase ↓ effect of methotrexate
Prednisone / Even though used with asparaginase, may cause ↑ toxicity
Vincristine / Even though used with asparaginase, may cause ↑ toxicity; ↑ hyperglycemic effect

Laboratory Test Interferences: ↑ Blood ammonia, BUN, glucose, uric acid, AST, ALT, alkaline phosphatase, bilirubin (direct and indirect). ↓ Serum calcium albumin, cholesterol, plasma fibrinogen. Interference with interpretation of thyroid function tests.

Dosage: IV, IM, *individualized.* **When used as sole agent: Adults and children,** 200 IU/kg/day **IV** for 28 days. **In combination with prednisone and vincristine: Asparaginase,** 1,000 IU/kg/day **IV** for 10 days beginning on day 22 of course of therapy; **vincristine:** 2 mg/m² **IV** once weekly on days 1, 8, and 15 of course of treatment (single dosage should not exceed 2 mg); **prednisone:** 40 mg/m²/day **PO** in 3 doses for 15 days; **then,** 20 mg/m² for 2 days, 10 mg/m² for 2 days, 5 mg/m² for 2 days, and 2.5 mg/m² for 2 days, followed by discontinuance of therapy.

Alternative regimen: Asparaginase, 6,000 IU/m² **IM** on days 4, 7, 10, 13, 16, 19, 22, 25, and 28 of course of treatment; **vincristine:** 1.5 mg/m² **IV** weekly on days 1, 8, 15, and 22 of course of treatment (maximum single dose should not exceed 2 mg); **prednisone:** 40 mg/m²/day **PO** in 3 divided doses for 28 days, followed by gradual discontinuation over a 2-week period.

NURSING CONSIDERATIONS

See also *Nursing Considerations* for *Antineoplastic Agents,* p. 88.

Administration/Storage

1. An intradermal skin test (0.1 ml of a 20-IU/ml solution) should be done at least 1 hr before initial administration of drug and when 1 week or more has elapsed between treatments.
2. A desensitization procedure, with increasing amounts of asparaginase, is sometimes carried out in clients hypersensitive to the drug.
3. Treatment should be initiated only in hospitalized clients.
4. Asparaginase should not be used as the sole induction agent unless a combined regimen is not possible due to toxicity or because the client is refractory.
5. For IV use, reconstitute the 10,000-unit vial with either 5 ml sterile water for injection or sodium chloride injection. The solution may be given by direct IV administration or by infusion. When infused, give over at least 30 min in side of arm; use an infusion of either sodium chloride injection or dextrose injection (5%).
6. When used IM, no more than 2 ml should be given at a single injection site.
7. Reconstitute for IM use by adding 2 ml sodium chloride injection to the 10,000-unit vial. Do not use after 8 hr following reconstitution.
8. The drug should be handled with care because it is a contact irritant.

Interventions

1. Have emergency equipment readily available during each administration of asparaginase because a severe hypersensitivity reaction is more likely to occur with this drug.
2. Obtain baseline serum amylase levels and check periodically during therapy to detect evidence of pancreatitis.
3. Monitor client for hyperglycemia, glycosuria, and polyuria, all of which may be precipitated by asparaginase.

4. Have IV fluids and regular insulin available to treat hyperglycemia. Anticipate discontinuation of asparaginase.
5. Monitor intake and output; assess client for any evidence of renal failure.
6. Observe client for peripheral edema due to hypoalbuminemia triggered by asparaginase.
7. Assess for shakiness or unusual body movements. A Parkinson-like condition may be precipitated by asparaginase.
8. If ordered, administer vincristine and prednisone before asparaginase to reduce the toxic effect.
9. Administration of asparaginase 9–10 days before or within 24 hr after methotrexate may be ordered to reduce the GI and hematologic effects of methotrexate.
10. Anticipate antiemetic administration prior to drug therapy.

Client/Family Teaching

1. Promptly report any stomach pain, nausea, and vomiting because these side effects may be symptoms of pancreatitis.
2. Report hyperthermia immediately
3. Encourage client to consume 3–4 L of fluid/day.
4. Caution that the drug may cause drowsiness, even several weeks after administration; therefore, the client should not drive a car or operate hazardous machinery.

Evaluation: Evaluate for:
- Improvement of hematologic parameters in clients with leukemia
- Absence of hypersensitivity reaction

Astemizole
(ah-**STEM**-ih-zohl)
Hismanil (Rx)

See also *Antihistamines,* p. 71.

Classification: Antihistamine, miscellaneous.

Action/Kinetics: Low to no sedative effect, antiemetic effect, or anticholinergic activity. The drug is metabolized in the liver to both active and inactive metabolites and is excreted through the feces. **t½:** About 1.6 days. **Onset:** 2–3 days. **Duration:** Up to several weeks. Over 95% is bound to plasma protein. Mainly excreted through the feces.

Special Concerns: Pregnancy category: C. Safety and efficacy have not been established in children less than 12 years of age.

Dosage: Tablets. Adults and children over 12 years, maintenance: 10 mg once daily; **pediatric, 6–12 years:** 5 mg once daily. The pharmacokinetics of the drug are proportional following single doses of 10–30 mg. Thus, to reduce the time required to reach steady state concentration, a single dose of 30 mg may be given on day 1, followed by 20 mg on day 2 and then on day 3, the recommended 10 mg daily dose may be given.

NURSING CONSIDERATIONS

See also *Nursing Considerations for Antihistamines,* p. 74.

Client/Family Teaching

1. Take medication on an empty stomach.
2. Do not eat until at least 1 hr after medication administration because food interferes with the drug absorption.

3. Take medication only as directed because desired effects may not be noticeable immediately.
4. Report any persistent side effects, including depression or weight gain, to the physician.

Evaluation: Evaluate client for subjective reports of a decrease in allergic symptoms.

Atenolol
(ah-**TEN**-oh-lohl)
Apo-Atenol✶, Novo-Atenol✶, Nu-Atenol✶, Tenormin (Rx)

See also *Beta-Adrenergic Blocking Agents,* p. 113.

Action/Kinetics: Predominantly beta-1 blocking activity. Has no membrane stabilizing activity or intrinsic sympathomimetic activity. Low lipid solubility. **Peak blood levels:** 2–4 hr. **t½:** 6–9 hr. 50% eliminated unchanged in the feces.

Uses: Hypertension (either alone or with other antihypertensives such as thiazide diuretics). Angina pectoris due to hypertension, coronary atherosclerosis, and acute myocardial infarction. *Investigational:* Prophylaxis of migraine, alcohol withdrawal syndrome, situational anxiety, ventricular arrhythmias, prophylactically to reduce incidence of supraventricular arrhythmias in coronary artery bypass surgery.

Special Concerns: Pregnancy category: C. Dosage has not been established in children.

Dosage: Tablets. *Hypertension:* **Initial,** 50 mg once daily, either alone or with diuretics; if response is inadequate, 100 mg once daily. Doses higher than 100 mg daily will not produce further beneficial effects. Maximum effects will usually be seen within 1–2 weeks. *Angina:* **Initial,** 50 mg once daily; if maximum response is not seen in 1 week, increase dose to 100 mg daily (some clients require 200 mg daily). *Alcohol withdrawal syndrome:* 100 mg daily. *Prophylaxis of migraine:* 50–100 mg daily. *Ventricular arrhythmias:* 50–100 mg daily. *Prior to coronary artery bypass surgery:* 50 mg daily started 72 hr prior to surgery. Adjust dosage in cases of renal failure to 50 mg daily if creatinine clearance is 15–35 ml/min/1.73 m² and to 50 mg every other day if creatinine clearance is less than 15 ml/min/1.73 m².

IV. *Acute myocardial infarction:* 5 mg over 5 min followed by a second 5 mg dose 10 min later. Treatment should begin as soon as possible after client arrives at the hospital. In clients who tolerate the full 10-mg dose, a 50-mg tablet should be given 10 min after the last IV dose followed by another 50-mg dose 12 hr later. **Then,** 100 mg once a day or 50 mg b.i.d. for 6–9 days (or until discharge from the hospital).

NURSING CONSIDERATIONS

See also *Nursing Considerations* for *Antihypertensive Agents,* p. 78 and *Beta-Adrenergic Blocking Agents,* p. 116.

Administration/Storage

1. For IV use, the drug may be diluted in sodium chloride injection, dextrose injection, or sodium chloride and dextrose injection.
2. For hemodialysis clients, 50 mg should be given in the hospital after each dialysis.

A

Assessment: Note any client history of diabetes mellitus, pulmonary disease, or cardiac failure.

Client/Family Teaching

1. Advise not to stop drug abruptly as this could precipitate an anginal attack.
2. Report any changes in mood or affect to the physician, especially severe depression.
3. Drug may enhance sensitivity to cold.

Evaluation: Evaluate for a positive clinical response as evidenced by:

- A ↓ in blood pressure
- Subjective reports of a decrease in the frequency of anginal attacks

---

Atracurium besylate
(ah-trah-**KYOUR**-ee-um)
Tracrium Injection (Rx)

See also *Neuromuscular Blocking Agents,* p. 183.

Classification: Nondepolarizing skeletal muscle relaxant.

Action/Kinetics: Atracurium prevents the action of acetylcholine by competing for the cholinergic receptor at the neuromuscular junction. It may also release histamine, leading to hypotension. **Onset:** Within 2 min. **Peak effect:** 1–2 min. **Duration:** 20–40 min with balanced anesthesia. Recovery occurs more quickly than with other nondepolarizing agents (e.g., *d*-tubocurarine). **t½:** 20 min. Drug is metabolized in the plasma.

Uses: Skeletal muscle relaxant during surgery; adjunct to general anesthesia; assist in endotracheal intubation. *Investigational:* Treat

seizures due to drugs or electrically induced.

Contraindications: In clients with myasthenia gravis, Eaton-Lambert syndrome, electrolyte disorders, bronchial asthma.

Special Concerns: Use with caution in pregnancy (category: C) and during labor and delivery. Safety and efficacy have not been determined during lactation. Children up to 1 month of age may be more sensitive to the effects of atracurium.

Additional Side Effects: *CV:* Bradycardia. Other side effects may be due to histamine release and include flushing, erythema, wheezing, urticaria, bronchial secretions, blood pressure and heart rate changes.

Additional Drug Interactions

Enflurane / ↑ Muscle relaxation
Halothane / ↑ Muscle relaxation
Isoflurane / ↑ Muscle relaxation
Lithium / ↑ Muscle relaxation
Phenytoin / ↓ Effect of atracurium
Succinylcholine / ↑ Onset and depth of muscle relaxation
Theophylline / ↓ Effect of atracurium
Trimethaphan / ↑ Muscle relaxation
Verapamil / ↑ Muscle relaxation

Dosage: IV only. Adults and children over 2 years, initial: 0.4–0.5 mg/kg as IV bolus; **maintenance:** 0.08–0.1 mg/kg. *Following use of succinylcholine for intubation under balanced anesthesia:* **Initial,** 0.3–0.4 mg/kg; if using potent inhalation anesthetics, further reductions may be required. *Use in cardiovascular disease or* *patients with history of asthma or anaphylaxis:* **Initial,** 0.3–0.4 mg/kg, given slowly over 1 min. *Use after steady-state enflurane or isoflurane anesthesia established:* 0.25–0.35/kg (about ⅓ less than the usual initial dose). *Use in infants 1 month to 2 years of age under halothane anesthesia:* 0.3–0.4 mg/kg.

Supplemental use: **IV,** 0.08–0.1 mg/kg 20–45 min after the initial dose; then q 15–25 min or as needed. *IV Infusion, balanced anesthesia:* **IV infusion,** 0.009–0.01 mg/kg until the level of neuromuscular blockade is re-established; **then,** rate of infusion is adjusted according to client needs (usually 0.005–0.009 mg/kg/min although some clients may require as little as 0.002 mg/kg/min and others as much as 0.015 mg/kg/min). *For cardiopulmonary bypass surgery in which hypothermia is induced:* **IV infusion,** Reduce rate of infusion by 50%.

NURSING CONSIDERATIONS

See also *Nursing Considerations for Neuromuscular Blocking Agents,* p. 184.

Administration/Storage

1. Initial dosage should be reduced to 0.25–0.35 mg/kg if drug is being used with steady-state enflurane or isoflurane (smaller reductions if halothane is being used).
2. Dosage should be reduced in clients with myasthenia gravis or other neuromuscular diseases, electrolyte disorders, or carcinomatosis.
3. Atracurium should not be mixed with alkaline solutions.
4. Maintenance doses can be given by continuous infusion of a diluted solution to clients 2 years of age to adulthood.
5. Solutions for infusion should be used within 24 hr.
6. To preserve potency, the drug should be refrigerated at 2°C–8°C (36°F–46°F).
7. IM administration may cause tissue irritation.

Interventions

1. Anticipate reduced dosage in clients with myasthenia gravis or other neuromuscular diseases, electrolyte disorders, or carcinomatosis.
2. Monitor heart rate. IV atropine may be used to treat bradycardia due to atracurium.

Evaluation: Evaluate client for desired level of skeletal muscle relaxation without adverse side effects.

Atropine sulfate
(AH-troh-peen)
Atropair, Atropine Minims✸, Atropine Sulfate S.O.P., Atropine-Care Ophthalmic, Atropisol Ophthalmic, Isopto Atropine Ophthalmic, I-Tropine, Ocu-Tropine (Rx)

See also *Cholinergic Blocking Agents,* p. 136.

Classification: Cholinergic blocking agent.

Action/Kinetics: Atropine blocks the action of acetylcholine on postganglionic cholinergic receptors in smooth muscle, cardiac muscle, exocrine glands, urinary bladder, and the artrioventricular (AV) and sinoatrial (SA) nodes in the heart. Ophthalmologically, atropine blocks the effect of acetylcholine on

A

the sphincter muscle of the iris and the accommodative muscle of the ciliary body. This results in dilation of the pupil (mydriasis) and paralysis of the muscles required to accommodate for close vision (cycloplegia). This enables the physician to examine the inner structure of the eye, including the retina. It also permits examination of refractive errors of the lens without the patient automatically accommodating. **Peak effect:** *Mydriasis,* 30–40 min; *cycloplegia,* 1–3 hr. **Recovery:** Up to 12 days. **Duration, oral:** 4–6 hr. **t½:** 2.5 hr. Metabolized by the liver although 30%–50% is excreted through the kidneys unchanged.

Uses: Oral: Adjunct in peptic ulcer treatment. Irritable bowel syndrome. Adjunct in treatment of spastic disorders of the biliary tract. Urologic disorders, urinary incontinence. During anesthesia to control salivation and bronchial secretions. Has been used for parkinsonism but more effective drugs are available.

    Parenteral: Antiarrhythmic, adjunct in GI radiography. Prophylaxis of arrhythmias induced by succinylcholine or surgical procedures. Reduce sinus bradycardia (severe) and syncope in hyperactive carotid sinus reflex. Prophylaxis and treatment of toxicity due to cholinesterase inhibitors, including organophosphate pesticides. Treatment of curariform block. As a preanesthetic or in dentistry to decrease secretions.

    Ophthalmologic: Cycloplegic refraction, treatment of uveitis. *Investigational:* Treatment and prophylaxis of posterior synechiae; pre- and postoperative mydriasis; treatment of malignant glaucoma.

Additional Contraindications: Ophthalmic use: Infants less than 3 months of age.

Special Considerations: Pregnancy category: C. Use with caution in infants, children, geriatric clients, diabetes, hypo- or hyperthyroidism, narrow anterior chamber angle.

Additional Side Effects: *Ophthalmologic:* Blurred vision, stinging, increased intraocular pressure, contact dermatitis. Long-term use may cause irritation, photophobia, eczematoid dermatitis, conjunctivitis, hyperemia, or edema.

Dosage: Tablets, Soluble Tablets. *Anticholinergic or antispasmodic.* **Adults:** 0.3–1.2 mg q 4–6 hr. **Pediatric, over 41 kg:** same as adult; **29.5–41 kg:** 0.4 mg q 4–6 hr; **18.2–29.5 kg:** 0.3 mg q 4–6 hr; **10.9–18.2 kg:** 0.2 mg q 4–6 hr; **7.3–10.9 kg:** 0.15 mg q 4–6 hr; **3.2–7.3 kg:** 0.1 mg q 4–6 hr. *Prophylaxis of respiratory tract secretions and excess salivation during anesthesia:* **Adults,** 2 mg. *Parkinsonism:* **Adults:** 0.1–0.25 mg q.i.d.

    IM, IV, SC. *Anticholinergic:* **Adults, IM, IV, SC,** 0.4–0.6 mg q 4–6 hr. **Pediatric, SC,** 0.01 mg/kg, not to exceed 0.4 mg (or 0.3 mg/m²). *Reverse curariform block:* **Adults, IV** 0.6–1.2 mg given at the same time or a few minutes before 0.5–2 mg neostigmine methylsulfate (use separate syringes). *Treatment of toxicity from cholinesterase inhibitors:* **Adults, IV, initial,** 2–4 mg; **then,** 2 mg repeated q 5–10 min until muscarinic symptoms disappear and signs of atropine toxicity begin to appear. **Pediatric, IM, IV, initial:** 1 mg; **then,** 0.5–1 mg q 5–10 min until muscarinic symptoms disappear and signs of atropine toxicity appear. *Treatment of mushroom poisoning due to muscarine:* **Adults, IM, IV,** 1–2 mg q hr until respiratory effects decrease. *Treatment of organophosphate poisoning:* **Adults, IM, IV, initial:** 1–2 mg; **then,** repeat in 20–30 min (as soon as cyanosis has disappeared). Dosage may be continued for up to 2 days until symptoms improve. *Arrhythmias:* **Pediatric, IV:** 0.01–0.03 mg/kg. *Prophylaxis of respiratory tract secretions, excessive salivation, succinylcholine- or surgical procedure-induced arrhythmias:* **Pediatric, SC:** Up to 3 kg, 0.1 mg; **7–9 kg:** 0.2 mg; **12–16 kg:** 0.3 mg; **20–27 kg:** 0.4 mg; **32 kg:** 0.5 mg; **41 kg:** 0.6 mg.

NURSING CONSIDERATIONS

See also *Nursing Considerations for Cholinergic Blocking Agents,* p. 138.

Administration/Storage: For ophthalmologic use, atropine sulfate is available in 0.5%–3% solutions or 1.0% ointment.

Assessment: Check for a history of angle-closure glaucoma, before administering the drug in the eye because atropine may precipitate an acute crisis.

Client/Family Teaching

1. Warn that when atropine is used in the eye, vision will be temporarily impaired. Therefore, close work, operating machinery, or driving a car should be avoided until the effects of the medication have worn off.
2. Drug impairs heat regulation; avoid strenuous activity in hot environments.

3. Males with prostatic hypertrophy may experience urinary retention and hesitancy.

Evaluation: Evaluate for a positive clinical response as evidenced by:
- ↑ in heart rate
- Dilatation of the pupils
- ↓ in GI activity
- Reversal of muscarinic effects

Auranofin
(or-**AN**-oh-fin)
Ridaura (Rx)

Classification: Oral gold compound for arthritis.

Action/Kinetics: Auranofin is a gold-containing (29%) compound that was developed for oral administration. The oral drug has fewer side effects than injectable gold products. Although the mechanism is not known, auranofin will improve symptoms of rheumatoid arthritis; it is most effective in the early stages of active synovitis and may act by inhibiting sulfhydryl systems. Other possible mechanisms include inhibition of phagocytic activity of macrophages and polymorphonuclear leukocytes, alteration of biosynthesis of collagen, and alteration of the immune response. Gold will not reverse damage to joints caused by disease. Approximately 25% of an oral dose is absorbed. **Plasma t½ of auranofin gold:** 26 days. **Onset:** 3–4 months (up to 6 months in certain clients). Approximately 3 months are required for steady state blood levels to be achieved. The drug is metabolized and excreted in both the urine and feces.

A

Uses: Adults and children with rheumatoid arthritis that has not responded to other drugs. Up to 6 months may be required for beneficial effects to occur. Auranofin should be part of a total treatment regimen for rheumatoid arthritis, including nondrug treatments.

Contraindications: History of gold-induced disorders including necrotizing enterocolitis, pulmonary fibrosis, exfoliative dermatitis, bone marrow aplasia, or other hematologic disorders. Use during lactation.

Special Concerns: Pregnancy category: C. Use with caution in renal or hepatic disease, skin rashes, or history of bone marrow depression. Although used in children, a recommended dosage has not been established.

Side Effects: *GI:* Nausea, vomiting, diarrhea (common), abdominal pain, metallic taste, stomatitis, glossitis, gingivitis, anorexia, constipation, flatulence, dyspepsia, dysgeusia. Rarely, melena, GI bleeding, dysphagia, ulcerative enterocolitis. *Dermatologic:* Skin rashes, pruritus, alopecia, urticaria, angioedema. *Hematologic:* Leukopenia, anemia, thrombocytopenia, hematuria, neutropenia, agranulocytosis. *Renal:* Proteinuria, hematuria. *Other:* Conjunctivitis, cholestatic jaundice, fever, interstitial pneumonia and fibrosis, peripheral neuropathy.

Symptoms of Overdose: Rapid appearance of hematuria, proteinuria, thrombocytopenia, granulocytopenia. Also, nausea, vomiting, diarrhea, fever, urticaria, papulovesicular lesions, exfoliative dermatitis, pruritus.

Laboratory Test Interference: ↑ Liver enzymes.

Dosage: Capsules. Adults: Initial, Either 6 mg once daily or 3 mg b.i.d. If response is unsatisfactory after 6 months, increase to 3 mg t.i.d. If response is still inadequate after 3 additional months, the drug should be discontinued. Dosages greater than 9 mg daily are not recommended. *Transfer from injectable gold:* Discontinue injectable gold and begin auranofin at a dose of 6 mg daily.

NURSING CONSIDERATIONS

Administration/Storage

1. This is the only gold compound administered orally.
2. A positive response should be noted after 6 months of therapy.
3. *Treatment of Overdose:* Discontinue and give dimercaprol. Supportive therapy should be provided for renal and hematologic symptoms. In acute overdosage, induction of emesis or gastric lavage should be performed immediately.

Assessment

1. Review client medical history and note any other severe systemic diseases such as renal disease, history of hepatic infections or heart disease.
2. Note the extent of the client's debilitation and ROM.
3. Inspect the client's skin prior to initiating therapy to determine if there are any skin eruptions.
4. Assess the client's gums and oral mucosa prior to therapy, noting any lesions or need for treatment of oral problems.

Interventions

1. Monitor and record intake and output and daily weights.

2. If the client complains of diarrhea, monitor electrolytes and report any evidence of abnormality to the physician.
3. Monitor liver and renal function studies. Send urine to test for evidence of protein and blood. Document and report results to the physician.
4. Observe client for the presence of peripheral neuropathy.
5. To encourage client to return for appropriate follow-up evaluation, provide the client with only a 2 week supply of medications.

Client/Family Teaching

1. Report any skin lesions or changes in the mucous membranes immediately to their physician.
2. Avoid sunlight. If exposure is necessary, wear long sleeves, a hat, keep legs covered, and apply a sunscreen.
3. Inspect mouth regularly. Advise clients on a regular program of oral hygiene. This should include regular brushing of the teeth, daily flossing, and mouth washes, avoiding those with alcohol or other drying ingredients.
4. Provide a printed list of the signs of toxicity that require immediate reporting and attention by the physician (skin rash, pruritus, metallic taste, stomatitis, diarrhea, leukopenia, and thrombocytopenia). Remind clients that side effects can occur at any time and must not be ignored.
5. Advise the client that it may take several weeks of therapy before improvement will be noticed.

6. Women of childbearing age who are sexually active may wish to use some form of birth control while they are receiving gold therapy.

Evaluation: Evaluate client for:
- Improved mobility and ROM
- Reports of a decrease in pain, swelling, and stiffness in joints

Aurothioglucose suspension

(or-oh-thigh-oh-**GLOO**-kohz)
Solganol (Rx)

Classification: Antirheumatic agent.
Note: For additional information regarding aurothioglucose, see *Gold Sodium Thiomalate,* p. 689.

Special Concerns: Pregnancy category: C.

Dosage: IM only. Adults: *Week 1:* 10 mg; *weeks 2 and 3:* 25 mg; **then,** 25–50 (maximum) mg weekly until a total of 0.8–1 g has been administered. If client tolerates the dose and has improved, 50 mg may be given q 3–4 week for several months. **Pediatric, 6–12 years:** *Week 1:* 2.5 mg; *weeks 2 and 3:* 6.25 mg; **then,** 12.5 mg q week until a total dose of 200–250 mg has been administered. **Maintenance:** 6.25–12.5 mg q 3–4 weeks.

NURSING CONSIDERATIONS

See also *Nursing Considerations for Gold Sodium Thiomalate,* p. 690.

Administration/Storage

1. The client should remain lying down for 10 min after the

injection and should be observed for 15 min following drug administration.

2. IM injections should be made only in the upper outer quadrant of the gluteal region; an 18-gauge, 1½-inch needle (or 2 inches for obese clients) should be used.

3. To obtain a uniform suspension, the vial should be shaken carefully before the dose is withdrawn.

4. Both the syringe and needle used to withdraw the dose should be dry.

5. The vial can be immersed in warm water to assist with withdrawing the appropriate dose of the suspension.

6. *Treatment of Overdose:* Discontinue and give dimercaprol. Supportive therapy should be provided for renal and hematologic symptoms. In acute overdosage, induction of emesis or gastric lavage should be performed immediately.

Evaluation: Evaluate client for reports of symptomatic improvement in joint pain, swelling, and stiffness.

Azathioprine

(ay-zah-**THIGH**-oh-preen)
Imuran (Rx)

Classification: Immunosuppressant.

Action/Kinetics: Antimetabolite that is quickly split to form mercaptopurine. To be effective, the drug must be given during the induction period of the antibody response. The precise mechanism in depressing the immune response is unknown, but it suppresses cell-mediated hypersensitivities, causing changes in antibody production. The drug inhibits synthesis of DNA, RNA, and proteins and may interfere with miosis and cellular metabolism. Is readily absorbed from the GI tract. The anuric client manifests increased effectiveness and toxicity (up to twofold). **Onset:** 6–8 weeks for rheumatoid arthritis. **t½:** 3 hr.

Uses: Prophylaxis to prevent rejection of kidney transplants. Rheumatoid arthritis (adults only). *Investigational:* Chronic ulcerative colitis, chronic active hepatitis, systemic lupus erythematosus, nephrotic syndrome, glomerulonephritis, biliary cirrhosis, inflammatory myopathy, myasthenia gravis, pemphigoid, pemphigus, systemic dermatomyositis.

Contraindications: Treatment of rheumatoid arthritis in pregnancy or in clients previously treated with alkylating agents. Pregnancy and lactation.

Side Effects: *Hematologic:* Leukopenia, thrombocytopenia. *GI:* Nausea, vomiting, diarrhea, steatorrhea. *Other:* Increased risk of carcinoma, severe infections, and hepatotoxicity are major side effects. Less frequent: Skin rashes, fever, alopecia, arthralgias, negative nitrogen balance.

Drug Interactions

Allopurinol / ↑ Pharmacologic effect of azathioprine due to ↓ breakdown in liver

Corticosteroids / With azathioprine, it may cause muscle wasting after prolonged therapy

Tubocurarine / Azathioprine ↓ effect of tubocurarine

Dosage: Tablets, IV. *Immunosuppression:* **Adults and children, initial,** 3–5 mg/kg (120 mg/m²), 1–3 days before or on the day of transplantation; **maintenance:** 1–2 mg/kg (45 mg/m²) daily. *Rheumatoid arthritis, systemic lupus erythematosus:* **Adults and children, tablets: initial,** 1 mg/kg; **then,** increase dose by 0.5 mg/kg/day after 6–8 weeks and thereafter every 4 weeks up to maximum of 2.5 mg/kg/day; **maintenance:** lowest effective dose. Dosage should be reduced in clients with renal dysfunction. *Investigational Uses:* **Adults and children, tablets, initial:** 1 mg/kg; **then,** increase the dose by 0.5 mg/kg daily after 6–8 weeks and q 4 weeks thereafter up to a maximum of 2.5 mg/kg daily.

NURSING CONSIDERATIONS

Administration/Storage: Reconstitute the drug with sterile water for injection and use within 24 hr.

Assessment

1. Take a drug history to determine if the client is taking any drugs with which azathioprine interacts unfavorably.
2. Determine that baseline liver and renal function studies have been performed.

Interventions

1. Observe the client for symptoms of hepatic dysfunction. If the client develops jaundice, discontinue the drug and report to the physician.
2. Monitor intake and output and weigh client daily.
3. Observe the client for any decreases in urine volume and creatinine clearance. These are symptoms of kidney transplant rejection.
4. Report any oliguria to the physician.
5. Encourage the client to increase fluid intake.

Client/Family Teaching

1. Advise to take only as directed and not to skip or stop medication without notifying physician.
2. Women of childbearing age should practice contraceptive methods during and for 4 months following therapy.
3. Provide a printed list of side effects that should be reported to the physician immediately such as bruising, bleeding, S&S of infection, abdominal pain, itching and/or clay colored stools.
4. Explain that in order to prevent transplant rejection the client must take this medication for life.
5. Avoid contact with any person who has taken oral poliovirus vaccine recently or persons with active infections.

Evaluation

1. Assess for a positive clinical response to drug therapy in the prevention of kidney transplant rejections.
2. When used for rheumatoid arthritis, subjective reports of symptomatic improvement of joint pain, swelling and stiffness. The client should be considered refractory if no beneficial effect is noted after 12 weeks of therapy.
3. Monitor appropriate lab data to

determine effectiveness of drug therapy and to detect any early evidence of adverse effects.

Azithromycin

(az-**zith**-roh-**MY**-sin)
Zithromax (Rx)

Classification: Antibiotic, azalide.

Action/Kinetics: Azithromycin is an azalide antibiotic (subclass of macrolides) derived from erythromycin. The drug acts by binding to the 50S ribosomal subunit of susceptible organisms, thus interfering with microbial protein synthesis. It is rapidly absorbed and distributed widely throughout the body. Food decreases the absorption of azithromycin. $t^{1/2}$, **terminal:** 68 hr. A loading dose will achieve steady state levels more quickly. The major route of elimination is biliary excretion of unchanged drug with a small amount being excreted through the kidneys.

Uses: Mild to moderate infections in clients 16 years of age or older as described below. Acute bacterial exacerbations of chronic obstructive pulmonary disease due to *Hemophilus influenzae, Morazella catarrhalis,* or *Streptococcus pneumoniae.* Pneumonia due to *S. pneumoniae* or *H. influenzae.* As an alternative to first-line therapy to treat streptococcal pharyngitis or tonsillitis due to *Streptococcus pyogenes.* Uncomplicated skin and skin structure infections due to *Staphylococcus aureus, S. pyogenes,* or *S. agalactiae.* Nongonococcal urethritis and cervicitis due to *Chlamydia trachomatis.*

Contraindictions: Hypersensitivity to azithromycin, any macrolide antibiotic, or erythromycin.

Special Concerns: Pregnancy category: B. Use with caution in clients with impaired hepatic or renal function and during lactation. Safety and effectiveness have not been determined in children less than 16 years of age.

Side Effects: *GI:* Nausea, vomiting, diarrhea, abdominal pain, dyspepsia, flatulence, melena, cholestatic jaundice, pseudomembranous colitis. *CNS:* Dizziness, headache, somnolence, fatigue, vertigo. *CV:* Chest pain, palpitations. *GU:* Monilia, nephritis, vaginitis. *Allergic:* Angioedema, photosensitivity, rash. *Hematologic:* Leukopenia, neutropenia, decreased platelet count.

Drug Interactions: See also *Drug Interactions* for *Erythromycins,* p. 145.

Aluminum- and magnesium-containing antacids will ↓ the peak serum levels of azithromycin but not the total amount absorbed.

Laboratory Test Interferences: ↑ Serum creatine phosphokinase, potassium, ALT, GGT, AST, serum alkaline phosphatase, bilirubin, BUN, creatinine, blood glucose, LDH, and phosphate.

Dosage: Capsules. *Upper and lower respiratory tract infections, uncomplicated skin and skin structure infections:* **Adults and children over 16 years of age:** 500 mg as a single dose on day 1 followed by 250 mg once daily on days 2 through 5 for a total dose of 1.5 g. *Nongonococcal urethritis and cervicitis due to C. trachomatis:* 1 g given as a single dose.

NURSING CONSIDERATIONS

See also *General Nursing Considerations* for *All Anti-Infectives*, p. 83.

Administration/Storage: The drug should be given at least 1 hr prior to a meal or at least 2 hr after a meal.

Assessment

1. Determine any history of sensitivity to erythromycins.
2. Note any previous experience with macrolide antibiotics and results.
3. Obtain baseline liver and renal function studies.
4. Determine if client is currently prescribed warfarin or theophylline. Azithromycin may cause an increase in serum concentrations of these drugs so levels should be monitored throughout therapy.
5. Obtain documentation that clients with sexually transmitted cervicitis or urethritis are tested for gonorrhea and syphilis at the time of diagnosis. Ensure that appropriate drug therapy is instituted if necessary.

Client/Family Teaching

1. Do not administer with meals because food decreases absorption.
2. Avoid ingesting aluminum- or magnesium-containing antacids simultaneously with azithromycin.
3. Advise client to encourage sexual partner to seek medical evaluation and treatment to prevent reinfections (when being treated for a STD). Condoms should be used throughout therapy in this event.

Evaluation: Evaluate client for:

- Resolution of signs and symptoms of infection
- Laboratory confirmation of negative culture reports

Aztreonam for injection

(as-**TREE**-oh-nam)

Azactam for Injection (Rx)

See also *Anti-Infectives*, p. 80.

Classification: Monobactam antibiotic.

Action/Kinetics: Aztreonam belongs to a new class of antibiotics called *monobactams*. It is a synthetic drug that is bactericidal against gram-negative aerobic pathogens. The drug acts by inhibiting cell wall synthesis. It is effective against *Escherichia coli, Klebsiella, Enterobacter, Pseudomonas, Proteus, Citrobacter, Serratia marcescens,* and *Hemophilus influenzae*. $t\frac{1}{2}$: 1.5–2 hr. The $t\frac{1}{2}$ is prolonged in clients with impaired renal function.

Uses: Infections due to gram-negative aerobic organisms may be treated, including urinary tract, lower respiratory tract, skin and skin structures, intra-abdominal, gynecologic, and septicemia.

Contraindications: Allergy to aztreonam.

Special Concerns: Pregnancy category B. Use in pregnancy only if clearly needed. Safety and effectiveness have not been determined in children and infants. Use with caution in clients allergic to penicillins or cephalosporins and in those with impaired hepatic or renal function.

Side Effects: *GI:* Nausea, vomiting,

abdominal cramps, *Clostridium difficile*-associated diarrhea or GI bleeding. *CNS:* Confusion, seizures, vertigo, paresthesia, insomnia, dizziness. *Hematologic:* Anemia, neutropenia, thrombocytopenia, leukocytosis, thrombocytosis, pancytopenia. *Dermatologic:* Rash, purpura, erythema multiforme, urticaria, petechiae, pruritus, diaphoresis, exfoliative dermatitis. *CV:* Hypotension, transient ECG changes. *Miscellaneous:* Anaphylaxis, headache, weakness, fever, malaise, hepatitis, jaundice, muscle aches, tinnitus, diplopia, nasal congestion, halitosis, altered taste, mouth ulcers, sneezing, vaginal candidiasis, vaginitis, breast tenderness.

Drug Interactions: Antibiotics that increase levels of beta-lactamase (e.g., cefoxitin, imipenem) may inhibit the activity of aztreonam.

Laboratory Test Interferences: ↑ AST, ALT, alkaline phosphatase, serum creatinine, prothrombin time. Positive Coombs' test.

Dosage: IM, IV. *Urinary tract infections:* 0.5–1 g q 8–12 hr, not to exceed 8 g daily. *Moderate to severe systemic infections:* 1–2 g q 8–12 hr, not to exceed 8 g daily. *Severe systemic or life-threatening infections:* 2 g q 6–8 hr, not to exceed 8 g daily.

NURSING CONSIDERATIONS

See also *General Nursing Considerations For All Anti-Infectives,* p. 83.

Administration/Storage

1. The IV route should be used for doses greater than 1 g or in clients with septicemia.
2. Therapy should be continued for at least 48 hr after the client becomes asymptomatic or until laboratory tests indicate that the infection has been eradicated.
3. An IV bolus injected slowly over 3–5 min may be used to initiate therapy.
4. For IM use, the drug should be given in a large muscle mass.
5. For use as a bolus, the 15-ml vial should be diluted with 6–10 ml sterile water for injection. For IM use, the 15-ml vial should be diluted with at least 3 ml of either sterile water for injection, sodium chloride injection, bacteriostatic water for injection, or bacteriostatic sodium chloride injection.
6. Aztreonam is incompatible with cephradine, nafcillin sodium, and metronidazole. Data for other drugs are not available.
7. *Treatment of Overdose:* Hemodialysis or peritoneal dialysis to reduce serum levels.

Interventions

1. Obtain baseline liver and renal function studies and monitor throughout therapy.
2. Anticipate reduced dosage in clients with impaired renal function (see package insert).

Client/Family Teaching

1. Reassure client that during therapy a slightly itchy, red rash and nasal congestion may occur.
2. Advise that a taste alteration may be experienced during IV therapy.

B

Bacampicillin hydrochloride
(bah-kam-pih-**SILL**-in)
Penglobe✿, Spectrobid (Rx)

See also *Anti-Infectives,* p. 80, and *Penicillins,* p. 197.

Classification: Antibiotic, penicillin.

Action/Kinetics: Bacampicillin is a semisynthetic, acid-resistant penicillin that is hydrolyzed to the active ampicillin in the GI tract. Food does not affect absorption of the drug. The drug is 98% absorbed from the GI tract and is approximately 20% plasma protein bound. **Peak serum levels:** Obtained in 0.9 hr are approximately 3 times those seen with equivalent doses of ampicillin. Seventy-five percent is excreted in the urine as active ampicillin within 8 hr.

Uses: Upper and lower respiratory tract infections caused by beta-hemolytic streptococcus, *Staphylococcus pyogenes,* pneumococci, non-penicillinase-producing staphylococci, and *Hemophilus influenzae.* Urinary tract infections caused by *Escherichia coli, Proteus mirabilis,* and enterococci. Skin infections caused by streptococci and susceptible staphylococci. Acute uncomplicated urogenital infections caused by *Neisseria gonorrhoeae.*

Contraindications: History of penicillin allergy. Concomitant use with disulfiram (Antabuse).

Drug Interaction: Bacampicillin should not be used concomitantly with disulfiram.

Laboratory Test Interferences: False + reaction to Clinitest, Benedict's solution, and Fehling's solution. ↑ AST.

Dosage: Oral Suspension, Tablets. *Upper respiratory tract infections, otitis media, urinary tract infections, skin and skin structure infections:* **Adults (25 kg or more),** 400 mg q 12 hr; **pediatric:** 25 mg/kg/day in equally divided doses q 12 hr. Dose may be doubled in cases of lower respiratory tract infections, severe infections, or in treating less susceptible organisms. *Gonorrhea (males and females):* 1.6 g with 1 g probenecid as a single dose. No pediatric dosage has been established.

NURSING CONSIDERATIONS

See also *General Nursing Considerations For All Anti-Infectives,* p. 83.

Client/Family Teaching

1. Warn client not to start disulfiram therapy while taking bacampicillin.
2. Advise clients with diabetes to use Labstix, Clinistix, Tes-Tape, or Diastix for testing urine, as Benedict's and Fehling's solutions result in false + reactions. To enhance accuracy, do finger sticks.

Evaluation

1. Assess for a positive clinical response based on C&S results and subjective reports of improvement.
2. Evaluate client also on allopurinol for increased incidence of skin rash.

Bacitracin intramuscular

(bass-ih-**TRAY**-sin)

Bacitin ✽, Bacitracin Sterile (Rx)

Bacitracin ointment

(bass-ih-**TRAY**-sin)

Baciguent (OTC)

Bacitracin ophthalmic

(bass-ih-**TRAY**-sin)

AK-Tracin, Bacitracin Ophthalmic (Rx)

See also *Anti-Infectives,* p. 80.

Classification: Antibiotic, miscellaneous.

Action/Kinetics: This antibiotic is produced by *Bacillus subtilis.* The drug interferes with synthesis of cell wall, preventing incorporation of amino acids and nucleotides. Bacitracin is bactericidal, bacteriostatic, and active against protoplasts. It is not absorbed from the GI tract. When given parenterally, drug is well distributed in pleural and ascitic fluids.

Bacitracin has high nephrotoxicity. Its systemic use is restricted to infants (see *Uses*). Renal function must be carefully evaluated prior to, and daily, during use. **Peak plasma levels:** IM, 0.2–2 mcg/ml after 2 hr. From 10%–40% is excreted in the urine after IM administration.

Uses: Bacitracin is used locally during surgery for cranial and neurosurgical infections caused by susceptible organisms.

As an ointment (preferred) or solution, bacitracin is prescribed for superficial pyoderma-like impetigo and infectious eczematoid dermatitis, for secondary infected dermatoses (atopic dermatitis, contact dermatitis), and for superficial infections of the eye, ear, nose, and throat by susceptible organisms.

Parenteral use is limited to the treatment of staphylococcal pneumonia and staphylococcus-induced empyema in infants.

Contraindications: Hypersensitivity or toxic reaction to bacitracin. Pregnancy.

Side Effects: Nephrotoxicity due to tubular and glomerular necrosis, renal failure; toxic reactions; nausea, vomiting.

Drug Interactions

Aminoglycosides / Additive nephrotoxicity and neuromuscular blocking activity

Anesthetics / ↑ Neuromuscular blockade → possible muscle paralysis

Neuromuscular blocking agents / Additive neuromuscular blockade → possible muscle paralysis

Dosage: IM only. Infants, 2.5 kg and below: 900 units/kg/day in 2–3 divided doses; **infants over 2.5 kg:** 1,000 units/kg/day in 2–3 divided doses. **Ophthalmic ointment (500 units/g):** *Acute infections:* ½ inch in lower conjunctival sac q 3–4 hr. *Mild to moderate infections:* ½ inch b.i.d.–t.i.d. **Topical ointment (500 units/g):** Apply 1–5 times daily to affected area.

NURSING CONSIDERATIONS

See also *General Nursing Considerations For All Anti-Infectives,* p. 83.

Administration/Storage: Do not mix bacitracin with glycerin or other polyalcohols that cause drug to deteriorate. Bacitracin unguentin base is anhydrous, consisting of liquid and white petrolatum.

Interventions

1. Monitor and maintain adequate fluid intake and output with parenteral use of drug.
2. Withhold drug and consult with physician when fluid output is inadequate. Monitor renal function studies.
3. Test pH of urine daily because it should be kept at 6 or greater to decrease renal irritation.
4. Have sodium bicarbonate or another alkali available to administer if pH drops below 6.
5. Do not administer concurrently or sequentially with a topical or systemic nephrotoxic drug.
6. Cleanse area before applying bacitracin as a wet dressing or ointment.

Evaluation

1. Note status (presence/absence) of pretreatment symptoms and C&S results to determine effectiveness of treatment.
2. Evaluate client for evidence of toxicity or hypersensitivity.

Baclofen

(**BAK**-low-fen)
Alpha-Baclofen✹, Lioresal (Rx)

See also *Centrally Acting Skeletal Muscle Relaxants,* p. 130.

Classification: Centrally acting muscle relaxant.

Action/Kinetics: The mechanism of action of baclofen is not fully known, but the drug is known to inhibit both mono- and polysynaptic spinal reflexes. It may also act at certain brain sites. **Peak serum levels:** 2–3 hr. **Therapeutic serum levels:** 80–400 ng/ml.

t½: 3–4 hr. 70%–80% of the drug is eliminated unchanged by the kidney.

Uses: Multiple sclerosis (flexor spasms, pain, clonus, and muscular rigidity) and diseases and injuries of the spinal cord associated with spasticity. It is not effective for the treatment of cerebral palsy, stroke, parkinsonism, or rheumatic disorders. *Investigational:* Trigeminal neuralgia, tardive dyskinesia.

Contraindications: Hypersensitivity. Rheumatic disorders, spasm resulting from Parkinson's disease, stroke, cerebral palsy.

Special Concerns: Safe use in pregnancy or for children under 12 years of age has not been established. Use with caution in impaired renal function. Geriatric clients may be at higher risk for developing CNS toxicity, including mental depression, confusion, hallucinations, and significant sedation.

Side Effects: *CNS:* Drowsiness, dizziness, weakness, fatigue, confusion, headaches, insomnia. Hallucinations following abrupt withdrawal. *CV:* Hypotension. Rarely, chest pain, syncope, palpitations. *GI:* Nausea, constipation. *GU:* Urinary frequency. *Other:* Rash, pruritus, ankle edema, increased perspiration, weight gain, dyspnea, nasal congestion.

Drug Interactions: Concomitant use with CNS depressants → additive CNS depression.

Laboratory Test Interference: ↑ AST, alkaline phosphatase, blood glucose.

Dosage: Tablets. Adults: Initial, 5 mg t.i.d. for 3 days; **then,** 10 mg t.i.d. for 3 days, 15 mg t.i.d. for 3 days, and 20 mg t.i.d. Additional increases in dose may be required but should not exceed 20 mg q.i.d.

NURSING CONSIDERATIONS

See also *Nursing Considerations* for *Centrally Acting Skeletal Muscle Relaxants,* p. 130.

Administration/Storage

1. If beneficial effects are not noted, the drug should be withdrawn slowly.
2. Have gastric lavage equipment available in the event of drug overdosage. Maintain adequate respiratory exchange. Do not use respiratory stimulants.

Assessment

1. Assess clients with epilepsy for clinical signs and symptoms of their disease. Arrange for an EEG at regular intervals because baclofen has been associated with reduced seizure control.
2. Obtain liver and renal function studies prior to initiating therapy.
3. Note if the client has diabetes.

Interventions

1. Note any evidence of hypersensitivity reaction and report.
2. Notify physician of clients who require hypertonicity to stand upright, to maintain balance when walking, or to increase their function. Baclofen may be contraindicated in these instances because it interferes with this coping mechanism.
3. If clients complain of constipation, increase fluid intake and increase the roughage in the diet.

4. Monitor urinary output and test the urine for occult blood.
5. Monitor the client's weight, reporting any evidence of edema to the physician.
6. If improvement in the client's condition does not occur within 6–8 weeks, the drug should be withdrawn gradually.

Client/Family Teaching

1. Take the medication with meals or a snack to avoid gastric irritation. If GI symptoms are severe or persistent, notify the physician.
2. Reassure that it may take several weeks of therapy before physical improvement occurs.
3. Instruct clients how to monitor their own intake and output and keep a record of the frequency and amounts of each voiding.
4. If clients have diabetes mellitus, teach them how to monitor blood glucose levels and compare them with levels obtained at the onset of therapy.
5. Advise male clients of the potential for the drug to cause impotence. If this occurs, report the problem to the physician. A change of drug or dosage may be required. Clients should be warned, however, not to discontinue taking the drug without the physician's knowledge.

Evaluation: Evaluate client for:
- A positive clinical response to the drug therapy by week 8
- Reports of ↓ spasticity and pain
- Measurable improvement in the client's muscle tone and involuntary movements

Basic Aluminum Carbonate Gel

(ah-**LOO**-mih-num)
Basaljel (OTC)

See also *Antacids,* p. 37.

Classification: Antacid.

Action/Kinetics: The acid neutralizing capacity of the capsules, suspension, or tablets is 12–13 mEq/capsule, tablet, or 5 ml. The acid neutralizing capacity of the extra strength suspension is 22 mEq/5 ml.

Uses: Hyperacidity. With low-phosphorus diet to prevent phosphate urinary stones by reducing urinary phosphate levels.

Note: See *Aluminum Hydroxide Gel* for *Contraindications, Side Effects,* and *Additional Drug Interactions.*

Dosage: *Antacid:* 2 tablets or capsules, 2 teaspoons of regular strength suspension, or 1 teaspoon of extra strength suspension q 2 hr, if necessary, up to 12 times each day. *Hyperphosphatemia:* 2 capsules or tablets, 12 ml suspension, or 5 ml extra strength suspension t.i.d.–q.i.d. after meals.

NURSING CONSIDERATIONS

See also *Nursing Considerations* for *Aluminum Hydroxide Gel,* p. 289.

Administration/Storage

1. Dilute the liquid form in water or fruit juice.
2. Administer medication after meals and at bedtime.

Interventions: Monitor appropriate laboratory data. Prolonged use may lead to hypophosphatemia, reabsorption of calcium, and bone demineralization.

Evaluation: Evaluate client for:
- ↓ in gastric acidity
- ↓ in urinary phosphate levels

Beclomethasone dipropionate

(be-kloh-**METH**-ah-zohn))
Becloforte Inhaler✲, Aerosol: Beclovent, Vanceril (Rx). Intranasal: Beclodisk✲, Beconase AQ, Beconase Nasal Inhaler, Vancenase AQ, Vancenase Nasal Inhaler (Rx). Topical: Propaderm✲

See also *Adrenocorticosteroids and Analogs,* p. 8.

Classification: Adrenocorticosteroid, synthetic, glucocorticoid type.

Action/Kinetics: Rapidly inactivated, thereby resulting in few systemic effects.

Note: If a client is on systemic steroids, transfer to beclomethasone may be difficult because recovery from impaired renal function may be slow.

Uses: Inhalation therapy for chronic use in bronchial asthma. In glucocorticoid-dependent clients, beclomethasone often permits a decrease in the dosage of the systemic agent. Withdrawal of systemic corticosteroids must be carried out gradually.

Contraindications: Status asthmaticus, acute episodes of asthma, hypersensitivity to drug or aerosol ingredients.

Special Concerns: Safe use during pregnancy (category: C) and lactation and in children under 6 years of age not established.

B

Dosage: Inhalation Aerosol.

Asthma: **Adults,** 2 inhalations (total of 84 mcg beclomethasone) t.i.d.–q.i.d. In some clients, 4 inhalations (168 mcg) b.i.d. have been effective. *Severe asthma:* **Initial,** 12–16 inhalations (504–672 mcg beclomethasone) daily; **then,** decrease dose according to response. **Maximum daily dose:** 20 inhalations (840 mcg beclomethasone). **Pediatric, 6–12 years:** 1–2 inhalations (42–84 mcg) t.i.d.–q.i.d., not to exceed 10 inhalations (420 mcg) daily. In some clients, 2–4 inhalations (84–168 mcg) b.i.d. have been effective.

Nasal Aerosol or Spray. *Rhinitis:* **Adults and children over 12 years,** 1 inhalation (42 mcg) in each nostril b.i.d.–q.i.d. (i.e., total daily dose: 168–336 mcg daily). If no response after 3 weeks, discontinue therapy.

In clients also receiving systemic glucocorticosteroids, beclomethasone should be started when client's condition is relatively stable.

NURSING CONSIDERATIONS

See also *Nursing Considerations* for *Adrenocorticosteroids and Analogs,* p. 15.

Administration/Storage

1. To administer beclomethasone with an inhaler use the following procedure:
   - Shake metal canister thoroughly immediately prior to use.
   - Instruct clients to exhale as completely as possible.
   - Have clients place the mouthpiece of the inhaler into their mouth and tighten their lips around it.
   - Instruct clients to inhale deeply through their mouth while pressing the metal canister down with their forefinger.
   - Instruct clients to hold their breath for as long as possible.
   - Remove mouthpiece.
   - Instruct clients to exhale slowly.
2. A minimum of 60 sec must elapse between inhalations.
3. To prevent explosion of contents under pressure, do not store or use near heat or open flame, or throw into a fire or incinerator. Keep secure from children.

Assessment: Note any history of sensitivity to the drug.

Interventions

1. For clients who are receiving systemic steroid therapy, initiate beclomethasone therapy *very* slowly, withdrawing the systemic steroids as ordered by the physician.
2. Observe the client for subjective signs of adrenal insufficiency, such as muscular pain, lassitude, and depression. Document and report to the physician even if the client's respiratory function has improved.
3. Note objective signs of adrenal insufficiency, such as hypotension and weight loss. This is an indication that the dosage of systemic steroid should be boosted temporarily, and then withdrawn more gradually.

Client/Family Teaching

1. Instruct in the use and care of the inhaler. Caution the client to wash the mouth piece and sprayer and to dry it after each use.

2. Explain that the inhaler is not to be used for asthmatic attacks.
3. Stress the importance of complying with the prescribed drug therapy even though it may take 1–4 weeks for any improvement in respiratory function to be realized.
4. More than 1 mg in adults or more than 500 mcg in children may precipitate hypothalamic-pituitary axis depression, resulting in adrenal insufficiency. Therefore, advise clients not to overuse the inhaler.
5. Instruct the client to report any symptoms of localized fungal infections in the mouth. These must be reported immediately and will require antifungal medication and possibly discontinuation of the drug.
6. Advise clients also receiving bronchodilators by inhalation that they should use the bronchodilator for at least several minutes before using beclomethasone. This increases the penetration of steroid and reduces the potential toxicity from inhaled fluorocarbon propellants of both inhalers.
7. Once the client has had a systemic steroid withdrawn, the client should be provided with a supply of oral glucocorticoids. These are to be taken immediately if the client is subjected to unusual stress or is having an asthmatic attack. Notify the physician immediately after the steroids have been taken.
8. Instruct the client in relaxation techniques to practice during stressful situations.
9. Carry a card indicating the diagnosis, treatment, and the possible need for systemic glucocorticoids, in the event of exposure to unusual stress.

Evaluation: Evaluate client for subjective reports of improvement in the control of symptoms of asthma.

Benazepril hydrochloride
(beh-**NAYZ**-eh-prill)
Lotensin (Rx)

See also *ACE Inhibitors,* p. 33.

Classification: Antihypertensive, angiotensin-converting enzyme inhibitor.

Action/Kinetics: Benazepril inhibits angiotensin-converting enzyme (ACE), which is responsible for converting angiotensin I to angiotensin II (a powerful vasoconstrictor). Thus, inhibition of ACE leads to decreased vasopressor activity and decreased aldosterone secretion with a small increase in serum potassium. Both supine and standing blood pressure are reduced in clients with mild-to-moderate hypertension with no compensatory tachycardia. Benazepril also has an antihypertensive effect in clients with low-renin hypertension. Food does not affect the extent of absorption. Benazepril is almost completely converted to the active benazeprilat which has greater ACE inhibitor activity. **Peak plasma levels, benazepril:** 30–60 min. **Peak plasma levels, benazeprilat:** 1–2 hr if fasting and 2–4 hr if not fasting. **t½, benazeprilat:** 10–11 hr. **Peak effect with chronic therapy:** 1–2 weeks. The drug is excreted through the urine with about 20% of a dose excreted as benazeprilat.

Uses: Used alone or in combination with thiazide diuretics to treat hypertension.

Contraindications: Hypersensitivity to benazepril or any other ACE inhibitor.

Special Concerns: Pregnancy category: D; neonatal hypotension, renal failure, skull hypoplasia, oligohydramnios, and death have been reported. Safety and effectiveness have not been determined in children.

Side Effects: *CNS:* Headache, dizziness, fatigue, anxiety, insomnia, nervousness. *GI:* Nausea, vomiting, constipation, gastritis, melena. *CV:* Symptomatic hypotension, postural hypotension, syncope, angina pectoris, palpitations, peripheral edema. *Dermatologic:* Dermatitis, pruritus, rash, flushing. *GU:* Decreased libido, impotence, urinary tract infection. *Respiratory:* Cough, asthma, bronchitis, dyspnea, sinusitis. *Neuromuscular:* Paresthesia, arthralgia, arthritis, asthenia, myalgia. *Miscellaneous:* Angioedema which may be associated with involvement of the tongue, glottis, or larynx; sweating, hypertonia.

Drug Interactions

Diuretics / Excessive reduction of blood pressure
Lithium / ↑ Serum lithium levels with ↑ risk of lithium toxicity
Potassium-sparing diuretics, potassium supplements / ↑ Risk of hyperkalemia

Laboratory Test Interferences: ↑ Serum creatinine, BUN, serum potassium. ↓ Hemoglobin.

Dosage: Tablets. *Clients not receiving a diuretic:* **initial,** 10 mg once daily; **maintenance:** 20–40 mg daily given as a single dose or in 2 equally divided doses. Total daily doses greater than 80 mg have not been evaluated. *Clients receiving a diuretic:* **initial,** 5 mg once daily. *Creatinine clearance <30 ml/ min/1.73 m²:* The recommended starting dose is 5 mg once daily; **maintenance:** titrate dose upward until blood pressure is controlled or to a maximum total daily dose of 40 mg.

NURSING CONSIDERATIONS

See also *Nursing Considerations for ACE Inhibitors,* p. 35.

Administration/Storage

1. Dosage adjustment should be based on measuring peak (2–6 hr after dosing) and trough responses. If once daily dosing does not provide an adequate trough response, an increase in dose or giving divided doses should be considered.
2. If blood pressure cannot be controlled by benazepril alone, a diuretic can be added.
3. If a client is receiving a diuretic, the diuretic, if possible, should be discontinued 2–3 days before beginning benazepril therapy.
4. The drug may be taken without regard to food.

Assessment

1. Note any previous experience with this class of drugs.
2. Obtain baseline electrolytes and renal function studies and monitor throughout therapy.

Client/Family Teaching

1. Take only as directed.
2. Avoid concomitant administration of potassium supplements,

potassium salt substitutes, or potassium-sparing diuretics as these can lead to increases of serum potassium.

3. Advise that the side effects of headache, fatigue, dizziness, and cough have been associated with this drug therapy and if persistent or bothersome should be reported to the physician.

Special Concerns: The drug is well tolerated in geriatric clients.

Evaluation: Evaluate client for evidence of control of hypertension with a minimum of side effects.

Benzphetamine hydrochloride
(bens-FET-ah-meen)
Didrex (C-III) (Rx)

See also *Amphetamines and Derivatives,* p. 29.

Classification: Anorexiant.

Action/Kinetics: $t^{1/2}$: 6–12 hr.

Use: Short-term (8–12 weeks) treatment of exogenous obesity in conjunction with a weight reduction regimen such as exercise, restriction of calories, and behavior modification.

Additional Contraindication: Use in pregnancy (category: X).

Dosage: Tablets. Adults: initial, 25–50 mg once daily; **then,** increase dose according to response (dose ranges from 25–50 mg 1–3 times daily 1 hr before meals).

NURSING CONSIDERATIONS

See also *Nursing Considerations* for *Amphetamines and Derivatives,* p. 31.

Administration/Storage

1. It is preferable to administer a single dose in mid-morning or mid-afternoon, depending on the eating habits of the client.
2. Anorexiant effects occur within 1–2 hr and last approximately 4 hr.

Assessment

1. Note any history of glaucoma, advanced arteriosclerosis, cardiac disease, or mental instability. The drug is contraindicated in these instances.
2. Determine the possibility of the client being pregnant. Benzphetamine is toxic to the fetus and should not be administered to pregnant women or nursing mothers.
3. Assess client's willingness to comply with exercise program and reduce caloric intake.

Evaluation: Evaluate client for:
- Knowledge and understanding of disease and compliance with drug therapy
- Weight reduction

Benztropine mesylate
(BENS-troh-peen)
Apo-Benztropine✱, Cogentin, PMS Benztropine✱ (Rx)

See also *Cholinergic Blocking Agents,* p. 136.

Classification: Antiparkinson agent, synthetic anticholinergic.

Action/Kinetics: Benztropine is a synthetic anticholinergic possessing antihistamine and local anesthetic properties. **Onset, PO:** 1–2 hr; **IM, IV:** Within a few minutes. Its effects are cumulative, and it is long-acting

(24 hr). Full effects are manifested in 2–3 days. The drug produces a low incidence of side effects.

Uses: As adjunct in the treatment of parkinsonism (all types). Used to reduce severity of extrapyramidal effects in phenothiazine or other antipsychotic drug therapy (not effective in tardive dyskinesia).

Special Concerns: Pregnancy category: C. Not recommended for children under three years of age. Geriatric and emaciated clients cannot tolerate large doses. Certain drug-induced extrapyramidal symptoms may not respond to benztropine.

Dosage: Tablets, (rarely IV or IM). *Parkinsonism:* 1–2 mg daily (range: 0.5–6 mg daily). *Idiopathic parkinsonism:* **Initial,** 0.5–1 mg daily, increased gradually to 4–6 mg daily, if necessary. *Postencephalitic parkinsonism:* 2 mg daily in one or more doses. *Drug-induced extrapyramidal effects:* 1–4 mg 1–2 times daily. *Acute dystonic reactions:* **IM, IV, initial:** 1–2 mg; **then,** 1–2 mg PO b.i.d. usually prevents recurrence. Clients can rarely tolerate full dosage.

NURSING CONSIDERATIONS

See also *Nursing Considerations* for *Cholinergic Blocking Agents,* p. 138.

Administration/Storage

1. When used as replacement for or supplement to other antiparkinsonism drugs, substitute or add gradually.
2. For clients who have difficulty swallowing tablets, the tablets may be crushed and mixed with a small amount of food or liquid.
3. Some clients may benefit by taking the entire dose at bedtime while others are best treated by taking divided doses, b.i.d.–q.i.d.
4. Therapy should be initiated with a low dose (e.g., 0.5 mg) and then increased in increments of 0.5 mg at 5–6-day intervals. The maximum daily dose should not exceed 6 mg.
5. If the drug is to be administered IV, it may be given undiluted at a rate of 1 mg/min or less.

Assessment

1. When taking the client's drug history, note if phenothiazines or tricyclic antidepressants are being used. When taken with benztropine mesylate, these drugs can cause a paralytic ileus.
2. Assess for any evidence of medical conditions that would preclude beginning the drug therapy.
3. Note the age of the client. Anticipate that elderly clients will require a lower dosage.

Interventions

1. If the client develops excitation or vomiting, the drug may need to be withdrawn temporarily. When treatment is resumed the dosage should be lowered.
2. Monitor intake and output. Auscultate for bowel sounds. This is especially important if the client has limited mobility.
3. Inspect the client's skin at regular intervals for any evidence of skin changes.

Client/Family Teaching

1. Review the goals of therapy and the possible side effects.

2. Use caution when performing tasks that require mental alertness because drug has a sedative effect.
3. Remind clients that it usually takes 2–3 days for the drug to exert a desired effect. The drug should be taken as ordered unless side effects occur. These then should be reported to the physician before interrupting drug therapy.
4. Reassure that side effects usually subside with continued use of the drug.
5. Client's ability to tolerate heat will be reduced. Therefore, clients should avoid heat and plan rest periods during the day.
6. Report any difficulty in voiding or inadequate emptying of the bladder.
7. Avoid the use of alcoholic beverages.

Evaluation

1. Review goals of therapy with the client and family and assess the degree to which they have been attained.
2. Evaluate client for a reduction in muscle tremors and rigidity.

Bepridil hydrochloride
(**BEH**-prih-dill)
Vascor (Rx)

See also *Calcium Channel Blocking Drugs,* p. 118.

Classification: Calcium channel blocking drug, antianginal.

Action/Kinetics: Bepridil inhibits the transmembrane influx of calcium ions into cardiac and vascular smooth muscle. The drug increases the effective refractory period of the atria, AV node, His-Purkinje fibers, and ventricles. The drug dilates peripheral arterioles and reduces total peripheral resistance; it reduces heart rate and arterial pressure at rest and at a given level of exercise. The drug is rapidly and completely absorbed following oral use. **Onset:** 60 min. **Time to peak plasma levels:** 2–3 hr. Greater than 99% bound to plasma protein. Food does not affect either the peak plasma levels or the extent of absorption. **Therapeutic serum levels:** 1–2 ng/ml. **t½, distribution:** 2 hr; **terminal elimination:** 24 hr. Steady state blood levels do not occur for 8 days. The drug is metabolized in the liver and metabolites are excreted through both the kidney (70%) and the feces (22%).

Uses: Chronic stable angina (classic effort-associated angina) in clients who have failed to respond to other antianginal medications or who are intolerant to such medications. It may be used alone or with beta blockers or nitrates.

Contraindications: Clients with a history of serious ventricular arrhythmias, sick sinus syndrome, second- or third-degree heart block (except in the presence of a functioning ventricular pacemaker), hypotension (less than 90 mm Hg systolic), uncompensated cardiac insufficiency, congenital QT interval prolongation, and in those taking other drugs that prolong the QT interval (e.g., quinidine, procainamide, tricyclic antidepressants). Use in clients with myocardial infarction during the previous three months. During lactation.

Special Concerns: Pregnancy category: C. Safety and effectiveness have not been determined in children. Use with caution in clients with

CHF, left bundle block, sinus bradycardia (less than 50 beats/min), serious hepatic or renal disorders. New arrhythmias can be induced.

Side Effects: *CV:* Induction of new serious arrhythmias such as torsades de pointes type ventricular tachycardia, prolongation of QTc and QT interval, increased premature ventricular contraction rates, new sustained VT and VT/VF, sinus tachycardia, sinus bradycardia, hypertension vasodilation, palpitations. *GI:* Nausea (common), dyspepsia, GI distress, diarrhea, dry mouth, anorexia, abdominal pain, constipation, flatulence, gastritis, increased appetite. *CNS:* Nervousness, dizziness, drowsiness, insomnia, depression, vertigo, akathisia, anxiousness, tremor, tremor of hand, syncope, paresthesia. *Respiratory:* Cough, pharyngitis, rhinitis, dyspnea, respiratory infection. *Body as a whole:* Asthenia, headache, flu syndrome, fever, pain, superinfection. *Dermatologic:* Rash, skin irritation, sweating. *Miscellaneous:* Tinnitus, arthritis, blurred vision, taste change, loss of libido, impotence, agranulocytosis.

Drug Interactions

Cardiac glycosides / Exaggeration of the depression of AV nodal conduction
Digoxin / Possible ↑ in serum digoxin levels
Potassium-wasting diuretics / Hypokalemia, which causes an ↑ risk of serious ventricular arrhythmias
Procainamide / ↑ Risk of serious side effects due to exaggerated prolongation of the QT interval
Quinidine / ↑ Risk of serious side effects due to exaggerated prolongation of the QT interval

Tricyclic antidepressants / ↑ Risk of serious side effects due to exaggerated prolongation of the QT interval

Laboratory Test Interferences: ↑ ALT. Abnormal liver function tests.

Dosage: Tablets. Adults, initial: 200 mg once daily; after 10 days the dosage may be adjusted upward depending on the response of the client (e.g., ability to perform activities of daily living, QT interval, heart rate, frequency and severity of angina). **Maintenance:** 300 mg once daily, not to exceed 400 mg daily.

NURSING CONSIDERATIONS

See also *Nursing Considerations* for *Calcium Channel Blocking Agents,* p. 119.

Administration/Storage

1. Can be taken with meals or at bedtime if nausea occurs.
2. Bepridil should be taken at about the same time each day. If a dose is missed, the next dose should **not** be doubled.
3. Geriatric patients may require more frequent monitoring.

Assessment

1. Determine which antianginal agents have been used in the past and their effects.
2. Perform baseline CBC and ECG prior to initiating drug therapy.
3. List drugs currently prescribed to client to determine potential drug interactions.
4. Serum potassium should be checked before bepridil is prescribed.
5. QTc intervals should be checked prior to initiating therapy with bepridil, 1–3 weeks after

beginning therapy, and periodically thereafter, especially after any dosage adjustment. Clients with prolongation of QTc intervals may be at greater risk for developing serious ventricular arrhythmias.

6. Document any evidence of AV block, arrhythmias, MI, and implanted ventricular pacemaker.

Interventions

1. Clients requiring diuretics should take a potassium-sparing agent.
2. The physician should be notified if the client is taking any medications that prolong the QT interval (e.g., procainamide, quinidine, tricyclic antidepressants).
3. Monitor BP. Observe closely for evidence of new arrhythmias, especially torsades de pointes tachycardia.

Client/Family Teaching

1. Clients should be instructed to inform their physician of all medications being taken.
2. Advise clients to continue taking nitroglycerin, if prescribed by their physician.

Evaluation: Evaluate client for:
- Subjective reports of control of angina
- Therapeutic serum drug levels 1–2 ng/ml

Beractant
(beh-**RACK**-tant)
Survanta (Rx)

Classification: Lung surfactant.

Action/Kinetics: Beractant, derived from natural bovine lung extract, contains phospholipids, fatty acids, neutral lipids, and surfactant-associated proteins (to which colfosceril palmitate, tripalmitin, and palmitic acid are added). The proteins in the product—SP-B and SP-C—are hydrophobic, low molecular weight, and surfactant associated. Beractant replenishes pulmonary surfactant and restores surface activity to the lungs of premature infants to reduce respiratory distress syndrome. The drug is intended for intratracheal use only. Significant improvement is observed in the arterial-alveolar oxygen ratio and mean airway pressure. Beractant significantly decreases the incidence of respiratory distress syndrome, mortality due to respiratory distress syndrome, and air leak complications.

Uses: Prevention and treatment ("rescue") of respiratory distress syndrome (hyaline membrane disease) in premature infants.

Special Concerns: Beractant can quickly affect oxygenation and lung compliance; thus, it should only be used in a highly supervised setting with immediate availability of physicians experienced with intubation, ventilator management, and general care of premature infants.

Side Effects: Commonly, side effects are associated with the dosing procedure and include transient bradycardia, oxygen desaturation, endotracheal tube reflux, vasoconstriction, pallor, hypotension, hypertension, endotracheal tube blockage, hypocarbia, hypercarbia, and apnea. Other symptoms include intracranial hemorrhage, rales, moist breath sounds, and nosocomial sepsis.

Symptom of Overdose: Acute airway obstruction.

B **Dosage: Intratracheal only:** 4 ml/kg (100 mg phospholipids/kg birth weight).

NURSING CONSIDERATIONS

Administration/Storage

1. For prevention of respiratory distress syndrome in premature infants weighing less than 1,250 g at birth or with evidence of surfactant deficiency, beractant should be given as soon as possible, preferably within 15 min of birth.

2. To treat infants with confirmed respiratory distress syndrome and who require mechanical ventilation, beractant should be given as soon as possible, preferably within 8 hours of birth.

3. Four doses can be given within the first 48 hr of life; doses should be given no sooner than q 6 hr.

4. Beractant should be refrigerated at 2°–8°C (36°–46°F) and warmed at room temperature for at least 20 min or in the hand for at least 8 min before administration. The drug does not have to be reconstituted or sonicated before use. If a prevention dose is required, preparation should begin before the infant is born. The drug should not be warmed and then returned to the refrigerator for future use more than once.

5. Prior to administration the vial should be visually inspected for discoloration (beractant is off-white to light brown). If settling occurs during storage, the vial should be swirled gently (not shaken) to redisperse although some foaming may occur at the surface during handling.

6. Each vial is for single use only; any residual drug should thus be discarded.

7. Instill beractant through a 5 French end-hole catheter that has been inserted into the endotracheal tube of the infant with the tip of the catheter protruding just beyond the end of the endotracheal tube above the infant's carina. The length of the catheter should be shortened before inserting it through the endotracheal tube. The drug should not be given into a mainstem bronchus.

8. To ensure homogeneous distribution, each dose should be divided into four quarter-doses with each quarter-dose given with the infant in a different position—head and body inclined slightly down, head turned to the right; head and body inclined slightly down, head turned to the left; head and body inclined slightly up, head turned to the right; and, head and body inclined slightly up, head turned to the left.

9. For the first dose, determine the total dose based on the infant's birth weight and withdraw the entire contents of the vial into the plastic syringe using at least a 20-gauge needle. The premeasured 5 French end-hole catheter is attached to the syringe and the catheter filled with beractant. Any excess should be discarded through the catheter so that only the total dose to be given remains in the syringe. Before giving the drug, proper placement and patency of the endo-

tracheal tube must be ensured (the tube may be suctioned before giving the drug). The infant should be allowed to stabilize before proceeding with dosing.

10. If the first dose is to be used for prevention strategy, the dose should be administered to the stabilized infant as soon as possible after birth (preferably within 15 min). The infant is positioned appropriately and the first quarter-dose is gently injected through the catheter over 2–3 sec. After the first quarter-dose is given, the catheter is removed from the endotracheal tube. To prevent cyanosis, manually ventilate with sufficient oxygen using a hand-bag (ambu type) at a rate of 60 breaths/min with sufficient positive pressure to provide adequate air exchange and chest wall excursion.

11. If rescue strategy is to be undertaken, the first dose should be given as soon as possible after the infant is placed on a ventilator for management of hyaline membrane disease. Studies have been undertaken in which the infant's ventilator settings were changed to a rate of 60/min (inspiratory time 0.5 sec and FiO_2 1) immediately before instilling the first quarter-dose. The infant is positioned appropriately and the first quarter-dose is gently injected through the catheter over 2–3 sec. The catheter is removed from the endotracheal tube and the infant is returned to the mechanical ventilator.

12. When using both prevention and rescue strategies, the infant is ventilated for 20 sec or until stable. The infant is repositioned for instillation of the next quarter-dose. The remaining quarter-doses are given using the same procedures. After instillation of each quarter-dose, the catheter is removed and the infant is ventilated for 30 sec or until stabilized. After the final quarter-dose is instilled, the catheter is removed without flushing. The infant should not be suctioned for 1 hr after dosing unless signs of significant obstruction of the airway occur. After the dosing procedure is completed, usual ventilator management and clinical care should be resumed.

13. If repeat doses are necessary, the dose is also 100 mg phospholipids/kg with the dose based on the infant's birth weight (the infant should not be reweighed). Additional doses are determined by evidence of continuing respiratory distress. Repeat doses should not be given sooner than 6 hr after the preceding dose if the infant remains intubated and requires at least 30% inspired oxygen to maintain a PaO_2 less than or equal to 80 torr. Radiographic confirmation of respiratory distress syndrome should be made before giving additional doses to infants who received a prevention dose.

14. Repeat doses are given by the same procedure as described for prevention strategy. However, studies have used different ventilator settings. For repeat doses, the FiO_2 was increased by 0.2 or an amount sufficient

to prevent cyanosis. The ventilator delivered a rate of 30/min with an inspiratory time <1 sec. If the infant's pretreatment rate was greater than or equal to 30, it was left unchanged during instillation. Manual hand-bag ventilation should not be used to give repeat doses.

15. Unopened vials should be stored in the refrigerator at 2°–8°C (36°–46°F) and protected from light. Vials should be stored in the carton until ready for use.

16. Vials are for single use only. After opening, any unused drug should be discarded.

17. Ross Laboratories offers audiovisual instructional materials concerning administration procedures and dosing requirements.

Assessment

1. Note indications for medication therapy (prevention, rescue, or both).

2. The infant heart rate, color, chest expansion, facial expression, oximeter readings, and endotracheal tube patency and position should be documented and monitored carefully before and during beractant therapy.

3. Ascertain that the endotracheal tube tip is in the trachea and not in the esophagus or right or left mainstem bronchus, before inserting the 5 French end-hole catheter, to ensure appropriate drug dispersion to all lung areas.

4. Document baseline birth weight, arterial blood gases, chest X ray, and physical assessment findings.

Interventions

1. Follow administration guidelines carefully. Beractant is for intratracheal administration only. It should only be administered by trained personnel in a highly supervised environment permitting continuous client observation.

2. Auscultate lung fields frequently and avoid suctioning for 1 hr after dosing unless symptoms of significant airway obstruction are evident.

3. Monitor ECG, arterial BP, and transcutaneous oxygen saturation continuously. After beractant treatment, frequent ABGs should be measured to prevent postdosing hyperoxia and hypocarbia.

4. Monitor (during dosing) for any evidence of transient bradycardia and decreased oxygen saturation. If evident, the dosing procedure should be stopped and the client treated symptomatically until stabilized; then the dosing procedure may be resumed.

5. Observe closely for air leaks and mucous plugs. If mucous plug is unrelieved by suctioning, the endotracheal tube must be replaced immediately.

Evaluation: Evaluate client for:
- Clinical evidence of improved airway exchange and a reduction of pulmonary air leaks
- Oxygen saturation readings between 90% and 95% and improved pulmonary parameters more consistent with survival
- The prevention or successful treatment of respiratory distress syndrome

Betamethasone

(bay-tah-**METH**-ah-zohn)
Betnesol✺, Celestone (Rx)

Betamethasone benzoate

(bay-tah-**METH**-ah-zohn)
Topical: Beben✺, Uticort (Rx)

Betamethasone dipropionate

(bay-tah-**METH**-ah-zohn)
Topical: Alphatrex, Diprolene, Diprosone, Maxivate Occlucort✺, Topilene✺, Topisone✺ (Rx)

Betamethasone sodium phosphate

(bay-tah-**METH**-ah-zohn)
Betnesol✺, Celestone Phosphate, Cel-U-Jec, Selestoject (Rx)

Betamethasone sodium phosphate and Betamethasone acetate

(bay-tah-**METH**-ah-zohn)
Celestone Soluspan (Rx)

Betamethasone valerate

(bay-tah-**METH**-ah-zohn)
Topical: Betacort✺, Betaderm✺, Betagel✺, Betatrex, Beta-Val, Betnovate✺, Betnovate-1/2✺, Celestoderm-V✺, Celestoderm-V/2✺, Dermabet, Ectosone Mild✺, Ectosone Regular, Novo-Betamet✺, Prevex B✺, Rholosone✺, Valisone, Valisone Reduced Strength, Valnac (Rx)

See also *Adrenocorticosteroids and Analogs*, p. 8.

Classification: Adrenocorticosteroid, synthetic, glucocorticoid type.

Action/Kinetics: Causes low degree of sodium and water retention, as well as potassium depletion. The injectable form contains both rapid-acting and repository forms of betamethasone (mixture of betamethasone sodium phosphate and betamethasone acetate). Not recommended for replacement therapy in any acute or chronic adrenal cortical insufficiency because it does not have strong sodium-retaining effects. Long-acting. **t½:** over 300 min.

Additional Use: Prevention of respiratory distress syndrome in premature infants.

Special Concerns: Safe use during pregnancy and lactation have not been established.

Dosage: *Betamethasone.* **Syrup, Tablets.** 0.6–7.2 mg/day. *Betamethasone sodium phosphate:* **Parenteral (IV, local): initial,** up to 9 mg/day; **then,** adjust dosage at minimal level to reduce symptoms. *Betamethasone sodium phosphate and betamethasone acetate:* (contains 3 mg each of the acetate and sodium phosphate per ml). **IM: initial,** 0.5–9 mg/day (dose ranges are ⅓–½ the oral dose given q 12 hr. **Intra-articular, intrabursal, intradermal, intralesional.** *Bursitis, peritendinitis, tenosynovitis:* 1 ml. *Rheumatoid arthritis and osteoarthritis:* 0.25–2 ml, depending on size of the joint. *Dermatologic:* **Intradermally,** 0.2 ml/cm², not to exceed 1 ml/week. *Foot disorders, bursitis:* 0.25–0.5 ml under heloma durum or heloma molle; 0.5 ml under calcaneal spur or over hallux rigidus or digiti quinti varus. *Tenosynovitis or periostitis of cuboid:* 0.5 ml. *Acute gouty arthritis:* 0.5–1 ml.

Betamethasone benzoate, betamethasone dipropionate, betamethasone valerate: **Topical Aerosol, Cream, Gel, Lotion, Ointment:** Apply sparingly to affected areas and rub in lightly.

Betamethasone sodium phosphate: **Ophthalmic or Otic Solution:** 2–3 drops in the ear or 1–2 drops in the eye q 2–3 hr; dosage should be decreased as inflammation improves.

NURSING CONSIDERATIONS

See *Nursing Considerations* for *Adrenocorticosteroids and Analogs,* p. 15.

Administration/Storage: Avoid injection into deltoid muscle because SC atrophy of tissue may occur.

Evaluation: Evaluate clients for subjective reports of symptomatic improvement in condition that generated their original complaint.

Betaxolol hydrochloride

(beh-**TAX**-oh-lohl)
Betoptic, Kerlone (Rx)

See also *Beta-Adrenergic Blocking Agents,* p. 113.

Classification: Beta-adrenergic blocking agent.

Action/Kinetics: Inhibits beta-1 adrenergic receptors although beta-2 receptors will be inhibited at high doses. Has some membrane stabilizing activity but no intrinsic sympathomimetic activity. Low lipid solubility. When used in the eye, betaxolol reduces the production of aqueous humor, thus, reducing intraocular pressure. It has no effect on pupil size or accommodation.

$t^{1}/_{2}$: 14–22 hr. Metabolized in the liver with most excreted through the urine; about 15% is excreted unchanged.

Uses: PO: Hypertension, alone or with other antihypertensive agents (especially diuretics). **Ophthalmic:** Ocular hypertension and chronic open-angle glaucoma (used alone or in combination with other drugs).

Special Concerns: Pregnancy category: C. Use with caution during lactation. Safety and effectiveness have not been determined in children. Geriatric clients are at greater risk of developing bradycardia.

Dosage: Tablets. Initial: 10 mg once daily either alone or with a diuretic. If the desired effect is not reached, the dose can be increased to 20 mg although doses higher than 20 mg will not increase the therapeutic effect. In geriatric clients the initial dose should be 5 mg daily. **Ophthalmic Solution. Adults:** One gtt daily. If used to replace another drug, continue the drug being used and add 1 gtt of betaxolol b.i.d. The previous drug should be discontinued the following day. If transferring from several antiglaucoma drugs being used together, adjust one drug at a time at intervals of not less than 1 week. The antiglaucoma drug dosage can be decreased or discontinued depending on the response of the client.

NURSING CONSIDERATIONS

See also *Nursing Considerations* for *Beta-Adrenergic Blocking Agents,* p. 116.

Administration/Storage: PO

1. The full effect is usually observed within 7–14 days.

2. As the dose is increased, the heart rate decreases.
3. Drug therapy with betaxolol should be discontinued gradually over a 2-week period.

Evaluation: Evaluate client for:
- ↓ in blood pressure
- ↓ in intraocular pressure

Bethanechol chloride
(beh-**THAN**-eh-kohl)
Duvoid, Myotonachol, PMS-Bethanechol✿, Urecholine (Rx)

Classification: Cholinergic (parasympathomimetic), direct-acting.

Action/Kinetics: Directly stimulates cholinergic receptors, primarily muscarinic type. This results in stimulation of gastric motility, increases gastric tone, and stimulates the detrusor muscle of the urinary bladder. Bethanecol produces a slight transient fall of diastolic BP, accompanied by minor reflex tachycardia. The drug is resistant to hydrolysis by acetylcholinesterase, which increases its duration of action. **PO: Onset,** 30–90 min; **maximum:** 60–90 min; **duration:** up to 6 hr. **SC: Onset,** 5–15 min; **maximum:** 15–30 min; **duration:** 2 hr.

Uses: Postpartum or postoperative urinary retention, atony of the bladder with urinary retention. *Investigational:* Reflux esophagitis.

Contraindications: Hypotension, hypertension, coronary artery disease, coronary occlusion, AV conduction defects, vasomotor instability, bradycardia. Also, peptic ulcer, asthma (latent or active), hyperthyroidism, parkinsonism, epilepsy, obstruction of the bladder, if the strength or integrity of the GI or

bladder wall is questionable, peritonitis, GI spastic disease, inflammatory lesions of the GI tract, vagotonia. Not to be used IM or IV.

Special Concerns: Pregnancy category: C. Use with caution during lactation. Safety and effectiveness have not been determined in children.

Side Effects: Serious side effects are uncommon with oral dosage but more common following SC use. *GI:* Nausea, diarrhea, salivation, GI upset, involuntary defecation, cramps, colic, belching, rumbling/gurgling of stomach. *CV:* Hypotension with reflex tachycardia, vasomotor response. *CNS:* Headache, malaise. *Other:* Flushing, sensation of heat about the face, sweating, urinary urgency, attacks of asthma, bronchial constriction, miosis, lacrimation.

Symptoms of Overdose: Early signs include nausea, vomiting, abdominal discomfort, salivation, sweating, flushing.

Drug Interactions

Cholinergic inhibitors / Additive cholinergic effects
Ganglionic blocking agents / Critical hypotensive response preceded by severe abdominal symptoms
Procainamide / Antagonism of cholinergic effects
Quinidine / Antagonism of cholinergic effects

Dosage: Tablets: Adults, usual, 10–50 mg t.i.d.–q.i.d. to a maximum of 120 mg/day. The minimum effective dose can be determined by giving 5–10 mg initially and repeating this dose q 1–2 hr until a satisfactory response is observed or a maximum of 50 mg has been given. **Pediatric:** 0.2 mg/kg

(6.7 mg/m²) t.i.d. **SC: usual,** 5 mg t.i.d.–q.i.d. The minimum effective dose is determined by giving 2.5 mg initially and repeating this dose at 15–30 min intervals to a maximum of 4 doses or until a satisfactory response is obtained. **Pediatric:** 0.15–0.2 mg/kg (5–6.7 mg/m²) t.i.d. Never give IM or IV.

NURSING CONSIDERATIONS

Administration/Storage

1. To avoid nausea and vomiting, bethanechol tablets should be taken on an empty stomach. Usually, 1 hr before or 2 hr after meals.
2. Administer orally or subcutaneously only.
3. The client should be observed closely for 30–60 min after drug administration for possible severe side effects. A syringe containing atropine should be available to reverse the effects of bethanechol.
4. *Treatment of Overdose:* Atropine, 0.6 mg SC for adults; a dose of 0.01 mg/kg atropine SC (up to a maximum of 0.4 mg) is recommended for infants and children up to 12 years of age. IV atropine may be used in emergency situations.

Assessment

1. Take a complete nursing history.
2. Note the drugs the client is currently taking to determine if any are likely to interact with bethanecol.
3. Obtain baseline data concerning the client's intake and output when the drug is to be used to treat urinary tract problems.
4. If the drug is to be used to treat GI atony, obtain baseline data

concerning bowel sounds and habits.
5. If the client is taking antacids, investigate the reasons to determine if the client has a history of peptic ulcers.

Interventions

1. Monitor the client's vital signs, intake and output until it can be determined what the effects of the drug will be.
2. If the drug is to be administered SC, administer 2 hr before eating to reduce the potential for nausea.
3. Have atropine available during SC therapy to counteract manifestations of acute toxicity.
4. If the drug is being administered for GI atony, monitor for bowel sounds.
5. If the client complains of gnawing, aching, burning or epigastric pain in the left epigastric area, document and report to the physician for further investigation of the problem.
6. If the client complains of tightness in the region of the urinary bladder, monitor client intake and output closely. If the output is inadequate for the amount of intake, record and report to the physician immediately because the drug should be discontinued.

Evaluation: Evaluate client for subjective reports of improved bladder tone and function.

Biperiden hydrochloride
(bye-**PER**-ih-den)
Akineton Hydrochloride (Rx)

Biperiden lactate
(bye-**PER**-ih-den)
Akineton Lactate (Rx) (PC: C)

See also *Antiparkinson Agents,*
p. 99, and *Cholinergic Blocking
Agents,* p. 136.

Classification: Antiparkinson
agent, synthetic anticholinergic.

Action/Kinetics: Tolerance may
develop to this synthetic anticholinergic. Tremor may increase as spasticity is relieved. The drug has slight
respiratory and cardiovascular effects. **Time to peak levels:** 60–90
min. **Peak levels:** 4–5 mcg/L. **t½:**
About 18–24 hr.

Uses: Parkinsonism, especially of
the postencephalitic, arteriosclerotic, and idiopathic types. Drug-induced (e.g., phenothiazines) extrapyramidal manifestations.

Additional Contraindications:
Children under the age of 3 years.

Special Concerns: Pregnancy category: C. Use with caution in older
children.

Additional Side Effects: Muscle
weakness, inability to move certain
muscles.

**Dosage: Tablets (Hydrochlor-
ide).** *Parkinsonism,* **Adults:** 2 mg
t.i.d.–q.i.d., to a maximum of 16 mg
daily. *Drug-induced extrapyramidal effects:* 2 mg 1–3 times/day.
Maximum daily dose: 16 mg. **IM,
Slow IV (Lactate).** *Drug-induced
extrapyramidal effects:* **Adults,** 2
mg; repeat q 30 min until symptoms
improve, but not more than 4
doses/day. **Pediatric:** 0.04 mg/kg
(1.2 mg/m²); repeat q 30 min until
symptoms improve, but not more
than 4 doses/day.

NURSING CONSIDERATIONS

See also *Nursing Considerations*
for *Cholinergic Blocking Agents,*
p. 138.

Administration/Storage
1. Administer after meals to avoid
   gastric irritation.
2. If the drug is administered IM,
   assist the client in walking
   because of the possibility of
   transient incoordination.
3. If the drug is administered IV,
   have the client remain recumbent during the procedure and
   for 15 min after it is completed.
   Once the IV is finished, assist
   clients to get up by having
   them dangle their legs at the
   bedside prior to standing and
   walking, to lower the potential
   for hypotension, syncope, and
   falling.

Assessment
1. Note the client's age. Older
   clients should receive lower
   doses of the medication.
2. Record other drugs the client is
   taking and compare with the
   list of drugs with which biperiden lactate interacts.

Client/Family Teaching
1. Keep a record of stools. Encourage the client to increase
   the intake of fluids and fruit
   juices to avoid constipation.
2. Maintain a record of intake and
   output. Report any difficulty
   with urination.
3. Avoid overheating as drug ↓
   perspiration.
4. Do not use antacids or an
   antidiarrheal for 1–2 hr after
   taking medication.

B

Evaluation: Evaluate client for:
- Reports of ↓ rigidity and drooling
- Control of drug-induced (phenothiazines) extrapyramidal manifestations

Bisacodyl

(bis-ah-**KOH**-dill)

Apo-Bisacodyl ✦, Bisacodyl Uniserts, Bisacolax✦, Dulcagen, Dulcolax, Fleet Bisacodyl, Fleet Bisacodyl Prep, PMS-Bisacodyl ✦ (OTC)

Bisacodyl tannex

(bis-ah-**KOH**-dill)

Clysodrast (Rx)

See also *Laxatives,* p. 171.

Classification: Laxative, stimulant.

Action/Kinetics: Bisacodyl is a local chemical stimulant that acts by increasing the contraction of the muscles of the colon by stimulating the myenteric plexus; this results in an alteration of water and electrolyte secretion. Bisacodyl is not absorbed systemically and can be administered orally or as a rectal suppository or solution. It produces a gentle bowel movement with soft, formed stools. It usually acts within 6–10 hr after PO administration and 15–60 min after rectal administration.

Uses: Cleansing of colon preoperatively and postoperatively and for diagnostic procedures (radiology, barium enemas, proctoscopy), colostomies. Short-term treatment of constipation.

May be used during pregnancy or in the presence of cardiovascular, renal, or hepatic disease.

Contraindications: Acute surgical abdomen or acute abdominal pain. Children less than 6 years of age. Use of bisacodyl tannex in patients with ulcerative lesions of the colon or in children less than 10 years of age.

Special Concerns: Use bisacodyl tannex with caution when multiple enemas are given.

Additional Side Effects: Suppositories may cause burning sensation, proctitis, and inflammation.

Drug Interaction: Use of bisacodyl with antacids, milk, or cimetidine may result in premature dissolution of the enteric coating, leading to cramping and vomiting.

Dosage: Tablets. Adults: 10–15 mg at bedtime or before breakfast. *Preparation of lower GI tract:* Up to 30 mg; **Pediatric, over 6 years:** 5–10 mg at bedtime or before breakfast. **Rectal suppository, adults and children over 2 years:** 10 mg; **under 2 years:** 5 mg.

Bisacodyl tannex. **Cleansing enema:** 2.5 g (1 packet) in 1 L warm water. *Barium enema:* 2.5 or 5 g in 1 L barium suspension. **Note:** No more than 10 g should be given within a 3-day period. Also, the total dose for one examination of the colon should not exceed 7.5 g.

NURSING CONSIDERATIONS

See also *Nursing Considerations* for *Laxatives,* p. 172.

Administration/Storage

1. Bisacodyl tablets should be swallowed whole and should not be taken within 1 hr of milk or antacids.
2. Bisacodyl tablets should be taken either at bedtime for effectiveness in the morning or

before breakfast so as not to interfere with the client's rest at night. The tablets should be effective within 6 hr.

3. If the tablets are being given to prepare the client for surgery, radiography, or sigmoidoscopy, the drug should be taken orally the night before the procedure and by rectal suppository early that morning.

4. Bisacodyl tablets should be refrigerated at temperatures not to exceed 30°C (86°F).

5. Lubricate suppositories with warm water prior to administration.

Client/Family Teaching

1. Swallow the tablet whole. Do not crush or chew the tablets.

2. Children who cannot swallow tablets will be unable to take the laxative by mouth.

3. Advise the client not to take the laxative within 1 hr of ingesting milk or an antacid.

Evaluation: Evaluate client for:
• Relief of constipation
• Effective colon cleansing for bowel preps

Bitolterol mesylate
(bye-**TOHL**-ter-ohl)
Tornalate Aerosol (Rx)

See also *Sympathomimetic Drugs,* p. 218.

Classification: Bronchodilator.

Action/Kinetics: Bitolterol is considered a prodrug in that it is converted by esterases in the body to the active colterol. Colterol is said to combine with beta-2-adrenergic receptors, producing dilation of bronchioles. **Onset follow-**

ing inhalation: 3–4 min. **Time to peak effect:** 30–60 min. **Duration:** 6–7 hr.

Uses: Prophylaxis and treatment of bronchial asthma and bronchospasms. Treatment of bronchitis, emphysema, bronchiectasis, and chronic obstructive pulmonary disease. May be used with theophylline and/or steroids.

Special Concerns: Safety has not been established for use during pregnancy (category: C) and lactation and in children less than 12 years of age. Use with caution in ischemic heart disease, hypertension, hyperthyroidism, diabetes mellitus, cardiac arrhythmias, seizure disorders, or in those who respond unusually to beta-adrenergic agonists. There may be decreased effectiveness in steroid-dependent asthmatic clients.

Side Effects: *CNS:* Tremors, dizziness, lightheadedness, nervousness, headache, insomnia. *CV:* Palpitations, tachycardia, premature ventricular contractions, flushing. *Respiratory:* Cough, dyspnea, tightness in chest, bronchospasm. *Other:* Nausea, throat irritation.

Drug Interactions: Additive effects with other beta-adrenergic bronchodilators.

Laboratory Test Interference: ↑ AST. ↓ Platelets, WBCs. Proteinuria.

Dosage: Inhalation Aerosol. *Bronchodilation.* **Adults and children over 12 years,** 2 inhalations at an interval of 1–3 min q 8 hr (if necessary, a third inhalation may be taken). The dose should not exceed 3 inhalations q 6 hr or 2 inhalations q 4 hr. *Prophylaxis of bronchospasm.* **Inhalation:** 2 inhalations q 8 hr.

NURSING CONSIDERATIONS

See also *Nursing Considerations* for *Sympathomimetic Drugs,* p. 220.

Administration/Storage

1. Bitolterol is available in a metered-dose inhaler (MDI). With the inhaler in an upright position, the client should breathe out completely in a normal fashion. As the client is breathing in slowly and deeply, the canister and mouthpiece should be squeezed between the thumb and forefinger, activating the medication. The breath should be held for 10 sec and then slowly exhaled.
2. The medication should not be stored above 120°F.

Evaluation: Evaluate client for:
- Improved airway exchange
- Subjective reports of symptomatic relief of respiratory symptoms

---

Bleomycin sulfate

(blee-oh-**MY**-sin)

Blenoxane (Abbreviation: BLM) (Rx)

See also *Antineoplastic Agents,* p. 85.

Classification: Antineoplastic, antibiotic.

Action/Kinetics: Bleomycin is a glycopeptide antibiotic produced by *Streptomyces verticillus.* It is most effective in the G_2 and M phases of cell division although some activity is noted in noncycling cells. The action may be due to binding to DNA, inducing lability of the DNA structure and decreasing synthesis of DNA and to a lesser extent RNA and protein. Drug currently used is mostly a mixture of bleomycin A_2 and B_2. Drug has relatively low bone marrow depressant activity, localizes in certain tissues, and is an important component of some combination regimens. **Peak plasma levels** (after 4–5 days of therapy): 50 ng/ml. **$t^{1/2}$, after rapid IV and intrapleural, adults:** 24 min and 4 hr; **children, less than 3 years of age:** 54 min and 3 hr. **$t^{1/2}$, continuous IV, adults:** 79 min and 9 hr; **children, less than 3 years of age:** 2.3 hr (terminal phase). Two-thirds excreted in urine as active bleomycin. 60%–70% excreted in the urine unchanged.

Uses: Palliative treatment, either alone or in combination, for Hodgkin's and non-Hodgkin's lymphomas (including lymphosarcoma and reticulum cell sarcoma), testicular carcinomas, and squamous cell carcinomas (especially of the head and neck, larynx, paralarynx, penis, cervix, vulva, and skin). *Investigational:* Soft tissue sarcomas, osteosarcoma, malignant effusions (peritoneal, pleural), ovarian tumors. Also for severe, recalcitrant common warts (verruca vulgaris).

Additional Contraindications: Renal or pulmonary diseases. Pregnancy, lactation.

Additional Side Effects: Pulmonary fibrosis, especially in older clients. Mucocutaneous toxicity and hypersensitivity reactions. In approximately 1% of lymphoma clients, an idiosyncratic reaction manifested by hypotension, fever, chills, mental confusion, and wheezing has been reported.

Additional Drug Interaction: Bleomycin may ↓ plasma levels and renal excretion of digoxin.

Dosage: **SC, IM, IV.** *Hodgkin's disease, lymphosarcoma, reticulum cell sarcoma, testicular carcinoma, squamous cell carcinoma:* 0.25–0.5 units/kg (10–20 units/m^2) once or twice weekly. **Maintenance, IM or IV,** *Hodgkin's disease:* 1 unit/day or 5 units/week. *Squamous cell carcinoma of head, neck, or cervix:* **Regional arterial infusion,** 30–60 units/day over a period of 1–24 hr. *Warts:* **Intralesional,** 0.2–0.8 units (depending on the size) one or more times q 2–4 weeks (up to a maximum total dose of 2 units using a solution of 15 units of sterile bleomycin solution in 15 ml 0.9% saline or water for injection).

NURSING CONSIDERATIONS

See also *Nursing Considerations* for *Antineoplastic Agents,* p. 88.

Administration/Storage

1. For IM or SC use, the drug should be reconstituted with 1–5 ml sterile water for injection, 5% dextrose injection, sodium chloride for injection, or bacteriostatic water for injection.
2. Administer IV slowly over 10 min.
3. Hodgkin's disease and testicular tumors should respond within 2 weeks; squamous cell cancers require at least 3 weeks.
4. Bleomycin is stable for 24 hr at room temperature in sodium chloride, 5% dextrose solution, and 5% dextrose containing heparin, 100 or 1,000 units/ml.

Assessment: Assess client for basilar rales, cough, dyspnea on exertion, and tachypnea, all of which are dose-related symptoms of pulmonary toxicity.

Client/Family Teaching

1. Teach client and/or family the idiosyncratic reaction (see *Additional Side Effects*) that may occur in clients with lymphoma.
2. Advise that clients receiving digoxin should be monitored closely and have digoxin levels monitored during therapy with bleomycin.
3. Avoid vaccinations.
4. Practice safe form of contraception.
5. Report any abnormal oral or skin rashes.
6. Advise that smoking may aggravate pulmonary symptoms.

Evaluation: Evaluate for evidence of a decrease in tumor size and spread.

Bretylium tosylate
(breh-**TILL**-ee-um **TOZ**-ill-ayt)
Bretylate Parenteral✿, Bretylol (Rx)

Classification: Antiarrhythmic, type III.

Action/Kinetics: Bretylium inhibits catecholamine release at nerve endings by decreasing excitability of the nerve terminal. The drug also increases the duration of the action potential and the effective refractory period, which may assist in reversing arrhythmias. **Peak plasma concentration and effect:** 1 hr after IM injection. Antifibrillatory effect within a few minutes after IV use. Suppression of ventricular tachycardia and ventricular arrhythmias takes 20–120 min, whereas suppression of premature ventricular contractions does not occur for 6–9 hr. **Therapeutic serum lev-**

els: 0.5–1.5 mcg/ml. **t½:** 5–10 hr. Up to 90% of drug is excreted unchanged in the urine after 24 hr.

Uses: Life-threatening ventricular arrhythmias that have failed to respond to other antiarrhythmics. Prophylaxis and treatment of ventricular fibrillation. For short-term use only.

Contraindications: Severe aortic stenosis, severe pulmonary hypertension.

Special Concerns: Safe use during pregnancy and in children has not been established.

Side Effects: *CV:* Hypotension (including postural hypotension), transient hypertension, increased frequency of premature ventricular contractions, bradycardia, precipitation of anginal attacks, initial increase in arrhythmias, sensation of substernal pressure. *GI:* Nausea, vomiting (especially after rapid IV administration), diarrhea, abdominal pain, hiccoughs. *CNS:* Vertigo, dizziness, lightheadedness, syncope, anxiety, paranoid psychosis, confusion, mood swings. *Miscellaneous:* Renal dysfunction, flushing, hyperthermia, shortness of breath, nasal stuffiness, diaphoresis, conjunctivitis, erythematous macular rash, lethargy.

Drug Interactions

Digitoxin, Digoxin / Bretylium may aggravate digitalis toxicity due to initial release of norepinephrine
Procainamide, Quinidine / Concomitant use with bretylium ↓ inotropic effect of bretylium and ↑ hypotension

Dosage: IV. *Ventricular fibrillation:* 5 mg/kg of undiluted solution given rapidly. Can increase to 10 mg/kg and repeat as needed. **Maintenance, IV infusion:** 1–2 mg/min; or, 5–10 mg/kg q 6 hr of diluted drug infused over 10–30 min *Other ventricular arrhythmias:* **IV infusion:** 5–10 mg/kg of diluted solution over 10–30 min. **Maintenance:** 5–10 mg/kg q 6 hr or 1–2 mg/min of continuous IV infusion.

IM. *Other ventricular arrhythmias:* 5–10 mg/kg of undiluted solution followed, if necessary, by the same dose at 1–2 hr intervals; **then,** give same dosage q 6–8 hr.

NURSING CONSIDERATIONS

See also *Nursing Considerations for Antiarrhythmic Drugs,* p. 52.

Administration/Storage

1. For IV infusion, dilute the 10 ml ampule up to a minimum of 50 ml with either 5% dextrose injection or sodium chloride injection.
2. For IM injection, use the drug undiluted.
3. Rotate the injection sites so that no more than 5 ml of drug is given at any site. This avoids localized atrophy, necrosis, fibrosis, vascular degeneration, or inflammation.
4. The client should be placed on an oral antiarrhythmic medication as soon as possible.

Assessment: Note if client is taking digitalis. Bretylium tosylate may aggravate digitalis toxicity.

Interventions

1. To reduce nausea and vomiting, administer the IV drug over an 8 min period.
2. IV solutions should be administered with the client lying

down. BP should be monitored every 15 min along with cardiac rhythm strips.

3. Bretylium often causes a fall in supine blood pressure within 1 hr of IV administration. If the systolic pressure falls below 75 mm Hg, anticipate the need to use pressor agents.

4. Once the IV is finished, the client should continue to lie down until the blood pressure has stabilized.

5. Supervise clients once ambulation is permitted because they may develop lightheadedness and vertigo.

6. If clients develop side effects, stay with them, reassuring and reorienting as needed.

7. Remember that the dose of bretylium to be administered is titrated based on the client's response to therapy. Therefore, careful recording of the drug effects is important as well as consultation with the physician.

Evaluation: Assess for effectiveness of drug therapy as evidenced by termination of life-threatening ventricular arrhythmia.

────── COMBINATION DRUG ──────
Brevicon 21-Day and Brevicon 28-Day
(BREV-ih-kon)
(Rx)

See also *Oral Contraceptives,* p. 192.

Classification: Monophasic combination oral contraceptive.

Components: Each tablet of Brevicon 21-Day and the first 21 tablets of Brevicon 28-Day contains ethinyl estradiol, 35 mcg and northindrone, 0.5 mg (blue tablets); the 28s also contain 7 orange inert tablets.

Special Concerns: Pregnancy category: X.

NURSING CONSIDERATIONS

See *Oral Contraceptives,* p. 192.

Bromocriptine mesylate
(broh-moh-**KRIP**-teen)
Parlodel (Rx)

Classification: Prolactin secretion inhibitor; dopamine receptor agonist.

Action/Kinetics: Bromocriptine is a nonhormonal agent that inhibits the release of the hormone prolactin by the pituitary. The drug should be used only when prolactin production by pituitary tumors has been ruled out. Its effect in parkinsonism is due to a direct stimulating effect on dopamine type 2 receptors in the corpus striatum. Less than 30% of the drug is absorbed from the GI tract. **Onset, lower prolactin:** 2 hr; **antiparkinson:** 30–90 min; **decrease growth hormone:** 1–2 hr. **Peak plasma concentration:** 1–3 hr. **t½, plasma:** 3 hr; **terminal:** 15 hr. **Duration, lower prolactin:** 24 hr (after a single dose; **decrease growth hormone:** 4–8 hr. Significant first-pass effect. Metabolized in liver, excreted mainly through bile and thus the feces.

Uses: Short-term treatment of amenorrhea/galactorrhea associated with hyperprolactinemia. Prevention of physiologic lactation. Acromegaly. Parkinsonism. Female infertility associated with hyperprolactinemia. *Investigational:* Hyperprolactinemia due to pituitary adenoma; male infertility.

Contraindications: Sensitivity to ergot alkaloids. Pregnancy, lactation, children under 15 years of age. Peripheral vascular disease, ischemic heart disease.

Special Concerns: Geriatric clients may manifest more CNS effects. Use with caution in liver or kidney disease.

Side Effects: The type and incidence of side effects depends on the use of the drug. *When used for hyperprolactinemia. GI:* Nausea, vomiting, abdominal cramps, diarrhea, constipation. *CNS:* Headache, dizziness, fatigue, drowsiness, lightheadedness, psychoses. *Other:* Nasal congestion, mild hypotension.

When used to prevent physiologic lactation. GI: Nausea, vomiting, cramps, diarrhea. *CNS:* Headaches, dizziness, fatigue, syncope. *CV:* Decreased blood pressure (transient).

When used for acromegaly. GI: Nausea, vomiting, anorexia, dry mouth, dyspepsia, indigestion, GI bleeding. *CNS:* Dizziness, syncope, drowsiness, tiredness, headache; rarely, lightheadedness, lassitude, vertigo, sluggishness, paranoia, insomnia, decreased sleep requirement, delusional psychosis, visual hallucinations. *CV:* Orthostatic hypotension, digital vasospasm, worsening of Raynaud's syndrome; rarely, arrhythmias, ventricular tachycardia, bradycardia, vasovagal attack; *Other:* Rarely, potentiation of effects of alcohol, hair loss, shortness of breath, paresthesia, tingling of ears, muscle cramps, facial pallor, reduced tolerance to cold.

When used for parkinsonism. GI: Nausea, vomiting, abdominal discomfort, constipation, anorexia, dry mouth, dysphagia. *CNS:* Confusion, hallucinations, fainting, drowsiness, dizziness, insomnia, depression, vertigo, anxiety, fatigue, headache, lethargy, nightmares. *GU:* Urinary incontinence, urinary retention, urinary frequency. *Other:* Abnormal involuntary movements, asthenia, visual disturbances, ataxia, hypotension, shortness of breath, edema of feet and ankles, blepharospasm, erythromelalgia, skin mottling, nasal stuffiness, paresthesia, skin rash, signs and symptoms of ergotism.

Drug Interactions

Alcohol / ↑ Chance of GI toxicity; alcohol intolerance
Antihypertensives / Additive ↓ in blood pressure
Butyrophenones / ↓ Effect of bromocriptine because butyrophenones are dopamine antagonists
Diuretics / Should be avoided during bromocriptine therapy
Phenothiazines / ↓ Effect of bromocriptine because phenothiazines are dopamine antagonists

Laboratory Test Interference: ↑ BUN, AST, ALT, GGPT, CPT, alkaline phosphatase, uric acid.

Dosage: Capsules, Tablets. *Amenorrhea/galactorrhea/female or male infertility due to hyperprolactinemia:* **Adults, initial,** 1.25–2.5 mg daily with meals; **then,** increase dose by 2.5 mg q 3–7 days until optimum response observed (usual: 5–7.5 mg daily; range: 2.5–15 mg daily). For amenorrhea/galactorrhea, do not use for more than 6 months. *Prevention of physiologic lactation:* (begin no sooner than 4 hr after delivery) usual, 2.5 mg b.i.d. with meals; therapy should be continued for 14–21 days. *Parkinsonism:* **Initial,** 1.25

mg (one-half tablet) b.i.d. with meals while maintaining dose of levodopa, if possible. Dosage may be increased q 14–28 days by 2.5 mg/day with meals. Dose should not exceed 100 mg/day. *Acromegaly:* **Initial,** 1.25–2.5 mg for 3 days with food and on retiring; **then,** increased by 1.25–2.5 mg q 3–7 days until optimum response observed. Usual optimum therapeutic range: 20–30 mg daily, not to exceed 100 mg daily. Clients should be reevaluated monthly and dosage adjusted accordingly.

NURSING CONSIDERATIONS

Administration/Storage

1. Before administering the first dose of drug, have the client lie down because of the possibility of fainting or dizziness.
2. For doses less than 5 mg, tablets should be used.

Assessment

1. In taking a drug history, inquire about any sensitivity to ergot alkaloids.
2. Note the age of the client, if she is female and sexually active and likely to become pregnant.
3. If the client has any history of liver or kidney dysfunction, obtain baseline liver and renal function studies.
4. List other drugs the client is taking to determine the potential for drug interactions.

Interventions: Observe the client for complaints of fatigue, headache, nausea, drowsiness, cramps or diarrhea. Document and report these findings to the physician.

Client/Family Teaching

1. Take the drug with food to minimize GI upset.

2. Caution that drug may cause dizziness, drowsiness, or syncope. If clients experience syncope or dizziness, instruct them to lie down. Advise clients to avoid activities that require mental alertness.
3. If the client is using oral contraceptives, advise her to use other contraceptive measures while taking bromocriptine.
4. When a menstrual period is missed, schedule the sexually active client for pregnancy tests every 4 weeks during the period of amenorrhea and after resumption of menses.
5. Discuss with the client the signs and symptoms of pregnancy. If pregnancy is likely, advise withholding the drug and reporting to the physician. Explain that pregnancy tests may fail to diagnose early pregnancy and the medication may harm the fetus.

Evaluation: Evaluate client for:
- Resumption of normal menstrual cycle
- Decrease in breast engorgement and galactorrhea
- Prevention of physiologic lactation
- Reduction of growth hormone in acromegaly
- ↓ in muscle rigidity and tremor in Parkinson's disease

Brompheniramine maleate
(brohm-fen-**EAR**-ah-meen)
Brombay, Bromphen, Chlorphed, Codimal-A, Conjec-B, Cophene-B, Dehist, Diamine T.D., Dimetane, Dimetane Extentabs, Dimetane-Ten, Histaject

B

Modified, Nasahist B, ND Stat Revised, Oraminic II, Sinusol-B, Veltane (Rx; Dimetane and Dimetane Extentabs are OTC)

See also *Antihistamines,* p. 71.

Classification: Antihistamine, alkylamine type.

Action/Kinetics: Fewer sedative effects. **t½:** 25 hr. **Time to peak effect:** 3–9 hr. **Duration:** 4–25 hr.

Special Concerns: Pregnancy category: B. Use is not recommended for neonates. Geriatric clients may be more sensitive to the usual adult dose.

Dosage: Elixir, Tablets. Adults and children over 12: 4 mg q 4–6 hr, or 8–12 mg sustained-release b.i.d.–t.i.d., not to exceed 24 mg/day. **Pediatric, 6–12 years:** 2 mg q 4–6 hr, not to exceed 12 mg daily; **2–6 years:** 1 mg q 4–6 hr, not to exceed 6 mg daily. **Extended-release Tablets. Adults and children over 12:** 8 mg q 8–12 hr or 12 mg q 12 hr; **pediatric, 6–12 years:** 8–12 mg q 12 hr.

IM, IV, SC. Adults: usual, 10 mg (range: 5–20 mg) q 8–12 hr (maximum daily dose: 40 mg); **pediatric, under 12 years:** 0.125 mg/kg (3.75 mg/m^2) 3–4 times daily.

NURSING CONSIDERATIONS

See *Nursing Considerations* for *Antihistamines,* p. 74.

Administration/Storage

1. Do not use solutions containing preservatives for IV injection.
2. For children aged 6–12 years, sustained-release preparations require the supervision of a physician.
3. For IV administration, the 10 mg/ml preparations may be used undiluted or diluted 1:10 with sterile saline for injection.
4. The 10 mg/ml preparations may also be added to 5% glucose, normal saline, or whole blood.
5. The 100 mg/ml preparation is not recommended for IV use.
6. For IM or SC use, the drug may be used undiluted or diluted 1:10 with saline.

Evaluation: Client reports symptomatic improvement of allergic manifestations.

Buclizine hydrochloride
(BYOU-klih-zeen)
Bucladin-S Softabs (Rx)

See also *Antiemetics,* p. 70, and *Antihistamines,* p. 71.

Classification: Antiemetic, antihistamine, piperazine type.

Action/Kinetics: Buclizine suppresses nausea and vomiting through an action on the CNS to decrease vestibular stimulation and depress labyrinthine function. The drug may also act on the chemoreceptor trigger zone to decrease vomiting. **Duration:** 4–6 hr.

Uses: Nausea, vomiting, dizziness of motion sickness.

Additional Contraindications: Hypersensitivity to drug, pregnancy, lactation.

Special Concerns: Pregnancy category: B. Safe use in children not established. Geriatric clients may be more susceptible to the usual adult dose.

Side Effects: Drowsiness, dry mouth, headache, nervousness.

Dosage: Chewable   Tablets.

Adults: 50 mg 30 min before travel; dosage may be repeated after 4–6 hr. *Severe nausea:* Up to 150 mg daily.

NURSING CONSIDERATIONS

See *Nursing Considerations* for *Antiemetics,* p. 71, and *Antihistamines,* p. 74.

Administration/Storage

1. To prevent motion sickness, take medication 30 min before departure.
2. Tablets can be chewed, swallowed whole, or dissolved in the mouth.

Evaluation: Evaluate client for:
- ↓ in nausea and vomiting
- Prevention of motion sickness

Bumetanide

(byou-**MET**-ah-nyd)
Bumex (Rx)

See also *Diuretics,* p. 140.

Classification: Loop diuretic.

Action/Kinetics: Bumetanide inhibits reabsorption of both sodium and chloride in the ascending loop of Henle. It may also have some activity in the proximal tubule especially to promote phosphate excretion. **Onset, PO:** 30–60 min. **Peak effect, PO:** 1–2 hr. **Duration, PO:** 4–6 hr (dose-dependent). **Onset, IV:** Several minutes. **Peak effect, IV:** 15–30 min. **Duration, IV:** 3.5–4 hr. **t½:** 1–1.5 hr. Metabolized in the liver although 45% excreted unchanged in the urine.

Uses: Edema associated with congestive heart failure, nephrotic syndrome, hepatic disease. Adjunct to treat acute pulmonary edema. Espe-

cially useful in clients refractory to other diuretics. *Investigational:* In combination with other drugs to treat mild to moderate hypertension. Hypercalcemia.

Contraindications: Anuria, hepatic coma, severe electrolyte depletion, hypersensitivity to the drug.

Special Concerns: Safety during pregnancy (category: C) and lactation and children under 18 has not been established. Geriatric clients may be more sensitive to the hypotensive and electrolyte effects and are at greater risk in developing thromboembolic problems and circulatory collapse.

Side Effects: *Electrolyte and fluid changes:* Excess water loss, dehydration, electrolyte depletion including hypokalemia, hypochloremia, hyponatremia; hypovolemia, thromboembolism, circulatory collapse. *Otic:* Hearing loss, ear discomfort, tinnitus, ototoxicity. *GI:* Nausea, abdominal pain, vomiting, dry mouth, diarrhea, gastric upset, anorexia, jaundice, acute pancreatitis. *CNS:* Dizziness, headache, vertigo, blurred vision, asterixis, encephalopathy (with preexisting liver disease). *Allergic:* Pruritus, urticaria, rashes. *GU:* Premature ejaculation, difficulty in maintaining an erection, renal failure. *Hematologic:* Agranulocytosis, thrombocytopenia. *Miscellaneous:* Rash, pain following parenteral use, hypotension, hyperglycemia, ECG changes, joint and muscle pain, chest pain, sweating, hyperventilation, pruritus, hives, nipple tenderness. Cross-sensitivity may be seen in clients allergic to sulfonamides.

Symptoms of Overdose: Profound loss of water, electrolyte depletion, dehydration, decreased blood vol-

B

ume, circulatory collapse (possibility of vascular thrombosis and embolism). Symptoms of electrolyte depletion include: anorexia, cramps, weakness, dizziness, vomiting, and mental confusion.

Drug Interactions

Aminoglycosides / Additive ototoxicity

Antihypertensive drugs / Potentiation of antihypertensive effect

Cisplatin / ↑ Chance of ototoxicity

Digitalis glycosides / Bumetanide produces excess K loss with ↑ chance of cardiac arrhythmias

Indomethacin / ↓ Effect of bumetanide

Lithium / ↑ Risk of lithium toxicity due to ↓ renal excretion

Probenecid / ↓ Effect of bumetanide

Laboratory Test Interferences: Alterations in LDH, AST, ALT, alkaline phosphatase, creatinine clearance, total serum bilirubin, serum proteins.

Dosage: Tablets. Adults, 0.5–2 mg once daily; if response is inadequate, a second or third dose may be given at 4- to 5-hr intervals up to a maximum of 10 mg daily. **IV, IM:** 0.5–1 mg; if response is inadequate, a second or third dose may be given at 2- to 3-hr intervals up to a maximum of 10 mg daily. Oral dosing should be started as soon as possible.

NURSING CONSIDERATIONS

See also *Nursing Considerations* for *Diuretics,* p. 141.

Administration/Storage

1. Solutions for IM or IV use should be freshly prepared and used within 24 hr.

2. Ampules may be reconstituted with 5% dextrose in water, 0.9% sodium chloride, or lactated Ringer's solution.

3. IV solutions should be administered slowly over 1–2 min.

4. IV or IM administration should be reserved for clients in whom oral use is not practical or in whom absorption from the GI tract is impaired.

5. The recommended oral medication schedule is on alternate days or for 3–4 days with a 1- to 2-day rest period in between.

6. Bumetanide, at a 1:40 ratio of bumetanide:furosemide, may be ordered for clients allergic to furosemide.

7. *Treatment of Overdose:* Replace electrolyte and fluid losses and monitor urinary electrolyte levels as well as serum electrolytes. Emesis or gastric lavage. Oxygen or artificial respiration may be necessary. General supportive measures.

Interventions

1. Monitor BP and pulse regularly. Rapid diuresis may cause dehydration and circulatory collapse. Hypotension may also occur when drug is administered with antihypertensive drugs.

2. Observe for ototoxicity, especially if the client is receiving other ototoxic drugs.

3. Monitor hepatic and renal function studies as well as serum electrolyte levels.

Evaluation: Evaluate client for:
- ↓ in blood pressure and edema
- ↑ in urinary output

Buprenorphine hydrochloride

(byou-pren-**OR**-feen)

Buprenex (C-V, Rx)

See also *Narcotic Analgesics,* p. 174.

Classification: Narcotic agonist/antagonist.

Action/Kinetics: Semisynthetic opiate possessing both narcotic agonist and antagonist activity. It has limited activity at the mu receptor. **IM, onset:** 15 min; **Peak effect:** 1 hr; **Duration:** 6 hr. **t½:** 2–3 hr. May also be given IV with shorter onset and peak effect. Buprenorphine is about equipotent with naloxone as a narcotic antagonist.

Uses: Moderate to severe pain.

Special Concerns: Use during pregnancy (category: C) and lactation only if benefits outweigh risks. In children, safety and efficacy have not been established. Use with caution in clients with compromised respiratory function, in head injuries, in impairment of liver or renal function, Addison's disease, prostatic hypertrophy, biliary tract dysfunction, urethral stricture, myxedema, and hypothyroidism. Administration to individuals physically dependent on narcotics may result in precipitation of a withdrawal syndrome.

Side Effects: *CNS:* Sedation, dizziness, confusion, headache, euphoria, slurred speech, depression, paresthesia, psychosis, malaise, hallucinations, coma, dysphoria, agitation, seizures. *GI:* Nausea, vomiting, constipation, dyspepsia, loss of appetite, dry mouth. *Ophthalmologic:* Miosis, blurred vision, double vi-

sion, conjunctivitis. *CV:* Hypotension, bradycardia, tachycardia, Wenckebach block. *Respiratory:* Decreased respiratory rate, cyanosis, dyspepsia. *Dermatologic:* Sweating, rash, pruritus, flushing. *Other:* Urinary retention, chills, tinnitus.

Drug Interactions: Additive CNS depression with alcohol, general anesthetics, antianxiety agents, sedative-hypnotics, phenothiazines, and other narcotic analgesics.

Dosage: IM, Slow IV, over 13 years of age: 0.3 mg q 6 hr. Up to 0.6 mg may be given; doses greater than 0.6 mg not recommended.

NURSING CONSIDERATIONS

See also *Nursing Considerations* for *Narcotic Analgesics,* p. 177.

Administration/Storage

1. Buprenorphine may be mixed with isotonic saline, lactated Ringer's solution, and 5% dextrose and 0.9% saline.
2. Buprenorphine may be mixed with solutions containing haloperidol, glycopyrrolate, scopolamine hydrobromide, hydroxyzine chloride, or droperidol.
3. Buprenorphine should not be mixed with solutions containing diazepam or lorazepam.
4. Storage in excessive heat and light should be avoided.

Assessment

1. Determine if the client has evidence of respiratory depression and report to the physician because drug is contraindicated.
2. Note if the client has any head injuries and if so report immediately.

3. If the client has been receiving narcotics, observe for evidence of withdrawal effects and document on the chart.
4. Note any evidence of liver or renal dysfunction, diseases of the biliary tract, or prostatic hypertrophy.

Evaluation: Client reports effective control of pain.

Bupropion hydrochloride
(byou-**PROH**-pee-on)
Wellbutrin

Classification: Antidepressant, miscellaneous.

Action/Kinetics: Bupropion is an antidepressant whose mechanism of action is not known; the drug does not inhibit MAO and it only weakly blocks neuronal uptake of epinephrine, serotonin, and dopamine. **Peak plasma levels:** 2 hr. **t½:** 8–24 hr. Metabolized to both active and inactive metabolites. Excreted through both the urine (87%) and the feces (10%).

Uses: Short-term (6 weeks or less) treatment of depression.

Contraindications: Seizure disorders; presence or history of bulimia or anorexia nervosa. Concomitant use of an MAO inhibitor.

Special Concerns: Pregnancy category: B. Use with caution in clients with a history of seizures, cranial trauma, with drugs that lower the seizure threshold, and other situations that might cause seizures. Use with caution and in lower doses in clients with liver or kidney disease and in those with a recent history of myocardial infarction or unstable heart disease. Assess benefits versus risks during lactation. Safety and efficacy have not been established in clients less than 18 years of age.

Side Effects: *CNS:* Dose-dependent risk of seizures; agitation, sedation, headache or migraine, insomnia, decreased concentration, euphoria, delusions, hallucinations, psychoses, confusion, paranoia, anxiety, manic episodes in bipolar manic depression, suicide. *GI:* Nausea, vomiting, constipation, anorexia, weight loss (up to 2.3 kg), diarrhea, dyspepsia, increased appetite, weight gain, dry mouth, increased salivation. *Neurologic:* Akinesia, bradykinesia, tremor, sensory disturbances, pseudoparkinsonism, akathisia, muscle spasms. *CV:* Dizziness, tachycardia, hypertension, hypotension, palpitations, cardiac arrhythmias, syncope. *GU:* Impotence, menstrual irregularities, urinary frequency or retention. *Miscellaneous:* Excessive sweating, blurred vision, auditory disturbances, alteration in taste, rash, pruritus, fever, chills, arthritis, fatigue, upper respiratory problems, temperature disturbances of the skin.

Drug Interactions

Alcohol / Alcohol lowers seizure threshold; use with bupropion may precipitate seizures
Carbamazepine / Possible additive effect to ↑ drug metabolizing enzymes in the liver
Cimetidine / See *Carbamazepine*
Levodopa / ↑ Risk of side effects
MAO inhibitors / Acute toxicity to bupropion may be increased especially if used with phenelzine
Phenobarbital / See *Carbamazepine*
Phenytoin / See *Carbamazepine*

Dosage: Tablets. Adults, initial: 100 mg in the morning and evening for the first 3 days; **then,** 100 mg t.i.d., given in the morning, midday, and in the evening (6 hr should elapse between doses). If no response is observed after 4 weeks or longer, the dose may be increased to 450 mg daily with individual doses not to exceed 150 mg. Doses higher than 450 mg should not be administered. **Maintenance:** Lowest dose to control depression.

NURSING CONSIDERATIONS

Administration/Storage

1. To reduce the risk of seizures, the total daily dose should not exceed 450 mg, each single dose should not exceed 150 mg, and doses of drug should be increased gradually.
2. Several months of treatment may be necessary to control acute depression.
3. Review list of drugs with which this medication interacts.
4. *Treatment of Overdose:* Client should be hospitalized. If conscious, syrup of ipecac is given to induce vomiting followed by activated charcoal q 6 hr during the first 12 hr after ingestion. Both ECG and EEG should be monitored for 48 hr and fluid intake must be adequate. If the client is in a stupor, is comatose, or is convulsing, gastric lavage may be undertaken provided intubation of the airway has been performed. Seizures may be treated with IV benzodiazepines and other supportive procedures.

Assessment

1. Obtain baseline weight, ECG, liver and renal function studies.

Anticipate reduced dose with renal and/or liver dysfunction.
2. Determine if client has a history of seizures and/or recent myocardial infarction. Dose of bupropion may need to be reduced.
3. Note any client history of bulimia or anorexia nervosa.
4. Determine if the woman client is of childbearing age and lactating. Assess the benefits and risks and discuss with the physician. This information may serve as a guide when discussing the drug therapy with the client.

Client/Family Teaching

1. Discuss the side effects associated with drug therapy.
2. Explain the potential for a change in taste perceptions. The result could be loss of appetite and weight loss. These symptoms should be reported and an accurate accounting of weight loss should be recorded for the physician's review.
3. Young women should be informed about possible menstrual irregularities.
4. Men should be warned about possible symptoms of impotence. These symptoms should be reported.
5. The beneficial effects of the drug may not be noticed for 5–21 days. The client should continue taking the medication and not be discouraged by the delayed response.
6. Report any changes in urinary output. The client should be instructed how to record intake and output.
7. Dizziness may occur. Therefore, clients should not arise

from a supine position suddenly. If dizziness occurs during the day, the client should sit down until the sensation subsides. If it persists, notify the physician.

8 Report any bothersome or persistent side effects, especially marked weight loss or diarrhea.

9. Stress the importance of reporting for follow-up lab studies and medical visits so that drug therapy and dosage may be evaluated and adjusted as needed.

10. Report any mood swings or suicidal ideations.

Evaluation: Evaluate client for:
- Subjective reports of improvement in symptoms of depression
- Freedom from complications of drug therapy

Buspirone hydrochloride
(byou-**SPYE**-rohn)
BuSpar (Rx)

Classification: Antianxiety agent.

Action/Kinetics: The mechanism of action is unknown. Buspirone is not chemically related to the benzodiazepines; it does not manifest anticonvulsant or muscle relaxant properties. Significant sedation has not been observed. The drug binds to serotonin (5-HT$_{1A}$) and dopamine (D$_2$) receptors in the CNS; it is thus possible that dopamine-mediated neurologic disorders may occur. These include dystonia, Parkinson-like symptoms, akathisia, and tardive dyskinesia. **Peak plasma levels:** 1–6 ng/ml 40–90 min after a single oral dose of 20 mg. **t½:** 2–3 hr. The drug undergoes extensive first-pass metabolism and active and inactive metabolites are excreted in the urine and through the feces.

Uses: Anxiety disorders, short-term use to relieve symptoms of anxiety due to motor tension, apprehension, autonomic hyperactivity, or hyperattentiveness. Not usually indicated for treatment of anxiety and tension due to stress of everyday living.

Contraindications: Psychoses, severe liver or kidney impairment, lactation.

Special Concerns: Use with caution in pregnancy (category: B). Safety and efficacy in children less than 18 years of age not established. A decrease in dose may be necessary in geriatric clients due to age-related impairment of renal function.

Side Effects: *CNS:* Dizziness, drowsiness, insomnia, fatigue, nervousness, excitement, dream disturbances, dysphoria, noise intolerance, euphoria, depersonalization, akathisia, hallucinations, suicidal ideation, seizures, decreased concentration, confusion, anger or hostility, depression. *CV:* Nonspecific chest pain, hypotension, palpitations, tachycardia, syncope, hypertension. *GI:* Nausea, vomiting, diarrhea, constipation, abdominal distress, dry mouth, altered taste, increased appetite, irritable colon. *Ophthalmologic:* Redness and itching of eyes, conjunctivitis, photophobia, eye pain. *Dermatologic:* Skin rash, pruritus, dry skin, edema of face, acne, easy bruising, flushing. *Neurologic:* Paresthesia, tremor, numbness, incoordination. *GU:*

Urinary hesitancy or frequency, enuresis, amenorrhea, pelvic inflammatory disease. *Miscellaneous:* Tinnitus, sore throat, nasal congestion, altered smell, muscle aches or pains, skin rash, headache, sweating, hyperventilation, shortness of breath, hair loss, galactorrhea, decreased or increased libido, delayed ejaculation. *Symptoms of Overdose:* Dizziness, drowsiness, nausea, vomiting, gastric distress, miosis.

Drug Interactions: Use of MAO inhibitors may cause an increase in blood pressure.

Dosage: Tablets. Adults: 5 mg t.i.d. Dosage may be increased in increments of 5 mg/day every 2–3 days to achieve optimum effects; the total daily dose should not exceed 60 mg.

NURSING CONSIDERATIONS

Administration/Storage

1. Buspirone does not manifest cross-tolerance with other sedative-hypnotic drugs, including benzodiazepines.
2. Buspirone will not block the withdrawal syndrome, which may occur following cessation of sedative-hypnotics. Thus, clients on chronic sedative-hypnotic therapy should be withdrawn gradually prior to beginning buspirone therapy.
3. To date, buspirone has not manifested potential for abuse, tolerance, or either physical or psychologic dependence.
4. Up to 2 weeks may be required before beneficial antianxiety effects are manifested.
5. *Treatment of Overdose:* Immediate gastric lavage; general symptomatic and supportive measures.

Interventions

1. Note any client complaints of weakness, restlessness, nervousness, headaches, or feelings of depression. These should be reported to the prescribing physician.
2. Some clients may develop Parkinson-like symptoms or have suicide ideations. These should be reported immediately and anticipate that the physician will withdraw the drug.
3. Nausea is a common side effect that can be alleviated by advising the client to take the drug with a snack to lessen the effects. If the nausea persists or is severe, the physician should be notified.

Client/Family Teaching

1. Review the goals of therapy and the possible side effects. Advise the client to report any unexpected side effects.
2. The drug may cause drowsiness or dizziness. Use caution when operating a motor vehicle or performing tasks that require mental alertness.
3. Report any involuntary, repetitive movements of the face or neck muscles immediately.
4. Avoid the use of alcohol.
5. Discuss with the physician any decision to stop taking the drug. The client may experience withdrawal symptoms such as nausea, vomiting, dry mouth, nasal congestion, or sore throat. These symptoms may occur even with gradual withdrawal from the drug.
6. Caution the client to avoid using OTC preparations unless the physician has been consulted.

Evaluation: Evaluate for a positive clinical response as evidenced by subjective reports of a decrease in anxiety level.

Busulfan
(byou-**SUL**-fan)
Myleran (Abbreviation: Bus) (Rx)

See also *Antineoplastic Agents,* p. 85, and *Alkylating Agents,* p. 20.

Classification: Antineoplastic, alkylating agent.

Action/Kinetics: Busulfan is cell cycle-phase nonspecific and acts predominately against cells of the granulocytic type and is thought to act by alkylating cellular thiol groups. Cross-linking of nucleoproteins occurs. Busulfan may cause severe bone marrow depression. Leukocyte count drops during the second or third week. Thus, close medical supervision, including weekly laboratory tests, is mandatory. Resistance may develop and is thought to be due to the altered transport into the cell and/or increased intracellular inactivation. Rapidly absorbed from the GI tract; appears in serum 0.5–2 hr after PO administration. **t½:** 2.5 hr. It is slowly excreted by the kidney.

Increased appetite and sense of well-being may occur a few days after therapy is started. Sometimes administered with allopurinol to prevent symptoms of clinical gout.

Uses: Chronic myelogenous leukemia (granulocytic, myelocytic, myeloid). Less effective in individuals with chronic myelogenous leukemia who lack the Philadelphia (Ph[1]) chromosome. Not effective in individuals where the disease is in the "blastic" phase.

Contraindications: Use during lactation only if benefits outweigh risks.

Special Concerns: Pregnancy category: D.

Additional Side Effects: Pancytopenia (more severe than with other agents), bronchopulmonary dysplasia, interstitial pulmonary fibrosis, cataracts (after prolonged use), hyperpigmentation, adrenal insufficiency-like syndrome, gynecomastia, suppression of ovarian function, amenorrhea, cholestatic jaundice, myasthenia gravis. Cellular dysplasia in the adrenal glands, bone marrow, lymph nodes, liver, pancreas, and thyroid.

Symptoms of Overdose: Bone marrow toxicity.

Drug Interactions: Use with thioguanine may cause esophageal varices with abnormal liver function tests.

Laboratory Test Interference: ↑ Uric acid in blood and urine.

Dosage: Tablets. Individualized according to leukocyte count. *Chronic myelocytic leukemia:* **Adults, remission, induction, usual dose:** 4–8 mg daily until leukocyte count falls below 15,000/mm³; **maintenance:** 1–3 mg daily. Discontinue therapy if there is a precipitous fall in leukocyte count. **Children, induction:** 0.06–0.12 mg/kg or 1.8–4.6 mg/m² daily; **maintenance:** dosage is titrated to maintain a leukocyte count of 20,000/mm³.

NURSING CONSIDERATIONS

See also *Nursing Considerations* for *Antineoplastic Agents,* p. 88.

Administration/Storage

1. Busulfan should be taken at the same time each day.

2. Extra fluid intake may be required during therapy.
3. Busulfan should not be administered without supervision and the availability of facilities for weekly CBCs.
4. *Treatment of Overdose:* If ingestion is recent, gastric lavage or induction of vomiting followed by activated charcoal. Hematologic status must be monitored.

Assessment

1. Note previous experience with drug therapy and determine any resistance.
2. In clients with chronic myelogenous leukemia note presence of Philadelphia (Ph[1]) chromosome.
3. Document when disease is in "blastic" phase as drug is not effective.

Evaluation: Evaluate client for:
- Increased appetite and improved sense of well being
- ↓ leukocyte count to maintain leukocytes at 20,000/mm³
- In combination with allopurinol, prevention of symptoms of gout

---

Butoconazole nitrate
(byou-toe-**KON**-ah-zohl)
Femstat (Rx)

Classification: Antifungal agent.

Action/Kinetics: By permeating chitin in the fungal cell wall, butoconazole increases membrane permeability to intracellular substances, leading to reduced osmotic resistance and viability of the fungus. Approximately 5.5% of drug is absorbed following vaginal administration.

Uses: Vulvovaginal fungal infections caused by *Candida* species.

Contraindications: Use during first trimester of pregnancy.

Special Concerns: Pregnancy category: C (safe use in pregnancy has not been established). Pediatric dosage has not been established. Use with caution during lactation.

Side Effects: *GU:* Vaginal burning, vulvar burning or itching, discharge; soreness, swelling, and itching of the fingers.

Dosage: Vaginal cream. *During pregnancy, second and third trimesters only:* One applicatorful (about 5 g) of the cream intravaginally at bedtime for 6 days. *Nonpregnant:* One applicatorful (about 5 g) intravaginally at bedtime for 3 days (if necessary, may be used for up to 6 days).

NURSING CONSIDERATIONS

Administration/Storage

1. During pregnancy, use of a vaginal applicator may be contraindicated.
2. If there is no response, studies should be repeated to confirm the diagnosis before reinstituting antifungal therapy.
3. Not to be stored above 40°C (104°F).

Interventions

1. Determine if client is pregnant.
2. Obtain appropriate lab studies prior to initiating therapy.

Client/Family Teaching

1. Instruct in the appropriate technique for medication administration.

2. Continue therapy for pre-scribed regimen and during menstruation.
3. Insert cream high into the vagina.
4. Call the physician if irritation or burning occurs.
5. The use of sanitary napkins may prevent soiling and stain-ing of undergarments and clothing.
6. To prevent reinfection, the sexual partner should use a condom during intercourse.

Evaluation: Evaluate status (pres-ence/absence) of pretreatment symptoms as well as client's subjec-tive reports of improvement.

Butorphanol tartrate

(byou-**TOR**-fah-nohl)
Stadol, Stadol NS (Rx)

See also *Narcotic Analgesics,* p. 174.

Classification: Narcotic analge-sic—agonist-antagonist.

Action/Kinetics: Butorphanol has both narcotic agonist and antago-nist properties. Its analgesic poten-cy is said to be up to 7 times that of morphine and 30–40 times that of meperidine. Overdosage responds to naloxone. **Onset: IM,** 10 min; **IV,** rapid. **Duration:** 3–4 hr. **Peak analgesia:** 30–60 min following IM and more rapidly following IV ad-ministration. $t^{1/2}$: 2.5–4 hr. Butor-phanol is metabolized in the liver and excreted by the kidney. The drug has about 1/40 the narcotic antagonist activity as naloxone. A metered-dose nasal spray is now available for this drug.

Uses: Moderate to severe pain, especially after surgery. Also as preoperative medication (as part of balanced anesthesia). Postpartum pain.

Special Concerns: Safe use dur-ing pregnancy, during labor for premature infants, or in children under 18 years not established. Use with extreme caution in clients with acute myocardial infarction, ven-tricular dysfunction, and coronary insufficiency (morphine or meper-idine are preferred).

Additional Drug Interactions: Butorphanol may precipitate with-drawal in clients physically depen-dent on narcotics.

Dosage: IM: usual, 2 mg q 3–4 hr, as necessary; **range:** 1–4 mg q 3–4 hr. **IV: usual,** 1 mg q 3–4 hr; **range:** 0.5–2 mg q 3–4 hr. **Not recommended for use in child-ren.**

NURSING CONSIDERATIONS

See also *Nursing Considerations* for *Narcotic Analgesics,* p. 177.

Administration: If the drug is to be administered by direct IV infu-sion, it may be given undiluted. Administer it at a rate of 2 mg or less over a 3–5 min period of time.

Assessment

1. Determine if the client is likely to be dependent on narcotics. Butorphanol may precipitate withdrawal symptoms.
2. Note if the client has a history of cardiovascular problems. Document and report because morphine may be a preferred drug to use.

Evaluation: Client reports effec-tive control of pain.

C

Caffeine
(KAF-een)
Caffedrine, Dexitac, No Doz, Quick Pep, Tirend, Vivarin (OTC)

Caffeine, citrated
(KAF-een)
(OTC)

Caffeine and Sodium Benzoate injection
(KAF-een)
(Rx)

Classification: CNS stimulant, miscellaneous.

Note: Caffeine is found in a number of widely used combination drugs, including Fiorinal Plain and with Codeine, and Synalgos DC.

Action/Kinetics: Caffeine stimulates all levels of the CNS (cerebral cortex, medulla, and spinal cord). The mechanism of action includes competitive antagonism of central adenosine receptors. Caffeine is often used as an adjunct to analgesics used for headaches; the mechanism is thought to be due to constriction of blood vessels in the brain leading to a decrease in cerebral blood flow and oxygen tension of the brain. Caffeine may also help to relieve headache by enhancing the onset and effect of analgesics. Caffeine also possesses other pharmacologic activity, including dilation of coronary and peripheral blood vessels, constriction of cerebral blood vessels, increase in heart rate, stimulation of skeletal muscle, increased gastric acid secretion, and diuresis. **Peak plasma levels:** 15–45 min. **Therapeutic plasma levels:** 6–13 mcg/ml. **Levels above 20 mcg/ml produce toxic effects. $t\frac{1}{2}$, distribution:** 3.5 hr; **elimination:** 6 hr. The $t\frac{1}{2}$ is increased during pregnancy and during use of oral contraceptives. Approximately 17% bound to plasma protein. Metabolized primarily in liver and excreted by the kidneys. Sodium benzoate and citric acid increase the water solubility of caffeine.

Uses: Adjunct with nonnarcotic and narcotic analgesics to enhance pain relief; increased wakefulness by increasing mental alertness; adjunct in migraine headache therapy. Neonatal apnea. Although caffeine has been used to overcome hangover effects occurring during arousal from drug-induced coma such as that from intoxication with morphine, barbiturates, alcohol, and other CNS depressants, the use of caffeine for this purpose is neither advisable nor logical.

Contraindications: Use with caution in cardiovascular, renal, and ulcer disease, and in depression. Caffeine and sodium benzoate injection is not recommended for neonatal apnea due to the sodium benzoate content.

Special Concerns: Safety not established during pregnancy. Use with caution during lactation. Children are especially sensitive to the effects of caffeine, especially side effects; thus, use to relieve drowsiness is not recommended in children less than 12 years of age.

Side Effects: *CNS:* Symptoms of overexcitation including insomnia,

C

nervousness, lightheadedness, rest-lessness, headaches. *GI:* Nausea, vomiting, diarrhea, gastric upset. *GU:* Diuresis. **Note:** Large doses may cause anxiety neurosis with sensory disturbances, palpitations, tremors, arrhythmias, flushing, and other symptoms mentioned above. *Following abrupt withdrawal after use of 500–600 mg daily:* Withdrawal symptoms including anxiety, headache, muscle tension. *Symptoms of Overdose:* Insomnia, dyspnea, mild delirium followed by alternating states of consciousness, muscle twitching, diuresis, arrhythmias, hyperglycemia, seizures.

Drug Interactions

Cimetidine / ↑ Effect of caffeine due to ↓ breakdown by liver
MAO inhibitors / Excessive caffeine may cause hypertensive crisis; reduce intake of caffeine containing medication
Oral contraceptives / ↑ Effect of caffeine due to ↓ breakdown by liver
Propoxyphene / Caffeine given to patients taking large doses of propoxyphene may cause convulsions
Tobacco / ↑ Excretion of caffeine

Laboratory Test Interference: ↑ Urinary catecholamines.

Dosage: *Caffeine.* **Tablets.** *CNS Stimulant:* **Adults,** 100–200 mg q 3–4 hr. **Extended-release Capsules: Adults,** 200–250 mg no more often than q 3–4 hr. *Neonatal apnea:* **Initial,** 10 mg/kg; **maintenance:** 2.5 mg/kg daily beginning 48–72 hr after the initial dose. Dose may be increased as required up to 6 mg/kg b.i.d. to achieve a serum level of 8–20 mg/L.
Caffeine and sodium benzoate.

IM, IV. *CNS Stimulant:* **Adults,** Up to a maximum of 500 mg (250 mg anhydrous caffeine and 250 mg of sodium benzoate) per dose. Maximum daily dose: 1.25 g anhydrous caffeine and 1.25 g sodium benzoate.
Caffeine citrated. **Tablets.** *CNS Stimulant:* **Adults, initial** 65–325 mg (32–162 mg anhydrous caffeine) t.i.d. Up to 1 g anhydrous caffeine daily may be used. **Oral Solution, IV Injection.** *Neonatal apnea:* **Initial,** 20 mg (10 mg anhydrous caffeine and 10 mg anhydrous citric acid)/kg. **Maintenance:** 5 mg (2.5 mg anhydrous caffeine and 2.5 mg anhydrous citric acid)/kg beginning 48–72 hr after the initial dose; dose may be increased to 12 mg/kg b.i.d. to achieve a serum level of 8–20 mg/ liter.

NURSING CONSIDERATIONS

Administration/Storage

1. For neonatal apnea, caffeine tablets may be crushed and made into an oral suspension.
2. *Treatment of Overdose:* Treat symptoms. Gastric lavage followed by activated charcoal. Diazepam or phenobarbital to treat seizures.

Interventions

1. Assess for high caffeine intake, manifested by insomnia, irritability, tremors, cardiac irregularities, and gastritis.
2. Monitor intake, output, weight, and blood pressure. Document and report any unusual changes.

Client/Family Teaching: Avoid additional sources of caffeine such as coffee, tea, cocoa, and colas.

Calcitonin-human

(kal-sih-**TOH**-nin)

Cibacalcin (Rx)

Calcitonin-salmon

(kal-sih-**TOH**-nin)

Calcimar, Miacalcin (Rx)

Classification: Calcium regulator.

Action/Kinetics: Calcitonins are polypeptide hormones produced in mammals by the parafollicular cells of the thyroid gland. Calcitonin isolated from salmon has the same therapeutic effect as the human hormone, except for a greater potency per milligram and a somewhat longer duration of action. Calcitonin-human is a synthetic product that has the same sequence of amino acids as the naturally occurring calcitonin found in human beings. Calcitonin is ineffective when administered orally. Calcitonin is beneficial in Paget's disease of bone by reducing the rate of turnover of bone; the drug acts to both block initial bone resorption, decreasing alkaline phosphatase levels in the serum and urinary hydroxyproline excretion. Its effectiveness in treating osteoporosis or hypercalcemia is due to decreased serum calcium levels from direct inhibition of bone resorption. **Time to peak effect, calcitonin-salmon:** 2 hr for hypercalcemia. **Duration, calcitonin-salmon:** 6–8 hr for hypercalcemia. **t½:** 60 min for calcitonin-human and 70–90 min for calcitonin-salmon. The onset of calcitonin-human in reducing serum alkaline phosphatase level and urinary hydroxyproline excretion in Paget's disease may take 6–24 months. Calcitonin is metabolized to inactive compounds in the kidneys, blood, and peripheral tissues.

Uses: Moderate to severe Paget's disease characterized by polyostotic involvement with elevation of serum alkaline phosphatase and urinary excretion of hydroxyproline. For the early treatment of hypercalcemia. Calcitonin-salmon is used concomitantly with calcium and vitamin D to treat postmenopausal osteoporosis.

Contraindications: Allergy to calcitonin-salmon or its gelatin diluent.

Special Concerns: Use with caution during lactation and in pregnancy only if benefits outweigh risks (pregnancy category: C). Safe use in children not established.

Side Effects: *Allergic:* Due to foreign protein reaction to calcitonin or gelatin diluent. Skin rashes, systemic allergic reactions. *GI:* Nausea, vomiting, abdominal pain, diarrhea, anorexia, abdominal pain, salty taste. *Dermatologic:* Flushing of hands or face, inflammation at site of injection (salmon), foot edema. *CNS:* Headache, dizziness. *Other:* Antibody formation rendering the drug ineffective, increased urinary frequency, nocturia, eye pain, sensation of fever, chills, weakness, nasal congestion, shortness of breath, paresthesia. *Symptoms of Overdose:* Nausea and vomiting.

Laboratory Test Alteration: Reduction of alkaline phosphatase and 24-hr urinary excretion of hydroxyproline are indicative of successful therapy. Monitor urine for casts (indicative of kidney damage).

Dosage: SC. *Calcitonin-Human.*

Paget's disease, **Adults, initial,** 0.5 mg daily; **then,** depending on severity of disease, dosage may range from 0.5 mg 2–3 times weekly to 0.25 mg daily. **IM, SC.** *Calcitonin-Salmon. Paget's disease:* **Adults, initial,** 100 IU/day; **maintenance, usual:** 50 IU daily, every other day, or 3 times weekly. *Hypercalcemia;* **Adults, initial,** 4 IU/kg q 12 hr; **then,** increase the dose, if necessary, to 8 IU/kg q 12 hr up to a maximum of 8 IU/kg q 6 hr. *Postmenopausal osteoporosis:* **Adults,** 100 IU daily, once every other day, or 3 times a week given with calcium and vitamin D.

NURSING CONSIDERATIONS

Administration/Storage

1. Before initiating therapy, determine serum alkaline phosphatase level and urinary hydroxyproline excretion.
2. Repeat the above studies at the end of 3 months and every 3–6 months thereafter.
3. Store calcitonin-salmon at a temperature between 2°C–6°C (36°F–43°F).
4. Store calcitonin-human below 25°C (77°F).
5. When being used to treat Paget's disease, therapy for more than 1 year may be required to treat neurologic lesions.
6. Check for hypersensitivity reactions before administering either medication. Administer 1 IU in the forearm and observe for 15 min to ensure test is negative.
7. Have emergency drugs on hand for immediate use in the event of a hypersensitivity reaction.

Assessment: Note any history of client hypersensitivity to calcitonin-salmon or its gelatin diluent.

Interventions

1. Assess for systemic allergic reactions and be prepared to provide oxygen, epinephrine, and corticosteroids.
2. Report local inflammatory reactions at the site of injection.
3. Observe for facial flushing, document, and report to the physician.
4. Observe client for hypocalcemic tetany. Clients will exhibit muscular fibrillation, twitching, tetanic spasms, and may go into convulsions. Have calcium available for emergency use should any of these symptoms occur. Remain with clients following the injection and check them at least every 10 min for the next 30 min.
5. Check the client for evidence of hypercalcemia. Complaints of increased thirst, anorexia, polyuria, nausea, and vomiting should be reported to the physician.
6. Monitor the client for abdominal distress, anorexia, diarrhea, epigastric distress, or changes in taste perception. Monitor and record the weight, intake and output, and notify the physician if these symptoms persist.
7. If the client has a good initial clinical response and then has a relapse, evaluate for antibody formation in response to serum calcitonin.

Client/Family Teaching

1. Explain how to make appropriate assessments of the condi-

tion and to assess the response to therapy.

2. Review aseptic methods of reconstituting the solution, proper injection technique, and the importance of alternating and documenting injection sites.

3. Explain that nausea and vomiting may occur at the onset of therapy. However, the problem should subside as the treatment continues. If it persists, notify the physician.

4. Stress the importance of returning for periodic urine sedimentation tests to be sure there is no kidney damage.

5. Suggest that the client take the doses of medication in the evening to minimize the problem of flushing.

6. Refer to a dietitian for counselling concerning possible adjustments in the diet.

Evaluation: Evaluate client for:

- Laboratory evidence of a reduction in serum calcium, alkaline phosphatase, and 24-hr urinary excretion of hydroxyproline
- Subjective reports of a ↓ in bone pain
- Clinical evidence of a halt in the progression of postmenopausal osteoporosis

---

Calcium carbonate

(KAL-see-um KAR-bon-ayt)
Apo-Cal✹, Cal Carb-HD, Calci-Chew, Calciday-667, Calci-Mix, Calcite 500, Calcium 500✹, Calcium 600, Cal-Plus, Calsan✹, Caltrate 600, Caltrate Jr., Florical, Gencalc 600, Mega Cal✹, Neo-Cal 500✹, Nephro-Calci, Nu-Cal✹, Os-Cal 500, Os-Cal 500 Chewable, Oysco 500 Chewable, Oyst-Cal 500, Oystercal 500, Oyster Shell Calcium-500 (OTC)

See also *Calcium Salts,* p. 120, and *Antacids,* p. 37.

Classification: Calcium salt.

Uses: Mild hypocalcemia, antacid, antihyperphosphatemic.

Special Concerns: Dosage has not been established in children.

Dosage: Capsules, Suspension, Tablets, Chewable Tablets. *Treat hypoglycemia, nutritional supplement:* **Adults,** 1.25–1.5 g 1–3 times daily with or after meals. *Antihyperphosphatemic:* **Adults,** 5–13 g daily in divided doses with meals. **Note:** The preparation contains 40% elemental calcium and 400 mg elemental calcium/g (20 mEq/g). *Florical:* 1 capsule or tablet daily (also contains 8.3 mg sodium fluoride per capsule or tablet).

NURSING CONSIDERATIONS

See *Antacids,* p. 37, and *Calcium Salts,* p. 120.

Calcium carbonate precipitated

(KAL-see-um KAR-bon-ayt)
Alka-Mints, Amitone, Calcilac, Calglycine, Chooz, Dicarbosil, Equilet, Genalac, Glycate, Gustalac, Mallamint, Pama No. 1, Rolaids Calcium Rich, Titralac, Tums, Tums E-X Extra Strength, Tums Liquid Extra Strength (OTC)

See also *Antacids,* p. 37.

Classification: Antacid.

Action/Kinetics: Nonsystemic

antacid regarded by some as the antacid of choice. Since calcium carbonate is constipating, it is often alternated or even mixed with magnesium salts. Acid-neutralizing capacity: 8.25–10 mEq/tablet. Contains 40% calcium. Chronic use may lead to systemic effects. Rapid onset of action and relatively prolonged activity.

Uses: Antacid; adjunct in peptic ulcer therapy. Calcium deficiency.

Side Effects: *GI:* Constipation, rebound hyperacidity, flatulence, eructation, intestinal obstruction. *Milk-alkali syndrome:* Hypercalcemia, metabolic alkalosis, renal dysfunction.

Dosage: Chewing Gum, Oral Suspension, Tablets, Chewable Tablets. Adults, individualize, usual: 0.5–1 g as necessary (or 0.5–1.5 g q 2–4 hr).

NURSING CONSIDERATIONS

See also *Nursing Considerations* for *Antacids,* p. 38.

Administration/Storage: Tablets should be chewed before being swallowed.

Calcium chloride
(**KAL**-see-um **KLOH**-ryd)
Calciject ✹ 9Rx)

See also *Calcium Salts,* p. 120.

Classification: Calcium salt.

Uses: Mild hypocalcemia, latent tetany, severe hypocalcemic tetany, magnesium intoxication, cardiac resuscitation to reverse the harmful effects of hyperkalemia.

Special Concerns: Pregnancy category: C. Use usually restricted in children due to significant irritation

and possible tissue necrosis and sloughing caused by IV calcium chloride.

Additional Side Effects: Peripheral vasodilation with moderate decreases in blood pressure.

Dosage: IV only. *Hypocalcemia, replenish electrolytes:* **Adults,** 0.5–1 g q 1–3 days (given at a rate not to exceed 13.6–27.3 mg/min). **Pediatric:** 25 mg/kg given slowly. *Magnesium intoxication:* 0.5 g; observe for recovery before other doses given. *Cardiac resuscitation:* 0.5–1 g IV or 0.2–0.4 g injected into the ventricular cavity as a single dose. *Hyperkalemia:* Sufficient amount to return ECG to normal. **Never administer IM. Note:** The preparation contains 27.2% calcium and 272 mg calcium/g (13.6 mEq/g).

NURSING CONSIDERATIONS

See *Nursing Considerations* for *Calcium Salts,* p. 122.

Calcium citrate
(**KAL**-see-um **CIH**-trayt)
Citracal, Citracal Liquitab (OTC)

See also *Calcium Salts,* p. 120.

Additional Use: Renal osteodystrophy.

Special Concerns: Dosage has not been established in children.

Dosage: Tablets. *Treat hypocalcemia:* **Adults,** 0.9–1.9 g t.i.d.–q.i.d. after meals. *Nutritional supplement:* 3.8–7.1 g daily in 3–4 divided doses. Contains 21.1% elemental calcium and 211 mg calcium/g (10.5 mEq/g).

NURSING CONSIDERATIONS

See *Nursing Considerations* for *Calcium Salts,* p. 122.

Calcium glubionate

(**KAL**-see-um glue-**BYE**-oh-nayt)
Neo-Calglucon Calcium-Sandoz✹ (OTC)

See also *Calcium Salts,* p. 120.

Classification: Calcium salt.

Uses: Hypocalcemia, calcium deficiency, tetany of newborn, hypoparathyroidism, pseudohypoparathyroidism, osteoporosis, rickets, osteomalacia.

Special Concerns: Pregnancy category: C.

Dosage: Syrup. *Dietary supplement:* **Adults and children over 4 years,** 15 ml t.i.d.–q.i.d. **Pediatric (under 4 years):** 10 ml t.i.d. **Infants:** 5 ml 5 times/day. *Tetany of newborn:* On the basis of laboratory tests, usually 50–150 mg/kg/day in 3 or more divided doses. *Other calcium deficiencies:* **Adult:** 15–45 ml 1–3 times daily. **Note:** The preparation contains 6.5% elemental calcium and 65 mg calcium /g (3.2 mEq/g).

NURSING CONSIDERATIONS

See *Nursing Considerations* for *Calcium Salts,* p. 122.

Calcium gluceptate

(**KAL**-see-um **GLUE**-sep-tayt)
Calcium Zurich✹ (Rx)

See also *Calcium Salts,* p. 120.

Classification: Calcium salt.

Uses: Hypocalcemia, tetany, exchange transfusion in newborns. To replenish electrolytes. Antihypermagnesemic.

Special Concerns: Pregnancy category: C. Should only be given IM

to infants and children in emergency situations when the IV route is not possible.

Dosage: IM. *Treat hypocalcemia:* **Adults, IM,** 0.44–1.1 g; **IV,** 1.1–4.4 g given slowly at a rate not exceeding 36 mg calcium ion/min. **Pediatric, IM, IV:** 0.44–1.1 g; if used IV, give as a single dose at a rate not to exceed 36 mg of calcium ion/min. *Antihypermagnesemic:* **Adults,** 1.2–2.4 given slowly at a rate not to exceed 36 mg calcium ion/min. *Exchange transfusions in newborns:* **IV,** 0.11 g after every 100 ml blood exchanged. The elemental calcium content is 8.2% and there is 82 mg calcium/g (4.1 mEq/g).

NURSING CONSIDERATIONS

See also *Nursing Considerations* for *Calcium Salts,* p. 122.

Administration/Storage: In adults if more than 5 ml must be used IM, the dose should be given in the gluteal area.

Calcium gluconate

(**KAL**-see-um **GLUE**-koh-nayt)
H-F Antidote Gel✹, Kalcinate (Rx, injection; OTC, tablets)

See also *Calcium Salts,* p. 120.

Classification: Calcium salt.

Uses: Latent hypocalcemic tetany, severe hypocalcemic tetany. Replenish electrolytes, antihyperkalemic, antihypermagnesemic, cardiotonic.

Contraindications: Intramuscular, intramyocardial, or subcutaneous use due to severe tissue necrosis, sloughing, and abscess formation.

Dosage: Tablets. *Treatment of hypocalcemia:* **Adults,** 8.8–16.5 g daily in divided doses; **pediatric,** 0.5–0.72 g/kg daily in divided doses. *Nutritional supplement:* **Adults,** 8.8–16.5 g daily in divided doses. **IV only.** *Treatment of hypocalcemia:* **Adults,** 0.97 g given slowly at a rate not to exceed 47.5 mg calcium ion/min; dose may be repeated if necessary. **Pediatric:** 0.2–0.5 g given at the same rate as adults. *Replenish electrolyte:* **Adults,** 0.97 g given slowly at a rate not to exceed 47.5 mg calcium ion/min. *Antihyperkalemic, antihypermagnesemic:* **Adults,** 1–2 g administered slowly at a rate not to exceed 47.5 mg calcium ion/min. *Exchange transfusions in newborns:* 97 mg as a single dose administered slowly. **Note:** The preparation contains 9% calcium and 90 mg calcium/g (4.5 mEq/g).

NURSING CONSIDERATIONS

See *Nursing Considerations* for *Calcium Salts,* p. 122.

Calcium lactate
(**KAL**-see-um **LACK**-tayt)
(OTC)

See also *Calcium Salts,* p. 120.

Classification: Calcium salt.

Uses: Latent hypocalcemic tetany, hyperphosphatemia.

Dosage: Tablets. *Treatment of hypocalcemia:* **Adults:** 7.7 g daily in divided doses with meals. **Pediatric:** 0.34–0.5 g/kg daily in divided doses. **Note:** The preparation contains 13% calcium and 130 mg calcium/g (6.5 mEq/g).

NURSING CONSIDERATIONS

See *Nursing Considerations* for *Calcium Salts,* p. 122.

Capsaicin
(kap-**SAY**-ih-sin)
Axsain, Zostrix (Rx)

Classification: Topical drug used to relieve pain.

Action/Kinetics: Capsaicin is derived from natural sources from plants of the Solanaceae family. It is believed the drug depletes and prevents the reaccumulation of substance P, thought to be the main mediator of pain impulses from the periphery to the CNS. Two products are available: Axsain (0.075% cream) and Zostrix (0.025% cream).

Uses: *Axsain:* Relief of neuralgias due to painful diabetic neuropathy and postsurgical pain. *Zostrix:* Temporary relief of pain (neuralgia) after open skin lesions have healed following herpes zoster infections. *Investigational:* Possible use in psoriasis, intractable pruritus, reflex sympathetic dystrophy, postmastectomy, and postamputation neuroma.

Side Effects: *Skin:* Transient burning following application.

Dosage: Cream. Apply to affected area no more than 3–4 times daily.

NURSING CONSIDERATIONS
Client/Family Teaching
1. Advise that the drug is for external use only.
2. Avoid getting the medication in the eyes or on broken or irritated skin.
3. If clients apply the medication with the fingers, wash hands immediately after application.
4. Do not bandage the affected area tightly.
5. Consult the physician if the condition worsens, if symp-

toms persist more than 14–28 days, or if the symptoms clear but then recur within a few days.

Evaluation: Client reports effective control of pain.

Captopril
(KAP-toe-prill)
Apo-Captopril✶, Capoten, Syn-Captopril✶ (Rx)

See also *Angiotensin-Converting Enzyme Inhibitors,* p. 33.

Classification: Antihypertensive, inhibitor of angiotensin synthesis.

Action/Kinetics: Peak blood levels: 60–90 min; presence of food decreases absorption by 30%–40%. **Plasma protein binding:** 25%–30%. **Time to peak effect:** 60–90 min. **Duration:** 6–12 hr. $t^{1/2}$, **normal renal function:** 2 hr; $t^{1/2}$, **impaired renal function:** 3.5–32 hr. More than 95% of absorbed dose excreted in urine (40%–50% unchanged).

Uses: Antihypertensive, Step I therapy. Concomitant use with diuretic therapy may, however, cause precipitous hypotension. In combination with diuretics and digitalis in treatment of congestive heart failure not responding to conventional therapy. *Investigational:* Rheumatoid arthritis, hypertensive crisis, neonatal and childhood hypertension, hypertension related to scleroderma renal crisis, diagnosis of anatomic renal artery stenosis, diagnosis of primary aldosteronism, Raynaud's syndrome, hypertension of Takayasu's disease, idiopathic edema, prophylaxis of left ventricular function following myocardial infarction.

Special Concerns: Use with caution in cases of impaired renal function. Use in pregnancy only if potential benefits outweigh risks (pregnancy category: C). Use in children only if other antihypertensive therapy has proven ineffective in controlling BP. Use with caution during lactation.

Side Effects: *Dermatologic:* Rash with pruritus and occasionally fever, eosinophilia, and arthralgia. Alopecia, erythema multiforme, photosensitivity, exfoliative dermatitis, Stevens-Johnson syndrome, bullous pemphigus, onycholysis, flushing, pallor, scalded mouth sensation. *GI:* Nausea, vomiting, anorexia, constipation or diarrhea, gastric irritation, abdominal pain, dysgeusia, peptic ulcers, aphthous ulcers, dyspepsia, dry mouth, glossitis, pancreatitis. *Hepatic:* Jaundice, cholestasis, hepatitis. *CNS:* Headache, dizziness, insomnia, malaise, fatigue, paresthesias, confusion, depression, nervousness, ataxia, somnolence. *CV:* Hypotension, angina, myocardial infarction, Raynaud's phenomenon, chest pain, palpitations, tachycardia, cerebrovascular accident, congestive heart failure, cardiac arrest, orthostatic hypotension, rhythm disturbances, atrial fibrillation, bradycardia. *Renal:* Renal insufficiency or failure, proteinuria, urinary frequency, oliguria, polyuria, nephrotic syndrome, interstitial nephritis. *Respiratory:* Bronchospasm, cough, dyspnea, pulmonary embolism, pulmonary infarction. *Hematologic:* Agranulocytosis, neutropenia, thrombocytopenia, pancytopenia, aplastic or hemolytic anemia. *Other:* Decrease or loss of taste perception with weight loss (reversible), angioedema, asthenia, syncope, fever, myalgia, arthralgia, vasculitis, fever, blurred vision, impotence, hyperkalemia, hyponatremia, myasthenia, gynecomastia, rhinitis, eosinophilic pneumonitis.

Additional Drug Interactions

Probenecid / ↑ Blood levels of captopril due to ↓ renal excretion

Dosage: Tablets. *Hypertension:* **Adults, initial:** 25 mg b.i.d.–t.i.d. If unsatisfactory response after 1–2 weeks, increase to 50 mg b.i.d.–t.i.d.; if still unsatisfactory after another 1–2 weeks, thiazide diuretic should be added (e.g., hydrochlorothiazide, 25 mg/day). Dosage may be increased to 100–150 mg b.i.d.–t.i.d., not to exceed 450 mg daily. *Heart failure:* **Initial,** 25 mg t.i.d.; **then,** if necessary, increase dose to 50 mg t.i.d. and evaluate response; **maintenance:** 50–100 mg t.i.d., not to exceed 450 mg daily. **Note:** For adults, an initial dose of 6.25–12.5 mg (0.15 mg/kg t.i.d. in children) should be given b.i.d.–t.i.d. to clients who are sodium- and water-depleted due to diuretics, who will continue to be on diuretic therapy, and who have renal impairment. *Hypertensive crisis:* **initial,** 25 mg; **then,** 100 mg 90–120 min later, 200-300 mg daily for 2–5 days. *Rheumatoid arthritis:* 75–150 mg daily in divided doses. *Prophylaxis of left ventricular dysfunction following myocardial infarction:* 50–100 mg daily. For all uses, doses should be reduced in clients with renal impairment.

NURSING CONSIDERATIONS

See also *Nursing Considerations* for *Antihypertensive Agents,* p. 78.

Administration/Storage

1. In cases of overdosage, volume expansion with normal saline (IV) is the treatment of choice to restore BP.
2. Captopril should not be discontinued without the consent of a physician.

Assessment

1. Obtain baseline hematologic studies and renal and liver function tests prior to beginning therapy.
2. Determine if the client is taking nitroglycerin or other antianginal nitrates. These may act in synergism with captopril and may cause a more pronounced response.
3. Determine the potential for the client to understand and comply with the prescribed therapy.

Interventions

1. Observe client closely for a precipitous drop in BP within 3 hr after initial dose of captopril if a client has been on diuretic therapy and a sodium-restricted diet.
2. If BP falls rapidly, place the client in a supine position and be prepared to assist with an IV infusion of saline.
3. Check for proteinuria monthly after the onset of treatment and for at least 9 months.
4. Withhold potassium-sparing diuretics and consult with physician because hyperkalemia may result.
5. Be alert to hyperkalemia occurring several months after administration of spironolactone and captopril.

Client/Family Teaching

1. Take captopril 1 hr before meals, on an empty stomach.

Food interferes with the absorption of the drug.

2. Report fever, skin rash, sore throat, mouth sores, fast or irregular heartbeat, or chest pain to the physician.

3. Advise that some people may develop dizziness, fainting or lightheadedness. These symptoms usually disappear once the body adjusts to the medication. Encourage client to avoid sudden changes in posture to prevent dizziness and fainting.

4. Explain to clients that they may experience a loss of taste for the first 2–3 months. If this persists and interferes with nutrition, the physician should be notified. This usually disappears in 2–3 months.

5. Carry identification and a list of medications currently prescribed. Always inform any physician they may visit that they are taking captopril.

6. Call the physician if they have any questions concerning symptoms or about the effects of drug therapy. Remind them to not stop taking the medication without physician consent.

7. Insulin-dependent clients may experience hypoglycemia. Monitor blood sugar levels closely.

Evaluation: Evaluate client for:
- ↓ in blood pressure
- Improvement in symptoms of CHF

Carbamazepine
(kar-bah-**MAYZ**-eh-peen)
**Apo-Carbamazepine ✿,
Mazepine ✿, Epitol, Novo–**

Carbamaz ✿, Tegretol, Tegretol Chewtabs ✿, Tegretol CR ✿ (Rx)

See also *Anticonvulsants,* p. 61.

Classification: Anticonvulsant, miscellaneous.

Action/Kinetics: Carbamazepine is chemically similar to the cyclic antidepressants. It also manifests antimanic, antineuralgic, antidiuretic, anticholinergic, antiarrhythmic, and antipsychotic effects. The anticonvulsant action is not known but may involve depressing activity in the nucleus ventralis anterior of the thalamus. Due to the potentially serious blood dyscrasias, a benefit-to-risk evaluation should be undertaken before the drug is instituted. **Peak serum levels:** 4–5 hr. **t½** (serum): 12–17 hr with repeated doses. **Therapeutic serum levels:** 4–12 mcg/ml. Carbamazepine is metabolized in the liver to an active metabolite (epoxide derivative) with a half-life of 5–8 hr. Metabolites are excreted through the feces and urine.

Uses: Epilepsy, especially partial seizures with simple or complex symptomatology. Clonic-tonic seizures, psychomotor epilepsy, and diseases with mixed seizure patterns. Carbamazepine is often a drug of choice due to its low incidence of side effects. To treat pain associated with tic douloureux (trigeminal neuralgia) and glossopharyngeal neuralgia. *Investigational:* Neurogenic diabetes insipidus, alcohol and benzodiazepine withdrawal, cocaine withdrawal, herpes zoster, selected psychiatric disorders such as resistant schizophrenia, dyscontrol syndrome with limbic system dysfunction, bipolar disorders, explosive

C

disorder, borderline personality disorder, poststroke pain, restless leg syndrome.

Contraindications: History of bone marrow depression. Hypersensitivity to drug or tricyclic antidepressants. Lactation. In clients taking MAO inhibitors. Should not be used to relieve general aches and pains.

Special Concerns: Safe use during pregnancy (category: C) has not been established. Safety and effectiveness have not been established in children less than 6 years of age. Use with caution in glaucoma and in hepatic, renal, and cardiovascular disease. Use with caution in clients with mixed seizure disorder that includes atypical absence seizures (carbamazepine not effective). Use in geriatric clients may cause an increased incidence of confusion, agitation, AV heart block, syndrome of inappropriate antidiuretic hormone, and bradycardia.

Side Effects: *GI:* Nausea and vomiting (common), diarrhea, constipation, abdominal pain or upset, anorexia, glossitis, stomatitis, dryness of mouth and pharynx. *Hematologic:* Aplastic anemia, leukopenia, eosinophilia, thrombocytopenia, purpura, agranulocytosis, leukocytosis, pancytopenia, bone marrow depression. *CNS:* Dizziness, drowsiness and unsteadiness (common); headache, fatigue, confusion, speech disturbances, visual hallucinations, depression with agitation, talkativeness, hyperacusis, abnormal involuntary movements, behavioral changes in children. *CV:* Congestive heart failure, hypertension, hypotension, syncope, thrombophlebitis, worsening of angina, arrhythmias (including AV block). *GU:* Urinary frequency or retention, oliguria, impotence, renal failure, azotemia, albuminuria, glycosuria, increased BUN. *Dermatologic:* Pruritus, urticaria, photosensitivity, exfoliative dermatitis, erythematous rashes, alterations in pigmentation, alopecia, sweating, purpura, aggravation of toxic epidermal necrolysis (Lyell's syndrome), Stevens-Johnson syndrome, aggravation of systemic lupus erythematosus, alopecia, erythema nodosum or multiforme. *Ophthalmologic:* Nystagmus, double vision, blurred vision, oculomotor disturbances, conjunctivitis; scattered, punctate lens opacities. *Other:* Peripheral neuritis, paresthesias, tinnitus, fever, chills, joint and muscle aches and cramps, adenopathy or lymphadenopathy, dyspnea, pneumonitis, pneumonia, inappropriate antidiuretic hormone secretion syndrome. *Symptoms of Overdose:* Neuromuscular disturbances, irregular breathing, respiratory depression, tachycardia, hypo- or hypertension, conduction disorders, shock, seizures, impaired consciousness (deep coma possible), motor restlessness, muscle twitching or tremors, athetoid movements, ataxia, drowsiness, dizziness, nystagmus, mydriasis, psychomotor disturbances, hyperreflexia followed by hyporeflexia, opisthotonos, dysmetria, urinary retention, nausea, vomiting, anuria or oliguria.

Drug Interactions

Acetaminophen / ↑ Breakdown of acetaminophen → ↓ effect and ↑ risk of hepatotoxicity

Charcoal / ↓ Effect of carbamazepine due to ↓ absorption from GI tract

Cimetidine / ↑ Effect of carbamazepine due to ↓ breakdown by liver

Contraceptives, oral / ↓ Effect of

contraceptives due to ↑ breakdown by liver

Danazol / ↑ Effect of carbamazepine due to ↓ breakdown by liver

Desmopressin / ↑ Effect of desmopressin

Diltiazem / ↑ Effect of carbamazepine due to ↓ breakdown by liver

Doxycycline / ↓ Effect of doxycycline due to ↑ breakdown by liver

Erythromycin / ↑ Effect of carbamazepine due to ↓ breakdown by liver

Ethosuximide / ↓ Effect of ethosuximide due to ↑ breakdown by liver

Haloperidol / ↓ Effect of haloperidol due to ↑ breakdown by liver

Isoniazid / ↑ Effect of carbamazepine due to ↓ breakdown by liver; also, carbamazepine may ↑ risk of isoniazid-induced hepatotoxicity

Lithium / ↑ CNS toxicity

Lypressin / ↑ Effect of lypressin

MAO inhibitors / Exaggerated side effects of carbamazepine

Muscle relaxants, nondepolarizing / ↓ Effect of muscle relaxants

Nicotinamide / ↑ Effect of carbamazepine due to ↓ breakdown by liver

Phenobarbital / ↓ Effect of carbamazepine due to ↑ breakdown by liver

Phenytoin / ↓ Effect of carbamazepine due to ↑ breakdown by liver; also, phenytoin levels may ↑ or ↓

Primidone / ↓ Effect of carbamazepine due to ↑ breakdown by liver

Propoxyphene / ↑ Effect of carbamazepine due to ↓ breakdown by liver

Theophyllines / ↓ Effect of theophylline

Tricyclic antidepressants / ↓ Effect of tricyclic antidepressants due to ↑ breakdown by liver

Troleandomycin / ↑ Effect of carbamazepine due to ↓ breakdown by liver

Valproic acid / ↓ Effect of valproic acid due to ↑ breakdown by liver; half-life of carbamazepine may be ↑

Vasopressin / ↑ Effect of vasopressin

Verapamil / ↑ Effect of carbamazepine due to ↓ breakdown by liver

Warfarin sodium / ↓ Effect of anticoagulant due to ↑ breakdown by liver

Dosage: Oral Suspension, Tablets, Chewable Tablets, Extended-release Tablets. *Anticonvulsant.* **Adults and children over 12 years: initial,** 200 mg b.i.d. on day 1. Increase by 200 mg/day at weekly intervals until best response is attained. Divide total dose and administer q 6–8 hr. **Maximum dose, children 12–15 years:** 1,000 mg daily; **adults and children over 15 years:** 1,200 mg daily. **Maintenance:** decrease dose gradually to 800–1,200 mg daily. **Children, 6–12 years: initial,** 100 mg b.i.d. on day 1; **then,** increase slowly, at weekly intervals, by 100 mg/day; dose is divided and given q 6–8 hr. Daily dose should not exceed 1,000 mg. **Maintenance:** 400–800 mg daily. **Children, less than 6 years:** 10–20 mg/kg daily in 2–3 divided doses; dose can be increased slowly in weekly increments to maintenance levels of 250–300 mg daily (not to exceed 400 mg daily). *Trigeminal neuralgia:* **Initial,** 100 mg b.i.d. on day 1; increase by no more than 200 mg/day, using increments of 100 mg q 12 hr as needed, up to maximum of 1,200 mg daily. **Maintenance: Usual:** 400–800 mg daily (range: 200–1,200 mg daily). Attempt discontinuation of drug at least 1 time q 3 months.

NURSING CONSIDERATIONS

See also *Nursing Considerations* for *Anticonvulsants,* p. 63.

Administration/Storage

1. Do not administer for a minimum of 2 weeks after client has received MAO inhibitor drugs.
2. Protect tablets from moisture.
3. The drug should be taken with meals.
4. The therapy should be started gradually with the lowest doses of drug to minimize adverse reactions.
5. Carbamazepine should be added gradually to other anticonvulsant therapy. The other anticonvulsant dosage may be maintained or decreased except for phenytoin which may need to be increased.
6. *Treatment of Overdose:* Stomach should be irrigated completely even if more than 4 hr has elapsed following drug ingestion. Activated charcoal, 50–100 g initially, using a nasogastric tube (dose of 12.5 or more g/hr until client is symptom free). Diazepam or phenobarbital may be used to treat seizures (although they may aggravate respiratory depression, hypotension, and coma). Respirations should be monitored.

Assessment

1. Obtain baseline hematologic, liver, and renal function tests

prior to beginning therapy. Do not initiate therapy until significant abnormalities have been ruled out.
2. Obtain baseline eye examinations for evidence of opacities and baseline intraocular pressure measurement.
3. Assess if the client has a history of psychoses because drug may activate symptoms.

Interventions

1. CNS depression may impair client functions. If the client becomes agitated, side rails should be used.
2. Blood cell evaluation should be done on a weekly basis for the first 3 months of therapy, and monthly thereafter. The following guide should be used to determine the extent of bone marrow depression:
   - Erythrocyte count less than 4 million/mm³
   - Hematocrit less than 32%
   - Hemoglobin less than 11 g%
   - Leukocytes less than 4,000/mm³
   - Reticulocytes less than 0.3% of erythrocytes (20,000/mm³)
   - Serum iron greater than 150 mcg%
3. Carbamazepine should be discontinued slowly at the first sign of a blood cell disorder.
4. Monitor intake and output ratios and vital signs for evidence of fluid retention, renal failure, or cardiovascular complications during the period of dosage adjustment.
5. An EEG should be obtained periodically throughout the therapy.
6. If the drug has been quickly withdrawn from a client, use

seizure precautions. Quick withdrawal may precipitate status epilepticus.

Client/Family Teaching

1. Withhold drug and check with the physician if any of the following symptoms occur:
   - Fever, sore throat, mouth ulcers, easy bruising, petechial and purpuric hemorrhages. These are early signs of bone marrow depression.
   - Urinary frequency, acute urinary retention, oliguria, and sexual impotence. These are early signs of GU dysfunction.
   - Symptoms of congestive heart failure, syncope, collapse, edema, thrombophlebitis, or cyanosis. These are cardiovascular side effects that require immediate attention.
2. Use caution in operating an automobile or other dangerous machinery because the drug may interfere with vision and coordination.
3. Report any skin eruptions or changes in skin pigmentation. These may require withdrawal of the drug.
4. Avoid excessive sunlight and wear protective clothing and sunscreen because of the risk of photosensitivity.
5. Stress the importance of reporting for scheduled laboratory studies to assess for early organ dysfunction.

Evaluation: Evaluate client for:
   - A reduction in seizures among clients who have been unresponsive to other drug regimens
   - Subjective reports of a reduction of pain associated with trigeminal neuralgia

---

Carbenicillin indanyl sodium

(kar-ben-ih-**SILL**-in)

Geocillin, Geopen Oral✤, (Rx)

See also *Anti-Infectives,* p. 80, and *Penicillins,* p. 197.

Classification: Antibiotic, penicillin.

Action/Kinetics: The drug is acid stable. **Peak serum levels: PO:** 6.5 mcg/ml after 1 hr. **t½:** 60 min. Rapidly excreted unchanged in urine.

Uses: Upper and lower urinary tract infections or bacteriuria due to *Escherichia coli, Proteus vulgaris, P. mirabilis, Morganella morganii, Providencia rettgeri, Enterobacter, Pseudomonas,* and enterococci. Prostatitis due to *E. coli, S. faecalis* (enterococci), *P. mirabilis,* and *Enterobacter* species.

Additional Contraindications: Pregnancy.

Special Concerns: Safe use in children not established. Use with caution in clients with impaired renal function.

Additional Side Effects: Neurotoxicity in clients with impaired renal function.

Additional Drug Interactions: When used in combination with gentamicin or tobramycin for *Pseudomonas* infections, effect of carbenicillin may be enhanced.

Dosage: Tablets: *Urinary tract infections due to E. coli, Proteus, Enterobacter:* 382–764 mg q.i.d. *Urinary tract infections due to*

Pseudomonas and enterococci: 764 mg q.i.d. *Prostatitis due to E. coli, P. mirabilis, Enterobacter, and enterococcus:* 764 mg q.i.d.

NURSING CONSIDERATIONS

See also *Nursing Considerations for Penicillins,* p. 200.

Administration/Storage

1. Protect from moisture.
2. Store at temperature of 30°C or less.

Intervention: Provide frequent mouth care to minimize nausea and unpleasant aftertaste.

Evaluation

1. Assess client for a positive clinical response based on laboratory C&S results.
2. Assess client with impaired renal function for (a) neurotoxicity, manifested by hallucinations, impaired sensorium, muscular irritability, and seizures, and (b) hemorrhagic manifestations, such as ecchymosis, petechiae, and frank bleeding of gums and/or rectum.

Carbidopa
(**KAR**-bih-doh-pah)
Lodosyn (Rx)

—— *COMBINATION DRUG* ——
Carbidopa/Levodopa
(**KAR**-bih-doh-pah/
LEE-voh-doh-pah)
Sinemet-10/100, -25/100, or -25/250, Sinemet CR (Rx)

Classification: Antiparkinson agent.

Action/Kinetics: Carbidopa inhibits peripheral decarboxylation of levodopa but not central decarboxylation because it does not cross the blood-brain barrier. Since peripheral decarboxylation is inhibited, this allows more levodopa to be available for transport to the brain, where it will be converted to dopamine, thus relieving the symptoms of parkinsonism. It is recommended that both carbidopa and levodopa be given together (e.g., Sinemet). However, *the dosage of levodopa must be reduced by up to 80% when combined with carbidopa.* This decreases the incidence of levodopa-induced side effects. **Note:** Pyridoxine will not reverse the action of carbidopa/levodopa. **t½, carbidopa:** 1–2 hr; when given with levodopa, the t½ of levodopa increases from 1 hr to 2 hr (may be as high as 15 hr in some clients). About 30% carbidopa is excreted unchanged in the urine.

Uses: All types of parkinsonism (idiopathic, postencephalitic, following injury to the nervous system due to carbon monoxide and manganese intoxication). *Investigational:* Postanoxic intention myoclonus. See *Levodopa,* p. 791. **Warning:** Levodopa must be discontinued at least 8 hr before carbidopa/levodopa therapy is initiated. Also, clients taking carbidopa/levodopa must not take levodopa concomitantly, because the former is a combination of carbidopa and levodopa.

Contraindications: See *Levodopa,* p. 791. History of melanoma. MAO inhibitors should be stopped 2 weeks before therapy. Lactation.

Special Concerns: Use during pregnancy only if benefits outweigh risks. Safety and efficacy in children less than 18 years of age have not been determined. Lower doses may be necessary in geriatric clients due to aged-related decreases in peripheral dopa decarboxylase.

Side Effects: See *Levodopa,* p. 791. Also, because more levodopa reaches the brain, dyskinesias may occur at lower doses with carbidopa/levodopa than with levodopa alone. Clients abruptly withdrawn from levodopa may experience neuroleptic malignant-like syndrome including symptoms of muscular rigidity, hyperthermia, increased serum phosphokinase, and changes in mental status.

Drug Interactions: Use with tricyclic antidepressants may cause hypertension and dyskinesia.

Laboratory Test Interferences: ↓ Creatinine, BUN, and uric acid.

Dosage: Tablets. Individualized. *Clients not receiving levodopa:* **Initial,** 1 tablet of 10 mg carbidopa/ 100 mg levodopa t.i.d.–q.i.d. or 25 mg carbidopa/100 mg levodopa t.i.d.; **then,** increase by 1 tablet every 1–2 days until a total of 8 tablets/day is taken. If additional levodopa is required, substitute 1 tablet of 25 mg carbidopa/250 mg levodopa t.i.d.–q.i.d. *Clients receiving levodopa:* **Initial,** carbidopa/ levodopa dosage should be about 25% of prior levodopa dosage (levodopa dosage is discontinued 8 hr before carbidopa/levodopa is initiated); **then,** adjust dosage as required. Suggested starting dose is 1 tablet of 25 mg carbidopa/250 mg levodopa t.i.d.–q.i.d. for clients taking more than 1500 mg levodopa or 25 mg carbidopa/100 mg levodopa for clients taking less than 1500 mg levodopa. **Sustained-release tablets.** *Clients not receiving levodopa:* 1 tablet b.i.d. at intervals of not less than 6 hr. Depending on the response, dosage may be increased or decreased. Usual dose is 2–8 tablets daily in divided doses at intervals of 4–8 hr during waking hours (if divided doses are not equal, the smaller dose should be given at the end of the day). *Clients receiving levodopa:* 1 tablet b.i.d. Carbidopa is available alone for clients requiring additional carbidopa (i.e., inadequate reduction in nausea and vomiting); in such clients, carbidopa may be given at a dose of 25 mg with the first daily dose of carbidopa/levodopa. If necessary, additional carbidopa, at doses of 12.5 or 25 mg, may be given with each dose of carbidopa/ levodopa.

NURSING CONSIDERATIONS

Administration

1. Note any potential drug interactions prior to starting drug therapy.
2. Do not administer with levodopa.
3. Administration of the sustained release form of carbidopa/ levodopa with food results in increased availability of levodopa by 50% and increased peak levodopa levels by 25%
4. The sustained-release form of Sinemet should not be crushed or chewed but can be administered as whole or half tablets.
5. A minimum of three days should elapse between dosage adjustments of the sustained-release product.
6. If general anesthesia is necessary, therapy should be continued as long as oral fluids and other medication are allowed. Therapy should be resumed as soon as the client can take oral medication.

C

Assessment

1. Obtain baseline ECG, vital signs, respiratory assessment, and determine level of bladder function.
2. Note any history of cardiovascular disease, cardiac arrhythmias, or chronic obstructive pulmonary disease.
3. Determine the client's usual sleep patterns as baseline data against which to measure possible adverse effects of drug therapy.
4. Assess and document motor function, reflexes, gait, strength of grip, and amount of tremor.
5. Observe the extent of the tremors, muscle weakness, muscle rigidity, difficulty walking, or changing directions.

Interventions

1. Monitor blood pressure with the client supine and standing to facilitate the detection of postural hypotension.
2. Observe client closely during the dosage adjustment period. Note any involuntary movement that may require dosage reduction.
3. Assess for blepharospasm. This is an early sign of excessive dosage for some clients.
4. To facilitate the client's adjustment to changes in medication, administer the last dose of levodopa at bedtime and start carbidopa/levodopa when the client arises in the morning.

Client/Family Teaching

1. Review the side effects that may occur and advise the client to report these. The physician may reduce the dose of drug or temporarily discontinue the drug. They may also encourage the client to tolerate certain side effects because of the overall benefits gained with therapy.
2. Instruct that as clients improve with drug therapy, they may resume normal activity gradually. Also, remind clients that with increased activity, they must take other medical conditions into consideration.
3. Stress that antiparkinson drugs should not be withdrawn abruptly. When changing medication, one drug should be withdrawn slowly and the other started in small doses under medical supervision.
4. Advise that drug may discolor or darken urine and/or sweat.

Evaluation

1. Assess client for improvement in motor function, reflexes, gait, strength of grip, and amount of tremor.
2. Determine client's need for a drug "holiday" based on a decreased drug response.

Carboplatin for Injection

(KAR-boh-plah-tin)
Paraplatin (Rx)

See also *Antineoplastic Agents,* p. 85, and *Alkylating Agents,* p. 20.

Classification: Antineoplastic, alkylating agent.

Action/Kinetics: Related to cisplatin. Carboplatin acts by producing interstrand DNA cross-links and is thus thought to be cell-cycle nonspecific. $t^{1/2}$, **initial:** 1.1–2 hr; **postdistribution:** 2.6–5.9 hr. Carboplatin is not bound to plasma proteins although platinum from carboplatin is irreversibly bound to plasma protein with a slow half-life (5 days). The drug is eliminated unchanged in the urine at a rate related to creatinine clearance.

Uses: Initial treatment of advanced ovarian cancer in combination with other chemotherapeutic agents. Palliative treatment of recurrent ovarian cancer either initially or previously treated with chemotherapy, including cisplatin. *Investigational:* Small cell lung carcinoma (in combination with etoposide); advanced or recurrent squamous cell tumors of the head and neck (in combination with fluorouracil); seminoma of testicular cancer; advanced endometrial cancer; relapsed or refractory acute leukemia.

Additional Contraindications: History of severe allergy to mannitol or platinum compounds (including cisplatin). Severe bone marrow depression, significant bleeding, lactation.

Special Concerns: Pregnancy category: D.

Additional Side Effects: Bone marrow suppression may be severe. Vomiting is a frequent side effect. *Neurologic:* Central neurotoxicity, peripheral neuropathies (more common in ages 65 and over), ototoxicity. *GU:* Nephrotoxicity (including increased BUN and serum creatinine). *Electrolytes:* Loss of calcium, magnesium, potassium, sodium. *Allergic:* Rash, urticaria, pruritus, erythema; bronchospasm and hypotension (rare). *Miscellaneous:* Pain, alopecia, asthenia. Cardiovascular, respiratory, mucosal side effects, anaphylaxis. *Symptoms of Overdose:* Bone marrow suppression, hepatic toxicity.

Drug Interactions: Carboplatin can react with aluminum (e.g., needles, IV administration sets) causing formation of a precipitate and loss of potency.

Laboratory Test Interference: ↑ Alkaline phosphatase, AST, total bilirubin.

Dosage: **IV:** *Ovarian cancer, as a single agent:* 360 mg/m² q 4 weeks on day 1. Lower doses are recommended in clients with low creatinine clearances. *In combination with cyclophosphamide:* Carboplatin, 300 mg/m² plus cyclophosphamide, 600 mg/m², both on day 1 q 4 weeks.

NURSING CONSIDERATIONS

See also *Nursing Considerations for Antineoplastic Agents,* p. 88.

Administration/Storage

1. Single intermittent doses of carboplatin should not be repeated until the neutrophil count is at least 2,000/mm³ and the platelet count is 100,000/mm³.
2. The dose may be escalated by no more than 125% of the starting dose if platelet counts are greater than 100,000/mm³ and neutrophil counts are greater than 2,000/mm³. If platelet counts are less than 50,000/mm³ and neutrophil counts are less than 500/mm³, subsequent doses should be 75% of the prior dose.
3. The dose is administered by infusion lasting 15 min or longer.
4. For clients with impaired kidney function, the dose should be adjusted as follows: creatinine clearance of 41–59 ml/min, 250 mg/m² on day 1;

creatinine clearance of 16–40 ml/min, 200 mg/m². There is no recommended dose if the creatinine clearance is less than 15 ml/min.

5. Immediately before use, the drug should be reconstituted with either sterile water for injection, 5% dextrose in water, or sodium chloride injection to obtain a final concentration of 10 mg/ml. Carboplatin can be further diluted to concentrations as low as 0.5 mg/ml with 5% dextrose in water or sodium chloride injection.

6. Reconstituted solutions are stable for 8 hr at room temperature. Discard after this period of time because there is no antibacterial preservative in the formulation.

7. Unopened vials should be stored at room temperature, protected from light.

8. Should not be used with needles or IV administration sets containing aluminum.

9. *Treatment of Overdose:* Monitor bone marrow and liver function tests. Treat symptomatically.

Assessment

1. Note any evidence of kidney impairment.

2. Determine if client has a history of allergic responses to mannitol or platinum compounds.

3. Note any evidence of neurologic disorders as a means of determining if those that may occur at a later date are drug related or exacerbations of a prior condition.

4. Assess closely for drug-induced anemia, a frequent side effect of carboplatin therapy.

Interventions

1. Premedicate client with antiemetics because vomiting is a frequent side effect of drug therapy.

2. Anticipate reduced dose with impaired liver and/or renal function.

3. If the client has evidence of kidney impairment, give 1–2 L of water before starting therapy. This may be given over a period of time. Have diuretics available should the client begin to show signs of overhydration.

4. Drug dose is based on CBC and creatinine clearance results; monitor carefully.

5. Ascertain that alkaline phosphatase, AST, and total bilirubin have been done. These results serve as baseline data against which to measure client reactions to the drug therapy.

Client/Family Teaching

1. Warn that client may experience nausea and vomiting.

2. Instruct clients to alert the physician if they notice a rash, pruritus, redness of the skin or bronchospasm.

3. Maintain adequate fluid intake. Favorite fluids may be given, especially those with potassium and calcium, since these electrolytes may be lost in excess as a result of therapy.

4. Advise client to report any sore throat, fever, fatigue, or mouth sores. This may be an indication of bone marrow depres-

sion, which can be severe with this drug therapy.

Evaluation

1. Assess client color and any complaints that may be indications of anemia.
2. Observe for myelosuppression, which is usually most severe 21 days after the start of therapy; symptoms occur rapidly.
3. Assess client for evidence of a decrease in the size and spread of tumor.

Carisoprodol
(kar-eye-so-**PROH**-dohl)
Rela, Sodol, Soma, Soridol, Sporodol (Rx)

See also *Centrally Acting Skeletal Muscle Relaxants,* p. 130.

Classification: Centrally acting muscle relaxant.

Action/Kinetics: Carisoprodol may produce skeletal muscle relaxation by inhibiting synaptic reflexes in the descending reticular formation and spinal cord. Its sedative effects may also be responsible for muscle relaxation. **Onset:** 30 min. **Duration:** 4–6 hr. **Peak serum levels:** 4–7 mcg/ml. **t½:** 8 hr. The drug is metabolized in the liver and excreted in the urine.

Uses: As an adjunct to treat skeletal muscle disorders including bursitis, low back disorders, contusions, fibrositis, spondylitis, sprains, muscle strains, and cerebral palsy.

Contraindications: Porphyria. Hypersensitivity to carisoprodol or meprobamate. Children under 12 years of age.

Special Concerns: Use with caution during pregnancy (category: C). The drug may cause GI upset and sedation in the infant. Use with caution in impaired liver or kidney function.

Side Effects: *CNS:* Ataxia, dizziness, drowsiness, excitement, tremor, syncope, vertigo, insomnia. *GI:* Nausea, vomiting, gastric upset, hiccoughs. *CV:* Flushing of face, postural hypotension, tachycardia. *Allergic reactions:* Pruritus, skin rashes, erythema multiforme, eosinophilia, dizziness, angioneurotic edema, asthmatic symptoms, "smarting" of the eyes, weakness, hypotension, anaphylaxis.

Drug Interactions

Alcohol / Additive CNS depressant effects
Antidepressants, tricyclic / ↑ Effect of carisoprodol
Barbiturates / Possible ↑ effect of carisoprodol, followed by inhibition of carisoprodol
Chlorcyclizine / ↓ Effect of carisoprodol
CNS depressants / Additive CNS depression
MAO inhibitors / ↑ Effect of carisoprodol by ↓ breakdown by liver
Phenobarbital / ↓ Effect of carisoprodol by ↑ breakdown by liver
Phenothiazines / Additive depressant effects

Dosage: Tablets. Adults: 350 mg q.i.d. (take last dose at bedtime). **Pediatric:** 6.25 mg/kg q.i.d.

NURSING CONSIDERATIONS

See *Nursing Considerations* for *Centrally Acting Skeletal Muscle Relaxants,* p. 130.

Administration/Storage

1. If the client is unable to swallow tablets, mix drug with syrup, chocolate, or a jelly mixture.
2. Administer the drug with food if gastric upset occurs.

Assessment

1. Note any history of hypersensitivity to meprobamate or carisoprodol.
2. Record the extent of the client's skeletal muscular disorders as a baseline against which to compare the effects of the therapy.
3. Review drugs the client is currently taking to ensure that no drug interaction will occur.

Interventions

1. Observe client for evidence of ataxia or tremors and report.
2. If the client develops postural hypotension or tachycardia, report to the physician. These are adverse reactions that may necessitate taking the client off of the medication.

Client/Family Teaching

1. Provide a printed list of the potential side effects that should be reported to the physician, should they develop.
2. Assist the client in establishing a drug schedule so that the last dose of drug is taken at bedtime.
3. Due to the possibility of drug-induced dizziness or drowsiness, caution should be used when driving or undertaking other tasks requiring mental alertness.

Evaluation: Evaluate client for reports of symptomatic improvement in skeletal muscle pain and spasticity.

Carmustine
(kar-**MUS**-teen)
BiCNU (Abbreviation: BCNU) (Rx)

See also *Antineoplastic Agents,* p. 85, and *Alkylating Agents,* p. 20.

Classification: Antineoplastic, alkylating agent.

Action/Kinetics: Carmustine acts by alkylating DNA and RNA as well as by inhibiting several enzymes by carbamoylation of amino acids in proteins. It is cell-cycle nonspecific. The drug is not cross-resistant with other alkylating agents. Drug rapidly cleared from plasma and metabolized. Crosses blood-brain barrier (concentration in CSF at least 50% greater than in plasma). $t^{1/2}$: 15–30 min. Thirty percent excreted in urine after 24 hr, 60%–70% after 96 hr.

Uses: Alone or in combination with other antineoplastic agents for palliative treatment of primary (e.g., brainstem glioma, astrocytoma, glioblastoma, ependymoma) and metastatic brain tumors, multiple myeloma (in combination with prednisone). Advanced Hodgkin's disease and non-Hodgkin's lymphomas (not the drug of choice). *Investigational:* GI cancer, malignant melanoma, mycosis fungoides.

Special Concerns: Pregnancy category: D. Not recommended for use during lactation. Delayed bone marrow toxicity may be observed. Safety and effectiveness have not been established in children

Additional Side Effects: *GI:* Nausea and vomiting within 2 hr after administration, lasting 4–6 hr. *GU:* Renal failure, azotemia, decrease in kidney size. *Hepatic:* Reversible increases in alkaline phosphatase, bilirubin, and transaminase. *Other:* Rapid IV administration may produce transitory intense flushing of skin and conjunctiva (onset: after 2 hr; duration: 4 hr). Pulmonary fibrosis, ocular toxicity including retinal hemorrhage.

Drug Interactions

Cimetidine / Additive bone marrow suppression

Digoxin / ↓ Serum levels of digoxin → ↓ effect

Phenytoin / ↓ Serum levels of phenytoin → ↓ effect

Dosage: IV: *In previously untreated clients:* 150–200 mg/m² q 6–8 weeks as a single or divided dose (on consecutive days). Alternate dosing schedule: 75–100 mg/m² on 2 successive days q 6 weeks or 40 mg/m² on 5 successive days q 6 weeks. Subsequent dosage should be reduced if platelet levels are less than 100,000/mm³ and leukocyte levels are less than 4,000/mm³.

NURSING CONSIDERATIONS

See also *Nursing Considerations* for *Antineoplastic Agents,* p. 88.

Administration/Storage

1. Discard vials in which powder has become an oily liquid.
2. Store unopened vials at 2°C–8°C and protect from light. Store diluted solutions at 4°C and protect from light.
3. Reconstitute powder with absolute ethyl alcohol (provided); then add sterile water. For injection, these dilutions are stable for 24 hr when stored as noted above.
4. Stock solutions diluted to 500 ml with 0.9% sodium chloride for injection or with 5% dextrose for injection are stable for 48 hr when stored as noted above.
5. Administer by IV over 1- to 2-hr period; faster injection may produce intense pain and burning at site of injection.
6. Contact of reconstituted carmustine with skin may result in hyperpigmentation (transient). If contact occurs, the skin or mucosa should be washed thoroughly with soap and water.
7. *Do not use vial for multiple doses* because there is no preservative in vial.

Assessment: Determine baseline CBC and monitor for at least 6 weeks after a dose of carmustine because delayed bone marrow toxicity may develop.

Interventions

1. Check for extravasation if client complains of burning or pain at site of injection. Discomfort may be due to alcohol diluent.
2. If there is no extravasation, reduce rate of flow if client complains of burning at site of injection.
3. Slow rate of IV infusion and notify physician if client demonstrates intense flushing of skin and/or redness of conjunctiva.

Evaluation: Evaluate client for:
- A decrease in the extent and size of metastatic tumor process
- Platelet counts greater than 100,000/mm³ and leukocyte counts greater than 4,000/mm³

Carprofen
(kar-**PROH**-fen)
Rimadyl (Rx)

See also *Nonsteroidal Anti-Inflammatory Drugs,* p. 186.

Classification: Anti-inflammatory, nonsteroidal analgesic.

Action/Kinetics: t½: 6–17 hr. **Time to peak levels:** 1 hr.

Uses: Acute and chronic rheumatoid arthritis and osteoarthritis; acute gouty arthritis.

Special Concerns: Pregnancy category: C.

Additional Side Effects: Compared with other NSAIDs, carprofen causes increased incidence of rashes, lower urinary tract symptoms, and leukopenia. Also, there is a greater incidence of abnormalities in levels of transaminase and alkaline phosphatase.

Dosage: PO. *Chronic rheumatoid arthritis and osteoarthritis:* Not to exceed 150 mg b.i.d. or 100 mg t.i.d. *Acute gouty arthritis:* 600 mg daily in divided doses for 3–10 days. If ineffective after 2 days, the drug should be discontinued and other treatment started.

NURSING CONSIDERATIONS

See also *Nursing Considerations for Nonsteroidal Anti-Inflammatory Drugs,* p. 189.

Administration/Storage

1. When the client is to use the drug to treat chronic conditions, attempts should be made to reduce the dosage of drug after taking it for several weeks.
2. Lower doses of medication should be used for elderly clients and those with renal disease.

3. The maximum recommended dose is 300 mg daily.

Assessment: Determine that baseline transaminase, alkaline phosphatase, and renal function studies have been completed.

Interventions

1. Note if the client develops a rash during drug therapy and notify the physician.
2. Observe clients for evidence of lower urinary tract symptoms such as cystitis, nocturia, oliguria, anuria, or urinary frequency and report.

Client/Family Teaching

1. Notify the physician if no improvements are noted after 2 days of therapy.
2. Provide a list of side effects, such as GU reactions and skin rashes, which should be reported to the physician immediately.
3. Take with a full glass of water and remain upright.
4. Provide the names and addresses or phone numbers of local support groups that may assist clients in understanding and coping with chronic disorders.

Evaluation: Evaluate client for:
- Reports of effective relief of pain and discomfort
- Freedom from complications of drug therapy

Carteolol hydrochloride
(kar-**TEE**-oh-lohl)
Cartrol

See also *Beta-Adrenergic Blocking Agents,* p. 113.

Action/Kinetics: Carteolol has both beta-1 and beta-2 receptor blocking activity. The drug has no membrane stabilizing activity but does have moderate intrinsic sympathomimetic effects. Low lipid solubility. **t½:** 6 hr. Approximately 50%–70% excreted unchanged in the urine.

Uses: Hypertension. *Investigational:* Reduce frequency of anginal attacks.

Special Concerns: Pregnancy category: C. Dosage has not been established in children.

Dosage: Tablets. *Hypertension:* **Initial,** 2.5 mg once daily either alone or with a diuretic. In the event of an inadequate response, the dose may be increased gradually to 5 mg and then 10 mg daily as a single dose. **Maintenance:** 2.5–5 mg once daily. Doses greater than 10 mg daily are not likely to increase the beneficial effect and may decrease the response. The dosage interval should be increased in clients with renal impairment. *Reduce frequency of anginal attacks:* 10 mg daily.

NURSING CONSIDERATIONS

See also *Nursing Considerations* for *Beta-Adrenergic Blocking Agents,* p. 116.

Intervention: Anticipate reduced dose with impaired renal function.

Client/Family Teaching

1. Do not exceed prescribed dose because desired response may be altered.
2. Drug may cause increased sensitivity to cold.
3. Report any symptoms of bleeding, infection, dizziness, confusion, depression, or rash.

Evaluation: Evaluate client for:
- ↓ in blood pressure
- Reduction in the frequency of anginal attacks

Cascara sagrada

(kas-**KAR**-ah sah-**GRAD**-ah)
Cascara Sagrada Fluid Extract, Cascara Sagrada Aromatic Fluid Extract, Cascara Tablets (OTC)

See also *Laxatives,* p. 171.

Classification: Stimulant laxative.

Action/Kinetics: Cascara sagrada directly stimulates the intestinal mucosa and the myenteric plexus. The drug alters secretion of water and electrolytes. It produces stools within 6–10 hr. The drug is available in tablet form as well as an aromatic fluid extract.

Uses: Short-term treatment of constipation.

Additional Contraindication: The drug gets into breast milk and may cause diarrhea in the infant.

Additional Side Effects: Dark pigmentation of the mucosa of the colon (called melanosis coli), which is slowly reversed after the drug is discontinued. Acid urine may be colored yellowish brown while an alkaline urine may be colored pink, red, or violet.

Dosage: Aromatic fluid extract. Adults: 5 ml at bedtime; **pediatric, over 2 years of age:** 1–3 ml. **Fluid extract. Adults:** 1 ml at bedtime. **Tablets:** 1 tablet at bedtime.

NURSING CONSIDERATIONS

See also *Nursing Considerations* for *Laxatives,* p. 172.

Assessment: Determine how long

and how often the client has been using cascara.

Interventions: If the client has taken cascara over an extended period of time, monitor electrolyte levels.

Client/Family Teaching

1. Cascara sagrada may cause the urine to appear yellow-brown, violet, or reddish, but this should not cause alarm.
2. Read the bottle carefully to distinguish between the aromatic fluid extract and the fluid extract because the dosage is different.
3. If working with a pregnant client, advise her to consult with the physician prior to taking cascara.
4. Advise clients to use cascara for a short time only. Cascara sagrada can cause electrolyte imbalance, especially hypokalemia. This can be particularly dangerous for elderly clients.

Evaluation: Evaluate for relief of constipation.

Castor oil
(KAS-tor)
Kellogg's Castor Oil, Purge (OTC)

Castor oil, emulsified
(KAS-tor)
Alphamul, Emulsoil, Fleet Flavored Castor Oil, Neoloid, Ricifruit✶ (OTC)

See also *Laxatives,* p. 171.

Classification: Laxative, stimulant.

Action/Kinetics: The active ingredient is ricinoleic acid, which is liberated in the small intestine. This substance inhibits water and electrolyte absorption, leading to fluid accumulation and increased peristalsis. Prompt (within 2–6 hr) and complete evacuation of the bowel occurs, often with a watery stool.

Use: Short-term relief of constipation.

Contraindications: Pregnancy, menstruation, abdominal pain, and intestinal obstruction. Common constipation. Concomitantly with fat-soluble anthelmintics.

Side Effects: Severe diarrhea, abdominal pain and colic, altered mucosal permeability in the small intestine, dehydration, and changes in electrolyte balance, including hyperkalemia, acidosis, or alkalosis.

Dosage: *Castor oil:* 15–60 ml before diagnostic procedures; **infants:** 1–5 ml; **children over 2 years:** 5–15 ml. *Castor oil emulsified,* **PO:** 15–60 ml; **infants less than 2 years:** 1.25–7.5 ml; **children over 2 years:** 5–30 ml. Dose depends on strength of preparation.

NURSING CONSIDERATIONS

See also *Nursing Considerations for Laxatives,* p. 172.

Administration/Storage

1. Shake emulsions well prior to administering. They may be further diluted in water, juice or cola before administering unless otherwise indicated.
2. Regular castor oil does not mix well with water-based materials. Adding a small amount of sodium bicarbonate to castor oil immediately before administering it will cause the mixture to fizz, particularly

suspending the castor oil for a few minutes in the diluent. Discuss this with the physician prior to administering the laxative, unless the client's condition does not permit.

Client/Family Teaching

1. Clients usually prefer the more palatable oil-in-water emulsions that have been aromatized with flavoring agents.
2. Disguise the taste of plain castor oil by mixing with a glass of orange juice.

Evaluation: Evaluate client for reports of relief of constipation.

Cefaclor
(SEF-ah-klor)
Ceclor (Rx)

See also *Anti-Infectives,* p. 80, and *Cephalosporins,* p. 132.

Classification: Antibiotic, second-generation cephalosporin.

Action/Kinetics: Peak serum levels: 5–15 mcg/ml after 1 hr. **t½: PO,** 36–54 min. Well absorbed from GI tract. From 60%–85% excreted in urine within 8 hr.

Uses: Otitis media. Infections of the upper and lower respiratory tract, urinary tract, skin, and skin structures.

Special Concerns: Pregnancy category: B.

Additional Side Effects: Cholestatic jaundice, lymphocytosis.

Dosage: Capsules, Oral Suspension. Adult: 250 mg q 8 hr. Dose may be doubled in more severe infections or those caused by less susceptible organisms. Total daily dose should not exceed 4 g. **Children:** 20 mg/kg/day in divided doses q 8 hr. Dose may be doubled in more serious infections, otitis media, or for infections caused by less susceptible organisms. Total daily dose should not exceed 1 g. Safety for use in infants less than 1 month of age has not been established.

NURSING CONSIDERATIONS

See *Nursing Considerations* for *Cephalosporins,* p. 134.

Administration/Storage

1. The suspension should be refrigerated after reconstitution and discarded after 2 weeks.
2. The total daily dose for otitis media and pharyngitis can be divided and given q 12 hr.

Evaluation: Evaluate client for:
- Reports of improvement in symptoms of infection
- Laboratory evidence of resolution of infection

Cefadroxil monohydrate
(sef-ah-DROX-ill)
Duricef, Ultracef (Rx)

See also *Anti-Infectives,* p. 80, and *Cephalosporins,* p. 132.

Classification: Antibiotic, first-generation cephalosporin.

Action/Kinetics: Peak serum levels: PO, 15–33 mcg/ml after 90 min. **t½: PO,** 70–80 min. Ninety percent of drug is excreted unchanged in urine within 24 hr.

Uses: Pharyngitis, tonsillitis. Infections of the urinary tract, skin, and skin structures.

Special Concerns: Safe use in children and during pregnancy not established. (Pregnancy category: B.) Creatinine clearance determinations must be carried out in clients with renal impairment.

Dosage: Capsules, Oral Suspension, Tablets. Adults: *Pharyngitis, tonsillitis, skin and skin structure infections:* 1 g daily in single or divided two doses. *Urinary tract infections:* 1–2 g/day in single or two divided doses. **Children:** 30 mg/kg daily in divided doses q 12 hr. **For clients with creatinine clearance rates below 50 ml/min: Initial,** 1 g; **maintenance,** 500 mg at following dosage intervals: q 36 hr for creatinine clearance rates of 0–10 ml/min; q 24 hr for creatinine clearance rates of 10–25 ml/min; q 12 hr for creatinine clearance rates of 25–50 ml/min.

NURSING CONSIDERATIONS

See also *Nursing Considerations* for *Cephalosporins,* p. 134.

Administration/Storage

1. Cefadroxil can be given without regard to meals.
2. The suspension should be shaken well before using.
3. For beta-hemolytic streptococcal infections, treatment should be continued for 10 days.

Evaluation: Evaluate client for:
- Reports of symptomatic improvement
- Negative lab culture reports

Cefamandole nafate
(sef-ah-**MAN**-dole)
Mandol (Rx)

See also *Anti-Infectives,* p. 80, and *Cephalosporins,* p. 132.

Classification: Antibiotic, second-generation cephalosporin.

Action/Kinetics: Cefamandole nafate has a particularly broad spectrum of activity. **Peak serum levels: IM,** 12–36 mcg/ml after 30–120 min. **t½: IM,** 60 min; **IV,** 30 min. From 65%–85% excreted unchanged in urine.

Uses: Infections of the urinary tract, lower respiratory tract, bones, joints, skin, and skin structures. Mixed infections of the respiratory tract, skin, and in pelvic inflammatory disease. Peritonitis, septicemia, prophylaxis in surgery. Also, with aminoglycosides in gram-positive or gram-negative sepsis.

Special Concerns: Pregnancy category: B. Safety and effectiveness have not been determined in infants less than 1 month of age.

Additional Side Effects: Hypoprothrombinemia leading to bleeding and/or bruising; cholestatic jaundice, decreased creatinine clearance in clients with prior renal impairment.

Additional Drug Interaction: Concomitant use with ethanol produces a disulfiram-type reaction and hypotension.

Dosage: IV or deep IM injection only (in gluteus or lateral thigh to minimize pain). **Adult:** usual, 0.5–1 g q 4–8 hr. *Severe infections:* Up to 2 g q 4 hr. **Infants and children:** 50–100 mg/kg/day in equally divided doses q 4–8 hr. *Severe:* Up to 150 mg/kg/day (not to exceed adult dose) divided as above. *Preoperative:* **Adults: initial,** 1–2 g 30–60 min prior to surgery; **then,** 1–2 g q 6 hr for 1–2 days (3 days for prosthetic arthroplasty). For cesarean section, the first dose should be given just prior to surgery or just after the cord has been clamped. **Pediatric (3 months and older):** 50–100 mg/kg daily in divided doses, using same schedule as for adults. *Impaired renal function:* **Initial,** 1–2 g; then a maintenance dosage is given, depending on creatinine clearance, according to schedule provided by manufacturer.

NURSING CONSIDERATIONS

See *Nursing Considerations* for *Cephalosporins,* p. 134.

Administration/Storage

1. Review package insert for details on how to reconstitute drug.
2. Reconstituted solutions of cefamandole nafate are stable for 24 hr at room temperature and for 96 hr when stored in the refrigerator. Cefamandole solutions reconstituted with dextrose or sodium chloride are stable for 6 months when frozen immediately after reconstitution.
3. Carbon dioxide gas forms when reconstituted solutions are kept at room temperature. This gas does not affect the activity of the antibiotic and may be dissipated or used to aid in the withdrawal of the contents of the vial.
4. Use separate IV fluid containers and separate injection sites for each drug when cefamandole is administered concomitantly with another antibiotic such as an aminoglycoside.

Client/Family Teaching: Avoid alcohol and any medications containing alcohol as a disulfiram-type reaction may occur.

Cefazolin sodium
(sef-**AYZ**-oh-lin)
Ancef, Kefzol, Zolicef (Rx)

See also *Anti-Infectives,* p. 80, and *Cephalosporins,* p. 132.

Classification: Antibiotic, first-generation cephalosporin.

Action/Kinetics: Peak serum concentration: IM 17–76 mcg/ml after 1 hr. **t½: IM, IV:** 90–130 min. From 80%–100% excreted unchanged in urine.

Uses: Infections of the urinary tract, biliary tract, respiratory tract, bones, joints, soft tissue, and skin. Endocarditis, septicemia, prophylaxis in surgery.

Special Concerns: Pregnancy category: B.

Additional Side Effects: When high doses are used in renal failure clients: extreme confusion, tonic-clonic seizures, mild hemiparesis.

Dosage: IM, IV only. Adult: *Mild infections due to gram-positive cocci:* 250–500 mg q 8 hr; *moderate to severe infections:* 0.5–1 g q 6–8 hr. *Endocarditis, septicemia:* 1–1.5 g q 6 hr (rarely, up to 12 g daily). *Pneumococcal pneumonia:* 0.5 g q 12 hr. *Preoperative:* 1 g 30–60 min prior to surgery. *Acute, uncomplicated urinary tract infections:* 1 g q 12 hr. *Preoperative:* 1 g 30–60 min prior to surgery. *During surgery:* 0.5–1 g. *Postoperative:* 0.5–1 g q 6–8 hr for 24 hr (may be given up to 5 days, especially in open heart surgery or prosthetic arthroplasty). *Impaired renal function:* **Initial,** 0.5 g; **then,** maintenance doses are given, depending on creatinine clearance, according to schedule provided by manufacturer. **Children over 1 month:**

C

Mild to moderate infections: 25–50 mg/kg daily in 3–4 doses. *For severe infections,* up to 100 mg/kg daily may be used. Safety in infants under 1 month of age not determined.

NURSING CONSIDERATIONS

See *Nursing Considerations* for *Cephalosporins,* p. 134.

Administration/Storage

1. Dissolve the solute by shaking vial.
2. Discard reconstituted solution after 24 hr at room temperature and after 96 hr when refrigerated.
3. Note any evidence of renal dysfunction.

Cefixime oral

(seh-**FIX**-eem)
Suprax (Rx)

See also *Anti-Infectives,* p. 80, and *Cephalosporins,* p. 132.

Classification: Antibiotic, third-generation cephalosporin.

Action/Kinetics: Stable in the presence of beta-lactamase enzymes. **Peak serum levels:** 2–6 hr. **t½:** averages 3–4 hr. About 50% excreted unchanged in the urine and approximately 10% in the bile. In addition to the microorganisms listed under *Uses* for cephalosporins, cefixime is effective against *Moraxella catarrhalis, Streptococcus agalactiae, Haemophilus parainfluenzae, Pasteurella multocida, Salmonella* species, and *Shigella* species. The following microorganisms are resistant to cefixime: most strains of *Bacteroides fragilis* and clostridia, *Pseudomonas* species, strains of group *D. streptococci* including enterococci, *Listeria*

monocytogenes, and most strains of staphylococci and *Enterobacter.*

Uses: Uncomplicated urinary tract infections, otitis media, pharyngitis, tonsillitis, acute bronchitis, and acute exacerbations of chronic bronchitis caused by susceptible strains of microorganisms.

Special Concerns: Pregnancy category: B. Safe use in infants less than 6 months old has not been established.

Additional Side Effects: *GI:* Flatulence. *Hepatic:* Elevated alkaline phosphatase levels. *Renal:* Transient increases in BUN or creatinine.

Additional Laboratory Test Interference: False + test for ketones using nitroprusside test.

Dosage: Oral Suspension, Tablets. Adults: Either 400 mg once daily or 200 mg q 12 hr. **Children:** Either 8 mg/kg/day once daily or 4 mg/kg q 12 hr. Clients on renal dialysis or in whom creatinine clearance is 21–60 ml/min, the dose should be 75% of the standard dose (i.e., 300 mg daily). If the creatinine clearance is less than 20 ml/min, the dose should be 50% of the standard dose (i.e., 200 mg daily).

NURSING CONSIDERATIONS

See also *Nursing Considerations* for *Cephalosporins,* p. 134.

Administration/Storage

1. Therapy should be at least 10 days when treating *Streptococcus pyogenes.*
2. Children older than 12 years or weighing more than 50 kg should be given the adult dose.
3. Once reconstituted, the suspension should be kept at

room temperature where it maintains potency for 14 days.

Assessment

1. Take drug history, noting any prior sensitivity to cephalosporins or penicillins.
2. Assess client financial status and health care coverage because prescription cost may be prohibitive.

Interventions

1. Anticipate reduced dose with impaired renal function.
2. Use the suspension in children and when treating otitis media.
3. Cefixime may alter results of urine glucose and ketone testing; finger sticks may provide more accurate blood sugar recordings during drug therapy.

Client/Family Teaching

1. Cefixime may cause GI upset; report any bothersome side effects, especially persistent diarrhea.
2. Therapy requires only once-a-day dosing and should be taken at the same time each day.
3. Consult physician if child's condition does not improve after 48–72 hours of therapy or if condition deteriorates.

Evaluation: Note response to therapy, presence/absence of pretreatment symptoms, and results of follow-up C&S.

Cefmetazole sodium
(sef-**MET**-ah-zole)
Zefazone (Rx)

See also *Anti-Infectives*, p. 80, and *Cephalosporins*, p. 132.

Classification: Antibiotic, second-generation cephalosporin.

Uses: Urinary tract, lower respiratory tract, skin and skin structure, and intra-abdominal infections. Preoperatively to decrease incidence of postoperative infections following cesarean section, cholecystectomy (high risk), colorectal surgery, abdominal or vaginal hysterectomy.

Dosage: IV. *Infections:* 2 g q 6–12 hr for 5–14 days. *Prophylaxis, abdominal hysterectomy or high-risk cholecystectomy:* 1 g 30–90 min prior to surgery and again 8 and 16 hr following surgery. *Prophylaxis, vaginal hysterectomy:* 2 g 30–90 min prior to surgery or 1 g 30–90 min prior to surgery and again 8 and 16 hr following surgery. *Prophylaxis, cesarean section:* 2 g in a single dose after clamping cord or 1 g after clamping cord and again 8 and 16 hr later. *Prophylaxis, colorectal surgery:* 2 g 30–90 min prior to surgery or 2 g 30–60 min prior to surgery and again 8 and 26 hr following surgery.

NURSING CONSIDERATIONS

See also *Nursing Considerations* for *Cephalosporins*, p. 134.

Administration/Storage

1. The drug should be reconstituted with sterile water for injection, bacteriostatic water for injection, or 0.9% sodium chloride injection.
2. After reconstitution, the drug is stable for 24 hr at room temperature, for 7 days if refrigerated, and for 6 weeks if frozen.
3. If necessary, the reconstituted solution may be further diluted to concentrations of 1–20 mg/ml with 0.9% sodium chloride

injection, 5% dextrose injection, or lactated Ringer's injection. Such solutions are stable as described above.

4. Thawed solutions should not be refrozen.

5. Any unused solutions or frozen material should be discarded.

Interventions: Obtain baseline renal function studies and anticipate reduced dose and frequency of administration of cefmetazole with impaired renal function.

Cefonicid sodium
(seh-**FON**-ih-sid)
Monocid (Rx)

See also *Anti-Infectives*, p. 80, and *Cephalosporins*, p. 132.

Classification: Antibiotic, second-generation cephalosporin.

Uses: Infections of the lower respiratory tract, urinary tract, bones, joints, skin, and skin structures. Septicemia. Prophylaxis in surgery, especially colorectal surgery, vaginal hysterectomy, cholecystectomy, prosthetic arthroplasty, open heart surgery, cesarean section after the cord has been clamped.

Special Concerns: Pregnancy category: B.

Dosage: IV, Deep IM. Adults. *Uncomplicated urinary tract infections:* 0.5 g once/day. *Mild to moderate infections:* 1 g once/day. *Severe or life-threatening infections:* 2 g once/day. *Prophylaxis in surgery:* **Adults:** 1 g 1 hr prior to surgery; dosage may be repeated for 2 more days if required. *In renal impairment:* **Initial,** 7.5 mg/kg given **IV or IM; then,** follow schedule provided by manufacturer.

NURSING CONSIDERATIONS

See *Nursing Considerations* for *Cephalosporins*, p. 134.

Administration/Storage

1. If 2 g is required IM, half the dose should be given in different large muscle masses.

2. For IV bolus, cefonicid should be given slowly over 3–5 min either through IV tubing or directly, by the physician.

3. For IV infusion, reconstitute in 50–100 ml of appropriate diluent (see package insert). Solutions are stable for 24 hr at room temperature and 72 hr if refrigerated.

Cefoperazone sodium
(sef-oh-**PER**-ah-zohn)
Cefobid, Cefobine ✿ (Rx)

See also *Anti-Infectives*, p. 80, and *Cephalosporins*, p. 132.

Classification: Antibiotic, third-generation cephalosporin.

Action/Kinetics: Peak serum levels: 73–153 mcg/ml. **t½:** 102–156 min. Approximately 30% excreted unchanged in the urine.

Uses: Infections of skin, skin structures, urinary tract, and respiratory tract. Intra-abdominal infections including peritonitis. Bacterial septicemia, pelvic inflammatory disease, endometritis, other infections of the female genital tract.

Special Concerns: Pregnancy category: B. Use with caution in hepatic disease or biliary obstruction. Safety and effectiveness have not been determined in children.

Additional Side Effects: Hypoprothrombinemia resulting in bleeding and/or bruising.

Additional Drug Interaction:
Concomitant use with ethanol may cause an Antabuse-like reaction.

Dosage: IM, IV. Adult, usual: 2–4 g daily in divided doses q 12 hr (up to 12–16 g daily has been used in severe infections or for less sensitive organisms). **Note:** This drug is significantly excreted in the bile; thus, the daily dose should not exceed 4 g in hepatic disease or biliary obstruction.

NURSING CONSIDERATIONS

See also *Nursing Considerations* for *Cephalosporins,* p. 134.

Administration/Storage

1. Following reconstitution, the solution should be allowed to stand for dissipation of any foaming and to determine if complete solubilization has occurred. Vigorous shaking may be necessary to dissolve higher concentrations.
2. Reconstituted drug may be frozen; however, after thawing, any unused portion should be discarded.
3. The unreconstituted powder should be protected from light and stored in the refrigerator.
4. If used for neonates, cefoperazone should not be reconstituted with diluents containing benzyl alcohol.

Assessment

1. Obtain complete nursing history and assess for bruising, hematuria, black stools, or other evidence of bleeding.
2. If client receiving treatment for skin lesions, inspect lesions closely and note size, location, and extent of involvement.
3. Assess for any evidence/history of excessive use of alcohol.

Client/Family Teaching

1. Avoid ingesting alcohol and any medications containing alcohol for 72 hr after the last dose. An Antabuse-like reaction may occur with the ingestion of alcohol.
2. Review goals of therapy, note client/family understanding of infection for which client is being treated.
3. Explain the importance of reporting any evidence of bruising or bleeding immediately.

Evaluation: Evaluate client for:
- Decrease in the size and number of skin lesions
- Evidence of improved WBC and culture reports
- Resolution of S&S of infection

Ceforanide

(seh-**FOR**-ah-nyd)
Precef (Rx)

See also *Anti-Infectives,* p. 80, and *Cephalosporins,* p. 132.

Classification: Antibiotic, second-generation cephalosporin.

Action/Kinetics: $t^{1}/_{2}$: 2.5–3.5 hr. Over 80% is excreted unchanged in the urine.

Uses: Infections of the lower respiratory tract, urinary tract, bones, joints, skin, and skin structures. Endocarditis, prophylaxis in surgery, septicemia.

Special Concerns: Pregnancy category: B. Safety and effectiveness in children less than 1 year of age have not been determined.

Additional Side Effect: Elevated CPK following IM use.

C

Dosage: IM, IV. Adults: 0.5–1 g q 12 hr; **pediatric:** 20–40 mg/kg daily in equally divided doses q 12 hr. *Prophylaxis in surgery:* 0.5–1 g 60 min before surgery; may be repeated for 2 days after surgery. For all uses, dosage should be reduced in renal impairment.

NURSING CONSIDERATIONS

See *Nursing Considerations* for *Cephalosporins,* p. 134.

Administration/Storage

1. IM injections should be made into a deep muscle mass.
2. Ceforanide should be used IV in serious or life-threatening infections, such as septicemia.
3. Drug should be administered over 3–5 min if given by direct IV injection or over 30 min if IV infusion is used.

Evalation: Evaluate client for improvement in baseline lab data and symptoms of infection.

Cefotaxime sodium
(sef-oh-**TAX**-eem)
Claforan (Rx)

See also *Anti-Infectives,* p. 80, and *Cephalosporins,* p. 132.

Classification: Antibiotic, third-generation cephalosporin.

Action/Kinetics: Treatment should be continued for a minimum of 10 days for group A beta-hemolytic streptococcal infections to minimize the risk of glomerulonephritis or rheumatic fever. The IV route is preferable for clients with severe or life-threatening infections; for clients after surgery; or for those manifesting malnutrition, trauma, malignancy, heart failure, or diabetes, especially if shock is present or possible. $t^{1}/_{2}$: 1 hr. From 20%–36% is excreted unchanged in the urine.

Uses: Infections of the GU tract, lower respiratory tract (including pneumonia), skin, skin structures, bones, joints, and CNS (including ventriculitis and meningitis). Intra-abdominal infections (including peritonitis), gynecologic infections (including endometritis, pelvic cellulitis, pelvic inflammatory disease), septicemia, bacteremia, and prophylaxis in surgery. Used with aminoglycosides for gram-positive or gram-negative sepsis where the causative agent has not been identified.

Special Concerns: Pregnancy category: B.

Dosage: IV, IM. Adults. *Uncomplicated infections:* 1 g q 12 hr. *Moderate to severe infections:* 1–2 g q 8 hr. *Septicemia:* **IV,** 2 g q 6–8 hr. *Life-threatening infections:* **IV,** 2 g q 4 hr up to 12 g daily. *Gonorrhea:* **IM,** single dose of 1 g. *Preoperative prophylaxis:* 1 g 30–90 min prior to surgery. *Cesarean section:* **IV,** 1 g when the umbilical cord is clamped; **then,** give 1 g 6 and 12 hr after the first dose. **Pediatric, 1 month to 12 years, IM, IV:** 50–180 mg/kg daily in 4–6 divided doses; **1–4 weeks, IV:** 50 mg/kg q 8 hr; **0–1 week, IV:** 50 mg/kg q 12 hr. **Note:** Use adult dose in children 50 kg or over.

NURSING CONSIDERATIONS

See also *Nursing Considerations* for *Cephalosporins,* p. 134.

Administration/Storage

1. Cefotaxime should not be mixed with aminoglycosides

for continuous IV infusion. If they are to be given to the same client, each should be given separately.

2. Cefotaxime is maximally stable at a pH of 5–7; solutions should not be prepared with diluents having a pH greater than 7.5 (e.g., sodium bicarbonate injection).

3. Dry cefotaxime should be stored below 30°C and should be protected from excess heat and light to prevent darkening.

4. Add recommended amount of diluent, shake to dissolve, and observe for particles or discoloration of solution. Do not administer if particles are present or if solution is discolored. The normal color of solution ranges from light yellow to amber.

5. For IM use, reconstitute with sterile water for injection or bacteriostatic water for injection. Inject deeply into large muscle. Divide doses of 2 g and administer into different sites.

6. For intermittent IV administration, 1 or 2 g cefotaxime should be mixed with 10 ml sterile water for injection and administered over 3–5 min.

7. Discontinue IV administration of other solutions during administration of cefotaxime.

8. After reconstitution, the drug remains stable for 24 hr at room temperature, 5 days refrigerated, and 13 weeks frozen. Thaw frozen samples at room temperature before use. Do not refreeze unused portions.

9. Anticipate reduced dosage in clients with impaired renal function.

Assessment

1. For clients receiving therapy for joint infections, carefully assess the extent of their range of motion and freedom of movement.

2. In clients with gynecologic infections, determine how long symptoms have been evident and how extensive the infection is prior to treatment.

3. Obtain appropriate lab studies prior to initiating therapy.

Interventions

1. Maintain careful documentation of the type and extent of infection and subjective complaints.

2. Monitor and record intake and output.

Client/Family Teaching

1. Review the drugs being prescribed, their side effects, and the expected outcome of therapy.

2. Teach the person administering the drug the appropriate technique for administration and storage.

3. Monitor and record intake and output and report any reduction in urinary output to the physician.

4. Persistent diarrhea should be reported to the physician.

5. Reinforce the need to complete the course of therapy as prescribed despite feeling better.

6. Avoid alcohol in any form as a disulfiram-type reaction may occur.

Evaluation

1. Inspect site of injections for pain and redness. IM administration of these medications may cause thrombophlebitis.

2. Review lab data. Note any evidence of resistance to anti-infective drug therapy.
3. Note client reports of symptomatic improvement.

Cefotetan disodium
(sef-oh-**TEE**-tan)
Cefotan (Rx)

See also *Anti-Infectives,* p. 80, and *Cephalosporins,* p. 132.

Classification: Antibiotic, third-generation cephalosporin.

Action/Kinetics: Administered parenterally only. $t^{1/2}$: 3–4.6 hr. From 50%–80% is excreted unchanged in the urine.

Uses: Infections of the urinary tract, lower respiratory tract, skin and skin structures, bones, and joints. Also gynecologic and intra-abdominal infections. Prophylaxis of postoperative infections (e.g., due to abdominal or vaginal hysterectomy, transurethral surgery, GI or biliary tract surgery, cesarean section).

Special Concerns: Pregnancy category: B. Safety and effectiveness have not been determined in children.

Additional Side Effects: Concomitant use with ethanol produces a disulfiram-type reaction and hypotension.

Additional Laboratory Test Interference: The drug may affect measurement of creatinine levels by the Jaffe reaction.

Dosage: Adults, usual IV or IM: 1–2 g q 12 hr for 5–10 days. *Urinary tract infections,* **IV, IM:** Either 0.5 g q 12 hr, or 1–2 g q 12–24 hr. *Severe infections,* **IV:** 2 g q 12 hr. *Life-threatening infections,* **IV:** 3 g q 12 hr. *Prophylaxis of postoperative infection,* **IV:** 1–2 g 30–60 min prior to surgery.

NURSING CONSIDERATIONS

See also *Nursing Considerations* for *Cephalosporins,* p. 134.

Administration/Storage

1. Cefotetan disodium must be administered parenterally, because it is not absorbed from the GI tract.
2. IM injections should be made well within a large muscle (e.g., the gluteus maximus).
3. The IV route is preferred for clients with bacterial septicemia, bacteremia, or other severe or life-threatening infections. The IV route is also preferred for poor-risk clients as the result of malnutrition, surgery, diabetes, trauma, heart failure, malignancy, or if shock is present or impending.
4. Intermittent IV administration may be completed over 3–5 min following reconstitution in sterile water for injection.
5. For IM use, reconstitute with sterile water for injection, normal saline, bacteriostatic water for injection, or 0.5%–1% lidocaine HCl.
6. Reconstituted solutions maintain potency for 24 hr at room temperature, for 96 hr if refrigerated, and for 1 week if frozen.
7. Cefotetan should not be mixed with solutions containing aminoglycosides.
8. Dosage should be reduced in impaired renal function and depends on creatinine clearance.

Assessment

1. Assess for any evidence or history of excessive use of alcohol.
2. Obtain baseline coagulation studies and monitor during therapy as drug may cause hypoprothrombinemia.
3. Assess need for prophylactic vitamin K administration.

Client/Family Teaching

1. Avoid alcohol ingestion during and for 72 hr after cefotetan disodium therapy.
2. Report any side effects, such as diarrhea, bruising/bleeding, or decreased urine output, to the physician.

Cefoxitin sodium

(seh-**FOX**-ih-tin)
Mefoxin (Rx)

See also *Anti-Infectives*, p. 80, and *Cephalosporins*, p. 132.

Classification: Antibiotic, second-generation cephalosporin.

Action/Kinetics: Broad-spectrum cephalosporin that is penicillinase- and cephalosporinase-resistant and is stable in the presence of beta-lactamases. **Peak serum concentration: IM,** 20–30 min. $t^{1/2}$: **IM, IV,** 41–65 min; 85% of drug excreted unchanged in urine after 6 hr.

Uses: Infections of the urinary tract (including gonorrhea), bones, joints, lower respiratory tract (including lung abscesses and pneumonia), skin, and skin structures. Intra-abdominal infections (including intra-abdominal abscesses and peritonitis), gynecologic infections (including pelvic inflammatory disease, pelvic cellulitis, and endometritis), septicemia, and prophylaxis in surgery. **Note:** Many gram-negative infections resistant to certain cephalosporins and penicillins respond to cefoxitin.

Special Concerns: Pregnancy category: B.

Additional Side Effects: Higher doses have caused increased incidence of eosinophilia and increased AST levels in children over 3 months of age.

Additional Laboratory Test Interference: High concentrations may interfere with the measurement of creatinine by the Jaffe method.

Dosage: IM, IV. Adults. *Uncomplicated infections (cutaneous, pneumonia, urinary tract):* **IV, IM,** 1 g q 6–8 hr. *Severe infections:* **IV,** 1 g q 4 hr or 2 g q 6–8 hr. *Gas gangrene:* **IV,** 2 g q 4 hr or 3 g q 6 hr. *Gonorrhea:* 2 g IM with 1 g probenecid PO. *Prophylaxis in surgery:* **IV, IM,** 2 g 30–60 min before surgery followed by 2 g q 6 hr after first dose for 24 hr only (72 hr for prosthetic arthroplasty). *Cesarean section, prophylaxis:* 2 g **IV** when cord is clamped; **then,** give two additional doses IV or IM 4 and 8 hr later. Subsequent doses may be given q 6 hr for no more than 1 day. *Transurethral prostatectomy, prophylaxis:* 1 g before surgery; **then,** 1 g q 8 hr for up to 5 days. *Impaired renal function:* **Initial,** 1–2 g; **then,** follow maintenance schedule provided by manufacturer. **Children over 3 months:** 80–160 mg/kg daily in 4–6 divided doses. Total daily dosage should not exceed 12 g. *Prophylaxis:* 30–40 mg/kg q 6 hr.

NURSING CONSIDERATIONS

See also *Nursing Considerations for Cephalosporins,* p. 134.

C

Administration/Storage

1. Do not mix with other antibiotics during administration.
2. Reconstituted solutions are stable for 24 hr at room temperature, 1 week in the refrigerator, and 26 weeks when frozen.
3. Store drug vials below 30°C.
4. Reconstituted solutions are white to light amber. Color does not affect potency. Consult pharmacist if unsure of drug potency.
5. For IM injections, lidocaine hydrochloride 0.05% (without epinephrine) may be used as diluent, by physician's order, to reduce pain at injection site.
6. Do not administer cefoxitin rapidly, because it is irritating to veins.

Interventions

1. Monitor intake and output. Upon noting any significant reduction in urinary output, withhold medication, and report to physician.
2. Assess site of infusion for pain and redness, because medication can cause thrombophlebitis.

Ceftazidime

(sef-**TAY**-zih-deem)

Fortaz, Tazicef, Tazidime (Rx)

See also *Anti-Infectives*, p. 80, and *Cephalosporins*, p. 132.

Classification: Antibiotic, third-generation cephalosporin.

Action/Kinetics: Only for IM or IV use. **t½:** 2–3 hr. From 80%–90% is excreted unchanged in the urine.

Uses: Bacterial septicemia. Infections of the lower respiratory tract, skin and skin structures, bones and joints, CNS (including meningitis), and urinary tract. Also, intra-abdominal (including peritonitis) and gynecologic infections (including endometritis, pelvic cellulitis). Use with aminoglycosides, clindamycin, or vancomycin in severe or life-threatening infections or in the immunocompromised client.

Special Concerns: Pregnancy category: B. A sodium carbonate formulation should be used if the drug is indicated for children less than 12 years of age.

Dosage: IM, IV. Adults, usual: 1 g q 8–12 hr. *Urinary tract infections, uncomplicated,* **IM, IV:** 0.25 g q 12 hr. *Urinary tract infections, complicated,* **IM, IV:** 0.5 g q 8–12 hr. *Uncomplicated pneumonia, skin and skin structure infections,* **IM, IV:** 0.5–1 g q 8 hr. *Bone and joint infections,* **IV:** 2 g q 12 hr. *Serious gynecologic or intra-abdominal infections, meningitis, severe or life-threatening infections (especially in immunocompromised clients):* **IV:** 2 g q 8 hr. *Pseudomonal lung infections in cystic fibrosis clients:* **IV:** 30–50 mg/kg q 8 hr, not to exceed 6 g/day. **Neonates, 0–4 weeks, IV:** 30 mg/kg q 12 hr. **Infants and children, 1 month to 12 years, IV:** 30–50 mg/kg q 8 hr not to exceed 6 g/day.

NURSING CONSIDERATIONS

See also *Nursing Considerations* for *Cephalosporins*, p. 134.

Administration/Storage

1. Ceftazidime must be administered parenterally, because it is not absorbed from the GI tract.
2. If administering IM, use large muscle mass and inject deeply.
3. The IV route is preferred for clients with bacterial septicemia, peritonitis, bacterial men-

ingitis, or other severe or life-threatening infections. Also, IV should be used for clients considered to be poor risks due to malnutrition, surgery, diabetes, trauma, heart failure, malignancy, or if shock is present or imminent.

4. For direct intermittent IV administration, reconstitute in sterile water for injection and let physician administer over 3–5 min.

5. The drug may be given also via the tubing of an administration set (IVPB) and is compatible with 0.9% sodium chloride injection, Ringer's injection, lactated Ringer's injection, 5% or 10% dextrose injection, M/6 sodium lactate injection, 5% dextrose and 0.225%, 0.45%, or 0.9% sodium chloride injection, 10% invert sugar in water for injection. Sodium bicarbonate injection should not be used for reconstitution.

6. For IM administration, reconstitute in sterile water for injection, bacteriostatic water for injection, or 0.5%–1% lidocaine HCl injection.

7. Ceftazidime should not be added to solutions containing aminoglycosides.

8. Dosage must be reduced in clients with impaired renal function (see package insert).

Ceftizoxime sodium
(sef-tih-**ZOX**-eem)
Cefizox (Rx)

See also *Anti-Infectives,* p. 80, and *Cephalosporins,* p. 132.

Classification: Antibiotic, third-generation cephalosporin.

Action/Kinetics: t½: Approximately 1–2 hr. Approximately 80% excreted unchanged in the urine.

Uses: Infections of the urinary tract, lower respiratory tract, skin, skin structures, bones, and joints. Intra-abdominal infections, septicemia, meningitis (caused by *Hemophilus influenzae* or *Streptococcus pneumoniae),* gonorrhea (including uncomplicated cervical and urethral gonorrhea caused by *Neisseria*).

Special Concerns: Pregnancy category: B.

Additional Side Effects: Transient increased levels of eosinophils, AST, ALT, and CPK have been seen in children over 6 months of age.

Dosage: IM, IV. Adults. *Uncomplicated urinary tract and other infections:* 0.5 g q 12 hr. *Severe or resistant infections:* 1 g q 8 hr or 2 g q 8–12 hr. *Life-threatening infections:* Up to 3–4 g q 8 hr **IV**. *Uncomplicated gonorrhea:* 1 g as a single dose **IM. Pediatric, over 6 months:** 50 mg/kg q 6–8 hr up to 200 mg/kg daily (not to exceed the maximum adult dose). *Impaired renal function:* **Initial, IM, IV** 0.5–1 g; **then,** use maintenance schedule in package insert.

NURSING CONSIDERATIONS

See *Nursing Considerations* for *Cephalosporins,* p. 134.

Administration/Storage

1. For IM doses of 2 g, divide the dose equally and give in different large muscle masses.

2. For direct IV administration, give slowly over 3–5 min.

3. Reconstituted solutions are stable at room temperature for 8 hr and, if refrigerated, for 48 hr.

Ceftriaxone sodium

[sef-try-**AX**-ohn]

Rocephin (Rx)

See also *Anti-Infectives,* p. 80, and *Cephalosporins,* p. 132.

Classification: Antibiotic, third-generation cephalosporin.

Action/Kinetics: t½: Approximately 6–8 hr. Significantly protein bound. One-third to two-thirds excreted unchanged in the urine.

Uses: Infections of the lower respiratory tract, urinary tract, skin, skin structures, bones, joints, abdomen. Also, uncomplicated gonorrhea (cervical, urethral, rectal) including both penicillinase- and nonpenicillinase-producing strains of *Neisseria gonorrhoeae* and pharyngeal gonorrhea caused by nonpenicillinase-producing strains of *N. gonorrhoeae*. Pelvic inflammatory disease, meningitis, prophylaxis of infections in surgery, bacterial septicemia. *Investigational:* Neurologic complications, arthritis, and carditis associated with Lyme disease (infection caused by *Borrelia burgdorferi*) in clients refractory to penicillin G.

Special Concerns: Pregnancy category: B.

Additional Side Effects: Increase in serum creatinine, presence of casts in the urine, alteration of prothrombin times (rare).

Dosage: IV, IM. Adults: usual, 1–2 g daily in single or divided doses q 12 hr, not to exceed 4 g/day. Therapy is maintained for 4–14 days, depending on the infection. **Pediatric:** *Other than meningitis:* 50–75 mg/kg/day not to exceed total daily dose of 2 g given in divided doses q 12 hr. *Meningitis:* 100 mg/kg/day, not to exceed total daily dose of 4 g given in divided doses q 12 hr. A loading dose of 75 mg/kg may be used. *Prophylaxis of infection in surgery:* 1 g 30–120 min prior to surgery. *Uncomplicated gonorrhea:* **IM, Adults:** 250 mg as a single dose plus doxycycline. *Pharyngeal gonorrhea due to nonpenicillinase-producing strains of N. gonorrhoeae:* 250 mg as a single IM dose. *Gonococcal infections in children,* **less than 45 kg:** 125 mg given once. **Infants:** 25–50 mg/kg daily IV or IM in a single daily dose. *Acute inflammatory disease:* 250 mg IM plus doxycycline or tetracycline. *Lyme disease:* **IV,** 2–4 g daily for 14 days. Dosage adjustment is not required for renal or hepatic impairment; however, monitor blood levels in dialysis clients.

NURSING CONSIDERATIONS

See *Nursing Considerations* for *Cephalosporins,* p. 134.

Administration/Storage

1. IM injections should be deep into the body of a large muscle.
2. IV injections should be by infusing concentrations of 10–40 mg/ml.
3. The drug should not be mixed with other antibiotics.
4. Stability of solutions for IM or IV use varies depending on the diluent used; the package insert should be checked carefully.
5. Dosage should be maintained for at least 2 days after symptoms of infection have disappeared (usual course of therapy is 4–14 days, although complicated infections may require longer therapy).

6. Dosage should be continued for at least 10 days when treating *Streptococcus pyogenes* infections.

Assessment

1. Note if client has any history of GI disease, especially colitis, because drug should be used cautiously in this setting.
2. Obtain baseline coagulation studies and monitor as drug may alter prothrombin times.

Cefuroxime axetil
(sef-your-**OX**-eem)
Ceftin (Rx)

Cefuroxime sodium
(se-fyour-**OX**-eem)
Kefurox, Zinacef, Zinnat✤ (Rx)

See also *Anti-Infectives*, p. 80, and *Cephalosporins*, p. 132.

Classification: Antibiotic, second-generation cephalosporin.

Action/Kinetics: Cefuroxime axetil is used orally, whereas cefuroxime sodium is used either IM or IV. **IM, IV: t½:** 1–2 hr; 66%–100% is excreted unchanged in the urine.

Uses: PO. Pharyngitis, tonsillitis, otitis media, bronchitis, urinary tract infections, skin and skin structure infections. **IM, IV.** Infections of the urinary tract, lower respiratory tract (including pneumonia), skin and skin structures, bones joints. Septicemia, meningitis, gonorrhea. Prophylaxis in surgery.

Special Concerns: Pregnancy category: B.

Additional Side Effects: Decrease in hemoglobin and hematocrit.

Additional Laboratory Test In-terference: False (−) reaction in the ferricyanide test for blood glucose.

Dosage: Tablets. Adults and children over 12 years: 250 mg q 12 hr, up to 500 mg q 12 hr for severe infections or infections due to less susceptible organisms. *Uncomplicated urinary tract infections:* 125–250 mg q 12 hr. **Infants and children less than 12 years:** 125 mg b.i.d. *Otitis media:* **Less than 2 years:** 125 mg b.i.d.; **Over 2 years:** 250 mg b.i.d. **IM, IV. Adults.** *Uncomplicated infections, including urinary tract, pneumonia, disseminated gonococcal, skin and skin structure:* 0.75 g q 8 hr. *Severe, complicated, or life-threatening infections; bone and joint infections:* 1.5 g q 6–8 hr. *Bacterial meningitis:* Up to 3 g q 8 hr. *Gonorrhea (uncomplicated):* 1.5 g as a single IM dose. *Prophylaxis in surgery:* **IV,** 1.5 g 30–60 min before surgery; if procedure is of long duration, **IM, IV,** 0.75 g q 8 hr. *Open heart surgery, prophylaxis:* **IV,** 1.5 g when anesthesia is initiated; **then,** 1.5 g q 12 hr for a total of 6 g. **Pediatric, over 3 months.** *Uncomplicated infections:* 50–100 mg/kg daily in divided doses q 6–8 hr (not to exceed adult dose for severe infections). *Bacterial meningitis:* **Initial, IV,** 200–240 mg/kg daily in divided doses q 6–8 hr; **then,** after clinical improvement, 100 mg/kg daily **IV.** *Bone and joint infections:* 150 mg/kg daily in divided doses q 8 hr (not to exceed adult dose).

NURSING CONSIDERATIONS

See also *Nursing Considerations* for *Cephalosporins*, p. 134.

Administration/Storage

1. Use IV route for severe or life-threatening infections such as

septicemia or in poor-risk clients, especially in presence of shock.

2. For direct IV injection, give over 3–5 min; the drug may also be given through the tubing by which other IV solutions are being administered.

3. For IM use, inject deep into a large muscle mass.

4. Prior to reconstitution, protect the drug from light. The powder and reconstituted drug may darken without affecting potency.

5. Cefuroxime sodium should not be added to solutions of aminoglycosides; if both drugs are required, each should be given separately to the client.

6. Cefuroxime axetil for oral use is available only in tablet form. Crushed tablets (even mixed with food) have a strong, persistent, bitter taste; alternative therapy may be required in children who cannot ingest cefuroxime axetil reliably.

7. Therapy should be continued for at least 10 days in infections due to *Streptococcus pyogenes*.

8. Dosage in adults and children should be reduced in impaired renal function.

Assessment: Assess for any clinical and laboratory evidence of anemia.

Client/Family Teaching

1. Report signs of anemia to physician immediately.

2. Take tablets with food to enhance the absorption of the oral medication.

3. Crushed cefuroxime axetil tablets have a distinctive bitter taste even when hidden in foods. If unable to tolerate taste, notify physician so alternative drug therapy may be instituted.

Evaluation

1. Assess client for evidence of improvement in S&S of infection.

2. Review hemoglobin and hematocrit to ascertain if anemia is present.

Cephalexin hydrochloride monohydrate
(sef-ah-**LEX**-in)
Keftab (Rx)

Cephalexin monohydrate
(sef-ah-**LEX**-in)
Apo-Cephalex✽, Ceporex✽, Keflet, Keflex, Novo–Lexin✽, Nu-Cephalex✽ (Rx)

See also *Anti-Infectives,* p. 80, and *Cephalosporins,* p. 132.

Classification: Antibiotic, first-generation cephalosporin.

Action/Kinetics: Peak serum levels: PO, 9–39 mcg/ml after 1 hr. **t½, PO:** 30–72 min. Absorption delayed in children. The HCl monohydrate does not require conversion in the stomach before absorption. Ninety percent of drug excreted unchanged in urine within 8 hr.

Uses: Infections of the respiratory tract, skin, soft tissues, bones, and GU tract (including acute prostatitis). Otitis media.

Special Concerns: Pregnancy category: B. Safety and effectiveness of the HCl monohydrate have not been determined in children.

Additional Side Effects: Nephrotoxicity, cholestatic jaundice.

Dosage: Capsules, Oral Suspension, Tablets. Adult: Usual, 250 mg q 6 hr up to 4 g daily. *Infections of skin and skin structures, streptococcal pharyngitis, uncomplicated cystitis, over 15 years:* 500 mg q 12 hr. **Pediatric:** *Monohydrate,* 25–50 mg/kg daily in four equally divided doses. For streptococcal pharyngitis in children over 1 year and for skin and skin structure infections, the total daily dose should be divided and given q 12 hr. *Otitis media:* 75–100 mg/kg/day in four divided doses.

NURSING CONSIDERATIONS

See *Nursing Considerations* for *Cephalosporins,* p. 134.

Administration/Storage

1. After reconstitution, the drug should be refrigerated and the unused portion discarded after 14 days.
2. Treatment should be continued for at least 10 days for beta-hemolytic streptococcal infections.
3. Dosage may have to be reduced in clients with impaired renal function or increased for severe infections. Action of drug can be prolonged by the concurrent administration of oral probenecid.

Cephalothin sodium

(sef-**AL**-oh-thin)
Ceporacin✤, Keflin✤, Keflin Neutral (Rx)

See also *Anti-Infectives,* p. 80, and *Cephalosporins,* p. 132.

Classification: Antibiotic, first-generation cephalosporin.

Action/Kinetics: Poorly absorbed from GI tract; must be given parenterally. **Peak serum levels: IM,** 6–21 mcg/ml after 30 min. **t½ IM, IV:** 30–60 min. 55%–90% excreted unchanged in urine. Its low nephrotoxicity, ototoxicity, and neurotoxicity make the drug suitable for clients with impaired renal function.

Uses: Infections of the GU tract, GI tract, respiratory tract, skin, soft tissues, bones, and joints. Meningitis, septicemia (including endocarditis), and prophylaxis in surgery.

Special Concerns: Pregnancy category: B.

Additional Side Effects: Nephrotoxicity, severe phlebitis, hemolytic anemia, increased prothrombin time.

Laboratory Test Interferences: Large doses may produce false + results in urinary protein tests that use sulfosalicylic acid.

Dosage: Deep IM, IV. Adults: usual, 0.5–1 g q 4–6 hr. *Urinary tract infections, uncomplicated pneumonia, furunculosis with cellulitis:* 0.5 g q 6 hr (for severe infections increase the dose to 1 g or give 0.5 g q 4 hr). *Life-threatening infections:* 2 g q 4 hr (up to 12 g daily for bacteremia, septicemia). *Preoperative and during surgery:* 1–2 g 30–60 min prior to surgery and during surgery. *Postoperative:* 1–2 g q 6 hr for 24 hr. *Impaired renal function:* **Initial:** 1–2 g; **then,** use manufacturer's guidelines for maintenance doses. **Pediatric:** 80–160 mg/kg daily in divided doses. *Prophylaxis in surgery:* 20–30 mg/kg using adult schedule.

NURSING CONSIDERATIONS

See *Nursing Considerations* for *Cephalosporins,* p. 134.

Administration/Storage

1. Dilute according to directions on package insert.
2. Discard reconstituted solution after 12 hr at room temperature and after 96 hr when refrigerated.
3. Dissolve precipitate by warming vial in hand and shaking. Do not overheat.
4. Replace medication and IV solution after 24 hr.
5. For direct IV administration, add a small needle into larger veins.
6. Alter dose and follow manufacturer's guidelines for clients with impaired renal function.

serious or life-threatening infections. *Preoperatively:* 1–2 g 30–60 min before surgery. *During surgery:* 1–2 g. *Postoperatively:* 1–2 g q 6 hr for 24 hr. **Pediatric, over 3 months:** 40–80 mg/kg daily in four equally divided doses. In clients with impaired renal function, a dose of 7.5–15 mg/kg q 12 hr may be adequate.

NURSING CONSIDERATIONS

See *Nursing Considerations* for *Cephalosporins,* p. 134.

Administration/Storage: Discard after 12 hr when kept at room temperature and after 10 days when refrigerated at 4°C.

Cephapirin sodium
(sef-ah-**PIE**-rin)
Cefadyl (Rx)

See also *Anti-Infectives,* p. 80, and *Cephalosporins,* p. 132.

Classification: Antibiotic, first-generation cephalosporin.

Action/Kinetics: Peak serum levels: IM, 9.4 mcg/ml after 30 min. **t½, IM, IV:** 21–47 min. Virtually entirely excreted in the urine within 6 hr, with 41%–60% excreted unchanged.

Uses: Infections of the respiratory tract, urinary tract, skin, and skin structures. Septicemia, endocarditis, osteomyelitis, prophylaxis in surgery.

Special Concerns: Pregnancy category: B. Before use in children less than 3 months, assess benefits versus risks.

Additional Side Effects: Increase in serum bilirubin.

Dosage: IM, IV only. Adults: 0.5–1 g q 4–6 hr up to 12 g daily for

Cephradine
(**SEF**-rah-deen)
Anspor, Velosef (Rx)

See also *Anti-Infectives,* p. 80, and *Cephalosporins,* p. 132.

Classification: Antibiotic, first-generation cephalosporin.

Action/Kinetics: Similar to that of cephalexin. Rapidly absorbed from GI tract or IM injection site (30 min–2 hr); 60%–90% excreted after 6 hr. **Peak serum levels: PO,** 8–24 mcg/ml after 30–60 min; **IM,** 5.6–13.6 mcg/ml after 1–2 hr. **t½:** 42–120 min; 80%–95% excreted in urine unchanged.

Uses: Infections of the respiratory tract (including lobar pneumonia, tonsillitis, pharyngitis), urinary tract (including prostatitis and enterococcal infections), skin, skin structures, and bone. Otitis media, septicemia, prophylaxis in surgery, following cesarean section to prevent infection. In severe infections, therapy is usually initiated parenterally.

Special Concerns: Pregnancy category: B. Safe use during pregnancy has not been established. Safe use of the parenteral form in infants under 1 month of age and the oral form in children less than 9 months of age have not been established.

Additional Laboratory Test Interference: False + reactions using sulfosalicylic acid for urinary protein tests. High concentrations may interfere with measurement of creatinine by the Jaffe method.

Dosage: Capsules, Oral Suspension. Adults, usual, *Skin and skin structures, respiratory tract infections:* 250 mg q 6 hr or 500 mg q 12 hr. *Lobar pneumonia:* 500 mg q 6 hr or 1 g q 12 hr. *Uncomplicated urinary tract infections:* **Usual,** 500 mg q 12 hr; *more serious infections and prostatitis:* 500 mg q 6 hr or 1 g q 12 hr (severe, chronic infections may require up to 1 g q 6 hr). **Pediatric, over 9 months:** 25–50 mg/kg daily in equally divided doses q 6–12 hr (75–100 mg/kg/day for otitis media). **Deep IM, IV. Adults:** 2–4 g daily in equally divided doses q.i.d. *Surgical prophylaxis:* 1 g 30–90 min before surgery; **then,** 1 g q 4–6 hr for 1–2 doses (or up to 24 hr postoperatively). *Cesarean section, prophylaxis:* **IV,** 1 g when the umbilical cord is clamped; **then,** give two additional 1 g doses **IV or IM** 6 and 12 hr after the initial dose. **Pediatric, over 1 year:** 50–100 mg/kg/day in equally divided doses q.i.d.

NURSING CONSIDERATIONS

See also *Nursing Considerations* for *Cephalosporins,* p. 134.

Administration/Storage

1. Dilute according to directions on package insert.

2. Do not mix with lactated Ringer's solution.
3. Discard reconstituted solution after 10 hr at room temperature and after 48 hr when refrigerated at 5°C.
4. A slightly yellow solution may be retained for use; if unsure of solution potency, consult with pharmacist.
5. Be especially careful to inject into muscle, because sterile abscesses from accidental subcutaneous injection have occurred.
6. Before and after reconstitution, protect from excessive heat and light.
7. Replace medication infusion solution during prolonged IV administration every 10 hr.
8. Administer PO medication without regard to meals.
9. Reduce dose in clients with impaired renal function.
10. Rotate and document injection sites carefully.

Evaluation

1. Assess client for improvement in signs and symptoms of infection and lab culture reports.
2. During IM administration, assess injection sites for any evidence of abscess formation.

Chenodiol (Chenodeoxycholic acid)

(kee-noh-**DYE**-ohl)

Chenix (Rx)

Classification: Naturally occurring human bile acid.

Action/Kinetics: Chenodiol, by reducing hepatic synthesis of cholesterol and cholic acid, replaces both cholic and deoxycholic acids in the bile acid pool. This effect helps desaturation of biliary cholesterol and leads to dissolution of radiolucent cholesterol gallstones. The drug is ineffective on calcified gallstones or on radiolucent bile pigment stones. Fifty percent of clients have stone recurrence within 5 years. The drug also increases low-density lipoproteins and inhibits absorption of fluid from the colon. Chenodiol is well absorbed following oral administration. It is metabolized by bacteria in the colon to lithocholic acid, most of which is excreted in the feces.

Uses: Clients with radiolucent cholesterol gallstones in whom surgery is a risk due to age or systemic disease. The drug is ineffective in some clients and has potential liver toxicity. The best results have been seen in thin females with a serum cholesterol not higher than 227 mg/dl and who have a small number of radiolucent cholesterol gallstones.

Contraindications: Known hepatic dysfunction or bile ductal abnormalities. Colon cancer. Pregnancy or in those who may become pregnant (pregnancy category: X).

Special Concerns: Safety and efficacy in lactation and in children have not been established.

Side Effects: Hepatotoxicity including increased ALT in one-third of clients, intrahepatic cholestasis. *GI:* Diarrhea (common), anorexia, constipation, dyspepsia, flatulence, heartburn, cramps, epigastric distress, nausea/vomiting, abdominal pain. *Hematologic:* Decreased white cell count. Chenodiol may contribute to colon cancer in susceptible clients.

Drug Interactions

Antacids, aluminum / ↓ Effect of chenodiol due to ↓ absorption from GI tract
Cholestyramine / See *Antacids*
Clofibrate / ↓ Effect of chenodiol due to ↑ biliary cholesterol secretion
Colestipol / See *Antacids*
Estrogens, oral contraceptives / ↓ Effect of chenodiol due to ↑ biliary cholesterol secretion

Dosage: Tablets. Adults, initial: 250 mg b.i.d. for 2 weeks; **then,** increase by 250 mg weekly until maximum tolerated or recommended dose is reached (13–16 mg/kg/day in 2 divided doses morning and night with milk or food). **Note:** Doses less than 10 mg/kg are usually ineffective and may result in increased risk of cholecystectomy.

NURSING CONSIDERATIONS

Assessment

1. Obtain liver and renal function studies prior to initiating therapy.
2. Take a complete drug history, noting any potential drug interactions.
3. Determine if women in childbearing years are pregnant.

Interventions

1. Obtain periodic liver function tests such as serum aminotransferase levels, serum cholesterol, and monitor for stone dissolution.
2. Note any client complaint of severe, sudden upper quadrant pain that radiates to the shoulder, nonspecific abdominal

pain, nausea or vomiting. Report these symptoms to the physician immediately. These may be symptoms that the client has developed gallstone complications.

3. If the client develops diarrhea, the dose of medication may be reduced temporarily and antidiarrheal agents may be administered.

Client/Family Teaching

1. Advise that the drug may need to be taken for 24 months before gallstones are dissolved.
2. Discuss the likelihood that gallstones may recur even after successful treatment.
3. Pregnancy should be avoided during drug therapy. Oral contraceptives may decrease the effectiveness of chenodiol. Therefore, advise women of childbearing age to practice alternative methods of birth control.
4. Advise women to report to the physician if there is any possibility that conception has occurred.
5. Stress the importance of having periodic liver function tests performed and cholecystograms or gallbladder ultrasonography to evaluate the effectiveness of the drug therapy.
6. Consult with the physician if there is a need to use antacids. Most antacids have an aluminum base that absorbs the drug.
7. Report any incidence of diarrhea. This may be related to the dose of drug and can be relieved by appropriate changes in the dosage.
8. Discuss drug relationship to colon cancer and potential risks.

Evaluation: Evaluate client for:

- A reduction of radiolucent cholesterol gallstones
- Freedom from complications of drug therapy

C

Chloral hydrate

(**KLOH**-ral **HY**-drayt)

Aquachloral Supprettes, Noctec, Novo–Chlorhydrate✽ (C-IV, Rx)

Classification: Nonbarbiturate, nonbenzodiazepine sedative-hypnotic.

Action/Kinetics: Chloral hydrate is metabolized to trichloroethanol, which is the active metabolite causing CNS depression. Chloral hydrate produces only slight hangover effects and is said not to affect REM sleep. High doses lead to severe CNS depression, as well as depression of respiratory and vasomotor centers (hypotension). Both psychologic and physical dependence develop. **Onset:** Within 30 min. **Duration:** 4–8 hr. **t½, trichloroethanol:** 7–10 hr. The drug is readily absorbed from the GI tract and is distributed to all tissues; it passes the placental barrier and appears in breast milk as well. Metabolites excreted by kidney.

Uses: Short-term hypnotic. Daytime sedative and sedation prior to EEG procedures. Preoperative sedative and postoperative as adjunct to analgesics. Prevent or reduce symptoms of alcohol withdrawal.

Contraindications: Marked hepatic or renal impairment, severe cardiac disease, lactation. Drugs should not be given orally to clients with esophagitis, gastritis, or gastric or duodenal ulcer.

Special Concerns: Pregnancy category: C. Use by nursing mothers may cause sedation in the infant. A decrease in dose may be necessary in geriatric clients due to age-related decrease in both hepatic and renal function.

Side Effects: *CNS:* Paradoxical paranoid reactions. Sudden withdrawal in dependent clients may result in "chloral delirium." Sudden intolerance to the drug following prolonged use may result in respiratory depression, hypotension, cardiac effects, and possibly death. *GI:* Nausea, vomiting, diarrhea, bad taste in mouth, gastritis, increased peristalsis. *GU:* Renal damage, decreased urine flow and uric acid excretion. *Miscellaneous:* Skin reactions, hepatic damage, allergic reactions, leukopenia, eosinophilia.

Chronic toxicity is treated by gradual withdrawal and rehabilitative measures such as those used in treatment of the chronic alcoholic. Poisoning by chloral hydrate resembles acute barbiturate intoxication; the same supportive treatment is indicated (see *Barbiturates,* p. 101).

Drug Interactions

Anticoagulants, oral / ↑ Effect of anticoagulants by ↓ plasma protein binding
CNS depressants / Additive CNS depression. Concomitant use may lead to drowsiness, lethargy, stupor, respiratory collapse, coma, or death
Furosemide (IV) / Concomitant use results in diaphoresis, tachycardia, hypertension, flushing

Laboratory Test Interferences: ↑ 17-Hydroxycorticosteroids. Interference with fluorescence tests for catecholamines and copper sulfate test for glucose.

Dosage: Capsules,   Syrup. Adults: *Daytime sedative:* 250 mg t.i.d. after meals. *Preoperative sedative:* 0.5–1.0 g 30 min before surgery. *Hypnotic:* 0.5–1 g 15–30 min before bedtime. **Pediatric:** *Daytime sedative:* 8.3 mg/kg (250 mg/m²) up to a maximum of 500 mg t.i.d. after meals. *Hypnotic:* 50 mg/kg (1.5 g/m²) at bedtime (up to 1 g may be given as a single dose). *Premedication prior to EEG procedures:* 20–25 mg/kg.
    Suppositories, rectal. Adults: *Daytime sedative:* 325 mg t.i.d. *Hypnotic:* 0.5–1 g at bedtime. **Pediatric:** *Daytime sedative:* 8.3 mg/kg (250 mg/m²) t.i.d. *Hypnotic:* 50 mg/kg (1.5 g/m²) at bedtime (up to 1 g as a single dose).

NURSING CONSIDERATIONS

See also *Nursing Considerations* for *Barbiturates,* p. 104.

Administration/Storage

1. PO: give capsules after meals with a full glass of water. Give the syrup with half a glass of juice, water, or ginger ale.
2. Oral syrups have an unpleasant taste, which can be reduced by chilling the syrup before administration.
3. Have emergency drugs and equipment available should the client require supportive, physiologic treatment of acute poisoning.

Assessment

1. Assess client alertness and response to stimuli; document sleep patterns.

2. Note any history of cardiac disease, liver or renal dysfunction.

Interventions

1. Note the level of alertness of the client and compare with the premedication history.
2. Observe client respiratory and cardiac responses. Note any evidence of vasomotor depression and dilatation of cutaneous blood vessels.
3. Periodically perform liver and renal function studies to determine any evidence of impairment.
4. Observe client for psychologic and physical dependence. Symptoms of dependence resemble those of acute alcoholism, but with more severe gastritis. These should be documented and reported.
5. Offer measures to promote comfort and relaxation.
6. Protect client from injury. Assist with ambulation, side rails up, call bell within reach, and night light on at night.

Evaluation: Evaluate client for reports of effective sedation and improved sleep patterns.

Chlorambucil
(klor-**AM**-byou-sill)
Leukeran (Abbreviation: CHL) (Rx)

See also *Antineoplastic Agents,* p. 85, and *Alkylating Agents,* p. 20.

Classification: Antineoplastic, alkylating agent.

Action/Kinetics: Chlorambucil is cell-cycle nonspecific although it is also cytotoxic to nonproliferating cells. The drug forms an unstable ethylenimmonium ion which binds (alkylates) with intracellular substances such as nucleic acids. The cytotoxic effect is due to cross-linking of strands of DNA and RNA and inhibition of protein synthesis. The drug also has immunosuppressant activity. Is rapidly absorbed from the GI tract. **Peak plasma levels:** 1 hr. Plasma $t\frac{1}{2}$: about 60 min. Chlorambucil is 99% bound to plasma proteins, especially albumin. Is extensively metabolized by the liver and at least one metabolite is active. Sixty percent of the drug is excreted through the urine 24 hr after drug administration, and 40% is bound to tissues, including fat.

Uses: Palliation in chronic lymphocytic leukemia, malignant lymphomas (including lymphosarcoma), giant follicular lymphomas, and Hodgkin's disease. *Investigational:* Ovarian and testicular cancer, hairy cell leukemia, polycythemia vera, in combination with prednisone for nephrotic syndrome in adults and children unresponsive to other therapy.

Special Concerns: Pregnancy category: D. Use during lactation only if benefits outweigh risks. Safety and efficacy have not been established in children. The drug is carcinogenic in humans and may be both mutagenic and teratogenic in humans. It also affects fertility.

Additional Side Effects: *Hepatic:* Hepatotoxicity with jaundice. *Pulmonary:* Pulmonary fibrosis, bronchopulmonary dysplasia. *CNS:* Children with nephrotic syndrome have an increased risk of seizures. *Miscellaneous:* Keratitis, drug fever, sterile cystitis, interstitial pneumonia, peripheral neuropathy. Cross-sensitivity (skin rashes) may occur with other alkylating agents. *Symp-*

C

toms of Overdose: Pancytopenia (reversible), ataxia, agitated behavior, clonic-tonic seizures.

Laboratory Test Interference: ↑ Uric acid levels in serum and urine.

Dosage: Tablets: *Leukemia, lymphomas: Individualized* according to response of patient; **Adults, children, initial dose:** 0.1–0.2 mg/kg body weight (or 4–10 mg) daily in single or divided doses for 3–6 weeks; **maintenance:** 0.03–0.1 mg/kg daily depending on blood counts. **Alternative for chronic lymphocytic leukemia: Initial,** 0.4 mg/kg; **then,** repeat this dose every 2 weeks increasing by 0.1 mg/kg until either toxicity or control of condition is observed. *Nephrotic syndrome, immunosuppressant:* **Adults, children,** 0.1–0.2 mg/kg body weight daily for 8–12 weeks.

NURSING CONSIDERATIONS

See also *Nursing Considerations* for *Antineoplastic Agents,* p. 88.

Administration/Storage: *Treatment of Overdose:* General supportive measures. Blood should be carefully monitored; blood transfusions may be required.

Client/Family Teaching

1. The drug should be taken 1 hr before breakfast or 2 hr after the evening meal.
2. Monitor and record intake; 80–96 oz of fluid should be consumed each day.
3. During drug therapy, contraception should be practiced. Advise that drug may affect fertility.
4. Provide a printed list of adverse side effects. Advise that skin rash may be a result of cross-

sensitivity with other alkylating agents and should be reported if present.
5. Stress that drug is carcinogenic and may also be mutagenic and teratogenic. Explain what this means and the associated risks of this form of drug therapy. Stress the importance of practicing birth control during therapy.

Evaluation: Evaluate for a positive tumor response as evidenced by a decrease in tumor size and spread.

Chloramphenicol
(klor-am-**FEN**-ih-kohl)
Chloromycetin (Cream, Kapseals, and Otic), Chloroptic✲, Fenicol✲, Mychel, Nova-Phenicol✲, Novo–Chlorocap✲, Pentamycetin✲ (Rx)

Chloramphenicol ophthalmic
(klor-am-**FEN**-ih-kohl)
AK Chlor, Chloromycetin Ophthalmic, Chloroptic Ophthalmic, Chloroptic S.O.P. Ophthalmic, Ophthochlor, Ophtho-Chloram✲, Pentamycetin✲, Sopamycetin✲ (Rx)

Chloramphenicol palmitate
(klor-am-**FEN**-ih-kohl)
Chloromycetin Palmitate (Rx)

Chloramphenicol sodium succinate
(klor-am-**FEN**-ih-kohl)
Chloromycetin Sodium Succinate, Mychel-S (Rx)

See also *Anti-Infectives,* p. 80.

General Statement: This antibiotic was originally isolated from *Streptomyces venezuellae* and is now produced synthetically. The antibiotic can be extremely toxic (due to protein synthesis inhibition in rapidly proliferating cells, as in bone marrow) and should not be used for trivial infections.

Action/Kinetics: Chloramphenicol inhibits protein synthesis in bacteria by binding to ribosomes (50S subunit, an essential link in the protein synthesis machinery of the cell), thus interfering with peptide bond synthesis. Therapeutic serum concentrations: *peak,* 10–20 mcg/ml; *trough:* 5–10 mcg/ml (less for neonates). **Peak serum concentration: IM,** 2 hr. $t^{1/2}$: 4 hr. Drug is metabolized in the liver; 75%–90% of drug excreted in urine within 24 hr, as parent drug (8%–12%) and inactive metabolites. The drug is mostly bacteriostatic. Chloramphenicol is well absorbed from the GI tract and is distributed to all parts of the body, including CSF, pleural, and ascitic fluids; saliva; milk; and aqueous and vitreous humors.

Uses: *Not to be used for trivial infections, prophylaxis of bacterial infections, or to treat colds, flu, or throat infections.* **Systemic Use.** Treatment of choice for typhoid fever but not for typhoid carrier state. Serious infections caused by *Salmonella, Rickettsia, Chlamydia,* and lymphogranuloma-psittacosis group. Meningitis due to *Hemophilus influenzae.* Brain abscesses due to *Bacteroides fragilis.* Cystic fibrosis anti-infective. Meningococcal or pneumococcal meningitis. **Topical Use.** Otitis externa. Prophylaxis of infection in minor cuts, wounds, skin abrasions, burns; promote healing in superficial infections of the skin. **Ophthalmic Use.** Superficial ocular infections due to *Staphylococcus aureus; Streptococcus* species, including *S. pneumoniae* and beta-hemolytic streptococci; *Escherichia coli, Hemophilus influenzae, Klebsiella* species, *Neiserria* species, *Enterobacter* species, *Moraxella lacunata,* and *Pseudomonas aeruginosa.*

Contraindications: Hypersensitivity to chloramphenicol; pregnancy, especially near term and during labor; nursing mothers. Avoid simultaneous administration of other drugs that may depress bone marrow. Ophthalmically in the presence of dendritic keratitis, vaccinia, varicella, mycobacterial or fungal eye infections, or following removal of a corneal foreign body. Topical products should not be used near or in the eye.

Special Concerns: Use with caution in clients with intermittent porphyria or glucose-6-phosphate dehydrogenase deficiency. Ophthalmic ointments may retard corneal epithelial healing.

Side Effects: *Hematologic* (most serious): Aplastic anemia, thrombocytopenia, granulocytopenia, hemolytic anemia, pancytopenia. *Hematologic studies should be undertaken before and every 2 days during therapy. GI:* Nausea, vomiting, diarrhea, glossitis, stomatitis, unpleasant taste, enterocolitis, pruritus ani. *Allergic:* Fever, skin rashes, angioedema, macular and vesicular rashes, hemorrhages of the skin, intestine, bladder, mouth. Anaphylaxis. *CNS:* Headache, delirium, confusion, mental depression. *Neurologic:* Optic neuritis, peripheral neuritis. *Following topical use:*

Burning, itching, irritation, redness of skin. Hypersensitive clients may exhibit angioneurotic edema, urticaria, vesicular and maculopapular dermatoses. *Miscellaneous:* Superinfection. Jaundice (rare). Herxheimer-like reactions when used for typhoid fever (may be due to release of bacterial endotoxins). *Gray syndrome in infants:* Rapid respiration, ashen gray color, failure to feed, abdominal distention with or without vomiting, progressive pallid cyanosis, vasomotor collapse, death. Can be reversed when drug is discontinued. **Note:** *Neonates should be observed closely, since the drug accumulates in the bloodstream and the infant is thus subject to greater hazards of toxicity.*

Drug Interactions

Acetaminophen / ↑ Effect of chloramphenicol due to ↑ serum levels

Anticoagulants, oral / ↑ Effect of anticoagulants due to ↓ breakdown by liver

Antidiabetics, oral / ↑ Effect of antidiabetics due to ↓ breakdown by liver

Barbiturates / ↑ Effect of barbiturates due to ↓ breakdown by liver

Chlorpropamide / ↑ Effect due to ↓ breakdown by liver

Chymotrypsin / Chloramphenicol will inhibit chymotrypsin

Cyclophosphamide / ↑ Effect of cyclophosphamide due to ↓ breakdown by liver

Dicumarol / ↑ Effect due to ↓ breakdown by liver

Iron preparations / Chloramphenicol ↓ response to iron therapy

Penicillins / Possible ↓ effect of penicillins

Phenobarbital / ↑ Effect due to ↓ breakdown by liver

Phenytoin / ↑ Effect of phenytoin due to ↓ breakdown by liver

Rifampin / ↓ Effect of chloramphenicol due to ↑ breakdown by liver

Tolbutamide / ↑ Effect due to ↓ breakdown by liver

Vitamin B_{12} / ↓ Response to vitamin B_{12} therapy

Dosage: Capsules, Oral Suspension, IV. Chloramphenicol, chloramphenicol palmitate. **Adults:** 50 mg/kg daily in four equally divided doses q 6 hr. Can be increased to 100 mg/kg daily in severe infections, but dosage should be reduced as soon as possible. **Neonates and children with immature metabolic function:** 25 mg/kg daily in divided doses q 12 hr. **Pediatric:** 50–75 mg/kg daily in divided doses q 6 hr (50–100 mg/kg daily in divided doses q 6 hr for meningitis). **Newborns:** 25 mg/kg daily in four divided doses (after 2 weeks of life, up to 50 mg/kg daily can be given in four divided doses). **Neonates, less than 2 kg:** 25 mg/kg once daily. **Neonates, over 2 kg, over 7 days of age:** 50 mg/kg daily q 12 hr in divided doses. **Neonates, over 2 kg, from birth to 7 days of age:** 50 mg/kg once daily. **Note:** Carefully follow dosage for premature and newborn infants less than 2 weeks of age because blood levels differ significantly from those of other age groups.

Chloramphenicol sodium succinate—**IV only**—same dosage as above; switch to **PO** as soon as possible.

Chloramphenicol Ophthalmic Ointment 1%: 0.5-inch ribbon placed in lower conjunctival sac q 3–4 hr for acute infections and b.i.d.–t.i.d. for mild to moderate infections.

Chloramphenicol Ophthalmic Solution 0.5%: 1–2 drops in lower conjunctival sac 2–6 times daily (or more for acute infections).

Chloramphenicol Otic Solution 0.5%: 2–3 drops in ear t.i.d.

Chloramphenicol Topical Cream 1%: Apply 1–4 times daily.

NURSING CONSIDERATIONS

See also *General Nursing Considerations For All Anti-Infectives,* p. 83.

Administration/Storage

1. Administer IV as a 10% solution over at least a 60-sec interval.
2. When used for skin infections, a sterile bandage may be used if necessary.

Assessment

1. Note any history of hypersensitivity to chloramphenicol.
2. If client is a nursing mother, transmission of the drug to breast milk can result in the infant receiving the drug as well. Infants have underdeveloped capacity to metabolize chloramphenicol.
3. Take a complete client history. Clients who are diabetic and taking oral hypoglycemic agents may have to use insulin during treatment with chloramphenicol.
4. Chloramphenicol may produce a false + reaction with Fehling's or Benedict's solutions, both of which contain copper sulfate. In diabetic clients, use Lab-Stix to test the urine or, if available, do finger sticks for enhanced accuracy of glucose determinations.
5. If client is concomitantly receiving drugs that cause bone marrow depression, use of chloramphenicol is contraindicated.
6. Be certain that baseline hematologic studies are completed before drug treatment begins.

Interventions

1. Anticipate reduced dosage in clients with impaired renal function and in newborn infants.
2. Arrange for hematologic studies to be conducted every 2 days to detect early signs of bone marrow depression.
3. Become familiar with drugs that enhance the effects of chloramphenicol and monitor closely for evidence of severe toxicity in clients on concurrent therapy.
4. Client should receive the drug only as necessary; avoid repeated courses of therapy with chloramphenicol because the drug is highly toxic.

Client/Family Teaching

1. The drug should be taken at regularly spaced intervals *around the clock* to be most effective.
2. Chloramphenicol should be taken 1 hr before or 2 hr after meals; however, if GI upset occurs, it can be taken with food.
3. Avoid the use of alcohol during therapy.
4. Review the signs of hypersensitivity, such as rash, and stress the importance of reporting to physician.
5. Report any incidents of vaginal or rectal itching or diarrhea.
6. Report the development of sore throat, unusual fatigue, or

bleeding immediately because drug may need to be discontinued.

7. Ophthalmic solutions may cause blurred vision immediately after instillation; this should clear.

Evaluation

1. Assess client for bone marrow depression characterized by weakness, fatigue, sore throat, and bleeding. Review hematologic studies because discontinuation of the drug may be indicated.

2. Assess for optic neuritis, characterized by bilaterally reduced visual acuity, an indication to discontinue the drug immediately.

3. Assess for peripheral neuritis, characterized by pain and disturbance of sensation, both of which are indications to discontinue the drug immediately.

4. Development of gray syndrome in premature and newborn infants is characterized by rapid respiration, failure to feed, abdominal distention with or without vomiting, loose green stools, progressive cyanosis, and vasomotor collapse. Withhold drug and notify physician if any such symptoms are noted.

5. Assess for toxic and irritative effects, such as nausea, vomiting, unpleasant taste, diarrhea, and perineal irritation following PO administration. Differentiation of drug-induced diarrhea from that caused by a superinfection is critical and may be accomplished by assessment and analysis of all presenting symptoms.

Chlordiazepoxide

(klor-dye-**AYZ**-eh-**POX**-eyed)

Apo-Chlordiazepoxide✿, Libritabs, Librium, Lipoxide, Mitran, Novo–Poxide✿, Reposans-10, Solium✿ (C-IV, Rx)

See also *Benzodiazepines,* p. 108.

Classification: Antianxiety agent, benzodiazepine.

Action/Kinetics: Onset: PO, 30–60 min; **IM,** 15–30 min (absorption may be slow and erratic); **IV,** 3–30 min. **Peak plasma levels (PO):** 0.5–4 hr. **Duration:** $t^{1/2}$: 5–30 hr. Is metabolized to four active metabolites: desmethylchlordiazepoxide, desmethyldiazepam, oxazepam, and demoxepam. Chlordiazepoxide has less anticonvulsant activity and is less potent than diazepam.

Special Concerns: Pregnancy category: D.

Uses: Anxiety, acute withdrawal symptoms in chronic alcoholics. Sedative-hypnotic. Preoperatively to reduce anxiety and tension. Tension headache. Antitremor agent (PO). Antipanic (parenteral).

Additional Side Effects: Jaundice, acute hepatic necrosis, hepatic dysfunction.

Laboratory Test Interferences

1. *Interference with test methods:* ↑ 17-Hydroxycorticosteroids, 17-ketosteroids.

2. *Caused by pharmacologic effects:* ↑ Alkaline phosphatase, bilirubin, serum transaminase, porphobilinogen. ↓ Prothrombin time (clients on coumarin).

Dosage: **Capsules/Tablets.**
Adults: *Anxiety and tension,* 5–10

mg t.i.d.–q.i.d. (up to 20–25 mg t.i.d.–q.i.d. in severe cases). Reduce dose to 5 mg b.i.d.–q.i.d. in geriatric or debilitated clients. **Pediatric, over 6 years, initial,** 5 mg b.i.d.–q.i.d. May be increased to 10 mg b.i.d.–q.i.d. *Preoperatively:* 5–10 mg t.i.d.–q.i.d. on day before surgery. *Alcohol withdrawal/Sedative-hypnotic:* 50–100 mg; may be increased to 300 mg/day; **then,** reduce to maintenance levels.

   IM, IV (not recommended for children under 12 years): *Acute/severe agitation/anxiety:* **Initial,** 50–100 mg; **then,** 25–50 mg t.i.d.–q.i.d. *Preoperatively:* **IM,** 50–100 mg 1 hr before surgery. *Alcohol withdrawal:* **IM, IV,** 50–100 mg; repeat in 2–4 hr if necessary. Dosage should not exceed 300 mg/day. *Antipanic:* **Adults, initial:** 50–100 mg; dose may be repeated in 4–6 hr if needed.

NURSING CONSIDERATIONS

See also *Nursing Considerations* for *Benzodiazepines,* p. 111.

Administration/Storage

1. **IM:** Prepare solution immediately before administration by adding diluent, which is provided, to ampule. Shake until dissolved. Discard any unused solution. Inject slowly into upper, outer quadrant of gluteal muscle.
2. **IV:** Prepare immediately before administration by diluting with 5 ml of sterile water for injection or sterile 0.9% sodium chloride solution. Inject directly into vein over 1-min period. Do not add to IV infusion because of instability of drug. Do not use IV solution for IM.

Evaluation: Evaluate client for:
- Decrease in the frequency and strength of tremors
- Reports of a decrease in the symptoms of anxiety

Chloroquine hydrochloride
(KLOR-oh-kwin)
Aralen HCl (Rx)

Chloroquine phosphate
(KLOR-oh-kwin)
Aralen Phosphate, Novo-Chloroquine✤ (Rx)

See also *4-Aminoquinolines,* p. 27.

Classification: 4-Aminoquinoline, antimalarial, amebicide.

Special Concerns: Use during pregnancy only if benefits outweigh risks.

Additional Side Effects: Chloroquine may exacerbate psoriasis and precipitate an acute attack.

Drug Interactions

Cimetidine / ↓ Oral clearance rate and metabolism of chloroquine
Kaolin / ↓ Effect of chloroquine due to ↓ absorption from GI tract
Magnesium trisilicate / ↓ Effect of chloroquine due to ↓ absorption from GI tract

Dosage: Tablets. *Acute malarial attack.* **Adults: initial,** 1 g; **then,** 500 mg after 6–8 hr and 500 mg/day for next 2 days. **Children:** Total dose of 41.7 mg/kg given over a 3-day period as follows, **initial:** 16.7 mg/kg (not to exceed a single dose of 1 g); **then,** 8.3 mg/kg (not to exceed a single dose of 500 mg) given 6, 24, and 48 hr after the first dose. *Suppression (prophylaxis) of malaria.* **Adults:** 500 mg/week (on same day each week). If therapy has not been initiated 14 days before exposure, an initial loading dose of 1 g may be given in 500 mg doses 6 hr apart. **Children:** 8.3 mg/kg (not to exceed the adult dose) per week (on same day each week). If therapy has not been initiated 14 days before exposure, an initial loading dose of 16.7 mg/kg may be given in 2 divided doses 6 hr apart.

Amebiasis. **Adults,** 250 mg q.i.d. for 2 days; **then,** 250 mg b.i.d. for 2–3 weeks (combine with an intestinal amebicide). **Children:** 10 mg/kg (not to exceed 500 mg) daily for 3 weeks.

IM. *Acute malarial attack.* **Adults, initial,** 200–250 mg; repeat dosage in 6 hr if necessary. Total daily dose in first 24 hr should not exceed 1 g. Begin PO therapy as soon as possible. **IM, SC. Children and infants:** 6.25 mg/kg repeated in 6 hr; dose should not exceed 12.5 mg/kg/day. **IV infusion, initial:** 16.6 mg/kg over 8 hr; **then,** 8.3 mg/kg q 6–8 hr by continuous infusion.

IM. *Amebiasis:* **Adults,** 200–250 mg daily for 10–12 days. Begin PO therapy as soon as possible. **Children:** 7.5 mg/kg daily for 10–12 days.

NURSING CONSIDERATIONS

See *Nursing Considerations* for *4-Aminoquinolines,* p. 28.

Assessment

1. Determine if client has a history of psoriasis because drug may exacerbate condition and precipitate an acute attack.
2. Note drugs client currently prescribed to assess the pos-

sibility of any unfavorable drug interactions.

Client/Family Teaching

1. Take only as directed and complete prescribed full course of therapy.
2. Avoid activities that require mental alertness until drug effects realized as drug may cause dizziness.
3. Avoid direct sun exposure. Wear protective clothing, sunglasses and sunscreens.
4. Urine may be discolored dark yellow or reddish brown.
5. Review appropriate methods for protection against mosquitoes, i.e., wear long pants and long-sleeved shirts, apply repellents, and use netting or screens as indicated.
6. Avoid ingestion of alcohol in any form.

Evaluation: Evaluate client for:
* Reports of symptomatic improvement
* Negative culture reports

Chlorothiazide
(klor-oh-**THIGH**-ah-zyd)
Diuril (Rx)

Chlorothiazide sodium
(klor-oh-**THIGH**-ah-zyd)
Sodium Diuril (Rx)

See also *Diuretics,* p. 140, and *Thiazide and Related Diuretics,* p. 231.

Classification: Diuretic, thiazide type.

Action/Kinetics: Onset: 1–2 hr; **Peak effect:** 4 hr; **Duration:** 6–12 hr. **t½:** 13 hr. Incompletely absorbed from the GI tract. Produces a greater diuretic effect if given in divided doses. Also found in Diupres.

Special Concerns: Pregnancy category: C. Geriatric clients may be more sensitive to the usual adult dose.

Dosage: Oral Suspension, Tablets, IV. *Antidiuretic, diabetes insipidus,* **Adults,** 250 mg q 6–12 hr. *Antihypertensive:* **Adults, PO,** 250 mg–1 g daily in one or more divided doses; **Adults, IV,** 0.5–1 g daily in one or more divided doses. **Pediatric, 6 months and older:** 10–20 mg/kg daily in a single dose or in 2 divided doses; **6 months and younger:** 10–30 mg/kg daily in a single dose or in 2 divided doses.

NURSING CONSIDERATIONS

See *Nursing Considerations* for *Diuretics,* p. 141, and *Antihypertensive Agents,* p. 78.

Administration/Storage

1. To obtain an isotonic solution for injection, add 18 ml sterile water for injection to 500 mg powder.
2. IV use is not recommended for children and should be reserved for those adults unable to take oral medication or in emergency situations.
3. Unused reconstituted solutions should be discarded after 24 hr.
4. Simultaneous administration of whole blood or derivatives with chlorothiazide should be avoided.
5. The IV solution is compatible with sodium chloride or dextrose solutions.
6. Extravasation into SC tissues should be avoided.

Evaluation: Evaluate client for:
- ↓ blood pressure and edema
- ↑ urinary output

Chlorotrianisene
(klor-oh-try-**AN**-ih-seen)
Tace (Rx)

See also *Estrogens,* p. 147.

Classification: Estrogen, synthetic, nonsteroidal.

Action/Kinetics: The long-lasting effect of this synthetic estrogen is attributed to its storage in adipose tissue, which then acts as a reservoir.

Dosage: Capsules. *Prostatic cancer:* 12–25 mg daily (given chronically). *Breast engorgement:* The following regimens are used: (a) 12 mg q.i.d. for 7 days or (b) 50 mg q 6 hr for 6 doses. For each regimen, the first dose should be given within 8 hr after delivery. *Atrophic vaginitis, kraurosis vulvae:* 12–25 mg daily given cyclically for 30–60 days. *Female hypogonadism:* 12–25 mg/day cyclically for 21 days; give PO progestin for last 5 days of therapy or IM progesterone (100 mg). Begin next course on day 5 of menstrual flow. *Vasomotor symptoms associated with menopause:* 12–25 mg daily given cyclically for 30 days; additional courses of treatment may be necessary.

NURSING CONSIDERATIONS

See *Nursing Considerations* for *Estrogens,* p. 150.

Chlorpheniramine maleate
(klor-fen-**EAR**-ah-meen)
Syrup, Tablets, Chewable

C

Tablets: Aller-Chlor, Chlo-Amine, Chlorate, Chlor-Niramine, Chlortab 4, Chlor-Trimeton, Chlor-Tripolon✤, Genallerate, Novo–Pheniram✤,Pfeiffer's Allergy, Phenetron, Trymegen. Extended-release Capsules, Extended-release Tablets: Chlorspan-12, Chlortab 8, Chlor-Trimeton Repetabs, Chlor-Tripolon✤, Phenetron Telachlor, Teldrin. Injectables: Chlor-100, Chlor-Pro, Chlor-Pro 10, Chlor-Trimeton. (OTC and Rx)

See also *Antihistamines,* p. 71.

Classification: Antihistamine, alkylamine type.

Action/Kinetics: Sedation less pronounced. **t½:** 21–27 hr. **Time to peak effect:** 6 hr. **Duration:** 4–8 hr.

Additional Contraindication: Not recommended for children under 6 years of age.

Special Concerns: Pregnancy category: B. Geriatric clients may be more sensitive to the adult dose. The parenteral route is not recommended for neonates.

Dosage: Syrup, Tablets, Chewable Tablets. Adults: 4 mg q 6 hr as needed; **pediatric, 6–12 years:** 2 mg t.i.d.–q.i.d., not to exceed 12 mg daily. **Extended-release Capsules, Extended-release Tablets. Adults:** 8–12 mg q 8–12 hr as needed; **pediatric, 12 years and older:** 8 mg q 12 hr as needed.

IM, IV, SC. Adults: 5–40 mg as a single dose as needed, up to 40 mg daily; **pediatric, SC:** 0.0875 mg/kg (2.5 mg/m²) q 6 hr as needed.

NURSING CONSIDERATIONS

See *Nursing Considerations* for *Antihistamines,* p. 74.

Administration/Storage

1. If administered with food, the absorption of drug is delayed.
2. The injection containing 10 mg/ml may be administered IV, IM, or SC.
3. The injection containing 100 mg/ml should only be administered IM or SC.
4. Expect the onset of action to occur within 15–30 min and to last 3–6 hr.

Evaluation: Evaluate client for reports of a reduction in allergic manifestations.

Chlorpromazine
(klor-**PROH**-mah-zeen)
Chlorpromanyl✤, Largactil✤, Novo-Chlorpromazine✤, Thorazine (Rx)

Chlorpromazine hydrochloride
(klor-**PROH**-mah-zeen)
Chlorpromanyl-20 and -40✤, Largactil✤, Novo-Chlorpromazine✤, Ormazine, Thorazine, Thor-Prom (Rx)

See also *Phenothiazines,* p. 201.

Classification: Antipsychotic, dimethylamino-type phenothiazine.

Action/Kinetics: Chlorpromazine has significant antiemetic, hypotensive, and sedative effects; moderate to strong anticholinergic effects and weak to moderate extrapyramidal effects. **Peak plasma levels:** 2–3 hr after both PO and IM administration. **t½ (after IV, IM): Initial,** 4–5 hr; **final,** 3–40 hr. Chlorpromazine is extensively metabolized in the intestinal wall and liver; certain of the metabolites are active. **Steady-state plasma levels** (in psychotics): 10–1,300 ng/ml. After 2–3 weeks of therapy, plasma levels decline, possibly because of reduction in drug absorption and/or increase in drug metabolism.

Uses: Acute and chronic psychoses, including schizophrenia; manic phase of manic-depressive illness. Acute intermittent porphyria. Preanesthetic, adjunct to treat tetanus, intractable hiccoughs, severe behavioral problems in children, neuroses, nausea and vomiting. Treatment of choreiform movements in Huntington's disease.

Special Concerns: Use during pregnancy only if benefits outweigh risks. Oral dosage for psychoses and nausea/vomiting have not been established in children less than 6 months of age.

Additional Drug Interactions

Epinephrine / Chlorpromazine ↓ peripheral vasoconstriction and may reverse action of epinephrine

Norepinephrine / Chlorpromazine ↓ pressor effect and eliminates bradycardia due to norepinephrine

Valproic acid / ↑ Effect of valproic acid due to ↓ clearance

Dosage: Extended-release Capsules, Oral Concentrate, Syrup, Tablets. *Psychotic disorders:* **Adults and adolescents,** 10–25 mg (of the base) b.i.d.–q.i.d.; dosage may be increased by 20–50 mg a day q 3–4 days as needed. Or, 30–300 mg (of the base) using the extended-release capsules 1–3 times daily (the 300 mg extended-release capsules are used only in severe neuropsychiatric situations). **Pediatric:** 0.55 mg/kg (15 mg/m²) q 4–6 hr. *Nausea and vomiting:* **Adults and adolescents,** 10–25 mg (of the base) q 4 hr; dosage may

be increased as needed. **Pediatric:** 0.55 mg/kg (15 mg/m²) q 4–6 hr. *Preoperative sedation:* **Adults and adolescents,** 25–50 mg (of the base) 2–3 hr before surgery. **Pediatric:** 0.55 mg/kg (15 mg/m²) 2–3 hr before surgery. *Hiccoughs or porphyria:* **Adults and adolescents,** 25–50 mg (of the base) t.i.d.–q.i.d.

    IM. *Severe psychoses,* **Adults,** 25–50 mg (of the base) repeated in 1 hr if needed; **then,** repeat the dose q 3–4 hr as needed and tolerated (the dose may be increased gradually over several days). **Pediatric, over 6 months:** 0.55 mg/kg (15 mg/m²) q 6–8 hr as needed. *Nausea and vomiting:* **Adults,** 25 mg (base) as a single dose; **then,** increase to 25–50 mg q 3–4 hr as needed until vomiting ceases. **Pediatric:** 0.55 mg/kg q 6–8 hr as needed. *Nausea and vomiting during surgery:* **Adults,** 12.5 mg (base) as a single dose; repeat in 30 min if needed. **Pediatric,** 0.275 mg/kg; repeat in 30 min if needed. *Preoperative sedative:* **Adults,** 12.5–25 mg (base) 1–2 hr before surgery. **Pediatric:** 0.55 mg/kg 1–2 hr before surgery. *Hiccoughs:* **Adults,** 25–50 mg (base) t.i.d.–q.i.d. *Porphyria:* **Adults,** 25 mg (base) q 6–8 hr until patient can take PO therapy. *Tetanus:* **Adults,** 25–50 mg (base) t.i.d.–q.i.d. (dose can be increased as needed and tolerated).

    IV. *Nausea and vomiting during surgery:* **Adults,** 25 mg (base) diluted to 1 mg/ml with 0.9% sodium chloride injection given at a rate of no more than 2 mg q 2 min. **Pediatric:** 0.275 mg/kg diluted to 1 mg/ml with 0.9% sodium chloride injection given at a rate of no more than 1 mg q 2 min. *Tetanus:* **Adults,** 25–50 mg (base) diluted to 1 mg/ml with 0.9% sodium chloride injection and given at a rate of 1 mg/min. **Pediatric:** 0.55 mg/kg diluted to 1 mg/ml with 0.9% sodium chloride injection and given at a rate of 1 mg/2 min.

Suppositories. *Nausea and vomiting:* **Adults and adolescents,** 50–100 mg q 6–8 hr as needed up to a maximum of 400 mg daily. **Pediatric:** 1 mg/kg q 6–8 hr as needed (the 100 mg suppository should not be used in children).

NURSING CONSIDERATIONS

See also *Nursing Considerations* for *Phenothiazines,* p. 205.

Administration/Storage

1. Chlorpromazine should not be used to treat nausea and vomiting in children less than 6 months of age.
2. The maximum daily oral and parenteral dose for adults and adolescents should be 1 g of the base.
3. The maximum IM dose should be 40 mg daily for children up to 5 years of age and 75 mg daily for children 5–12 years of age.
4. Sustained-release capsules should be swallowed whole.
5. Solutions of chlorpromazine may cause contact dermatitis; thus, medical personnel should avoid getting solution on hands or clothing.
6. When used IV in children for tetanus, the preparation should be diluted to 1 mg/ml and given at a rate of 1 mg/2 min.
7. The concentrate (to be used in hospitals only) can be mixed with 60 ml or more of fruit or tomato juice, orange or simple syrup, milk, carbonated drinks, coffee, tea, water, or semisolid foods (e.g., soup, pudding).

8. Slight discoloration of injection or oral solutions will not affect the action of the drug.
9. Solutions with marked discoloration should be discarded. Consult with pharmacist if unsure of drug potency.
10. When administering the drug IM, select a large, well-developed muscle mass. Use the dorsogluteal site or rectus femoris in adults and the vastus lateralis in children.
11. Document and rotate injection sites.

Assessment

1. Note any history of seizure disorders as the drug is contraindicated in these instances.
2. Conduct baseline studies of liver and kidney function.
3. Determine age of male clients and assess for prostatic hypertrophy.

Client/Family Teaching

1. Provide a printed list of side effects and advise client to immediately report any extrapyramidal symptoms.
2. Advise that urine may become discolored pinkish to brown.

Evaluation: Evaluate client for:
- Improved patterns of behavior
- ↓ in nausea
- Cessation of hiccoughs

Chlorpropamide
(klor-**PROH**-pah-myd)
**Apo-Chlorpropamide ✤,
Diabinese, Glucamide, Novo–
Propamide ✤ (Rx)**

See also *Antidiabetic Agents, Oral,* p. 65.

Classification: First-generation sulfonylurea.

Action/Kinetics: Chlorpropamide may be effective in clients who do not respond well to other antidiabetic agents. **Onset:** 1 hr. **t½:** 35 hr. **Time to peak levels:** 2–4 hr. **Duration:** 24–48 hr (due to slow excretion). Eighty percent metabolized in liver; 80%–90% excreted in the urine.

Additional Use: *Investigational:* Neurogenic diabetes insipidus.

Special Concerns: Pregnancy category: C. If the client is susceptible to fluid retention or has impaired cardiac function, frequent monitoring is necessary.

Additional Side Effects: Occur frequently with chlorpropamide. Severe diarrhea is occasionally accompanied by bleeding in the lower bowel. Severe GI distress may be relieved by dividing total daily dose in half. In older clients, hypoglycemia may be severe. May cause inappropriate antidiuretic hormone secretion, leading to hyponatremia, water retention, low serum osmolality, and high urine osmolality.

Additional Drug Interactions

Ammonium chloride / ↑ Effect of chlorpropamide due to ↓ excretion by kidney
Disulfiram / More likely to interact with chlorpropamide than other oral antidiabetics
Probenecid / ↑ Effect of chlorpropamide
Sodium bicarbonate / ↓ Effect of chlorpropamide due to ↑ excretion by kidney

Dosage: PO. Adults, middle-aged clients, initial: 250 mg daily as a single or divided dose; **geriatric: initial,** 100–125 mg daily. **All**

clients, maintenance: 100–250 mg daily as single or divided doses. Severe diabetics may require 500 mg daily; doses greater than 750 mg daily are not recommended. *Neurogenic diabetes insipidus:* 125–250 mg daily, up to a maximum of 500 mg daily.

NURSING CONSIDERATIONS

See *Nursing Considerations* for *Antidiabetic Agents, Oral,* p. 68.

Assessment

1. Note the age of the client. Elderly clients tend to be more sensitive to hypoglycemic agents and exhibit more side effects.
2. Determine if the client is pregnant. The drug is contraindicated in pregnancy.
3. Note any allergy to sulfa drugs.

Interventions

1. Monitor weight and blood pressure and assess for evidence of the inappropriate secretion of antidiuretic hormone. Clients may appear confused, complain of feeling dizzy, depressed, and complain of nausea.
2. Monitor the client's serum electrolytes and urine osmolality. Record intake and output.

Evaluation: Evaluate client for the maintenance of blood sugar within the desired range.

Chlorprothixene
(klor-proh-**THICKS**-een)
Taractan, Tarasan✹ (Rx)

Classification: Antipsychotic, thioxanthene derivative.

Action/Kinetics: The antipsychotic effect of chlorprothixene is thought to be manifested by blocking postsynaptic dopamine receptors in the brain. Chlorprothixene causes significant sedation and orthostatic hypotension and antiemetic effects with moderate anticholinergic and extrapyramidal effects. It is a more potent inhibitor of postural reflexes and motor coordination than is chlorpromazine, but has less pronounced antihistaminic effects. The drug also produces alpha-adrenergic blockade and depresses the release of most hypothalamic and hypophyseal hormones. **IM, Onset:** 30 min; **duration:** up to 12 hr.

Uses: Neurosis, depression, schizophrenia, antiemesis, alcohol withdrawal. Adjunct in electroshock therapy. Drug may be effective in clients resistant to other psychotherapeutic drugs.

Special Concerns: Use during pregnancy only if benefits outweigh risks. Use with caution during lactation. Children are more prone to develop neuromuscular and extrapyramidal side effects (especially dystonias). Oral dosage has not been established in children less than 6 years of age and IM dosage has not been established in children less than 12 years of age. Adolescents may experience a higher incidence of hypotensive and extrapyramidal reactions than adults. Geriatric clients may be more prone to orthostatic hypotension and manifest an increased sensitivity to tardive dyskinesia and Parkinson-like symptoms. Geriatric or debilitated clients usually require a lower starting dose.

Side Effects: Drowsiness, lethargy, orthostatic hypotension, tachycardia, dizziness, and dry mouth occur especially frequently.

Drug Interactions: May cause additive hypotensive effects with methyldopa or reserpine.

Laboratory Test Interferences: False + immunologic urine pregnancy test.

Dosage: Oral Suspension, Tablets. *Antipsychotic:* **Adults and children over 12 years:** 25–50 mg t.i.d.–q.i.d. up to a maximum of 600 mg daily. **Pediatric, 6–12 years:** 10–25 mg t.i.d.–q.i.d. **IM.** *Antipsychotic:* **Adults and children over 12 years:** 25–50 mg t.i.d.–q.i.d. Doses exceeding 600 mg/day are rarely needed. Switch to oral dosage when feasible. **Geriatric or debilitated clients, initial:** 10–25 mg t.i.d.–q.i.d.

NURSING CONSIDERATIONS

See *Nursing Considerations* for *Phenothiazines,* p. 205.

Administration/Storage

1. Oral products should not be given to children less than 6 years of age, and parenteral products should not be given to children less than 12 years of age.
2. Inject deeply into large muscle mass.
3. Client should be supine during administration because of postural hypotension.
4. Protect from light.
5. The concentrate may be given undiluted or mixed with fruit juice, coffee, carbonated beverages, milk, or water.

Evaluation: Evaluate client for:
- Evidence of improved coping behaviors
- Reports of symptomatic improvement

Chlorthalidone
(klor-**THAL**-ih-dohn)
Apo-Chlorthalidone✿, Hygroton, Novo-Thalidone✿, Thalitone (Rx)

See also *Diuretics,* p. 140, and *Thiazide and Related Diuretics,* p. 231.

Classification: Diuretic, thiazide.

Action/Kinetics: Onset: 2 hr. **Peak effect:** Within 2–6 hr. **Duration:** 24–72 hr. **t½:** 35–50 hr.

Additional Uses: Particularly good for potentiating and reducing dosage of other antihypertensive agents.

Special Concerns: Pregnancy category: B. Geriatric clients may be more sensitive to the usual adult dose.

Dosage: Tablets. *Antidiuretic:* **Adults,** 25–100 mg daily or 100–200 mg 3 times/week. **Maximum daily dose:** 200 mg. **Pediatric:** all uses, 2 mg/kg (60 mg/m²) 3 times weekly. *Hypertension:* **Initial,** 25–50 mg once daily up to 100 mg daily; **maintenance;** usually lower than initial dose but determined by client response.

NURSING CONSIDERATIONS

See *Nursing Considerations* for *Diuretics,* p. 141, and *Thiazide and Related Diuretics,* p. 233.

Administration/Storage: Administer in the morning with food.

Chlorzoxazone
(klor-**ZOX**-ah-zohn)
Paraflex, Parafon Forte DSC (Rx)

See also *Centrally Acting Skeletal Muscle Relaxants,* p. 130.

Classification: Centrally acting muscle relaxant.

Action/Kinetics: Chlorzoxazone inhibits polysynaptic reflexes at both the spinal cord and subcortical areas of the brain. Its effect may also be due to the sedative properties of the drug. **Onset:** 1 hr. **Time to peak blood levels:** 1–2 hr. **Peak serum levels:** 10–30 mcg/ml (after 750 mg dose). **Duration:** 3–4 hr. **t½:** 1–2 hr. The drug is metabolized in the liver and inactive metabolites excreted in the urine.

Uses: As adjunct therapy for acute, painful musculoskeletal conditions (e.g., muscle spasms, sprains, muscle strain).

Special Concerns: Use during pregnancy only if benefits clearly outweigh risks.

Side Effects: *CNS:* Dizziness, drowsiness, malaise, lightheadedness, stimulation. *Dermatologic:* Skin rashes, petechiae, ecchymoses (rare). *Miscellaneous:* GI upset, angioneurotic edema, anaphylaxis (rare), discoloration of urine, liver damage.

Dosage: Tablets. Adults: 250–750 mg t.i.d.–q.i.d. with meals and at bedtime; **pediatric:** 125–500 mg t.i.d.–q.i.d. (or, 20 mg/kg in 3–4 divided doses daily).

NURSING CONSIDERATIONS

See also *Nursing Considerations* for *Centrally Acting Skeletal Muscle Relaxants,* p. 130.

C

Administration/Storage

1. Administer the drug with meals to minimize gastric irritation.
2. The drug may be mixed with food or beverages for administration to children.

Assessment: Assure that liver function studies have been conducted to serve as a baseline against which to compare liver function after the client has been taking the drug.

Intervention: If the client develops any evidence of hepatic dysfunction, order liver function studies and compare with pretreatment values.

Client/Family Teaching

1. The drug may cause the urine to have an orange or purple-red color when exposed to the air.
2. Do not operate dangerous machinery or drive a car because the drug causes drowsiness.

Evaluation: Evaluate client for reports of effective control of pain and discomfort.

Cholestyramine resin
(koh-less-TEER-ah-meen)
Cholybar, Questran, Questran Light (Rx)

Classification: Hypocholesterolemic agent, bile acid sequestrant.

Action/Kinetics: Cholestyramine binds sodium cholate (bile salts) in the intestine; thus, the principal precursor of cholesterol is not absorbed due to formation of an insoluble complex, which is excreted in the feces. The drug decreases cholesterol and LDL and has either no effect or increases triglycerides, VLDL, and HDL. Also, itching is relieved as a result of removing irritating bile salts. The antidiarrheal effect results from the binding and removal of bile acids. **Onset, to reduce plasma cholesterol:** Within 24–48 hr but levels may continue to fall for 1 yr; **to relieve pruritus:** 1–3 weeks; **relief of diarrhea associated with bile acids:** 24 hr. Cholesterol levels return to pretreatment levels 2–4 wks after discontinuance. Fat-soluble vitamins (A, D, K) and possibly folic acid may have to be administered IM during long-term therapy because cholestyramine binds these vitamins in the intestine.

Uses: Pruritus associated with partial biliary obstruction. Hyperlipoproteinemia (type IIA). Diarrhea due to bile acids. *Investigational:* Treatment of poisoning by chlordecone (Kepone), antibiotic-induced *Pseudomonas* colitis, digitalis toxicity, postvagotomy diarrhea, and hyperoxaluria.

Contraindications: Complete obstruction or atresia of bile duct.

Special Concerns: Use during pregnancy only if benefits outweigh risks. Use with caution during lactation and in children. Geriatric clients may be more likely to manifest GI side effects as well as adverse nutritional effects.

Side Effects: *GI:* Constipation (may be severe), nausea, vomiting, diarrhea, heartburn, GI bleeding, anorexia, flatulence, belching, abdominal distention, aggravation of hemorrhoids. Fecal impaction in elderly clients. Large doses may cause steatorrhea. *Other:* Bleeding tendencies (due to hypoprothrombinemia). Osteoporosis, electrolyte imbalance, and CNS and musculoskeletal manifestations. Prolonged administration may interfere with absorption of fat-soluble vitamins. Irritation and rash of skin, tongue, and perianal area.

Drug Interactions

Acetaminophen / ↓ Effect of acetaminophen due to ↓ absorption from GI tract

Amiodarone / ↓ Effect of amiodarone due to ↓ absorption from GI tract

Anticoagulants, oral / ↓ Anticoagulant effect due to ↓ absorption from GI tract

Cephalexin / ↓ Absorption of cephalexin from GI tract

Chenodiol / ↓ Effect of chenodiol due to ↓ absorption from GI tract

Chlorothiazide / ↓ Effect of chlorothiazide due to ↓ absorption from GI tract

Clindamycin / ↓ Absorption of clindamycin from GI tract

Corticosteroids / ↓ Effect of corticosteroids due to ↓ absorption from GI tract

Digitalis glycosides / Cholestyramine binds digitoxin in the intestine and ↓ its half-life

Iron preparations / ↓ Effect of iron preparations due to ↓ absorption from GI tract

Lovastatin / Effects may be additive

Naproxen / ↓ Effect of naproxen due to ↓ absorption from GI tract

Penicillin G / ↓ Effect of penicillin G due to ↓ absorption from GI tract

Phenobarbital / ↓ Absorption of phenobarbital from GI tract

Phenylbutazone / Absorption of phenylbutazone delayed by cholestyramine—may ↓ effect

Piroxicam / ↓ Effect of piroxicam due to ↓ absorption from GI tract

Propranolol / ↓ Effect of propranolol due to ↓ absorption from GI tract

Tetracyclines / ↓ Effect of tetracyclines due to ↓ absorption from GI tract

Thiazide diuretics / ↓ Effect of thiazides due to ↓ absorption from GI tract

Thyroid hormones / ↓ Effect of thyroid hormones due to ↓ absorption from GI tract

Trimethoprim / ↓ Effect of trimethoprim due to ↓ absorption from GI tract

Ursodiol / ↓ Effect of ursodiol due to ↓ absorption from GI tract

Warfarin / ↓ Effect of warfarin due to ↓ absorption from GI tract

Note: These drug interactions may also be observed with colestipol.

Dosage: Bar, Powder. Adults: 4 g 1–6 times daily of either the powder or the bar. After relief of pruritus, dosage may be reduced. Doses greater than 24 g daily result in an increased incidence of side effects. **Pediatric, 6–12 years:** 80 mg (anhydrous cholestyramine)/kg (2.35 g/m²) t.i.d. The adult dose should be used in children older than 12 years. Not recommended for children less than 6 years of age.

NURSING CONSIDERATIONS

Administration/Storage

1. Always mix powder with 60–180 ml water or noncarbonated beverage before administering because resin may cause esophageal irritation or blockage. Highly liquid soups

C

or pulpy fruits such as applesauce or crushed pineapple may also be used.

2. After placing contents of one packet of resin on the surface of 4–6 oz of fluid, allow it to stand without stirring for 2 min, occasionally twirling the glass, and then stir slowly (to prevent foaming) to form a suspension.

3. Avoid inhaling the powder while mixing as it may be irritating to mucous membranes.

4. The bar should be chewed thoroughly and taken with plenty of fluids.

Assessment

1. Note color of client's skin and eyes for evidence of jaundice.

2. Determine onset of pruritus and level of bile acid.

3. Perform baseline liver function studies.

Interventions

1. Anticipate that vitamins A, D, K, and folic acid will be administered during long-term therapy. These may be administered in a water-miscible form when the client is receiving medication.

2. Note client complaints of constipation, abdominal pain, or abdominal bloating. Encourage a fluid intake of 2,500–3,000 ml/day, and encourage an increased intake of citrus fruits, fruit juices and high fiber foods as preventive measures. Also, a stool softener may be indicated.

3. Encourage clients to increase their daily exercise as a method to avoid constipation.

4. If symptoms are severe or if they persist, discuss a change in dosage of drug or change of medication with the physician.

5. If the client complains of diarrhea, monitor intake, output, electrolytes, and weight. Note any evidence of dehydration and/or electrolyte imbalance.

6. Monitor the client's serum cholesterol and triglyceride levels. Clients should also have frequent serum transaminase and other liver function tests conducted routinely.

7. To ensure that the clients are not developing anemia, leukopenia, eosinophilia, potential anticoagulant effects, or renal dysfunction, blood counts and renal function tests should be done routinely.

8. If clients develop bleeding from any orifice or develop purpura, they should receive parenteral vitamin K.

Client/Family Teaching

1. Other prescribed medications should be taken at least 1 hr before or 4 hr after taking antihyperlipidemic medication. These drugs interfere with the absorption of other medications.

2. Discuss the constipating effects the drug may have and ways to control this problem. Drink extra fluids and include extra roughage in the diet.

3. If the client has problems with persistent constipation despite efforts to avoid the problem, a stool softener may be required.

4. Report tarry stools or any abnormal bleeding. These symptoms may indicate a need for vitamin K supplement.

5. Pruritus may subside 1–3 weeks after taking the drug but may return after the medication is discontinued. Corn starch or oatmeal baths may assist to alleviate this discomfort.

Evaluation: Evaluate client for:
- Reports of a decrease in pruritus
- ↓ in cholesterol levels
- Reduction in diarrheal stools

Chorionic gonadotropin (HCG)
(kor-ee-**ON**-ik go-**NAD**-oh-troh-pin)
A.P.L., Chorex-5 and -10, Chorigon, Choron 10, Corgonject-5, Follutein, Glukor, Gonic, Pregnyl, Profasi HP (Rx)

Classification: Gonadotropic hormone.

Action/Kinetics: The actions of human chorionic gonadotropin (HCG), produced by the trophoblasts of the fertilized ovum and then by the placenta, resemble those of luteinizing hormone (LH). In males, HCG stimulates androgen production by the testes, the development of secondary sex characteristics, and testicular descent when no anatomic impediment is present. In women, HCG stimulates progesterone production by the corpus luteum and completes expulsion of the ovum from a mature follicle.

Uses: *Males:* Prepubertal cryptorchidism, hypogonadism due to pituitary insufficiency. *Females:* Infertility (together with menotropins).

Contraindications: Precocious puberty, prostatic cancer or other androgen-dependent neoplasm, hypersensitivity to drug. Development of precocious puberty is cause for discontinuance of therapy.

Special Concerns: Pregnancy category: C. Since HCG increases androgen production, drug should be used with caution in clients in whom androgen-induced edema may be harmful (epilepsy, migraines, asthma, cardiac or renal diseases).

Side Effects: *CNS:* Headache, irritability, restlessness, depression, fatigue. *Miscellaneous:* Edema, precocious puberty, gynecomastia, pain at injection site.

Dosage: IM only. *Prepubertal cryptorchidism, not due to anatomical obstruction:* Various regimens including (1) 4,000 USP units 3 times/week for 3 weeks; (2) 5,000 USP units q other day for 4 injections; (3) 15 injections over a period of 6 weeks of 500–1,000 units/injection; (4) 500 USP units 3 times/week for 4–6 weeks; may be repeated after 1 month using 1,000 USP units. *Hypogonadism in males:* The following regimens may be used: (1) 500–1,000 USP units 3 times/week for 3 weeks; **then,** same dose twice weekly for 3 weeks; (2) 4,000 USP units 3 times/week for 6–9 months; then, 2,000 USP units 3 times/week for 3 more months; (3) 1,000–2,000 USP 3 times weekly. *Induction of ovulation (used with menotropins):* 5,000–10,000 USP units one day after the last dose of menotropins. *Stimulation of spermatogenesis (used with menotropins):* 5,000 units 3 times a week for 4–6 weeks; reduce dose of 2,000 units twice weekly when menotropin therapy is begun.

NURSING CONSIDERATIONS

Administration/Storage

1. Reconstituted solutions are stable for 1–3 months, depending on manufacturer, when stored at 2°C–8°C (35.6°F–46.4°F).
2. Have emergency drugs and equipment available in the event of an acute allergic response.

Assessment

1. Note any client history of hypersensitivity to the drug.
2. Assess the prepubescent male client for the appearance of secondary sex characteristics. The drug is contraindicated in this instance.

Interventions

1. Once started on the therapy, periodically examine the client for the beginning of secondary sex characteristics. This is an indication of sexual precocity and the drug should be withdrawn.
2. Note client complaints of headache, easy fatigue, and restlessness, or if the family complains that the client has become increasingly irritable and depressed. Note if there is any change in the client's attention to physical appearance. Document and report these to the physician because the drug may have to be withdrawn.
3. When treating clients for cryptorchidism, examine them once a week for testicular descent to evaluate the response to therapy.
4. Because edema is common, monitor the client's weight and extent of edema at regular intervals and report to the physician.

5. Observe the client for gynecomastia and offer emotional support. This is especially important for young male clients.
6. In female clients being treated for corpus luteum deficiency, question about the occurrence of bleeding after the 15th day of therapy. If bleeding occurs, hold the drug and notify the physician.

Client/Family Teaching

1. Teach how to assess for edema and advise clients to report any occurrence to the physician.
2. Explain that delayed menses, excessive menstrual bleeding, pain in the pelvic region, weakness, and fatigue are signs and symptoms of ectopic pregnancy and should be reported to the physician immediately.
3. Discuss the possibility of multiple births when the drug is used with menotropins.
4. Encourage the client to return for scheduled follow-up visits to monitor the effectiveness of the drug therapy.
5. Warn client that medication may cause pain at the site of injection.

Evaluation: Evaluate client for:
- Testicular descent
- Improved hormone production

Chymopapain for injection

(**KYE**-moh-pah-payn)
Chymodiactin (Rx)

Classification: Proteolytic enzyme.

Action/Kinetics: Chymopapain is

a proteolytic enzyme derived from the crude latex of *Carica papaya*. The nanoKatal (nKat) is used as the unit of chymopapain activity (1 mg of chymopapain is equivalent to at least 0.52 nKat units). The preparation also contains sodium L-cysteinate hydrochloride as a reducing agent to keep the sulfur in the sulfhydryl form. Chymopapain is injected into the herniated lumbar intervertebral disc (nucleus pulposus), where it hydrolyzes the noncollagenous proteins or polypeptides that maintain the structure of the chondromucoprotein of the nucleus pulposus. As a result of hydrolysis, the osmotic activity is decreased, leading to a decreased fluid absorption, thus reducing intradiscal pressure. Although chymopapain acts locally in the disc, it does appear in the plasma, where it is inactivated. Small amounts are excreted in the urine.

Uses: Chymopapain should be used only in a hospital setting by physicians and supportive personnel trained in the diagnosis and treatment of herniated lumbar intervertebral disc disease that has not responded to more conservative therapy.

Contraindications: Sensitivity to chymopapain, papaya, or its derivatives. Severe spondylolisthesis, significant spinal stenosis, spinal cord tumor or a cauda equina lesion, or in progressing paralysis manifested by rapidly progressing neurologic dysfunction. Clients previously treated with chymopapain. Injection into any location other than lumbar area.

Special Concerns: Use during pregnancy only when benefits outweigh risks (pregnancy category: C). Safety and efficacy have not been established for use in children.

Side Effects: *Neuromuscular:* Back pain, stiffness, soreness, back spasm, paraplegia, acute transverse myelitis or myelopathy characterized by onset of paraplegia or paraparesis (without prior symptoms) within 2–3 weeks. Also, sacral burning, leg pain, hyperalgesia, leg weakness, tingling/numbness in legs/toes, cramping in both calves, paresthesia, pain in opposite leg, postinjection pain, bacterial and aseptic discitis. *Allergic:* Anaphylaxis (more common in females). Complications secondary to anaphylaxis including staphylococcal meningitis with disc abscess. Rash, itching, urticaria, pilomotor erection, vasomotor rhinitis, conjunctivitis, angioedema, GI disturbances. *Other:* Cerebral hemorrhage, nausea, itching, paralytic ileus, urinary retention, headache, dizziness.

Drug Interactions: Possible arrhythmias if used with halothane or epinephrine.

Dosage: A single injection of 2–4 nKat units/disc (usual is 3 nKat units/disc in a volume of 1.5 ml). Maximum dose with multiple disc herniation is 10 nKat units.

NURSING CONSIDERATIONS

Administration/Storage

1. An open IV line must always be available in the event of anaphylaxis. Epinephrine is the drug of choice to treat anaphylaxis.
2. Sterile water for injection should be used for reconstitution, as bacteriostatic water for injection inactivates the enzyme. The reconstituted

drug must be used within 2 hr. Any unused, reconstituted drug should be discarded promptly.

3. Automatic filling syringes should not be used since a residual vacuum is present in the vial.

4. Alcohol should be used to cleanse the vial stopper before inserting the needle; since alcohol inactivates the enzyme, it should be allowed to *dry* before continuing with reconstitution.

5. The package literature should be consulted for the specific procedures for administration.

6. Prior to use, the client should be treated with histamine receptor H_1 and H_2 antagonists to decrease the severity of an anaphylactic reaction (e.g., cimetidine, 300 mg PO, q 6 hr and diphenhydramine, 50 mg PO, q 6 hr, both for 24 hr prior to therapy).

Assessment

1. Note onset of injury and pain and lumbar discs involved.

2. Determine if therapy with chymopapain has been used previously because additional treatments are contraindicated.

Interventions

1. Monitor the client's blood pressure and respiratory status. The drug can cause hypotension and bronchospasms.

2. Perform neurovascular checks postprocedure and document any progressive dysfunction.

Client/Family Teaching

1. Back pain and muscle spasms may occur within several days to several weeks following treatment.

2. Discuss the possibility of paraplegia and paresis occurring suddenly, several weeks after treatment. This should be reported immediately to the physician.

3. Report to the physician if leg weakness, tingling or numbness of the legs and/or toes, or cramping in the calves of the legs occurs.

4. Advise client that responses are not immediately evident. Prepare them for a lack of or poor response as surgery may be necessary in this event.

Evaluation: Evaluate client for:
- Reduced intradiscal pressure
- Reports of symptomatic improvement
- Freedom from complications of drug administration

Ciclopirox olamine
(sye-kloh-**PEER**-ox)
Loprox (Rx)

Classification: Antifungal, topical.

Action/Kinetics: This broad-spectrum fungicide is effective against dermatophytes, yeast, *Malassezia furfur, Trichophyton rubrum, T. mentagrophytes, Epidermophyton floccosum, Microsporum canis,* and *Candida albicans.* At lower concentrations the drug blocks the transport of amino acids into the cell, whereas at higher concentrations the cell membrane of the fungus is altered so that intracellular material leaks out. The drug may also inhibit synthesis of RNA, DNA, and protein in growing fungal cells. A small amount of drug is absorbed through the skin; it also penetrates to the sebaceous glands and dermis as well as into the hair.

Uses: Tinea pedis, tinea corporis, tinea cruris, tinea versicolor, candidiasis.

Contraindications: Use in or around the eyes.

Special Concerns: Safety and efficacy in pregnancy (category: B), in lactation, and in children under 10 years of age not established.

Side Effects: *Dermatologic:* Irritation, redness, burning, pain, skin sensitivity, pruritus at application site.

Dosage: Topical cream. Massage gently into the affected area and surrounding skin morning and evening. If no improvement after 4 weeks, diagnosis should be reevaluated.

NURSING CONSIDERATIONS

Assessment: If drug is used for suspected *M. furfur* infection, assist with establishing diagnosis by describing lesions and obtaining scraping of lesion because a technique for culture of organism does not exist.

Client/Family Teaching

1. Cleanse skin with soap and water and dry thoroughly.
2. Occlusive dressings or wrappings should not be used. Adult incontinence pads are an occlusive dressing and should not be used during therapy.
3. Even though symptoms have improved, the drug should be used for the full prescribed time.
4. Shoes and socks should be changed at least once daily. Shoes should be well-fitted and ventilated.
5. Notify care provider if the area of application shows evidence of blistering, burning, itching, oozing, redness, or swelling.

Evaluation: Observe infected area for positive response to treatment and any evidence of increased irritation.

Cimetidine
(sye-**MET**-ih-deen)
Apo-Cimetidine✹, Novo–Cimetidine✹, Nu-Cimet✹, Peptol✹, Tagamet (Rx)

See also *Histamine H_2 Blocking Agents,* p. 154.

Classification: Histamine H_2-receptor blocking agent.

Action/Kinetics: Cimetidine decreases the acidity of the stomach by blocking the action of histamine, a substance involved in triggering gastric acid secretion. Cimetidine blocks the action of histamine by competitively occupying the histamine (H_2) receptors in the gastric mucosa. This, in turn, inhibits the release of gastric (hydrochloric) acid. Cimetidine reduces postprandial daytime and nighttime gastric acid secretion by about 50%–80%. It is well absorbed from GI tract. The drug may increase gastromucosal defense and healing in acid-related disorders (e.g., stress-induced ulcers) by increasing production of gastric mucus, increasing mucosal secretion of bicarbonate and gastric mucosal blood flow as well as increasing endogenous mucosal synthesis of prostaglandins. It also inhibits cytochrome P-450 and P-448, which will affect metabolism of drugs. Cimetidine also possesses antiandrogenic activity and will increase prolactin levels following an IV bolus injection. **Peak plasma**

C

level, PO: 45–90 min. **Time to peak effect, after PO:** 1–2 hr. **Duration, nocturnal:** 6–8 hr; **basal:** 4–5 hr. **t½:** 2 hr, longer in presence of renal impairment. After PO use, most metabolized in liver; after parenteral use, about 75% of drug excreted unchanged in the urine.

Uses: Short-term (up to 8 weeks) and maintenance treatment of active duodenal ulcers; short-term (6 weeks) treatment of benign gastric ulcers. Management of gastric acid hypersecretory states (Zollinger-Ellison syndrome, systemic mastocytosis). Gastroesophageal reflux disease. Prophylaxis of upper GI bleeding in critically ill hospitalized clients. *Investigational:* Prior to surgery to prevent aspiration pneumonitis, secondary hyperparathyroidism in chronic hemodialysis clients, prophylaxis of stress-induced ulcers, hyperparathyroidism, dyspepsia, herpes virus infections, tinea capitis, prevent gastric damage due to NSAIDs, hirsute women, chronic idiopathic urticaria, dermatologic anaphylaxis, acetaminophen overdosage.

Contraindications: Children under 16, nursing mothers. Cirrhosis, impaired liver and renal function.

Special Concerns: Pregnancy category: B. In geriatric clients with impaired renal or hepatic function, confusion is more likely to occur.

Side Effects: *GI:* Diarrhea, pancreatitis, hepatitis, hepatic fibrosis. *CNS:* Dizziness, sleepiness, headache, confusion, delirium, hallucinations, double vision, dysarthria, ataxia. Severely ill clients may manifest agitation, anxiety, depression, disorientation, hallucinations, mental confusion, and psychosis. *CV:* Hypotension and arrhythmias following rapid IV administration. *Hematologic:* Agranulocytosis, thrombocytopenia, hemolytic or aplastic anemia, granulocytopenia. *GU:* Impotence (high doses for prolonged periods of time), gynecomastia (long-term treatment). *Other:* Arthralgia, myalgia, rash, vasculitis, galactorrhea, alopecia, bronchoconstriction.

Drug Interactions

Antacids / ↓ Effect of cimetidine due to ↓ absorption from GI tract

Anticholinergics / ↓ Effect of cimetidine due to ↓ absorption from GI tract

Benzodiazepines / ↑ Effect of benzodiazepines due to ↓ breakdown by liver

Beta-adrenergic blocking drugs / ↑ Effect of beta blockers due to ↓ breakdown by liver

Caffeine / ↑ Effect of caffeine due to ↓ breakdown by liver

Calcium channel blockers / ↑ Effect of calcium channel blockers due to ↓ breakdown by liver

Carbamazepine / ↑ Effect of carbamazepine due to ↓ breakdown by liver

Carmustine / Additive bone marrow depression

Chloroquine / ↑ Effect of iron due to ↓ breakdown by liver

Chlorpromazine / ↓ Effect of chlorpromazine due to ↓ absorption from GI tract

Digoxin / ↓ Serum levels of digoxin

Flecainide / ↑ Effect of flecainide

Fluconazole / ↓ Effect of fluconazole due to ↓ absorption from GI tract

Fluorouracil / ↓ Serum levels of fluorouracil

Indomethacin / ↓ Effect of indomethacin due to ↓ absorption from GI tract

Iron salts / ↓ Effect of iron due to ↓ absorption from GI tract

Ketoconazole / ↓ Effect of ketoconazole due to ↓ absorption from GI tract

Lidocaine / ↑ Effect of lidocaine due to ↓ breakdown by liver

Metoclopramide / ↓ Effect of cimetidine due to ↓ absorption from GI tract

Metronidazole / ↑ Effect of metronidazole due to ↓ breakdown by liver

Moricizine / ↑ Effect of moricizine due to ↓ breakdown by liver

Narcotics / Possible ↑ toxic effects (respiratory depression) of narcotics

Pentoxifylline / ↑ Effect of pentoxifylline due to ↓ breakdown by liver

Phenytoin / ↑ Effect of phenytoin due to ↓ breakdown by liver

Procainamide / ↑ Effect of procainamide due to ↓ excretion by kidney

Propafenone / ↑ Effect of propafenone due to ↓ breakdown by liver

Quinidine / ↑ Effect of quinidine due to ↓ breakdown by liver

Quinine / ↑ Effect of quinine due to ↓ breakdown by liver

Succinylcholine / ↑ Neuromuscular blockade → respiratory depression and extended apnea

Sulfonylureas / ↑ Effect of sulfonylureas due to ↓ breakdown by liver

Tetracyclines / ↓ Effect of tetracyclines due to ↓ absorption from GI tract

Theophyllines / ↑ Effect of theophyllines due to ↓ breakdown by liver

Tocainide / ↓ Effect of tocainide

Triamterene / ↑ Effect of triamterene due to ↓ breakdown by liver

Tricyclic antidepressants / ↑ Effect of tricyclic antidepressants due to ↓ breakdown by liver

Warfarin / ↑ Effect of anticoagulant due to ↓ breakdown by liver

Dosage: Tablets, Oral Solution. Adults: *Duodenal ulcers, short-term:* 800 mg h.s. Alternate dosage: 300 mg q.i.d. with meals and at bedtime for 4–6 weeks (administer with antacids, staggering the dose of antacids) or 400–600 mg b.i.d. (in the morning and evening). **Maintenance:** 400 mg h.s. *Active benign peptic ulcers:* 800 mg h.s. (preferred regimen) or 300 mg q.i.d. with meals and at bedtime for no more than 8 weeks. *Pathological hypersecretory conditions:* 300 mg q.i.d. with meals and at bedtime up to a maximum of 2,400 mg daily. *Erosive gastroesophageal reflux:* **Adults,** 800 mg b.i.d. or 400 mg q.i.d. for 12 weeks. *Upper GI bleeding:* 300 mg q 6 hr or 600 mg b.i.d. in the morning and at bedtime. *Dyspepsia:* 400 mg b.i.d. **Pediatric, all uses:** 20–40 mg/kg daily in divided doses q.i.d. with meals and at bedtime. **IM, IV, IV infusion.** *Duodenal ulcer, gastric ulcer, hypersecretory conditions, upper GI bleeding:* **Adults:** 300 mg (as the base) q 6–8 hr, not to exceed 2,400 mg daily. *Prophylaxis of stress ulcers:* **Adults:** 300 mg (base) q 6 hr (or more frequently to maintain the gastric pH above 4). *Prophylaxis of aspiration pneumonitis:* **Adults, IM:** 300 mg (base) 1 hr before induction of anesthesia and 300 mg (base) IM or IV q 4 hr until client is conscious. **Pediatric, all uses:** 5–10 mg/kg q 6–8 hr.

NURSING CONSIDERATIONS

Administration/Storage

1. For IV injections, dilute in 0.9% sodium chloride injection (or other compatible solution) to a total volume of 20 ml. Inject over a period of 1–2 min.
2. For intermittent IV infusion, dilute 300 mg in at least 50 ml of 5% dextrose injection (or other compatible solution) and infuse over 15–20 min.
3. For continuous IV infusion, give a loading dose of 150 mg (by intermittent IV infusion); then, administer 37.5 mg/hr (900 mg daily) in 0.9% sodium chloride injection, 5% or 10% dextrose injection, 5% sodium bicarbonate injection, lactated Ringer's solution, or as part of total parenteral nutrition.
4. Cimetidine is incompatible with aminophylline and barbiturates in IV solutions. Also, it is incompatible in the same syringe with pentobarbital sodium and a pentobarbital sodium/atropine sulfate combination.
5. For IM use, cimetidine can be given undiluted.
6. Administer oral medication with meals and a snack at bedtime.
7. If antacids are to be used, stagger the dose with that of cimetidine.
8. In impaired renal function, a dose of 300 mg q 8–12 hr may be necessary.

Assessment

1. Note the general over-all condition of the client. Clients receiving radiation therapy or myelosuppressive drugs may have their action potentiated by cimetidine.
2. Review the list of drug interactions prior to administering the drug. Determine if any of the drugs the client is taking may interact unfavorably with cimetidine.
3. Assess location and extent of abdominal pain. Note any blood in emesis, stool, or gastric aspirate.

Interventions

1. Be alert to mood swings that may occur. These are more common among the elderly than among people in other age groups. Report any new symptoms of confusion immediately.
2. Note if the client appears to have an increased susceptibility to infections. Clients taking cimetidine may develop agranulocytosis, thrombocytopenia, or anemia and should have periodic hematologic evaluations.
3. For the elderly, severely ill client or one who has renal impairment, monitor renal function, fluid intake, and output for the duration of the therapy.
4. Some clients develop diarrhea. Monitor the frequency of the episodes, their severity and persistence. Help the client to maintain adequate hydration, monitor the electrolytes, and if the problem persists, notify the physician.
5. Inspect the skin routinely for rashes or other skin changes. Document and report any abnormalities to the physician.

6. May alter response to skin tests with allergenic extracts. Discontinue drug 24 hr prior to skin testing.

Client/Family Teaching

1. Review the goals of the prescribed therapy and explain the need to continue taking the drug even though the symptoms may have disappeared.
2. Discuss other drugs that have been ordered and establish an appropriate schedule to assure compliance with drug therapy.
3. Discuss any required dietary modifications, especially if the client is being treated for GI problems. Evaluate carefully because it may be necessary to have a dietitian work with the client.
4. Instruct clients about the symptoms of gynecomastia or galactorrhea and advise them to report these side effects to the physician should they occur.
5. Report immediately if they have abdominal pain, bloody stools, or other indications that the ulcer has been reactivated.
6. Avoid alcohol, spicy foods, and aspirin-containing products, all of which may enhance GI irritation.
7. Advise that smoking may alter the drug's response. Offer assistance in smoking cessation.
8. Do not perform tasks that require mental alertness until drug effects are realized.

Evaluation: Evaluate client for:
- Reports of a reduction in abdominal pain
- Evidence of a reduction in GI irritation and bleeding
- Negative occult blood findings in GI secretions and stools

Cinoxacin
(sin-**OX**-ah-sin)
Cinobac Pulvules (Rx)

See also *Anti-Infectives*, p. 80.

Classification: Urinary anti-infective.

Action/Kinetics: Cinoxacin acts by inhibiting DNA replication, resulting in a bactericidal action. It is rapidly absorbed after oral administration; a 500-mg dose results in a urine concentration of 300 mcg/ml during the first 4-hr period and 100 mcg/ml during the second 4-hr period. Within 24 hr, 97% is excreted in the urine, 60% unchanged. **Mean serum t$^{1}/_{2}$:** 1.5 hr. Food decreases peak serum levels by approximately 30%.

Uses: Initial and recurrent urinary tract infections caused by *Escherichia coli, Proteus mirabilis, P. vulgaris, Klebsiella,* and *Enterobacter* species. **Note:** Cinoxacin is ineffective against *Pseudomonas,* staphylococci, and enterococci infections. Prophylaxis of urinary tract infections.

Contraindications: Hypersensitivity. Infants and prepubertal children. Anuric clients. Lactation.

Special Concerns: Pregnancy category: C. Use with caution in clients with hepatic or kidney disease.

Side Effects: *GI:* Nausea, vomiting, anorexia, cramps, diarrhea. *CNS:* Headache, dizziness, insomnia, confusion, nervousness. *Dermatologic:* Rash, pruritus, urticaria, edema. *Other:* Tingling sensation, photophobia, perineal burning, tinnitus.

Drug Interaction: Probenecid ↓ excretion of cinoxacin → ↓ concentration in the urine.

Laboratory Test Interference: ↑ BUN, AST, ALT, serum creatinine, and alkaline phosphatase.

Dosage: Capsules. Adults: 1 g/day in 2–4 divided doses for 7–14 days. *In clients with impaired renal function:* **Initial,** 500 mg; **then,** dosage schedule based on creatinine clearance (see package insert). *Prophylaxis of infections:* 250 mg at bedtime for up to 5 months.

NURSING CONSIDERATIONS

See also *General Nursing Considerations For All Anti-Infectives,* p. 83.

Assessment

1. Ascertain that renal and hepatic function tests are completed before initiating therapy.
2. Determine if client is anuric; if so do not administer.

Ciprofloxacin hydrochloride

(sip-row-**FLOX**-ah-sin)

Ciloxan Ophthalmic, Cipro, Cipro I.V. (Rx)

See also *Fluoroquinoline Antibiotics,* p. 152.

Classification: Antibacterial, fluoroquinolone derivative.

Action/Kinetics: Ciprofloxacin is effective against the following gram-positive organisms: staphylococci including *S. aureus, S. epidermidis,* and *S. hemolyticus;* streptococci including *S. pyogenes, S. pneumoniae, S. faecalis.* Also, ciprofloxacin is effective against a large number of gram-negative organisms, including: *Escherichia coli, Klebsiella* (including *K. pneumoniae, Proteus mirabilis, P. vulgaris, Enterobacter, Citrobacter, Salmonella, Shigella, Campylobacter, Providencia stuartii, P. rettgeri, P. alcalifaciens, Serratia, Morganella morganii, Acinetobacter, Pseudomonas aeruginosa, P. fluorescens, Hemophilus influenzae, H. ducreyi, H. parainfluenzae, Neisseria gonorrhoeae, N. meningitidis, Brucella melitensis, Pasturella, Legionella, Listeria monocytogenes,* and others. **Maximum serum levels:** 1–2 hr. **t½:** 4 hr. Peak serum levels above 5 mcg/ml should be avoided. Food delays absorption of the drug. About 40%–50% of an oral dose is excreted unchanged in the urine.

Uses: Systemic. Genitorurinary tract infections including pyelonephritis, complicated urinary tract infections, polycystic kidney disease, prostatitis. Respiratory infections including nosocomial pneumonia, cystic fibrosis in adults, bronchiectasis and COPD (adults). Not a drug of first choice in the treatment of presumed or confirmed pneumococcal pneumonia. Skin and soft tissue infections including wound infections, infections of the extremities in diabetes mellitus, puncture wounds of the feet, atypical mycobacteria. Sexually transmitted diseases such as chancroid and gonorrhea. Bone and joint infections as gram-negative arthritis, osteomyelitis. Traveler's diarrhea. **Ophthalmic.** Superficial ocular infections due to *Staphylococcus* species, *Streptococcus* species (including *S. pneumoniae, S. pyogenes*), *Escherichia coli, Hemophilus dureyi, H. influenzae, Klebsiella pneumoniae, Neisseria gonorrhoeae, Proteus* species, *Acinetobacter calcoaceticus, Enterobacter aerogenes, Pseudomonas aeruginosa,* and *Chlamydia trachomatis.*

Contraindications: Hypersensitivity to quinolones. Use in children. During lactation, consideration should be given either to discontinuing nursing or the drug. Ophthalmic use in the presence of dendritis keratitis, varicella, vaccinia, mycobacterial and fungal eye infections, and after removal of foreign bodies from the cornea.

Special Concerns: Pregnancy category: C. Safety and effectiveness of ophthalmic or IV use has not been determined in children.

Side Effects: *GI:* Nausea, vomiting, diarrhea, oral candidiasis, dysphagia, intestinal perforation, dyspepsia, heartburn, anorexia, pseudomembranous colitis, flatulence, abdominal discomfort, GI bleeding, oral mucosal pain, dry mouth, bad taste. *CNS:* Headache, restlessness, insomnia, nightmares, hallucinations, tremor, lightheadedness, confusion, seizures, ataxia, mania, weakness, drowsiness, dizziness, psychotic reactions, malaise, depression, depersonalization, paresthesia. *GU:* Nephritis, crystalluria, hematuria, cylindruria, renal failure, urinary retention, polyuria, vaginitis, urethral bleeding, acidosis, renal calculi, interstitial nephritis, vaginal candidiasis. *Skin:* Rashes, urticaria, photosensitivity, flushing, pruritus, erythema nodosum, cutaneous candidiasis, hyperpigmentation, edema (of lips, neck, face, conjunctivae, hands), angioedema, toxic epidermal necrolysis, exfoliative dermatitis, Stevens-Johnson syndrome. *Ophthalmic:* Blurred or disturbed vision, double vision, eye pain. *CV:* Hypertension, syncope, angina pectoris, palpitations, atrial flutter, myocardial infarction, cerebral thrombosis, ventricular ectopy, cardiopulmonary arrest, postural hypotension. *Respiratory:* Dyspnea, bronchospasm, pulmonary embolism, edema of larynx or lungs, hemoptysis, hiccoughs, epistaxis. *Hematologic:* Eosinophilia, pancytopenia, leukopenia, neutropenia, anemia, leukocytosis, agranulocytosis, bleeding diathesis. *GU:* Crystalluria, cylinduria, candiduria, hematuria, glucosuria, pyuria, albuminuria, proteinuria, vaginitis. *Miscellaneous:* Superinfections; fever; chills; tinnitus; joint pain or stiffness; back, neck or chest pain; flare-up of gout; flushing; hyperpigmentation; worsening of myasthenia gravis; hepatic necrosis; cholestatic jaundice; hearing loss. *After ophthalmic use:* Irritation burning, itching, angioneurotic edema, urticaria, maculopapular and vesicular dermatitis, crusting of lid margins, conjunctival hyperemia, bad taste in mouth, corneal staining, keratitis, keratopathy, allergic reactions, photophobia, decreased vision, tearing, lid edema. Also, a white, crystalline precipitate in the superficial part of corneal defect (onset within 1–7 days after initiating therapy; lasts about 2 weeks and does not affect continued use of the medication).

Additional Drug Interactions

Azlocillin ↓ excretion of ciprofloxacin → possible ↑ effect.

Laboratory Test Interferences: ↑ ALT, AST, alkaline phosphatase, serum bilirubin, LDH, serum creatinine, BUN, serum gamma-glutamyltransferase, serum amylase, uric acid, blood monocytes, potassium, prothrombin time, triglycerides, cholesterol. ↓ Hemoglobin/hematocrit. Either ↑ or ↓ blood glucose, platelets.

Dosage: Tablets. *Urinary tract infections:* 250 mg (mild) to 500 mg (severe) q 12 hr for 7–14 days. *Infectious diarrhea:* 500 mg q 12 hr for 5–7 days. *Skin, skin structures, respiratory tract, bone and joint infections:* 500 mg (mild) to 750 mg (severe or complicated) q 12 hr for 7–14 days. Treatment may be required for 4–6 weeks in bone and joint infections. Dose must be reduced in clients with a creatinine clearance less than 50 ml/min. **IV Infusion.** *Urinary tract infections:* 200 mg (mild) to 400 mg (severe or complicated) q 12 hr for 7–14 days. *Skin, skin structures, respiratory tract, bone and joint infections:* 400 mg (for mild to moderate infections) q 12 hr for 7–14 days. **Ophthalmic Solution.** *Acute infections:* **intial,** 1–2 gtt q 15–30 min; **then,** reduce dosage as infection improves. *Moderate infections:* 1–2 gtt 4–6 (or more) times daily.

NURSING CONSIDERATIONS

See also *General Nursing Considerations For All Anti-Infectives,* p. 83.

Administration/Storage

1. Although food delays the absorption of the drug, it may be taken with or without meals. The recommended time for dosing is 2 hr after a meal.
2. Clients on theophylline or probenecid require close observation and potential medication adjustments.
3. Do not administer to children.
4. Following instillation of the ophthalmic solution, light finger pressure should be applied to the lacrimal sac for 1 min.
5. The IV solution dose should be given over a period of 60 min.
6. The IV product can be diluted with 0.9% sodium chloride injection or 5% dextrose injection. Such dilutions are stable

up to 14 days at refrigerated or room temperatures and should not be frozen.

Client/Family Teaching

1. Take medication 2 hr after meals because food may delay absorption.
2. Avoid ingestion of antacids containing magnesium or aluminum within 2 hr of taking drug because antacids may interfere with absorption.
3. Stress the importance of drinking increased amounts of fluids and keeping the urine acidic to minimize the risk of crystalluria.
4. The medication may cause dizziness; use caution in any activity that requires mental alertness or coordination.
5. Report any persistent GI symptoms such as diarrhea, vomiting, or abdominal pain to the physician.
6. Provide a printed list of side effects stressing those that should be reported immediately.

Evaluation: Evaluate for a positive response as characterized by:
- Reduction of fever
- Decrease in WBCs
- Increased appetite
- Reports of symptomatic improvement
- Negative laboratory culture reports

Cisplatin

(sis-**PLAH**-tin)
**Platinol, Platinol-AQ
(Abbreviation: CDDP) (Rx)**

See also *Antineoplastic Agents,* p. 85.

Classification: Antineoplastic, alkylating agent.

Action/Kinetics: Cisplatin, a heavy metal inorganic coordination complex, acts similarly to alklyating agents in that it produces interstrand and intrastrand crosslinks in DNA. The drug is cell-cycle nonspecific. **t½: Initial,** 25–49 min; **postdistribution,** 58–73 hr. Incomplete urinary excretion (only 27%–43% after 5 days). Drug concentrates in liver, kidneys, large and small intestines, with low penetration of CNS. The drug is over 90% bound to plasma protein.

Uses: Treatment of metastatic testicular (in combination with bleomycin and vinblastine) and ovarian (in combination with doxorubicin) tumors in clients with prior radiotherapy or surgery. Advanced bladder cancer unresponsive to other treatment. *Investigational:* Cancer of the adrenal cortex, head and neck, breast, cervix, endometrium, stomach, lung, prostate. Neuroblastoma. Germ cell tumors of the ovary and in children. Osteosarcoma.

Additional Contraindications: Preexisting renal impairment, bone marrow suppression, hearing impairment, and allergic reactions to platinum. Lactation.

Special Concerns: Safe use during pregnancy has not been established.

Additional Side Effects: *Renal:* Severe cumulative renal toxicity, including renal tubular damage and renal insufficiency. *Electrolytes:* Low levels of calcium, magnesium, potassium, phosphate, and sodium. *Neurologic:* Seizures, taste loss, peripheral neuropathies. Neurotoxicity may occur 4–7 months after prolonged therapy. *Otic:* Ototoxicity characterized by tinnitus, especially in children. *Ophthalmologic:* Papilledema, cerebral blindness, optic neuritis. High doses have resulted in blurred vision and altered color perception. *Miscellanous:* Anaphylactic reactions, hyperuricemia.

C

Additional Drug Interactions

Aminoglycosides / Cumulative nephrotoxity
Anticonvulsants / Plasma levels of anticonvulsants may become subtherapeutic
Loop diuretics / Additive ototoxcity
Phenytoin / ↓ Effect of phenytoin due to ↓ plasma levels

Laboratory Test Interferences: ↑ Plasma iron levels. Nephrotoxicity results in ↑ serum uric acid, BUN, and creatinine and ↓ creatinine clearance.

Dosage: IV. *Metastatic testicular tumors, remission induction:* **Usual dosage,** cisplatin, 20 mg/m² daily for 5 days q 3 weeks for 3 courses; bleomycin sulfate, **IV (rapid infusion):** 30 units weekly (on day 2 of each week) for 12 consecutive weeks; vinblastine sulfate, **IV:** 0.15–0.2 mg/kg twice weekly (days 1 and 2) q 3 weeks for 4 courses (i.e., 8 doses total). *Metastatic ovarian tumor, as single agent:* 100 mg/m² once q 4 weeks. *In combination with doxorubicin hydrochloride,* cisplatin: 50 mg/m² once q 3 weeks (on day 1); doxorubicin hydrochloride: 50 mg/m² once q 3 weeks (on day 1). The drugs are given sequentially. *Advanced bladder cancer:* 50–70 mg/m² once q 3–4 weeks as a single agent. **Note:** Repeat courses should not be administered until (1) serum creatinine is below 1.5 mg/dl and/or the BUN is below 25 mg/dl; (2) platelets are equal to or greater than 100,000/mm³ and leukocyte count is equal to or greater than 4,000/mm³; and (3) auditory activity is within the normal range.

NURSING CONSIDERATIONS

See also *Nursing Considerations* for *Antineoplastic Agents,* p. 88.

Administration/Storage

1. Store unopened vials of dry powder in refrigerator at 2°C–8°C to maintain stability for 2 years.
2. Reconstitute 10- and 50-mg vials with 10 or 50 ml of sterile water for injection as instructed on package insert.
3. Do not refrigerate reconstituted vials because a precipitate will form. Reconstituted solution is stable at room temperature for 20 hr.
4. Use of a 0.45-μm filter is advised.
5. Before administration of cisplatin, hydrate client with 1–2 L of fluid by IV over a period of 8–12 hr.
6. Add dosage recommended from reconstituted vial to 2 L of 5% dextrose in one-half or one-third normal saline containing 37.5 g mannitol. Infuse over a period of 6–8 hr. Furosemide is ordered by some practitioners instead of mannitol.
7. Do not use any equipment with aluminum for preparing or administering because a black precipitate will form and loss of potency will occur.
8. Platinol-AQ is a sterile, multidose vial without preservatives.

Unopened containers should be stored between 15°–25°C protected from light. Once opened, the solution is stable for 28 days protected from light or for 7 days under fluorescent room light.

9. Have emergency equipment readily available to treat any occurrence of an anaphylactic reaction to cisplatin.

Interventions

1. *During therapy assess closely*
   - for facial edema, bronchoconstriction, tachycardia, and shock.
   - for tremors that may progress to seizures due to hypomagnesemia.
   - for tetany, confusion, or signs of hypocalcemia associated with hypomagnesemia; monitor Ca and Mg levels.
2. Ascertain that baseline renal tests are performed before therapy is instituted because cisplatin may cause severe cumulative renal toxicity.
3. Hydrate well and monitor for adequate hydration and output for 24 hr after treatment. Report oliguria.
4. Anticipate that additional doses of cisplatin will not be administered until the client's renal function has returned to baseline value.
5. Recommend client for audiometry before initiating therapy and before administering subsequent doses, to ascertain that client's hearing has not been affected.
6. Be alert to complaints of ringing in ears, difficulty in hearing, edema of lower extremities,

and decreased urination and report.

Evaluation: Evaluate client for evidence of a ↓ in tumor size and spread.

Clarithromycin
(klah-rith-roh-**MY**-sin)
Biaxin (Rx)

Classification: Antibiotic, macrolide.

Action/Kinetics: Clarithromycin is a macrolide antibiotic that acts by binding to the 50S ribosomal subunit of susceptible organisms, thus interfering with microbial protein synthesis. The drug is rapidly absorbed from the GI tract although food slightly delays the onset of absorption as well as the formation of the active metabolite but does not affect the extent of the bioavailability. **Peak serum levels:** 2 hr when fasting. **Steady state peak serum levels:** 1 mcg/ml within 2–3 days after 250 mg q 12 hr and 2–3 mcg/ml after 500 mg q 12 hr. Clarithromycin and 14-OH clarithromycin (active metabolite) are readily distributed to body tissues and fluids. **t½, elimination:** 3–7 hr (depending on the dose) for clarithromycin and 5–6 hr for 14-OH clarithromycin. Up to 30% of a dose is excreted unchanged in the urine.

Uses: Mild to moderate infections caused by susceptible strains of the following: Pharyngitis/tonsillitis due to *Streptococcus pyogenes* and acute maxillary sinusitis due to *S. pneumoniae*. Acute bacterial exacerbation of chronic bronchitis due to *Hemophilus influenzae*, *Moraxella catarrhalis*, or *S. pneu-*

moniae. Pneumonia due to *Mycoplasma pneumoniae* or *S. pneumoniae*. Uncomplicated skin and skin structure infections due to *Staphylococcus aureus* or *S. pyogenes*. The active metabolite, 14-OH clarithromycin, has significant activity (twice the parent compound) against *Hemophilus influenzae*.

Contraindications: Hypersensitivity to clarithromycin, other macrolide antibiotics, or erythromycin.

Special Concerns: Pregnancy category: C. Use with caution in severe renal impairment with or without concomitant hepatic impairment and during lactation. Safety and effectiveness in children less than 15 years of age have not been determined.

Side Effects: *GI:* Diarrhea, nausea, abnormal taste, dyspepsia, abdominal discomfort or pain, pseudomembranous colitis. *CNS:* Headache. *Hematologic:* Decreased white blood count, elevated prothrombin time.

Drug Interactions

See also Drug Interactions for
    Erythromycins, p. 145.
    Carbamazepine / ↑ Blood
    levels of carbamazepine
Theophylline / ↑ Serum levels of
    theophylline

Laboratory Test Interferences: ↑ ALT, AST, GGT, alkaline phosphatase, LDH, total bilirubin, BUN, serum creatinine.

Dosage: Tablets, adults and children over 15 years of age. *Pharyngitis, tonsillitis, chronic bronchitis due to S. pneumoniae or H. influenzae, pneumonia, skin and skin structure infections:* 250 mg q 12 hr. *Acute maxillary sinusitis, chronic bronchitis due to H. influenzae:* 500 mg q 12 hr.

NURSING CONSIDERATIONS

See also *General Nursing Considerations* for *All Anti-Infectives*, p. 83.

Administration/Storage

1. The drug may be given with or without meals.
2. Decreased doses or prolonging the dosing interval should be considered in clients with severe renal impairment with or without coexisting impaired hepatic function.
3. Drug may cause bitter taste.

Assessment

1. Note any sensitivity to erythromycin or any of the macrolide antibiotics.
2. Obtain baseline liver and renal function studies.
3. Determine that appropriate laboratory cultures are done prior to initiation of drug therapy.
4. List drugs client currently prescribed noting any potential interactions.

Interventions: Monitor I&O and observe client for any evidence of persistent diarrhea. Report this finding as an antibiotic-associated colitis may be precipitated by *Clostridium difficile* and require alternative management.

Evaluation: Evaluate client for:
- Clinical evidence and reports of symptomatic improvement
- Laboratory evidence of negative culture reports

Clindamycin hydrochloride hydrate

(klin-dah-**MY**-sin)

Cleocin Hydrochloride, Dalacin C 🌸 (Rx)

Clindamycin palmitate hydrochloride

(klin-dah-**MY**-sin)

Cleocin Pediatric, Dalacin C Palmitate 🌸 (Rx)

Clindamycin phosphate

(klin-dah-**MY**-sin)

Cleocin Phosphate, Cleocin T, Dalacin C Phosphate🌸, Dalacin T Topical🌸 (Rx)

See also *Anti-Infectives*, p. 80.

Classification: Antibiotic, clindamycin and lincomycin.

General Statement: Clindamycin is a semisynthetic antibiotic. Its spectrum resembles that of the erythromycins and includes a variety of gram-positive organisms, particularly staphylococci, streptococci, and pneumococci, and some gram-negative organisms. Should not be used for trivial infections.

Action/Kinetics: Suppresses protein synthesis by microorganism by binding to ribosomes (50S subunit) and preventing peptide bond formation. Is both bacteriostatic and bactericidal. **Peak serum concentration: PO,** 2.5 mcg/ml after 45 min. **t½:** 2.4 hr. In serious infections the rate of IV administration is adjusted to maintain appropriate serum drug concentrations: 4–6 mcg/ml.

Uses: Serious respiratory tract infections (e.g., empyema, lung abscess, pneumonia) caused by staphylococci, streptococci, and pneumococci. Serious skin and soft tissue infections, septicemia, intraabdominal infections, pelvic inflammatory disease, female genital tract infections. May be the drug of choice for *Bacteroides fragilis.* In combination with aminoglycosides for mixed aerobic and anaerobic bacterial infections. Staphylococci-induced acute hematogenous osteomyelitis. Adjunct to surgery for chronic bone/joint infections. Used topically for inflammatory acne vulgaris.

Contraindications: Hypersensitivity to either clindamycin or lincomycin. Not for use in treating viral and minor bacterial infections.

Special Concerns: Safe use during pregnancy has not been established. Use with caution in infants up to 1 month of age. Use with caution in clients with GI disease, liver or renal disease, history of allergy or asthma.

Side Effects: *GI:* Nausea, vomiting, diarrhea, abdominal pain, tenesmus, flatulence, bloating, anorexia, weight loss, esophagitis. Nonspecific colitis, pseudomembranous colitis (may be severe). *Allergic:* Morbilliform rash (most common). Also, maculopapular rash, urticaria, pruritus, fever, hypotension. Rarely, polyarteritis, anaphylaxis, erythema multiforme. *Hematologic:* Leukopenia, neutropenia, eosinophilia, thrombocytopenia, agranulocytosis. *Miscellaneous:* Superinfection. Also sore throat, fatigue, urinary frequency, headache. *Following IV use:* Thrombophlebitis, erythema, pain, swelling. *Following IM use:* Pain, induration, sterile abscesses. *Following topical use:* Erythema, irritation, dryness, peeling, itching, burning, oiliness. **Note:** The injection contains benzyl alcohol, which has been associated with a fatal gasping syndrome in infants.

Drug Interactions

Antiperistaltic antidiarrheals (opiates, Lomotil) / ↑ Diarrhea due to ↓ removal of toxins from colon
Ciprofloxacin HCl / Additive antibacterial activity
Erythromycin / Cross-interference → ↓ effect of both drugs
Kaolin (e.g., Kaopectate) / ↓ Effect due to ↓ absorption from GI tract
Neuromuscular blocking agents / ↑ Effect of blocking agents

Laboratory Test Interferences: ↓ Levels of AST, ALT, NPN, alkaline phosphatase, bilirubin, BSP retention, and ↓ platelet count.

Dosage: PO only: Capsules, Oral Solution. Adults: Clindamycin HCl, Clindamycin palmitate HCl: 150–450 mg q 6 hr, depending on severity of infection. **Pediatric:** Clindamycin HCl hydrate: 8–20 mg/kg daily divided into 3–4 equal doses; clindamycin palmitate HCl: 8–25 mg/kg daily divided into 3–4 equal doses. **Children less than 10 kg:** Minimum recommended dose is 37.5 mg t.i.d. **IV.** Clindamycin phosphate. **Adults:** 0.6–2.7 g daily in 2–4 equal doses depending on severity of infection. *Life-threatening infections:* 4.8 g. **Pediatric over 1 month:** 15–40 mg/kg daily in 3–4 equal doses depending on severity of infections. *Severe infections:* No less than 300 mg daily, regardless of body weight. *Acute pelvic inflammatory disease:* **IV,** 600 mg q.i.d. plus gentamicin, 2 mg/kg IV; **then,** gentamicin, 1.5 mg/kg t.i.d. IV therapy should be continued for 2 days after client improves. The 10- to 14-day treatment cycle should be completed using clindamycin, **PO,** 450 mg q.i.d. **Topical Gel or Solution:** Apply thin film b.i.d. to affected areas.

NURSING CONSIDERATIONS

See also *General Nursing Considerations For All Anti-Infectives,* p. 83.

Administration/Storage

1. Give parenteral clindamycin only to hospitalized clients.
2. Dilute IV injections to maximum concentration of 12 mg/ml, with no more than 1,200 mg administered in 1 hr.
3. Single IM injections greater than 600 mg are not advisable. Inject deeply into muscle to prevent induration, pain, and sterile abscesses.
4. Do not refrigerate; otherwise, solution may become thickened.
5. Administer IV over a period of 20–60 min, depending on dose and therapeutic serum concentration to be attained.
6. Dosage should be reduced in severe renal impairment.

Assessment

1. Take full history to determine extensiveness of respiratory tract infections.
2. Note presence of serious skin and soft tissue infections, septicemia, and evidence of infection of the female genital tract.
3. Note any client complaints indicative of pelvic inflammatory disease or intra-abdominal infections.
4. Note any client history of liver or renal disease, allergies, or history of GI problems.
5. Obtain baseline liver and renal function studies.

Interventions

1. Be prepared to manage pseudomembranous colitis, which can occur 2–9 days or several weeks after initiation of therapy. Provide fluids, electrolytes, protein supplements, systemic corticosteroids, and vancomycin as ordered.
2. Do not administer, and caution client against using, antiperistaltic agents if diarrhea occurs because these can prolong or aggravate the condition.
3. Do not administer kaolin concomitantly because this will reduce absorption of antibiotic. If kaolin is required, administer 3 hr before antibiotic.
4. Do not use any acne or topical mercury preparations containing a peeling agent in an area affected by medication because severe irritation may occur.
5. Administer on an empty stomach to ensure optimum absorption. Drug should be administered only as long as necessary.
6. During IV administration observe for hypotension and keep client in bed for 30 min following therapy. Advise that a bitter taste may also be evident.
7. Observe for drug interactions caused by concurrent administration of neuromuscular blocking agents. Be alert to hypotension, bronchospasms, cardiac disturbances, hyperthermia, and respiratory depression.
8. Observe closely for:
   - Skin rash because this is the most frequently reported side effect
   - Clients with renal and/or hepatic impairment and

newborns for organ dysfunction
- GI disturbances, such as abdominal pain, diarrhea, anorexia, nausea, vomiting, bloody or tarry stools, and excessive flatulence. Discontinuation of drug may be indicated.

Client/Family Teaching

1. Take oral medication with a full glass of water to prevent esophageal ulceration.
2. If client has slight GI disturbance, the drug may be taken with food because food does not affect the rate of absorption to any significant extent.
3. Report any side effects such as persistent vomiting, diarrhea, fever, or abdominal pain and cramping.
4. Review symptoms of colitis that may be severe and should be reported immediately to the physician, especially when working with the frail elderly.

Evaluation: Evaluate for:

- Client/family knowledge and understanding of illness, response to therapy, and teaching
- Subjective reports of symptomatic improvement
- Status (presence/absence) of pretreatment symptoms and C&S results to determine effectiveness of treatment

---

Clofazimine
(kloh-**FAYZ**-ih-meen)
Lamprene (Rx)

Classification: Leprostatic.

Action/Kinetics: This drug is thought to exert a bactericidal effect on the mycobacterium; the drug inhibits mycobacterial growth and binds to mycobacterial DNA. Cross-resistance with rifampin or dapsone is not observed. The drug is concentrated in fatty tissues and the reticuloendothelial system. **t½:** 70 days. The drug is excreted in the feces via the bile, as well as in sputum, sweat, and sebum.

Uses: Lepromatous leprosy (including dapsone-resistant leprosy and leprosy complicated by erythema nodosum leprosum). In combination with other drugs to prevent resistance in multibacillary leprosy.

Special Concerns: Pregnancy category: C. Use with caution in clients with abdominal pain or diarrhea. Use during lactation only if benefits outweigh risks. Safety and efficacy have not been determined in children.

Side Effects: *GI:* Nausea, vomiting, diarrhea, abdominal or epigastric pain. Rarely, GI bleeding, intestinal obstruction, anorexia, constipation, liver enlargement. *Dermatologic:* Pink to brownish black pigmentation of skin, ichthyosis, dryness of skin, pruritus, rash. *Ophthalmologic:* Pigmentation of conjunctiva and cornea (due to clofazimine crystals), phototoxicity, decreased vision, eye irritation, burning, itching, or dryness. *CNS:* Headache, dizziness, drowsiness, neuralgia, fatigue, depression. *Miscellaneous:* Jaundice, weight loss, hepatitis, anemia, thromboembolism, bone pain, edema, cystitis, fever, vascular pain, lymphadenopathy, eosinophilia, hypokalemia. Discoloration of urine, feces, sweat, or sputum.

Laboratory Test Interferences: ↑ AST, serum bilirubin, albumin.

Dosage: Capsules. *Leprosy resistant to dapsone:* 100 mg daily together with one or more other leprostatic drugs for a period of 3 years; **maintenance:** clofazimine alone, 100 mg daily. *Erythema nodosum leprosum:* Dosage depends on severity of symptoms, but doses greater than 200 mg daily are not recommended. Goal is 100 mg daily.

NURSING CONSIDERATIONS

Administration/Storage

1. Clofazimine should be given with one or more other leprostatic agents to prevent the development of resistance to each drug.
2. *Treatment of Overdose:* Gastric lavage or induction of vomiting. General supportive measures.

Client/Family Teaching

1. Take medication as ordered and with food to minimize GI irritation.
2. Report any increased GI distress, depression, and/or unusual side effects immediately.
3. Although reversible, clofazimine will cause pink to brownish black skin discoloration, which may persist after therapy.
4. Do not be alarmed because all body fluids become discolored during therapy.
5. Oil baths and frequent lotion application may minimize itchy, dry skin formation.

Evaluation: Evaluate for a positive clinical response as evidenced by:

- Subjective reports of symptomatic improvement
- Decrease in the size and number of skin lesions

Clofibrate
(kloh-**FYE**-brayt)
Atromid-S, Claripex✹, Novo–Fibrate✹ (Rx)

Classification: Antihyperlipidemic agent.

Action/Kinetics: Clofibrate decreases triglycerides, VLDL, and, cholesterol and either does not change or increases HDL and does not change or decreases LDL. The mechanism is not known with certainty but may be due to increased catabolism of VLDL to LDL and decreased synthesis of VLDL by the liver. The higher the cholesterol level, the more effective the drug. The drug may also increase the release of antidiuretic hormone from the posterior pituitary. **Peak plasma levels:** 2–6 hr. **t½:** 6–25 hr. **Therapeutic effect: Onset,** 2–5 days; **maximum effect:** 3 weeks. Triglycerides return to pretreatment levels 2–3 weeks after therapy is terminated. Clofibrate is hydrolyzed to the active p-chlorophenoxyisobutyric acid (CPIB) which is further metabolized and excreted in the urine. The drug may concentrate in fetal blood. Liver function tests should be performed during therapy.

Uses: As adjunct treatment for type III hyperlipidemia in clients with a significant risk of coronary heart disease who have not responded to diet or other measures. Limited use in type II hyperlipidemia. *Investigational:* Partial central diabetes insipidus in clients with some residual posterior pituitary function.

Contraindications: Impaired hepatic or renal function, primary biliary cirrhosis, pregnancy or expectation thereof, lactation, children.

Special Concerns: Use with caution in clients with gout and peptic ulcer. Reduced dosage may be required in geriatric clients due to age-related decreases in renal function. Dosage has not been established in children.

Side Effects: *GI:* Nausea, dyspepsia, weight gain, gastritis, vomiting, bloating, flatulence, abdominal distress, stomatitis, loose stools, hepatomegaly. *CNS:* Headaches, dizziness, fatigue, weakness, drowsiness. *CV:* Changes in blood-clotting time, arrhythmias, increased or decreased angina, thrombophlebitis, swelling and phlebitis at xanthoma site, pulmonary embolism. *Skeletal muscle:* Myositis, asthenia, myalgia, weakness, muscle aches, cramps. *GU:* Impotence, dysuria, hematuria, decreased urine output, decreased libido, proteinuria. *Hematologic:* Anemia, leukopenia, eosinophilia. *Dermatologic:* Urticaria, skin rash, dry skin, pruritus, dry brittle hair, alopecia. *Enzyme changes:* ↑ Creatine phosphokinase, increased serum transaminase (if levels continue to increase after maximum therapeutic response has been achieved, therapy should be discontinued). *Other:* Increased incidence of gallstones, dyspnea, polyphagia.

Drug Interactions

Anticoagulants / Clofibrate ↑ anticoagulant effect by ↓ plasma protein binding

Antidiabetics (sulfonylureas) / Clofibrate ↑ effect of antidiabetics

Furosemide / Concurrent use may ↑ effects of both drugs

Insulin / Clofibrate ↑ effect of insulin

Probenecid / ↑ Effect of clofibrate due to ↓ breakdown by liver and ↓ kidney excretion

Rifampin / ↓ Effect of clofibrate due to ↑ breakdown by liver

Dosage: Capsules. Adults: *Antihyperlipidemic,* 500 mg q.i.d. Therapeutic response may take several weeks to become apparent. Drug must be administered on a continuous basis because lowered levels of cholesterol and other lipids will return to elevated state within several weeks after administration is stopped. Discontinue after 3 months if response is poor.

NURSING CONSIDERATIONS

Assessment: If client is of childbearing age, determine if pregnant.

Client/Family Teaching

1. Nausea usually decreases with continued therapy or reduced dosage. Drug may be taken with food if GI upset occurs.
2. Observe for bleeding from any orifice or for purpura if client is also receiving anticoagulant therapy. A reduction in anticoagulant drug dosage is customary if clofibrate therapy is instituted.
3. Report symptoms of hypoglycemia because of possible drug interactions when taking oral antidiabetics.
4. Use contraception if appropriate because clofibrate may be teratogenic.
5. Do not discontinue contraception for several months after discontinuing drug therapy, if pregnancy is planned.
6. The drug must be taken as ordered to be effective.

7. Report any adverse side effects so that drug therapy can be evaluated.

Evaluation

1. Assess client compliance and side effects that may require a change in therapy.
2. Assess for ↓ in serum cholesterol and lipid levels.

Clomiphene citrate
(**KLOH**-mih-feen)
Clomid, Milophene, Serophene (Rx)

Classification: Ovarian stimulant.

Action/Kinetics: The drug acts by combining with estrogen receptors, thus decreasing the number of available receptor sites. Through negative feedback, the hypothalamus and pituitary are thus stimulated to increase secretion of LH and FSH. Under the influence of increased levels of these hormones, an ovarian follicle develops, followed by ovulation and corpus luteum development. Most women ovulate after the first course of therapy. Further treatment may be inadvisable if pregnancy fails to occur after ovulatory responses. It is readily absorbed from the GI tract and is excreted in the feces. $t^{1}/_{2}$: 5–7 days. **Time to peak effect:** 4–10 days after the last day of treatment for ovulation.

Uses: Selected cases of female infertility in which normal endogenous estrogen levels have been observed. *Investigational:* Male infertility, insufficiency of the corpus luteum, diagnosis of hypothalamic-pituitary-gonadal axis function in males and in ovarian function studies.

Contraindications: Pregnancy, liver disease or history thereof, abnormal bleeding of undetermined origin. Ovarian cysts. The absence of neoplastic disease should be established before treatment is initiated. Therapy is ineffective in clients with ovarian or pituitary failure.

Side Effects: *Ovarian:* Ovarian overstimulation and/or enlargement and subsequent symptoms resembling those of premenstrual syndrome. *Ophthalmologic:* Blurred vision, spots, or flashes, probably due to intensification of after images. *GI:* Abdominal distention, pain, or soreness; nausea, vomiting. *GU:* Abnormal uterine bleeding, breast tenderness. *CNS:* Insomnia, nervousness, headache, depression, fatigue, lightheadedness, dizziness. *Other:* Hot flashes, increased urination, allergic symptoms, weight gain, alopecia (reversible).

Laboratory Test Interferences: ↑ Serum thyroxine and thyroxine-binding globulin.

Dosage: Tablets. *First course:* 25–50 mg daily for 5 days. *Second course:* Same dosage if ovulation has occurred. In absence of ovulation, dose may be increased to 100 mg/day for 5 days (some clients may require up to 250 mg daily to induce ovulation).

NURSING CONSIDERATIONS

Administration

1. Therapy may be started any time in clients who have had no recent incidence of uterine bleeding.
2. If the client has had recent uterine bleeding, start the therapy on the fifth day of the cycle.
3. If the client has had a previous

course of therapy to which she did not respond, start the new therapy after 30 days have elapsed.

Note: Most clients will respond following the first course of therapy. Further therapy is not recommended if pregnancy does not result following 3 or 4 ovulatory responses.

Assessment

1. Note if the client has a history of hepatic dysfunction.
2. Determine if the client has had a history of abnormal bleeding of undetermined origin.
3. If the client is sexually active, determine the possibility of pregnancy.

Client/Family Teaching

1. Teach client to take basal body temperature and chart temperature on a graph to determine if ovulation has occurred.
2. If pain in the pelvic area or abdominal distention occur, she should discontinue the drug and report the symptoms to the physician. These symptoms indicate ovarian enlargement and the possible presence of an ovarian cyst.
3. If she develops blurred vision or has spots or flashes in the eyes, the retina of the eye may be affected. Discontinue taking the medication and report for an ophthalmologic examination.
4. Avoid performing hazardous tasks involving body coordination or mental alertness because the drug may cause lightheadedness, dizziness, or visual disturbances.
5. Discontinue taking the medication and check with the phy-

sician if pregnancy is suspected because the drug may have teratogenic effects.

Evaluation: Assess client for a positive clinical response as evidenced by ↑ in levels of FSH and LH with resultant ovulation and pregnancy.

Clomipramine hydrochloride
(kloh-**MIP**-rah-meen)
Anafranil (Rx)

See also *Tricyclic Antidepressants,* p. 239.

Classification: Antidepressant, tricyclic.

Action/Kinetics: Clomipramine possesses a high degree of anticholinergic and sedative effects as well as moderate orthostatic hypotension. **t½:** 19–37 hr. **Effective plasma levels:** 80–100 ng/ml. The drug is metabolized to the active desmethylclomipramine.

Uses: Treatment of obsessive-compulsive disorder in which the obsessions or compulsions cause marked distress, significantly interfere with social or occupational activities, or are time-consuming. Also, to treat panic attacks and cataplexy associated with narcolepsy.

Contraindications: To relieve symptoms of depression.

Special Concerns: Safety has not been established for use during pregnancy and lactation. Safety has not been established in children less than 10 years of age.

Additional Side Effects: Hyperthermia, especially when used with other drugs. Increased risk of seizures. Aggressive reactions, asthenia, anemia, eructation, failure to ejaculate, laryngitis, vestibular disorders, muscle weakness.

Dosage: Capsules. Adult, initial: 25 mg daily; **then,** increase gradually to approximately 100 mg during the first 2 weeks (depending on client tolerance). The dose may then be increased slowly to a maximum of 250 mg daily over the next several weeks. **Adolescents, children, initial:** 25 mg daily; **then,** increase gradually during the first 2 weeks to a maximum of 100 mg or 3 mg/kg, whichever is less. The dose may then be increased to a maximum daily dose of 3 mg/kg or 200 mg, whichever is less.

NURSING CONSIDERATIONS

See also *Nursing Considerations for Tricyclic Antidepressants,* p. 242.

Administration/Storage

1. Initially, the daily dosage should be divided and given with meals to reduce GI side effects.
2. After the optimum dose is determined, the total daily dose can be given at bedtime to minimize daytime sedation.
3. The dose for all ages should be adjusted to the lowest effective dose and be evaluated periodically to determine the continued need for treatment.
4. Although the efficacy of clomipramine has not been determined after 10 weeks of therapy, clients have successfully used the drug for up to 1 year without loss of beneficial effects.

Evaluation: Assess client for reports of symptomatic improvement in the frequency and duration of depressive episodes.

Clonazepam
(kloh-**NAY**-zeh-pam)

Klonopin, Rivotril✶ (C-IV) (Rx)

See also *Anticonvulsants,* p. 61, and *Benzodiazepines,* p. 108.

Classification: Anticonvulsant, miscellaneous.

Action/Kinetics: Benzodiazepine derivative. Clonazepam increases presynaptic inhibition and suppresses the spread of seizure activity. **Peak plasma levels:** 1–2 hr. **$t^{1/2}$:** 18–50 hr. **Peak serum levels:** 20–80 ng/ml. The drug is more than 80% bound to plasma protein; it is metabolized almost completely in the liver to inactive metabolites, which are excreted in the urine.

Even though a benzodiazepine, clonazepam is used only as an anticonvulsant. However, contraindications, side effects, and so forth are similar to those for diazepam.

Uses: Absence seizures (petit mal) including Lennox-Gastaut syndrome, akinetic and myoclonic seizures. Some effectiveness in clients resistant to succinimide therapy. *Investigational:* Parkinsonian dysarthria, acute manic episodes of bipolar affective disorder, leg movements (periodic) during sleep, adjunct in treating schizophrenia, neuralgias, multifocal tic disorders.

Contraindications: Sensitivity to benzodiazepines. Severe liver disease, acute narrow-angle glaucoma. Pregnancy.

Additional Side Effects: In clients in whom different types of seizure disorders exist, clonazepam may elicit or precipitate grand mal seizures.

Drug Interactions

CNS depressants / Potentiation of CNS depressant effect of clonazepam

Phenobarbital / ↓ Effect of clonazepam due to ↑ breakdown by liver

Phenytoin / ↓ Effect of clonazepam due to ↑ breakdown by liver

Valproic acid / ↑ Chance of absence seizures

Dosage: Tablets. *Seizure disorders:* **Adults: initial,** 0.5 mg t.i.d. Increase by 0.5–1 mg daily q 3 days until seizures are under control or side effects become excessive; **maximum:** 20 mg/day. **Pediatric up to 10 years or 30 kg:** 0.01–0.03 mg/kg/day in 2–3 divided doses up to a maximum of 0.05 mg/kg/day. Increase by increments of 0.25–0.5 mg q 3 days until seizures are under control or maintenance of 0.1–0.2 mg/kg is attained.

Parkinsonian dysarthria: 0.25–0.5 mg daily. *Acute manic episodes of bipolar affective disorder:* 0.75–16 mg daily. *Periodic leg movements during sleep:* 0.5–2 mg nightly. *Adjunct to treat schizophrenia:* 0.5–2 mg daily. *Neuralgias:* 2–4 mg daily. *Multifocal tic disorders:* 1.5–12 mg daily.

NURSING CONSIDERATIONS

See *Nursing Considerations* for *Benzodiazepines,* p. 111, and *Anticonvulsants,* p. 63.

Administration/Storage

1. Approximately one-third of clients show some loss of anticonvulsant activity within 3 months; adjustment of dose may reestablish effectiveness.
2. Adding clonazepam to existing anticonvulsant therapy may increase the depressant effects.
3. The daily dose should be divided into 3 equal doses; if doses can not be divided equally, the largest dose should be given at bedtime.

Evaluation: Evaluate client for reports of a decrease in the number and frequency of seizures.

Clonidine hydrochloride

(**KLOH**-nih-deen)

Apo-Clonidine✢, Catapres, Catapres-TTS-1, -2, and -3, Dixarit✢ (Rx)

Classification: Antihypertensive, centrally acting antiadrenergic.

Action/Kinetics: Stimulates alpha-adrenergic receptors of the CNS, which results in inhibition of the sympathetic vasomotor centers and decreased nerve impulses. Thus, bradycardia and a fall in both systolic and diastolic blood pressure occurs. Plasma renin levels are decreased, while peripheral venous pressure remains unchanged. The drug has few orthostatic effects. Although sodium chloride excretion is markedly decreased, potassium excretion remains unchanged. Tolerance to the drug may develop. **Onset, PO:** 30–60 min; **transdermal:** 2–3 days. **Peak plasma levels, PO:** 3–5 hr; **transdermal:** 2–3 days. **Maximum effect, PO:** 2–4 hr. **Duration, PO:** 12–24 hr; **transdermal:** 7 days (with system in place). $t^{1/2}$: 12–16 hr. Approximately 50% excreted unchanged in the urine; 20% excreted through the feces.

The transdermal dosage form contains the following levels of drug: Catapres-TTS-1 contains 2.5 mg clonidine (surface area 3.5 cm^2), with 0.1 mg released daily; Catapres-TTS-2 contains 5 mg clonidine (surface area 7 cm^2), with 0.2 mg released daily; and Catapres-TTS-3 contains 7.5 mg clonidine (surface area 10.5 cm^2), with 0.3 mg released daily.

Uses: Mild to moderate hypertension. A diuretic or other antihypertensive drugs, or both, are often used concomitantly. *Investigational:* Diabetic diarrhea, alcohol withdrawal, treatment of Gilles de la Tourette syndrome, detoxification of opiate dependence, constitutional growth delay in children, hypertensive urgency (diastolic > 120 mm Hg), menopausal flushing, diagnosis of pheochromocytoma, facilitate cessation of smoking, ulcerative colitis, postherpetic neuralgia, reduce allergen-induced inflammation in clients with extrinsic asthma.

Special Concerns: Pregnancy category: C. Use with caution in presence of severe coronary insufficiency, recent myocardial infarction, cerebrovascular disease, or chronic renal failure. Use with caution during lactation. Safe use in children not established. Geriatric clients may be more sensitive to the hypotensive effects; a decreased dosage may also be necessary in these clients due to age-related decreases in renal function.

Side Effects: *CNS:* Drowsiness (common), sedation, dizziness, headache, fatigue, malaise, nightmares, nervousness, restlessness, anxiety, mental depression, increased dreaming, insomnia, hallucinations, delirium, agitation. *GI:* Dry mouth (common), constipation, anorexia, nausea, vomiting, parotid pain, weight gain. *CV:* Congestive heart failure, Raynaud's phenomenon, abnormalities in ECG, palpitations, tachycardia and bradycardia, orthostatic symptoms, conduction disturbances, sinus bradycardia. *Dermatologic:* Urticaria, skin rashes, angioneurotic edema, pruritus, thinning of hair, alopecia. *GU:* Impotence, urinary retention, decreased sexual activity, loss of libido, nocturia, difficulty in urination. *Musculoskeletal:* Muscle or joint pain, leg cramps, weakness. *Other:* Gynecomastia, increase in blood glucose (transient), increased sensitivity to alcohol, dryness of mucous membranes of nose; itching, burning, dryness of eyes; skin pallor, fever.

Transdermal products: Localized skin reactions, pruritus, erythema, allergic contact sensitization and contact dermatitis, localized vesiculation, hyperpigmentation, edema, excoriation, burning, papules, throbbing, blanching, generalized macular rash.

Note: Rebound hypertension may be manifested if clonidine is withdrawn abruptly.

Symptoms of Overdose: Hypotension, bradycardia, respiratory and CNS depression, hypoventilation, hypothermia, apnea, miosis, agitation, irritability, lethargy, seizures, cardiac conduction defects, arrhythmias, transient hypertension, diarrhea, vomiting.

Drug Interactions

Alcohol / ↑ Depressant effects
Beta-adrenergic blocking agents /
   Paradoxical hypertension;

also, ↑ severity of rebound hypertension following clonidine withdrawal

CNS depressants / ↑ Depressant effect

Levodopa / ↓ Effect of levodopa

Tolazoline / Blocks antihypertensive effect

Tricyclic antidepressants / Blocks antihypertensive effect

Laboratory Test Interferences: Transient ↑ of blood glucose and serum creatinine phosphokinase. Weakly + Coombs' test. Alteration of electrolyte balance.

Dosage: Tablets. *Hypertension:* **Initial,** 0.1 mg b.i.d.; **then,** increase by 0.1–0.2 mg/day until desired response is attained; **maintenance:** 0.2–0.6 mg/day in divided doses (maximum: 2.4 mg/day). Tolerance necessitates increased dosage or concomitant administration of a diuretic. Gradual increase of dosage after initiation minimizes side effects. **Note:** In hypertensive clients unable to take oral medication, clonidine may be administered sublingually at doses of 0.2–0.4 mg daily. **Pediatric:** 5–25 mcg/kg daily in divided doses q 6 hr; increase dose at 5–7 day intervals.

Transdermal, initial: Use 0.1 mg system; **then,** if after 1–2 weeks adequate control has not been achieved, can use another 0.1 mg system or a larger system. The antihypertensive effect may not be seen for 2–3 days. The system should be changed every 7 days.

Investigational Uses. Gilles de la Tourette syndrome: 0.15–0.2 mg/day. *Withdrawal from opiate dependence:* 15–16 mcg/kg daily. *Alcohol withdrawal:* 0.3–0.6 mg q 6 hr. *Diabetic diarrhea:* 0.15–1.2 mg daily or 0.3 mg/24 hr patch. *Consti-*

tutional growth delay in children: 0.0375–0.15 mg/m^2 daily. *Hypertensive urgency:* **Initial:** 0.1–0.2 mg; **then,** 0.05–0.1 mg q hr to a maximum of 0.8 mg. *Menopausal flushing:* 0.1–0.4 mg daily or 0.1 mg/24 hr patch. *Diagnosis of pheochromocytoma:* 0.3 mg. *Postherpetic neuralgia:* 0.2 mg daily. *Reduce allergen-induced inflammation in extrinsic asthma:* 0.15 mg for 3 days. *Facilitate cessation of smoking:* 0.15–0.4 mg daily or 0.2 mg/24 hr patch. *Ulcerative colitis:* 0.3 mg t.i.d.

NURSING CONSIDERATIONS

Administration/Storage

1. If the transdermal system is used, apply the medication to a hairless area of skin, such as upper arm or torso changing the system every 7 days.
2. Use a different site with each application.
3. It may take 2–3 days to achieve effective blood levels using the transdermal system. Therefore, any prior drug dosage should be reduced gradually.
4. If the drug is to be taken orally, administer the last dose of the day at bedtime to ensure overnight control of blood pressure.
5. Clients with severe hypertension may require antihypertensive drug therapy in addition to transdermal clonidine.
6. If the drug is to be discontinued, it should be done gradually over a period of 2–4 days.
7. Have IV tolazoline readily available to treat acute toxicity caused by clonidine.
8. *Treatment of Overdose:* Maintain respiration; perform gastric lavage followed by activat-

ed charcoal. Magnesium sulfate may be used to hasten the rate of transport through the GI tract. IV atropine sulfate (0.6 mg for adults; 0.01 mg/kg for children), epinephrine, tolazoline, or dopamine to treat persistent bradycardia. IV fluids and elevation of the legs are used to reverse hypotension; if unresponsive to these measures, dopamine (2–20 mcg/kg/min) or tolazoline (1 mg/kg IV, up to a maximum of 10 mg/dose) may be used. To treat hypertension, diazoxide, IV furosemide, or an alpha-adrenergic blocking drug may be used.

Assessment: Note the client's occupation. This drug may interfere with the client's ability to work and should be noted.

Interventions

1. Monitor BP closely during the initial therapy. A decrease in BP occurs within 30–60 min after administration of clonidine and may persist for 8 hrs.
2. Weigh the client daily, in the morning, in clothing of the same weight, to determine if there is edema caused by sodium retention. Any fluid retention should disappear after 3–4 days.
3. Note any fluctuations in BP to determine whether it is preferable to use clonidine alone or concomitantly with a diuretic. A stable BP reduces orthostatic effects of postural changes.
4. Observe for a paradoxical hypertensive response if client is also receiving propranolol.
5. Note any evidence of depression that may be precipitated by the drug, especially in those clients with a history of mental depression.
6. If the client is concomitantly receiving tolazoline or a tricyclic antidepressant, be aware that these drugs may block the antihypertensive action of clonidine. An increased dosage of clonidine may be indicated.
7. Note any side effects clients experience. These can be minimized by increasing the dosage of clonidine gradually until the desired effects are obtained.
8. Drug dosage is based on the client's BP and tolerance to therapy. Therefore, side effects should be recorded and reported even if they may seem minor.

Client/Family Teaching

1. Do not engage in activities that require mental alertness, such as operating machinery or driving a car, because the drug may cause drowsiness.
2. Do not discontinue medication abruptly or without medical supervision. Also do not initiate any change in the medication regimen until this has been cleared by the physician.
3. If the drug is to be withdrawn, explain the need for gradual withdrawal to prevent rebound hypertension.
4. If the client has Parkinson's disease and is controlled with levodopa, advise to report any increase in signs and symptoms of the disease. Clonidine may reduce the effect of levodopa.

Evaluation

1. Assess client/family knowledge and understanding of illness

and response to prescribed therapy as well as teaching.

2. Evaluate client for effective control of blood pressure.
3. Assess client for freedom from complications of drug therapy.

Clorazepate dipotassium

(klor-**AYZ**-eh-payt)

Apo-Clorazepate ✹, Gen-Xene, Novo–Clopate ✹, Tranxene, Tranxene-SD, Tranxene-SD Half (C-IV, Rx)

See also *Benzodiazepines,* p. 108.

Classification: Antianxiety agent, benzodiazepine type; anticonvulsant.

Action/Kinetics: Peak plasma levels: 1–2 hr. $t^{1/2}$: 30–100 hr. Clorazepate is hydrolyzed in the stomach to desmethyldiazepam, the active metabolite. Oxazepam is also an active metabolite. $t^{1/2}$, **desmethyldiazepam:** 30–100 hr; $t^{1/2}$, **oxazepam:** 5–15 hr. **Time to peak plasma levels:** 0.5–2 hr. The drug is slowly excreted by the kidneys.

Uses: Anxiety, tension. Acute alcohol withdrawal, as adjunct in treatment of seizures. Adjunct for treating partial seizures.

Additional Contraindications: Depressed clients, nursing mothers. Give cautiously to clients with impaired renal or hepatic function.

Special Considerations: Pregnancy category: D.

Dosage: Capsules/Tablets. *Anxiety:* **Initial,** 7.5–15 mg b.i.d.–q.i.d.; **maintenance:** 15–60 mg/day in divided doses. **Elderly or debilitated clients: initial,** 7.5–15 mg/day. **Alternative: Single daily dosage: Adult, initial,** 15 mg; **then,** 11.25–22.5 mg once daily. *Acute alcohol withdrawal: Day 1,* **initial,** 30 mg; **then,** 15 mg b.i.d.–q.i.d. the first day; *day 2,* 45–90 mg/day; *day 3,* 22.5–45 mg/day; *day 4,* 15–30 mg/day. Thereafter, reduce to 7.5–15 mg/day and discontinue as soon as possible. *Anticonvulsant, adjunct:* **Adults and children over 12 years: initial,** 7.5 mg t.i.d.; increase no more than 7.5 mg/week to maximum of 90 mg/day. **Children (9–12 years): initial,** 7.5 mg b.i.d.; increase no more than 7.5 mg/week to maximum of 60 mg/day. Not recommended for children under 9 years of age.

NURSING CONSIDERATIONS

See *Nursing Considerations* for *Benzodiazepines,* p. 111.

Assessment

1. Note any evidence of depression because drug is contraindicated.
2. Determine in clients with excessive alcohol intake when they had their last drink.

Evaluation: Evaluate client for:
- Reports of a reduction in anxiety and tension levels
- Control of alcohol withdrawal seizures

Clotrimazole

(kloh-**TRY**-mah-zohl)

Canesten ✹, Canestin 1 ✹, Canestin 3 ✹, Canestin 10% Cream ✹, Clotrimaderm ✹, Gyne-Lotrimin, Lotrimin, Lotrimin AF, Mycelex, Mycelex-G, Mycelex OTC, Myclo ✹, Neo-Zol (OTC, Rx)

See also *Anti-Infectives,* p. 80.

Classification: Antifungal.

Action/Kinetics: Depending on concentration, this drug may be fungistatic or fungicidal. The drug acts by inhibiting the biosynthesis of sterols, resulting in damage to the cell wall and subsequent loss of essential intracellular elements due to altered permeability. Clotrimazole may also inhibit oxidative and peroxidative enzyme activity and inhibit the biosynthesis of triglycerides and phospholipids by fungi. When used for *Candida albicans,* the drug inhibits transformation of blastophores into the invasive mycelial form. It is poorly absorbed from the GI tract and metabolized in the liver to inactive compounds that are excreted through the feces. **Duration:** up to 3 hr.

Uses: Broad-spectrum antifungal effective against *Malassezia furfur, Trichophyton rubrum, T. mentagrophytes, Epidermophyton floccosum, Microsporum canis, Candida albicans. Oral troche:* Oropharyngeal candidiasis. *Topical OTC products:* Topically to treat tinea pedis, tinea cruris, and tinea corporis. *Topical prescription products:* Same as OTC plus candidiasis and tinea versicolor. *Vaginal products:* Vulvovaginal candidiasis.

Contraindications: Hypersensitivity. First trimester of pregnancy.

Special Concerns: Pregnancy category: C for systemic use and B for topical/vaginal use. Use with caution during lactation.

Side Effects: *Skin:* Irritation including rash, stinging, pruritus, urticaria, erythema, peeling, blistering, edema. *Vaginal:* Lower abdominal cramps; urinary frequency; bloating; vaginal irritation, itching or burning; dyspareunia. *Hepatic:* Abnormal liver function tests. *GI:* Nausea and vomiting following use of troche.

Dosage: Troche: One troche 5 times daily for 14 consecutive days. **Topical Cream, Lotion, Solution:** Massage into affected skin and surrounding areas b.i.d. in morning and evening. Diagnosis should be reevaluated if no improvement occurs in 4 weeks. **Vaginal tablets:** One 100-mg tablet/day at bedtime for 7 days or two 100-mg tablets at bedtime for 3 days. One 500-mg tablet can be inserted once at bedtime. **Vaginal cream:** 5 g (one applicatorful)/day at bedtime for 7–14 consecutive days.

NURSING CONSIDERATIONS

See also *General Nursing Considerations For All Anti-Infectives,* p. 83.

Administration/Storage

1. Mycelex-G vaginal cream can be stored at 2°C–30°C (36°F–86°F). Mycelex-G, 100-mg vaginal tablets should not be stored above 35°C (95°F); the 500 mg vaginal tablets should be stored below 30°C (86°F).
2. The troche should be slowly dissolved in the mouth.
3. Topical products should not come in contact with the eyes.

Client/Family Teaching

1. Review goals of therapy and appropriate method for administration.
2. Unless directed by physician to do otherwise, apply only after cleaning the affected area.
3. When treating vaginal infections, the client should not engage in intercourse; or, to

prevent infection, the partner should wear a condom.

4. To prevent staining of clothes, a sanitary napkin should be used with vaginal tablets or cream.

Evaluation: Evaluate for a positive clinical response based on laboratory findings and subjective reports of symptomatic improvement.

Cloxacillin sodium

(klox-ah-**SILL**-in)
**Apo-Cloxi✶, Cloxapen, Novo–
Cloxin✶, Orbenin✶, Tegopen
(Rx)**

See also *Anti-Infectives,* p. 80, and *Penicillins,* p. 197.

Classification: Antibiotic, penicillin.

Action/Kinetics: Resistant to penicillinase and is acid stable. **Peak plasma levels:** 7–15 mcg/ml after 30–60 min. **t½:** 30 min. Protein binding: 88%–96%. Well absorbed from GI tract. Mostly excreted in urine, but some excreted in bile.

Uses: Infections caused by penicillinase-producing staphylococci, including pneumococci, group A beta-hemolytic streptococci, and penicillin G-sensitive staphylococci.

Dosage: Capsules, Oral Solution. *Skin and soft tissue infections, mild to moderate upper respiratory tract infections:* **Adults and children over 20 kg:** 250 mg q 6 hr; **pediatric, less than 20 kg:** 50 mg/kg daily in divided doses q 6 hr. *Lower respiratory tract infections or disseminated infections:* **Adults and children over 20 kg:** 0.5 g q 6 hr; **pediatric, less than 20 kg:** 100 (or more) mg/kg daily in divided doses q 6 hr. Alternatively, a dose of 50–100 mg/kg daily (up to a maximum of 4 g/day) divided q 6 hr may be used for infants and children.

NURSING CONSIDERATIONS

See also *Nursing Considerations* for *Penicillins,* p. 200.

Administration/Storage

1. Add amount of water stated on label in 2 portions; shake well after each addition.
2. Shake well before pouring each dose.
3. Refrigerate reconstituted solution and discard unused portion after 14 days.
4. Administer 1 hr before or 2 hr after meals, because food interferes with absorption of drug.

Evaluation

1. Assess client closely for wheezing and sneezing because these side effects are more likely to occur with this drug.
2. Assess client for subjective reports of symptomatic improvement.
3. Note ↓ in fever, ↓ WBCs, and negative laboratory culture reports.

Clozapine

(**KLOH**-zah-peen)
Clozaril (Rx)

Classification: Antipsychotic.

Action/Kinetics: Clozapine interferes with the binding of dopamine to both D-1 and D-2 receptors; it is more active at limbic than at striatal dopamine receptors. Thus, it is relatively free from extrapyramidal side effects and it does not induce catalepsy. The drug also acts as an antagonist at adrenergic, cholinergic, histaminergic, and serotonergic receptors. Clozapine increases the amount of time spent in REM sleep. Food does not affect the bioavailability of clozapine. **Peak plasma levels:** 2.5 hr. **Average maximum concentration at steady state:** 122 ng/ml plasma after 100 mg b.i.d. Highly bound to plasma proteins. **t½:** 12 hr. Metabolized in the liver to inactive compounds and excreted through the urine (50%) and feces (30%).

Uses: Severely ill schizophrenic clients who do not respond adequately to conventional antipsychotic therapy, either because of ineffectiveness or intolerable side effects from other drugs. Due to the possibility of development of agranulocytosis and seizures, continued use should be avoided in patients failing to respond.

Contraindications: Myeloproliferative disorders. Use in conjunction with other agents known to suppress bone marrow function. Severe CNS depression or coma due to any cause. Lactation.

Special Concerns: Pregnancy category: B. Use with caution in clients with known cardiovascular disease, prostatic hypertrophy, narrow angle glaucoma, hepatic or renal disease.

Side effects: *Hematologic:* Agranulocytosis, leukopenia, neutropenia, eosinophilia. *CNS:* Seizures (appear to be dose dependent), drowsiness or sedation, dizziness, vertigo, headache, tremor, restlessness, nightmares, hypokinesia, akinesia, agitation, akathisia, confusion, rigidity, fatigue, insomnia, hyperkinesia, weakness, lethargy, slurred speech, ataxia, depression, anxiety, epileptiform movements. *CV:* Orthostatic hypotension (especially initially), tachycardia, syncope, hypertension, angina, chest pain, cardiac abnormalities, changes in ECG. *Neuroleptic malignant syndrome:* Hyperpyrexia, muscle rigidity, altered mental status, irregular pulse or blood pressure, tachycardia, diaphoresis, cardiac dysrhythmias. *GI:* Constipation, nausea, heartburn, abdominal discomfort, vomiting, diarrhea, anorexia. *GU:* Urinary abnormalities, incontinence, abnormal ejaculation, urinary frequency or urgency, urinary retention. *Musculoskeletal:* Muscle weakness, pain (back, legs, neck), muscle spasm, muscle ache. *Respiratory:* Dyspnea, shortness of breath, throat discomfort, nasal congestion. *Miscellaneous:* Salivation, sweating, visual disturbances, fever (transient), dry mouth, rash, weight gain, numb or sore tongue. *Symptoms of Overdose:* Drowsiness, delirium, tachycardia, respiratory depression, hypotension, hypersalivation, seizures, coma.

Drug Interactions

Anticholinergic drugs / Additive anticholinergic effects

Antihypertensive drugs / Additive hypotensive effects

Benzodiazepines / Possible respiratory depression and collapse

Digoxin / ↑ Effect of digoxin due to ↓ binding to plasma protein

Epinephrine / Clozapine may reverse effects if epinephrine is given for hypotension

Warfarin / ↑ Effect of warfarin due to ↓ binding to plasma protein

Dosage: PO, initial: 25 mg 1–2 times daily; **then,** if drug is tolerated, the dose can be increased by 25–50 mg/day to a dose of 300–450 mg/day at the end of 2 weeks.

Subsequent dosage increments should occur no more often than once or twice a week in increments not to exceed 100 mg. **Usual maintenance dose:** 300–600 mg/day (although doses up to 900 mg/day may be required in some patients). Total daily dose should not exceed 900 mg.

NURSING CONSIDERATIONS

Administration

1. Clozapine is no longer available through the "Clozaril Patient Management System." Rather, clozapine is now available through independent "Clozaril treatment systems" based upon a plan developed by physicians and pharmacists to ensure safe use of the drug with respect to weekly blood monitoring, data reporting, and drug dispensing. Prescriptions are limited to 1-week supplies and the drug may only be dispensed following receipt, by the pharmacist, of weekly white blood cell test results that fall within the established limits. All weekly blood test results must be reported by participating pharmacists to the Clozaril National Registry.
2. If the drug is effective, the lowest maintenance doses possible should be sought to maintain remission.
3. If termination of therapy is planned, the dose should be gradually reduced over a 1–2 week period. If cessation of therapy is abrupt due to toxicity, the client should be observed carefully for recurrence of psychotic symptoms.
4. Clozapine therapy may be initiated immediately upon discontinuation of other antipsychotic

medication; however, a 24-hr "washout period" is desirable.
5. *Treatment of Overdose:* An airway should be established and maintained with adequate oxygenation and ventilation. Give activated charcoal and sorbitol. Cardiac and vital signs should be monitored. General supportive measures.

Assessment

1. Observe and document client's behavior to determine baseline information against which to measure postmedication responses.
2. Obtain lab studies, including CBC, prior to initiating therapy.
3. Note any history of seizure disorder.
4. Obtain baseline vital signs and ECG.

Interventions

1. Periodically reassess the client to determine continued need for the drug.
2. If white blood cell counts fall below 2,000/mm^3 or granulocyte counts fall below 1,000/mm^3, the drug should be discontinued. Such clients should *not* be restarted on clozapine therapy.
3. Monitor vital signs and note any irregular pulse, tachycardia, hyperpyrexia, and hypotension and report to the physician.

Client/Family Teaching

1. Avoid driving or other potentially hazardous activity while taking clozapine due to the possibility of seizures.
2. Report immediately to the physician symptoms of lethargy, weakness, fever, sore throat,

malaise, mucous membrane ulceration, or other signs of infection.

3. Because of a risk of orthostatic hypotension, especially during initial dosing, use care when rising from a supine or sitting position.

4. Women of childbearing age should notify the physician if they become pregnant or intend to become pregnant during therapy.

5. Do not breast-feed when taking clozaril.

6. Do not take any prescription, OTC drugs or alcohol without the permission of the physician.

7. Stress the importance of periodic lab studies to monitor for the occurrence of agranulocytosis.

Evaluation

1. Observe for evidence of positive behaviors and compliance with prescribed drug therapy.

2. Review hematologic profile and note any evidence of bone marrow suppression because this is an indication to discontinue drug therapy.

------ *COMBINATION DRUG* ------
CoAdvil
(koh-**AD**-vil)
(OTC)

Classification/Content: Each tablet contains: *Nonsteroidal anti-inflammatory drug:* Ibuprofen, 200 mg. *Decongestant:* Pseudoephedrine HCl, 30 mg. See also information on individual components.

Uses: Temporary relief of symptoms associated with the common cold, flu, or sinusitis including fever, headache, nasal congestion, body aches, and pains.

Contraindications: Clients sensitive to aspirin. Hypertension, heart disease, diabetes, thyroid disease, difficulty in urination due to enlarged prostate. During the last 3 months of pregnancy. Should not be taken for more than 7 days for a cold or for more than 3 days for fever.

Special Concerns: Use with caution during lactation. Use in children under 12 years of age only on the advice of a physician.

Side Effects: *Higher doses:* Nervousness, dizziness, or sleeplessness. See also individual drugs.

Dosage: Tablets. 1 caplet q 4–6 hr while symptoms persist. If no response, dose can be increased to 2 caplets but the total dose should not exceed 6 caplets in 24 hr, unless directed otherwise by a physician.

NURSING CONSIDERATIONS

See *Nursing Considerations* for individual components.

Administration/Storage: The drug can be taken with food or milk if mild heartburn, stomach upset, or stomach pain occurs.

Evaluation: Assess client for subjective reports of improvement of cold and flu symptoms.

Codeine phosphate
(**KOH**-deen)
Paveral✣ (C-II, Rx)

Codeine sulfate
(**KOH**-deen)
(C-II, Rx)

See also *Narcotic Analgesics,* p. 174.

Classification: Narcotic analgesic, morphine type.

Action/Kinetics: Codeine resembles morphine pharmacologically but produces less respiratory depression, nausea, and vomiting. It is moderately habit-forming and constipating. Dosages over 60 mg often cause restlessness and excitement and irritate the cough center. However, in lower doses, it is a potent antitussive and is an ingredient in many cough syrups. **Onset:** 10–30 min. **Peak effect:** 30–60 min. **Duration:** 4–6 hr. **t½:** 3–4 hr. Codeine is 2/3 as effective orally as parenterally.

It is often used to supplement the effect of nonnarcotic analgesics such as aspirin and acetaminophen. Codeine is also found in many combination cough/cold products.

Uses: Relief of mild to moderate pain. Antitussive.

Special Concerns: Pregnancy category: C. May increase the duration of labor.

Additional Drug Interaction: Combination with chlordiazepoxide may induce coma.

Dosage: Tablets, IM, IV, SC. *Analgesia:* **Adults:** 15–60 mg q 4–6 hr, not to exceed 360 mg a day. **Pediatric, over 1 year:** 0.5 mg/kg q 4–6 hr. IV should not be used in children. *Antitussive:* **Adults:** 10–20 mg q 4–6 hr, up to maximum of 120 mg/day. **Pediatric, 2–6 years:** 2.5–5 mg orally q 4–6 hr, not to exceed 30 mg/day; **6–12 years:** 5–10 mg q 4–6 hr, not to exceed 60 mg/day.

NURSING CONSIDERATIONS

See also *Nursing Considerations for Narcotic Analgesics,* p. 177.

Client/Family Teaching: Clients taking codeine syrups to suppress coughs should be discouraged from overuse. Productive coughing is suppressed and may result in additional congestion.

Evaluation: Evaluate client for:
- Effective relief of pain
- Control of coughing with improved sleeping patterns

Colchicine
(KOHL-chih-seen)
(Rx)

Classification: Antigout agent.

Action/Kinetics: Colchicine, an alkaloid, does not increase the excretion of uric acid (not uricosuric), but it is believed to reduce the crystal-induced inflammation by reducing lactic acid production by leukocytes (resulting in a decreased deposition of sodium urate), by inhibiting leukocyte migration, and by reducing phagocytosis. The drug may also inhibit the synthesis of kinins and leukotrienes. **t½,** (IV, biphasic), initial: 20 min; final (in leukocytes): 60 hr. **Onset, IV:** 6–12 hr; **PO:** 12 hr. **Time to peak levels, PO:** 0.5–2 hr. Colchicine is metabolized in the liver and mainly excreted in the feces with 10%–20% excreted unchanged through the urine.

Uses: Prophylaxis and treatment of acute attacks of gout, either spontaneous or induced by allopurinol or uricosuric agents. Diagnosis of gout. *Investigational:* To slow progression of chronic progressive multiple sclerosis, to decrease frequency and severity of fever and to prevent amyloidosis in familiar Mediterranean fever, primary biliary cirrhosis, hepatic cirrhosis, adjunct in the treatment of primary amyloidosis, Behcet's disease, progressive systemic sclerosis, pseudogout due to chondrocalcinosis, dermatologic disorders including dermatitis herpetiformis, psoriasis, and palmo-plantar pustulosis.

Contraindications: Blood dyscrasias. Serious GI, hepatic, cardiac, or renal disorders.

Special Concerns: Pregnancy categories: C (oral) or D (parenteral). Use with caution during lactation. Dosage has not been established for children. Geriatric clients may be at greater risk of developing cumulative toxicity. Use with extreme caution for elderly, debilitated clients, especially in the presence of chronic renal, hepatic, GI, or cardiovascular disease. May impair fertility.

Side Effects: The drug is toxic; thus clients must be carefully monitored. *GI:* Nausea, vomiting, diarrhea, abdominal cramping. *Hematologic:* Aplastic anemia, agranulocytosis, or thrombocytopenia following long-term therapy. *Miscellaneous:* Peripheral neuritis, purpura, myopathy, neuropathy, alopecia, reversible azoospermia, dermatoses, hypersensitivity, liver dysfunction. If such symptoms appear, discontinue drug at once and wait at least 48 hr before reinstating drug therapy.

Symptoms of Acute Intoxication: Characterized at first by violent GI tract symptoms such as nausea, vomiting, abdominal pain, and diarrhea. The latter may be profuse, watery, bloody, and associated with severe fluid and electrolyte loss. Also, burning of throat and skin, hematuria and oliguria, rapid and weak pulse, general exhaustion, muscular depression, and CNS involvement. Death is usually caused by respiratory paralysis.

Drug Interactions

Acidifying agents / Inhibit the action of colchicine
Alkalinizing agents / Potentiate the action of colchicine
CNS depressants / Clients on colchicine may be more sensitive to CNS depressant effect of these drugs
Sympathomimetic agents / Enhanced by colchicine
Vitamin B$_{12}$ / Colchicine may interfere with absorption from the gut

Laboratory Test Interferences: Alters liver function tests. ↑ Alkaline phosphatase, AST. False + for hemoglobin or red blood cells in urine.

Dosage: Tablets. Adults: *Acute attack of gout,* Initially 1–1.2 mg followed by 0.5–1.3 mg q 1–2 hr until pain is relieved or nausea, vomiting, or diarrhea occurs. **Total amount required:** 4–8 mg. *Prophylaxis for gout:* 0.5–0.65 mg daily for 3–4 days a week if the client has less than one attack/year or 0.5–0.65 mg daily if the client has more than one attack/year. *Prophylaxis for surgical clients:* 0.5–0.65 mg t.i.d. for 3 days before and 3 days after surgery.

IV: Adults, initial, *acute attack of gout:* 2 mg; **subsequently,** 0.5 mg q 6 hr until pain is relieved; give up to 4 mg. (Some physicians recommend a single IV dose of 3 mg.) *Prophylaxis:* **PO:** 0.5–1 mg 1–2 times daily for 3–4 days/week. Usually, oral route is used exclusively.

NURSING CONSIDERATIONS

Administration/Storage

1. Store in tight, light-resistant containers.
2. Parenteral administration is only by the IV route. Drug causes severe local irritation if given SC or IM.
3. *Treatment of Acute Poisoning:* Gastric lavage, symptomatic support, including atropine and morphine, artificial respiration, hemodialysis, peritoneal dialysis, and treatment of shock.

Assessment

1. Note age and general physical condition of the client.
2. Obtain baseline CBC and hepatic studies prior to initiating therapy.
3. Document joint involvement noting pain, swelling, and degree of mobility.

Interventions

1. If the client develops nausea, vomiting, or diarrhea, notify the physician and discontinue the drug. These are early signs of toxicity.
2. If severe diarrhea occurs, anticipate the use of paregoric.
3. If the drug is administered IV, have atropine readily available to counteract adverse effects.
4. Assess the client for evidence of liver damage such as jaundice and a change in stool color. Monitor liver function studies and report any abnormal results.

Client/Family Teaching

1. If the physician has prescribed colchicine for use in acute attacks of gout, instruct the client to always have colchicine available.
2. Start or increase the dosage of colchicine as ordered at the first sign of joint pain or any other symptom of an impending attack of gout.

Evaluation: Evaluate client for:
- Effective relief of symptoms of gout attack with a ↓ in pain and swelling
- Freedom from complications of drug therapy

Colestipol hydrochloride
(koh-**LESS**-tih-poll)
Colestid (Rx)

Classification: Hypocholesterolemic, bile acid sequestrant.

Action/Kinetics: Colestipol, an anion exchange resin, binds bile acids in the intestine, forming an insoluble complex excreted in the feces. The loss of bile acids results in increased oxidation of cholesterol to bile acids and a decrease in LDL and serum cholesterol. Colestipol does not affect (or may increase) triglycerides or HDL and may increase VLDL. The drug is not absorbed from the GI tract. **Onset:** 1–2 days; **maximum effect:** 1 month. Return to pretreatment cholesterol levels after discontinuance of therapy: 1 month.

Uses: Primary hypercholesterolemia (type IIa hyperlipidemia) with a significant risk of coronary artery disease in clients who have not responded to diet or other measures. *Investigational:* Digitalis toxicity, pruritus associated with partial biliary obstruction, diarrhea due to bile acids, hyperoxaluria.

Contraindications: Complete obstruction or atresia of bile duct.

Special Concerns: Use during pregnancy only if benefits outweigh risks. Use with caution during lactation and in children. Children may be more likely to develop hyperchloremic acidosis although dosage has not been established. Clients over 60 years of age may be at greater risk of GI side effects and adverse nutritional effects.

Side Effects: *GI:* Constipation (may be severe), nausea, vomiting, diarrhea, heartburn, GI bleeding, anorexia, flatulence, belching, abdominal distention, aggravation of hemorrhoids. Fecal impaction in elderly clients. Large doses may cause steatorrhea. *Other:* Bleeding tendencies (due to hypoprothrombinemia). Osteoporosis, electrolyte imbalance, and CNS and musculoskeletal manifestations. Prolonged administration may interfere with absorption of fat-soluble vitamins. Irritation and rash of skin, tongue, and perianal area.

Drug Interactions: See *Cholestyramine,* p. 440.

Dosage: Oral Suspension. Adults: *Antihyperlipidemic:* 15–30 g daily before meals in 2–4 equally divided doses. *Digitalis toxicity:* 10 g followed by 5 g q 6–8 hr.

NURSING CONSIDERATIONS

Administration/Storage

1. Always mix with fluid before administering because resin may cause esophageal irritation or blockage.
2. Disguise unpalatable taste of drug by mixing it with fruit juice, soup, milk, water, applesauce, pureed fruit, or carbonated beverages.
3. Take other drugs 1 hr before or 4 hr after colestipol to reduce interference with their absorption.

Evaluation: Evaluate for:
- Client understanding of illness and response to therapy
- Decrease in serum cholesterol and LDL levels

Colfosceril palmitate (Dipalmitoylphosphatidylcholine, DPPC)

(kohl-**FOSS**-sir-ill)

Exosurf Neonatal (Rx)

Classification: Lung surfactant.

Action/Kinetics: Colfosceril contains dipalmitoylphosphatidylcholine (DPPC), which reduces surface tension in the lungs, as well as cetyl alcohol, which acts as a spreading agent for DPPC on the air–fluid surface. The product also contains tyloxapol, which is a nonionic surfactant that assists in dispersion of DPPC and cetyl alcohol, and sodium chloride to adjust osmolality. The drug can rapidly affect oxygenation and lung compliance. DPPC is reabsorbed from the alveoli into lung tissue where it is broken down and reutilized for further phospholipid synthesis and secretion.

Uses: Prophylaxis of respiratory distress syndrome in infants with birth weights of less than 1350 g and in infants with birth weights greater than 1350 g who manifest pulmonary immaturity. Treatment of infants who have developed respiratory distress syndrome. Such infants should be on mechanical ventilation and should have been diagnosed as having respiratory distress syndrome.

Special Concerns: Use of colfosceril should be undertaken only by medical personnel trained and experienced in airway and clinical management of unstable premature infants. Although colfosceril is effective in reducing mortality due to premature birth, infants may still develop severe complications resulting in either death or survival but with permanent handicaps. Benefits versus risks should be carefully assessed before using colfosceril in infants weighing 500–700 g.

Side Effects: *Respiratory:* Pulmonary hemorrhage, pulmonary air leak (pneumothorax, pneumomediastinum, pneumopericardium, pulmonary interstitial emphysema), mucous plugs in the endotracheal tube, apnea, congenital pneumonia, nosocomial pneumonia. *CV:* Intraventricular hemorrhage, patent ductus arteriosus, hypotension, bradycardia, tachycardia, exchange transfusion, persistent fetal circulation. *Changes in blood gases:* Fall or rise in oxygen saturation, fall or rise in transcutaneous pO_2, fall or rise in transcutaneous pCO_2. *Miscellaneous:* Necrotizing enterocolitis, major anomalies, hyperbilirubinemia, gagging, thrombocytopenia, seizures.

Dosage: Intratracheal. *Prophylaxis:* 5 ml/kg (as two 2.5 ml/kg half-doses) as soon as possible after birth. A second and third dose should be given 12 and 24 hr later to infants who are still on mechanical ventilation. *Rescue treatment:* 5 ml/kg (as two 2.5 ml/kg half-doses) as soon as possible after the diagnosis of respiratory distress syndrome

is confirmed. A second 5 ml/kg dose is given after 12 hr to infants who are still on mechanical ventilation. The safety and effectiveness of additional doses is not known.

NURSING CONSIDERATIONS
Administration/Storage

1. The drug should be reconstituted, according to the directions provided by the manufacturer, immediately prior to use with the diluent provided (preservative-free sterile water for injection). The reconstituted product is a milky white suspension.
2. The reconstituted suspension should be uniformly dispersed before administration. If the vial contains large flakes or particulate matter, it should not be used.
3. Five different-sized endotracheal tube adapters are provided with each vial of colfosceril. The adapters are clean but not sterile. The adapters should be used according to the instructions provided by the manufacturer.
4. Colfosceril is administered directly into the trachea through the sideport on the special endotracheal tube adapter without interruption of mechanical ventilation.
5. Each half-dose is given slowly over 1–2 min in small bursts timed with inspiration.
6. The first 2.5 ml/kg dose is given with the infant in the midline position; after the first half-dose is given, the infant's head and torso are first turned 45° to the right for 30 sec and then 45° to the left for 30 sec while continuing mechanical ventilation. This allows for

gravity to help with lung distribution of the drug.

7. Refluxing of colfosceril into the endotracheal tube may occur if the drug is given rapidly. If reflux is noted, administration of the drug should be stopped and the peak inspiratory pressure should be increased on the ventilator by 4–5 cm water until the endotracheal tube clears.

8. Colfosceril administration should be undertaken only by experienced neonatologists and other individuals experienced at neonatal intubation and ventilatory management.

Assessment

1. The infant heart rate, color, chest expansion, facial expression, oximeter readings, and endotracheal tube patency and position should be documented and monitored carefully before and during colfosceril dosing.

2. Ascertain that the endotracheal tube tip is in the trachea and not in the esophagus or right or left mainstem bronchus to ensure drug dispersion to all lung areas.

3. Document baseline weight, arterial blood gases, chest X ray, and physical assessment findings.

4. Review indications for drug therapy to ensure that infant meets criteria and document as rescue or prophylactic treatment.

Interventions

1. Confirm brisk and symmetrical chest movement and equal breath sounds in the two axillae with each mechanical inspiration prior to and at the conclusion of each dosing.

2. The infant should be suctioned before administration of the drug but not for 2 hr after colfosceril administration (unless clinically necessary).

3. It is essential that continuous monitoring of ECG, arterial BP, and transcutaneous oxygen saturation be undertaken during dosing. After either prophylactic or rescue treatment, frequent ABGs should be measured to prevent postdosing hyperoxia and hypocarbia.

4. The volume of the 5 ml/kg dose may cause a transient impairment of gas exchange due to physical blockage of the airway. Thus, infants may show a decrease in oxygen saturation during dosing, especially if they are on low ventilator settings prior to dosing. If this occurs, the peak inspiratory pressure on the ventilator should be increased by 4–5 cm water for 1–2 min. Also, the fraction of oxygen inspired should be increased for 1–2 min.

5. If chest expansion improves significantly after dosing, the peak ventilator inspiratory pressure should be reduced immediately. Failure to do this may cause lung overdistention and fatal pulmonary air leak.

6. If the infant becomes pink and transcutaneous oxygen saturation is more than 95%, the fraction of inspired oxygen should be reduced in small, but repeated steps until saturation is 90%–95%. Failure to do this may cause hyperoxia.

7. If arterial or transcutaneous CO_2 levels are less than 30 mg

Hg, the ventilator rate must be reduced immediately. Failure to do this can result in significant hypocarbia, which reduces brain blood flow.

8. After the dose has been administered, the position of the endotracheal tube should be confirmed by listening for equal breath sounds in the two axillae. Particular attention should be paid to chest expansion, color, transcutaneous saturation, and ABGs (samples should be taken frequently). The nurse should remain at the bedside for at least 30 min after dosing.

9. Observe closely for air leaks and mucus plugs. If mucus plug is unrelieved by suctioning, the endotracheal tube must be replaced immediately.

Evaluation: Evaluate client for:
- Oxygen saturation between 90% and 95% and improved pulmonary parameters more consistent with survival
- Reduction of pulmonary air leaks
- Freedom from complications of drug therapy

Collagenase
(koh-**LAJ**-eh-nace)
Biozyme-C, Santyl (Rx)

Classification: Topical enzyme.

Action/Kinetics: Collagenase digests collagen, which accounts for 75% of the dry weight of skin; thus, it is effective to remove tissue debris. Collagenase assists in the formation of granulation tissue and subsequent epithelialization of dermal ulcers and severely burned areas. The drug may also reduce the incidence of hypertrophic scarring. Collagen in healthy tissue or newly formed granulation is not affected.

Uses: Reduces pus, odor, necrosis, and inflammation in chronic dermal ulcers and severely burned areas.

Contraindications: Local or systemic hypersensitivity to collagenase.

Side Effects: No allergic sensitivity or toxic reactions have been noted.

Drug Interactions: Detergents, benzalkonium chloride, hexachlorophene, nitrofurazone, tincture of iodine, and certain heavy metal ions used in some antiseptics (e.g., mercury, silver) inhibit the activity of collagenase.

Dosage: Ointment: Apply once daily (more frequently if the dressing becomes soiled).

NURSING CONSIDERATIONS
Administration/Storage

1. If any of the agents listed under drug interactions have been used, the area should be cleaned thoroughly with repeated washings using normal saline before collagenase ointment is applied.

2. The action of the enzyme may be stopped by applying Burrow's solution (pH 3.6–4.4) to the lesion.

3. Before applying the ointment, the site should be cleansed of debris and other material by gently rubbing with a gauze pad saturated with hydrogen peroxide or Dakin's solution followed by sterile normal saline.

4. If infection is present, a topical

antibiotic powder should be applied to the lesion before collagenase is applied. If the infection does not respond, collagenase therapy should be discontinued until the infection is in remission.

5. Apply collagenase ointment to deep lesions using a wooden tongue depressor or spatula; for shallow lesions, a sterile gauze pad may be applied to the area and then properly secured.

6. Crosshatching thick eschar with a #10 blade allows more surface area for the collagenase to come in contact with necrotic tissue. As much loosened debris as possible should be removed with forceps and scissors.

7. All excess ointment should be removed each time the dressing is changed.

8. Collagenase ointment therapy should be terminated when debridement of necrotic tissue is complete and granulation tissue is well established.

Assessment

1. Document cause and describe area of tissue disruption.

2. Assess area to be treated noting wound size, depth, color, presence of eschar, any evidence of drainage, swelling, or odor and document.

Client/Family Teaching

1. Review the appropriate method for tissue preparation (described under administration) and demonstrate collagenase application. Observe a return demonstration to generate questions and to assess for problems in administration.

2. Explain the importance of frequent position changes, methods to reduce pressure to bony prominences, proper body alignment, proper skin care, adequate nutrition, and clean, dry linens in the overall goal to reduce the size and spread of the disrupted tissue, whether from an ulcer or from a burn.

3. Stress the importance of returning for follow-up evaluations to determine the effectiveness of prescribed therapy.

Evaluation: Evaluate for a positive clinical response as evidenced by the formation of new granulation tissue and re-epithelialization in the wound.

Corticotropin injection (Adrenocorticotropic hormone)
(kor-tih-koh-**TROH**-pin)
ACTH, Acthar (Rx)

Corticotropin repository injection (ACTH gel, Corticotropin gel)
(kor-tih-koh-**TROH**-pin)
ACTH -40 and -80 Acthar Gel (H.P.)✦, H.P. Acthar Gel (Rx)

Corticotropin zinc hydroxide
(kor-tih-koh-**TROH**-pin)
Cortrophin-Zinc (Rx)

See also *Adrenocorticosteroids and Analogs,* p. 8.

Classification: Anterior pituitary hormone.

Action/Kinetics: Corticotropin is extracted from the anterior pituitary gland. The hormone stimulates the functional adrenal cortex to secrete its entire spectrum of hormones, including the corticosteroids.

Thus, the overall physiologic effects of corticotropin are similar to those of cortisone. Since the latter is more easily obtainable, is more predictable, and has more prolonged activity, it is usually used for therapeutic purposes. Corticotropin is, however, useful for the diagnosis of Addison's disease and other conditions in which the functionality of the adrenal cortex is to be determined. *Corticotropin cannot elicit a hormonal response from a nonfunctioning adrenal gland.* **Peak plasma levels (corticotropin injection):** 1 hr. **t½:** 15 min. The respository injection contains ACTH in a gelatin base to delay the rate of absorption and increase the duration. Corticotropin zinc hydroxide also has a slow absorption rate and increased duration. **Duration** (repository and zinc hydroxide forms): Up to 3 days.

Uses: Diagnosis of adrenal insufficiency syndromes, nonsuppurative thyroiditis, hypercalcemia associated with cancer, tuberculous meningitis with subarachnoid block or impending block (with tuberculostatic drugs). *Investigational:* Infant spasm, multiple sclerosis. For same diseases as glucocorticosteroids.

Additional Contraindications: Cushing's syndrome, psychotic or psychopathic clients, active TB, active peptic ulcers. Lactation.

Special Concerns: Pregnancy category: C. Use with caution in clients who have diabetes and hypotension.

Additional Side Effects: In the treatment of myasthenia gravis, corticotropin may cause severe muscle weakness 2–3 days after initiation of therapy. Equipment for respiratory assistance must be on hand for such emergencies. Muscle strength returns and increases 2–7 days after cessation of treatment, and improvement lasts for about 3 months.

Laboratory Test Interferences: ↓ I^{131} uptake and suppress skin test reactions. False ↓ levels of estradiol and estriol using the Brown method. False (−) estrogens using colorimetric or fluorometric tests.

Dosage: SC, IM, or slow IV drip. *Highly individualized.* **Usual** (*aqueous solution*), **IM or SC:** 20 units q.i.d. **IV:** 10–25 units of aqueous solution in 500 ml 5% dextrose injection over period of 8 hr. Infants and young children require larger dose per body weight than do older children or adults. *Acute exacerbation of multiple sclerosis:* **IM,** 80–120 units/day for 2–3 weeks. *Infantile spasms:* **IM,** 20–40 units/day or 80 units q other day for 3 months (or 1 month after cessations of seizures).

Repository gel (IM, SC) or aqueous suspension with zinc hydroxide (IM only): 40–80 units q 24–72 hr. A dose of 12.5 units q.i.d. causes little metabolic disturbance; 25 units q.i.d. causes definite metabolic alterations.

As a general rule, clients are started on 10–12.5 units q.i.d. If no clinical effect is noted in 72–96 hr, dosage is increased by 5 units q few days to a final maximum of 25 units q.i.d.

NURSING CONSIDERATIONS

See also *Nursing Considerations* for *Adrenocorticosteroids and Analogs,* p. 15.

Administration/Storage

1. Check label carefully for IV administration. **The label must say that the product is for IV use.** IV administration should be slow, taking 8 hr.
2. Corticotropin zinc products should be injected deeply into the gluteal muscle.

Assessment: Before administering IV corticotropin, make sure that the client allergic to porcine proteins has been tested for any sensitivity to the brand of corticotropin to be used.

Interventions

1. Anticipate that the potassium requirements will be increased during IV administration of ACTH. Therefore, monitor serum potassium and sodium levels.
2. Observe the client for exaggerated euphoria and nervousness or client complaints of insomnia and depression. These are indications that the dosage should be reduced or discontinued and the symptoms should be reported to the physician.
3. Sedatives may be ordered p.r.n.
4. Monitor BP, intake and output, and weight for any marked changes. Document and report these to the physician.

Evaluation: Evaluate client for:
* Differential diagnosis of adrenal insufficiency syndrome
* Reduction in serum calcium levels

Cortisone acetate (Compound E)

(KOR-tih-zohn)
Cortone ✜, Cortone Acetate, Cortone Acetate Sterile Suspension (Rx)

See also *Adrenocorticosteroids and Analogs,* p. 8.

Classification: Adrenocorticosteroid, naturally occurring; glucocorticoid-type.

Action/Kinetics: Possesses both glucocorticoid and mineralocorticoid activity. Short-acting. **$t^{1/2}$, plasma:** 30 min; **$t^{1/2}$, biologic:** 8–12 hr.

Uses: Primarily used for replacement therapy in chronic cortical insufficiency. Also inflammatory or allergic disorders, but only for short-term use because the drug has a strong mineralocorticoid effect. The sterile suspension is used to treat children suffering from congenital adrenal hyperplasia.

Special Concerns: Use during pregnancy only if benefits outweigh risks.

Dosage: Tablets, initial *or during crisis:* 25–300 mg daily. Decrease gradually to lowest effective dose. *Anti-inflammatory:* 25–150 mg daily, depending on severity of the disease. *Acute rheumatic fever:* 200 mg b.i.d. day 1, thereafter, 200 mg daily. *Addison's disease:* **maintenance, PO:** 0.5–0.75 mg/kg daily.

NURSING CONSIDERATIONS

See also *Nursing Considerations* for *Adrenocorticosteroids and Analogs,* p. 15.

Administration/Storage: Single course of therapy should not exceed 6 weeks. Rest periods of 2–3 weeks are indicated between treatments.

Cosyntropin
(koh-SIN-troh-pin)
Cortrosyn, Synacthen ✹ (Rx)

See also *Adrenocorticosteroids and Analogs, p. 8.*

Classification: Synthetic ACTH derivative.

Action/Kinetics: Cosyntropin is a synthetic ACTH derivative that causes effects similar to those of ACTH although fewer hypersensitivity reactions have been noted. The activity of 0.25 mg cosyntropin is equal to 25 units of ACTH.

Uses: Diagnosis of adrenocortical insufficiency.

Special Concerns: Pregnancy category: C.

Dosage: IM, rapid IV, IV infusion. Adults, usual, IM: 0.25 mg dissolved in sterile saline. Range: 0.25–0.75 mg. Pediatric, under 2 years: 0.125 mg.

NURSING CONSIDERATIONS

See also *Nursing Considerations* for *Adrenocorticosteroids and Analogs, p. 15.*

Administration/Storage

1. When given by IV infusion, 0.25 mg cosyntropin is added to dextrose or saline solution, and 40 mcg/hr is administered over 6 hr.
2. For IM use, the drug (usually 0.25 mg) should be dissolved in sterile saline.

Cromolyn sodium
(CROH-moh-lin)
Gastrocrom, Intal, Nalcrom ✹, Nasalcrom, Opticrom 4%, Rynacrom ✹, Vistacrom ✹ (Rx)

Classification: Antiasthmatic, antiallergic drug.

Action/Kinetics: Cromolyn sodium appears to act locally on the lung mucosa, preventing the release of histamine, slow-reacting substance of anaphylaxis, and other endogenous substances causing hypersensitivity reactions. The drug, when effective, reduces the number and intensity of asthmatic attacks. The drug has no antihistaminic, anti-inflammatory, or bronchodilator effects and has no role in terminating an acute attack of asthma. After inhalation, some of the drug is absorbed systemically. It is excreted about equally in urine and bile (feces). $t\frac{1}{2}$: 81 min; from lungs: 60 min. About 50% excreted unchanged through the urine and 50% through the bile. When used in the eye, approximately 0.03% is absorbed. Onset, ophthalmic: Several days. Onset, nasal: Less than 1 week. Time to peak effect, nasal: Up to 4 weeks.

Uses: *Inhalation:* Prophylactic and adjunct in the management of severe bronchial asthma in selected patients. Prophylaxis of exercise-induced bronchospasms and bronchospasms due to allergens, cold dry air, or environmental pollutants. *Ophthalmologic:* Treat allergic ocular disorders, including allergic keratoconjunctivitis, giant papillary conjunctivitis, vernal keratoconjunctivitis, vernal conjunctivitis, and vernal keratitis. *Nasal:* Prophylaxis and treatment of allergic rhinitis.

Oral: Mastocytosis (improves symptoms including diarrhea, flushing, headaches, vomiting, urticaria, nausea, abdominal pain, and itching). *Investigational:* Orally to treat food allergies.

Contraindications: Hypersensitivity. Acute attacks and status asthmaticus. Soft contact lenses should not be worn if the drug is used in the eye. For mastocytosis in premature infants.

Special Concerns: Safe use in pregnancy not established (pregnancy category: B). Dosage of the ophthalmic product has not been established in children less than 4 years of age; dosage of the nasal product has not been established in children less than 6 years of age. Use with caution for long periods of time or in the presence of renal or hepatic disease.

Side Effects: *Respiratory:* Bronchospasm, cough, laryngeal edema (rare), eosinophilic pneumonia. *CNS:* Dizziness, drowsiness, headache. *Allergic:* Urticaria, rash, angioedema, serum sickness, anaphylaxis. *Other:* Nausea, urinary frequency, dysuria, joint swelling and pain, lacrimation, swollen parotid gland.
    Following nebulization: Sneezing, wheezing, itching, nose bleeds, burning, nasal congestion. **Following nasal solution:** Burning, stinging, irritation of nose; sneezing, nose bleeds, headache, bad taste in mouth, postnasal drip. **Following ophthalmic use:** Stinging and burning after use.
    Following oral use: *GI:* Diarrhea, taste perversion, spasm of esophagus, flatulence, dysphagia, burning of mouth and throat. *CNS:*

Headache, dizziness, fatigue, migraine, paresthesia, anxiety, depression, psychosis, behavior changes, insomnia, hallucinations, lethargy, lightheadedness after eating. *Dermatologic:* Flushing, angioedema, urticaria, skin burning, skin erythema. *Musculoskeletal:* Arthralgia, stiffness and weakness in legs. *Miscellaneous:* Altered liver function test, dyspnea, dysuria, polycythemia, neutropenia.

Dosage: Capsules or Solution for Inhalation. *Prophylaxis of bronchial asthma:* **Adults:** 20 mg q.i.d. at regular intervals. Adjust dosage as required. *Prophylaxis of bronchospasm:* **Adults:** 20 mg as a single dose just prior to exposure to the precipitating factor. If used chronically, 20 mg q.i.d, up to a maximum of 160 mg daily.
    Ophthalmic Solution. Adults and children over 4 years: 1–2 gtt of the 4% solution 4–6 times daily at regular intervals.
    Nasal Solution. Adults and children over 6 years: 2.6 mg in each nostril six times daily or 5.3 mg in each nostril 3–4 times daily at regular intervals.
    Oral Capsules (for mastocytosis). Adults: 200 mg q.i.d. 30 min before meals and at bedtime. **Pediatric, term to 2 years:** 20 mg/kg daily in four divided doses; should be used in this age group only in severe incapacitating disease where benefits outweigh risks. **Pediatric, 2–12 years:** 100 mg q.i.d. 30 min before meals and at bedtime. If relief is not seen within 2–3 weeks, dose may be increased, but should not exceed 40 mg/kg daily for adults and children over 2 years of age and 30 mg/kg daily for children 6 months–2 years.

NURSING CONSIDERATIONS
Administration/Storage

1. Institute only after acute episode is over, when airway is clear and client can inhale adequately.
2. Corticosteroid dosage should be continued when initiating cromolyn therapy. However, if improvement occurs, the steroid dosage may be tapered slowly. Steroid therapy may have to be reinstituted if cromolyn inhalation is impaired, in times of stress, or in adrenocortical insufficiency.
3. One drop of the ophthalmic solution contains 1.6 mg cromolyn sodium.
4. The ophthalmic solution should be protected from direct sunlight and, once opened, should be discarded after 4 weeks.

Client/Family Teaching

1. Provide written guidelines concerning the prescribed method of medication administration.
2. When the medication is administered by inhaler, the following procedure should be used:
   • Demonstrate how to load the capsule into the inhaler.
   • Instruct the client to inhale and exhale fully and then to introduce the mouthpiece between the lips.
   • Tilt head back and inhale deeply and rapidly through the inhaler. This causes the propeller to turn rapidly and to supply more medication in one breath.
   • Remove inhaler, hold breath a few seconds, and exhale slowly.
   • Repeat this procedure until the powder is completely administered.
   • Do not wet powder with breath while exhaling.
3. When used orally, the following procedure should be used to prepare the solution in water:
   • Open the capsule (which is oversized to prevent spilling of powder when opened) and pour the powder into one-half glass of hot water.
   • Stir the mixture until the powder is completely dissolved and the solution is clear.
   • While stirring, add an equal quantity of cold water.
   • The drug should **not** be mixed with milk, foods, or fruit juice.
   • The entire glass of liquid should be consumed.
4. When used in the eye advise client not to wear soft contacts until drug therapy is completed.
5. Encourage the client to continue self-administration of medication as ordered. It may take up to 4 weeks for frequency of asthmatic attacks to decrease.
6. If the client wishes to discontinue medication, stress the importance of notifying the physician. Rapid withdrawal of the drug may precipitate an asthmatic attack, and concomitant corticosteroid therapy may require adjustment.

Evaluation: Evaluate client for:
   • Improved airway exchange
   • Reports of symptomatic improvement with a notable ↓

- in the number and frequency of asthma attacks
- Improved symptoms of conjunctivitis

Crystalline Amino Acid Infusion

(ah-ME-no AH-sid)

Aminosyn 3.5%, 3.5%M, 5%, 7%, 8.5%, and 10%; Aminosyn (pH 6) 7% and 8.5%, 10%; Aminosyn 7% and 8.5% with Electrolytes; Aminosyn II 3.5%, 3.5%M, 5%, 7%, 8.5%, 10%; Aminosyn II 7%, 8.5%, or 10% with Electrolytes; Aminosyn II 3.5% with 5% Dextrose; Aminosyn II 4.25% in 10% or 20% Dextrose; Aminosyn II 3.5%, 4.25%, or 5% in 25% Dextrose; Aminosyn II 3.5% or 4.25% with Electrolytes in 25% Dextrose; Aminosyn-PF 10%; Freamine III 8.5% and 10%; Freamine III 3% or 8.5% with Electrolytes; Novamine 11.4% or 15%; Procalamine; Travasol 10%; Travasol 5.5% with Electrolytes; Travasol 5.5% without Electrolytes; 3.5% and 5.5% Travasol with Electrolytes; TrophAmine 6%, 10% (Rx)

See information on *Intravenous Nutritional Therapy,* p. 168.

Classification: Nutritional agent.

Action/Kinetics: These products are hypertonic solutions containing both essential and nonessential amino acids as well as various electrolytes. Dextrose, IV fat emulsion, vitamins, and minerals may be added as required. Percentage refers to the amino acid concentration. The amino acids present in the products either conserve protein or induce protein synthesis by providing the necessary amino acids.

Special Concerns: Pregnancy category: C.

Dosage: *Peripheral protein sparing:* 1–1.7 g/kg/day through a peripheral vein. *Peripheral vein administration:* Mix with low concentrations of dextrose solutions (5% or 10%) with fat emulsions. *Central vein administration:* 500 ml mixed with 500 ml concentrated dextrose injection, vitamins, or electrolytes given over 8 hr.

NURSING CONSIDERATIONS

See also *Nursing Considerations* for *Intravenous Nutritional Therapy,* p. 170.

Administration/Storage: The initial rate of infusion should not exceed 2 ml/min. The rate may then be increased slowly depending on laboratory values of urinary and blood glucose.

Cyanocobalamin (Vitamin B$_{12}$)

(sye-an-oh-koh-BAL-ah-min)

Oral: Kaybovite. Parenteral: Anacobin✽, Bedoz✽, Berubigen, Kaybovite-1000, Redisol, Rubion✽, Rubramin✽, Rubramin PC (OTC, Rx)

Cyanocobalamin crystalline

(sye-an-oh-koh-BAL-ah-min)

Classification: Vitamin B$_{12}$.

Action/Kinetics: Cyanocobalamin (vitamin B$_{12}$) is a cobalt-containing vitamin essential to growth. The vitamin can also be isolated from liver and is identical to that of the antianemic factor of liver. This vitamin is required for hematopoiesis, cell reproduction, nucleoprotein and myelin synthesis. Plasma vitamin B_{12} levels: 150–750 pg/ml.

Intrinsic factor is required for adequate absorption of oral vitamin B_{12} and in pernicious anemia and malabsorption diseases intrinsic factor is administered simultaneously. This vitamin is rapidly absorbed following IM or SC administration. Following absorption, vitamin B_{12} is carried by plasma proteins to the liver where it is stored until required for various metabolic functions.

Products containing less than 500 mcg vitamin B_{12} are nutritional supplements and are not to be used for the treatment of pernicious anemia. **t½:** 6 days (400 days in the liver). **Time to peak levels, after PO:** 8–12 hr.

Uses: Vitamin B_{12} deficiency due to pernicious anemia, cancer of the bowel or pancreas, sprue, total or partial gastrectomy, accompanying folic acid deficiency, GI surgery or pathology, gluten enteropathy, fish tapeworm infestation, bacterial overgrowth of the small intestine.

Also, in conditions with an increased need for vitamin B_{12} such as thyrotoxicosis, hemorrhage, malignancy, pregnancy, and in liver and kidney disease. Vitamin B_{12} is particularly suitable for the treatment of clients allergic to liver extract.

Investigational: Diagnosis of vitamin B_{12} deficiency.

Note: Folic acid is not a substitute for vitamin B_{12} although concurrent folic acid therapy may be required.

Contraindications: Hypersensitivity to cobalt, Leber's disease.

Special Concerns: Pregnancy category: C. Use with caution in clients with gout.

Side Effects: Manifested following parenteral use. *Allergic:* Urticaria, itching, exanthema, anaphylaxis, shock, death. *CV:* Peripheral vascular thrombosis, congestive heart failure, pulmonary edema. *Other:* Polycythemia vera, optic nerve atrophy in clients with hereditary optic nerve atrophy, diarrhea, hypokalemia, body feels swollen.

Note: Benzyl alcohol, which is present in certain products, may cause a fatal "gasping syndrome" in premature infants.

Drug Interactions

Alcohol / ↓ Vitamin B_{12} absorption
Aminosalicylic acid / ↓ Vitamin B_{12} absorption
Chloramphenicol / ↓ Response to vitamin B_{12} therapy
Cholestyramine / ↓ Vitamin B_{12} absorption
Cimetidine / ↓ Digestion and release of vitamin B_{12}
Colchicine / ↓ Vitamin B_{12} absorption
Neomycin / ↓ Vitamin B_{12} absorption
Potassium, timed-release / ↓ Vitamin B_{12} absorption

Laboratory Test Interferences: Antibiotics may interfere with the microbiologic assay for serum and erythrocyte vitamin B_{12}.

Dosage: Tablets, Soluble Tablets. *Nutritional supplement:* **Adults:** 1 mcg daily (up to 25 mcg for increased requirements). **Pediatric, up to 1 year:** 0.3 mcg daily; **over 1 year:** 1 mcg daily.

IM, Deep SC. *Treatment of deficiency:* **Adults:** 100 mcg daily for 6–7 days; **then,** 100 mcg every other day for 7 doses. If improvement is noted along with a reticulocyte response, 100 mcg q 3–4 days for 2–3 weeks; **maintenance, IM:** 100–200 mcg once a month. **Pediatric, initial:** 30–50 mcg daily for 2 or more weeks (total dose of 1–5 mg); **maintenance:** 100 mcg once a month. *Diagnosis of vitamin B_{12} deficiency:* **Adults, IM:** 1 mcg/day for 10 days plus low dietary folic acid and vitamin B_{12}. Loading dose for the Schilling test is 1,000 mcg given IM.

NURSING CONSIDERATIONS

Administration/Storage

1. Protect cyanocobalamin crystalline injection from light.
2. The medication should not be frozen.
3. Have epinephrine, antihistamines, and steroids available in the event of an adverse drug reaction.
4. Note that if the client is being treated for pernicious anemia, the drug cannot be administered orally.

Assessment

1. Determine if the client is allergic to cobalt.
2. Note if the client has been taking chloramphenicol. This drug antagonizes the hematopoietic response to vitamin B_{12}.
3. Determine if the client is taking any other drugs that could cause an unfavorable response to vitamin B_{12}.
4. Perform a baseline assessment of the client's peripheral pulses.

Interventions

1. Observe for urticaria, complaints of itching, and evidence of anaphylaxis. Report these findings to the physician immediately.
2. If clients complain of diarrhea, monitor the frequency and consistency of their stools. If the diarrhea is severe or persists, a change in drug may be required.
3. Monitor serum potassium levels if the client is being treated for megaloblastic anemia.

Client/Family Teaching

1. If the client is being treated for pernicious anemia, stress that vitamin B_{12} replacement *must* be taken for life.
2. When repository vitamin B_{12} is used, it will provide medication for at least 4 weeks.
3. Explain that the stinging, burning sensation that may occur after injection is transitory. However, remind the client that if the burning sensation occurs anywhere except where the needle is, to call it to the nurse's attention immediately. The needle should be withdrawn and a different site selected for injection.
4. If vitamin B_{12} therapy is the result of dietary deficiency, discuss diet with the client. Provide printed material concerning appropriate foods (such as meats, fermented cheeses, egg yolks, and seafood) and review with clients methods of achieving a balance in their diet. Refer to a dietitian for additional assistance as needed.
5. Avoid alcohol while taking vitamin B_{12} because it will interfere with the absorption of the medication.

Evaluation: Evaluate for:
- Client knowledge and understanding of underlying cause and associated symptoms of vitamin B$_{12}$ deficiency state
- Improvement in symptoms of vitamin B$_{12}$ deficiency following replacement therapy

Cyclizine hydrochloride
(SYE-klih-zeen)
Marezine, Marzine✹ (OTC)

Cyclizine lactate
(SYE-klih-zeen)
Marezine, Marzine✹ (Rx)

See also *Antihistamines,* p. 71.

Classification: Antihistamine, antiemetic.

Action/Kinetics: The mechanism for the antiemetic effect is not known with certainty but may be due to central anticholinergic effects to cause reduced labyrinthine function and decreased vestibular stimulation. This action is thought to be mediated through pathways to the vomiting center from the chemoreceptor trigger zone or peripheral nerve pathways. **Onset:** 30–60 min. **Duration:** 4–6 hr.

Uses: Nausea, vomiting, dizziness of motion sickness. *Investigational:* Postoperative vomiting.

Contraindications: Pregnancy and lactation.

Special Concerns: Safety for use in children less than 12 years of age has not been determined; children may be more sensitive to the anticholinergic effects of the drug.

Geriatric clients may experience a greater incidence of constipation, dry mouth, and urinary retention (i.e., due to the anticholinergic effects).

Side Effects: *CNS:* Drowsiness, excitation, nervousness, restlessness, insomnia, euphoria, vertigo, hallucinations (auditory or visual). *GI:* Nausea, vomiting, diarrhea, constipation, anorexia). *GU:* Urinary frequency or retention; difficulty in urination. *CV:* Hypotension, tachycardia, palpitations. *Miscellaneous:* Dry nose and throat, blurred or double vision, tinnitus, rash, urticaria.

Dosage: Tablets, Injection (IM). *Motion sickness:* **Adults,** 50 mg 30 min before leaving and q 4–6 hr thereafter, not to exceed 200 mg/day; **pediatric, 6–12 years:** 1 mg/kg (33 mg/m^2) t.i.d. or 25 mg 30 min before travel and repeated in 6–8 hr if needed, not to exceed 75 mg daily. *Postoperative vomiting:* **Adults, IM:** 50 mg 30 min before end of surgery; may be repeated t.i.d. during first few postoperative days. **Pediatric, 6–12 years:** 25 mg 30 min before end of surgery and repeated t.i.d. during first few postoperative days; **Less than 6 years:** 12.5 mg given same as for older children.

NURSING CONSIDERATIONS

See also *Nursing Considerations* for *Antihistamines,* p. 74.

Client/Family Teaching
1. Take 30 min before travel.
2. Drug may cause dizziness so use caution.
3. Avoid alcohol.

Evaluation: Evaluate client for:
- A decrease in the frequency

and intensity of nausea and vomiting
- Reports of symptomatic improvement of the dizziness from motion sickness
- Freedom from complications of adverse side effects of drug therapy

Cyclobenzaprine hydrochloride

(sye-kloh-**BENZ**-ah-preen)

Flexeril (Rx)

See also *Centrally Acting Skeletal Muscle Relaxants,* p. 130.

Classification: Centrally acting muscle relaxant.

Action/Kinetics: Structurally and pharmacologically, cyclobenzaprine is related to the tricyclic antidepressants and possesses both sedative and anticholinergic properties. In contrast to many skeletal muscle relaxants, cyclobenzaprine hydrochloride is thought to act mainly at the level of the brain stem (compared to the spinal cord) to inhibit reflexes by reducing tonic somatic motor activity. **Onset:** 1 hr. **Time to peak plasma levels:** 3–8 hr. **Therapeutic plasma levels:** 20–30 ng/ml. **Duration:** 12–24 hr. $t\frac{1}{2}$: 1–3 days. The drug is highly bound to plasma protein. Inactive metabolites are excreted in the urine.

Uses: Adjunct to rest and physical therapy for relief of muscle spasms associated with acute and/or painful musculoskeletal conditions. It is not indicated for the treatment of spastic diseases or for cerebral palsy.

Contraindications: Hypersensitivity. Arrhythmias, heart block, CHF, or soon after myocardial infarctions. Hyperthyroidism. Concomitant use of MAO inhibitors.

Special Concerns: Safe use during pregnancy (category: B) and lactation and in children under age 15 has not been established. Due to atropine-like effects, use with caution in situations where cholinergic blockade is not desired. Geriatric clients may be more sensitive to cholinergic blockade.

Side Effects: Symptoms of cholinergic blockade including dry mouth, dizziness, tachycardia, blurred vision, urinary retention. Also, drowsiness, weakness, dyspepsia, paresthesia, unpleasant taste, insomnia. Since cyclobenzaprine resembles tricyclic antidepressants, side effects to these drugs should also be noted.

Physostigmine salicylate, 1–3 mg IV, may be used to reverse symptoms of severe cholinergic blockade.

Drug Interactions

Anticholinergics / Additive anticholinergic side effects
CNS depressants / Additive depressant effects
Guanethidine / Cyclobenzaprine may block effect
MAO inhibitors / Hypertensive crisis, severe convulsions
Tricyclic antidepressants / Additive side effects

Dosage: Tablets. Adults: 20–40 mg daily in 3–4 divided doses (usual: 10 mg t.i.d.), up to a maximum of 60 mg daily in divided doses.

NURSING CONSIDERATIONS

See also *Nursing Considerations* for *Tricyclic Antidepressants,* p. 242, and *Centrally Acting Skeletal Muscle Relaxants,* p. 130.

Administration/Storage

1. Cyclobenzaprine should be used only for 2–3 weeks.
2. If the client has been taking an MAO inhibitor, do not administer cyclobenzaprine for at least 2 weeks after discontinuing the MAO inhibitor.
3. Review the list of drugs with which cyclobenzaprine interacts.

Assessment

1. Take a complete drug history, noting any evidence of hypersensitivity.
2. Check the client's cardiovascular system for evidence of cardiac arrhythmias. Note if the client has a history of recent myocardial infarction.
3. Obtain a CBC and liver profile prior to starting therapy to serve as baseline data.
4. Document the extent of the client's acute or painful musculoskeletal condition.
5. Determine if the client has any spasticity. This drug is contraindicated in the treatment of spastic conditions.

Intervention: Should the client complain of itchy skin or show evidence of yellow sclera or skin, withhold drug and evaluate liver function studies.

Client/Family Teaching

1. Report any unusual fatigue, unexplained fever, easy bruising or bleeding, or sore throat. These symptoms could indicate a blood dyscrasia and require the discontinuation of drug therapy.
2. Report nausea or abdominal pain because this could indicate hepatic toxicity and require the termination of therapy.
3. Symptoms such as dry mouth, blurred vision, dizziness, tachycardia, or urinary retention should also be reported so that therapy can be evaluated.
4. Due to drug-induced drowsiness, dizziness, or blurred vision, caution should be observed if the client drives or performs other activities requiring mental alertness.
5. Do not extend drug therapy beyond 3 weeks. Longer periods of therapy with this drug are contraindicated.

Evaluation: Evaluate client for:
- Reports of relief of muscle spasms
- Freedom from complications of drug therapy

Cyclophosphamide
(sye-kloh-**FOS**-fah-myd)
Cytoxan, Cytoxan Lyophilized, Neosar, Procytox✽ (Abbreviation: CYC) (Rx)

See also *Antineoplastic Agents,* p. 85, and *Alkylating Agents,* p. 20.

Classification: Antineoplastic, alkylating agent.

Action/Kinetics: Cyclophosphamide is metabolized in the liver to both active antineoplastic alkylating agents and inactive metabolites. The active metabolites alkylate nucleic acids, thus interfering with the growth of neoplastic and normal tissues. The cytotoxic action is due to cross-linking of strands of DNA and RNA and inhibition of protein synthesis. The drug also possesses immunosuppressive activity. **t½:** 3–12 hr, but remnants of drug and/

C

or metabolites detectable in serum after 72 hr; in children, the **t½** averages 4.1 hr. Metabolites are excreted through the urine with up to 20% of cyclophosphamide excreted unchanged. Cyclophosphamide is also excreted in milk.

Uses: Often used in combination with other antineoplastic drugs. Multiple myeloma. Malignant lymphomas: Hodgkin's disease, follicular lymphoma, lymphocytic lymphosarcoma, reticulum cell sarcoma, lymphoblastic lymphosarcoma, Burkitt's lymphoma. Mycosis fungoides. Leukemias: Chronic lymphocytic and granulocytic leukemia, acute myelogenous and monocytic leukemia, acute lymphoblastic leukemia in children. Neuroblastoma, adenocarcinoma of ovary, retinoblastoma. Carcinoma of breast. *Investigational:* Rheumatic diseases including rheumatoid arthritis and lupus erythematosus, multiple sclerosis, polyarteritis nodosa, Ewing's sarcoma, osteosarcoma, soft tissue sarcomas, prophylaxis of rejection in organ transplants. Also, cancer of the cervix, lung, endometrium, bladder, prostate and testes; Wilms' tumor.

Contraindications: Lactation. Severe bone marrow depression.

Special Concerns: Pregnancy category: D. Use with caution in clients with thrombocytopenia, leukopenia, previous radiation therapy, bone marrow infiltration of tumor cells, previous therapy causing cytotoxicity, and impaired liver and kidney function. May interfere with wound healing.

Additional Side Effects: Acute hemorrhagic cystitis. Bone marrow depression appears frequently during 9th to 14th day of therapy.

Alopecia occurs more frequently than with other drugs. Secondary neoplasia (especially of urinary bladder), pulmonary fibrosis, cardiotoxicity, darkening of skin or fingernails. Interference with oogenesis and spermatogenesis

Drug Interactions

Allopurinol / ↑ Chance of bone marrow toxicity
Anticoagulants / ↑ Effect of anticoagulants
Chloramphenicol / ↓ Metabolism of cyclophosphamide to active metabolites → ↓ pharmacologic effect
Doxorubicin / Cardiotoxicity due to doxorubicin is ↑
Insulin / ↑ Hypoglycemia
Phenobarbital / ↑ Rate of metabolism of cyclophosphamide in liver
Succinylcholine / ↑ Succinylcholine-induced apnea due to ↓ breakdown in plasma
Thiazide diuretics / ↑ Chance of leukopenia

Laboratory Test Interference: ↑ Uric acid in blood and urine; false + Pap test; ↓ serum pseudocholinesterase. Suppression of certain skin tests.

Dosage: IV. For malignancies; Adults, loading dose: 40–50 mg/kg in divided doses over 2–5 days. Alternative therapy: 10–15 mg/kg q 7–10 days, 3–5 mg/kg twice weekly, or 1.5–3 mg/kg daily. **Children, induction:** 2–8 mg/kg (or 60–250 mg/m² daily in divided doses for 6 or more days); **maintenance:** 10–15 mg/kg q 7–10 days or 30 mg/kg q 3–4 weeks (or when bone marrow recovery occurs).

   Oral Solution, Tablets: Malignancies: Adults: 1–5 mg/kg depending on client tolerance. **Main-**

tenance (various schedules): **PO:** 1–5 mg/kg/day. **Children, induction:** 2–8 mg/kg (or 60–250 mg/m² in divided doses for 6 or more days); **maintenance:** 2–5 mg/kg (or 50–150 mg/m²) twice a week. Attempt to maintain leukocyte count at 3,000–4,000/mm³. Dosage should be adjusted for kidney or liver disease. *Nephrotic syndrome in children:* **PO:** 2.5–3 mg/kg daily for 60–90 days.

NURSING CONSIDERATIONS

See also *Nursing Considerations* for *Antineoplastic Agents,* p. 88.

Administration/Storage

1. IV/IM: Dissolve 100 mg cyclophosphamide in 5 ml sterile water for injection or bacteriostatic water.
2. Solutions may be given IV, IM, intraperitoneally, or intrapleurally. Also, they may be infused IV with 5% dextrose injection, 5% dextrose and 0.9% sodium chloride injection, 5% dextrose and Ringer's injection, lactated Ringer's injection, 0.45% sodium chloride injection, or 1/6M sodium lactate injection.
3. The reconstituted solution may be stored at room temperature for 24 hr and for 6 days if refrigerated at 2°C–8°C (36°F–46°F).
4. An oral solution may be prepared by dissolving injectable cyclophosphamide in aromatic elixir.
5. PO: Administer preferably on empty stomach. Give with meals in case of GI disturbance.
6. Fluid intake should be increased before, during, and for 24 hr after cyclophosphamide administration.
7. The initial loading dose may

need to be reduced by 1/3–1/2 in clients who have previously received cytotoxic drugs or radiation therapy.
8. *Treatment of Overdose:* General supportive measures. Dialysis.

Assessment

1. Note any client history of prior radiation therapy and/or chemotherapy because this is an indication for dose reduction of cyclophosphamide.
2. Assess skin condition and integrity. Document evidence of breakdown.

Interventions

1. Keep client well hydrated to help prevent hemorrhagic cystitis due to excessive concentration of drug in urine.
2. Administer the drug in the morning so that kidneys can eliminate the drug before bedtime. Encourage frequent voiding.
3. Observe for any evidence of dysuria and hematuria.
4. Monitor for cardiotoxicity; client complaints of shortness of breath, presence of pulmonary crackles, or tachycardia.
5. Observe for increased coughing or shortness of breath. Obtain periodic chest X-rays and pulmonary function tests.
6. See *Nursing Considerations* for *Neuromuscular Blocking Agents,* p. 184, if client is also receiving succinylcholine because apnea may be induced.

Client/Family Teaching

1. Take medication on an empty stomach unless otherwise ordered.

2. Increase consumption of fluids during and for 24 hr after cyclophosphamide therapy.
3. Reassure client with alopecia that hair should grow back when drug is stopped or when a maintenance dosage is given.
4. Advise women that drug may cause a false + Pap test.
5. Contraception should be practiced by both men and women during therapy.
6. Advise diabetic client that signs and symptoms of hypoglycemia may be precipitated by drug interactions with insulin. Instruct to monitor sugars closely and to consult with physician for possible insulin dosage adjustment.
7. Report any evidence of injury or delayed healing of wounds.

Evaluation: Evaluate client for:
- Improved hematologic counts
- ↓ in tumor size and spread
- Freedom from complications of drug therapy

Cyclosporine
(sye-kloh-**SPOR**-een)
Sandimmune (Rx)

Classification: Immunosuppressant.

Action/Kinetics: Cyclosporine is an immunosuppressant thought to act by inhibiting the immunocompetent lymphocytes in the G_o or G_1 phase of the cell cycle. T-lymphocytes are specifically inhibited; both the T-helper cell and the T-suppressor cell may be affected. Cyclosporine also inhibits interleukin 2 or T-cell growth factor production and release. **Peak plasma levels:** 3.5

hr. Food may both delay and impair absorption of the drug. **t½:** Approximately 19 hr for adults and 7 hr in children. Metabolized by the liver. Inactive metabolites are excreted mainly through the bile.

Uses: In combination with corticosteroids for prophylaxis of rejection in kidney, liver, and heart transplants. Treatment of chronic rejection in clients previously treated with other immunosuppressants.

A number of other diseases have been treated with cyclosporine including aplastic anemia, myasthenia gravis, atopic dermatitis, Crohn's disease, Graves ophthalmology, severe psoriasis, multiple sclerosis, polymyositis, dermatomyositis, uveitis, biliary cirrhosis, and others.

Contraindications: Hypersensitivity to cyclosporine or polyoxyethylated castor oil. Lactation. Use of potassium-sparing diuretics.

Special Concerns: Use with caution during pregnancy (category: C), and in clients with impaired renal or hepatic function. Safety and efficacy have not been established in children. Clients with malabsorption may not achieve therapeutic levels following oral use.

Side Effects: *GI:* Nausea, vomiting, diarrhea, gum hyperplasia, anorexia, gastritis, hiccoughs, peptic ulcer, abdominal discomfort, upper GI bleeding, pancreatitis, constipation, mouth sores, difficulty in swallowing. *Hematologic:* Leukopenia, lymphoma, thrombocytopenia, microangiopathic hemolytic anemia syndrome. *Allergic:* Anaphylaxis (rare). *CV:* Hypertension, edema, myocardial infarction. *CNS:* Headache, tremor, confusion, fever, seizures, anxiety, depression, weakness, lethargy, ataxia, hallucinations, mania, encephalopathy, sleep disturbances. *Miscellaneous:* Nephrotoxicity, hepatotoxicity, acne, hirsutism, flushing, paresthesia, sinusitis, gynecomastia, conjunctivitis, brittle fingernails, hearing loss, tinnitus, hyperglycemia, hyperkalemia, hyperuricemia, muscle pain, infections, hematuria, blurred vision, cramps, weight loss, chest and joint pain, conjunctivitis, fever, night sweats. *Symptoms of Overdose:* Transient hepatotoxicty and nephrotoxicity.

Drug Interactions

Aminoglycosides / ↑ Risk of nephrotoxicity

Amphotericin B / ↑ Risk of nephrotoxicity.

Azathioprine / ↑ Imnmunosuppression due to suppression of lymphocytes → possible infection and malignancy

Carbamazepine / ↓ Plasma level of cyclosporine due to ↑ breakdown by liver

Cimetidine / ↑ Plasma level of cyclosporine due to ↓ breakdown by liver

Corticosteroids / ↑ Immunosuppression due to suppression of lymphocytes → possible infection and malignancy

Cyclophosphamide / ↑ Immunosuppression due to suppression of lymphocytes → possible infection and malignancy

Danazol / ↑ Plasma level of cyclosporine due to ↓ breakdown by liver

Digoxin / ↑ Digoxin levels → toxicity

Diltiazem / ↑ Plasma level of cyclosporine due to ↓ breakdown by liver

Erythromycin / ↑ Plasma level of cyclosporine due to ↓ breakdown by liver and ↓ biliary excretion

Fluconazole / ↑ Plasma level of cyclosporine due to ↓ breakdown by liver

Imipenem-cilastatin / ↑ Plasma level of cyclosporine due to ↓ breakdown by liver

Isoniazid / ↓ Plasma level of cyclosporine due to ↑ breakdown by liver

Ketoconazole / ↑ Plasma level of cyclosporine due to ↓ breakdown by liver

Melphalan / ↑ Risk of nephrotoxicity

Methylprednisolone / ↑ Risk of seizures

Metoclopramide / ↑ Plasma level of cyclosporine due to ↑ absorption from GI tract

Nephrotoxic drugs / Additive nephrotoxicity

Nicardipine / ↑ Plasma level of cyclosporine due to ↓ breakdown by liver

Nondepolarizing muscle relaxants / ↑ Neuromuscular blockade

Nonsteroidal anti-inflammatory drugs / ↑ Risk of nephrotoxicity

Oral contraceptives / ↑ Plasma level of cyclosporine due to ↓ breakdown by liver

Phenobarbital / ↓ Plasma level of cyclosporine due to ↑ breakdown by liver

Phenytoin / ↓ Plasma level of cyclosporine due to ↑ breakdown by liver

Prednisolone / ↑ Plasma level of cyclosporine due to ↓ breakdown by liver

Rifampin / ↓ Plasma level of cyclosporine due to ↑ breakdown by liver

Sulfamethoxazole and/or trimethoprim / ↑ Risk of nephrotoxicity; also, ↓ serum levels of cyclosporine → possible rejection

Sulfatrimethoprim / ↓ Plasma level of cyclosporine due to ↑ breakdown by liver

Verapamil / ↑ Degree of immunosuppression

Laboratory Test Interferences: ↑ Serum creatinine, BUN, total bilirubin, alkaline phosphatase, serum potassium. Possibly ↑ cholesterol, LDL, and apolipoprotein B.

Dosage: Capsules, Oral Solution. Adults and children, initial: 14–18 mg/kg/day given 4–12 hr prior to transplantation (usual was 15 mg/kg/day); **then,** 15 mg/kg/day postoperatively for 1–2 weeks followed by 5% decrease in dose per week to maintenance dose of 5–10 mg/kg/day. **IV (only in clients unable to take PO medication):** 5–6 mg/kg/day 4–12 hr prior to transplantation and postoperatively until patient can be switched to PO dosage. **Note:** Steroid therapy must be used concomitantly.

NURSING CONSIDERATIONS

Administration/Storage

1. The oral solution may be diluted with milk, chocolate milk, or juice immediately before being administered. The oral solutions should not be stored in the refrigerator; contents should be used within 2 months after being opened.
2. Due to variable absorption of the oral solution, blood levels of cyclosporine should be monitored.
3. The IV concentration should be diluted 1 ml in 20–100 ml 0.9% sodium chloride injection or 5% dextrose injection. The IV solution is given by slow IV infusion over 2–6 hr.
4. The polyoxyethylated castor oil found in the concentrate for IV infusion may cause phthalate stripping from PVC.
5. The IV solution should be protected from light.
6. Due to the possibility of anaphylaxis, clients receiving IV cyclosporine should be closely monitored for 30 min following the initiation of the infusion. Epinephrine (1:1,000) should be available at the bedside for treating anaphylaxis.
7. Clients with malabsorption from the GI tract may not achieve appropriate blood levels.
8. *Treatment of Overdose:* Induction of vomiting (up to 2 hr after ingestion). General supportive measures.

Assessment

1. List all drugs the client is currently taking and note the potential for any drug interactions.
2. Obtain baseline CBC, white cell differential, and platelet count.
3. Prior to administration, obtain a liver profile, BUN, and creatinine levels.

Interventions

1. Monitor the client's blood pressure and pulse. Document and report to the physician any changes from the baseline data.
2. Observe the client for complaints of fatigue, malaise, unexplained bleeding or bruising, bleeding from the gums, nosebleeds or hematuria. Monitor CBC, white cell differential,

and platelet count. Document and report any deviation from baseline data.

3. If client finds the oral medication unpalatable, mix with milk or juice. Mix the medication in a glass container to minimize adherence to the container. The medication should be taken immediately after mixing.

4. Monitor the client for jaundice, fever, and other signs of hepatotoxicity. Assess drug levels and monitor liver and renal function studies throughout drug therapy.

5. Routinely inspect the client's teeth and gums. Note any signs of changes in dentition.

6. Anticipate that clients will receive concomitant administration of adrenal corticosteroids.

Client/Family Teaching

1. Demonstrate and explain how to measure the dose of medication accurately.

2. Explain the importance of following the written guidelines for medication therapy explicitly. Call the physician with questions or if problems arise. Reinforce that the drug must be taken throughout one's lifetime to prevent transplant rejection.

3. Review the side effects of drug therapy. Because this drug is so important to transplant clients in preventing rejection, the client and family should be provided a written list of all possible side effects of drugs and know which side effects need to be reported to the physician.

4. Keep an account of daily weight. Discuss the importance

of reporting any persistent diarrhea, nausea, and vomiting and of recording the intake and output.

5. Advise client that taking the drug with food may reduce nausea and associated GI upset.

6. Do not stop the drug abruptly. If the drug must be discontinued, it should be done gradually.

7. Stress the importance of using nystatin swish and swab as directed to prevent the development of thrush. Frequent oral care and dental exams should be routine.

8. Warn clients that they may develop acne and hirsutism as a side effect. This should be reported to the physician because a dermatologist referral may be necessary.

Evaluation

1. In clients with organ transplants, prevent rejection.

2. Assess client closely for adverse side effects that may require drug adjustment.

Cyproheptadine hydrochloride

(sye-proh-**HEP**-tah-deen)
Periactin (Rx)

See also *Antihistamines,* p. 71.

Classification: Antihistamine, piperidine-type.

Action/Kinetics: Cyproheptadine also possesses antiserotonin activity. **Duration:** 8 hr.

Additional Uses: Cold urticaria. *Investigational:* Cluster headaches, appetite stimulant in underweight clients and those with anorexia nervosa.

Additional Contraindications: Glaucoma, urinary retention.

Special Concerns: Pregnancy category: B. Geriatric clients may be more sensitive to the usual adult dose.

Additional Side Effect: Increased appetite.

Laboratory Test Interferences: ↑ Serum amylase and prolactin if given with thyroid-releasing hormone.

Dosage: Syrup, Tablets. *Antihistaminic:* **Adults, initial:** 4 mg q 8 hr; **then,** 4–20 mg daily, not to exceed 0.5 mg/kg daily. **Pediatric, 2–6 years:** 2 mg q 8–12 hr, not to exceed 12 mg daily; **6–14 years:** 4 mg q 8–12 hr, not to exceed 16 mg daily. *Appetite stimulant:* **Adults,** 4 mg t.i.d. with meals. **Pediatric, 6–14 years, initial:** 2 mg t.i.d.–q.i.d. with meals; **then,** reduce dose to 4 mg t.i.d. **Pediatric, 2–6 years, initial:** 2 mg t.i.d. with meals; **then,** dose may be increased to a total of 8 mg daily.

NURSING CONSIDERATIONS

See *Nursing Considerations* for *Antihistamines,* p. 74.

Administration/Storage

1. Drug should not be given more than 6 months to adults and 3 months to children for appetite stimulation.
2. Anticipate the onset of action to occur within 15–30 min and to last from 3–6 hr.

Evaluation: Evaluate client for:
- Reports of symptomatic improvement of allergic manifestations
- Weight gain

Cytarabine (ARA-C, Cytosine Arabinoside)

(sye-**TAIR**-ah-been)

Cytosar❦, Cytosar-U, (Rx)

See also *Antineoplastic Agents,* p. 85.

Classification: Antineoplastic, antimetabolite.

Action/Kinetics: Cytarabine is thought to act by inhibiting DNA polymerase as well as by being incorporated into both DNA and RNA. The drug is cell-phase specific, acting in the S phase and also blocking the progression of cells from the G_1 phase to the S phase. Cytarabine may also decrease the immune response. After oral administration, cytarabine is rapidly broken down by the GI mucosa and liver, resulting in systemic availability of less than 20%. **$t\frac{1}{2}$ after IV:** distribution, 10 min; elimination, 1–3 hr. The drug is metabolized in the liver to uracil arabinoside, which is excreted in the urine. Crosses blood-brain barrier. Eighty percent eliminated in urine in 24 hr.

Uses: Induction and maintenance of remission in acute myelocytic leukemia in adults and children, acute lymphocytic leukemia, chronic myelocytic leukemia, erythroleukemia, and meningeal leukemia. In combination with other drugs for non-Hodgkin's lymphoma in children. *Investigational:* Hodgkin's lymphomas, myelodysplastic syndrome.

Contraindications: Use during lactation. Anaphylaxis has occurred causing acute cardiopulmonary arrest. Use with caution in impaired hepatic function.

Special Concerns: Pregnancy category: D. Anaphylaxis has occurred, causing acute cardiopulmonary arrest. Use with caution in clients with impaired renal function.

Additional Side Effects: "Cytarabine syndrome" (6–12 hr following drug administration) manifested by bone pain, fever, myalgia, maculopapular rash, conjunctivitis, chest pain, or malaise. Nephrotoxicity, neuritis, skin ulceration, sepsis, acute pancreatitis (in clients previously treated with l-asparaginase), pneumonia, hyperuricemia. Thrombophlebitis at injection site.

The incidence of side effects (nausea and vomiting for several hours) is higher in clients receiving rapid IV injection than in those receiving drug by IV infusion. Intrathecal administration may result in systemic side effects including nausea, vomiting, fever, and rarely neurotoxicity and paraplegia. *Symptoms of Overdose:* CNS toxicity.

Drug Interactions: Absorption of digoxin may be impaired when cytarabine is used with other antineoplastics.

Dosage: Note: Cytarabine is frequently used in combination with other drugs; thus, dosage varies and must be carefully checked. *Acute myelocytic leukemia, acute lymphocytic leukemia:* **IV infusion:** 100–200 mg/m² as a continuous infusion over 24 hr or in divided doses (by rapid injection) for 5–10 days; repeat every 2 weeks. *Acute nonlymphocytic leukemia (in combination with other drugs):* 100 mg/m²/day by continuous IV infusion (days 1–7) or 100 mg/m² q 12 hr (days 1–7). *Meningeal leukemia:* **Intrathecal, usual:** 30 mg/m² every

4 days with hydrocortisone sodium succinate and methotrexate, each at a dose of 15 mg/m², until CSF findings are normal, followed by one additional dose. *Refractory acute leukemia:* **IV:** 3 g/m² q 12 hr for 4–12 doses; repeat at 2–3 wk intervals.

The drug should be discontinued if platelet level falls to 50,000/mm³ or less or polymorphonuclear granulocyte level falls to 1,000/mm³ or less.

NURSING CONSIDERATIONS

See also *Nursing Considerations* for *Antineoplastic Agents,* p. 88.

Administration/Storage

1. Cytarabine may be given SC, IV infusion, or IV injection. It is ineffective orally.
2. The 100-mg vial of cytarabine should be reconstituted with 5 ml bacteriostatic water for injection with benzyl alcohol (0.9%) with the resultant solution containing 20 mg/ml. The 500 mg vial should be reconstituted with 10 ml of bacteriostatic water for injection with benzyl alcohol (0.9%) with the resultant solution containing 50 mg/ml cytarabine. Benzyl alcohol should not be used for reconstitution if the drug will be used intrathecally; rather, 0.9% saline or Elliott's B solution should be used.
3. Reconstituted solution should be stored at room temperature and used within 48 hr.
4. Discard hazy solution.
5. Assess closely during drug administration for evidence of anaphylactic reaction. Have appropriate resuscitative drugs and equipment readily available.

6. *Treatment of Overdose:* General supportive measures.

Assessment

1. Determine baseline CBC, platelets and liver function. Note any history of impaired hepatic function.
2. Document any previous therapy for leukemia.

Interventions

1. Observe closely 6–12 hr following drug administration for the development of "cytarabine syndrome."

2. Monitor VS and intake and output during therapy.
3. Obtain written laboratory parameters that would necessitate the interruption of drug therapy.

Evaluation

1. Anticipate that systemic toxicity may result from intrathecal use of cytarabine.
2. Evaluate client for:
   • ↓ in tumor size and spread
   • Improved hematologic parameters
   • Evidence of a remission

D

Dacarbazine
(dah-**KAR**-bah-zeen)
DTIC✹, DTIC-Dome, Imidazole Carboxamide (Abbreviation: DTIC) (Rx)

See also *Antineoplastic Agents,* p. 85, and *Alkylating Agents,* p. 20.

Classification: Antineoplastic, alkylating agent.

Action/Kinetics: The drug is thought to act by three mechanisms including: alkylation by an activated carbonium ion, antimetabolite to inhibit DNA synthesis, and by combining with protein sulfhydryl groups. The drug is cell-cycle nonspecific. **t½, biphasic, initial,** 19 min; **terminal,** 5 hr. Drug probably localizes in liver. Limited amounts (14% of plasma level) enter CSF. Approximately 40% of drug excreted in urine unchanged within 6 hr. Dacarbazine is secreted through the kidney tubules rather than filtered through the glomeruli.

Uses: Metastatic malignant melanoma. Hodgkin's disease (with other agents).

Contraindications: Use during lactation.

Special Concerns: Pregnancy category: C. Dosage has not been established in children.

Additional Side Effects: Especially serious (fatal) hematologic toxicity. More than 90% of clients develop nausea, vomiting, and anorexia 1 hr after initial administration, which persists for 12–48 hr. Rarely, diarrhea, stomatitis, and intractable nausea. Also, flu-like syndrome, severe pain along injected vein, facial flushing, alopecia, photosensitivity. Elevation of AST, ALT, and other enzymes, CNS symptoms.

Dosage: IV only. *Malignant melanoma:* 2–4.5 mg/kg daily for 10 days; may be repeated at 4-week intervals; or 250 mg/m²/day for 5 days; may be repeated at 3-week intervals. *Hodgkin's disease:* 150 mg/m²/day for 5 days; or 375 mg/m² on day 1, with other drugs repeated every 15 days.

NURSING CONSIDERATIONS

See also *Nursing Considerations* for *Antineoplastic Agents,* p. 88.

Administration/Storage

1. To minimize adverse GI effects, antiemetics, fasting, and limited fluid intake (4–6 hr preceding treatment) have been suggested.
2. Extreme care should be taken to avoid extravasation.
3. Drug can be given by IV push over 1-min period or further diluted and administered by IV infusion (preferred) over 15- to 30-min period.
4. Protect dry vials from light and store at 2°C–8°C.
5. Reconstituted solutions are stable for up to 72 hr at 4°C or for 8 hr at 20°C. More dilute solutions for IV infusions are stable for 24 hr when stored at 2°C–8°C.
6. *Treatment of Overdose:* Monitor blood cell counts; supportive treatment.

Interventions

1. Ascertain how physician wishes to handle fluid status (have client fast for 4–6 hr before treatment to reduce emesis or allow client to have fluids up to 1 hr before administration to minimize dehydration following treatment).

2. Anticipate antiemetic administration before and throughout therapy. Report nausea and vomiting because these side effects may last for 1–12 hr after injection.
3. Have phenobarbital and/or prochlorperazine available for palliation of vomiting following administration of dacarbazine.
4. Clients may develop flu-like symptoms with fever, aches, fatigue, usually starting 7–10 days after dose of drug. Administer antipyretics and analgesics as needed.
5. Monitor client and laboratory studies closely for evidence of bone marrow depression, liver toxicity, or hypersensitivity reaction.

Client/Family Teaching

1. Reassure client that after the first 1–2 days of dacarbazine therapy, vomiting ceases because tolerance develops to the drug.
2. Report to physician any flu-like symptoms (fever, myalgia, and malaise) that may occur after treatment.
3. Avoid prolonged exposure to sun or ultraviolet light, as photosensitivity reaction may occur.

Evaluation: Evaluate client for:
- Decrease in tumor size and spread
- Control of nausea and vomiting

Dactinomycin
(dack-tin-oh-**MY**-sin)
Actinomycin D, Cosmegen (Rx)

See also *Antineoplastic Agents,* p. 85.

Classification: Antineoplastic, antibiotic.

Action/Kinetics: Chromopeptide antibiotic produced by *Streptomyces parvullus*. Dactinomycin acts by intercalating into the purine–pyrimidine base pair, thereby inhibiting synthesis of messenger RNA. The activity is cell-cycle nonspecific although the maximum number of cells are destroyed in the G_1 phase. The drug is cleared from the blood within 2 min and concentrated in nucleated cells. $t\frac{1}{2}$: 36 hr. The drug does not cross the blood-brain barrier and is excreted mainly unchanged.

During therapy, leukocyte counts should be performed daily, and platelet counts q 3 days. Frequent liver and kidney function tests are recommended. Appearance of toxic manifestations may be delayed by several weeks. Irreversible bone marrow depression may occur in clients with preexisting renal, hepatic, or bone marrow impairment. The drug is corrosive to soft tissue.

Uses: In combination with vincristine, surgery and/or irradiation for treatment of Wilms' tumor (nephroblastoma) and its metastases. In combination with methotrexate to treat metastatic and nonmetastatic choriocarcinoma. In combination with cyclophosphamide, doxorubicin, and vincristine to treat rhabdomyosarcoma. Nonseminomatous testicular carcinoma. With cyclophosphamide and radiotherapy to treat Ewing's sarcoma. In combination with radiotherapy to treat sarcoma botryoides. Endometrial carcinoma. *Investigational:* Ovarian cancer, Kaposi's sarcoma, osteosarcoma, malignant melanoma.

Contraindications: Concurrent infection with chickenpox or herpes zoster (death may result). Lactation. Infants less than 6–12 months of age.

Special Concerns: Pregnancy category: C. When used with X-ray therapy, erythema is seen in normal skin and the buccal and pharyngeal mucosa.

Additional Side Effects: Anaphylaxis. Due to corrosiveness, extravasation causes severe damage to soft tissues. Hypocalcemia. When combined with radiation, increased severity of skin reactions, GI toxicity, and bone marrow depression.

Laboratory Test Interference: Interferes with bioassay tests used to determine antibacterial drug levels.

Dosage: IV, individualized. Adults, usual, 0.5 mg/m² once weekly for 3 weeks; or, 0.01–0.015 mg/kg daily for a maximum of 5 days q 4–6 weeks. **Pediatric:** 10–15 mcg/kg (0.45 mg/m²) daily for 5 days; **alternatively,** a total dose of 2.4 mg/m² over 1 week. Total daily dosage for both adults and children should not exceed 15 mcg/kg over a 5-day period. Course of treatment may be repeated after 3 weeks unless contraindicated due to toxicity. If no toxicity, second course can be given after 3 weeks. *Ewing's sarcoma/sarcoma botryoides,* **Isolation-perfusion:** 0.05 mg/kg for pelvis and lower extremities and 0.035 mg/kg for upper extremities.

NURSING CONSIDERATIONS

See also *Nursing Considerations for Antineoplastic Agents,* p. 88.

Administration/Storage

1. For IV use, dactinomycin is available in a lyophilized dactinomycin-mannitol mixture that

turns a gold color upon reconstitution with sterile water. Use only sterile water without a preservative to reconstitute the drug for IV use, as it will precipitate. Solutions should not be exposed to direct sunlight.

2. *The drug is extremely corrosive.* It is most safely administered through the tubing of a running IV (e.g., 5% dextrose or sodium chloride). It may be given directly into the vein, but the needle used to draw up the solution should be discarded and another sterile needle attached, before injection, to prevent subcutaneous reaction and thrombophlebitis.

3. Extreme care should be exercised in reconstituting and administering dactinomycin so that the dust or vapors are not inhaled or come in contact with skin or mucous membranes. Special care should be exercised to prevent contact with the eyes.

4. Any portion of the solution not used for the injection should be discarded.

Assessment

1. Assess and report if client is pregnant, lactating, or infected with herpes, all of which are contraindications for dactinomycin therapy.

2. Determine baseline CBC and monitor closely throughout therapy for evidence of bone marrow depression.

Interventions

1. Report erythema of the skin, which can lead to desquamation and sloughing, particularly in areas previously affected by radiation. Erythema may be seen in normal skin and the buccal and pharyngeal mucosa.

2. Warn client of the possibility of delayed toxic reactions and stress importance of returning for blood tests.

3. Anticipate that dactinomycin may be administered intermittently if nausea and vomiting persist even when an antiemetic is given.

4. Anticipate that penicillin will not be used if client contracts an infection because dactinomycin inhibits the action of penicillin.

5. Drug interferes with bioassay test used to measure antibacterial drug levels; monitor client response to antibiotic therapy carefully.

Evaluation: Evaluate client for a positive tumor response with a minimum of adverse side effects.

Danazol
(**DAN**-ah-zohl)
Cyclomen✦, Danocrine (Rx)

Classification: Gonadotropin inhibitor.

Action/Kinetics: This synthetic androgen inhibits the release of gonadotropins (FSH and LH) by the anterior pituitary. In women this action arrests ovarian function, induces amenorrhea, and causes atrophy of normal and ectopic endometrial tissue. Has weak androgenic effects. **Onset, fibrocystic disease:** 4 weeks. **Time to peak effect, amenorrhea and anovulation:** 6–8 weeks; **fibrocystic disease:** 2–3 months to eliminate breast pain and tenderness and 4–6 months for elimination of nodules. **t½:** 4.5 hr. **Duration:** Ovulation and menstruation usually resume 60–90 days after cessation of therapy.

Uses: Endometriosis amenable to hormonal management in clients who cannot tolerate or who have not responded to other drug therapy. Fibrocystic breast disease. Hereditary angioedema in males and females. *Investigational:* Gynecomastia, menorrhagia, precocious puberty.

Contraindications: Undiagnosed genital bleeding, markedly impaired hepatic, renal, and cardiac function, pregnancy and lactation.

Special Concerns: Use with caution in children treated for hereditary angioedema due to the possibility of virilization in females and precocious sexual development in males. Geriatric clients may have an increased risk of prostatic hypertrophy or prostatic carcinoma.

Side Effects: *Androgenic:* Acne, decrease in breast size, oily hair and skin, weight gain, deepening of voice and hair growth, clitoral hypertrophy, testicular atrophy. *Estrogen deficiency:* Flushing, sweating, vaginitis, nervousness, changes in emotions. *GI:* Nausea, vomiting, constipation, gastroenteritis. *Hepatic:* Jaundice, dysfunction. *CNS:* Fatigue, tremor, headache, dizziness, sleep problems, paresthesia, anxiety, depression, appetite changes. *Miscellaneous:* Allergic reactions, muscle cramps or spasms, joint swelling or lock-up, hematuria, increased blood pressure, chills, pelvic pain, carpal tunnel syndrome, hair loss, change in libido.

Drug Interactions

Insulin / Danazol ↑ insulin requirements
Warfarin / Danazol ↑ prothrombin time in warfarin-stabilized clients

Dosage: Capsules. *Endometriosis:* 400 mg b.i.d. (moderate to severe) or 100–200 mg b.i.d. (mild) for 3–6 months (up to 9 months may be required in some clients). Begin therapy during menses, if possible, to be sure that client is not pregnant. *Fibrocystic breast disease:* 50–200 mg b.i.d. beginning on day 2 of menses. *Hereditary angioedema:* **Initial,** 200 mg b.i.d.–t.i.d.; after desired response, decrease dosage by 50% (or less) at 1- to 3-month intervals. Subsequent attacks can be treated by giving up to 200 mg/day. No more than 800 mg daily should be given to adults.

NURSING CONSIDERATIONS

Assessment

1. Discuss with the client the presence of undiagnosed genital bleeding and determine onset, frequency, extent, and any precipitating factors.
2. Obtain renal and hepatic function studies to serve as baseline data.
3. If the client is female, sexually active, and of child-bearing age, determine if she is pregnant.
4. Note any evidence or history of cardiac dysfunction.
5. Document subjective reports of endometrial pain. Note breast pain, tenderness, and presence of nodules.
6. Attempt to identify factors that precipitate angioedema.

Interventions

1. Observe the client closely for signs of virilization such as

hirsutism, reduced breast size, deepening of the voice, acne, increased oiliness of the skin, and clitoral enlargement. Some androgenic side effects may not be reversible and may require a change in drug dosage or discontinuation of the drug.

2. Observe clients with a history of epilepsy, migraines, cardiac or renal dysfunction for fluid retention. Danazol may cause fluid retention with resultant edema and if this occurs it may be necessary to have the drug discontinued.

Client/Family Teaching

1. Take with meals to decrease GI upset.
2. Describe the signs of virilization that may occur with drug therapy (e.g., abnormal hair growth, deepening of the voice). Report these symptoms to the physician so that the dosage of drug can be adjusted.
3. Explain that the hypoestrogenic side effects usually disappear after the therapy is discontinued.
4. Ovulation will resume 60–90 days after the drug has been discontinued.
5. Wearing cotton underwear and paying careful attention to hygiene may diminish the incidence of vaginitis associated with danazol therapy.
6. Stress the importance of practicing birth control.
7. Advise that several months of therapy may be required before any improvements may be noted.
8. Continue to perform self breast exams (SBE) and report any changes.

Evaluation: Evaluate client for:
- Reports of control of endometrial pain (usually requires 3–6 months of therapy)
- A decrease in breast tenderness and pain (usually after 2–3 months)
- Improved allergic responses R/T angioedema

Dantrolene sodium
(DAN-troh-leen)
Dantrium, Dantrium IV (Rx)

See also *Centrally Acting Skeletal Muscle Relaxants,* p. 130.

Classification: Centrally acting muscle relaxant.

Action/Kinetics: Dantrolene is a hydantoin derivative and, as such, is chemically unrelated to other skeletal muscle relaxants. It acts directly on skeletal muscle, probably by dissociating the excitation-contraction coupling mechanism as a result of interference of release of calcium from the sarcoplasmic reticulum. This action results in a decreased force of reflex muscle contraction and a reduction of hyperreflexia, spasticity, involuntary movements, and clonus. Its effectiveness in malignant hyperthermia is due to an inhibition of release of calcium from the sarcoplasmic reticulum. This results in prevention or reduction of the increased myoplasmic calcium ion concentration that activates the acute catabolic processes associated with malignant hyperthermia. Absorption is slow and incomplete, but consistent. **Peak plasma levels:** 4–6 hr. **t½: oral,** 8.7 hr; **t½: IV,** 5 hr. There is significant plasma protein binding of the drug.

Uses: Muscle spasticity associated with severe chronic disorders, such as multiple sclerosis, cerebral palsy, spinal cord injury, and stroke. Muscle pain due to exercise. Malignant hyperthermia due to hypermetabolism of skeletal muscle. *Investigational:* Exercise-induced muscle pain, heat stroke, and neuroleptic malignant syndrome.

Contraindications: Rheumatic diseases, pregnancy, lactation, or children under 5 years of age. Acute hepatitis and cirrhosis of the liver.

Special Concerns: (Pregnancy category: C—parenteral use). Use with caution in clients with impaired pulmonary function.

Side Effects: Following PO use: Side effects are dose-related and decrease with usage. Fatal and nonfatal hepatotoxicity. *CNS:* Drowsiness, dizziness, weakness, malaise, lightheadedness, headaches, insomnia, seizures, speech disturbances, fatigue, confusion, depression, nervousness. *GI:* Diarrhea (common), anorexia, gastric upset, cramps, GI bleeding. *Musculoskeletal:* Backache, myalgia. *Dermatologic:* Rashes, photosensitivity, pruritus, urticaria, hair growth, sweating. *CV:* Blood pressure changes, phlebitis, tachycardia. *GU:* Urinary retention, hematuria, crystalluria, nocturia, impotence. *Miscellaneous:* Visual disturbances, chills, fever, tearing, feeling of suffocation, pleural effusion with pericarditis.

Following IV use: Pulmonary edema, thrombophlebitis, urticaria, erythema.

Dosage: Capsules. *Spastic conditions.* **Adults: initial,** 25 mg/day; **then,** increase to 25 mg b.i.d.–q.i.d.; dose may then be increased by 25-mg increments up to 100 mg b.i.d.–q.i.d. (doses in excess of 400 mg/day not recommended). **Pediatric: initial,** 0.5 mg/kg b.i.d.; **then,** increase to 0.5 t.i.d.–q.i.d.; dose may then be increased by increments of 0.5 mg/kg to 3 mg/kg b.i.d.–q.i.d. (doses should not exceed 400 mg/day). *Malignant hyperthermia, preoperatively.* **Adults and children, PO:** 4–8 mg/kg daily in 3–4 divided doses 1–2 days before surgery. *Postmalignant hyperthermic crisis:* 4–8 mg/kg daily in four divided doses for 1–33 days.

   IV infusion. *Malignant hyperthermia, crisis treatment:* **Adults and children, initial,** 2.5 mg/kg 60 min prior to surgery and infused over 1 hr. **IV push: Initial,** At least 1 mg/kg; continue administration until symptoms decrease or a cumulative dose of 10 mg/kg has been administered.

NURSING CONSIDERATIONS

See also *Nursing Considerations* for *Centrally Acting Skeletal Muscle Relaxants,* p. 130.

Administration/Storage

1. If the drug is to be administered IV, the powder should be reconstituted by adding 60 ml of sterile water for injection.
2. Reconstituted solutions should be protected from light and used within 6 hr.
3. When administered orally, the drug can be mixed with fruit juice or other liquid vehicle.
4. If the drug is being administered to counteract spasticity, beneficial effects may not be noted for a week. The drug should be discontinued after 6 weeks if beneficial effects are not evident.

5. Due to potential hepatotoxicity, long-term benefits must be evaluated for each client.

6. *Treatment of Overdose:* Immediate gastric lavage. Maintain airway and have artificial resuscitation equipment available. Large quantities of IV fluids to prevent crystalluria. Monitor ECG.

Assessment

1. Note the client's mental status and general appearance.

2. Obtain baseline liver function studies prior to initiating drug therapy. Impaired hepatic function is more likely to occur in women over 35 years of age.

3. Auscultate lung and heart sounds prior to beginning therapy and record these findings for use as baseline data.

4. Note any evidence of impaired pulmonary function, cardiac disorders, or history of the client having either benign or malignant breast tumors. Dantrolene may increase the incidence of mammary tumors.

5. Note the extent of the client's spasticity, involuntary movements, and clonus. Record these findings for use as baseline data against which to compare the results of the drug therapy.

Interventions

1. Auscultate respiratory and heart sounds at regular intervals during the therapy. Note any changes.

2. Inspect the client's skin to detect any changes.

3. Routinely perform liver function studies throughout therapy. Withhold drug and notify physician of any abnormal findings.

4. Monitor intake and output and note any evidence of blood in the urine. Document and report to the physician as drug therapy may need to be discontinued.

5. Monitor stools for diarrhea and/or any evidence of blood.

6. If clients develop diplopia, reassure them that this and many of the other bothersome side effects associated with drug therapy may lessen with the continued use of the drug.

Client/Family Teaching

1. Since this drug causes drowsiness, clients should be instructed not to operate dangerous machinery or drive a car.

2. Report any increased muscle weakness or impaired physical ability.

3. Reassure the client that several weeks of therapy may be required before improvements in the client's condition will be noted. Insomnia and depression should be reported to the physician.

4. Teach client how to take and monitor BP, check stools for the presence of occult blood, and keep a record of urinary output. Report any marked changes in BP and any evidence of diarrhea or blood in the urine or stool.

5. If client develops slurred speech, drooling, inability to perform usual physical functions, or enuresis, the drug may require withdrawal.

6. Encourage female clients to have mammograms and to do breast self-examinations to de-

tect any occurrence of lumps since this drug has the potential to cause the development of these problems. This is especially important in women with a family history of malignant or benign breast tumors.

7. Explain to male clients the potential for impotence. Report this side effect to the physician.

Evaluation

1. Evaluate client for:
   - Reduction in spasticity and/or muscle pain
   - Reduction in exercise-induced muscle pain
   - Evidence of rebound spasticity or hallucinations after withdrawal of the drug therapy
   - Decrease in temperature in malignant hyperthermia due to hypermetabolism of skeletal muscle

2. Drug should be discontinued if improvement is not evident after 45 days.

Dapiprazole hydrochloride

(dah-**PIP**-rah-zol)
Rev-Eyes (Rx)

Classification: Ophthalmic alpha-adrenergic blocking agent.

Action/Kinetics: Dapiprazole produces miosis by blocking the alpha-adrenergic receptors on the dilator muscle of the iris. The drug does not have significant action on ciliary muscle contraction; thus, it does not cause changes in the depth of the anterior chamber of the thickness of the lens. Dapiprazole does not alter the intraocular pressure either in normal eyes or in eyes with elevated intraocular pressure. The rate of pupillary constriction may be slightly slower in clients with brown irides than in clients with blue or green irides.

Uses: To reverse diagnostic mydriasis induced by adrenergic (e.g., phenylephrine) or parasympatholytic (e.g., tropicamide) agents.

Contraindications: Acute iritis or other conditions where miosis is not desirable. To reduce intraocular pressure or to treat open angle glaucoma.

Special Concerns: Pregnancy category: B. Use with caution during lactation. Safety and effectiveness have not been determined in children.

Side Effects: *Ophthalmic:* Conjunctival injection lasting 20 min, burning on instillation, ptosis, lid erythema, itching, lid edema, chemosis, corneal edema, punctate keratitis, photophobia, tearing and blurring of vision, dryness of eyes. *Miscellaneous:* Headaches, browache.

Dosage: Ophthalmic solution: 2 gtt followed in 5 min by 2 more gtt applied to the conjunctiva of the eye after ophthalmic examination.

NURSING CONSIDERATIONS

Administration/Storage

1. The drug should not be used in the same client more frequently than once a week.

2. To prepare the solution, the aluminum seals and rubber plugs should be removed and discarded from both the drug and diluent vials. After pouring the diluent into the drug vial, the dropper assembly should

be removed from its sterile wrapping and attached to the drug vial. The container should be shaken for several minutes to ensure adequate mixing.

3. Reconstituted eye drops may be stored at room temperature for 21 days.

4. Any solution that is not clear and colorless should be discarded.

Assessment

1. Determine any hypersensitivity to alpha-adrenergic blocking agents.

2. Note eye color. Pupillary constriction may be slightly slower in clients with brown irides as opposed to those with blue or green irides.

Evaluation: Evaluate client for evidence of successful reversal of drug-induced mydriasis.

Dapsone (DDS)

(DAP-sohn)
Avlosulfon ✸ (Rx)

Classification: Sulfone, leprostatic.

Action/Kinetics: Dapsone is a synthetic agent with both bacteriostatic and bactericidal activity, especially against *Mycobacterium leprae* (Hansen's bacillus). Although the exact mechanism is not known, dapsone is thought to act similarly to sulfonamides in that it interferes with the metabolism of the infectious organism. Widely distributed throughout the body. **Peak plasma levels:** 4–8 hr. Doses of 200 mg daily for 8 days will lead to a plateau plasma level of 0.1–7 mcg/ml. **t½:** About 28 hr. The drug is acetylated

in the liver and metabolites are excreted in the urine.

Uses: Lepromatous and tuberculoid types of leprosy, dermatitis herpetiformis, and for prophylaxis of malaria. *Investigational:* Relapsing polychondritis.

Contraindications: Advanced amyloidosis of kidneys. Lactation.

Special Concerns: Pregnancy category: C.

Side Effects: *Hematologic:* Hemolytic anemia, methemoglobinemia. *GI:* Nausea, vomiting, anorexia, abdominal discomfort. *CNS:* Headache, insomnia, vertigo, paresthesia, psychoses, peripheral neuropathy. *Dermatologic:* Photosensitivity, lupus-like syndrome. *Hypersensitivity:* Severe skin reactions including exfoliative dermatitis, erythema multiforme, urticaria, erythema nodosum, toxic erythema, toxic epidermal necrolysis, morbilliform and scarlatiniform reactions. *Miscellaneous:* Muscle weakness, hypoalbuminemia, albuminuria, nephrotic syndrome, renal papillary necrosis, blurred vision, tinnitus, male infertility, fever, tachycardia, mononucleosis-type syndrome.

A leprosy-reactional state may occur in large numbers of clients during therapy with dapsone. Type 1 occurs soon after therapy is initiated. Clients manifest an enhanced delayed hypersensitivity syndrome, leading to swelling of existing nerve and skin lesions with possible neuritis. However, this is not an indication to discontinue therapy. Steroids, analgesics, and surgical decompression of swollen nerve trunks may be used to reduce symptoms. Type 2 occurs in nearly 50% of clients during the first year of therapy. Symptoms include fever, erythematous skin nodules, joint swelling, neuritis, orchitis, malaise, depression, iritis, or epistaxis. Usually therapy is continued with the use of analgesics, steroids, or clofazimine to suppress the reaction. *Symptoms of Overdose:* Nausea, vomiting, hyperexcitability (up to 24 hr after ingestion of an overdose). Methemoglobin-induced depression, seizures, severe cyanosis, headache, hemolysis.

Drug Interactions

Para-aminobenzoic acid / ↓ Effect of dapsone
Probenecid / ↑ Effect of dapsone due to inhibition of renal excretion
Pyrimethamine / ↑ Risk of hematologic reactions
Rifampin / ↓ Effect of dapsone due to ↑ plasma clearance

Laboratory Test Interference: Altered liver function tests.

Dosage: Tablets. *Leprosy:* **Adults:** 50–100 mg/day. The full dose should be initiated and continued without interruption. *Leprosy, bacteriologically negative tuberculoid and indeterminate type:* **Adults:** 100 mg daily with rifampin, 600 mg daily for 6 months; **then,** continue dapsone for a minimum of 3 years. *Leprosy, lepromatous and borderline clients:* 100 mg daily for at least 10 years. *Dermatitis herpetiformis:* **Adults, initial:** 50 mg/day; dosage may be increased to 300 mg/day or higher, if necessary. **Maintenance:** Reduce dosage to minimum maintenance dose as soon as possible; maintenance dosage may be reduced or eliminated in clients on a gluten-free diet. Dosage should be correspondingly less in children.

NURSING CONSIDERATIONS

See also *General Nursing Considerations For All Anti-Infectives,* p. 83.

Administration/Storage

1. For tuberculoid and indeterminate clients, dosage should be continued for at least 3 years.
2. For lepromatous clients, full dosage may be necessary for life.
3. Possible resistance to dapsone should be carefully evaluated, especially if lepromatous or borderline lepromatous clients relapse. If there is no response to dapsone therapy within 3–6 months, dapsone resistance can be confirmed.
4. *Treatment of Overdose:* Gastric lavage. In normal and methemoglobin-reductase deficient clients, give methylene blue, 1–2 mg/kg by slow IV (may need to be repeated if methemoglobin reaccumulates). In nonemergencies, methylene blue may be given orally, 3–5 mg/kg q 4–6 hr.

Assessment

1. Obtain baseline CBC, liver and renal function studies, and monitor throughout therapy.
2. Document size, extent, and location of lesions.

Interventions

1. Anticipate that dosage is increased slowly during initiation period.
2. Check whether physician wishes client to receive hematinics.
3. Use strict medical asepsis because client may have leukopenia.
4. Observe clients in whom there are other concurrent chronic

conditions particularly closely and anticipate reduction in dosage of sulfones.

5. Assess for symptoms of anemia. Report RBC count below 2,500,000/mm³ or if it remains low during first 6 weeks of therapy. Also note when WBC falls below 5,000/mm³.

Client/Family Teaching

1. Instruct lactating mothers to report cyanosis of nursing infant because this indicates high sulfone levels, and withdrawal of drug may be indicated.
2. Take medication exactly as ordered.
3. Follow their diet as prescribed (e.g., gluten-free). Refer to dietitian as needed for additional counseling and instruction.
4. Provide a printed list of side effects. Note any evidence of psychoses, GI disturbances, lepra reaction, headaches, dizziness, lethargy, severe malaise, tinnitus, paresthesias, deep aches, neuralgic pains, and ocular disturbances should be reported to physician.
5. Stress the importance of reporting for scheduled lab studies and follow-up visits to evaluate effectiveness of therapy.
6. Identify local support groups that may assist the client to understand and cope with chronic disease states.

Evaluation: Evaluate client for:
- ↓ in the size and extent of lesions
- Improvement of inflammation and ulceration of the mucous membranes during the first 3–6 months of therapy. Lack of response may

indicate a need for other therapy.
- Allergic dermatitis, which usually appears before the tenth week of therapy. Allergic dermatitis may develop into fatal exfoliative dermatitis.

D

------ *COMBINATION DRUG* ------
Darvocet-N 50 and Darvocet-N 100
(**DAR**-voh-set)
(Rx)

Classification/Content: *Nonnarcotic analgesic:* Acetaminophen, 325 (Darvocet-N 50) or 650 mg (Darvocet-N 100). *Analgesic:* Propoxyphene napsylate, 50 or 100 mg.

Uses: Mild to moderate pain (may be used if fever is present).

Special Concerns: Use during pregnancy only if benefits outweigh risks.

Dosage: Tablets. Two Darvocet-N 50 tablets or one Darvocet-N 100 tablet q 4 hr. Maximum daily dose of propoxyphene napsylate should not exceed 600 mg. Total daily dose should be reduced in clients with impaired hepatic or renal function.

NURSING CONSIDERATIONS

See *Nursing Considerations* for *Acetaminophen,* p. 252, and *Propoxyphene napsylate,* p. 1101.

------ *COMBINATION DRUG* ------
Darvon Compound 65
(**DAR**-von)
(Rx)

Classification/Content: Darvon Compound 65: Propoxyphene HCl, 65 mg; aspirin, 389 mg; and caffeine, 32.4 mg.

Propoxyphene and aspirin are analgesics, whereas caffeine is a CNS stimulant. See also information on individual components.

Uses: Mild to moderate pain, with or without accompanying fever.

Special Concerns: Use during pregnancy only if benefits outweigh risks.

Dosage: Capsules. One capsule q 4 hr of Darvon Compound 65. Total daily dose of propoxyphene HCl should not exceed 390 mg. Total daily dosage should be decreased in clients with hepatic or renal impairment.

NURSING CONSIDERATIONS

See also *Nursing Considerations* for *Aspirin,* p. 264, and *Caffeine,* p. 378.

Client/Family Teaching

1. Advise to use caution when performing tasks that require mental alertness because drug may cause dizziness and sedation.
2. Do *not* ingest alcohol.
3. Keep out of reach of children.
4. Use cautiously because psychological and physical dependence may occur.

Evaluation: Evaluate client for reports of effective control of pain and discomfort.

Daunorubicin

(daw-noh-**ROO**-bih-sin)
Cerubidine (Abbreviation: DNR) (Rx)

See also *Antineoplastic Agents,* p. 85.

Classification: Antineoplastic, antibiotic.

Action/Kinetics: Anthracycline antibiotic produced by *Streptomyces coeruleorubidus.* Daunorubicin is most active in the S phase of cell division but is not cell-cycle specific. The drug inhibits synthesis of nucleic acid by inserting into the double helix of DNA. Daunorubicin also possesses immunosuppressive, cytotoxic, and antimitotic activity. Rapidly cleared from the plasma. Metabolized to the active daunorubicinol. **t½:** daunorubicin, 18.5 hr; daunorubicinol, 27 hr. Drug rapidly taken up by heart, kidneys, lung, liver, and spleen. Chiefly excreted in bile (40%) and unchanged in urine (25%). Does not pass blood-brain barrier.

Uses: Acute nonlymphocytic leukemia in adults (myelogenous, erythroid, monocytic). When combined with cytarabine, effectiveness is increased. Acute lymphocytic leukemia in children (increased effectiveness when combined with vincristine and prednisone). *Investigational:* Ewing's sarcoma, chronic myelocytic leukemia, neuroblastoma, non-Hodgkin's lymphomas, Wilms' tumor.

Special Concerns: Pregnancy category: D. Not recommended for use during lactation. Use with caution in preexisting heart disease or bone marrow depression, renal or hepatic failure.

Additional Side Effects: *Myocardial toxicity:* Potentially fatal congestive heart failure especially if total dosage exceeds 550 mg/m² for adults, 300 mg/m² for children more than 2 years of age, and 10 mg/kg for children less than 2 years of age. Mucositis (3–7 days after administration), red-colored urine, hyperuricemia. Severe tissue necrosis if extravasation occurs. Cross-resistance with doxorubicin (produced by similar microorganism) and vinca alkaloids. Hyperuricemia may occur due to lysis of leukemic cells; allopurinol should be given as a precaution, before starting antileukemic therapy.

Dosage: IV infusion (rapid).
Acute nonlymphocytic leukemia.
Adults: *daunorubicin,* 45 mg/m²/day on days 1, 2, and 3 of first course and days 1 and 2 of additional courses; *cytosine arabinoside (Ara-c),* **IV infusion,** 100 mg/m²/day for 7 days during first course and for 5 days during any additional courses of treatment. Some recommend reducing the dose of daunorubicin to 30 mg/m² in clients 60 years of age and older. Up to 3 courses may be required.
Acute lymphocytic leukemia:
adults: daunorubicin, 45 mg/m², **IV,** on days 1, 2, and 3; vincristine, **IV,** on days 1, 8, and 15; prednisone, **PO,** 40 mg/m² daily for days 1–22 and then taper between days 22–29; and, L-asparaginase, **IV,** 500 IU/kg/day on days 22–32.
Acute lymphocytic leukemia:
Children: daunorubicin, 25 mg/m², and vincristine, 1.5 mg/m² each **IV** on day 1 every week with prednisone, 40 mg/m² **PO** daily. Usually 4 courses will induce remission.
Note: Calculate the dose on the basis of mg/kg if the child is less than 2 years of age or the body surface is less than 0.5 m².
Acute nonlymphocytic leukemia:
Geriatric clients: 30 mg/m² on days 1, 2, and 3 of the first course and days 1 and 2 of the second course in combination with cytarabine.
Dosage should be reduced in clients with renal or hepatic disease.

NURSING CONSIDERATIONS

See also *Nursing Considerations* for *Antineoplastic Agents,* p. 88.

Administration/Storage

1. Dilute in vial with 4 ml sterile water for injection USP. Agitate gently until dissolved (solution contains 5 mg daunorubicin/ml). Withdraw desired dose into syringe containing 10–15 ml isotonic saline; inject into tubing of rapidly flowing 5% glucose or normal saline IV. *Never administer daunorubicin IM or SC.*
2. Reconstituted solution stable for 24 hr at room temperature; for 48 hr when refrigerated.
3. Protect from sunlight.
4. Do not mix with other drugs or heparin.
5. Extravasation may cause severe local tissue necrosis.

Interventions

1. Assess client during and after termination of therapy for myocardial toxicity, manifested by changes in baseline ECG, edema, dyspnea, and cyanosis. Clients with a cardiac history who receive doses above 550 mg/m² are more susceptible to congestive heart failure.
2. Have digitalis preparations and diuretics readily available to treat congestive heart failure.
3. Anticipate that allopurinol will be administered prior to antileukemic therapy as drug may precipitate hyperuricemia.

Client/Family Teaching

1. Review side effects and have client report any signs and symptoms of cardiac toxicity.
2. Urine may appear red for sev-

eral days following therapy with daunorubicin.

3. Record intake and output and report any altered elimination patterns.

4. Avoid foods high in purines and avoid alcohol.

Evaluation: Assess client for improved hematological parameters with a minimum of adverse side effects.

—— *COMBINATION DRUG* ——
Deconamine SR capsules
(deh-**KON**-ah-meen)
(Rx)

Deconamine syrup and tablets
(deh-**KON**-ah-meen)
(Rx)

Classification/Content: Syrup. *Antihistamine:* Chlorpheniramine maleate, 2 mg/5 ml and *Decongestant:* Pseudoephedrine sulfate, 30 mg/5 ml. **Tablets.** *Antihistamine:* Chlorpheniramine maleate, 4 mg and *Decongestant:* Pseudoephedrine sulfate, 60 mg. The SR capsules contain twice the amount of each drug in each capsule.

See also information on individual components.

Uses: Nasal congestion due to hay fever and other allergies, the common cold, sinusitis, allergic and vasomotor rhinitis, blockage of eustachian tubes.

Special Concerns: Pregnancy category: C. Should not be used for children less than 2 years of age unless directed by a physician.

Dosage: Extended-release Capsules, Syrup, Tablets. Adults and children over 12 years: 1 tablet t.i.d.–q.i.d. or 1 SR capsule q 12 hr, or 5–10 ml syrup t.i.d.–q.i.d. **Pediatric, 6–12 years:** 2.5–5 ml t.i.d.–q.i.d., not to exceed 20 ml daily; **2–6 years:** 2.5 ml t.i.d.–q.i.d., not to exceed 10 ml daily.

NURSING CONSIDERATIONS

See *Nursing Considerations* for *Antihistamines*, p. 74, and *Sympathomimetics*, p. 220.

—— *COMBINATION DRUG* ——
Demulen 1/35–21 and Demulen 1/35–28
(**DEM**-you-len)
(Rx)

Demulen 1/50–21 and Demulen 1/50–28
(**DEM**-you-len)
(Rx)

See also *Oral Contraceptives*, p. 192.

Classification: Monophasic combination oral contraceptive.

Components: Each tablet of Demulen 1/35–21 and the first 21 tablets of Demulen 1/35–28 contains ethinyl estradiol, 35 mcg and ethynodiol diacetate, 1 mg (white tablets); the 28s also contain 7 inert blue tablets. Each tablet of Demulen 1/50–21 and the first 21 tablets of Demulen 1/50–28 contains ethinyl estradiol, 50 mcg and ethynodiol diacetate, 1 mg (white tablets); the 28s also contain 7 inert pink tablets.

Special Concerns: Pregnancy category: X.

NURSING CONSIDERATIONS

See *Nursing Considerations* for *Oral Contraceptives*, p. 195.

Desipramine hydrochloride
(dess-**IP**-rah-meen)
Norpramin, Pertofrane (Rx)

See also *Tricyclic Antidepressants,* p. 239.

Classification: Antidepressant, tricyclic.

Action/Kinetics: Has minimal anticholinergic and sedative effects and slight ability to cause orthostatic hypotension. **Effective plasma levels:** 125–300 ng/ml. **t½:** 12–24 hr. Clients who will respond to drug usually do so within the first week.

Uses: Symptoms of depression. Bulimia nervosa. To decrease craving and depression during cocaine withdrawal. To treat severe neurogenic pain. Cataplexy associated with narcolepsy. Attention deficit disorders with or without hyperactivity in children over 6 years of age.

Additional Side Effects: Bad taste in mouth, hypertension during surgery.

Dosage: Capsules, Tablets. *Antidepressant:* **initial,** 100–200 mg in single or divided doses. **Maximum daily dose:** 300 mg. **Maintenance:** 50–100 mg given once daily. **Geriatric clients:** 25–50 mg/day in divided doses up to a maximum of 150 mg daily. **Children, 6–12 years:** 10–30 mg daily (1–5 mg/kg) in divided doses. **Adolescents:** 25–50 mg daily in divided doses up to a maximum of 100 mg. *Cocaine withdrawal:* 50–200 mg daily.

NURSING CONSIDERATIONS

See also *Nursing Considerations* for *Tricyclic Antidepressants,* p. 242.

Administration/Storage

1. Clients requiring 300 mg daily should have treatment initiated in a hospital setting.
2. Maintenance doses should be given for at least 2 months following a satisfactory response.
3. Administration of a single daily dose or any increases in the dosage should be administered at bedtime in order to reduce daytime sedation.

Evaluation: Evaluate client for:
• Reports of symptomatic improvement of depression
• Serum drug levels within therapeutic range (125–300 ng/ml)

Deslanoside
(dez-**LAN**-oh-syd)
Cedilanid✻, Cedilanid-D (Rx)

See also *Cardiac Glycosides,* p. 123.

Action/Kinetics: Onset, IV: 10–30 min. **Peak effect:** 1–3 hr. **t½:** About 36 hr. **Duration:** 2–5 days. Low protein binding (25%). Is excreted mainly unchanged by the kidneys.

Uses: Rapid digitalization in emergency situations or when cardiac glycosides cannot be taken orally.

Dosage: IV. Adults, *digitalization:* 1.6 mg as a single dose or 0.8 mg initially and repeated after 4 hr. **IM. Adults,** *digitalization:* 0.8 mg given at each of two injection sites.
IV, IM. Pediatric, 3 years or older: *digitalization,* 0.0225 mg/kg divided into 2–3 equal doses and given at 3–4-hr intervals (may be given as a single dose in emergencies). **Children, 2 weeks–3**

years: 0.025 mg/kg divided into 2–3 equal doses and given at 3–4-hr intervals (may be given as a single dose in emergencies). **Premature, full-term neonates, clients with reduced renal function or myocarditis:** 0.022 mg/kg divided into 2–3 equal doses and given at 3–4-hr intervals (may be given as a single dose in emergencies).

NURSING CONSIDERATIONS

See also *Nursing Considerations* for *Cardiac Glycosides,* p. 126.

Administration/Storage

1. The injection vehicle contains ethyl alcohol and glycerin.
2. The product should be protected from light.

Desoxycorticosterone acetate

(des-ox-ee-kor-tih-koh-**STEER**-ohn)

DOCA Acetate (Rx)

Desoxycorticosterone pivalate

(des-ox-ee-kor-tih-koh-**STEER**-ohn)

Percorten Pivalate (Rx)

See also *Adrenocorticosteroids and Analogs,* p. 8.

Classification: Adrenocorticosteroid, naturally occurring; mineralocorticoid type.

Action/Kinetics: Desoxycorticosterone, a mineralocorticoid, increases sodium and water retention and promotes potassium excretion by altering reabsorption by the renal tubules. It also decreases the sodium content of saliva, sweat, and gastric juices. By normalizing electrolyte balance and plasma volume, the hormone increases cardiac output, increases BP, increases fat and glucose absorption from the GI tract, and decreases nitrogen retention. Desoxycorticosterone does not affect protein or carbohydrate metabolism or skin pigmentation. **Duration:** 1–2 days for the acetate and 4 weeks for the pivalate product.

Uses: Primary and secondary adrenocortical insufficiency in Addison's disease and salt-losing adrenogenital syndrome.

Contraindication: Use with caution in clients with hypertension.

Special Concerns: Pregnancy category: C.

Side Effects: Serious adverse effects may result from excessive dosage or prolonged treatment. These include increased blood volume, edema, increased blood pressure, enlargement of heart, headaches, arthralgia, ascending paralysis, and low potassium syndrome (sudden attacks of weakness, changes in ECG).

Dosage: IM, maintenance: 2–5 mg daily with either hydrocortisone (10–30 mg daily) or cortisone (10–37.5 mg daily). Also available as a long-acting suspension (25–100 mg IM, q 4 weeks) or as implantable pellets lasting 8–12 months. The latter are implanted surgically under aseptic conditions.
Acute crisis: 10–15 mg b.i.d. for 1 or 2 days; supportive measures (whole adrenal cortical extract, cortisone or hydrocortisone, infusions of dextrose in isotonic sodium chloride solution, whole blood or plasma) may also be indicated.
Drug requirements and salt intake are inversely related. The higher the sodium intake, the lower are the requirements for the drug.

Most clients need 3 mg of the drug when ingesting 3–6 g of sodium chloride in addition to a normal diet. Potassium intake has no effect.

NURSING CONSIDERATIONS

See also *Nursing Considerations* for *Adrenocorticosteroids and Analogs,* p. 15.

Administration/Storage: IM: Use a 20-gauge needle and inject into upper, outer quadrant of buttock.

Dexamethasone
(dex-ah-**METH**-ah-zohn)
Oral: Decadron, Deronil✱, Dexameth, Dexamethasone Intensol, Dexasone✱, Dexone, Hexadrol (Rx). Topical: Aeroseb-Dex, Decaderm, Decaspray (Rx). Ophthalmic: Maxidex Ophthalmic (Rx)

See also *Adrenocorticosteroids and Analogs,* p. 8.

Classification: Adrenocorticosteroid, synthetic; glucocorticoid type.

Action/Kinetics: Long-acting. Low degree of sodium and water retention. Diuresis may ensue when clients are transferred from other corticosteroids to dexamethasone. Not recommended for replacement therapy in adrenal cortical insufficiency. **t½:** 110–210 min.

Additional Uses: In acute allergic disorders, oral dexamethasone may be combined with dexamethasone sodium phosphate injection. This combination is used for 6 days. Used to test for adrenal cortical hyperfunction. Cerebral edema due to brain tumor, craniotomy, or head injury. *Investigational:* Diagnosis of depression. Antiemetic in cisplatin-induced vomiting. Prophylaxis or treatment of acute mountain sick-

ness. Decrease hearing loss in bacterial meningitis. Bronchopulmonary dysplasia in preterm infants. Hirsutism.

Special Concerns: Use during pregnancy only if benefits outweigh risks.

Additional Drug Interaction: Ephedrine ↓ the effect of dexamethasone due to ↑ breakdown by the liver.

Dosage: Oral Solution, Tablets. Initial: 0.75–9 mg/day; **maintenance:** gradually reduce to minimum effective dose (0.5–3 mg/day). *Suppression test for Cushing's syndrome:* 0.5 mg q 6 hr for 2 days for 24-hr urine collection (or 1 mg at 11 P.M. with blood withdrawn at 8 A.M. for blood cortisol determination). *Suppression test to determine cause of pituitary ACTH excess:* 2 mg q 6 hr for 2 days (for 24-hr urine collection). *Acute allergic disorders or acute worsening of chronic allergic disorders:* **Day 1,** dexamethasone sodium phosphate injection, 4–8 mg IM; **Days 2 and 3,** 3 mg in 2 divided doses (use 0.75 mg tablets); **Day 4,** 1.5 mg in 2 divided doses; **Days 5 and 6:** 0.75 mg; **Day 7:** no treatment; **Day 8:** follow-up visit with physician.

Topical Aerosol, Cream, Gel: Apply sparingly as a light film to affected area b.i.d.–t.i.d.

Ophthalmic Ointment, Solution: 1–2 gtt in the conjunctival sac q hr during day and q 2 hr during night until a satisfactory response obtained; **then,** 1 gtt q 4 hr and finally 1 qtt q 6–8 hr.

For allergic disorders, either self-limited or acute worsening of chronic conditions: Combination of oral and parenteral therapy. **Day 1:** 4–8 mg of dexamethasone sodium phosphate, **IM. Days 2 and 3:**

Two 0.75 mg dexamethasone tablets b.i.d. **Day 4:** One 0.75-mg dexamethasone tablet b.i.d. **Days 5 and 6:** One 0.75-mg dexamethasone tablet. **Day 8:** Follow-up visit to physician.

NURSING CONSIDERATIONS

See also *Nursing Considerations* for *Adrenocorticosteroids and Analogs,* p. 15.

Evaluation: Evaluate client for:
- ↓ in symptoms of allergic response
- Reduction in cerebral edema
- Prevention of mountain sickness

Dexamethasone acetate

(dex-ah-**METH**-ah-zohn)

Dalalone D.P., Dalalone LA., Decadron-LA, Decaject-LA., Dexacen LA-8, Dexasone LA, Dexone LA, Solurex LA (Rx)

See also *Adrenocorticosteroids and Analogs,* p. 8.

Classification: Adrenocorticosteroid, synthetic; glucocorticoid type.

Action/Kinetics: This ester of dexamethasone is practically insoluble and provides the prolonged activity suitable for repository injections, although it has a prompt onset of action. Not for IV use.

Special Concerns: Use during pregnancy only if benefits outweigh risks.

Dosage: Repository injection. IM: 8–16 mg q 1–3 weeks, if necessary. **Intralesional:** 0.8–1.6 mg. **Soft tissue and intra-articular:** 4–16 mg repeated at 1- to 3-week intervals.

NURSING CONSIDERATIONS

See *Nursing Considerations* for *Adrenocorticosteroids and Analogs,* p. 15.

Dexamethasone sodium phosphate

(dex-ah-**METH**-ah-zohn)

Systemic: Dalalone, Decadron Phosphate, Decaject, Dexacen-4, Dexasone, Dexone, Hexadrol Phosphate, Oradexon✽, Solurex (Rx). Inhaler: Decadron Phosphate Respihaler (Rx). Nasal: Decadron Phosphate Turbinaire (Rx). Ophthalmic: AK-Dex, Baldex, Decadron Phosphate, Dexair, Dexotic, I-Methasone, Maxidex, Ocu-Dex, PMS-Dexamethasone Sodium Phosphate✽, Spersadex✽ (Rx). Otic: AK-Dex, Decadron, I-Methasone (Rx). Topical: Decadron Phosphate (Rx)

See also *Adrenocorticosteroids and Analogs,* p. 8.

Classification: Adrenocorticosteroid, synthetic; glucocorticoid type.

Additional Uses: For IV or IM use in emergency situations when dexamethasone cannot be given PO. Has a rapid onset and a short duration of action. Routes of administration include inhalation (especially for bronchial asthma), ophthalmic, topical, intrasynovial, and intra-articular. Intranasally for nasal polyps, allergic or inflammatory nasal conditions.

Contraindications: Acute infections, persistent positive sputum cultures of *Candida albicans.* Lactation.

Special Concerns: Use during

pregnancy only if benefits outweigh risks.

Side Effects: *Following inhalation:* Nasal and nasopharyngeal irritation, burning, dryness, stinging, headache.

Dosage: IM, IV. Range: 0.5–9 mg daily (⅓–½ the oral dose q 12 hr). *Cerebral edema:* **Adults, initial, IV:** 10 mg; **then, IM,** 4 mg q 6 hr until maximum effect obtained (usually within 12–24 hr). Switch to oral therapy (1–3 mg t.i.d.) as soon as feasible and then slowly withdraw over 5–7 days. *Shock, unresponsive:* **IV, initial,** either 1–6 mg/kg or 40 mg; **then,** repeat IV dose q 2–6 hr as long as necessary. *Intralesional, intra-articular, soft tissue injections:* 0.4–6 mg, depending on the site (e.g., small joints: 0.8–1 mg; large joints: 2–4 mg; soft tissue infiltration: 2–6 mg; ganglia: 1–2 mg; bursae: 2–3 mg; tendon sheaths: 0.4–1 mg.

Inhalation: *Bronchial asthma:* **Adults, initial,** 3 inhalations (84 mcg dexamethasone/inhalation) t.i.d.–q.i.d.; **maximum:** 3 inhalations/dose; 12 inhalations/day. **Pediatric: initial,** 2 inhalations t.i.d.–q.i.d.; **maximum:** 2 inhalations/dose; 8 inhalations/day.

Intranasal: *Allergies, nasal polyps:* **Adults,** 2 sprays (total of 168 mcg dexamethasone) in each nostril b.i.d.–t.i.d. (maximum: 12 sprays/day); **pediatric, 6–12 years:** 1–2 sprays (total of 84–168 mcg dexamethasone) in each nostril b.i.d. (maximum: 8 sprays/day).

Ophthalmic Ointment, Solution: Instill a small amount into the conjunctival sac t.i.d.–q.i.d. As response is obtained, reduce the number of applications. **Ophthalmic solution:** Instill 1–2 drops into the conjunctival sac q hr during

the day and q 2 hr at night until response obtained; **then,** reduce to 1 gtt q 6–8 hr.

Otic Solution: 3–4 drops into the ear canal b.i.d.–t.i.d.

Topical cream: Apply sparingly to affected areas and rub in.

NURSING CONSIDERATIONS

See also *Nursing Considerations* for *Adrenocorticosteroids and Analogs,* p. 15.

Administration/Storage

1. Do not use preparation containing lidocaine IV.
2. For intranasal use, some clients are controlled using 1 spray in each nostril twice daily.

Dexchlorpheniramine maleate
(dex-klor-fen-**EAR**-ah-meen)
Dexchlor, Poladex T.D., Polaramine, Polargen (Rx)

See also *Antihistamines,* p. 71.

Classification: Antihistamine, alkylamine type.

Action/Kinetics: Less severe sedative effects. **Duration:** 8 hr.

Special Concerns: Pregnancy category: B. Extended-release tablets should not be used in children. Geriatric clients may be more sensitive to the usual adult dose.

Dosage: Syrup, Tablets. Adults: 2 mg q 4–6 hr as needed. **Pediatric, 5–12 years:** 1 mg q 4–6 hr as needed; **2–5 years:** 0.5 mg q 4–6 hr as needed. **Extended-release Tablets. Adults:** 4–6 mg q 8–12 hr as needed.

NURSING CONSIDERATIONS

See *Nursing Considerations* for *Antihistamines,* p. 74.

Dextroamphetamine sulfate

(dex-troh-am-**FET**-ah-meen)
Dexedrine, Ferndex, Oxydess II, Spancap No. 1 (C-II) (Rx)

See also *Amphetamines and Derivatives,* p. 29.

Classification: CNS stimulant, amphetamine type.

Action/Kinetics: Dextroamphetamine has stronger CNS effects and weaker peripheral action than does amphetamine; thus, dextroamphetamine manifests fewer undesirable cardiovascular effects. After PO administration, completely absorbed in 3 hr. **Duration: PO,** 4–24 hr; **t½, adults:** 10–12 hr; **children:** 6–8 hr. Excreted in urine. Acidification will increase excretion, while alkalinization will decrease it.

Uses: Attention deficit disorders in children, narcolepsy.

Additional Contraindications: Lactation. Use for obesity.

Special Concerns: Use in pregnancy only if benefits outweigh risks (pregnancy category: C). Use of extended-release capsules for attention deficit disorders in children less than 6 years of age and the elixir or tablets for attention deficit disorders in children less than 3 years of age is not recommended. Dosage for narcolepsy has not been determined in children less than 6 years of age.

Dosage: Elixir, Tablets. *Attention deficit disorders in children:* **3–5 years, initial:** 2.5 mg/day; increase by 2.5 mg/day at weekly intervals until optimum dose is achieved (usual range 0.1–0.5 mg/kg/dose each morning). **6 years and older, initial:** 5 mg 1–2 times/day; increase in increments of 5 mg weekly until optimum dose is achieved (rarely over 40 mg/day). *Narcolepsy:* **Adults:** 5–60 mg in divided doses daily. **Children over 12 years, initial:** 10 mg daily; increase in increments of 10 mg/day at weekly intervals until optimum dose is reached. **Children, 6–12 years, initial:** 5 mg daily; increase in increments of 5 mg at weekly intervals until optimum dose is reached (maximum is 60 mg daily).

Extended-Release Capsule. *Narcolepsy:* **Adults:** 5–30 mg once daily. **Children, 6–12 years:** 5–15 mg once daily; **12 years and older:** 10–15 mg once daily. *Attention deficit disorders:* **Children, 6 years and older:** 5–15 mg once daily.

NURSING CONSIDERATIONS

See also *Nursing Considerations* for *Amphetamines and Derivatives,* p. 31.

Administration/Storage

1. Long-acting products may be used for once-a-day dosing in attention deficit disorders and narcolepsy.
2. When tablets or the elixir are used for attention deficit disorders or narcolepsy, the first dose should be given on awakening with additional one or two doses given at intervals of 4–6 hr. If possible, the last dose should be given 6 hr before bedtime.
3. If the client is already receiving an MAO inhibitor, a period of at least 14 days should elapse before dextroamphetamine is initiated.

Evaluation: Evaluate client for:
- Improved attention span
- ↓ occurrences of narcolepsy

Dextromethorphan hydrobromide

(dex-troh-meth-**OR**-fan)

Anti-Cough Syrup✲, Balminil D.M. Syrup✲, Benylin DM, Broncho-Grippol-DM✲, Congespirin For Children, Cremacoat 1, Delsym, DM Cough, D-M No Sugar✲, Hold, Koffex Syrup✲, Mediquell, Neo-DM✲, Ornex-DM✲, Pedia Care 1, Pertussin Cough Suppressant, Pertussin 8 Hour Cough Formula, Robidex Syrup✲, St. Joseph For Children, Sedatuss✲, Sucrets Cough Control Formula, Vick's Children's Cough Syrup✲ (OTC)

Classification: Nonnarcotic antitussive.

Action/Kinetics: Dextromethorphan selectively depresses the cough center in the medulla, and its antitussive activity is about equal to that of codeine. It is a common ingredient of nonprescription cough medications; it does not produce physical dependence or respiratory depression. Well absorbed from GI tract. **Onset:** 15–30 min. **Duration:** 3–6 hr.

Use: Symptomatic relief of nonproductive cough due to colds or inhaled irritants.

Contraindications: Persistent or chronic cough. Use during first trimester of pregnancy unless directed otherwise by physician.

Special Concerns: Use is not recommended in children less than 2 years of age. Use with caution in

clients with nausea, vomiting, high fever, rash, or persistent headache.

Side Effects: *CNS:* Dizziness, drowsiness. *GI:* Nausea, vomiting, stomach pain.

Drug Interaction: Contraindicated with MAO inhibitors.

Dosage: Syrup, Lozenges, Chewable Tablets. Adults and children over 12: 10–20 mg q 4–8 hr or 30 mg q 6–8 hr, not to exceed 120 mg/day; **pediatric, 6–12 years:** either 5–10 mg q 4 hr or 15 mg q 6–8 hr, not to exceed 60 mg/day; **pediatric, 2–6 years:** either 2.5–5 mg q 4 hr or 7.5 mg q 6–8 hr, not to exceed 30 mg/day. **Controlled-release Oral Suspension. Adults:** 60 mg q 12 hr. **Pediatric, 6–12 years:** 30 mg q 12 hr, not to exceed 60 mg daily; **pediatric, 2–6 years:** 15 mg q 12 hr, not to exceed 30 mg daily.

NURSING CONSIDERATIONS

Administration/Storage

1. Increasing the dose of dextromethorphan will not increase its effectiveness but will increase the duration of action.
2. The lozenges should not be given to children under 6 years of age.

Assessment

1. Note the length of time the client has had the cough. Document sputum production, color, amount, and if an odor is evident. If the cough persists, dextromethorphan should not be given.
2. In taking the client's history, note if the client has had nausea, vomiting, persistent headache, or a high fever.
3. If the client is pregnant, de-

termine if she is in the first trimester of pregnancy. The drug is contraindicated in this instance.

Client/Family Teaching

1. Do not perform any tasks that require mental alertness until drug effects realized.
2. Avoid alcohol in any form.
3. Humidity should be added to a dry environment.
4. Advise that smoke, dust, and chemical fumes are irritants that may aggravate underlying condition.
5. Symptoms that persist for more than a week require medical intervention; record onset and response to therapy.

Evaluation: Evaluate client for control of cough with improved sleep patterns.

Dextrose and electrolytes

(DEX-trohs)
Lytren, Pedialyte, Rehydralyte, Resol (Rx)

Classification: Electrolyte replenisher.

Action/Kinetics: These oral products containing varying amounts of sodium, potassium, chloride, citrate, and dextrose (Lytren and Resol contain 20 g/L whereas Pedialyte and Rehydralyte contain 25 g/L). In addition, Resol contains magnesium, calcium, and phosphate. **Time to peak effect:** 8–12 hr.

Uses: Diarrhea. Prophylaxis and treatment of electrolyte depletion in diarrhea or in continuing fluid loss. Maintenance of hydration.

Contraindications: Anuria, oliguria. Severe dehydration including severe diarrhea (IV therapy is necessary for prompt replacement of fluids and electrolytes). Malabsorption of glucose. Severe and sustained vomiting when the client is unable to drink. Intestinal obstruction, perforated bowel, paralytic ileus.

Special Concerns: Use with caution in premature infants.

Side Effects: Overhydration indicated by puffy eyelids. Hypernatremia, vomiting (usually shortly after treatment has started).

Dosage: Oral Solution. *Mild dehydration:* **Adults and children over 10 years, initial:** 50 ml/kg over 4–6 hr; **maintenance:** 100–200 ml/kg over 24 hr until diarrhea stops. *Moderate dehydration:* **Adults and children over 10 years, initial:** 100 ml/kg over 6 hr; **maintenance:** 15 ml/kg q hr until diarrhea stops. *Moderate to severe dehydration:* **Pediatric, 2–10 years, initial:** 50 ml/kg over the first 4–6 hr followed by 100 ml/kg over the next 18–24 hr; **less than 2 years, initial:** 75 ml/kg during the first 8 hr and 75 ml/kg during the next 16 hr.

NURSING CONSIDERATIONS

Administration/Storage

1. No more than 1,000 ml/hr should be given to adults and no more than 100 ml of fluid should be given to children over a 20-min period.
2. The amount and rate of solution should be adjusted depending on need, thirst, and response.
3. Infants and small children should be assisted in drinking

the solution slowly and frequently in small quantities and, if necessary, being fed by a spoon.

4. Rehydration solutions should not be diluted with water.

Client/Family Teaching

1. Soft foods such as bananas, cereal, cooked peas, beans, and potatoes should be given to maintain nutrition.
2. Explain that if output of fluid exceeds intake, if there is no weight gain, or if clinical symptoms of dehydration persist, client should be seen by the physician immediately.
3. If vomiting occurs after oral therapy is initiated, continue therapy but use small amounts of solution administered frequently and slowly.
4. If dehydration is severe, instruct parents and client to seek medical attention immediately. IV fluids and electrolytes should be started since the onset of action of oral solution is too slow. Explain that the oral solution should not be discarded because it can be used for maintenance.

Evaluation: Evaluate client for:
- Maintenance of adequate hydration
- Prevention of electrolyte depletion

Dextrothyroxine sodium

(dek-stroh-thigh-**ROX**-een)

Choloxin (Rx)

Classification: Antihyperlipidemic.

Action/Kinetics: Dextrothyroxine (the dextro isomer of thyroid hormone) increases the rate at which cholesterol is metabolized in the liver; excretion of cholesterol and metabolites is increased, leading to decreased serum levels of cholesterol and LDL; there is no change in levels of triglycerides or HDL. Dextrothyroxine has little effect on the basal metabolic rate (BMR) but is otherwise similar physiologically to levothyroxine. The effectiveness increases as cholesterol levels increase. Approximately 25% is absorbed from the GI tract; almost completely bound to plasma proteins. $t\frac{1}{2}$: 18 hr. **Duration:** Serum lipid levels return to pretreatment levels from 6–12 weeks after termination of drug therapy. Eliminated through both the kidneys and feces.

Uses: Only for clients with primary hypercholesterolemia (type IIa hyperlipidemia) who are at a significant risk for coronary artery disease and who have not responded to diet or other measures.

Contraindications: Euthyroid clients with hypertensive organic heart disease, including angina pectoris, history of myocardial infarction, cardiac arrhythmias or tachycardia, rheumatic disease, CHF, decompensated or borderline compensated cardiac status, hypertension (other than mild, labile, systolic). Pregnancy, lactation, advanced liver or kidney disease, or a history of hypersensitivity to iodine.

Special Concerns: Use with caution in impaired liver and kidney function. Clients intolerant to lactose, milk, or milk products may be intolerant to the tablet since it also contains lactose. Geriatric clients may be more sensitive to the effects of dextrothyroxine.

Side Effects: *CNS:* Insomnia, nervousness, fever, headache, decreased sensorium, paresthesia, dizziness, malaise, tiredness, psychic changes, tremors. *CV:* Angina pectoris, increase in heart size, ischemic myocardial changes (ECG changes), arrhythmias including ectopic beats, supraventricular tachycardia, extrasystoles, worsening of peripheral vascular disease, possibility of fatal or nonfatal myocardial infarction (relationship to drug uncertain). *GI:* Nausea, vomiting, diarrhea, constipation, anorexia, dyspepsia, weight loss, bitter taste, GI hemorrhages. *Other:* Drooping eyelids, changes in libido, sweating, hair loss, diuresis, menstrual irregularities, hoarseness, tinnitus, peripheral edema, visual disturbances, muscle pain, gallstones, increases in blood sugar of diabetic clients, skin rashes, itching, flushing.

Aggravation of existing cardiac disease is cause for discontinuation. *Symptoms of Overdose:* Hyperthyroidism, diarrhea, cramps, vomiting, nervousness, twitching, tachycardia, and weight loss.

Drug Interactions

Anticoagulants, oral / ↑ Effect of anticoagulants by ↑ hypoprothrombinemia
Antidiabetics, oral / ↓ Diabetic control as dextrothyroxine ↑ blood glucose
Beta-adrenergic blocking agents / Dextrothyroxine ↓ effect of beta-blockers
Cholestyramine / ↓ Effect of dextrothyroxine due to ↓ absorption from GI tract
Colestipol / ↓ Effect of dextrothyroxine due to ↓ absorption from GI tract

Digitalis / Additive stimulation of myocardium
Epinephrine / In coronary artery disease, concomitant use → coronary insufficiency
Insulin / ↓ Diabetic control as dextrothyroxine ↑ blood glucose
Thyroid drugs / ↑ Sensitivity of hypothyroid clients to thyroid drugs
Tricyclic antidepressants / Use with dextrothyroxine → CNS stimulation, ↑ heart rate, cardiac arrhythmias, nervousness

Dosage: Tablets. Adults, initial: 1–2 mg daily. Daily dosage can be increased every 4 weeks by 1–2 mg; **maintenance:** 4–8 mg daily. **Maximum daily dosage:** 8 mg. It may take 2–4 weeks for the therapeutic response to become manifested. **Pediatric, initial:** 0.05 mg/kg (1.5 mg/m^2) daily. Increase by 0.05 mg/kg every month, up to maximum of 4 mg daily, until satisfactory control is established. **Maintenance:** 0.1 mg/kg (3 mg/m^2) daily. Withdraw drug 2 weeks before surgery.

NURSING CONSIDERATIONS

Assessment

1. Note any client history of coronary artery disease. Use should be discontinued if symptoms of cardiac disease develop.
2. Obtain a baseline ECG prior to starting the client on therapy.
3. Determine if the client is taking cardiac glycosides or oral anticoagulants as dextrothyroxine may enhance the action of these agents.

Interventions

1. Assess for and note client complaints of chest pain or any attacks of angina.
2. Monitor pulse and if it remains greater than 120 beats/min,

withhold the dosage (unless otherwise indicated) and report to the physician.

3. If the client complains of nausea or a decrease in appetite, taking the drug with meals may reduce the gastric irritation and ensure better compliance with the drug regimen.

4. With diabetes, dextrothyroxine may increase blood glucose levels. Monitor serum glucose levels as the client may require an adjustment in oral hypoglycemic agents if on oral medication or an adjustment in insulin dosage.

5. Check eyes routinely for exophthalmos.

Client/Family Teaching

1. Provide a printed list of drug side effects. Advise client to report any new signs or changes to the physician to ensure that serious side effects are not developing.

2. Stress the importance of continuing to follow prescribed exercise program and dietary guidelines.

3. Report for all scheduled laboratory studies so the drug effectiveness can be evaluated.

Evaluation: Evaluate client for:
- Reduction in the serum levels of cholesterol and LDL
- Freedom from complications of drug therapy

Dezocine
(DEZ-oh-seen)
Dalgan (Rx)

See also *Narcotic Analgesics,* p. 174.

Classification: Narcotic agonist–antagonist analgesic.

Action/Kinetics: Dezocine is a parenteral narcotic analgesic possessing both agonist and antagonist activity. It is similar to morphine with respect to analgesic potency and onset and duration of action. However, there is less risk of abuse due to the mixed agonist–antagonist properties of the drug. The narcotic antagonist activity is greater than that of pentazocine. **Onset:** Approximately 30 min after IM and approximately 15 min after IV. **Peak effect:** 30–150 min. **Peak plasma levels:** 10–38 ng/ml after a 10-mg dose. **Duration:** 2–4 hr. **t½, after IV:** 2.4 hr. Approximately two-thirds of a dose is excreted in the urine mostly as the glucuronide conjugate.

Uses: Analgesic when use of a narcotic is desirable.

Contraindications: Lactation. Individuals dependent on narcotics. SC administration.

Special Concerns: Pregnancy category: C. Use in labor and delivery only if benefits outweigh risks. Safety and effectiveness have not been determined in children less than 18 years of age. Use with caution in clients with impaired renal or hepatic function. Use with caution in clients with head injury or increased intracranial pressure, in chronic obstructive pulmonary disease, and in biliary surgery. Geriatric clients are at an increased risk for depressed respiration, reduced ventilatory drive, alteration of mental status, and delirium. Dezocine should not be used in clients who are tolerant to opiate drugs since there is a risk of precipitating an acute withdrawal syndrome.

Side Effects: *CNS:* Sedation (common), dizziness, vertigo, confusion, anxiety, crying, sleep disturbances, delusions, headache, depression, delirium. *Respiratory:* Respiratory depression, atelectasis. *CV:* Hypotension, irregular heart or pulse, hypertension, chest pain, pallor, thrombophlebitis. *GI:* Nausea, vomiting, dry mouth, constipation, abdominal pain, diarrhea. *Dermatologic:* Reactions at the injection site, pruritus, rash, erythema. *EENT:* Diplopia, blurred vision, congestion in ears, tinnitus. *GU:* Urinary frequency, retention, or hesitancy. *Miscellaneous:* Sweating, chills, edema, flushing, low hemoglobin, muscle cramps or aches, muscle pain, slurred speech.

Drug Interactions: Additive depressant effect when used with general anesthetics, sedatives, antianxiety drugs, hypnotics, alcohol, and other opiate analgesics.

Dosage: IM. Adults: 5–20 mg (usual is 10 mg) as a single dose; dose may be repeated q 3–6 hr with dosage adjusted, if necessary, depending on the status of the client. **IV. Adults:** 2.5–10 mg (usual initial dose is 5 mg) repeated q 2–4 hr.

NURSING CONSIDERATIONS

See also *Nursing Considerations* for *Narcotic Analgesics,* p. 177.

Administration/Storage

1. The maximum single dose should not exceed 20 mg and the maximum daily dose should not exceed 120 mg.
2. Dezocine can be stored at room temperature protected from light.
3. The solution should not be used if it contains a precipitate.
4. *Treatment of Overdose:* Naloxone IV with appropriate supportive measures including oxygen, IV fluids, vasopressors, and artificial respiration.

Assessment

1. Note any client sulfite sensitivity because drug contains sodium metabisulfite.
2. Determine any history or current use of opiate drugs because dezocine may precipitate an acute withdrawal syndrome.
3. Note any evidence of impaired renal or liver function; obtain pretreatment lab values.
4. Assess for any evidence of head injury or increased intracranial pressure.

Interventions

1. Monitor for any evidence of allergic reaction.
2. Record vital signs and assess respiratory patterns.
3. Anticipate reduced dosage in clients with renal or hepatic dysfunction.
4. Geriatric clients should receive reduced doses and be individually evaluated for subsequent dose levels.
5. If dezocine is administered with CNS depressants anticipate the dose of one or both agents should be reduced.

Client/Family Teaching

1. Provide a printed list of drug side effects and instruct client to report those that are bothersome or persistent.
2. Caution clients not to drive or operate dangerous machinery until the effects of the drug have worn off.
3. Avoid the use of any unprescribed sedatives, hypnotics, or antianxiety agents during therapy with dezocine.

4. Do not ingest alcohol during drug therapy.

Special Concerns: Elderly clients should be observed closely because they are at an increased risk for altered respiratory patterns and mental changes.

Evaluation: Satisfactory pain management is achieved as evidenced by increased activity, improved appetite, and subjective reports of effective pain control.

Diazepam
(dye-**AYZ**-eh-pam)
Apo-Diazepam✶, Diazemuls✶, Diazepam Intensol, Novo–Dipam✶, Rival✶, Valium, Valrelease, Vivol✶, Zetran (C-IV, Rx)

See also *Benzodiazepines,* p. 108.

Action/Kinetics: Onset: PO, 30–60 min; **IM,** 15–30 min; **IV,** more rapid. **Peak plasma levels: PO,** 0.5–2 hr; **IM,** 0.5–1.5; **IV,** 0.25 hr. **Duration:** 3 hr. **t½:** 20–70 hr. Diazepam is broken down in the liver to the active metabolites desmethyldiazepam, oxazepam, and temazepam. Diazepam and metabolites are excreted through the urine.

Uses: Anxiety, tension (more effective than chlordiazepoxide), alcohol withdrawal, muscle relaxant, adjunct to treat seizure disorders, antipanic drug. Used prior to gastroscopy and esophagoscopy, pre-operatively and prior to cardioversion. In dentistry to induce sedation. Treatment of status epilepticus. Adjunct in cerebral palsy, paraplegia, or tetanus. Relieve spasms of facial muscles in occlusion and temporomandibular joint

disorders. IV to treat status epilepticus and severe recurrent seizures.

Additional Contraindications: Narrow-angle glaucoma, children under 6 months, and parenterally in children under 12 years. During lactation.

Special Concerns: Pregnancy category: D.

Additional Drug Interactions

1. Diazepam potentiates antihypertensive effects of thiazides and other diuretics.
2. Diazepam potentiates muscle relaxant effects of *d*-tubocurarine and gallamine.
3. Ranitidine ↓ GI absorption of diazepam.
4. Isoniazid ↑ half-life of diazepam.
5. Fluoxetine ↑ half-life of diazepam.

Dosage: Tablets, Oral Solution. Adults: *Antianxiety, anticonvulsant, adjunct to skeletal muscle relaxants:* 2–10 mg b.i.d.–q.i.d. **Elderly, debilitated clients:** 2–2.5 mg 1–2 times daily. May be gradually increased to adult level. **Pediatric, over 6 months: initial,** 1–2.5 mg (0.04–0.2 mg/kg or 1.17–6 mg/m²) t.i.d.–b.i.d. *Alcohol withdrawal:* 10 mg t.i.d.–q.i.d. during the first 24 hr; **then,** decrease to 5 mg t.i.d.–q.i.d. as required.

   Extended-release   Capsules. Adults: *Antianxiety, skeletal muscle relaxant:* 15–30 mg once daily. To be used in children over 6 months of age only if the dose has been determined to be 5 mg t.i.d. (use one 15-mg capsule daily).

   IM, IV. Adults: IM, *Preoperative or diagnostic use:* 10 mg 5–30 min before procedure. *Adjunct to treat skeletal muscle spasm:* 5–10 mg initially; **then,** repeat in 3–4 hr if needed (larger doses may be required for tetanus). *Moderate anxiety:* 2–5 mg q 3–4 hr if necessary. *Severe anxiety, muscle spasm:* 5–10 mg q 3–4 hr, if necessary. *Acute alcohol withdrawal:* **initial,** 10 mg; **then,** 5–10 mg q 3–4 hr. *Preoperatively:* **IM,** 10 mg prior to surgery. *Endoscopy:* **IV,** 10 mg or less although doses up to 20 mg can be used; **IM,** 5–10 mg 30 min prior to procedure. *Cardioversion:* **IV,** 5–15 mg 5–10 min prior to procedure. *Tetanus in children,* **IM, IV, over 1 month:** 1–2 mg, repeated q 3–4 hr as necessary; **5 years and over:** 5–10 mg q 3–4 hr. **IV,** *Status epilepticus:* **Adults,** 5–10 mg initially; **then,** dose may be repeated at 10–15 min intervals up to a maximum dose of 30 mg. Dosage may be repeated after 2–4 hr. **Children, 1 month–5 years:** 0.2–0.5 mg q 2–5 min, up to maximum of 5 mg. Can be repeated in 2–4 hr. **5 years and older:** 1 mg q 2–5 min up to a maximum of 10 mg; dose can be repeated in 2–4 hr, if needed.

Elderly or debilitated clients should not receive more than 5 mg parenterally at any one time.

NURSING CONSIDERATIONS

See *Nursing Considerations* for *Benzodiazepines,* p. 111.

Administration/Storage

1. One 15-mg sustained-release diazepam capsule may be used if the daily dosage is 5 mg t.i.d.
2. The Intensol solution should be mixed with beverages such as water, soda, and juices, or soft foods such as applesauce or puddings. Only the calibra-ted dropper provided with the product should be used to withdraw the medication. Once the medication is withdrawn and mixed, it should be used immediately.
3. To reduce reactions at the site of IV administration, diazepam should be given slowly (5 mg/min). Also, small veins or intra-arterial administration should be avoided.
4. When administering the drug IV, have emergency equipment and drugs available.
5. Due to the possibility of precipitation and instability, diazepam should not be infused. Also, the drug should not be mixed or diluted with other solutions or drugs in the syringe or infusion flask.
6. Diazepam interacts with plastic; therefore, introducing diazepam into plastic containers or administration sets will decrease availability of the drug.
7. Except for the deltoid muscle, absorption from IM sites is slow and erratic.
8. Review the drug interaction chart before administering the drug.
9. The IV route is preferred in the convulsing client.

Assessment

1. Obtain a CBC, platelet count, liver and renal profiles as baseline data.
2. Note if the client has diabetes and the type of agent used for testing the urine as diazepam interferes with many of these agents. Have client convert to finger sticks for a more accurate blood glucose determination.

3. Determine any history of depression or drug abuse.

Interventions

1. Parenteral administration may cause bradycardia, respiratory or cardiac arrest. Monitor vital signs and client closely.
2. Elderly clients may experience adverse reactions more quickly than younger clients. Therefore, anticipate a lower dose of drug to be ordered in this group.
3. Simultaneous use of CNS depressants should be avoided.
4. Anticipate a gradual reduction of drug to avoid withdrawal symptoms such as anxiety, tremors, anorexia, insomnia, weakness, headache, nausea, and vomiting.

Evaluation: Evaluate client for:
- Reports of improvement in the number and frequency of anxiety and tension episodes
- Alcohol withdrawal without symptoms of delirium tremens
- Interruption and control of seizures
- ↓ in frequency and occurrences of panic attacks
- Effective sedation

Diazoxide
(dye-az-**OX**-eyed)
Hyperstat IV (Rx)

Classification: Antihypertensive, direct action on vascular smooth muscle.

Action/Kinetics: Diazoxide is thought to exert a direct action on vascular smooth muscle to cause

arteriolar vasodilation and decreased peripheral resistance. **Onset:** 1–5 min. **Time to peak effect:** 2–5 min. **Duration** (variable): usual, 3–12 hr. Excreted through the kidney (50% unchanged).

Uses: May be the drug of choice for hypertensive crisis (malignant and nonmalignant hypertension). Often given concomitantly with a diuretic. Especially suitable for clients with impaired renal function, hypertensive encephalopathy, hypertension complicated by left ventricular failure, and eclampsia. Ineffective for hypertension due to pheochromocytoma.

Contraindications: Hypersensitivity to drug or thiazide diuretics.

Special Concerns: Pregnancy category: C. A decrease in dose may be necessary in geriatric clients due to age-related decreases in renal function.

Side Effects: *CV:* Hypotension (may be severe), sodium and water retention, arrhythmias, cerebral or myocardial ischemia, palpitations, bradycardia. *CNS:* Headache, dizziness, drowsiness, lightheadedness. Confusion, seizures, paralysis, unconsciousness, numbness (all due to cerebral ischemia). *Respiratory:* Tightness in chest, cough, dyspnea, sensation of choking. *GI:* Nausea, vomiting, diarrhea, anorexia, parotid swelling, change in sense of taste, salivation, dry mouth, ileus, constipation. *Other:* Hyperglycemia (may be serious enough to require treatment), sweating, flushing, sensation of warmth, tinnitus, hearing loss, retention of nitrogenous wastes, acute pancreatitis. Pain, cellulitis, phlebitis at injection site. *Symptoms of Overdose:* Hypotension, excessive hyperglycemia.

D

Drug Interactions

Anticoagulants, oral / ↑ Effect of oral anticoagulants due to ↓ plasma protein binding

Nitrites / ↑ Hypotensive effect

Phenytoin / Diazoxide ↓ anticonvulsant effect of phenytoin

Reserpine / ↑ Hypotensive effect

Thiazide diuretics / ↑ Hyperglycemic, hyperuricemic, and antihypertensive effect of diazoxide

Vasodilators, peripheral / ↑ Hypotensive effect

Laboratory Test Interference: False + or ↑ uric acid.

Dosage: IV push (30 sec or less): **Adults:** 1–3 mg/kg up to a maximum of 150 mg; may be repeated at 5- to 15-min intervals until adequate blood pressure response obtained. Drug may then be repeated at 4- to 24-hr intervals for 4–5 days or until oral antihypertensive therapy can be initiated. **Pediatric:** 1–3 mg/kg (30–90 mg/m²) using the same dosing intervals as adults.

NURSING CONSIDERATIONS

Administration/Storage

1. Do not administer IM or SC. Medication is highly alkaline.
2. Inject rapidly (30 sec) undiluted into a peripheral vein to maximize response.
3. Protect from light, heat, and freezing.
4. *Treatment of Overdose:* Use the Trendelenberg maneuver to reverse hypotension.

Assessment

1. Note client history for hypersensitivity to thiazide diuretics, sulfa drugs, or to diazoxide.
2. Particularly note if client has diabetes mellitus. Diazoxide can cause serious elevations in blood sugar levels.

Interventions

1. Inspect the IV line to ensure patency before administering the medication.
2. Have a sympathomimetic drug, such as norepinephrine, available to treat severe hypotension should it occur.
3. Explain to client the need to remain in a recumbent position during and for 30 min after injection to avoid orthostatic hypotension.
4. Maintain the client in a recumbent position for 8–10 hr if furosemide is added and administered as part of the therapy.
5. Monitor BP after injection until it has stabilized and then every hour thereafter until hypertensive crisis is resolved.
6. Obtain final BP of client upon arising after injection.
7. Note client complaints of sweating, flushing, or evidence of hyperglycemia and be prepared to treat.
8. Assess the site of insertion for signs of irritation or extravasation. If extravasation should occur, apply ice packs.
9. Obtain uric acid level and assess for evidence of hyperuricemia.

Evaluation: Evaluate client for a decrease in BP during hypertensive crisis.

Diazoxide oral
(dye-az-**OX**-eyed)
Proglycem (Rx)

Classification: Insulin antagonist, hypotensive agent.

Action/Kinetics: Diazoxide inhibits the release of insulin from beta islet cells of the pancreas, leading to an increase in blood glucose levels. Effect is dose related. Diazoxide causes sodium, potassium, uric acid, and water retention. **Onset:** 1 hr. **t½:** 28 hr (up to 53 hr in clients with anuria). **Duration:** 8 hr. Metabolized in the liver although 50% is excreted through the kidneys unchanged.

Uses: Hypoglycemia caused by insulin overdosage or overproduction of insulin by malignant beta cells. The drug is used parenterally as an antihypertensive agent (see *Diazoxide,* p. 533).

Contraindications: Functional hypoglycemia, hypersensitivity to diazoxide or thiazides.

Special Concerns: Safe use during pregnancy not established (pregnancy category: C). Infants are particularly prone to development of edema. Use with extreme caution in clients with history of gout and in those in whom edema presents a risk (cardiac disease).

Side Effects: *CV:* Sodium and fluid retention (common), palpitations, increased heart rate, hypotension, transient hypertension. *Metabolic:* Hyperglycemia, glycosuria, diabetic ketoacidosis, hyperosmolar nonketotic coma. *GI:* Nausea, vomiting, diarrhea, transient taste loss, anorexia, ileus, abdominal pain. *CNS:* Weakness, headache, insomnia, extrapyramidal symptoms, dizziness, paresthesia, fever. *Hematologic:* Thrombocytopenia, purpura, eosinophilia, neutropenia, decreased hemoglobin. *Dermatologic:* Skin rashes, hirsutism, herpes, loss of hair from scalp, monilial dermatitis. *GU:* Hematuria, proteinuria, decrease in urine production, nephrotic syndrome (reversible). *Ophthalmologic:* Blurred or double vision, lacrimation, transient cataracts, ring scotoma, subconjunctival hemorrhage. *Other:* Pancreatitis, pancreatic necrosis, galactorrhea, gout, premature aging of bone, polyneuritis, enlargement of lump in breast. *Symptoms of Overdose:* Hypotension; excessive hyperglycemia.

Drug Interactions

Alpha-adrenergic blocking agents / ↓ Effect of diazoxide
Anticoagulants, oral / ↑ Effect of anticoagulant due to ↓ plasma protein binding
Antihypertensives / Excessive ↓ blood pressure due to additive effects
Phenytoin / ↓ Effect of phenytoin due to ↑ breakdown by liver
Sulfonylureas / ↓ Effect of both drugs
Thiazide diuretics / ↑ Hypoglycemic and hyperuricemic effects

Laboratory Test Interferences: ↑ Serum uric acid, AST, alkaline phosphatase; ↓ creatinine clearance.

Dosage: Capsules, Oral Suspension. Dosage is individualized on the basis of blood glucose level and response of patient. **Adults and children, usual, initial:** 1 mg/kg q 8 hr (adjust according to response); **maintenance:** 3–8 mg/kg/day divided into 2 or 3 equal doses q 8–12 hr. **Infants and newborns, initial:** 3.3 mg/kg q 8 hr (adjust according to response); **maintenance:** 8–15 mg/kg/day divided into 2 or 3 equal doses q 8–12 hr.

NURSING CONSIDERATIONS

Administration/Storage

1. Blood glucose levels and urinary glucose and ketones must be monitored carefully until the client has stabilized, which usually takes 1 week. The drug is discontinued if a satisfactory effect has not been established within 2–3 weeks.
2. Have available insulin and IV fluids to counteract possible ketoacidosis.
3. *Treatment of Overdose:* Insulin to treat hyperglycemia; use Trendelenberg maneuver to reverse hypotension.

Interventions

1. If the client has a history of congestive heart failure, observe carefully for fluid retention, which could precipitate heart failure.
2. If the client is already taking an antihypertensive agent, monitor blood pressure for potentiation of antihypertensive effect.
3. Monitor the client for ecchymosis, the development of petechiae, or frank bleeding. These symptoms should be reported to the physician and may require discontinuation of the drug.
4. If the client has had an overdosage of drug, observe closely for the first 7 days until blood sugar level is again within normal limits (80–120 mg/100 ml).
5. If the client develops hirsutism, reassure that the condition should subside once the drug is discontinued.

Evaluation: Evaluate client for:
- Return of serum glucose to desired range

- Freedom from adverse effects of drug therapy

Dibasic calcium phosphate dihydrate (OTC)

See also *Calcium Salts,* p. 120.

Classification: Calcium salt.

Uses: Calcium deficiency states, dietary supplement.

Special Concerns: Increased risk of hypoparathyroidism or hyperphosphatemia in clients with renal insufficiency.

Dosage: Tablets. *Treatment of hypocalcemia:* **Adults:** 4.4 g daily in divided doses with or after meals; **pediatric:** 0.2–0.28 g/kg daily in divided doses with or after meals. **Note:** This preparation contains 23% calcium and 230 mg calcium/g (11.5 mEq/g).

NURSING CONSIDERATIONS

See also *Nursing Considerations* for *Calcium Salts,* p. 122.

Administration/Storage: Should be taken with meals in clients with achlorhydria or hypochlorhydria.

Diclofenac sodium
(dye-**KLOH**-fen-ack)
Apo-Diclo✲, Novo–Difenac✲, Nu-Diclo✲, Voltaren (Rx)

See also *Nonsteroidal Anti-Inflammatory Drugs,* p. 186.

Classification: Nonsteroidal anti-inflammatory analgesic.

Action/Kinetics: Diclofenac sodium is a phenylacetic acid derivative. **Peak plasma levels:** 2–3 hr. **t½:** 1–2 hr. Food will affect the rate, but not the amount, of drug absorbed from the GI tract. The drug is metabolized in the liver and excreted by the kidneys.

Uses: *Orally:* Rheumatoid arthritis, osteoarthritis, ankylosing spondylitis. *Investigational:* Mild to moderate pain, juvenile rheumatoid arthritis, acute painful shoulder, sunburn. *Ophthalmic:* Postoperative inflammation following cataract extraction.

Contraindications: Ophthalmically in clients who wear soft contact lenses.

Special Concerns: Pregnancy category: B. Use with caution during lactation. Safety and effectiveness has not been determined in children. When used ophthalmically, may cause increased bleeding of ocular tissues in conjunction with ocular surgery. Healing may be slowed or delayed.

Side Effects: *Following ophthalmic use:* Keratitis, increased intraocular pressure, ocular allergy, nausea, vomiting, anterior chamber reaction, viral infections, transient burning and stinging upon administration.

Dosage: Enteric-coated Tablets. *Rheumatoid arthritis:* 150–200 mg daily in 2–4 divided doses. *Osteoarthritis:* 100–150 mg daily in 2–3 divided doses. *Ankylosing spondylitis:* 25 mg q.i.d. with an extra 25 mg dose at bedtime, if necessary. **Ophthalmic Solution.** 1 gtt of the 0.1% solution in the affected eye q.i.d. beginning 24 hr after cataract surgery and for 2 weeks thereafter.

NURSING CONSIDERATIONS

See also *Nursing Considerations* for *Nonsteroidal Anti-Inflammatory Drugs,* p. 189.

Administration/Storage

1. May be taken with meals, a full glass of water or milk if GI upset occurs.
2. Up to 3 weeks may be required for beneficial effects to be realized when used for rheumatoid arthritis or osteoarthritis.
3. The delayed-release tablets should not be crushed or chewed.

Interventions: Monitor liver and renal function studies on a routine basis.

Evaluation: Assess client for subjective reports of symptomatic improvement in joint pain and mobility.

Dicloxacillin sodium
(dye-klox-ah-**SILL**-in)
Dycill, Dynapen, Pathocil (Rx)

See also *Anti-Infectives,* p. 80, and *Penicillins,* p. 197.

Classification: Antibiotic, penicillin.

Action/Kinetics: This drug is penicillinase-resistant and acid resistant. **Peak serum levels: IM, PO,** 4–20 mcg/ml after 1 hr. **t½:** 40 min. Chiefly excreted in urine.

Uses: Resistant staphylococcal infections. To initiate therapy in any suspected staphylococcal infection. Infections due to *Streptococcus pneumoniae.*

Contraindications: Treatment of meningitis.

Dosage: Capsules, Oral Suspension. *Skin and soft tissue infections, mild to moderate upper respiratory tract infections:* **Adults and children over 40 kg:** 125 mg q 6 hr; **pediatric:** 12.5 mg/kg/day in 4 equal doses given q 6 hr. *Lower respiratory tract infections or disseminated infections:* **Adults and children over 40 kg:** 250 mg q 6 hr, up to a maximum of 4 g daily; **pediatric:** 12–25 mg/kg daily in 4 equal doses given q 6 hr. Dosage not established for the newborn.

NURSING CONSIDERATIONS

See also *Nursing Considerations* for *Penicillins,* p. 200.

Administration/Storage

1. To prepare oral suspension, shake container to loosen powder, measure water for reconstitution as indicated on label, add half of the water, and immediately shake vigorously because usual handling may cause lumps. Add the remainder of the water and again shake vigorously.
2. Shake well before pouring each dose.
3. The reconstituted oral solution is stable for 7 days at room temperature, 10 days if refrigerated, and 21 days if frozen.
4. Give at least 1 hr before meals or no sooner than 2–3 hr after a meal.

Dicyclomine hydrochloride
(dye-**SYE**-kloh-meen)
Antispas, A-Spas, Bentyl, Bentylol✳, Byclomine, Dibent, Di-Cyclonex, Dilomine, Di-Spaz, Formulex✳, Lomine✳, Neoquess, Or-Tyl, Spasmoban✳, Spasmoject (Rx)

See also *Cholinergic Blocking Agents,* p. 136.

Classification: Cholinergic blocking agent.

Action/Kinetics: t½, initial: 1.8 hr; **secondary:** 9–10 hr.

Uses: Hypermotility and spasms of GI tract associated with irritable colon and spastic colitis, mucous colitis.

Additional Contraindications: Use for peptic ulcer.

Special Concerns: Pregnancy category: C. Pediatric dosage of the injectable form has not been established. Use of capsules and tablets in children less than 6 years of age not recommended; use of the syrup in children less than 6 months of age not recommended.

Additional Side Effects: Brief euphoria, slight dizziness, feeling of abdominal distention. **Use of the syrup in infants less than 3 months of age:** Seizures, syncope, respiratory symptoms, fluctuations in pulse rate, asphyxia, muscular hypotonia, coma.

Dosage: Capsules, Syrup, Tablets. Adults: 10–20 mg t.i.d.–q.i.d.; **then,** may increase to total daily dose of 160 mg (only oral dose shown to be effective) if side effects do not limit this dosage. **Pediatric, 6 years and older, capsules or tablets:** 10 mg t.i.d.–q.i.d.; adjust dosage to need and incidence of side effects. **Pediatric, 6 months–2 years, syrup:** 5–10 mg t.i.d.–q.i.d.; **2 years and older:** 10 mg t.i.d.–q.i.d. The dose should be adjusted to need and incidence of side effects.

   IM. Adults: 20 mg q 4–6 hr. **Not for IV use.**

NURSING CONSIDERATIONS

See also *Nursing Considerations* for *Cholinergic Blocking Agents,* p. 138.

Administration/Storage: Drug can be administered to clients with glaucoma.

Special Concerns

1. Anticipate reduced dose in the elderly.
2. Elderly clients may be more inclined to develop confusion, agitation, excitement, or drowsiness.

Evaluation: Evaluate client for reports of symptomatic improvement in abdominal pain and for a reduction in diarrhea.

Didanosine (ddI, dideoxyinosine)
(die-DAN-oh-seen)
Videx (Rx)

Classification: Antiviral.

Action/Kinetics: Didanosine is a nucleoside analog of deoxyadenosine. After entering the cell, it is converted to the active dideoxyadenosine triphosphate (ddATP) by cellular enzymes. Due to the chemical structure of ddATP, its incorporation into viral DNA leads to chain termination and therefore inhibition of viral replication. ddATP also inhibits viral replication by interfering with the HIV–RNA-dependent DNA polymerase by competing with the natural nucleoside triphosphate for binding to the active site of the enzyme. Didanosine has shown in vitro antiviral activity in a variety of HIV-infected T cell and monocyte/macrophage cell cultures. Didansosine is broken down quickly at acidic pH; therefore, oral products contain buffering agents to increase the pH of the stomach. Food will decrease the rate of absorption of the drug. **t½, elimination:** 1.6 hr for adults and 0.8 hr for children. The drug is metabolized in the liver and excreted mainly through the urine.

Uses: Advanced HIV infection in adult and pediatric (over 6 months of age) clients who are intolerant of zidovudine therapy or who have demonstrated decreased effectiveness of zidovudine therapy. Zidovudine should be considered as initial therapy for the treatment of advanced HIV infection, unless contraindicated.

Contraindications: Lactation.

Special Concerns: Pregnancy category: B. Administer with caution in clients with renal and hepatic impairment and in those on sodium-restricted diets. Clients may continue to develop opportunistic infections and other complications of HIV infection and should thus remain under close observation.

Side Effects: Commonly pancreatitis and peripheral neuropathy (manifested by tingling, burning, pain, or numbness in the hands or feet).

In adults. *GI:* Diarrhea, nausea, vomiting, abdominal pain, constipation, stomatitis, loss of taste, altered taste, dry mouth, dyspepsia, flatulence, GI hemorrhage, dysphagia, colitis, esophagitis, sialadenitis, oral moniliasis. *CNS:* Headache, insomnia, CNS depression, dizziness, seizures, confusion, anxiety, nervousness, abnormal thinking, hypertonia, dementia, agitation, ataxia, amnesia, speech disorder. *Hematologic:* Leukopenia, granulocytopenia, thrombocytopenia, anemia. *Dermatologic:* Rash, pruritus, sweating, acne, herpes. *Musculoskeletal:* Asthenia, myalgia, arthritis.

Body as a whole: Pain, alopecia, pneumonia, infection, anorexia, weight loss, sepsis, ascites, enlarged abdomen, facial edema, flu syndrome. *CV:* Hypertension, edema, syncope, congestive heart failure, pericardial effusion, vasodilation, cardiomyopathy, palpitation, cerebrovascular disorder. *Respiratory:* Cough, dyspnea, pharyngitis, apnea, sinusitis, bronchitis, pleural effusion, rhinitis, pneumothorax. *Miscellaneous:* Liver abnormalities, hyperlipemia, increase in CPK, kidney failure, polyuria, amblyopia, deafness, eye disorder.

In children. *GI:* Diarrhea, nausea, vomiting, melena, oral thrush, abdominal pain, constipation, dry mouth, stomatitis, mouth sores, pancreatitis. *CNS:* Headache, nervousness, insomnia, poor coordination, lethargy, dizziness, seizures. *Hematologic:* Granulocytopenia, leukopenia, thrombocytopenia, anemia, ecchymosis, hemorrhage, petechiae. *Dermatologic:* Rash, pruritus, alopecia, eczema, skin disorder, sweating, excoriation, erythema, impetigo. *Musculoskeletal:* Asthenia, muscle atrophy, arthritis, myalgia, decreased strength. *Body as a whole:* Malaise, chills, fever, anorexia, pain, failure to thrive, flu syndrome, pneumonia, dehydration, pain, weight loss, changes in appetite. *CV:* Vasodilation, arrhythmia. *Respiratory:* Cough, rhinitis, asthma, dyspnea, pharyngitis, epistaxis, rhinorrhea, hypoventilation, rhonchi, rales, sinusitis, congestion. *Miscellaneous:* Liver abnormalities, otitis, ear pain, photophobia, strabismus, impaired vision, urinary frequency, diabetes mellitus, diabetes insipidus.

Symptoms of Overdose: Pancreatitis, peripheral neuropathy, diarrhea, hyperuricemia, hepatic dysfunction.

Drug Interactions

Ketoconazole / ↓ Absorption of ketoconazole due to gastric pH change caused by buffering agents in didanosine
Pentamidine (IV) / ↑ Risk of pancreatitis
Quinolone antibiotics / ↓ Plasma levels of quinolone antibiotics
Ranitidine / ↓ Absorption of ranitidine due to gastric pH change caused by buffering agents in didanosine
Tetracyclines / ↓ Absorption of tetracyclines from the stomach

Laboratory Test Interferences: ↑ AST, ALT, alkaline phosphatase, bilirubin, uric acid, amylase.

Dosage: Chewable/Dispersible Buffered Tablets, Buffered Powder for Oral Solution, Pediatric Powder for Oral Solution. Adults, initial, weight over 75 kg: Two 150 mg tablets q 12 hr; **weight between 50–74 kg:** Two 100 mg tablets q 12 hr; **weight between 35–49 kg:** one 100 mg and one 25 mg tablet q 12 hr. **Pediatric, over 6 months, body surface area 1.1–1.4 m²:** Two 50 mg tablets q 12 hr; **body surface area 0.8–1.0 m²:** One 50 and one 25 mg tablet q 12 hr. **body surface area 0.5–0.7 m²:** Two 25 mg tablets q 12 hr; **body surface area less than 0.4 m²:** One 25 mg tablet q 12 hr.

NURSING CONSIDERATIONS

Administration/Storage

1. Didanosine should be administered on an empty stomach.
2. To prevent gastric acid degradation, adult and pediatric (over 1 year) clients should take a two-tablet dose. Pediatric clients under 12 months of age should receive a one-tablet dose.

3. Tablets should not be swallowed whole. Tablets may be chewed or crushed thoroughly before taking or tablets may be dispersed in at least 1 oz of drinking water (stir thoroughly and drink immediately).

4. To prepare the buffered powder for oral solution, the contents should be mixed with 4 oz of drinking water; the powder should not be mixed with fruit juice or other acid-containing beverages. The mixture should be stirred until the powder dissolves completely (about 2–3 min). The entire solution should be consumed immediately.

5. To prepare the pediatric powder for oral solution, the dry powder must be mixed with purified water to an initial concentration of 20 mg/ml. The resulting solution is then mixed with antacid to a final concentration of 10 mg/ml. This admixture must be shaken thoroughly prior to use and may be stored in a tightly closed container in the refrigerator for up to 30 days.

6. *Treatment of Overdose:* There are no antidotes; treatment should be symptomatic.

Assessment

1. Document all previous experience with zidovudine therapy and the outcome listing reasons for transfer to didanosine.

2. Obtain baseline CBC, CD4 counts, liver and renal function studies and monitor throughout therapy.

3. Note baseline vital signs and weight.

Interventions

1. Anticipate reduced dose with liver and renal impairment. Monitor I&O and laboratory parameters.

2. Assess clients on sodium-restricted diets as sodium content is more in the single dose packet than in the two-tablet dose.

3. Observe for evidence of diarrhea and/or hyperuricemia as drug dosage, in this event, requires adjustment.

4. Any changes in vision should be documented and evaluated with an ophthalmic examination.

Client/Family Teaching

1. Tablets should be chewed or crushed; follow administration guidelines carefully.

2. Food decreases the rate of drug absorption so take on an empty stomach.

3. Advise clients with symptoms of neuropathy (numbness, burning, or tingling in the hands or feet) to report these to the physician as drug should be discontinued until symptoms subside. Client may tolerate a reduced dose of didanosine once these symptoms have been resolved.

4. Report any symptoms of abdominal pain, nausea, and vomiting immediately as these may be clinical signs of pancreatitis. The drug should be stopped immediately and the client evaluated with dosing resumed only after pancreatitis has been ruled out.

5. Advise client to avoid alcohol and any other drugs that may

exacerbate the toxicity of didanosine.

6. Remind client and family that didanosine is not a cure, but it alleviates the symptoms of HIV infections. Stress that clients may continue to acquire opportunistic infections.

7. Stress that didanosine therapy has not been shown to reduce the risk of transmission of HIV to others through sexual contact or blood contamination and that appropriate precautions should continue to be taken.

8. Provide referrals to local support groups that may assist client/family to understand and cope with the disease.

Evaluation

1. Evaluate for the control and treatment of symptoms of AIDS, ARC, and opportunistic infections in clients with HIV who are intolerant to or have clinically deteriorated during therapy with zidovudine.

2. Evaluate client for evidence of freedom from further complications related to drug therapy.

Diethylpropion hydrochloride

(dye-eth-ill-**PROH**-pee-on)
M-Orexic, Tenuate, Tenuate Dospan, Tepanil, Tepanil Ten-Tab (C-IV) (Rx)

See also *Amphetamines and Derivatives,* p. 29.

Classification: Anorexiant.

Action/Kinetics: Duration, tablets: 4 hr; **extended-release tablets:** 12 hr.

Use: Short-term (8–12 weeks) treatment of exogenous obesity in conjunction with a weight reduction regimen including exercise, reduced caloric intake, and behavior modification.

Special Concerns: Pregnancy category: B. Use with caution during lactation.

Additional Side Effects: May cause increased risk of seizures in epileptics.

Dosage: Tablets. Adults: 25 mg t.i.d. 1 hr before meals. **Extended-release Tablets. Adults:** 75 mg at midmorning.

NURSING CONSIDERATIONS

See also *Nursing Considerations* for *Amphetamines and Derivatives,* p. 31.

Administration/Storage

1. Give extended-release tablets in the mid-morning.
2. The drug may be taken in the mid-evening to reduce night hunger.

Assessment

1. Note any history of seizure disorder.
2. Assess client life-style and willingness to change negative behaviors.

Evaluation: Evaluate client for a reduction in weight and for evidence of compliance with overall weight loss program.

Diethylstilbestrol

(dye-eth-ill-still-**BESS**-trohl)
(Abbreviation: DES) (Rx)

Diethylstilbestrol diphosphate

(dye-eth-ill-still-**BESS**-trohl)

Honvol✹, Stilboestrol✹, Stilphostrol (Abbreviation: DES) (Rx)

See also *Estrogens,* p. 147, and *Antineoplastic Agents,* p. 85.

Classification: Estrogen, synthetic, nonsteroidal.

Action/Kinetics: Synthetic estrogen, which competes with androgen receptors, thereby preventing androgen from inducing further growth of the neoplasm. Diethylstilbestrol also binds to cytoplasmic receptor protein. The estrogen–receptor complex translocates to the nucleus, where metabolic alterations ensue. Metabolized in the liver.

Uses: Postcoital contraceptive (emergency use only). Palliative treatment of inoperable, progressive prostatic cancer.

Contraindications: Known or suspected breast cancer, estrogen-dependent neoplasia, active thrombophlebitis, thromboembolic disease, markedly impaired liver function. **Not to be used during pregnancy because of the possibility of vaginal cancer in female offspring (pregnancy category: X).** The diphosphate is not to be used to treat any disorder in women.

Special Concerns: Use with caution in presence of hypercalcemia, epilepsy, migraine, asthma, cardiac and renal disease. Use with caution in children in whom bone growth is incomplete.

Side Effects: *CV:* Thrombophlebitis, pulmonary embolism, cerebral thrombosis, neuro-ocular lesions. *GI:* Nausea, vomiting, anorexia. *CNS:* Headaches, malaise, irritability. *Skin:* Allergic rash, itching. *GU:* Gynecomastia, changes in libido. *Other:* Porphyria, backache, pain and sterile abscess at injection site, postinjection flare.

Dosage: *Diethylstilbestrol.* **Tablets.** *Menopausal symptoms, atrophic vaginitis, kraurosis vulvae:* 0.2–0.5 mg up to 2 mg daily, given cyclically. *Estrogen deficiency states:* 0.2–0.5 mg daily, given cyclically. *Breast cancer in males and females:* 15 mg daily. *Prostatic cancer:* **initial,** 1–3 mg; **then,** increase as needed but later reduce dose to 1 mg daily. *Postcoital contraceptive (emergency treatment only):* 25 mg b.i.d. for 5 consecutive days, beginning within 24 hr (and not later than 72 hr) after exposure.

Diethylstilbestrol diphosphate. Palliative treatment of prostatic carcinoma: **Tablets:** 50 mg t.i.d. up to 200 mg t.i.d., not to exceed 1 g daily. **IV:** 500 mg (in 250 ml 5% dextrose or saline) on day 1 followed by 1 g (in 250–500 ml 5% dextrose or saline) daily for 5 days. **Maintenance, IV:** 250–500 mg 1 to 2 times weekly. Maintenance dose may also be given orally.

NURSING CONSIDERATIONS

See also *Nursing Considerations* for *Antineoplastic Agents,* p. 88, and *Estrogens,* p. 150.

Administration/Storage

1. Administer the diphosphate slowly by drip (20–30 drops/ min for first 10–15 min); then adjust flow for a total administration period of 1 hr.

D

2. The diphosphate solution is stable for 5 days at room temperature if stored away from direct light. Do not use if solution appears cloudy or if a precipitate has formed.

Assessment

1. Assess client with poor cardiac function for edema.
2. The effect of the steroid and osteolytic metastases may result in hypercalcemia. Assess for symptoms of hypercalcemia: insomnia, lethargy, anorexia, nausea, vomiting, coma, and vascular collapse.
3. During pregnancy, the drug is not administered because of the high incidence of genital tumors in offspring.

Interventions

1. Withhold drug and report high serum calcium levels.
2. Monitor vital signs and I&O. Encourage high fluid intake to minimize hypercalcemia.
3. Be prepared to assist with administration of IV fluids, diuretics, adrenocorticosteroids, and phosphate supplements for severe hypercalcemia.
4. Closely monitor clients who resume therapy after drug-induced hypercalcemia is corrected.
5. Anticipate that gynecomastia in men may be prevented by low doses of radiation before therapy with diethylstilbestrol is initiated.
6. The diphosphate should not be used to treat any disorder in women.
7. Observe closely for evidence of thrombic disorders or visual changes.

Client/Family Teaching

1. Report any nausea, vomiting, abdominal pain, and painful swelling of breasts to physician. Identify symptoms that require immediate reporting.
2. Instruct client that solid foods often relieve nausea.
3. Be alert for increased complications and/or edema in clients with poor cardiac function.

Evaluation: Evaluate client for:
- Reports of improvement in menopausal symptoms
- ↓ in tumor size and spread with metastatic breast or prostate cancer

—— *COMBINATION DRUG* ——

Difenoxin hydrochloride with Atropine sulfate
(dye-fen-**OX**-in **AH**-troh-peen)
Motofen (Rx)

Classification: Antidiarrheal.

Action/Kinetics: Difenoxin is related chemically to meperidine; thus, atropine sulfate is incorporated to prevent deliberate overdosage. Difenoxin is the active metabolite of diphenoxylate and is effective at one-fifth the dosage of diphenoxylate. Difenoxin slows intestinal motility by a local effect on the GI wall. **Peak plasma levels:** 40–60 min. The drug and its inactive metabolites are excreted through both the urine and feces.

Uses: Management of acute nonspecific diarrhea and acute episodes of chronic functional diarrhea.

Contraindications: Diarrhea

caused by *Escherichia coli, Salmonella,* or *Shigella;* pseudomembranous colitis caused by broad-spectrum antibiotics; jaundice; children less than 2 years of age.

Special Concerns: Pregnancy category: C. Use with caution in ulcerative colitis, liver and kidney disease, lactation, and in clients receiving dependence-producing drugs or in those who are addiction prone. Safety and effectiveness in children less than 12 years of age have not been determined.

Side Effects: *GI:* Nausea, vomiting, dry mouth, epigastric distress, constipation. *CNS:* Lightheadedness, dizziness, drowsiness, headache, tiredness, nervousness, confusion, insomnia. *Ophthalmic:* Blurred vision, burning eyes.

Symptoms of Overdose: Initially include dry skin and mucous membranes, hyperthermia, flushing, and tachycardia. These are followed by hypotonic reflexes, nystagmus, miosis, lethargy, coma, and respiratory depression (may occur up to 30 hr after overdose taken).

Drug Interactions

Antianxiety agents / Potentiation or addition of CNS depressant effects
Barbiturates / Potentiation or addition of CNS depressant effects
Ethanol / Potentiation or addition of CNS depressant effects
MAO inhibitors / Precipitation of hypertensive crisis
Narcotics / Potentiation or addition of CNS depressant effects

Dosage: Tablets. Adults, initial: 2 tablets (2 mg difenoxin); **then,** 1 tablet (1 mg difenoxin) after each loose stool or 1 tablet q 3–4 hr as needed. Total dose during a 24-hr period should not exceed 8 mg (i.e., 8 tablets).

NURSING CONSIDERATIONS
Administration/Storage

1. Continued administration beyond 48 hr is not recommended, if clinical improvement is not noted.
2. Treatment beyond 48 hr is usually not necessary for acute diarrhea or acute exacerbation of functional diarrhea.
3. *Treatment of Overdose:* Naloxone may be used to treat respiratory depression.

Assessment

1. Note the onset and frequency of diarrhea.
2. Discuss the possible precipitating factors, e.g., travel, food, medication regimens.
3. Note evidence of dehydration such as weakness, weight loss, sunken eyes, poor skin turgor, elevated temperature, rapid weak pulse, or decreased urinary output.
4. Assess for evidence of electrolyte imbalance such as weakness, irritability, anorexia, nausea, and dysrhythmias.
5. Note the client's skin and sclera color for evidence of hepatic disease.

Interventions

1. If the client has a history of heart disease, monitor closely and report any adverse effects to the physician immediately.
2. Monitor intake and output. Keep a record of the number and consistency of the stools. If the diarrhea persists, consult with the physician.
3. Monitor the client for changes

in electrolyte balance. Document and report to the physician.

4. Check the client's gums for swelling and the extremities for numbness.

5. If the client is also receiving Lomotil and other narcotics or barbiturates observe closely for the potentiation of CNS depression.

6. If the client has a history of liver disease, observe for signs of impending coma, such as increased drowsiness, mental aberrations, motor disturbances, or a flapping tremor of the hands. Monitor liver function studies as drug may precipitate hepatic coma in clients with abnormal liver function.

7. Difenoxin contains atropine sulfate as an active ingredient; closely observe Down syndrome children receiving this drug for symptoms of atropinism.

8. Do not administer to clients receiving MAO inhibitors as concomitant use may precipitate hypertensive crisis.

9. Difenoxin has the potential to become addictive; monitor accordingly.

10. Overdosed clients should be hospitalized for observation since latent (12–30 hr later) respiratory depression may occur.

Client/Family Teaching

1. Provide printed instructions concerning the recommended dosage schedule and side effects to be reported to the physician.

2. Do not perform tasks that require mental alertness until drug effects are realized.

3. Take only as directed and do not share medications with anyone, no matter what the symptoms.

4. Suck on ice chips, chew sugarless gum, or suck on hard, sugarless candy if dry mouth is a problem.

5. Keep out of reach of children as drug may be fatal if ingested by children.

6. Drug should *not* be taken by mothers who are breast-feeding.

7. Avoid alcohol or any other unprescribed CNS depressants.

8. Advise that treatment may take 24–36 hr before effects are evident.

Evaluation

1. Evaluate client for a reduction in the frequency and number of diarrheal stools.

2. Check laboratory culture reports to determine if therapy is appropriate.

Diflunisal
(dye-**FLEW**-nih-sal)
Dolobid (Rx)

Classification: Nonsteroidal analgesic, anti-inflammatory, antipyretic.

Action/Kinetics: Diflunisal is a salicylic acid derivative although it is not metabolized to salicylic acid. Its mechanism is not known although it is thought to be an inhibitor of prostaglandin synthetase. **Onset:** 1 hr. **Peak plasma levels:** 2–3 hr. **Peak effect:** 2–3 hr. **t½:** 8–12 hr. Ninety-nine percent protein bound. Metabolites excreted in urine.

Uses: Analgesic, rheumatoid arthritis, osteoarthritis, ankylosing spondylitis, psoriatic arthritis, musculo-skeletal pain. Prophylaxis and treatment of vascular headaches.

Contraindications: Hypersensitivity to diflunisal, aspirin, or other anti-inflammatory drugs. Acute asthmatic attacks, urticaria, or rhinitis precipitated by aspirin. During lactation and in children less than 12 years of age.

Special Concerns: Pregnancy category: C. Use with caution in presence of ulcers or in clients with a history thereof, in clients with hypertension, compromised cardiac function, or in conditions leading to fluid retention. Use with caution in only first two trimesters of pregnancy. Geriatric clients may be at greater risk of GI toxicity.

Side Effects: *GI:* Nausea, dyspepsia, GI pain and bleeding, diarrhea, vomiting, constipation, flatulence, peptic ulcer, eructation, anorexia. *CNS:* Headache, fatigue, fever, malaise, dizziness, somnolence, insomnia, nervousness, vertigo, depression, paresthesias. *Dermatologic:* Rashes, pruritus, sweating, Stevens-Johnson syndrome, dry mucous membranes, erythema multiforme. *CV:* Palpitations, syncope, edema. *Other:* Tinnitus, asthenia, chest pain, hypersensitivity reactions, anaphylaxis, dyspnea, dysuria, muscle cramps, thrombocytopenia. *Symptoms of Overdose:* Drowsiness, nausea, vomiting, diarrhea, tachycardia, hyperventilation, stupor, disorientation, diminished urine output, coma, cardiorespiratory arrest.

Drug Interactions

Acetaminophen / ↑ Plasma levels of acetaminophen

Antacids / ↓ Plasma levels of diflunisal

Anticoagulants / ↑ Prothrombin time

Furosemide / ↓ Hyperuricemic effect of furosemide

Hydrochlorothiazide / ↑ Plasma levels and ↓ hyperuricemic effect of hydrochlorothiazide

Indomethacin / ↓ Renal clearance of indomethacin → ↑ plasma levels

Naproxen / ↓ Urinary excretion of naproxen and metabolite

Dosage: Tablets. *Mild to moderate pain:* **initial,** 1,000 mg; **then,** 250–500 mg q 8–12 hr. *Rheumatoid arthritis, osteoarthritis:* 250–500 mg b.i.d. Doses in excess of 1,500 mg/day are not recommended. For some clients, an initial dose of 500 mg followed by 250 mg q 8–12 hr may be effective. Dosage should be reduced in clients with impaired renal function.

NURSING CONSIDERATIONS

Administration/Storage

1. When given for analgesic or antipyretic effect, expect the onset of action to occur within 20 min and to last for 4–6 hr.
2. If administering the drug to counteract the pain and swelling of arthritis, expect maximum relief to occur in 2–3 weeks.
3. Diflunisal may be given with water, milk, or meals to reduce gastric irritation.
4. Do not give acetaminophen or aspirin with diflunisal.
5. Tablets should not be crushed or chewed.
6. Serum salicylate levels are not used as a guide to dosage or toxicity because the drug is not hydrolyzed to salicylic acid.
7. *Treatment of Overdose:* Supportive measures. To empty the

stomach, induce vomiting or perform gastric lavage. Hemodialysis may not be effective since the drug is significantly bound to plasma protein.

Assessment

1. Note any client history of hypersensitivity to salicylates or other anti-inflammatory drugs.
2. Review the client's history, noting whether or not the client has had peptic ulcers, hypertension, or any evidence of compromised cardiac function.
3. If the client is female, of childbearing age and sexually active question her concerning the possibility of pregnancy. The drug should be avoided or used with extreme caution during the first two trimesters of pregnancy.
4. If the client is on anticoagulant therapy, have prothrombin and coagulation times checked prior to administering drug.

Interventions

1. Assess clients for increased tendencies of bleeding when receiving high doses of diflunisal. This drug may inhibit platelet aggregation.
2. If the client is on oral anticoagulant therapy, observe for any increase in bleeding tendencies. The prothrombin time may be increased due to drug interactions.
3. If the client is elderly, note complaints of diarrhea. This can cause an electrolyte imbalance and should be corrected. Document and report to the physician.

Client/Family Teaching

1. Antacids may lower plasma levels of diflunisal, reducing the effectiveness of the drug. Therefore, consult the physician before using an antacid to prevent gastric irritation.
2. To minimize gastric irritation, take the medication with meals, milk, or a snack. If these measures do not work, consult the physician concerning the use of an antacid.
3. Taking the medication on a regular basis is necessary to sustain the anti-inflammatory effect of the drug. Therefore, compliance with the prescribed regimen is of utmost importance.
4. Urge the client to report for medical follow-up and supervision on a regular basis. The medication needs to be adjusted according to the client's age, condition, and changes in disease activity.
5. The medication may cause dizziness or drowsiness; use care when operating machinery or driving an automobile.
6. Advise parents to avoid aspirin or salicylates when treating children with a fever, children infected with varicella, or children who have influenza-like symptoms. Stress the importance of consulting with the child's physician before administering any OTC or unprescribed drugs.

Evaluation: Evaluate client for:
- Subjective reports of symptomatic improvement in pain and mobility of involved joints
- Prevention of vascular headaches

Digitoxin
(dih-jih-**TOX**-in)
Digitaline ✽ (Rx)

See also *Cardiac Glycosides,* p. 123.

Classification: Cardiac glycoside.

Action/Kinetics: Most potent of the digitalis glycosides. Its slow onset of action makes it unsuitable for emergency use. Almost completely absorbed from GI tract. **Onset: PO,** 1–4 hr; maximum effect: 8–12 hr. **t½:** 5–9 days; **Duration:** 2 weeks. Significant protein binding (over 90%). Metabolized by the liver and excreted as inactive metabolites through the urine. **Therapeutic serum levels:** 14–26 ng/ml. Withhold drug and check with physician if serum level exceeds 35 ng/ml, indicating toxicity.

Use: Drug of choice for maintenance in congestive heart failure.

Special Concerns: Pregnancy category: C. Digitalis tablets may not be suitable for small children; thus, other digitalis products should be considered.

Additional Drug Interactions

Aminoglutethimide / ↓ Effect of digitoxin due to ↑ breakdown by liver
Barbiturates / ↓ Effect of digitoxin due to ↑ breakdown by liver
Diltiazem / May ↑ serum levels of digitoxin
Phenylbutazone / ↓ Effect of digitoxin due to ↑ breakdown by liver
Phenytoin / ↓ Effect of digitoxin due to ↑ breakdown by liver
Quinidine / May ↑ serum levels of digitoxin

Rifampin / ↓ Effect of digitoxin due to ↑ breakdown by liver
Verapamil / May ↑ serum levels of digitoxin

Dosage: Tablets. Adults. Digitalizing dose: Rapid, 0.6 mg followed by 0.4 mg in 4–6 hr; **then,** 0.2 mg q 4–6 hr until therapeutic effect achieved. **Digitalizing dose: Slow,** 0.2 mg b.i.d. for 4 days. **Maintenance dose: PO,** 0.05–0.3 mg/day (**usual:** 0.15 mg/day).

NURSING CONSIDERATIONS

See also *Nursing Considerations* for *Cardiac Glycosides,* p. 126.

Administration/Storage

1. Incompatible with acids and alkali.
2. Protect from light.

Evaluation: Evaluate client for:
- Control of signs and symptoms of CHF
- Serum digitoxin level within therapeutic range (14–26 ng/ml)

Digoxin
(dih-**JOX**-in)
Lanoxicaps, Lanoxin, Novo–Digoxin ✽ (Rx)

See also *Cardiac Glycosides,* p. 123.

Classification: Cardiac glycoside.

Action/Kinetics: Action prompter and shorter than that of digitoxin. **Onset: PO,** 0.5–2 hr; **time to peak effect:** 2–6 hr. **Duration:** 6 days. **Onset, IV:** 5–30 min; **time to peak effect:** 1–4 hr. **Duration:** 6 days. **t½:** 35 hr. **Therapeutic serum level:** 0.5–2.0 ng/ml. Serum levels above 2.5 ng/ml indicate toxicity. 50%–70% is excreted unchanged by the kidneys. Bioavailability depends on the dosage form: tablets (60%–80%), capsules (90%–100%), and elixir (70%–85%). Thus, changing dosage forms may require dosage adjustments.

Uses: May be drug of choice for congestive heart failure because of rapid onset, relatively short duration, and ability to be administered PO or IV.

Special Concerns: Pregnancy category: A.

Additional Drug Interactions

1. The following drugs increase serum digoxin levels, leading to possible toxicity: Aminoglycosides, amiodarone, anticholinergics, benzodiazepines, captopril, diltiazem, erythromycin, esmolol, flecainide, hydroxychloroquine, ibuprofen, indomethacin, nifedipine, quinidine, quinine, tetracyclines, tolbutamide, verapamil.
2. Disopyramide may alter the pharmacologic effect of digoxin.
3. Penicillamine decreases serum digoxin levels.

Dosage: Capsules. Adults, Digitalization: Rapid, 0.4–0.6 mg initially followed by 0.1–0.3 mg q 6–8 hr until desired effect achieved. **Digitalization: Slow,** a total of 0.05–0.35 mg daily divided in two doses for a period of 7–22 days to reach steady-state serum levels. **Maintenance:** 0.05–0.35 mg once or twice daily. **Pediatric. Digitalizing dosage is divided into 3 or more doses with the initial dose being about one-half the total dose; doses are given q 4–8 hr. Children, 10 years and older:** 0.008–0.012 mg/kg. **5–10 years:** 0.015–0.03 mg/kg. **2–5 years:** 0.025–0.035 mg/kg. **1 month–2 years:** 0.03–0.05 mg/kg. **Neonates, full-term:** 0.02–0.03 mg/kg. **Neonates, premature:** 0.015–0.025 mg/kg. **Maintenance, premature neonates:** 20%–30% of total digitalizing dose divided and given in 2–3 daily doses. **Maintenance, neonates to 10 years:** 25%–35% of the total digitalizing dose divided and given in 2–3 daily doses.

Elixir, Tablets. Adults, Digitalization: Rapid, a total of 0.75–1.25 mg divided into 2 or more doses each given at 6–8-hr intervals. **Digitalization: Slow,** 0.125–0.5 mg once daily for 7 days. **Maintenance:** 0.125–0.5 mg daily. **Pediatric. Digitalizing dose is divided into 2 or more doses and given at 6–8-hr intervals. Children, 10 years and older, rapid or slow:** Same as adult dose. **5–10 years:** 0.02–0.035 mg/kg. **2–5 years:** 0.03–0.05 mg/kg. **1 month–2 years:** 0.035–0.06 mg/kg. **Premature and newborn infants to 1 month:** 0.02–0.035 mg/kg. **Maintenance:** one-fifth to one-third the total digitalizing dose daily. **Note:** An alternate regimen (referred to as the "small-dose" method) is 0.017 mg/kg daily. This dose causes less toxicity.

IV. Adults, digitalization: Same as Capsules. **Maintenance:** 0.125–0.5 mg daily in divided doses or as a single dose. **Pediatric:** Same as Capsules.

NURSING CONSIDERATIONS

See also *Nursing Considerations* for *Cardiac Glycosides,* p. 126.

Administration/Storage

1. IV injections should be given over 5 min (or longer) either

undiluted or diluted fourfold or greater with sterile water for injection, 0.9% sodium chloride injection, lactated Ringer's injection, or 5% dextrose injection.

2. Lanoxicaps gelatin capsules are more bioavailable than tablets. Thus, the 0.05 mg capsule is equivalent to the 0.0625 mg tablet; the 0.1 mg capsule is equivalent to the 0.125 mg tablet and the 0.2 mg capsule is equivalent to the 0.25 mg tablet.

3. Differences in bioavailability have been noted between products; thus, clients should be monitored when changing from one product to another.

4. Protect from light.

5. *Treatment of Overdose:* Use digoxin immune Fab (see below).

Evaluation: Evaluate client for:

- Control of signs and symptoms of CHF with resultant ↑ in cardiac output
- Serum digoxin level within therapeutic range (0.5–2.0 ng/ml

Digoxin Immune Fab (Ovine)

(dih-**JOX**-in)

Digibind (Rx)

Classification: Digoxin antidote.

Action/Kinetics: Digoxin immune Fab are antibodies that bind to digoxin. The antibody is produced in sheep by immunization with digoxin bound to human albumin. In cases of digoxin toxicity, the antibodies can bind to digoxin and the complex is excreted through the kidneys. As serum levels of digoxin decrease, digoxin bound to tissue is released into the serum to maintain equilibrium and this is then bound and excreted. The net result is a decrease in both tissue and serum digoxin. **Onset:** Less than 1 min. **t½:** 15–20 hr (after IV administration). Each vial contains 40 mg of pure digoxin immune Fab, which will bind approximately 0.6 mg digoxin or digitoxin.

Uses: Life-threatening digoxin or digitoxin toxicity or overdosage. Symptoms of toxicity include severe sinus bradycardia, second- or third-degree heart block which does not respond to atropine, ventricular tachycardia, ventricular fibrillation.

Note: Cardiac arrest can be expected if a healthy adult ingests more than 10 mg digoxin or a healthy child ingests more than 4 mg. Also, steady-state serum concentrations of digoxin greater than 10 ng/ml or potassium concentrations greater than 5 mEq/L as a result of digoxin therapy require use of digoxin immune Fab.

Special Concerns: Use with caution during pregnancy (category: C) and lactation. Use in infants only if benefits outweigh risks. Clients sensitive to products of sheep origin may also be sensitive to digoxin immune Fab.

Side Effects: *CV:* Worsening of congestive heart failure or low cardiac output, atrial fibrillation (all due to withdrawal of the effects of digoxin). *Other:* Hypokalemia.

Dosage: **IV.** Dosage depends on the serum digoxin concentration. A large dose has a faster onset but there is an increased risk of allergic or febrile reactions. The package insert should be carefully consulted.

NURSING CONSIDERATIONS

Administration/Storage

1. The lyophilized material should be reconstituted with 4 ml of sterile water for injection to give a concentration of 10 mg/ml. If small doses are required (e.g., in infants), reconstituted antibody can be further diluted with 36 ml sterile isotonic saline to obtain a concentration of 1 mg/ml.
2. The reconstituted antibody should be used immediately. However, it may be stored for up to 4 hr at 2°C–8°C (36°F–46°F).
3. The dose should be administered over a 30-min period through a 0.22 μm membrane filter. A bolus injection may be used if there is immediate danger of cardiac arrest.
4. The total number of vials of antibody needed can be determined by dividing the total body load (in mg) by the amount of digoxin bound by each vial (0.6 mg).
5. If acute digoxin ingestion results in severe symptoms and a serum concentration is not known, 800 mg (20 vials) of digoxin immune Fab may be given. However, volume overload must be monitored in small children.
6. The dosage in infants should be administered with a tuberculin syringe.

Assessment

1. Evaluate laboratory data for electrolyte imbalance and correct.

2. Note the presence of hypokalemia or evidence of increased congestive heart failure and document.
3. Determine pretreatment digoxin or digitoxin levels.

Interventions

1. In the event of a hypersensitivity reaction, have epinephrine (1:1,000) immediately available.
2. Monitor vital signs and cardiac rhythm in a monitored environment. Have emergency drugs and equipment readily available.
3. Clients with known allergy to sheep proteins should be appropriately identified and this information should be documented in their records. Do not administer digoxin immune Fab to these persons.

Evaluation

1. Assess client for return of baseline cardiac rhythm.
2. Repeat serum digoxin level to evaluate response to therapy.

Dihydroergotamine mesylate

(dye-hy-droh-er-**GOT**-ah-meen)
D.H.E. 45, Dihydroergotamine-Sandoz (Rx)

Classification: Alpha-adrenergic blocking agent.

Action/Kinetics: Dihydroergotamine manifests alpha-adrenergic receptor blocking activity as well as a direct stimulatory action on vascular smooth muscle of peripheral and cranial blood vessels, resulting in vasoconstriction, thus preventing the onset of a migraine attack.

Dihydroergotamine manifests greater adrenergic blocking activity, less pronounced vasoconstriction, less nausea and vomiting, and less oxytocic properties than does ergotamine. It is more effective when given early in the course of a migraine attack. **Onset: IM,** 15–30 min; **IV,** less than 5 min. **Duration: IM,** 3–4 hr. **t½: initial,** 1.4 hr; **final,** 18–22 hr. Metabolized in liver and excreted in feces with less than 10% excreted through the urine.

Uses: Migraine, migraine variant, histaminic cephalalgia, and cluster headaches. Especially useful when rapid effect is desired or when other routes of administration are not possible. *Investigational:* Adjunct in prophylaxis of deep venous and pulmonary thrombosis.

Contraindications: Lactation. Peripheral vascular disease, coronary heart disease, hypertension, impaired hepatic or renal function, sepsis, hypersensitivity, or malnutrition, severe pruritus, presence of infection. Not recommended for prophylaxis of migraine attack.

Special Concerns: Pregnancy category: X. Geriatric clients may be more affected by peripheral vasoconstriction that results in hypothermia.

Side Effects: *CV:* Precordial pain, transient tachycardia or bradycardia. Large doses may cause increased blood pressure, vasoconstriction of coronary arteries, and bradycardia. *GI:* Nausea, vomiting, diarrhea. *Other:* Numbness and tingling of fingers and toes, muscle pain in extremities, weakness in legs, localized edema, and itching. *Prolonged use:* Gangrene, ergotism. *Symptoms of Overdose:* Nausea, vomiting, diarrhea, severe thirst, formication, chest pain, hypo- or hypertension, bradycardia or tachycardia, seizures, confusion, cutaneous hypoperfusion, sensory loss, coma.

Drug Interactions: Oral nitroglycerin ↑ bioavailability of hydro-ergotamine.

Dosage: IM. *Suppress vascular headache:* **initial,** 1 mg at first sign of headache; repeat every 1–2 hr to a total of 3 mg/attack or 6 mg/week. **IV.** *Suppress vascular headache:* Similar to IM but to a maximum of 2 mg/attack or 6 mg weekly. **SC.** *Prophylaxis of thrombosis:* 0.5 mg 2 hr prior to surgery concurrently with heparin; **then,** repeat dose q 12 hr for 5–7 days.

NURSING CONSIDERATIONS

Administration/Storage

1. Adjust the dosage if the client complains of severe headaches. This dose should then be used when subsequent headaches begin.
2. *Treatment of Overdose:* Maintain adequate circulation. IV nitroglycerin and nitroprusside to treat vasospasm. IV heparin and low molecular weight dextran to minimize thrombosis.

Assessment

1. Obtain a thorough nursing, diet, and drug history.
2. Note any history of prior adverse reactions to ergotamine.
3. Determine if the client is taking nitroglycerin. Dihydroergotamine interacts with nitroglycerin and should be avoided.
4. Determine the severity of the client's headaches, how long they last and what, if any, medications have been effective in relieving them in the past.

5. If the client is of childbearing age and is sexually active, note the possibility of pregnancy. Ergotamine has an oxytocic effect and therefore is contraindicated in this setting.

Client/Family Teaching

1. Take the drug at the onset of a migraine headache. This drug is most effective when administered early in an attack.
2. Seek bed rest in a darkened room for 1–2 hr after drug ingestion.
3. Teach client alternative methods for dealing with stress, such as relaxation techniques.
4. Report any bothersome side effects. To avoid gangrene, any evidence of cold extremities, numbness or tingling of the extremities should be reported immediately to the physician.
5. Take the drug only as directed. Do not stop taking the drug abruptly or without the physician's knowledge.

Evaluation: Evaluate client for:
- Prevention or termination of migraine headaches
- Effectiveness in preventing postoperative complication of thrombosis

Dihydroxyaluminum sodium carbonate

(dye-hy-**drox**-ee-ah-**LOO**-mih-num)

Rolaids Antacid (OTC)

See also *Antacids,* p. 37.

Classification: Antacid.

Action/Kinetics: Nonsystemic antacid with adsorbent and protective properties similar to those of aluminum hydroxide but reported to act more rapidly. Acid-neutralizing capacity: 7 mEq/tablet. **Note:** See *Aluminum Hydroxide Gel* for Uses, Contraindications, Side Effects, and Drug Interactions.

Dosage: Chewable Tablets. Adults: 1–2 tablets chewed after meals and at bedtime; 1–2 tablets chewed q 2–4 hr may be required to alleviate severe discomfort.

NURSING CONSIDERATIONS

See *Nursing Considerations* for *Antacids,* p. 38.

Diltiazem hydrochloride

(dill-**TIE**-ah-zem)

Apo-Diltiaz✣, Cardizem, Cardizem CD, Cardizem Injectable, Cardizem-SR, Novo-Diltazem✣, Nu-Diltiaz✣, Syn-Diltiazem✣ (Rx)

See also *Calcium Channel Blocking Agents,* p. 118.

Classification: Calcium channel blocking agent (antianginal, antihypertensive).

Action/Kinetics: Decreases SA and AV conduction and prolongs AV node effective and functional refractory periods. The drug also decreases myocardial contractility and peripheral vascular resistance. **Tablets: Onset,** 30–60 min; **time to peak plasma levels:** 2–3 hr; **t½, first phase:** 20–30 min; **second phase:** about 3–4.5 hr (5–8 hr with high and repetitive doses); **duration:** 4–8 hr. **Extended-release Capsules: Onset,** 2–3 hr; **time to peak plasma levels:** 6–11 hr; **t½:** 5–7 hr; **duration:** 12 hr. **Therapeutic serum levels:** 0.05–0.2 mcg/ml. Metabolized to desacetyldiltiazem, which manifests

25%–50% of the activity of diltiazem. Excreted through both the bile and urine.

Uses: Tablets. Vasospastic angina (Prinzmetal's variant); chronic stable angina (especially in clients who cannot use beta-adrenergic blockers or nitrates or who remain symptomatic after clinical doses of these agents). *Sustained-release form:* Only used to treat essential hypertension. **Parenteral.** Atrial fibrillation or flutter. Paroxysmal supraventricular tachycardia. *Investigational:* Prophylaxis of reinfarction of non-Q wave myocardial infarction; tardive dyskinesia, Raynaud's syndrome.

Contraindications: Hypotension, second- or third-degree AV block, sick sinus syndrome. Acute myocardial infarction, pulmonary congestion.

Special Concerns: Use during pregnancy only if benefits outweigh risks (pregnancy category: C). Safety and effectiveness in children have not been determined. Excreted in breast milk. The half-life may be increased in geriatric clients. Use with caution in hepatic disease and in congestive heart failure. Abrupt withdrawal may cause an increase in the frequency and duration of chest pain.

Side Effects: *CV:* AV block, bradycardia, congestive heart failure, hypotension, syncope, palpitations, peripheral edema, arrhythmias, angina, tachycardia, abnormal ECG, ventricular extrasystoles. *GI:* Nausea, vomiting, diarrhea, constipation, anorexia, abdominal discomfort, cramps, dry mouth, dysgeusia. *CNS:* Weakness, nervousness, dizziness, lightheadedness, headache, depression, psychoses, hallucinations, disturbances in sleep, somno-lence, insomnia, amnesia, abnormal dreams. *Dermatologic:* Rashes, dermatitis, pruritus, urticaria, erythema multiforme, Stevens-Johnson syndrome. *Other:* Photosensitivity, joint pain or stiffness, flushing, nasal or chest congestion, dyspnea, shortness of breath, nocturia/polyuria, sexual difficulties, weight gain, paresthesia, tinnitus, tremor, asthenia, gynecomastia, gingival hyperplasia, petechiae, ecchymosis, purpura, bruising, hematoma, leukopenia, double vision, epistaxis, eye irritation, thirst, alopecia, bundle branch block, abnormal gait, hyperglycemia.

Additional Drug Interactions

Carbamazepine / ↑ Effect of diltiazem due to ↓ breakdown by liver

Cyclosporine / ↑ Effect of cyclosporine possibly leading to renal toxicity

Lithium / ↑ Risk of neurotoxicity

Laboratory Test Interferences: ↑ Alkaline phosphatase, CPK, LDH, AST, ALT.

Dosage: Tablets, initial: 30 mg q.i.d. before meals and at bedtime; **then,** increase gradually to total daily dose of 180–360 mg given in 3–4 divided doses q 1–2 days. **Capsules, sustained-release (Cardizem-SR), initial:** 60–120 mg b.i.d.; **then,** when maximum antihypertensive effect is reached (approximately 14 days), adjust dosage to a range of 240–360 mg daily. **IV bolus: initial.** 0.25 mg/kg (average 20 mg) given over 2 min. **then,** if response is inadequate, a second bolus dose may be given after 15 min. The second bolus dose is 0.35 mg/kg (average 25 mg) given over 2 min. **IV infusion.** *Atrial fibrillation/flutter:* 10 mg/hr following IV bolus dose(s) of 0.25 mg/kg or 0.35 mg/kg. Some clients may require 5 mg/hr while others may require 15 mg/hr.

NURSING CONSIDERATIONS

See also *Nursing Considerations* for *Calcium Channel Blocking Agents,* p. 119.

Administration/Storage

1. Sublingual nitroglycerin may be taken concomitantly for acute angina.
2. Diltiazem may be taken together with long-acting nitrates.
3. Use with beta-blockers or digitalis is usually well tolerated but the effects of concomitant administration cannot be predicted.
4. The infusion may be maintained for up to 24 hr. Use for more than 24 hr is not recommended.
5. For IV infusion, the drug may be mixed with normal saline, 5% dextrose, or 5% dextrose and 0.45% NaCl.

Assessment

1. Note any evidence of edema.
2. Review lab test results especially those that are indicative of hepatic and/or renal dysfunction and document.
3. Assess ECG for evidence of AV block.

Interventions

1. Anticipate reduced dosage of diltiazem in clients with impaired renal or hepatic function.
2. The plasma half-life of the drug may be prolonged in elderly clients. Therefore, monitor these clients closely.

Client/Family Teaching

1. Drug may cause drowsiness or dizziness.
2. Review the symptoms of postural hypotension and advise client to rise slowly from a lying to a sitting and to a standing position.
3. The client may experience constipation, unusual tiredness, or weakness. Advise to report any persistent and bothersome side effects.
4. Continue carrying short-acting nitrites (nitroglycerin) at all times and use as directed by the physician.

Evaluation: Evaluate client for:
- Reports of symptomatic improvement in the frequency and intensity of vasospastic anginal attacks
- Reduction in blood pressure

Dimenhydrinate
(dye-men-**HY**-drih-nayt)
Elixir, Syrup, Tablets, Chewable Tablets: Apo-Dimenhydrinate✤, Calm-X, Dimentabs, Dramamine, Gravol✤, Marmine, Motion-Aid, Nauseatol✤, Novo–Dimenate✤, Travamine, Travel-Aid✤, Travel Eze✤, Travel Tabs✤, Triptone (OTC). Injection: Dimenhydrinate Injection✤, Dinate, Dommanate, Dramamine, Dramanate, Dramilin, Dramocen, Dramoject, Dymenate, Gravol✤, Hydrate, Marmine, Reidamine, Wehamine (Rx)

See also *Antihistamines,* p. 71, and *Antiemetics,* p. 70.

Classification: Antiemetic/antihistamine.

Action/Kinetics: Dimenhydrinate contains both diphenhydramine and chlorotheophylline. The precise mechanism for the antiemetic effect is not known but the drug does depress labyrinthine and vestibular function. The drug may mask ototoxicity due to aminoglycosides. Possesses anticholinergic activity. **Duration:** 3–6 hr.

Uses: Motion sickness, especially to relieve nausea, vomiting, or dizziness. Treat vertigo.

Special Concerns: Pregnancy category: B. Use of the injectable form is not recommended in neonates. Geriatric clients may be more sensitive to the usual adult dose.

Dosage: Elixir, Syrup, Tablets, Chewable Tablets. Adults: 50–100 mg q 4 hr not to exceed 400 mg/day. **Pediatric, 6–12 years:** 25–50 mg q 6–8 hr, not to exceed 150 mg/day; **2–6 years:** 12.5–25 mg q 6–8 hr, not to exceed 75 mg/day. **Extended-release Capsules. Adults:** 1 capsule q 12 hr. Use is not recommended in children. **IM, IV. Adults:** 50 mg as required. **Pediatric, over 2 years:** 1.25 mg/kg (37.5 mg/m²) q.i.d., not to exceed 300 mg/day. **IV. Adults:** 50 mg in 10 ml sodium chloride injection given over 2 min; may be repeated q 4 hr as needed. **Pediatric:** 1.25 mg/kg (37.6 mg/m²) in 10 ml of 0.9% sodium chloride injection given slowly over 2 min; may be repeated q 6 hr, not to exceed 300 mg daily. **Suppositories. Adults:** 50–100 mg q 6–8 hr. **Pediatric, 12 years and older:** 50 mg q 8–12 hr; **8–12 years:** 25–50 mg q 8–12 hr; **6–8 years:** 12.5–25 mg q 8–12 hr. Dosage not established in children less than 6 years of age.

NURSING CONSIDERATIONS

See also *Nursing Considerations* for *Antihistamines,* p. 74, and *Antiemetics,* p. 71.

Evaluation: Evaluate client for:
- Reports of improvement in symptoms of nausea and vomiting caused by motion sickness
- Control of vertigo
- Any evidence of vestibular damage when administered with antihistamines

—— *COMBINATION DRUG* ——
Dimetane Decongestant Elixir and Tablets
(DYE-meh-tayn)
(OTC)

Classification/Content: *Antihistamine:* Brompheniramine maleate, 4 mg/tablet or 2 mg/5 ml elixir. *Decongestant:* Phenylephrine HCl, 10 mg/tablet or 5 mg/5 ml elixir. Also see information on individual components.

Uses: Relief of symptoms due to the common cold, hay fever, sinusitis, or other upper respiratory tract allergies including sneezing, itchy nose or throat, runny nose, itchy and watery eyes.

Special Concerns: May cause stimulation, especially in children.

Dosage: Tablets. Adults and children over 12 years: One tablet q 4 hr not to exceed 6 tablets daily; **pediatric, 6–12 years:** ½ tablet q 4 hr, not to exceed three whole tablets daily. **Elixir. Adults and children over 12 years:** 10 ml q 4 hr, not to exceed 60 ml daily; **pediatric, 6–12 years:** 5 ml q 4 hr, not to exceed 30 ml daily.

NURSING CONSIDERATIONS

See *Nursing Considerations* for *Antihistamines,* p. 74.

—— COMBINATION DRUG ——
Dimetapp Elixir and Tablets, Dimetapp Plus Caplets

(**DYE**-meh-tap)
(OTC)

Classification/Content: Each Dimetapp tablet contains: *Antihistamine:* Brompheniramine maleate, 4 mg. *Decongestant:* Phenylpropanolamine HCl, 25 mg. The long-acting tablets contain three times the amount of the above drugs while 5 ml of the elixir contains one-half the amount of the above drugs. Each Dimetapp Plus Caplet contains: *Nonnarcotic analgesic:* Acetaminophen, 500 mg. *Antihistamine:* Brompheniramine maleate, 2 mg. *Decongestant:* Phenylpropanolamine HCl, 12.5 mg. See also information on individual components.

Uses: Relief of symptoms due to the common cold, hay fever, sinusitis, or other upper respiratory tract allergies including sneezing, itchy nose or throat, runny nose, or itchy and watery eyes. Dimetapp Plus is indicated for the previous conditions where there is also need for temporary relief of aches and pains, fever, and headache.

Dosage: Tablets. Adults and children over 12 years: One tablet q 4 hr; **pediatric, 6–12 years:** ½ tablet q 4 hr. Dosage for adults should not exceed six tablets daily. **Long-acting tablets. Adults and children over 12 years:** One tablet q 12 hr, not to exceed two tablets in a 24-hr period. **Elixir.**

Adults and children over 12 years: 10 ml q 4 hr, not to exceed 60 ml daily; **pediatric, 6–12 years:** 5 ml q 4 hr, not to exceed 30 ml daily. Consult physician if elixir is indicated in children less than 6 years of age. **Dimetapp Plus Caplets. Adults and children over 12 years:** 2 caplets q 6 hr, not to exceed 8 caplets in a 24-hr period.

NURSING CONSIDERATIONS

See also *Nursing Considerations* for *Antihistamines,* p. 74.

Evaluation: Assess client for subjective reports of symptomatic improvement of allergic manifestations and/or of cold symptoms.

Diphenhydramine hydrochloride

(dye-fen-**HY**-drah-meen)
Allerdryl✱, AllerMax, Beldin Cough, Belix, Bena-D, Bena-D 50, Benadryl, Benadryl Complete Allergy, Benahist 10 and 50, Ben-Allergin-50, Benoject-10 and -50, Benylin Cough, Benaphen, Bydramine Cough, Clear Caladryl Spray✱, Diahist, Dihydrex, Diphenacen-10 and -50, Diphenadryl, Diphen Cough, Fenylhist, Fynex, Hydramine, Hydramine Cough, Hydril, Hyrexin-50, Noradryl, Nordryl, Nordryl Cough, PMS-Diphenhydramine✱, Tusstat, Valdrene, Wehdryl (OTC and Rx). Sleep-Aids: Compoz, Dormarex 2, Insomnal✱, Nervine Nighttime Sleep-Aid, Nytol with DPH, Sleep-Eze 3, Sominex 2, Twilite (OTC)

See also *Antihistamines,* p. 71, *Antiemetics,* p. 70, and *Antiparkinson Agents,* p. 99.

Classification: Antihistamine, antiemetic (ethanolamine-type).

Additional Uses: Treatment of parkinsonism in geriatric clients unable to tolerate more potent drugs. Also for mild parkinsonism in other age groups. Drug-induced extrapyramidal symptoms. Motion sickness, antiemetic, as a sleep-aid. Coughs, including those due to allergy.

Special Concerns: Pregnancy category: B.

Dosage: Capsules, Elixir, Syrup, Tablets. *Antihistamine, antiemetic, antimotion sickness, parkinsonism:* **Adults,** 25–50 mg t.i.d.–q.i.d.; **pediatric, over 9.1 kg:** 12.5–25 mg t.i.d.–q.i.d. (or 5 mg/kg/day not to exceed 300 mg daily). *Sleep aid:* **Adults,** 50 mg at bedtime. *Antitussive:* **Adults,** 25 mg q 4 hr, not to exceed 150 mg daily; **pediatric, 6–12 years:** 12.5 mg q 4 hr, not to exceed 75 mg daily; **pediatric, 2–6 years:** 6.25 mg q 4 hr, not to exceed 25 mg daily. **IV, deep IM, Adults,** 10–50 mg up to 100 mg, not to exceed 400 mg daily; **pediatric:** 5 mg/kg/day, not to exceed 300 mg daily.

NURSING CONSIDERATIONS

See also *Nursing Considerations* for *Antihistamines,* p. 74, *Antiemetics,* p. 71, and *Antiparkinson Agents,* p. 99.

Administration/Storage

1. When using for motion sickness, the full prophylactic dose should be administered 30 min prior to travel.
2. Similar doses should also be taken with meals and at bedtime.
3. Determine client symptoms that necessitate drug adminis-

tration and note as drug has multiple indications.

——— *COMBINATION DRUG* ———

Diphenoxylate hydrochloride with Atropine

(dye-fen-**OX**-ih-layt, **AH**-troh-peen)
Lofene, Logen, Lomanate, Lomodix, Lomotil, Lonox, Low-Quel (C-V) (Rx)

Classification: Antidiarrheal agent, systemic.

Action/Kinetics: Diphenoxylate is a systemic constipating agent chemically related to the narcotic analgesic drug meperidine but without the analgesic properties. Diphenoxylate inhibits GI motility and has a constipating effect. This product may aggravate diarrhea due to organisms that penetrate the intestinal mucosa (e.g., *Escherichia coli, Salmonella, Shigella*) or in antibiotic-induced pseudomembranous colitis. High doses over prolonged periods can, however, cause euphoria and physical dependence. The preparation also contains small amounts of atropine sulfate, which is not present in sufficient quantities to decrease GI motility. However, the atropine will prevent abuse by deliberate overdosage. **Onset:** 45–60 min. **t½, diphenoxylate:** 2.5 hr; **diphenoxylic acid:** 12–24 hr. **Duration:** 2–4 hr. Diphenoxylate is metabolized in the liver to the active diphenoxylic acid and excreted through the urine.

Uses: Symptomatic treatment of chronic and functional diarrhea. Also, diarrhea associated with gastroenteritis, irritable bowel, regional enteritis, malabsorption syndrome, ulcerative colitis, acute infections, food poisoning, postgastrectomy, and drug-induced diarrhea. Therapeutic results for control of acute diarrhea are inconsistent. Also used in the control of intestinal passage time in clients with ileostomies and colostomies.

Contraindications: Obstructive jaundice, liver disease, diarrhea associated with pseudomembranous enterocolitis after antibiotic therapy or enterotoxin-producing bacteria, children under the age of 2.

Special Concerns: Use with caution during pregnancy (category: C) and lactation and in clients in whom anticholinergics may be contraindicated. Use with caution in those with advanced hepatic-renal disease or abnormal renal functions. Children (especially those with Down syndrome) are susceptible to atropine toxicity. Children and geriatric clients may be more sensitive to the respiratory depressant effects of diphenoxylate. Dehydration, especially in young children, may cause a delayed diphenoxylate toxicity.

Side Effects: *GI:* Nausea, vomiting, anorexia, abdominal discomfort, paralytic ileus, megacolon. *Allergic:* Pruritus, angioneurotic edema, swelling of gums. *CNS:* Dizziness, drowsiness, malaise, restlessness, headache, depression, numbness of extremities, respiratory depression, coma. *Topical:* Dry skin and mucous membranes, flushing. *Other:* Tachycardia, urinary retention, hyperthermia. *Symptoms of Overdose:* Dry skin and mucous membranes, flushing, hyperthermia, mydriasis, restlessness, tachycardia followed by miosis, lethargy, hypotonic reflexes, nystagmus, coma, severe (and possibly fatal) respiratory depression.

Drug Interactions

Alcohol / Additive CNS depression
Antianxiety agents / Additive CNS depression
Barbiturates / Additive CNS depression
MAO inhibitors / ↑ Chance of hypertensive crisis
Narcotics / ↑ Effect of narcotics

Dosage: Oral Solution, Tablets. Adults, initial: 2.5–5 mg (of diphenoxylate) t.i.d.–q.i.d.; **maintenance:** 2.5 mg b.i.d.–t.i.d. **Pediatric, 2–12 years:** 0.3–0.4 mg/kg/day (of diphenoxylate) in divided doses. Contraindicated in children under 2 years of age. See also below.

Pediatric / Dose

2–3 years / 0.75–1.5 mg q.i.d.
3–4 years / 1–1.5 mg q.i.d.
4–5 years / 1–2 mg q.i.d.
5–6 years / 1.25–2.25 mg q.i.d.
6–9 years / 1.25–2.5 mg q.i.d.
9–12 years / 1.75–2.5 mg q.i.d.

Based on 4 ml/tsp or 2 mg of diphenoxylate. Each tablet or 5 ml of liquid preparation contains 2.5 mg diphenoxylate hydrochloride and 25 mcg of atropine sulfate. Dosage should be maintained at initial levels until symptoms are under control; then reduce to maintenance levels.

NURSING CONSIDERATIONS

See also *Nursing Considerations* for *Difenoxin HCl with Atropine sulfate,* p. 545.

Administration/Storage

1. For liquid preparations, use only the plastic dropper supplied by the manufacturer to measure the dosage of drug.

2. If clinical improvement is not seen after 10 days with a maximum dose of 20 mg daily, further use will not likely control symptoms.
3. *Treatment of Overdose:* Gastric lavage, induce vomiting, establish a patent airway, and assist respiration. Activated charcoal (100 g) given as a slurry. IV administration of a narcotic antagonist. Administration may be repeated after 10–15 min. Observe client and readminister antagonist if respiratory depression returns.

Assessment

1. Note any evidence of hepatic or renal dysfunction.
2. Determine fluid and electrolyte status. Dehydration in young children may cause a delayed diphenoxylate toxicity.

Evaluation

1. Assess client for a decrease in the number and frequency of diarrheal stools.
2. Review laboratory culture reports to determine if drug is appropriate therapy for diarrhea especially if it is not effective within 24–36 hr after administration.

Dipyridamole
(dye-peer-**ID**-ah-mohl)
Apo-Dipyridamole✿, Dipimol, Dipridacot, Novo–Dipiradol✿, Persantine, Persantine IV, Pyridamole (Rx)

Classification: Adjunct to coumarin anticoagulants.

Action/Kinetics: Dipyridamole inhibits platelet adhesion by mechanisms that might include inhibition of uptake of adenosine, an inhibitor of platelet adhesion; inhibition of thromboxane A_2, a stimulator of platelet activity; or, inhibition of phosphodiesterase which increases cyclic-3',5'-AMP within platelets. **Peak plasma levels after PO:** 75 min. **t½, initial:** 40 min; **terminal:** 10 hr. Highly protein bound. Dipyridamole is metabolized in the liver to inactive compounds which are excreted through the bile.

Uses: In combination with warfarin to prevent thromboembolism in clients with prosthetic heart valves. IV to evaluate coronary artery disease (as an alternative to exercise in thallium myocardial perfusion in those who cannot exercise appropriately). *Investigational:* In combination with aspirin to prevent myocardial infarction and coronary bypass graft occlusion. **Note:** Although used in the past to treat chronic angina, this combination is no longer recommended because it is no more effective than aspirin alone.

Contraindications: Sensitivity to dipyridamole.

Special Concerns: Pregnancy category: B. Use with caution in clients with hypotension and during lactation. Safety and efficacy have not been demonstrated in children less than 12 years of age.

Side Effects: PO. *CNS:* Headaches, dizziness, weakness, or syncope. *GI:* Nausea, GI distress. *Other:* Flushing, skin rashes pruritus. Rarely, aggravation of angina pectoris. **IV:** *CV:* Fatal and nonfatal myocardial infarction, symptomatic ventricular tachycardia, ventricular fibrillation, transient cerebral ischemia. Palpitation, bradycardia, AV block, ortho-

D

static hypotension, atrial fibrillation, supraventricular tachycardia, cardiomyopathy, edema. *CNS:* Anxiety, vertigo, nervousness, hypothesia, tremor, hypertonia, dysphoria, sleepiness, migraine, abnormal coordination. *GI:* Dyspepsia, dry mouth, abdominal pain, flatulence, vomiting, dysphagia, increased appetite, tenesmus. *Respiratory:* Bronchospasms, pharyngitis, rhinitis, hyperventilation, coughing, pleural pain. *Musculoskeletal:* Myalgia, back pain, asthenia, arthralgia. *EENT:* Earache, tinnitus, vision abnormalities, eye pain. *Miscellaneous:* Diaphoresis, reaction at injection site, rigor, dysgeusia, thirst, depersonalization, renal pain, perineal pain, breast pain, leg cramping, intermittent claudication. *Symptom of Overdose:* Hypotension.

Drug Interactions

Alteplase / ↑ Risk of bleeding
Aspirin / ↑ Anticoagulant effect
Theophylline / ↓ Coronary
  vasodilation caused by
  dipyridamole → false (−)
  results of thallium imaging

Dosage: Tablets. *Adjunct to prevent thromboembolism after cardiac valve replacement:* 75–100 mg q.i.d. with warfarin. A dose of 100 mg daily when given with 1 g aspirin daily. **Note:** Differences in bioavailability between products may occur. **IV infusion.** *Platelet aggregation inhibitor:* 250 mg daily at a rate of 10 mg/hr. **IV,** *Diagnosis of coronary artery disease:* 0.142 mg/kg/min (0.57 mg/kg total) infused over 4 min. Dilute in 1:2 ratio with 0.5 N or 1 N sodium chloride injection or 5% dextrose injection. Thallium should be injected within 5 min after the infusion of dipyridamole.

NURSING CONSIDERATIONS

Administration/Storage: *Treatment of Overdose:* A vasopressor may be used if necessary.

Assessment

1. Determine if client is taking or receiving any drugs such as aspirin, theophylline or alteplase that may interact with dipyridamole.
2. Obtain baseline ECG and note any evidence of abnormal cardiac status.
3. Document baseline vital signs and bleeding times (PT/PTT).

Client/Family Teaching

1. Do not take any unprescribed drugs, such as aspirin, without first consulting the physician.
2. Do not switch brands without physician approval since there may be differences in drug bioavailability.
3. Report any symptoms such as weakness, dizziness, or faintness. These may have been potentiated by the medication and may indicate a need to change the drug regimen.
4. Clinical responses to drug therapy may be delayed from 1–3 months. Therefore, clients need to be encouraged to continue to comply with the drug regimen even if discouraged by this delay.
5. Provide a printed list of adverse drug effects. Stress those that require immediate reporting such as palpitations, chest pain, confusion, and respiratory difficulty.
6. Avoid alcohol and tobacco products because of hypotensive vasoconstrictive effects.

Evaluation: Evaluate client for:

- Prevention of thromboembolism (with warfarin) following valve replacement
- Prevention of coronary bypass graft occlusion (with ASA) and prevention of AMI

Disopyramide

(dye-so-**PEER**-ah-myd)

Napamide, Norpace, Norpace CR, Rythmodan✻, Rythmodan-LA✻ (Rx)

Classification: Antiarrhythmic, type IA.

Action/Kinetics: Disopyramide reduces the excitability of cardiac muscle to electrical stimulation and prolongs the refractory period. It manifests anticholinergic effects although it has fewer side effects than quinidine. The drug does not affect blood pressure significantly and it can be used in digitalized and nondigitalized clients. **Onset:** 30 min. **Peak plasma levels:** 2 hr. **Duration:** average of 6 hr (range 1.5–8 hr). **t½:** 5–8 hr. **Therapeutic serum levels:** 2–8 mcg/ml. Serum levels should not be used to adjust the dose because of variance in protein binding and potential toxicity of unbound drug. **Protein binding:** 40%–60%. Both unchanged drug (50%) and metabolites (30%) are excreted through the urine. Approximately 15% is excreted through the bile.

Uses: Prevention, recurrence, and control of unifocal, multifocal, and paired premature ventricular contractions. Arrhythmias in coronary artery disease. *Investigational:* Ventricular arrhythmias in emergency conditions, paroxysmal supraventricular tachycardia.

Contraindications: Hypersensitivity to drug. Cardiogenic shock, heart failure, heart block, especially preexisting second- and third-degree AV block, glaucoma, urinary retention.

Special Concerns: Safe use during pregnancy (category: C), childhood, labor, and delivery has not been established. Geriatric clients may be more sensitive to the anticholinergic effects of this drug.

Side Effects: *CV:* Hypotension, congestive heart failure, edema, weight gain, cardiac conduction disturbances, hypotension, shortness of breath, syncope, chest pain. *Anticholinergic:* Dry mouth, urinary retention, constipation, blurred vision, dry nose, eyes, and throat. *GU:* Urinary frequency and urgency. *GI:* Nausea, pain, flatulence, anorexia, diarrhea, vomiting. *CNS:* Headache, nervousness, dizziness, fatigue, depression, insomnia, psychoses. *Dermatologic:* Rash/dermatoses. *Other:* Fever, respiratory problems, gynecomastia, anaphylaxis, malaise, muscle weakness, numbness, tingling, angle-closure glaucoma. *Symptoms of Overdose:* Apnea, loss of consciousness, cardiac arrhythmias (widening of QRS complex and QT interval, conduction disturbances), hypotension, bradycardia, anticholinergic symptoms, death.

Drug Interaction: Phenytoin and rifampin ↓ effect due to ↑ breakdown by liver.

Dosage: Capsules. *Individualized.* **Initial loading dose:** 300 mg (200 mg if client weighs less than 50 kg); **maintenance:** 400–800 mg/day in 4 divided doses (usual: 150 mg q 6 hr). *For clients less than 50 kg:* **maintenance:** 100 mg q 6

hr. If controlled-release form used, administer q 12 hr. *Severe refractory tachycardia:* up to 400 mg q 6 hr may be required. *Cardiomyopathy:* do not administer a loading dose; give 100 mg q 6 hr. For all uses, dosage must be decreased in clients with renal or hepatic insufficiency. *Moderate renal failure or hepatic failure:* 100 mg q 6 hr (or 200 mg q 12 hr of sustained-release form). *Severe renal failure:* 100 mg q 8–24 hr depending on severity.
Capsules, extended-release. *Arrhythmias:* 300 mg q 12 hr (200 mg q 12 hr if client weighs less than 50 kg).

NURSING CONSIDERATIONS

See also *Nursing Considerations* for *Antiarrhythmic Drugs,* p. 52.

Administration/Storage

1. Administer drug only after ECG assessment has been done.
2. Administer with caution to clients who are receiving or who have recently received other antiarrhythmic agents.
3. The extended-release capsule should not be used for initial dosage. These are intended for maintenance therapy.
4. When the client is being transferred from the regular oral capsule, the first extended-release capsule should be given 6 hr after the last regular dose.
5. *Treatment of Overdose:* Induction of vomiting, gastric lavage, or a cathartic followed by activated charcoal. Monitor ECG. IV isoproterenol, IV dopamine, cardiac glycosides, diuretics, intraaortic balloon counterpulsation, artificial respiration, hemodialysis. Use endocardial pacing to treat AV block and neostigmine to treat anticholinergic symptoms.

Assessment

1. Determine if client has been taking other antiarrhythmic agents and document the response to that therapy.
2. Check client history for any evidence of hypersensitivity to the drug.
3. Note any client complaint of dribbling, frequency of voiding, or sensation of bladder fullness. The condition may worsen once the client begins taking disopyramide.
4. Determine serum potassium levels and, if low, take corrective measures before initiating therapy.

Interventions

1. Clients who have been receiving other antiarrhythmic agents and who are now being placed on disopyramide therapy need to be monitored closely for anticholinergic side effects.
2. Monitor BP frequently for hypotensive effect. Clients with poor left ventricular function are more likely to develop hypotension and require close monitoring.
3. If the client is receiving the drug in the hospital, monitor ECG for QRS widening and QT prolongation. If this occurs, the drug should be discontinued.
4. Note symptoms of congestive heart failure, such as cough, dyspnea, moist rales, and cyanosis.
5. Monitor serum potassium levels to ensure effective response to disopyramide. Hyperkalemia increases drug toxicity.

6. Assess intake and output. Question clients about urinary hesitancy, difficulty voiding, or a sense of not completely emptying the bladder. This is particularly important in men with hypertrophy of the prostate and elderly clients who have had prior urinary tract problems. Palpate the bladder if hesitancy is severe.
7. Weigh client daily and record.
8. If the ECG shows a new onset of first-degree heart block, do not administer the drug. Report the incident to the physician and anticipate the dosage of drug will be reduced.

Client/Family Teaching

1. Instruct clients how to take their own BP and assist to develop a method to maintain a written record for physician evaluation and review.
2. Increase intake of fruit juices and other bulk foods to prevent constipation.
3. For complaints of dry mouth suggest using frequent mouth rinses, chewing gum, or sucking on hard candy (use sugarfree varieties).
4. Avoid using alcohol.
5. Review the symptoms of congestive heart failure (edema, cough, sudden weight gain, dyspnea) and stress the importance of reporting these findings immediately to the physician.
6. Change positions slowly and avoid hot showers, temperature extremes, exposure to the sun, or prolonged standing.
7. Report any evidence of mental confusion.
8. Take only as prescribed. Do not omit drug doses.

Evaluation: Evaluate for:
- A decrease in the frequency and occurrence of ventricular arrhythmias
- Client response and tolerance to drug as well as side effects to determine appropriate drug dose

Disulfiram
(dye-**SUL**-fih-ram)
Antabuse (Rx)

Classification: Treatment of alcoholism.

Action/Kinetics: Disulfiram produces severe hypersensitivity to alcohol. It is used as an adjunct in the treatment of alcoholism. The toxic reaction to disulfiram appears to be due to the inhibition of liver enzymes that participate in the normal degradation of alcohol. When alcohol and disulfiram are both present, acetaldehyde accumulates in the blood. High levels of acetaldehyde produce a series of symptoms referred to as the disulfiram-alcohol reaction or syndrome. The specific symptoms are listed under *Side Effects*. The symptoms vary individually, are dose-dependent with respect to both alcohol and disulfiram, and persist for periods ranging from 30 min to several hours. A single dose of disulfiram may be effective for 1–2 weeks. **Onset:** May be delayed up to 12 hr because disulfiram is initially localized in fat stores.

Uses: To prevent further ingestion of alcohol in chronic alcoholics. Disulfiram should be given only to cooperating clients fully aware of the consequences of alcohol ingestion.

Contraindications: Alcohol intoxication. Severe myocardial or occlusive coronary disease. Use of paraldehyde or alcohol-containing products such as cough syrups. If client is exposed to ethylene dibromide.

Special Concerns: Use in pregnancy only if benefits outweigh risks. Use with caution in narcotic addicts or clients with diabetes, goiter, epilepsy, psychosis, hypothyroidism, hepatic cirrhosis, or nephritis.

Side Effects: In the absence of alcohol, the following symptoms have been reported: Drowsiness (most common), headache, restlessness, fatigue, psychoses, peripheral neuropathy, dermatoses, hepatotoxicity, metallic or garlic taste, arthropathy, impotence. **In the presence of alcohol,** the following symptoms may be manifested. *CV:* Flushing, chest pain, palpitations, tachycardia, hypotension, syncope, arrhythmias, cardiovascular collapse, myocardial infarction, acute congestive heart failure. *CNS:* Throbbing headaches, vertigo, weakness, uneasiness, confusion, unconsciousness, seizures, death. *GI:* Nausea, severe vomiting, thirst. *Respiratory:* Respiratory difficulties, dyspnea, hyperventilation, respiratory depression. *Other:* Throbbing in head and neck, sweating. In the event of an Antabuse–alcohol interaction, measures should be undertaken to maintain blood pressure and treat shock. Oxygen, antihistamines, ephedrine, and/or vitamin C may also be used.

Drug Interactions

Anticoagulants, oral / ↑ Effect of anticoagulants by ↑ hypoprothrombinemia

Barbiturates / ↑ Effect of barbiturates due to ↓ breakdown by liver

Chlordiazepoxide, diazepam / ↑ Effect of chlordiazepoxide or diazepam due to ↓ plasma clearance

Isoniazid / ↑ Side effects of isoniazid (especially CNS)

Metronidazole / Acute toxic psychosis or confusional state

Paraldehyde / Concomitant use produces Antabuse-like effect

Phenytoin / ↑ Effect of phenytoin due to ↓ breakdown by liver

Tricyclic antidepressants / Acute organic brain syndrome

Dosage: Tablets. Adults, initial (after alcohol-free interval of 12–48 hr): 500 mg daily for 1–2 weeks; **maintenance: usual,** 250 mg daily (range: 120–500 mg daily). Dose should not exceed 500 mg/day.

NURSING CONSIDERATIONS

Administration/Storage

1. Tablets can be crushed or mixed with liquid.
2. Clients should always carry appropriate identification indicating disulfiram is being taken.
3. Have oxygen, pressor agents, and antihistamines available to treat disulfiram-alcohol reactions.

Client/Family Teaching

1. Emphasize to the family that disulfiram should never be given to the client without client's knowledge.
2. Explain the effects of disulfiram and emphasize the need for close medical and psychiatric supervision.
3. If the client experiences CNS

side effects, explain that these will lessen as the drug is continued.

4. Explain that ingesting as little as 30 ml of 100-proof alcohol (e.g., one shot) while on disulfiram therapy may cause severe symptoms and possibly death.

5. Advise the client to avoid alcohol in any form, in foods, sauces, or other medications, such as cough syrups or tonics. Clients should also be advised to avoid vinegar, paregoric, liniments, or lotions containing alcohol.

6. Instruct the client to read carefully all labels on foods before consuming them to avoid those that may contain alcohol.

7. Discuss with clients the fact that they may feel tired, experience drowsiness, headaches and develop a metallic or garlic-like taste. These side effects tend to subside after about 2 weeks of therapy.

8. Explain to male clients that they may have occasional impotence. This is usually transient. Remind clients that they should discuss this problem with the physician before discontinuing the medication.

9. If skin eruptions occur, advise the client to consult the physician since an antihistamine may be prescribed.

10. Advise clients to carry an identification card stating that they are taking disulfiram and describing the symptoms and treatment if clients have a disulfiram reaction. Included should be the name of the physician treating the client and a telephone number where the physician may be reached. (Cards may be obtained from the Wyeth-Ayerst Laboratories, PO Box 8299, Philadelphia, PA 19101-1245; attention: Professional Services.)

11. Advise the client and family to attend meetings of local support groups such as Alcoholics Anonymous (AA) and Al-Anon to gain a better understanding of the disease. These groups offer the support, structure, referral, and encouragement that may help the client in the quest for an alcohol-free life.

Evaluation

1. Evaluate client knowledge and understanding of disease and compliance with drug therapy.

2. Note side effects that may necessitate adjustment in drug dosage.

3. Assess for freedom from alcohol and its effects with resultant sobriety.

Divalproex sodium

(dye-**VAL**-proh-ex)
Depakote, Epival✢ (Rx)

See *Valproic Acid,* p. 1260.

Dobutamine hydrochloride

(doh-**BYOU**-tah-meen)
Dobutrex (Rx)

See also *Sympathomimetic Drugs,* p. 218.

Classification: Direct-acting adrenergic (sympathomimetic) agent, cardiac stimulant.

Action/Kinetics: Stimulates beta-1 receptors (in the heart), increasing cardiac function, cardiac output, and stroke volume, with minor effects on heart rate. The drug decreases after load reduction although systolic blood pressure and pulse pressure may remain unchanged or increase (due to increased cardiac output). Dobutamine also decreases elevated ventricular filling pressure and helps AV node conduction. **Onset:** 1–2 min. **Peak effect:** 10 min. **t½:** 2 min. **Therapeutic plasma levels:** 40–190 ng/ml. Metabolized by the liver and excreted in urine.

Uses: Short-term treatment of cardiac decompensation secondary to depressed contractility due to organic heart disease or cardiac surgical procedures.

Contraindications: Idiopathic hypertrophic subaortic stenosis.

Special Concerns: Safe use during pregnancy, childhood, or after acute myocardial infarction not established.

Side Effects: *CV:* Marked increase in heart rate, BP, and ventricular ectopic activity. Anginal and nonspecific chest pain, palpitations. *Other:* Nausea, headache, and shortness of breath.

Additional Drug Interactions: Concomitant use with nitroprusside causes ↑ cardiac output and ↓ pulmonary wedge pressure.

Dosage: IV infusion: *individualized,* **usual,** 2.5–15 mcg/kg/min (up to 40 mcg/kg/min). Rate of administration and duration of therapy depend on response of client, as determined by heart rate, presence of ectopic activity, BP, and urine flow.

NURSING CONSIDERATIONS

See also *Nursing Considerations* for *Sympathomimetic Drugs,* p. 220.

Administration/Storage

1. Reconstitute solution according to directions provided by manufacturer. Dilution process takes place in two stages.
2. The more concentrated solution may be stored in refrigerator for 48 hr and at room temperature for 6 hr.
3. Before administration, the solution is diluted further according to the fluid needs of the client. This more dilute solution should be used within 24 hr.
4. Dilute solutions of dobutamine may darken. This does not affect the potency of the drug when used within the time spans detailed above.
5. The drug is incompatible with alkaline solutions.
6. Have available IV equipment to infuse volume expanders before therapy with dobutamine is started.
7. Medication should be administered utilizing an electronic infusion device. Carefully reconstitute and calculate dosage according to the client's weight.

Interventions

1. Be prepared to monitor central venous pressure to assess vascular volume and efficiency of cardiac pumping on the right side of the heart. The normal range is 5–10 cm water.
2. An elevated central venous pressure generally indicates disruption of cardiac output, as in pump failure or pulmonary edema. A low central venous pressure (CVP) may indicate hypovolemia.
3. Be prepared to monitor pul-

monary artery wedge pressure (PACWP) to determine the pressures in the left atrium and left ventricle and to measure the efficiency of cardiac output. The usual wedge pressure range is 4–12 mm Hg.

4. Monitor ECG and blood pressure continuously during drug administration.

5. Obtain written parameters for systolic blood pressure and titrate infusion as ordered.

6. Monitor and record intake and output.

Evaluation: Evaluate client for:

• Improved cardiac output based on CVP and/or PACWP readings

• Systolic blood pressure greater than 90 mm Hg

• Increased urinary output

Docusate calcium (Dioctyl calcium sulfosuccinate)

(DEW-kyou-sayt)

Calax✹, DC Softgels, Doxate-C✹, Novo–Docusate Calcium✹, PMS Docusate Calcium✹, Pro-Cal-Sof, Sulfalax Calcium, Surfak✹, Surfak Liquigels (OTC)

Docusate potassium (Dioctyl potassium sulfosuccinate)

(DEW-kyou-sayt)

Dialose, Diocto-K, Kasof (OTC)

Docusate sodium (Dioctyl sodium sulfosuccinate)

(DEW-kyou-sayt)

Colace, Diocto, Dioeze, Disonate, DOK, DOS Softgel,

Doxate-S✹, Doxinate, D-S-S, Modane Soft, Novo–Docusate✹, Pro-Sof, Pro-Sof Liquid Concentrate Regulex✹, Regulax SS, Regulex✹, Regutol, Selax✹ (OTC)

See also *Laxatives,* p. 171.

Classification: Laxative, emollient.

Action/Kinetics: These laxatives promote defecation by softening the feces. Useful when it is desirable to keep the feces soft or when straining at stool is undesirable. They act by lowering the surface tension of the feces and promoting their penetration by water and fat, thus increasing the softness of the fecal mass. Docusate is not absorbed systemically and does not seem to interfere with the absorption of nutrients. **Onset:** 24–72 hr.

Uses: To lessen strain of defecation in persons with hernia or cardiovascular diseases or other diseases in which straining at stool should be avoided. Megacolon or bedridden clients. Constipation associated with dry, hard stools.

Contraindications: Nausea, vomiting, abdominal pain, and intestinal obstruction.

Special Concerns: Pregnancy category: C.

Drug Interactions: Docusate may ↑ absorption of mineral oil from the GI tract.

Dosage: *Docusate calcium.* **Capsules. Adults:** 240 mg daily until bowel movements are normal; **pediatric, over 6 years:** 50–150 mg daily. *Docusate potassium.* **Capsules. Adults,** 100–300 mg daily; **pediatric, over 6 years:** 100 mg at bedtime. *Docusate sodium.* **Capsules, Oral Solution, Syrup,**

Tablets. **Adults and children over 12 years:** 50–500 mg; **pediatric, under 3 years:** 10–40 mg; **3–6 years:** 20–60 mg; **6–12 years:** 40–120 mg. **Rectal Solution.** *Flushing or retention enema:* 50–100 mg.

NURSING CONSIDERATIONS

See also *Nursing Considerations* for *Laxatives,* p. 172.

Administration/Storage

1. Administer oral solutions of docusate sodium with milk or fruit juices to help mask the bitter taste.
2. If docusate sodium is to be used in enemas, add 50–100 mg (5–10 ml) to a retention or flushing enema.
3. A glass of water should be consumed with each oral dose of docusate sodium.
4. Because docusate salts are minimally absorbed, it may require 1–3 days to soften fecal matter.

Evaluation: Evaluate client for elimination of a soft formed stool with a minimum of effort.

——— COMBINATION DRUG ———
Donnatal capsules, elixir, tablets
(DON-nah-tal)
(Rx)

Classification/Content: Each tablet, capsule, or 5-ml elixir contains: *Anticholinergic:* Atropine sulfate, 0.0194 mg. *Anticholinergic:* Hyoscyamine sulfate, 0.1037 mg. *Anticholinergic:* Scopolamine hydrobromide, 0.0065 mg. *Sedative:* Phenobarbital, 16.2 mg. **Note:** The Extentabs contain three times the amount of drugs found in tablets.

Uses: Possibly effective as an adjunct in the treatment of irritable colon, spastic colon, mucous colitis, and acute enterocolitis. Has also been used in the treatment of duodenal ulcer.

Special Concerns: Pregnancy category: C. It is not known with certainty whether or not anticholinergic drugs aid in the healing in duodenal ulcer or decrease the rate of recurrence or prevent complications.

Dosage: Capsules, Elixir, Tablets. Adults, usual: 1–2 tablets or capsules t.i.d.–q.i.d. (or one Extentab q 12 hr). If the elixir is used, **adult, usual:** 5–10 ml t.i.d.–q.i.d. **Pediatric:** Use elixir as follows: **4.5–9.0 kg:** 0.5 ml q 4 hr or 0.75 ml q 6 hr; **9.1–13.5 kg:** 1.0 ml q 4 hr or 1.5 ml q 6 hr; **13.6–22.6 kg:** 1.5 ml q 4 hr or 2.0 ml q 6 hr; **22.7–33.9 kg:** 2.5 ml q 4 hr or 3.75 ml q 6 hr. **34.1–45.3 kg:** 3.75 ml q 4 hr or 5 ml q 6 hr; **45.4 kg:** 5 ml q 4 hr or 7.5 ml q 6 hr.

NURSING CONSIDERATIONS

See *Nursing Considerations* for *Cholinergic Blocking Agents,* p. 138, and *Barbiturates,* p. 104.

Dopamine hydrochloride
(DOH-pah-meen)
Intropin, Revimine✦ (Rx)

See also *Sympathomimetic Drugs,* p. 218.

Classification: Direct and indirect-acting adrenergic (sympathomimetic) agent, cardiac stimulant and vasopressor.

Action/Kinetics: Dopamine is the immediate precursor of epinephrine in the body. Exogenously administered, dopamine produces direct stimulation of beta-1 receptors and variable (dose-dependent) stimulation of alpha receptors (peripheral vasoconstriction). Also, dopamine will cause a release of norepinephrine from its storage sites. These actions result in increased myocardial contraction, cardiac output, and stroke volume, as well as increased renal blood flow and sodium excretion. Exerts little effect on diastolic BP and induces fewer arrhythmias than are seen with isoproterenol. **Onset:** 5 min. **Duration:** 10 min. **t½:** 2 min. Metabolized in liver and excreted in urine.

Uses: Cardiogenic shock, especially in myocardial infarctions associated with severe CHF. Also shock associated with trauma, septicemia, open heart surgery, renal failure, and CHF. Especially suitable for clients who react adversely to isoproterenol. Poor perfusion of vital organs; hypotension due to poor cardiac output. CHF in clients refractory to digitalis and diuretics. Cardiac output may be increased if dopamine is combined with dobutamine, isoproterenol, or sodium nitroprusside.

Additional Contraindications: Pheochromocytoma, uncorrected tachycardia or arrhythmias. Pediatric clients.

Special Concerns: Use in pregnancy only if benefits outweigh risks (pregnancy category: C). Dosage has not been established in children. Dosage may have to be adjusted in geriatric clients with occlusive vascular disease.

Additional Side Effects: *CV:* Ectopic heartbeats, tachycardia, anginal pain, palpitations, vasoconstriction, hypotension, hypertension. *Other:* Dyspnea, headache, mydriasis.

Additional Drug Interactions

Diuretics / Additive or potentiating effect
Phenytoin / Hypotension and bradycardia
Propranolol / ↓ Effect of dopamine

Dosage: IV infusion: Initial, 1–5 mcg/kg/min; **then,** increase in increments of 1–4 mcg/kg/min at 10–30 min intervals until desired response is obtained. *Severely ill clients:* **initial,** 5 mcg/kg/min; **then,** increase rate in increments of 5–10 mcg/kg/min up to 20–50 mcg/kg/min as needed.

NURSING CONSIDERATIONS

See also *Nursing Considerations for Sympathomimetics,* p. 220.

Administration/Storage

1. Drug must be diluted before use—see package insert.
2. Dilute solution is stable for 24 hr. Protect from light.
3. To prevent overloading system with excess fluid, clients receiving high doses of dopamine may receive more concentrated solutions than average.
4. Medication should be administered utilizing an electronic infusion device. Carefully reconstitute and calculate dosage according to the client's weight.
5. Check infusion site frequently for extravasation. Sloughing and necrosis may occur. If extravasation occurs, local subcutaneous administration of diluted phentolamine may decrease the sloughing (see package insert).

Interventions

1. Monitor blood pressure and ECG continuously during drug administration.
2. Obtain written parameters for systolic blood pressure and titrate the infusion as ordered.
3. Monitor intake and output. If medication is being administered for renal perfusion, infuse as ordered, usually less than 5 mcg/kg/min.
4. Be prepared to monitor central venous pressure and pulmonary artery wedge pressures.
5. Monitor the client for ectopic heart beats, palpitations, anginal pain or vasoconstriction. If these side effects occur, document and report them to the physician.

Evaluation: Evaluate client for:

- Systolic BP greater than 90 mm Hg
- Improved organ perfusion as evidenced by increased urinary output

---

Doxacurium chloride
(dox-ah-**KYOUR**-ee-um **KLOR**-ide)
Neuromax (Rx)

Classification: Neuromuscular blocking agent.

Action/Kinetics: Doxacurium binds to cholinergic receptors on the motor end-plate to block the action of acetylcholine; this results in a blockade of neuromuscular transmission. Doxacurium is up to three times more potent than pancuronium and up to twelve times more potent than metocurine. The time to maximum neuromuscular blockade during balanced anesthesia is dose-dependent and ranges from 9.3 min (following doses of 0.025 mg/kg) to 3.5 min (following doses of 0.08 mg/kg). The time to 25% recovery from blockade following balanced anesthesia ranges from 55 min for doses of 0.025 mg/kg to 160 min for doses of 0.08 mg/kg. **t½, elimination:** Dose-dependent, ranging from 86–123 min. The half-life is prolonged in kidney transplant clients. Children require higher doses on a mg/kg basis than adults to achieve the same level of blockade. Also, the onset, time, and duration of block are shorter in children than adults. The blockade may be reversed by anticholinesterase agents. The drug is excreted unchanged through the urine and bile.

Uses: Adjunct to general anesthesia to provide skeletal muscle relaxation during surgery. Skeletal muscle relaxation for endotracheal intubation.

Special Concerns: Pregnancy category: C. Use with caution during lactation. Safety and effectiveness have not been determined in children less than 2 years of age. The duration of action may be up to twice as long for clients over 60 years of age and those who are obese (more than 30% more than ideal body weight for height). Malignant hyperthermia may occur in any client receiving a general anesthetic.

Side Effects: *Neuromuscular:* Skeletal muscle weakness, profound and prolonged skeletal muscle paralysis causing respiratory insufficiency and apnea; difficulty in reversing the neuromuscular blockade. *CV:* Hypotension, flushing, ventricular fibrillation, myocardial infarction. *Respiratory:* Wheezing, bronchospasm. *Dermatologic:* Urticaria, reaction at injection site. *Miscellaneous:* Fever, diplopia.

Symptoms of Overdose: Prolonged neuromuscular block.

Drug Interactions

Aminoglycosides / ↑ Duration of action of doxacurium

Bacitracin / ↑ Duration of action of doxacurium

Carbamazepine / ↑ Onset of effects and shortens the duration of action of doxacurium

Clindamycin / ↑ Duration of action of doxacurium

Colistin / ↑ Duration of action of doxacurium

Enflurane / ↓ Amount of doxacurium necessary to cause blockade and ↑ the duration of action

Halothane / ↓ Amount of doxacurium necessary to cause blockade and ↑ the duration of action

Isoflurane / ↓ Amount of doxacurium necessary to cause blockade and ↑ the duration of action

Lincomycin / ↑ Duration of action of doxacurium

Lithium / ↑ Duration of action of doxacurium

Local anesthetics / ↑ Duration of action of doxacurium

Magnesium salts / ↑ Effects of doxacurium

Phenytoin / ↑ Onset of effects and shortens the duration of action of doxacurium

Polymyxins / ↑ Duration of action of doxacurium

Procainamide / ↑ Duration of action of doxacurium

Quinidine / ↑ Duration of action of doxacurium

Tetracyclines / ↑ Duration of action of doxacurium

Dosage: IV only. Individualized. *As a component of thiopental/narcotic induction-intubation, to produce neuromuscular blockade of long-duration:* **Adults, initial,** 0.05 mg/kg. *If administered during steady-state enflurane, halothane, or isoflurane anesthesia:* Reduce dose by one-third. *Used with succinylcholine to facilitate endotracheal intubation:* 0.025 mg/kg will provide approximately 60 min of effective blockade. **Maintenance doses:** Required about 60 min after an initial dose of 0.025 mg/kg or 100 min after an initial dose of 0.05 mg/kg during balanced anesthesia. Maintenance doses between 0.005–0.01 mg/kg provide an average of 30 min and 45 min, respectively, of additional neuromuscular blockade.

Children. *Administered during halothane anesthesia:* **initially,** 0.03 mg/kg for blockade lasting about 30 min or 0.05 mg/kg for blockade lasting about 45 min. Maintenance doses are required more frequently in children.

NURSING CONSIDERATIONS

See also *Nursing Considerations for Neuromuscular Blocking Agents,* p. 184.

Administration/Storage

1. The dose should be reduced in debilitated clients, in clients with neuromuscular disease, severe electrolyte abnormalities, and carcinomatosis.

2. The dose may need to be increased in burn clients.

3. The dose for obese clients is determined using the ideal body weight (IBW) calculated as follows:
   - For men: IBW (kg) = (106 + [6 x inches in height above 5 feet])/2.2

- For women: IBW (kg) = (106 + [5 x inches in height above 5 feet])/2.2

4. Doxacurium may not be compatible with alkaline solutions with a pH more than 8 (e.g., barbiturates).

5. Doxacurium may be mixed with 5% dextrose injection, 5% dextrose and 0.9% sodium chloride injection, 0.9% sodium chloride injection, lactated Ringer's injection, and 5% dextrose and lactated Ringer's injection. The drug is also compatible with alfentanil, fentanyl, and sufentanil.

6. Doxacurium diluted 1:10 with 5% dextrose injection or 0.9% sodium chloride injection is stable for 24 hr if stored in polypropylene syringes at 5°–25°C (41°–77°F). However, immediate use of the drug, if diluted, is preferable.

7. Any unused portion of diluted doxacurium should be discarded after 8 hr.

8. *Treatment of Overdose:* Maintain a patent airway and use controlled ventilation if necessary until recovery of normal neuromuscular function. Once recovery begins, it can be facilitated by giving neostigmine, 0.06 mg/kg.

Assessment

1. Determine any history of neuromuscular disease as doxacurium may have profound effects in clients with neuromuscular diseases such as myasthenia gravis.

2. Obtain baseline weight and serum electrolytes.

3. Note any drugs client is currently prescribed that may interact unfavorably with doxacurium.

4. Identify burn victims and anticipate altered requirements of drug as these clients tend to develop a resistance to doxacurium.

Interventions

1. The drug should only be given if there are facilities for intubation, artificial respiration, and oxygen therapy, and the availability of an antagonist.

2. The drug should be administered only by those experienced with skeletal muscle relaxants.

3. A peripheral nerve stimulator should be used to monitor drug response.

4. Since doxacurium has no effect on consciousness, pain threshold, or cerebration, it generally should not be administered before unconsciousness, to avoid client stress.

5. Determine client need for additional medication for anxiety and for sedation.

6. Explain all procedures and provide emotional support. Reassure clients that they will be able to talk and move once the drug effects are reversed.

7. Position the client for comfort and so that the body is in proper alignment. Turn client and perform mouth care and eye care frequently.

8. Provide continuous ventilatory support. Make certain that the ventilator alarms are set and on at all times. Assess the client's airway at frequent intervals. Have a suction machine readily available.

9. Monitor and record vital signs, I&O.

Evaluation: Evaluate client for evidence of desired level of skeletal muscle relaxation/paralysis and for suppression of the twitch response when tested with a peripheral nerve stimulator.

Doxapram hydrochloride
(DOX-ah-pram)
Dopram (Rx)

Classification: CNS stimulant, analeptic.

Action/Kinetics: Doxapram increases the rate and depth of respiration by stimulating carotid chemoreceptors. Higher doses also stimulate respiratory centers in the medulla with progressive stimulation of other CNS centers as well (toxic doses may induce tonic-clonic convulsions). An increase in blood pressure may also occur due to increased cardiac output. The drug will antagonize respiratory depression, but not analgesia, induced by narcotics. An increased salivation and release of both gastric acid and catecholamines may be seen. **Onset** (after IV): 20–40 sec. **Peak effect:** 1–2 min. **Duration:** 5–12 min. **t½:** Approximately 2.5–4 hr. Doxapram is metabolized in the liver and is excreted in the urine.

Uses: Respiratory stimulant in mild to moderate drug overdose, drug-induced postanesthetic respiratory depression, apnea not associated with muscle relaxants, acute respiratory insufficiency in chronic obstructive pulmonary disease (used for 2 hr). The analeptic agents are no longer considered drugs of choice in the treatment of CNS depression caused by a severe overdosage of sedatives and hypnotics. Current therapy for overdose of sedative-hypnotics relies largely on supportive therapy, such as establishing a patent airway, administering oxygen, assisting or controlling respiration when necessary, and maintaining blood pressure and blood volume.

Contraindications: Epilepsy, convulsive states, respiratory incompetence due to muscle paresis, flail chest, pneumothorax, pulmonary fibrosis, acute bronchial asthma, extreme dyspnea, severe hypertension, and cerebrovascular accidents. Hypersensitivity. Use in newborns or immature infants (the benzoyl alcohol present may cause a fatal toxic reaction).

Special Concerns: Pregnancy category: B. Use with caution during lactation. Safety and efficacy have not been established in children less than 12 years of age. Use with caution in clients with cerebral edema, asthma, severe cardiovascular disease, hyperthyroidism, and pheochromocytoma (cancer of adrenals), peptic ulcer, or gastric surgery.

Side Effects: *CNS:* Excess stimulation including hyperactivity, clonus, convulsions. Headache, apprehension, dizziness, disorientation. *Autonomic:* Flushing, sweating, paresthesia, feeling of warmth, burning, or hot sensation in area of perineum and genitalia, mydriasis. *GI:* Nausea, vomiting, diarrhea, urge to defecate. *Respiratory:* Bronchospasm, dyspnea, cough, hiccoughs, rebound hypoventilation, laryngospasm, tachypnea. *CV:* Arrhythmias, abnormal ECG, tightness in chest or chest pain, phlebitis, change in heart rate, increase in blood pressure. *GU:* Spontaneous micturition, urinary retention, proteinuria. *Miscellaneous:* Muscle spasms, involuntary movements, pruritus, increased deep tendon reflexes, pyrexia. *Symptoms of Overdose:* Respiratory alkalosis and hypocapnia (too little CO_2 in blood) with tetany and apnea. Also excessive stimulation of CNS, which may result in convulsions. Hypertension, tachycardia, hyperactivity of skeletal muscle, enhanced deep tendon reflexes.

Drug Interactions

Anesthetics, general / Since doxapram increases epinephrine release, do not give until 10 min after anesthetic discontinued if halothane, cyclopropane, or enflurane used to minimize cardiac arrhythmias

MAO inhibitors / Additive pressor effects

Muscle relaxants / Doxapram may mask effects of muscle relaxants

Sympathomimetic amines / Additive pressor effects

Laboratory Test Interferences: ↓ Hemoglobin, hematocrit, RBCs. ↑ BUN, proteinuria.

Dosage: IV. *After anesthesia:* **Single IV injection:** 0.5–1.0 mg/kg, not to exceed 1.5–2.0 mg/kg; may be given in several injections at 5-min intervals. **IV infusion:** 1 mg/ml of dextrose or saline solution, initially at a rate of 5 mg/min; **then,** 1–3 mg/min. Total recommended dose: 4 mg/kg (approximately 300 mg). *Chronic obstructive lung disease with acute hypercapnia:* **IV infusion,** 1–2 mg/min up to maximum of 3 mg/min for no longer than 2 hr. *Drug-induced CNS depression:* **IV injection, initial:** 1–2 mg/kg as a single dose; repeat in 5 min and every 1–2 hr to a maximum of 3 g daily. **Intermittent IV infusion, initial:** 2 mg/kg; **then,** if client not responsive, continue supportive treatment for 1–2 hr and repeat doxapram dose to a maximum of 3 g daily. If response occurs, infuse 1 mg/ml at a rate of 1–3 mg/min. The infusion should be discontinued at the end of 2 hr or if the client awakens.

NURSING CONSIDERATIONS

Administration/Storage

1. Allow a minimum of 10 min between the discontinuation of anesthetic and the administration of doxapram.
2. Children under 12 years of age should not receive doxapram.
3. *Treatment of Overdose:* Have short-acting barbiturates, oxygen, and resuscitative equipment available.

Assessment

1. Note any client history of epilepsy or other convulsive disorders.
2. Obtain a complete baseline assessment of the CNS and ECG prior to the client receiving therapy.
3. Note the age of clients. Elderly people and debilitated clients may be unable to tolerate the increase in respirations caused by doxapram.
4. Obtain baseline arterial blood gases, BP, heart rate, and deep tendon reflexes.
5. Review drugs the client is taking that may interact adversely with doxapram and note on the client's record.

Interventions

1. Drug should only be administered in a closely monitored environment.
2. Frequently assess the client's responses to doxapram as compared with their baseline parameters to detect signs of overdosage and to provide a guide for adjusting the rate of infusion.
3. For at least ½–1 hr after the client is alert, assess for possible poststimulation respiratory depression.
4. Position clients so that, in the event of vomiting, they will not aspirate.
5. Monitor intake and output. If the client has not voided in 2–4 hr, palpate the bladder to detect urinary retention. Catheterization may be required.
6. If the client has persistent diarrhea or vomiting, notify the physician.
7. Ensure a patent airway. Administer oxygen along with the drug to clients suffering from chronic pulmonary insufficiency.
8. Follow seizure precautions after administration of drug. Have available IV diazepam.

Doxazosin mesylate
(dox-AYZ-oh-sin)
Cardura (Rx)

Classification: Antihypertensive.

Action/Kinetics: Doxazosin is a quinazoline compound that blocks the alpha-1 (postjunctional) adrenergic receptors resulting in a decrease in systemic vascular resistance and a corresponding decrease in blood pressure. **Peak plasma levels:** 2–3 hr. **Peak effect:** 2–6 hr. Significantly bound (98%) to plasma proteins. Metabolized in the liver to active and inactive metabolites, which are excreted through the feces and urine. **t½:** 22 hr.

Uses: Alone or in combination with diuretics or beta-adrenergic blocking drugs for the treatment of hypertension.

Contraindications: Use in clients allergic to prazosin or terazosin.

Special Concerns: Pregnancy category: B. Use with caution during lactation. Safety and effectiveness have not been demonstrated in children. Due to the possibility of severe hypotension, the 2-, 4-, and 8-mg tablets are not to be used for initial therapy. Use with caution in clients with impaired hepatic function or in those who are taking drugs known to influence hepatic metabolism.

Side Effects: *CV:* Dizziness (most frequent), syncope, vertigo, lightheadedness, edema, palpitation, arrhythmia, postural hypotension, tachycardia, peripheral ischemia. *CNS:* Fatigue, headache, paresthesia, kinetic disorders, ataxia, somnolence, nervousness, depression, insomnia. *Musculoskeletal:* Arthralgia, arthritis, muscle weakness, muscle cramps, myalgia, hypertonia. *GU:* Polyuria, sexual dysfunction, urinary incontinence, urinary frequency. *GI:* Nausea, diarrhea, dry mouth, constipation, dyspepsia, flatulence, abdominal pain, vomiting. *Respiratory:* Fatigue or malaise, rhinitis, epistaxis, dyspnea. *Miscellaneous:* Rash, pruritus, flushing, abnormal vision, conjunctivitis, eye pain, tinnitus, chest pain, asthenia, facial edema, generalized pain, slight weight gain. *Symptom of Overdose:* Hypotension.

Dosage: Tablets. Adults: initial, 1 mg once daily at bedtime; **then,** depending on the response (client's standing blood pressure both 2–6 hr and 24 hr after a dose), the dose may be increased to 2 mg daily. A maximum of 16 mg daily may be required to control blood pressure.

NURSING CONSIDERATIONS

Administration/Storage

1. To minimize the possibility of severe hypotension, initial dosage should be limited to 1 mg daily.
2. The drug should be given once daily at bedtime.
3. Increasing the dose higher than 4 mg daily increases the possibility of severe syncope, postural dizziness, vertigo, and postural hypotension.
4. *Treatment of Overdose:* IV fluids.

Assessment

1. Note any allergy to prazosin or terazosin as drug is a quinazoline derivative.
2. Determine hepatic function and note any history of liver failure.
3. List drugs client prescribed to ensure there will be no drug interactions.

Client/Family Teaching

1. Instruct client to take BP and to maintain a written record for review at each medical appointment.
2. Show client how to assess for edema and advise to record weight three times a week.
3. Provide a printed list of side

effects and advise client to notify physician if any are persistent or bothersome.
4. Review signs and symptoms of postural hypotension and advise client to rise slowly to a sitting position before attempting to stand.
5. Explain that postural effects are most likely to occur 2–6 hr after a dose.
6. Driving and hazardous tasks should be avoided for 24 hr after the first dose.
7. Provide recommendations concerning appropriate diet and activity schedules to follow.

Evaluation: Evaluate client for:
- Knowledge and understanding of illness as well as level of compliance
- Control of hypertension by maintaining a diastolic pressure of less than 90 mm Hg

---

Doxepin hydrochloride

(**DOX**-eh-pin)

Adapin, Sinequan, Triadapin ✤ (Rx)

See also *Tricyclic Antidepressants,* p. 239.

Classification: Antidepressant, tricyclic.

Action/Kinetics: Doxepin is metabolized to the active metabolite, desmethyldoxepin. It has moderate anticholinergic effects and ability to cause orthostatic hypotension and high sedative effects. **Minimum effective plasma level of both doxepin and desmethyldoxepin:** 100–200 ng/ml. **t½:** 8–24 hr.

Uses: Symptoms of depression. Antianxiety agent, depression accompanied by anxiety and insomnia, depression in clients with manic-depressive illness. Depression or anxiety due to organic disease or alcoholism. Chronic, severe neurogenic pain. Peptic ulcer disease. Dermatologic disorders including chronic urticaria, angioedema, and nocturnal pruritus due to atopic eczema.

Additional Contraindications: Glaucoma or a tendency for urinary retention.

Special Concerns: Safety has not been determined in pregnancy. Not recommended for use in children less than 12 years of age.

Additional Side Effects: Doxepin has a high incidence of side effects, including a high degree of sedation, decreased libido, extrapyramidal symptoms, dermatitis, pruritus, fatigue, weight gain, edema, paresthesia, breast engorgement, insomnia, tremor, chills, tinnitus, and photophobia.

Dosage: Capsules, Oral Solution. *Antidepressant, mild to moderate anxiety or depression:* **Adults:** 25 mg t.i.d. (or up to 150 mg can be given at bedtime); **then,** adjust dosage to individual response (usual optimum dosage: 75–150 mg/day). **Geriatric clients, initially:** 25–50 mg daily; dose can be increased as needed and tolerated. *Severe symptoms:* **Initial,** 50 mg t.i.d.; **then,** gradually increase to 300 mg/day. *Emotional symptoms with organic disease:* 25–50 mg daily. *Antipruritic:* 10–30 mg at bedtime.

NURSING CONSIDERATIONS

See also *Nursing Considerations* for *Tricyclic Antidepressants,* p. 242.

Administration/Storage: Oral concentrate is to be diluted with 4 oz water, fruit juice, or milk just before ingestion. The concentrate should not be mixed with carbonated beverages or grape juice.

Evaluation: Evaluate client for:
- Reports of ↓ symptoms of anxiety and depression
- Evidence of improved sleeping patterns
- Effective control of chronic neurogenic pain
- Improvement in symptoms of dermatologic disorders

Doxorubicin hydrochloride (ADR)
(dox-oh-**ROO**-bih-sin)
Adriamycin PFS, Adriamycin RDF, Rubex (Rx)

See also *Antineoplastic Agents,* p. 85.

Classification: Antineoplastic, antibiotic.

Action/Kinetics: Anthracycline antibiotic produced by *Streptomyces peucetius*. Doxorubicin is cell-cycle specific for the S phase of cell division. Its antineoplastic activity may be due to binding to DNA by intercalating between base pairs resulting in inhibition of synthesis of DNA and RNA by template disordering and steric obstruction. The drug is metabolized in the liver to the active adriamycinol as well as inactive metabolites, which are excreted through the bile. **t½, doxorubicin: biphasic, initial:** 0.6 hr; **final,** 16.7 hr.

Uses: Acute lymphoblastic leukemia, acute myeloblastic leukemia, Wilms' tumor, soft tissue and osteogenic sarcomas, neuroblastoma, cancer of the breast, ovaries, lungs, bladder, and thyroid, lymphomas (Hodgkin's and non-Hodgkin's), bronchogenic carcinoma (especially small cell histologic type). *Investigational:* Cancer of the head and neck, cervix, liver, pancreas, prostate, testes, and endometrium.

Additional Contraindications: Lactation. Depressed bone marrow or cardiac disease. IM or SC use.

Special Concerns: Use in pregnancy only if benefits outweigh risks. Use with caution in impaired hepatic function and necrotizing colitis.

Additional Side Effects: *Myocardial toxicity:* Potentially fatal congestive heart failure. Mucositis, lacrimation, conjunctivitis. Hyperpigmentation of nail beds. Facial flushing if injection is too rapid. Hyperuricemia, red-colored urine (initially). Extravasation may cause severe cellulitis and tissue necrosis. Drug may reactivate previous cardiac, skin, mucosal, and liver radiation damage. Cross-resistance with daunorubicin. Severe myelo-suppression. When combined with cytarabine, necrotizing colitis may occur. *Symptoms of Overdose:* Mucositis, leukopenia, thrombocytopenia. Increased risk of cardiomyopathy and subsequent congestive heart failure with chronic overdosage.

Drug Interactions

Barbiturates / ↑ Plasma clearance of doxorubicin
Cyclophosphamide / ↑ Risk of hemorrhagic cystitis
Digoxin / ↓ Digoxin plasma levels and renal excretion
6-Mercaptopurine / ↑ Risk of hepatotoxicity

Dosage: IV only. *Adults, highly*

individualized: 60–75 mg/m² q 21 days, or 25–30 mg/m² for 3 successive days q 3–4 weeks, or 20 mg/m² every week. Total dose should not exceed 550 mg/m² (440 mg/m² in clients with previous chest irradiation or medications increasing cardiotoxicity). **Pediatric:** 30 mg/m² on 3 successive days q 4 weeks. Use reduced dosage in clients with hepatic dysfunction, depending on serum bilirubin level. If bilirubin is 1.2–3 mg/100 ml, give 50% of usual dose; if it is greater than 3 mg/100 ml, give 25% of usual dose.

NURSING CONSIDERATIONS

See also *Nursing Considerations* for *Antineoplastic Agents,* p. 88.

Administration/Storage

1. Initiate therapy only in hospitalized clients.
2. The drug should be reconstituted with saline to give a final concentration of 2 mg/ml (e.g., dilute 10-mg vial with 5 ml). The reconstituted solution is stable for 24 hr at room temperature and 48 hr if stored at 2°C–8°C (36°F–46°F).
3. If the powder or solution comes in contact with the skin or mucous membranes, wash with soap and water thoroughly.
4. *Do not administer SC or IM because severe necrosis of tissue may result.* To minimize danger of extravasation, inject slowly into tubing of free-flowing IV infusion of either 5% dextrose or sodium chloride injection.
5. Should not be mixed with heparin, dexamethasone sodium phosphate, or cephalothin because a precipitate may form. Mixing with aminophylline or 5-fluorouracil will result

in a change from red to blue-purple indicating decomposition.

6. *Treatment of Overdose:* If the client is myelosuppressed, antibiotics and platelet and granulocyte transfusions may be necessary. Treat symptoms of mucositis.

Interventions

1. Observe client for cardiac arrhythmias and/or respiratory difficulties indicative of cardiac toxicity.
2. Monitor IV administration carefully. Stinging, burning, or edema at injection site indicates extravasation. Administration should be stopped and injection site moved to avoid tissue necrosis.
3. Be prepared with an injectable corticosteroid for local infiltration and flood site with normal saline. Examine area frequently for ulceration that may necessitate early wide excision followed by plastic surgery.

Client/Family Teaching

1. If medication reactivates previous radiotherapy damage, such as erythema, edema, and desquamation, reassure the client that these symptoms should disappear after 7 days.
2. Inform the client that urine will turn red-brown for 1–2 days after initiation of therapy.
3. Advise the client that alopecia may occur but hair will grow back 2–3 months after discontinuation of therapy.
4. Report any flu-like symptoms immediately because drug causes severe myelosuppression.

Evaluation: Evaluate client for:
- Decrease in tumor size and growth
- Improved hematologic parameters

Doxycycline calcium
(dox-ih-**SYE**-kleen)
Vibramycin (Rx)

Doxycycline hyclate
(dox-ih-**SYE**-kleen)
Apo-Doxy ✱, Doryx, Doxy 100 and 200, Doxy-Caps, Doxycin ✱, Doxychel Hyclate, Neo-Vibrin ✱, Novo–Doxylin ✱, Vibramycin, Vibramycin IV, Vibra-Tabs, Vivox (Rx)

Doxycycline monohydrate
(dox-ih-**SYE**-kleen)
Monodox, Vibramycin (Rx)

See also *Anti-Infectives,* p. 80, and *Tetracyclines,* p. 222.

Classification: Antibiotic, tetracycline.

Action/Kinetics: More slowly absorbed, and thus more persistent, than other tetracyclines. Preferred for clients with impaired renal function for treating infections outside the urinary tract. From 80%–95% is bound to serum proteins. **t½:** 14.5–22 hr; 30%–40% excreted unchanged in urine.

Additional Uses: Orally for uncomplicated gonococcal infections in adults (except anorectal infections in males); acute epididymo-orchitis caused by *Neisseria gonorrhoeae* and *Chlamydia trachomatis;* gonococcal arthritis-dermatitis syndrome; nongonococcal urethritis caused by *C. trachomatis* and *Ureaplasma urealyticum.* Prophylaxis of malaria in those intolerant to mefloquine or where drug is contraindicated.

Contraindications: Prophylaxis of malaria in pregnant individuals and in children less than 8 years old. Use during the last half of pregnancy and in children up to 8 years of age (tetracycline may cause permanent discoloration of the teeth). Lactation.

Special Concerns: Safety for IV use in children less than 8 years of age has not been established.

Additional Drug Interaction: Carbamazepine, phenytoin, and barbiturates ↓ effect of doxycycline by ↑ breakdown of doxycycline by the liver.

Dosage: Capsules, Delayed-release Capsules, Oral Suspension, Tablets. IV. Adult: First day, 100 mg q 12 hr; **maintenance:** 100–200 mg daily, depending on severity of infection. **Children, over 8 years (45 kg or less): First day,** 4.4 mg/kg in 1–2 doses; **then,** 2.2–4.4 mg/kg daily in divided doses depending on severity of infection. Children over 45 kg should receive the adult dose. **PO.** *Acute gonorrhea:* 200 mg at once; **then,** 100 mg h.s. (at bedtime) on first day, followed by 100 mg b.i.d. for 3 days. Alternatively, 300 mg immediately followed in 1 hr with 300 mg. *Syphilis (primary/secondary):* 300 mg daily in divided doses for 10 days. *Chlamydia trachomatis infections:* 100 mg b.i.d. for minimum of 7 days. *Prophylaxis of "traveler's diarrhea":* 100 mg daily. *Prophylaxis of malaria:* **Adults,** 100 mg once daily; **Pediatric,** 2 mg/kg daily up to 100 mg/day. **IV.** *Endometritis, parametritis, peritonitis, salpingitis:* 100 mg b.i.d. with 2 g cefoxitin, IV, q.i.d. continued for

at least 4 days or 2 days after improvement observed. This is followed by doxycycline, PO, 100 mg b.i.d. for 10–14 days of total therapy. **Note:** The Centers for Disease Control have established treatment schedules for sexually transmitted diseases.

NURSING CONSIDERATIONS

See also *Nursing Considerations for Tetracyclines,* p. 224, and *General Nursing Considerations For All Anti-Infectives,* p. 83.

Administration/Storage

1. Powder for suspension has expiration date of 12 months from date of issue.
2. Solution stable for 2 weeks when stored in refrigerator.
3. Follow directions on vial for dilution. Concentrations should be no lower than 0.1 mg/ml and no higher than 1.0 mg/ml.
4. During infusion protect solution from light.
5. Complete administration of solutions diluted with NaCl injection, D5W, Ringer's injection, and 10% invert sugar within 12 hr.
6. Complete administration of solutions diluted with lactated Ringer's injection or 5% dextrose in lactated Ringer's injection within 6 hr.
7. Prophylaxis for malaria can begin 1–2 days before travel begins, during travel, and for 4 weeks after leaving the malarious area.

Client/Family Teaching

1. May take with food. To prevent esophageal ulceration take with a full glass of water.

2. Avoid direct exposure to sunlight and wear protective clothing and sunscreens when exposure is necessary.

Evaluation

1. Assess client for reports of symptomatic improvement.
2. Review laboratory culture data to determine efficacy of drug therapy.

—— *COMBINATION DRUG* ——
Drixoral
(drix-**OR**-al)
(OTC)

Classification/Content: *Antihistamine:* Brompheniramine maleate, 2 mg/5 ml elixir or 6 mg/ sustained-release tablet. *Decongestant:* Pseudoephedrine sulfate, 30 mg/5 ml elixir or 120 mg/sustained-release tablet. See also information on individual components.

Uses: Symptoms of the common cold, allergic rhinitis (i.e., hay fever), or other upper respiratory allergies with symptoms of nasal congestion, runny nose, sneezing, itchy nose or throat, itchy and watery eyes.

Dosage: Sustained-release Tablets. Adults and children over 12 years: One tablet q 12 hr, not to exceed 2 tablets in 24 hr. **Syrup. Adults and children over 12 years:** 10 ml q 4–6 hr; **pediatric, 6–12 years:** 5 ml q 4–6 hr. No more than four doses should be given in 24 hr.

NURSING CONSIDERATIONS

See *Nursing Considerations* for *Antihistamines,* p. 74, and *Sympathomimetic Drugs,* p. 220.

Dronabinol (Delta-9-tetrahydro-cannabinol)
(droh-**NAB**-ih-nohl)
Marinol (C-II, Rx)

Classification: Antinauseant.

Action/Kinetics: Dronabinol is the active component in marijuana and, as such, will manifest significant psychoactive effects. These include euphoria, anxiety, panic, depression, paranoia, decrement in memory and cognitive performance, decreased ability to control drives and impulses, and distortion in perception including time. In therapeutic doses, the drug also causes conjunctival injection and an increased heart rate. The antiemetic effect is thought to be due to inhibition of the vomiting center in the medulla. **Peak plasma levels:** 2–3 hr. Significant first-pass effect. The 11-hydroxytetrahydrocannabinol metabolite is active. **t½, biphasic:** 4 hr and 25–36 hr. **t½, 11-hydroxy-THC:** 15–18 hr. Metabolized in the liver and mainly excreted in the feces. Cumulative toxicity using clinical doses may occur.

Use: Nausea and vomiting associated with cancer chemotherapy, especially in clients who have not responded to other antiemetic treatment. Stimulate appetite and prevent weight loss in AIDS patients.

Contraindications: Nausea and vomiting from any cause other than cancer chemotherapy. Lactation. Hypersensitivity to sesame oil.

Special Concerns: Pregnancy category: B. Pediatric and geriatric clients should be monitored carefully due to an increased risk of psychoactive effects. Use with caution in clients with hypertension, heart disease, mania, depression, schizophrenia, and concomitantly with other psychoactive drugs.

Side Effects: *CNS:* Side effects are due mainly to the psychoactive effects of the drug and, in addition to those listed above, include dizziness, muddled thinking, coordination difficulties, irritability, weakness, headache, ataxia, paresthesia, hallucinations, visual distortions, depersonalization, confusion, nightmares, disorientation, and confusion. *CV:* Syncope, postural hypotension, tachycardia. *GI:* Diarrhea, dry mouth, fecal incontinence. *Other:* Facial flushing, tinnitus, speech difficulty, muscle pains. *Symptoms of Overdose:* Extension of the pharmacologic effects including anxiety reactions, hallucinations, psychotic episodes, respiratory depression, coma.

Drug Interactions

CNS depressants / Additive CNS depressant effects
Ethanol / During subchronic dronabinol use, lower and delayed peak alcohol blood levels

Dosage: Capsules. Adults and children, initial: 5 mg/m² 1–3 hr before chemotherapy; **then,** 5 mg/m² q 2–4 hr for a total of 4–6 doses/day. If ineffective, this dose may be increased by 2.5 mg/m² to a maximum of 15 mg/m²/dose. However, the incidence of serious psychoactive side effects increases dramatically at these higher dose levels.

NURSING CONSIDERATIONS

Administration/Storage

1. Due to its CNS effects, dronabinol should be used only when the client can be under close supervision.
2. Dronabinol has the potential for abuse. Therefore, prescriptions should be limited to one course of chemotherapy (i.e., several days) and reordered as needed to ensure the client receives the benefit of therapy.
3. *Treatment of Overdose:* Place client in a quiet environment and provide supportive treatment, including reassurance.

Assessment

1. Note if the client has any history of allergic responses to sesame oil or seeds.
2. Determine if the client's nausea and vomiting are caused by anything other than cancer chemotherapy.

Interventions: If clients develop serious psychoactive side effects, they should be placed in a quiet environment and provided with supportive care. Monitor vital signs and reassure clients.

Client/Family Teaching

1. Discuss the anticipated benefits to be derived from the therapy.
2. Take the medication 1–3 hr before the scheduled cancer chemotherapy.
3. Use caution when sitting or standing suddenly because dizziness may occur.
4. Do not drive or perform hazardous tasks requiring mental acuity.
5. Discuss the potential for psychoactive symptoms, visual dis-

tortions, and mental confusion. Advise the family that these symptoms may be minimized by providing a quiet, supportive environment.

6. Keep medication out of reach of children and do not share medications with anyone, no matter what their symptoms.

Evaluation: Evaluate client for:
• Relief of the symptoms of nausea and vomiting associated with cancer chemotherapy
• Improved appetite and prevention of weight loss in clients with AIDS

────── *COMBINATION DRUG* ──────
Dyazide
(**DYE**-ah-zyd)
(Rx)

Classification/Content: This drug is a combination of hydrochlorothiazide and a potassium-sparing diuretic (triamterene). *Antihypertensive/diuretic:* Hydrochlorothiazide, 25 mg. *Diuretic:* Triamterene, 50 mg. See also individual components, p. 718, and p. 1234.

Uses: Hypertension or edema in clients who develop hypokalemia on hydrochlorothiazide alone. May be used alone or with beta-adrenergic blocking agents.

Contraindications: Initial therapy of edema or hypertension except in clients where the development of hypokalemia cannot be risked. Use with other potassium-conserving diuretics. Use (unless in severe cases of hypokalemia) with potassium supplements.

Special Concerns: Use during pregnancy only if benefits outweigh risks. Use in children not recommended. Geriatric clients may be more sensitive to the usual adult dose.

Dosage: Capsules. Individualized. Adults, usual: 1–2 capsules b.i.d. after meals, not to exceed 4 capsules daily.

NURSING CONSIDERATIONS

See also *Nursing Considerations* for *Diuretics,* p. 141.

Administration/Storage

1. If another antihypertensive drug is to be used concurrently, the dose of the other antihypertensive should be one-half the usual dose.
2. If potassium supplements are being used with other diuretics, they should be discontinued when using Dyazide due to the potassium-sparing effects of triamterene.
3. Some clients may be maintained on one capsule of Dyazide daily or every other day.

Evaluation: Evaluate client for:
• Improved diuresis
• ↓ in blood pressure
• Reduction in edema
• Decrease in body weight R/T edema

E

Econazole nitrate

(ee-**KON**-ah-zohl)

Ecostatin✿, Spectazole (Rx)

Classification: Antifungal, topical.

Action/Kinetics: This drug may be fungistatic or fungicidal, depending on concentration. The drug inhibits the synthesis of sterols that damages the cell membrane and increases the permeability, resulting in a loss of essential intracellular elements. It may also inhibit biosynthesis of triglycerides and phospholipids and inhibit oxidative and peroxidative enzyme activity. Effective concentrations are found in the stratum corneum, epidermis, and the dermis. Systemic absorption is low.

Uses: Broad-spectrum fungicide effective against *Microsporum audouinii, M. canis, M. gypseum, Epidermophyton floccosum, Trichophyton mentagrophytes, T. rubrum, T. tonsurans, Candida albicans, Malassezia furfur,* and some gram-positive bacteria. Used to treat tinea cruris, tinea corporis, tinea pedis, tinea versicolor, cutaneous candidiasis.

Contraindications: Hypersensitivity. Ophthalmic use.

Special Concerns: Pregnancy category: C. Use with caution in pregnancy and lactation.

Side Effects: *Topical:* Burning, erythema, itching, stinging.

Dosage: Topical cream. *Tinea cruris, tinea corporis, tinea pedis, tinea versicolor:* Apply sufficient cream to cover the affected areas once daily. *Cutaneous candidiasis:* Apply b.i.d. in the morning and evening. If no improvement is noted after recommended treatment period, diagnosis should be reevaluated.

NURSING CONSIDERATIONS

See also *General Nursing Considerations For All Anti-Infectives,* p. 83.

Client/Family Teaching

1. Review goals of therapy and the appropriate method for administration.
2. The skin should be cleansed with soap and water and dried thoroughly. Cream should be applied as directed after cleaning the affected area.
3. For athlete's foot, the shoes and socks should be changed at least once daily. Shoes should be well-fitted and ventilated.
4. To reduce chance of reinfection, tinea pedis should be treated for 1 month and tinea cruris, tinea corporis, and candidal infections should be treated for 2 weeks.
5. The drug should be used for the full prescribed time even though symptoms have improved.
6. The physician should be notified if condition worsens or symptoms of burning, itching, redness, and stinging occur.

Evaluation: Evaluate client for:
- Knowledge and understanding of illness and level of compliance
- Status   (presence/absence)

of pretreatment symptoms and overall condition of treatment area

Edrophonium chloride

(ed-roh-**FOH**-nee-um)

Enlon, Reversol, Tensilon (Rx)

For additional information, see *Neostigmine,* p. 926.

Classification: Indirectly acting cholinergic-acetylcholinesterase inhibitor.

Action/Kinetics: Edrophonium is a short-acting agent mostly used for diagnosis and not for maintenance therapy. By increasing the duration of action at the motor end plate, edrophonium causes a transient increase in muscle strength in myasthenia gravis clients and either no change or a slight weakness in muscle strength in clients with other disorders. **Onset: IM,** 2–10 min; **IV,** less than 1 min. **Duration: IM,** 5–30 min; **IV,** 10 min. Eliminated through the kidneys.

Uses: Diagnosis of myasthenia gravis, adjunct to treat respiratory depression due to curare and similar nondepolarizing agents such as gallamine, pancuronium, and tubocurarine. *Investigational:* Treatment of supraventricular tachycardia.

Special Concerns: Pregnancy category: C.

Dosage: IM, IV. *Diagnosis of myasthenia gravis.* **IV, Adults:** 2 mg initially over 15–30 sec; with needle in place, wait 45 sec; if no response occurs after 45 sec inject an additional 8 mg. If a reaction is obtained following 2 mg, test is discontinued and atropine, 0.4–0.5 mg, is given IV. The test may be repeated in 30 min. **Pediatric, up to 34 kg, IV:** 1 mg; if no response after 45 sec, can give up to 5 mg. **Pediatric, over 34 kg, IV:** 2 mg; if no response after 45 sec, can give up to 10 mg in 1 mg increments q 30–45 sec. **Infants:** 0.5 mg. If IV injection is not feasible, IM can be used. **IM, Adults:** 10 mg; if hyperreactivity occurs, retest after 30 min with 2 mg IM to rule out false (−). **Pediatric, up to 34 kg:** 2 mg; **more than 34 kg:** 5 mg. (There is a 2–10 min delay in reaction with IM route.)

To evaluate treatment needs in myasthenic clients: 1 hr after PO administration of drug used to treat myasthenia, give edrophonium IV, 1–2 mg (**Note:** Response will be myasthenic in undertreated clients, adequate in controlled clients, and cholinergic in overtreated clients.)

Curare antagonist: **Slow IV:** 10 mg over 30–45 sec; repeat if necessary to maximum of 40 mg. *Treat supraventricular tachycardia:* **Adults, IV, initial:** 5–10 mg repeated in 10 min if necessary. **Pediatric, IV:** 2 mg given slowly.

NURSING CONSIDERATIONS

See also *Nursing Considerations* for *Neostigmine,* p. 928.

Administration/Storage

1. Edrophonium should not be given before curare or curarelike drugs.
2. Have IV atropine sulfate available to use as an antagonist.

Interventions

1. Observe the client closely in a monitored environment during drug administration.
2. Monitor vital signs, intake and output at least every 4 hr.

3. Observe the client for side effects such as increased salivation, bronchial spasm, bradycardia, and cardiac arrhythmia. This is particularly important when working with elderly clients. Document and report these symptoms to the physician immediately.
4. When the drug is being administered as an antidote for curare, assess the client for the effects of each dose of drug. Do not administer the next dose of drug unless the prior effects have been observed and recorded. Larger doses of medication may potentiate effects.
5. Evaluate the client's respiratory effort and provide assisted ventilation as needed.
6. Clients in cholinergic crisis should have their state of consciousness monitored closely.

Evaluation: Evaluate client for:

- Diagnosis of myasthenia gravis based on drug responses (transient ↑ in muscle strength)
- ↓ respiratory depression following administration of anesthetic agents

Eflornithine hydrochloride

(ee-**FLOR**-nih-theen)
Ornidyl (Rx)

See also *Anti-Infectives*, p. 80.

Classification: Anti-infective, antiprotozoal.

Action/Kinetics: Eflornithine inhibits the enzyme ornithine decarboxylase; this enzyme decarboxylates ornithine, which is a necessary step in the biosynthesis of poly-amines such as putrescine, sperimidine, and spermine. These polyamines are thought to play an important function in cell division and differentiation. The drug crosses the blood-brain barrier. **$t\frac{1}{2}$, terminal elimination:** 3 hr. Approximately 80% of an IV dose is excreted unchanged in the urine within one day.

Uses: Treatment of the meningoencephalitic stage of African trypanosomal infections due to *Trypanosoma brucei gambiense*.

Contraindications: Use during lactation.

Special Concerns: Pregnancy category: C. Safety and effectiveness have not been determined in children. Use with caution in clients with impaired renal function. Clients should be carefully monitored for 24 months to ensure that therapy is reinstituted if relapses occur.

Side Effects: *Hematologic:* Anemia (over 50% of clients), leukopenia (over one-third of clients), thrombocytopenia, eosinophilia. *GI:* Diarrhea, vomiting, anorexia, abdominal pain. *CNS:* Seizures, headache, dizziness. *Miscellaneous:* Alopecia, hearing impairment, asthenia, facial edema.

Dosage: Injection Concentrate. Adult: 100 mg/kg q 6 hr by IV infusion for 14 days.

NURSING CONSIDERATIONS

See also *General Nursing Considerations For All Anti-Infectives*, p. 83.

Administration/Storage

1. The infusion should be given over a minimum of 45 consecutive minutes.
2. Other drugs should not be

given during IV infusion of eflornithine.

3. The concentrate must be diluted with sterile water for injection before being infused.
4. To prepare the infusion, withdraw the entire contents of each 100-ml vial using strict aseptic technique. Inject 25 ml into each of four IV diluent bags, each bag containing 100 ml sterile water. This results in an eflornithine concentration of 40 mg/ml.
5. The diluted drug must be used within 24 hr of preparation and should be stored at 4°C (39°F). The undiluted vial may be stored at room temperature, preferably below 30°C (86°F).
6. The dose should be reduced in clients with impaired renal function depending on the serum creatinine level.

Assessment

1. Document dates and location of suspected exposure.
2. Obtain baseline CBC, platelets, liver and renal function studies.
3. Perform baseline audiogram and assess periodically throughout eflornithine therapy.

Interventions

1. Observe closely for seizure activity resulting from drug therapy and incorporate appropriate precautions.
2. Monitor hematologic studies throughout therapy, documenting any evidence of anemia, myelosuppression, leukopenia, or thrombocytopenia as the dosage may require modification or interruption if severe.
3. At the conclusion of therapy stress the importance of a 24-

month medical follow-up to evaluate for relapses as therapy then must be reinstituted.

Evaluation: Evaluate client for a positive clinical response based on appropriate laboratory culture results..

─── *COMBINATION DRUG* ───
Empirin with Codeine
(**EM**-pih-rin, **KOH**-deen)
(C-III, Rx)

See also *Narcotic Analgesics,* p. 174, and *Aspirin,* p. 260.

Classification/Content: *Nonnarcotic analgesic:* Aspirin, 325 mg (in all tablets). *Narcotic analgesic:* Codeine, 15 mg (No. 2), 30 mg (No. 3), 60 mg (No. 4).

Uses: Relief of mild, moderate, or moderate-severe pain.

Special Concerns: Pregnancy category: C.

Dosage: Tablets. Individualized. Adults, usual: 1–2 tablets of No. 2 or No. 3 q 4 hr as needed; 1 tablet of No. 4 q 4 hr.

NURSING CONSIDERATIONS

See *Nursing Considerations* for *Narcotic Analgesics,* p. 177, and *Aspirin,* p. 264.

Client/Family Teaching

1. Take with food, milk, or water to decrease gastric irritation.
2. This product may be habit-forming; advise to take only as directed.
3. The dose is adjusted according to the severity of the pain and the response of the client. The dose may exceed the recommended dosage if pain is severe or tolerance to the analgesic effect has developed.

Evaluation: Evaluate client for reports of effective control and symptomatic relief of pain.

Enalapril maleate

(en-**AL**-ah-prill)

Vasotec, Vasotec I.V. (Rx)

See also *Angiotensin-Converting Enzyme Inhibitors,* p. 33.

Classification: Antihypertensive, angiotensin-converting enzyme inhibitor.

Action/Kinetics: Enalapril is converted in the liver by hydrolysis to the active metabolite, enalaprilat. The parenteral product is enalaprilat injection. **Onset, PO:** 1 hr; **IV,** 15 min. **Time to peak action, PO:** 4–6 hr; **IV,** 1–4 hr. **Duration, PO:** 24 hr; **IV,** About 6 hr. Approximately 50%–60% is protein bound. **t½, PO:** 1 hr; **IV,** 15 min. Enalapril is excreted unchanged through the kidneys.

Use: Alone or in combination with a thiazide diuretic for the treatment of hypertension (Step I therapy). As adjunct with digitalis and diuretic in acute and chronic congestive heart failure. *Investigational:* Hypertension in children, hypertension related to scleroderma renal crisis, diabetic nephropathy.

Special Concerns: Pregnancy category: D. Use with caution during lactation. Safety and effectiveness have not been determined in children.

Side Effects: *CV:* Palpitations, hypotension, chest pain, syncope, angina, cerebrovascular accident, myocardial infarction, orthostatic hypotension, disturbances in rhythm, tachycardia, cardiac arrest.

GI: Nausea, vomiting, diarrhea, abdominal pain, alterations in taste, anorexia, dry mouth, constipation, dyspepsia, glossitis, ileus, melena, stomatitis. *CNS:* Insomnia, headache, fatigue, dizziness, paresthesias, nervousness, sleepiness, ataxia, confusion, malaise, depression, vertigo. *Hepatic:* Hepatitis, hepatocellular or cholestatic jaundice, pancreatitis, elevated liver enzymes. *Respiratory:* Bronchitis, cough, dyspnea, bronchospasm, upper respiratory infection, pneumonia, asthma. *Renal:* Renal dysfunction, transient increases in creatinine and BUN. *Hematologic:* Rarely, neutropenia, thrombocytopenia, bone marrow depression, decreased hemoglobin and hematocrit in hypertensive or congestive heart failure clients. *Dermatologic:* Rash, pruritus, alopecia, flushing, erythema multiform, exfoliative dermatitis, photosensitivity, urticaria, increased sweating, Stevens-Johnson syndrome, herpes zoster, toxic epidermal necrolysis. *Other:* Angioedema, muscle cramps, asthenia, impotence, blurred vision, fever, arthralgia, arthritis, vasculitis, eosinophilia, tinnitus, myalgia, rhinorrhea, sore throat, hoarseness, conjunctivitis, tearing, dry eyes, loss of sense of smell, hearing loss.

Additional Drug Interactions: Rifampin may ↓ the effects of enalapril.

Explain that drug should not be discontinued without first reporting this side effect to the physician.

Dosage: Tablets. *In clients not taking diuretics:* **Initial:** 5 mg once daily; **then,** adjust dosage according to response (range: 10–40 mg daily in 1–2 doses). *In clients taking diuretics:* **Initial:** 2.5 mg. Since hypotension may occur following the initiation of enalapril, the diuretic should be discontinued, if possible, for 2–3 days before initiating enalapril. If blood pressure is not maintained with enalapril alone, diuretic therapy may be resumed. Dosage should be decreased in clients with a creatinine clearance less than 30 ml/min and a serum creatinine level greater than 3 mg/dl. *Heart failure:* **Initial:** 2.5 mg 1–2 times daily; **then,** depending on the response, 5–20 mg/day in two divided doses. Dose should not exceed 40 mg daily. Dosage must be adjusted in clients with renal impairment or hyponatremia.

IV. *Hypertension:* 1.25 mg over a 5-min period; repeat q 6 hr. *In clients taking diuretics:* **Initial:** 0.625 mg over 5 min; if an adequate response is seen after 1 hr, administer another 0.625-mg dose. Thereafter, 1.25 mg q 6 hr.

NURSING CONSIDERATIONS

See also *Nursing Considerations* for *Antihypertensive Agents,* p. 78, and *Captopril,* p. 386.

Administration/Storage

1. Following IV administration, the peak effect after the first dose may not be observed for 4 hr (whether or not the client is on a diuretic). For subsequent doses, the peak effect is usually within 15 min.
2. Enalapril should be given as a slow IV infusion (over 5 min) either alone or diluted up to 50 ml with an appropriate diluent. Any of the following can be used: 5% dextrose injection, 5% dextrose in lactated Ringer's injection, Isolyte E, 0.9% sodium chloride injection, or 0.9% sodium chloride injection in 5% dextrose.

3. To convert from IV to PO therapy in clients on a diuretic, begin with 2.5 mg once daily for clients responding to a 0.625-mg IV dose. Thereafter, 2.5 mg once daily may be given.
4. To convert from PO to IV enalapril therapy in clients not on a diuretic, use the recommended IV dose (i.e., 1.25 mg q 6 hr). To convert from IV to PO therapy, begin with 5 mg once daily.
5. Anticipate lowered dosage for clients receiving diuretics.

Assessment

1. Obtain CBC, serum electrolytes, liver and renal function studies as baseline data and monitor.
2. Identify drugs the client may be taking that would interact unfavorably with enalapril and note on the client's record.
3. Document baseline vital signs and weight.

Client/Family Teaching

1. Stress the importance of keeping scheduled laboratory and physician appointments.
2. If there is a conflict, clients should be advised to reschedule the appointment as soon as possible.
3. Report any weight loss that may result from the client's loss of taste.
4. Any flu-like symptoms should be reported immediately.
5. Emphasize the importance of maintaining a healthy diet, of limiting their intake of caffeine, and avoiding the use of alcoholic beverages.
6. Stress the importance of re-

porting for laboratory tests and physician appointments as scheduled. If there needs to be a change, the lab and/or physician should be notified.

Evaluation: Evaluate client for:
- Evidence of control of lethal ventricular arrhythmias
- Therapeutic serum drug level of 0.1–0.3 mcg/ml
- A positive clinical response as evidenced by a lowering of diastolic BP and improvement in cardiac output

—— *COMBINATION DRUG* ——
Enalapril maleate and Hydrochlorothiazide
(en-**AL**-ah-prill/
high-droh-**KLOR**oh-**THIGH**-ah-zyd)
Vaseretic (Rx)

See also *Enalapril maleate*, p. 590, and *Hydrochlorothiazide*, p. 718.

Classification/Content: *Angiotensin-converting enzyme inhibitor:* Enalapril, 10 mg. *Diuretic:* Hydrochlorothiazide, 25 mg.

Uses: Hypertension in clients in whom combination therapy is appropriate.

Contraindications: Use for initial therapy of hypertension. Anuria or severe renal dysfunction. History of angioedema related to use of angiotensin-converting enzyme inhibitors. Lactation.

Special Concerns: Pregnancy category: D. Excessive hypotension may be observed in clients with severe salt or volume depletion such as those treated with diuretics or on dialysis. Significant hypotension may also be seen in clients with severe congestive heart failure, with or without associated renal insufficiency. A significant fall in blood pressure may result in myocardial infarction or cerebrovascular accident in clients with ischemic heart or cerebrovascular disease.

Safety and effectiveness have not been established in children.

Dosage: Tablets. Adults: 1–2 of the 10-25 tablets once daily.

NURSING CONSIDERATIONS

See also *Nursing Considerations* for *Enalapril*, p. 591, and *Thiazides and Related Diuretics*, p. 233.

Administration/Storage

1. The dose of Vaseretic must be individualized and is determined by the titration of the individual components. Once the client has been successfully titrated with the individual components, Vaseretic (1 or 2 of the 10-25 tablets) may be given once daily if the titrated doses are the same as those in the fixed combination.
2. The daily dose should not exceed 2 tablets.
3. In clients who are being treated with hydrochlorothiazide, hypotension may occur following the initial dose of enalapril. Thus, if possible, the diuretic should be discontinued for 2–3 days before beginning therapy with enalapril. If the diuretic cannot be discontinued, an initial dose of 2.5 mg enalapril should be used under close medical supervision for at least 2 hr and until blood pressure has stabilized for at least 1 additional hr.
4. Administration of potassium supplements, potassium salt substitutes, or potassium-sparing drugs may increase serum potassium levels.

5. The usual dose of Vaseretic is recommended for clients with a creatinine clearance greater than 30 ml/min.

Assessment

1. Document baseline BP, CBC, electrolytes, liver, and renal function.
2. Note any evidence of heart failure or cerebrovascular disease.
3. Document any history of gout, elevated cholesterol levels, or diabetes.

Evaluation: Evaluate client for evidence of effective control of hypertension with a minimum of drug side effects.

—— COMBINATION DRUG ——
Entex LA
(EN-tex)
(Rx)

Classification/Content: *Expectorant:* Guaifenesin, 400 mg. *Decongestant:* Phenylpropanolamine HCl, 75 mg.
See also information on individual components.

Uses: Nasal congestion and viscous mucus in the lower respiratory tract accompanying bronchitis, sinusitis, pharyngitis, coryza.

Special Concerns: Pregnancy category: C.

Dosage: Tablets. Adults and children over 12 years: 1 tablet q 12 hr; **children, 6–12 years:** one-half tablet q 12 hr. Not recommended for children under 6 years of age.

NURSING CONSIDERATIONS

See also *Nursing Considerations* for *Sympathomimetics,* p. 220.

Administration/Storage: Tablets should not be crushed or chewed before swallowing, although they may be broken in half for ease of administration.

Evaluation: Assess client for reports of symptomatic improvement of nasal congestion and mucus production.

E

Ephedrine sulfate
(eh-**FED**-rin)
Nasal decongestants: Efedron Nasal, Vatronol Nose Drops (OTC). Systemic: Ephed II (Rx: Injection; OTC: Oral dosage forms)

See also *Sympathomimetic Drugs,* p. 218, and *Nasal Decongestants,* p. 182.

Classification: Direct- and indirect-acting adrenergic agent.

Action/Kinetics: Releases norepinephrine from synaptic storage sites. Has direct effects on alpha, beta-1, and beta-2 receptors, causing increased blood pressure due to arteriolar constriction and cardiac stimulation, bronchodilation, relaxation of GI tract smooth muscle, nasal decongestion, mydriasis, and increased tone of the bladder trigone and vesicle sphincter. It may also increase skeletal muscle strength, especially in myasthenia clients. Ephedrine is more stable and longer-lasting than epinephrine. **Onset, IM:** 10–20 min; **PO:** 15–60 min. **Duration, IM, SC, IV:** 30–60 min; **PO:** 3–5 hr. Excreted mostly unchanged through the urine (rate dependent on urinary pH–increased in acid urine).

Uses: Bronchial asthma and reversible bronchospasms associated with obstructive pulmonary diseases; narcolepsy, angioneurotic edema, hay fever. Enuresis and myasthenia gravis (has been replaced by more effective agents). Topically as a nasal decongestant. Parenterally as a vasopressor.

Special Concerns: Use during pregnancy only if clearly needed (pregnancy category: C). Geriatric clients may be at higher risk to develop prostatic hypertrophy.

Additional Side Effects: Precordial pain, urinary retention, painful urination, decrease in urine formation, pallor, respiratory difficulty.

Drug Interactions

Dexamethasone / Ephedrine ↓ effect of dexamethasone
Diuretics / Diuretics ↓ response to sympathomimetics
Guanethidine / ↓ Effect of guanethidine by displacement from its site of action
Methyldopa / Effect of ephedrine ↓ in methyldopa-treated clients

Dosage: Capsules, Syrup, Tablets. *Bronchodilator, systemic nasal decongestant, CNS stimulant:* **Adults:** 25–50 mg q 3–4 hr. **Pediatric:** 3 mg/kg (100 mg/m²) daily in 4–6 divided doses. *Enuresis:* 25–50 mg at bedtime. *Myasthenia gravis:* 25 mg t.i.d.–q.i.d.

SC, IM, slow IV. *Bronchodilator:* **Adult:** 12.5–25 mg; subsequent doses determined by client response. *Vasopressor:* **Adults:** 25–50 mg (IM or SC) or 5–25 mg (IV) repeated in 5 min if necessary. **Pediatric (SC, IM, IV):** 3 mg/kg (100 mg/m²) daily in 4–6 divided doses. **Topical** (0.5% drops, 0.5% jelly): **Adults and children over 6 years:** 2–3 drops of solution or small amount of jelly in each nostril q 4 hr. Should not be used topically for more than 3 or 4 consecutive days. Not to be used in children under 6 years of age unless so ordered by physician.

NURSING CONSIDERATIONS

See also *Nursing Considerations* for *Sympathomimetic Drugs,* p. 220, and *Nasal Decongestants,* p. 182.

Assessment

1. Conduct a careful examination of the client's mental status and document prior to beginning drug therapy.
2. Take a baseline BP and pulse before initiating therapy. If the drug is being administered for hypotension, monitor frequently until the blood pressure has stabilized.

Interventions

1. If the client has used ephedrine for prolonged periods of time, observe the client for drug resistance. Allow the client to rest without medication for 3–4 days, then resume drug therapy. The client will usually respond to the drug again. If there is no further response, document and report the incident to the physician.
2. Monitor the client's mental status regularly. Note any signs of depression, lack of interest in personal appearance, or client complaints of insomnia or anorexia. Report these symptoms to the physician.
3. Monitor intake and output. Elderly men may have difficulty and pain on urination. Be alert for urinary retention and report any difficulty in voiding to the physician.

Client/Family Teaching

1. Teach the client and family how to take and maintain a written record of radial pulse readings. Instruct the client to report to the physician an elevated or irregular pulse rate.
2. Advise male clients to report any difficulty with voiding. This may be caused by drug-induced urinary retention.

Evaluation: Evaluate client for:

- Reports of improved airway exchange
- ↓ in congestion and mucus production and ↓ in allergic responses
- ↓ frequency of narcolepsy

Epinephrine
(ep-ih-**NEF**-rin)
Adrenalin Chloride Solution, Bronkaid Mist, Bronkaid Mistometer✱, Epipen ✱, Epipen Jr.✱, Primatene Mist Solution, Sus-Phrine (Both Rx and OTC)

Epinephrine bitartrate
(ep-ih-**NEF**-rin)
Asthmahaler, Bronitin Mist, Bronkaid Mist Suspension, Epitrate, Medihaler-Epi, Primatene Mist Suspension (OTC)

Epinephrine borate
(ep-ih-**NEF**-rin)
Epinal Ophthalmic, EPPY/N 1/2%, 1%, 2% Ophthalmic Solutions (Rx)

Epinephrine hydrochloride
(ep-ih-**NEF**-rin)
Adrenalin Chloride, Asthma Nefrin, Dey-Dose Epinephrine, Dysne-Inhal✱, Epifrin, Glaucon, Micro Nefrin, S-2 Inhalant, Vaponefrin (Both Rx and OTC)

See also *Sympathomimetic Drugs*, p. 218, and *Nasal Decongestants*, p. 182.

Classification: Direct-acting adrenergic agent.

Action/Kinetics: Epinephrine, a natural hormone produced by the adrenal medulla, induces marked stimulation of alpha, beta-1, and beta-2 receptors, causing sympathomimetic stimulation, pressor effects, cardiac stimulation, bronchodilation, and decongestion. **Extreme caution must be taken never to inject 1:100 solution intended for inhalation—injection of this concentration has caused death. SC: Onset,** 6–15 min; **duration:** less than 1–4 hr. **Inhalation: Onset,** 3–5 min; **duration:** 1–3 min; **duration:** 1–3 hr. **IM, Onset:** variable; **duration:** less than 1–4 hr. Epinephrine is ineffective when given orally.

Uses: Cardiac arrest, Stokes-Adams syndrome, low cardiac output following extracorporeal cardiopulmonary bypass. To prolong the action of local anesthetics. As a hemostatic during ocular surgery; treatment of conjunctival congestion during surgery; to induce mydriasis during surgery; treat ocular hypertension during surgery. Topically to control bleeding. Acute bronchial asthma, bronchospasms due to emphysema, chronic bronchitis, or other pulmonary diseases. Treatment of anaphylaxis, angioedema, anaphylactic shock, drug-induced allergic reactions, transfusion reactions, insect bites or stings. As an adjunct in the treatment of open-angle glaucoma. To produce mydriasis, to treat conjunctivitis.

Additional Contraindications: Narrow-angle glaucoma. Lactation.

Special Concerns: Pregnancy category: C (may cause anoxia in the fetus). Administer parenteral epinephrine to children with caution. Syncope may occur if epinephrine is given to asthmatic children.

Additional Side Effects: *CV:* Fatal ventricular fibrillation, cerebral or subarachnoid hemorrhage, obstruction of central retinal artery. *GU:* Decreased urine formation, urinary retention, painful urination. *At injection site:* Bleeding, urticaria, wheal formation. *Ophthalmic:* Transient stinging when administered, conjunctival hyperemia, brow ache, headache, blurred vision, photophobia, poor night vision, eye ache, eye pain. Prolonged ophthalmic use may cause deposits of pigment in the cornea, lids, or conjunctiva.

Additional Drug Interaction: Epinephrine, 1:100, will inactivate chymotrypsin in 60 min.

Laboratory Test Interferences: False + or ↑ BUN, fasting glucose, lactic acid, urinary catecholamines, glucose (Benedict's), ↓ coagulation time. The drug may affect electrolyte balance.

Dosage: Inhalation Aerosol, Bitartrate Inhalation Aerosol. Adults and children over 4 years of age: *Bronchodilation,* 0.2–0.275 mg (1 inhalation) of the Aerosol or 0.16 mg (1 inhalation) of the Bitartrate Aerosol; may be repeated after 1–2 min if needed. At least 3 hr should elapsed before subsequent doses. Dosage not established in children less than 4 years of age. **Inhalation Solution.**

Adults and children over 6 years of age: *Bronchodilation,* 1 inhalation of the 1% solution (of the base); may be repeated after 1–2 min.

Injection: IM, IV, SC. *Bronchodilation:* **Adults:** 0.2–0.5 mg SC repeated q 20 min–4 hr as needed; dose may be increased to 1 mg/dose. **Pediatric:** 0.01 mg/kg (0.3 mg/m^2) SC up to a maximum of 0.5 mg/dose; may be repeated q 15 min for 2 doses and then q 4 hr as needed. *Anaphylaxis:* **Adults:** 0.2–0.5 mg SC q 10–15 min as needed, up to a maximum of 1 mg/dose if needed. **Pediatric:** 0.01 mg/kg (0.3 mg/m^2) up to a maximum of 0.5 mg/dose; may be repeated q 15 min for 2 doses and then q 4 hr as needed. *Vasopressor:* **Adults, IM or SC, initial:** 0.5 mg repeated q 5 min if needed; **then,** give 0.025–0.050 mg IV q 5–15 min as needed. **Adults, IV, initial:** 0.1–0.25 mg given slowly. May be repeated q 5–15 min as needed. Or, use IV infusion beginning with 0.001 mg/min and increasing the dose to 0.004 mg/min if needed. **Pediatric, IM, SC:** 0.01 mg/kg, up to a maximum of 0.3 mg repeated q 5 min if needed. **Pediatric, IV:** 0.01 mg/kg q 5–15 min if an inadequate response to IM or SC administration is observed. *Cardiac stimulant:* **Adults, intracardiac or IV:** 0.1–1 mg repeated q 5 min if needed. **Pediatric, intracardiac or IV:** 0.005–0.01 mg/kg (0.15–0.3 mg/m^2) repeated q 5 min if needed; this may be followed by IV infusion beginning at 0.0001 mg/kg/min and increased in increments of 0.0001 mg/kg/min up to a maximum of 0.0015 mg/kg/min. *Adjunct to local anesthesia:* **Adults and children:** 0.1–0.2 mg in a 1:200,000–1:20,000 solution. *Ad-*

junct with intraspinal anesthetics: **Adults:** 0.2–0.4 mg added to the anesthetic spinal fluid. *Antihemorrhagic, mydriatic, decongestant:* **Adults and children, intracameral or subconjunctival:** 0.01%– 0.1% solution. *Topical antihemorrhagic:* **Adults and children:** 0.002%–0.1% solution.

Sterile Suspension. *Bronchodilation:* **Adults, SC, initial:** 0.5 mg; **then,** 0.5–1.5 mg no more often than q 6 hr. **Pediatric, SC, initial:** 0.025 mg/kg (0.625 mg/ m²); dose may be repeated but no more often than q 6 hr.

Ophthalmic Solution, Bitartrate Ophthalmic Solution, Borate Ophthalmic Solution. Adults: 1 drop up to 2 times daily. Dosage has not been established in children.

NURSING CONSIDERATIONS

See also *Nursing Considerations* for *Sympathomimetic Drugs,* p. 220, and *Nasal Decongestants,* p. 182.

Administration/Storage

1. *Never administer* 1:100 solution IV. Use 1:1,000 solution for IV administration.
2. Preferably use a tuberculin syringe to measure epinephrine, as the parenteral doses are small and the drug is potent. An error in measurement may be disastrous.
3. Administer epinephrine IV by a double bottle setup (piggyback) so that the rate of administration may be easily adjusted.
4. For IV administration to adults, the drug must be well diluted as a 1:1,000 solution and quantities of 0.05–0.1 ml of solution should be injected cautiously and slowly, taking about 1 min

for each injection, noting the response of the client (BP and pulse). Dose may be repeated several times if necessary.

5. Administer infusions with an electronic infusion device for safety and accuracy.
6. Briskly massage site of SC or IM injection to hasten the action of the drug. Do not expose epinephrine to heat, light, or air, as this causes deterioration of the drug.
7. Discard if solution is reddish brown in color and after expiration date.
8. Because of the presence of sodium bisulfite as a preservative in the topical preparation, there may be slight stinging after administration.
9. The topical preparation should not be used in children under 6 years of age.

Assessment

1. Note any history of sulfite sensitivity.
2. Obtain baseline recordings of client blood pressure and pulse rate prior to beginning drug therapy.

Interventions

1. Closely monitor the client receiving solutions of IV epinephrine. Keep the environment as peaceful as possible.
2. Monitor the client's blood pressure and pulse every minute until the desired effect from the drug has been achieved. Then take it every 2–5 min until the client's condition has stabilized. Once stable, monitor BP every 15–30 min as indicated.
3. Note if the client has any evi-

dence of shock such as cold, clammy skin, cyanosis, and loss of consciousness.

4. If the client goes into hypovolemic shock, be prepared to assist with administering additional IV flt

Evaluation: Evaluate client for:
- Return of cardiac activity following cardiac arrest
- Improved cardiac output following E.C. bypass
- ↓ intraocular pressures
- Reversal of signs and symptoms of anaphylaxis
- Improved airway exchange following asthma attack

Epoetin alfa recombinant
(ee-**POH**-ee-tin)
Epogen, Procrit (Rx)

Classification: Recombinant human erythropoietin.

Action/Kinetics: Epoetin alfa is a 165 amino acid glycoprotein made by recombinant DNA technology; it has the identical amino acid sequence and same biological effects as endogenous erythropoietin (which is normally synthesized in the kidney and stimulates red blood cell production). Epoetin alfa will elevate or maintain the red blood cell level, decreasing the need for blood transfusions. **t½:** 4–13 hr in clients with chronic renal failure. **Peak serum levels after SC:** 5–24 hr.

Uses: Treatment of anemia associated with chronic renal failure, including clients on dialysis (end-stage renal disease) or not on dialysis. AZT-induced anemia in HIV-infected clients. *Investigational:* Reverse anemia in cancer clients receiving chemotherapy. To increase the procurement of autologous blood in clients undergoing elective surgery (i.e., to decrease the need for homologous blood transfusions).

Contraindications: Uncontrolled hypertension, hypersensitivity to mammalian cell-derived products, hypersensitivity to human albumin. Use in clients with uncontrolled hypertension.

Special Concerns: Pregnancy category: C. Safety and efficacy have not been established in children. The safety and efficacy of epoetin alfa are not known in clients with a history of seizures or underlying hematologic disease (e.g., hypercoagulable disorders, myelodysplastic syndromes, sickle cell anemia). Use with caution in clients with porphyria, during lactation, and preexisting vascular disease.

Side Effects: In Chronic Renal Failure Clients (symptoms may be due to the disease). *CV:* Hypertension, tachycardia, edema, myocardial infarction, cardiovascular accident, transient ischemic attack, clotted vascular access. *CNS:* Headache, fatigue, dizziness, seizures. *GI:* Nausea, diarrhea, vomiting. *Miscellaneous:* Shortness of breath, hyperkalemia, arthralgias, chest pain, skin reaction at administration site, asthenia.

In AZT-Treated HIV-Infected Clients. *CNS:* Pyrexia, fatigue, headache, dizziness. *Respiratory:* Cough, respiratory congestion, shortness of breath. *GI:* Diarrhea, nausea. *Miscellaneous:* Rash, asthenia, reaction at injection site, allergic reactions.

Symptom of Overdose: Polycythemia.

Dosage: *Chronic renal failure:* **IV, initial (dialysis or nondialysis clients), SC (nondialysis clients), initial:** 50–100 units/kg 3 times weekly. The rate of increase of hematocrit depends on both dosage and client variation. **Maintenance:** Individualize (usual: 25 U/kg 3 times weekly).

AZT-treated, HIV-infections: **IV, SC, initial:** 100 U/kg 3 times a week for 8 weeks (in clients with serum erythropoietin levels less than or equal to 500 mU/ml who are receiving less than or equal to 4,200 mg/week of AZT). If a satisfactory response is obtained, the dose can be increased by 50–100 U/kg 3 times a week. The response should be evaluated q 4–8 weeks thereafter with dosage adjusted by 50–100 U/kg increments 3 times a week. If clients have not responded to 300 U/kg 3 times a week, it is likely they will not respond to higher doses.

NURSING CONSIDERATIONS

Administration/Storage

1. During hemodialysis, clients treated with epoetin alfa may require increased anticoagulation with heparin to prevent clotting of the artificial kidney.
2. The hematocrit should be determined twice weekly until it has stabilized in the target range and the maintenance dose of epoetin alfa has been determined. Also, after any dosage adjustment, the hematocrit should be monitored twice weekly for 2–6 weeks.
3. The dose of epoetin alfa should be reduced by about 25 U/kg 3 times weekly when the target range (30%–33%) is reached. Maintenance doses must then be individually determined.
4. If the hematocrit exceeds 36%, the drug should be withheld temporarily until the hematocrit decreases to 30%–33%. Upon re-initiation of therapy, the dose should be reduced by about 25 U/kg 3 times weekly.
5. The dose of epoetin alfa should be reduced immediately if the hematocrit increases more than 4 points in any 2-week period. After reduction, the hematocrit should be monitored twice a week for 2–6 weeks with maintenance doses individually determined.
6. The dose of epoetin alfa should be increased in increments of 25 U/kg 3 times weekly if the hematocrit does not increase by 5–6 points after 8 weeks of therapy. Further increases of 25 U/kg 3 times weekly may be made at 4–6-week intervals until a desired response is observed.
7. The preparation should not be shaken because shaking will denature the glycoprotein, making it biologically inactive.
8. Vials showing particulate matter or discoloration should not be used.
9. Only one dose per vial should be withdrawn and any unused portion should be discarded. The product contains no preservative.
10. The drug should be stored at 2°–8°C (36°–46°F).
11. Epoetin alfa should not be given with any other drug solutions.

Assessment

1. During the nursing history, note if client has any history of hypersensitivity to mammalian cell-derived products or human albumin.
2. Determine client iron stores prior to initiating therapy. Transferrin saturation should be at least 20% and serum ferritin should be at least 200 ng/ml. It may be necessary to provide supplemental iron to increase or maintain transferrin saturation to levels required to support stimulation of erythropoiesis by epoetin alfa.
3. Obtain baseline CBC and platelet count before starting therapy.
4. Note history of hypertension and perform baseline readings.
5. In clients infected with HIV, note when AZT therapy was instituted and the onset of anemia.

Interventions

1. Monitor CBC and platelet count throughout therapy and report to the physician. Drug dose may need to be adjusted frequently.
2. Assess BP and monitor throughout epoetin alfa therapy. Hypertension should be controlled prior to initiation of drug therapy.
3. Monitor renal function studies, electrolytes, phosphorous and uric acid levels especially in clients with chronic renal failure.

Client/Family Teaching

1. Advise clients and family that over 95% of clients with chronic renal failure manifested significant increases in hematocrit and nearly all clients were transfusion-independent within 2 months after beginning epoetin alfa therapy.
2. Explain that the desired drug response may take as long as 6 weeks.
3. Stress the importance of reporting for scheduled lab studies because drug dose must be adjusted based on these results.
4. Provide a printed list of drug side effects. Instruct client to report any persistent and/or bothersome side effects of epoetin alfa therapy to the physician.
5. Explain the importance of the client continuing to follow the prescribed dietary and dialysis recommendations.
6. Caution client not to perform any tasks that require mental alertness during the first 90 days of therapy with epoetin alfa.

Evaluation

1. Assess hematocrit twice weekly to determine a clinically significant response to epoetin alfa, which may not be observed for 2 weeks and may require up to 6 weeks in some clients.
2. Evaluate client for freedom from complications of side effects related to drug therapy.

———— *COMBINATION DRUG* ————

Equagesic

(eh-kwah-**JEE**-sik)

(Rx)

Classification/Content: *Nonnarcotic Analgesic:* Aspirin, 325 mg. *Antianxiety agent:* Meprobamate, 200 mg.

See also information on individual components.

Uses: Treatment (short-term only) of pain due to musculoskeletal disease accompanied by anxiety and tension.

Additional Contraindications: Pregnancy. Children under 12 years of age. Use for longer than 4 months.

Dosage: Tablets. Adults: 1–2 tablets t.i.d.–q.i.d.

NURSING CONSIDERATIONS

See also *Aspirin,* p. 264, and *Benzodiazepines,* p. 111.

Evaluation: Assess client for reports of symptomatic improvement of pain and a reduction in anxiety levels.

Ergonovine maleate
(er-**GON**-oh-veen)
Ergotrate Maleate (Rx)

Classification: Oxytocic agent.

Action/Kinetics: Ergonovine is a natural alkaloid obtained from ergot (a fungus that grows on rye). The drug stimulates the rate, tone, and amplitude of uterine contractions. The uterus becomes more sensitive to the drug toward the end of pregnancy. Ergonovine also stimulates smooth muscle surrounding certain blood vessels by interacting with adrenergic, dopaminergic, and tryptaminergic receptors. **Onset** (uterine contractions): **PO,** 5–15 min; **IM,** 2–3 min; **IV,** 60 sec. **Duration: PO, IM,** 3 or more hr; **IV,** 45 min.

Uses: Management and prevention of postpartum and postabortal hemorrhage by producing firm uterine contractions and decreasing uterine bleeding. Migraine headaches. *Investigational:* Ergonovine has been used to diagnose Prinzmetal's angina (variant angina).

Contraindications: Pregnancy, toxemia, hypertension. Ergot hypersensitivity. Should be given with caution in sepsis, obliterative vascular disease, impaired renal or hepatic function. To induce labor or threatened spontaneous abortions. Administration prior to delivery of the placenta.

Side Effects: *GI:* Nausea, vomiting, diarrhea. *Miscellaneous:* Allergic reactions, headache, increased blood pressure. *Ergotism:* In overdosage. Nausea, vomiting, diarrhea, changes in blood pressure, chest pain, hypercoagulability, numb and cold extremities, gangrene of fingers and toes, dyspnea, weak pulse, excitability to convulsions, delirium, hallucinations, death. Treatment is symptomatic and to decrease drug absorption.

Note: Use of ergonovine during labor may result in uterine tetany with rupture, cervical and perineal lacerations, embolism of amniotic fluid as well as hypoxia and intracranial hemorrhage in the infant.

Symptoms of Overdose: Nausea, vomiting, diarrhea, increase or decrease of blood pressure, numbness and coldness of extremities, dyspnea, weak pulse, chest pain, confusion, delirium, loss of consciousness, tingling, gangrene of fingers and toes, hypercoagulability, hallucinations, seizures, coma.

Dosage: *Uterine stimulant:* **IM, IV (emergencies only):** 0.2 mg no more often than q 2–4 hr, up to 5 doses. *Diagnosis of angina pectoris:* **IV:** 0.05 mg q 5 min until

E

chest pain occurs or a total dose of 0.4 mg has been given.

Tablets, oral or sublingual: 0.2–0.4 mg q 6–12 hr for 48 hr or until danger of uterine atony has passed. **Note:** Severe cramping is indicator of effectiveness. IV calcium salts may be required to enhance effectiveness in calcium-deficient clients.

NURSING CONSIDERATIONS

Administration/ Storage

1. Ergonovine ampules must be stored in a cold place away from light.
2. Since ergonovine loses its potency, if kept in the delivery room, it must be discarded after 60 days.
3. *Treatment of Overdose:* Give tap water, milk, or activated charcoal to delay absorption; remove by inducing vomiting or by gastric lavage followed by a cathartic. Treat symptoms (e.g., heparin to control hypercoagulability, nitroglycerin for coronary vasospasm, nitroprusside for severe vasospasm).

Assessment

1. Determine the location of the fundus, its height, and consistency.
2. Record the color, consistency, and amount of lochia.

Interventions

1. Note the character and amount of lochia; document and report to the physician if the amount is abnormal.
2. Monitor the uterus and palpate the fundus and note findings.
3. Monitor the blood pressure, pulse, and respirations. If there is any abnormal elevation or

decrease in blood pressure, or if the pulse and respirations assume a pattern unusual for the client, document and report to the physician.
4. If the client complains of severe cramping, report because this adverse effect suggests the need for a reduction in dosage of the drug.
5. Question the client about the presence of dizziness, headache, or ringing in the ears. Note if the client has nausea, complains of drowsiness, or has diarrhea, and if client appears to be confused. These are early signs of accidental ergotism; the drug is a derivative of lysergic acid. GI and CNS effects may occur before disturbances to the circulation of the hands and feet. Document and report to the physician immediately.
6. After administration, check the client's vital signs for evidence of shock or hypertension. Have emergency drugs available.

Evaluation: Evaluate client for:
- Prevention of postpartum hemorrhage
- Decrease in the amount and frequency of uterine bleeding
- Evidence of firm uterine contractions

Erythrityl tetranitrate
(er-**RIH**-thrih-till)
Cardilate (Rx)

See also *Antianginal Drugs,* p. 47.

Classification: Coronary vasodilator.

Action/Kinetics: Sublingual: Onset, 2–5 min; maximum effect:

30–45 min. **Duration:** 1–3 hr. **PO: Onset,** 20–40 min; maximum effect: 1–1.5 hr. **Duration:** 4–6 hr. **PO, Sustained-release, onset,** Up to 4 hr; **duration:** 6–8 hr. Tolerance may develop.

Uses: Prophylaxis and chronic treatment of angina. Diffuse esophageal spasm. May improve exercise tolerance. As a vasodilator in congestive heart failure.

Additional Contraindication: To treat acute attacks of angina pectoris.

Special Concerns: Pregnancy category: C. Dosage has not been established for children.

Dosage: Sublingual Tablets: 5–10 mg prior to physical or emotional stress. **Oral Tablets:** 10 mg before each meal as well as mid-morning and mid-afternoon. An additional dose may be given at bedtime if nocturnal attacks occur. Dose may be increased to 100 mg daily if necessary (chance of headache increases).

NURSING CONSIDERATIONS

See also *Nursing Considerations* for *Antianginal Drugs,* p. 49.

Interventions

1. Report symptoms of headaches and/or GI upset. These symptoms call for a reduction in dosage early in therapy.
2. Anticipate that analgesics will be ordered for headaches.

Client/Family Teaching

1. Explain that all restrictions on activity cannot be removed, even though drug may permit more normal activity.
2. Sublingual tingling sensations may be relieved by placing tablet in buccal pouch.

Evaluation: Evaluate client for:
- ↓ frequency and severity of anginal episodes
- Improved exercise tolerance
- Control of esophageal spasm

Erythromycin base
(eh-**rih**-throw-**MY**-sin)
Capsules/Tablets: Apo-Erythro Base✿, Apo-Erythro- EC✿, E-Base Caplets, E-Base Tablets, E-Mycin, Erybid✿, Eryc, Ery-Tab, Erythromid✿, Erythromycin Base Film-Tabs, Novo–Rythro✿, Novo–Rythro EnCap✿, PCE✿, PCE Dispertab, Robimycin. Gel, topical: Erygel. Ointment, topical: Akne-mycin. Ointment, ophthalmic: AK-Mycin, Ilotycin Ophthalmic. Pledgets: Erycette, T-Stat. Solution, topical: Akne-mycin, A/T/S, EryDerm, Erymax, ETS, Mythromycin, Staticin, T-Stat. (Rx)

See also *Erythromycins,* p. 144.

Classification: Antibiotic, erythromycin.

Uses: See *Erythromycins,* p. 144. *Ophthalmic solution:* Treatment of ocular infections (along with oral therapy) due to *Neisseria gonorrhoeae* and *Chlamydia trachomatis; Bacteroides* infections. *Topical solution:* Acne vulgaris. *Topical ointment:* Prophylaxis of infection in minor skin abrasions; treatment of superficial infections of the skin. Acne vulgaris.

Dosage: Delayed-Release Capsules, Enteric-Coated Tablets, Delayed-Release Tablets. *Respiratory tract infections due to Mycoplasma pneumoniae:* 500 mg q 6 hr for 5–10 days (up to 3 weeks for severe infections). *Intestinal amebi-*

asis due to Entamoeba histolytica:
Adults: 250 mg q.i.d. to 10–14 days; **pediatric:** 30–50 mg/kg daily in divided doses for 10–14 days. *Legionnaire's disease:* 500–1,000 mg q.i.d. for 3 weeks (or, 1–4 g/day in divided doses). *Bordetella pertussis:* 500 mg q.i.d. for 10 days (or, 40–50 mg/kg/day in divided doses for 5–14 days). *Infections due to Corynebacterium diphtheriae:* 500 mg q.i.d. for 10 days. *Erythrasma:* 250 mg t.i.d. for 3 wks.

Primary syphilis: 20 g in divided doses over 10 days. *Upper respiratory tract infections due to Streptococcus pneumoniae or group A beta-hemolytic streptococcus:* 250–500 mg q.i.d. *Lower respiratory tract infections due to Streptococcus pneumoniae or S. pyogenes:* 250–500 mg q 6 hr (or, 20–50 mg/kg daily in divided doses for 10 days). *Chlamydial infections:* **Infants:** 50 mg/kg daily in 4 divided doses for 14 (conjunctivitis)–21 (pneumonia) days; **adults:** 500 mg q.i.d. for 7 days. Mild to moderate skin and skin structure infections due to *Streptococcus pyogenes and Staphylococcus aureus:* 250–500 mg q 6 hr, to a maximum of 4 g daily. *Listeria monocytogenes infections:* 500 mg q 12 hr (or, 250 mg q 6 hr), up to maximum of 4 g daily.

Nongonococcal urethritis, Campylobacter fetus infections, chancroid, lymphogranuloma venereum: 500 mg q.i.d. for 7 days. *Pelvic inflammatory disease, acute Neisseria gonorrhoeae:* Erythromycin lactobionate, 500 mg IV q 6 hr for 3 days; **then,** 250 mg erythromycin base q 6 hr for 7 days. Alternatively for pelvic inflammatory disease, 500 mg, orally, q.i.d. for 10–14 days.

Prophylaxis of initial or recur-

rent rheumatic fever: 250 mg b.i.d. *Bacterial endocarditis due to alpha-hemolytic streptococcus:* **Adults,** 1 g 2 hr prior to the procedure; **then,** 500 mg 6 hr after the initial dose. **Pediatric,** 20 mg/kg 2 hr prior to the procedure; **then,** 10 mg/kg 6 hr after the initial dose.

Ophthalmic Ointment. *Mild to moderate infections:* 0.5 inch ribbon b.i.d.–t.i.d. *Acute infections:* 0.5 inch q 3–4 hr until improvement is noted. *Prophylaxis of neonatal gonococcal or chlamydial conjunctivitis:* 0.2–0.4 inch into each conjunctival sac.

Topical Solution. Apply morning and evening to affected areas. **Topical Ointment (2%).** Apply 1–5 times each day to affected area.

NURSING CONSIDERATIONS

See *Nursing Considerations* for *Erythromycins,* p. 146.

Administration/Storage

1. The ophthalmic ointment should not be washed from the eyes.
2. Before applying the topical solution, the affected areas should be washed, rinsed, and dried.
3. A sterile bandage may be used with the topical ointment.
4. Food does not affect absorption.

Erythromycin estolate
(eh-**rih**-throw-**MY**-sin)
Ilosone, Novo–Rythro ✲ (Rx)

See also *Erythromycins,* p. 144.

Classification: Antibiotic, erythromycin.

Action/Kinetics: Most active form of erythromycin, with relatively long-lasting activity.

Uses: See *Erythromycins,* p. 144.

Additional Contraindications: Cholestatic jaundice or preexisting liver dysfunction. Not recommended for treatment of chronic disorders such as acne or furunculosis or for prophylaxis of rheumatic fever.

Additional Side Effects: Hepatotoxicity.

Dosage: Capsules, Suspension, Tablets. See *Erythromycin base,* p. 603. Similar blood levels are achieved using erythromycin base, estolate, or stearate.

NURSING CONSIDERATIONS

See also *Nursing Considerations* for *Erythromycins,* p. 146.

Administration/Storage

1. Shake oral suspension well before pouring.
2. Do not store suspension longer than 2 weeks at room temperature.
3. Chewable tablets must be chewed or crushed.

Erythromycin ethylsuccinate

(eh-**rih**-throw-**MY**-sin)

Apo-Erythro-ES, E.E.S. 200 and 400, E.E.S. Granules, EryPed, EryPed 200, EryPed 400, EryPed Drops, Erythrocin✲ (Rx)

See also *Erythromycins,* p. 144.

Classification: Antibiotic, erythromycin.

Uses: See *Erythromycins,* p. 144.

Additional Contraindications: Preexisting liver disease.

Dosage: Oral Suspension, Tablets, Chewable Tablets. See *Erythromycin base,* p. 603. **Note:** 400 mg of erythromycin ethylsuccinate will achieve the same blood levels of erythromycin as 250 mg of the base, estolate, or stearate forms.

Hemophilus influenzae infections: Erythromycin ethylsuccinate, 50 mg/kg daily with sulfisoxazole, 150 mg/kg daily, both for a total of 10 days.

NURSING CONSIDERATIONS

See also *Nursing Considerations* for *Erythromycins,* p. 146.

Administration/Storage

1. Inject into large muscle mass.
2. Rotate site of injections.
3. Do not administer to infants, as muscle mass is too small.
4. Do not mix with other medications in same syringe.
5. Avoid accidental IV administration.
6. Refrigerate aqueous suspensions and store for maximum of 1 week.
7. Chewable tablets must be chewed or crushed.

Erythromycin gluceptate

(eh-**rih**-throw-**MY**-sin)

Ilotycin Gluceptate (Rx)

See also *Erythromycins,* p. 144.

Classification: Antibiotic, erythromycin.

Uses: Primarily for unconscious, vomiting, or gravely ill clients with serious infections of gram-positive

E

bacteria, especially hemolytic streptococci, pneumococci, staphylococci, and gonococci. Legionnaire's disease.

Drug Interactions: Drug for IV administration is incompatible with amikacin, aminophylline, cefazolin, cephalothin, metaraminol, novobiocin, oxytetracycline, pentobarbital, secobarbital, streptomycin, and tetracycline.

Dosage: IV only, Adults and children: 15–20 mg/kg daily (up to 4 g daily may be required for serious infections). *Acute pelvic inflammatory disease caused by gonorrhea:* 500 mg q 6 hr for 3 days, followed by 250 mg erythromycin stearate PO q 6 hr for 7 days. *Legionnaire's disease:* 1–4 g/day in divided doses.

NURSING CONSIDERATIONS

See also *Nursing Considerations* for *Erythromycins,* p. 146.

Administration/Storage

1. Follow directions on vial for dilution.
2. Concentrate (which must be diluted further before administration) will remain stable in refrigerator for 7 days.
3. Administer slowly over period of 20–60 min or infuse IV over 24 hr.

Erythromycin lactobionate

(eh-**rih**-throw-**MY**-sin)
Erythrocin Lactobionate IV (Rx)

See also *Erythromycins,* p. 144.

Classification: Antibiotic, erythromycin.

Uses: For seriously ill or vomiting clients with infections caused by susceptible organisms; acute pelvic inflammatory disease due to gonorrhea. Legionnaire's disease.

Additional Side Effect: Transient deafness.

Additional Drug Interaction: Some physicians recommend that no drugs be added to IV solutions of erythromycin lactobionate.

Dosage: IV, Adults and children: 15–20 mg/kg/day up to 4 g/day in severe infections. *Acute pelvic inflammatory disease caused by gonorrhea:* 500 mg q 6 hr for 3 days followed by 250 mg erythromycin stearate, **PO,** q 6 hr for 7 days. *Legionnaire's disease:* 1–4 g/day in divided doses. Change to oral therapy as soon as possible.

NURSING CONSIDERATIONS

See *Nursing Considerations* for *Erythromycins,* p. 146.

Administration/Storage:

1. Sterile water for injection is the preferred diluent. However, 5% dextrose injection or 5% dextrose and lactated Ringer's injection may also be used provided that they are first buffered with 4% sodium bicarbonate injection.
2. The initial reconstituted solution is stable for 2 weeks if refrigerated or for 24 hr at room temperature. However, the final diluted solution should be given within 8 hr. The reconstituted piggyback vial should be used within 24 hr if stored in the refrigerator or 8 hr if stored at room temperature.
3. If the reconstituted solution is frozen, it can be stored for 30 days. Once thawed, it should

be used within 8 hr. A thawed solution should not be refrozen.

Erythromycin stearate
(eh-**rih**-throw-**MY**-sin)

Apo-Erythro-S ✿, Eramycin, Erythrocin Stearate, Novorythro ✿, Wyamycin S (Rx)

See also *Erythromycins,* p. 144.

Classification: Antibiotic, erythromycin.

Uses: See *Erythromycins,* p. 144.

Additional Side Effects: Drug causes more allergic reactions (e.g., skin rash and urticaria) than other erythromycins. Hepatotoxicity.

Dosage: Tablets. See *Erythromycin base,* p. 603. Similar blood levels are achieved using erythromycin base, estolate, or stearate forms.

NURSING CONSIDERATIONS

See also *Nursing Considerations* for *Erythromycins,* p. 146.

Client/Family Teaching

1. Do not administer with meals because food decreases absorption.
2. Report any evidence of allergic reaction such as rash or itching.

Esmolol hydrochloride
(**EZ**-moh-lohl)

Brevibloc (Rx)

See also *Beta-Adrenergic Blocking Agents,* p. 113.

Classification: Beta-adrenergic blocking agent.

Action/Kinetics: Esmolol preferentially inhibits beta-1 receptors.

It has a rapid onset and a short duration of action. It has no membrane stabilizing or intrinsic sympathomimetic activity. Low lipid solubility. **t½:** 9 min. Is rapidly metabolized by esterases in red blood cells.

Uses: Supraventricular or noncompensatory tachycardia, sinus tachycardia.

Special Concerns: Pregnancy category: C. Dosage has not been established in children.

Addtional Side Effects: *Dermatologic:* Inflammation at site of infusion, flushing, pallor, induration, erythema, burning, skin discoloration, edema. *Other:* Urinary retention, midscapular pain, asthenia, changes in taste.

Additional Drug Interactions

Digoxin / Esmolol ↑ digoxin blood levels
Morphine / Morphine ↑ esmolol blood levels

Dosage: IV infusion. *Supraventricular tachycardia:* **Initial:** 500 mcg/kg/min for 1 min; **then,** 50 mcg/kg/min for 4 min. If after 5 min an adequate effect is not achieved, repeat the loading dose followed by a maintenance infusion of 100 mcg/kg/min for 4 min. This procedure may be repeated, increasing the maintenance infusion by 50 mcg/kg/min increments (for 4 min) until the desired heart rate or lowered blood pressure is approached. **Then,** omit the loading infusion and reduce incremental infusion rate from 50 to 25 mcg/kg/min or less. The interval between titrations may be increased from 5 to 10 min.

Once the heart rate has been

controlled, the client may be transferred to another antiarrhythmic agent. The infusion rate of esmolol should be reduced by 50% 30 min after the first dose of the alternative antiarrhythmic agent. If satisfactory control is observed for 1 hr after the second dose of the alternative agent, the esmolol infusion may be stopped.

NURSING CONSIDERATIONS

See also *Nursing Considerations* for *Beta-Adrenergic Blocking Agents,* p. 116.

Administration/Storage

1. Infusions of esmolol may be necessary for 24–48 hr.
2. Esmolol HCl is not intended for direct IV push administration.
3. The concentrate should not be diluted with sodium bicarbonate.
4. To minimize venous irritation and thrombophlebitis, infusion concentrations should not be greater than 10 mg/ml.
5. Diluted esmolol is compatible with 5% dextrose injection, 5% dextrose in Ringer's injection, 5% dextrose and 0.9% sodium chloride injection, 5% dextrose and 0.45% sodium chloride injection, 0.45% sodium chloride injection, or lactated Ringer's injection.

Interventions

1. Monitor client closely for evidence of hypotension and/or bradycardia. Interrupt infusion if values for blood pressure and heart rate fall below critical levels and notify physician immediately.
2. Infusions should be administered in a monitored environ-

ment and with an electronic infusion device.
3. Have emergency drugs and equipment readily available.

Evaluation: Evaluate client for evidence of conversion of supraventricular arrhythmias to a controlled rate rhythm.

Estazolam

(es-**TAYZ**-oh-lam)
ProSom (C-IV, Rx)

See also *Benzodiazepines,* p. 108.

Classification: Hypnotic, benzodiazepine.

Action/Kinetics: Peak plasma levels: 2 hr. $t^{1/2}$: 10–24 hr. The clearance is increased in smokers compared with nonsmokers. Metabolized in the liver and excreted mainly in the urine. Two metabolites–4'-hydroxy estazolam and 1-oxo-estazolam–have minimal pharmacologic activity although at the levels present they do not contribute significantly to the hypnotic effect of estazolam.

Uses: Short-term use for insomnia characterized by difficulty in falling asleep, frequent awakenings, and/or early morning awakenings.

Contraindications: Pregnancy (category: X). Use during labor and delivery and during lactation.

Special Concerns: Use with caution in geriatric or debilitated clients, in those with impaired renal or hepatic function, in those with compromised respiratory function, and in those with depression or who show suicidal tendencies. Safety and efficacy have not been determined in children less than 18 years of age.

Side Effects: *CNS:* Hypokinesia, dizziness, anxiety, incoordination, somnolence, nervousness, hangover, confusion, depression, abnormal dreams, abnormal thinking, agitation, amnesia, apathy, emotional lability, euphoria, hostility, stupor, paresthesia, seizures, stupor. *GI:* Nausea, dyspepsia, abdominal pain, constipation, dry mouth, decreased or increased appetite, flatulence, gastritis, vomiting. *Respiratory:* Symptoms of a cold, pharyngitis. *CV:* Flushing, palpitation. *Musculoskeletal:* Asthenia, muscle stiffness, lower or upper extremity pain, back pain, neck pain, body pain. *EENT:* Abnormal vision, eye irritation, eye pain or swelling, photophobia, tinnitus, ear pain, altered taste. *GU:* Frequent urination, urinary hesitancy or urgency, vaginal discharge or itching, menstrual cramps. *Dermatologic:* Pruritus, rash, sweating, urticaria. *Miscellaneous:* Headache, chills, fever, chest pain, malaise, allergic reaction, thirst. Withdrawal symptoms of the sedative-hypnotic type have been noted after discontinuing doses higher than those recommended therapeutically.

Drug Interactions: Additive CNS depression when given with antianxiety drugs, anticonvulsants, antihistamines, alcohol, barbiturates, MAO inhibitors, narcotics, phenothiazines.

Dosage: Tablets. Adults: 1 mg at bedtime (although some clients may require 2 mg). The initial dose in small or debilitated geriatric clients is 0.5 mg. Prolonged use is not recommended or necessary.

NURSING CONSIDERATIONS

See also *Nursing Considerations* for *Benzodiazepines,* p. 111.

Assessment

1. Determine any history of depression or suicidal tendencies.
2. Obtain baseline liver and renal function studies and monitor if evidence of impairment.
3. Note any history or evidence of compromised respiratory status.

Interventions

1. Observe closely and anticipate reduced dosage in geriatric and debilitated clients and those with impaired renal and hepatic function.
2. Identify if client is a smoker because this may alter drug absorption.
3. Attempt to determine the underlying cause(s) for client's insomnia because alternative nonpharmacologic methods for sleep inducement may be useful.

Client/Family Teaching

1. Provide a printed list of adverse drug effects and stress those symptoms that require immediate reporting to the physician.
2. Instruct females of childbearing age to practice contraception. Advise client to discontinue the use of estazolam prior to becoming pregnant.
3. Do not perform tasks that require mental alertness until drug effects are realized. The ability to drive or operate dangerous machinery may be impaired.
4. Avoid alcohol during drug therapy and do not take any OTC medications without physician consent.
5. Take only as directed because

estazolam may produce psychological and physical dependence.

6. Do not stop taking the drug abruptly without physician knowledge. After prolonged treatment, gradual withdrawal is recommended.

E

Evaluation

1. Evaluate client for reports of enhanced duration and quality of sleep and less frequent awakenings.
2. Estazolam may enhance the duration and quality of sleep for up to 12 weeks. Carefully assess the need for continued therapy for insomnia after this period of time.

Esterified estrogens

(es-**TER**-ih-fyd **ES**-troh-jens)

Estratab, Menest, Neo-Estrone♣ (Rx)

See also *Estrogens,* p. 147.

Classification: Estrogen, natural.

Action/Kinetics: This product is a mixture of sodium salts of sulfate esters of natural estrogenic substances: 75%–85% estrone sodium sulfate and 6%–15% equilin sodium sulfate. Less potent than estrone.

Uses: Replacement therapy in primary ovarian failure, following castration, or hypogonadism. Prostatic or breast carcinoma. Vasomotor symptoms, atrophic vaginitis, and kraurosis vulvae due to menopause. Prophylaxis of osteoporosis.

Dosage: Tablets. *Menopausal symptoms:* 0.3–1.25 mg daily, up to 3.75 mg daily if necessary, given cyclically. *Atrophic vaginitis, kraurosis vulvae:* 0.3–1.25 mg/day; use cyclically for short-term. *Hypogonadism:* 2.5–7.5 mg/day in divided doses for 20–21 days, followed by a 7- to 10-day rest period. *Primary ovarian failure, castration:* 1.25 mg/day in divided doses for 20 days with the addition of a progestin the last 5 days. *Prostatic carcinoma:* 1.25–2.5 mg t.i.d. for several weeks. *Breast carcinoma in men and postmenopausal women:* 10 mg t.i.d. for 3 months. *Prophylaxis of osteoporosis:* 0.3–1.25 mg daily for 20 or 21 days (a progestin should be given concurrently for 10–14 days of each cycle).

NURSING CONSIDERATIONS

See *Nursing Considerations* for *Estrogens,* p. 150.

Estradiol transdermal system

(ess-trah-**DYE**-ohl)

Estraderm (Rx)

See also *Estrogens,* p. 147.

Classification: Estrogen.

Action/Kinetics: This transdermal system allows a constant low dose of estradiol to reach the systemic circulation directly. It is believed that this system overcomes certain of the problems associated with oral use, including first-pass hepatic metabolism, GI upset, and induction of liver enzymes. The system is available in surface areas of 10 cm^2 (4 mg estradiol with a release rate of 0.05 mg/24 hr) and 20 cm^2 (8 mg estradiol with a release rate of 0.1 mg/24 hr).

Uses: Menopausal symptoms, female hypogonadism or castration, atrophic vaginitis, kraurosis vulvae, primary ovarian failure. Prophylaxis and treatment of postmenopausal osteoporosis.

Dosage: Dermal System. Initial: One 0.05 mg system applied to the skin two times each week; **then,** dose is adjusted to control symptoms. Attempts should be made to decrease the dose or withdraw the medication every 3–6 months. *Prophylaxis of osteoporosis:* **initial,** one 0.05 mg system daily as soon as possible after menopause; **then,** adjust dose, if necessary, to control concurrent menopausal symptoms.

NURSING CONSIDERATIONS

See also *Nursing Considerations* for *Estrogens,* p. 150.

Administration/Storage

1. If the client has been taking oral estrogens, withdraw the oral therapy and wait 1 week before applying the system.
2. For clients who have not undergone a hysterectomy, the system is usually used for 3 weeks, followed by 1 week of rest.
3. Place the system on a clean, dry area of the skin on the trunk of the body (preferably the abdomen).
4. The system should not be applied to the breasts or the waistline.
5. The application site should be rotated. Allow at least a 1-week interval between reapplication to a particular site.
6. Addition of a progestin for 7 or more days may reduce the incidence of endometrial hyperplasia.

Client/Family Teaching

1. If the client is to use a transdermal patch, instruct her to cleanse the area, usually on the abdomen, and apply the patch.

2. Avoid using areas of the body with excessive amounts of hair.
3. Apply the system immediately after opening the pouch and removing the protective liner. Press the system firmly in place by holding for 10 sec.
4. If the patch falls off, it should be replaced by a new one and the days of dosage administration should be readjusted. If the client has difficulty following the instructions, stress the importance of contacting the nurse or physician to review the instructions.
5. The drug is usually prescribed to be used twice a week. Discuss the importance of administering the drug only as prescribed.
6. Explain the importance of rotating the patch sites and teach the client how to record them so that one area is not overused.

Evaluation: Evaluate client for:
- Reports of symptomatic relief of menopausal symptoms
- Therapeutic levels of estrogen

Estramustine phosphate sodium
(es-trah-**MUS**-teen)
Emcyt (Rx)

See also *Antineoplastic Agents,* p. 85.

Classification: Hormonal agent, alkylating agent.

Action/Kinetics: Estramustine is a water-soluble drug that combines estradiol and mechlorethamine (a nitrogen mustard). The estradiol facilitates uptake into cells containing the estrogen receptor while the nitrogen mustard acts as an alkylating agent. Chronic estramustine administration results in plasma levels and effects of estradiol similar to those of conventional estradiol therapy. It is well absorbed from the GI tract and dephosphorylated before reaching the general circulation. Metabolites include estromustine, estrone, and estradiol. **t½:** 20 hr. Major route of excretion is in the feces.

Uses: Palliative treatment of metastatic and/or progressive prostatic carcinoma.

Contraindications: Active thrombophlebitis or thromboembolic disease unless the tumor mass is causing the thromboembolic disorder. Allergy to nitrogen mustard or estrogen.

Special Concerns: Use with caution in presence of cerebrovascular disease, coronary artery disease, diabetes, hypertension, congestive heart failure, impaired liver or kidney function, and metabolic bone diseases associated with hypercalcemia.

Additional Side Effects: *CV:* Myocardial infarction, cardiovascular accident, thrombosis, congestive heart failure, increased blood pressure, thrombophlebitis, leg cramps, edema. *Respiratory:* Pulmonary embolism, dyspnea, upper respiratory discharge, hoarseness. *GI:* Flatulence, burning sensation of throat, thirst. *CNS:* Emotional lability, insomnia, anxiety, lethargy, headache. *Dermatologic:* Easy bruising, flushing, peeling of skin or fingertips. *Miscellaneous:* Chest pain, tearing of eyes, breast tenderness or enlargement, decreased glucose

tolerance. *Symptoms of Overdose:* Extensions of the side effects.

Laboratory Test Interferences: ↑ Bilirubin, AST, LDH. ↓ Glucose tolerance. Abnormal hematologic tests for leukopenia and thrombocytopenia.

Drug Interactions: Drugs or food containing calcium may ↓ absorption of estramustine phosphate sodium.

Dosage: Capsules: 14 mg/kg/day in 3–4 divided doses (range: 10–16 mg/kg/day) or 600 mg (base)/m² daily in 3 divided doses. Treat for 30–90 days before assessing beneficial effects; continue therapy as long as the drug is effective. Some clients have taken doses from 10 to 16 mg/kg/day for more than 3 years.

NURSING CONSIDERATIONS

See also *Nursing Considerations* for *Antineoplastic Agents,* p. 88.

Administration/Storage

1. Capsules should be stored in the refrigerator at 2°C–8°C (36°F–46°F), although they may be kept at room temperature up to 48 hr without affecting potency.
2. Capsules should be taken with water 1 hr before or 2 hr after meals.
3. *Treatment of Overdose:* Gastric lavage; treat symptoms. Monitor blood counts and liver profiles for at least 6 weeks.

Assessment

1. Note any history of client allergy to nitrogen mustard or estrogen.
2. Assess clients with diabetes for hyperglycemia because glucose tolerance may be de-

creased. Ask clients about their tests at home and any difficulties or changes they may have noted in their condition such as increased fatigue, weakness, etc.

3. Assess for symptoms of hypercalcemia: insomnia, lethargy, anorexia, nausea, vomiting, coma, and vascular collapse.

4. Ascertain that serum calcium levels are routinely done; assess results (normal: 4.5–5.5 mEq/L). The effect of the steroid and osteolytic metastases may result in hypercalcemia.

Interventions

1. Take client blood pressure at each visit and teach the client and/or family member to take the blood pressure. BP elevation occurs in conjunction with this therapy.

2. Explain to male clients that impotence resulting from previous estrogen therapy may be reversed.

3. Estramustine phosphate sodium may cause genetic mutation. Therefore, contraceptive measures should be practiced to prevent teratogenesis.

4. Withhold drug and report high serum calcium levels. Encourage high fluid intake to minimize hypercalcemia.

5. For severe hypercalcemia, be prepared to assist with administration of IV fluids, diuretics, adrenocorticosteroids, and phosphate supplements.

6. Closely monitor clients who resume therapy after drug-induced hypercalcemia is corrected.

Evaluation: Evaluate client for positive tumor response based on a decrease in size and spread of prostatic carcinoma.

Estrogenic substances, aqueous
(es-troh-**JEN**-ick)
Estroject-2, Gynogen, Kestrin Aqueous, Wehgen (Rx)

See also *Estrogens,* p. 147.

Classification: Estrogen, steroidal.

Action/Kinetics: These preparations contain a mixture of steroidal estrogens, mostly estrone, in an aqueous suspension.

Dosage: IM only. *Menopause, kraurosis vulvae, atrophic vaginitis:* 0.1–0.5 mg 2–3 times/week. *Hypogonadism, primary ovarian failure, castration:* **Initial:** 0.1–1 mg/week in single or divided doses. Up to 2 mg/week may be necessary. *Prostatic carcinoma (inoperable):* 2–4 mg 2–3 times/week. Response to therapy should become apparent within 3 months after initiation of therapy.

NURSING CONSIDERATIONS

See *Nursing Considerations* for *Estrogens,* p. 150.

Estrogens conjugated, oral (conjugated estrogenic substances)
(ES-troh-jens)
C.E.S. ✻, Congest ✻, Conjugated Estrogens C.S.D. ✻, Premarin, Progens (Rx)

Estrogens conjugated, parenteral
(ES-troh-jens)
Premarin IV (Rx)

Estrogens conjugated, vaginal

(ES-troh-jens)

Premarin (Rx)

See also *Estrogens,* p. 147, and *Esterified Estrogens,* p. 610.

Classification: Estrogen, natural.

Action/Kinetics: This preparation contains 50%–65% sodium estrone sulfate and 20%–35% sodium equilin sulfate.

Uses: Oral: Menopausal symptoms, atrophic vaginitis, kraurosis vulvae, hypogonadism in females, primary ovarian failure, female castration, palliation in mammary or prostatic carcinoma, osteoporosis, prophylaxis of postpartum breast engorgement. **Parenteral:** Abnormal bleeding due to imbalance of hormones and in the absence of disease. **Vaginal:** Atrophic vaginitis and kraurosis vulvae associated with menopause.

Dosage: Tablets. *Menopausal symptoms, primary ovarian failure, female castration:* 1.25 mg daily. *Atrophic vaginitis, kraurosis vulvae:* 0.3–1.25 mg daily (higher doses may be necessary, depending on the response). *Hypogonadism in females:* 2.5–7.5 mg daily in divided doses followed by a 10-day rest period. *Palliation of mammary carcinoma:* 10 mg t.i.d. for at least 90 days. *Palliation of prostatic carcinoma:* 1.25–2.5 mg t.i.d. *Prophylaxis of postpartum breast engorgement:* 3.75 mg q 4 hr for a total of 5 doses (alternate regimen: 1.25 mg q 4 hr for 5 days). *Prophylaxis of osteoporosis:* 0.625 mg daily (given cyclically).

IM, IV: 25 mg, which may be repeated after 6–12 hr if necessary.

Vaginal cream: 2–4 g daily given for 3 weeks on and 1 week off.

NURSING CONSIDERATIONS

See also *Nursing Considerations for Estrogens,* p. 150.

Administration/Storage

1. For all uses, except postpartum breast engorgement and palliation of mammary and prostatic carcinoma, oral conjugated estrogens are administered cyclically—3 weeks of hormone therapy and 1 week off.
2. Parenteral solutions of conjugated estrogens are compatible with normal saline, invert sugar solutions, and dextrose solutions.
3. Parenteral solutions are incompatible with acid solutions, ascorbic acid solutions, and protein hydrolysates.
4. Reconstituted parenteral solutions should be used within a few hours after mixing if kept at room temperatures. Put the date and time of reconstitution on the solution label.
5. If the solution is refrigerated it will remain stable for 60 days.
6. When used vaginally, the cream should be inserted high into the vagina (2/3 the length of the applicator).

Evaluation

1. Determine the serum phosphatase levels to evaluate the effectiveness in palliation of prostatic carcinoma.
2. Evaluate client for:
   - Control of abnormal uterine bleeding R/T hormonal imbalance
   - Reports of symptomatic relief of menopausal symptoms

Estropipate (Piperazine Estrone Sulfate)

(es-troh-**PIE**-payt)

Ogen (Rx)

See also *Estrogens,* p. 147.

Classification: Estrogen.

Action/Kinetics: This product contains solubilized crystalline estrone stabilized with piperazine.

Uses: Oral: Vasomotor symptoms, atrophic vaginitis, or kraurosis vulvae associated with menopause. Primary ovarian failure, female castration, female hypogonadism. **Vaginal:** Atrophic vaginitis and kraurosis vulvae associated with menopause.

Contraindications: Use during pregnancy.

Dosage: Tablets. *Vasomotor symptoms, atrophic vaginitis, kraurosis vulvae:* 0.625–5 mg/day for short-term therapy (give cyclically). *Hypogonadism, primary ovarian failure, castration:* 1.25–7.5 mg/day for first 3 weeks; **then,** rest period of 8–10 days. An oral progestin can be given during the third week if withdrawal bleeding does not occur. **Vaginal cream:** 2–4 g daily (depending on severity of condition) for 3 weeks followed by a 1-week rest period.

NURSING CONSIDERATIONS

See also *Nursing Considerations for Estrogens,* p. 150.

Administration/Storage

1. Administration should be cyclic–3 weeks on the medication and 1 week off.
2. Attempts should be made to taper or discontinue the medication at 3–6-month intervals.
3. When used to relieve vasomotor symptoms, cyclic administration is initiated on day 5 of bleeding if the client is menstruating. If the client has not menstruated within the last 2 months (or more), cyclic administration may be initiated at any time.
4. To deliver the vaginal cream, the end of the applicator (after the appropriate amount is introduced) should be inserted into the vagina and the plunger pushed all the way down.
5. Between uses the plunger of the applicator should be pulled out of the barrel and washed in warm, soapy water. The applicator should not be put in hot or boiling water.

Client/Family Teaching

1. Review appropriate method and frequency of administration, advising client to take medications at the same time each day.
2. Advise that nausea may be relieved during oral therapy by consuming solid foods.
3. Review side effects of drug therapy stressing those symptoms requiring immediate reporting such as thromboembolic events (headache, blurred vision, pain, swelling or tenderness in the extremities); fluid retention (weight gain, swelling of extremities); hepatic dysfunction (yellowing of skin or eyes, itching, dark urine, clay-colored stools); changes in mental status or any unusual bleeding.
4. During treatment with vaginal

preparations advise client to administer at bedtime remaining recumbent for 30 min. Protect clothing and bed linens by wearing a sanitary pad.

5. Avoid cigarette smoking; review added risks.

6. Drug may cause increased pigmentation of skin so advise to wear protective clothing and sunscreens when sunlight exposure is necessary; otherwise avoid prolonged exposure.

7. Stop therapy and notify physician if pregnancy is suspected.

8. Stress the importance of reporting for all follow-up lab studies and exams to assess drug effectiveness and to determine the need to continue therapy.

Evaluation: Evaluate client for:

- Reports of improvement in menopausal symptoms
- Clinical evidence and laboratory confirmation of restoration of hormonal balance in deficiency states

Ethacrynate sodium

(eth-ah-**KRIH**-nayt)
Sodium Edecrin (Rx)

Ethacrynic acid

(eth-ah-**KRIH**-nik **AH**-sid)
Edecrin (Rx)

See also *Diuretics,* p. 140.

Classification: Loop diuretic.

Action/Kinetics: Ethacrynic acid inhibits the reabsorption of sodium and chloride in the loop of Henle; the drug also decreases reabsorption of sodium and chloride and increases potassium excretion in the distal tubule. It also acts directly on the proximal tubule to enhance excretion of electrolytes. Large quantities of sodium and chloride and smaller amounts of potassium and bicarbonate ion are excreted during diuresis. **Onset: PO,** 30 min; **IV,** 5–15 min. **Peak: PO,** 2 hr; **IV,** 15–30 min. **Duration: PO,** 6–8 hr. **IV,** 2 hr. Metabolites are excreted through the urine. Diuresis and electrolyte loss are more pronounced with ethacrynic acid than with thiazide diuretics. Ethacrynic acid is often effective in clients refractory to other diuretics. Careful monitoring of the diuretic effects is necessary.

Uses: Of value in clients resistant to less potent diuretics. Congestive heart failure, pulmonary edema, edema associated with nephrotic syndrome, ascites due to idiopathic edema, lymphedema, malignancy. Short-term use for ascites as a result of malignancy, lymphedema, or idiopathic edema; also, for short-term use in pediatric clients (except infants) with congenital heart disease. *Investigational.* **Ethacrynic acid:** Nephrogenic diabetes insipidus unresponsive to vasopressin. In combination with other drugs to treat mild to moderate hypertension. **Ethacrynate sodium:** Hypercalcemia, bromide intoxication, and with mannitol in ethylene glycol poisoning.

Contraindications: Pregnancy. Not recommended for use in neonates. Anuria and severe renal damage. Clients with history of gout should be watched closely.

Special Concerns: Geriatric clients may be more sensitive to the usual adult dose. To be used with caution in diabetic clients and those with hepatic cirrhosis (who are particularly susceptible to electrolyte imbalance).

Side Effects: Electrolyte imbalance (hypokalemia). The drug may also cause dehydration, reduction in blood volume, vascular complications, tetany, and metabolic alkalosis. *GI* (frequent): Anorexia, nausea, diarrhea, vomiting, acute pancreatitis, jaundice, dysphagia. Severe, watery diarrhea is an indication for permanent discontinuance of drug. GI bleeding, especially in clients on IV therapy or receiving heparin concomitantly. *CNS:* Tinnitus, hearing loss (permanent), vertigo, headache, blurred vision, apprehension, confusion, fatigue, malaise, dizziness. *Hematologic:* Agranulocytosis, thrombocytopenia, neutropenia. *Miscellaneous:* Skin rashes, abnormal liver function tests in seriously ill clients, fever, chills, hematuria. Ethacrynic acid increases uric acid levels and may precipitate attacks of gout. The drug may also produce changes in glucose metabolism (hyperglycemia and glycosuria). *Symptoms of Overdose:* Profound water loss, electrolyte depletion (causes dizziness, weakness, mental confusion, vomiting, anorexia, lethargy, cramps), dehydration, reduction of blood volume, circulatory collapse (possibility of vascular thrombosis).

Drug Interactions

Alcohol / ↑ Orthostatic hypotension

Aminoglycoside antibiotics / Additive ototoxicity and nephrotoxicity

Anticoagulants, oral / ↑ Effect of anticoagulants by ↓ plasma protein binding

Antidiabetic agents / Ethacrynic acid antagonizes hypoglycemic effect of antidiabetics

Antihypertensive agents / ↑ Antihypertensive effect

Barbiturates / ↑ Orthostatic hypotension

Cephaloridine / ↑ Risk of ototoxicity and nephrotoxicity

Cisplatin / ↑ Risk of ototoxicity

Corticosteroids / Enhanced K loss due to K-losing properties of both drugs

Digitalis glycosides / Ethacrynic acid produces excess K and Mg loss with ↑ chance of cardiac arrhythmias

Furosemide / Combination may result in hypokalemia, tachycardia, deafness, hypotension—**do not use together**

Indomethacin / ↓ Effect of ethacrynic acid

Lithium / ↑ Risk of lithium toxicity due to ↓ renal clearance

Narcotics / ↑ Orthostatic hypotension

Skeletal muscle relaxants, nondepolarizing / ↑ Muscle relaxation

Warfarin / ↑ Effect of warfarin due to ↓ plasma protein binding

Dosage: Ethacrynic acid: Oral Solution, Tablets. Adults, initial: 50–100 mg daily in single or divided doses; can increase by 25–50 mg daily if needed. **Maintenance:** Usually 50–200 mg (up to a maximum of 400 mg) daily once dry weight is reached. **Pediatric, initial:** 25 mg daily; can increase by 25 mg daily if needed. **Maintenance:** Adjust dose to needs of patient. **Ethacrynate sodium: IV. Adults:** 50 mg (base) (or 0.5–1 mg/kg); may be repeated in 2–4 hr if needed; **then,** administer q 4–6 hr if client is responding, to a maximum of 100 mg daily. **Pediatric:** 1 mg/kg.

NURSING CONSIDERATIONS

See also *Nursing Considerations* for *Diuretics,* p. 141.

Administration/Storage

1. Due to local pain and irritation, the drug should not be given SC or IM.
2. IV administration should be at a slow rate over a 30-min period given either directly or through IV tubing.
3. If a second IV injection is necessary, a different site should be used to prevent thrombophlebitis.
4. When used orally, administer after meals.
5. Reconstitute the powder for injection by adding 50 ml of 5% dextrose injection or sodium chloride injection.
6. When reconstituted with 5% dextrose injection, the resulting solution may be hazy or opalescent. Such solutions should not be used. Also, this solution should not be mixed with whole blood or its derivatives.
7. Use reconstituted solutions within 24 hr.
8. Ammonium chloride or arginine chloride may be prescribed for clients who are at a higher risk of developing metabolic acidosis.
9. *Treatment of Overdose:* Replace electrolytes and fluid and monitor urine output and serum electrolyte levels. Induce emesis or perform gastric lavage. Artificial respiration and oxygen may be needed. Treat other symptoms.

Assessment

1. Note if the client has diabetes mellitus or hepatic cirrhosis.

2. Check the client's urinary output to determine that anuria has not occurred.
3. List the drugs the client is taking to identify any with which the drug interacts unfavorably.

Interventions

1. Observe the client for excessive diuresis or a weight loss of up to 0.9 kg daily because electrolyte imbalance may develop quickly.
2. Assess clients with rapid excessive diuresis for pain in their calves, in the pelvic area, or in the chest. Rapid hemoconcentration may cause thromboembolic effects.
3. Observe clients for GI effects that may necessitate discontinuing the drug. The drug should be withdrawn if the client manifests severe, watery diarrhea.
4. Monitor for blood in the urine and the stools.
5. Observe the client for vestibular disturbances. Do not administer the drug IV concomitantly with any other ototoxic agent.
6. Monitor the serum potassium levels and consult with the physician regarding the need for supplementary potassium.
7. Since ethacrynic acid has such a profound effect on sodium excretion, dietary salt restriction is not necessary; if sodium is restricted, hyponatremia may result.

Evaluation: Evaluate for a positive clinical response as evidenced by ↓ edema, ↓ weight, ↑ urine output, and/or ↓ abdominal girth.

Ethambutol hydrochloride

(eh-**THAM**-byou-tohl)

Etibi✿, Myambutol (Rx)

Classification: First-line antitubercular agent.

Action/Kinetics: Tuberculostatic. Inhibits the synthesis of metabolites resulting in impairment of cell metabolism, arrest of multiplication, and ultimately cell death. The drug is active against *Mycobacterium tuberculosis,* but not against fungi, other bacteria, or viruses. Readily absorbed after oral administration. Widely distributed in body tissues except CSF. **Peak plasma concentration:** 2–5 mcg/ml after 2–4 hr. **t½:** 3–4 hr. About 65% of metabolized and unchanged drug excreted in urine and 20%–25% unchanged drug excreted in feces. Drug accumulates in clients with renal insufficiency.

Uses: Pulmonary tuberculosis in combination with other tuberculostatic drugs.

Contraindications: Hypersensitivity to ethambutol, preexisting optic neuritis, and in children under 13 years of age.

Special Concerns: Should be used with caution and in reduced dosage in clients with gout, impaired renal function, and in pregnant women.

Side Effects: *Ophthalmologic:* Optic neuritis, decreased visual acuity, loss of color (green) discrimination, temporary loss of vision or blurred vision. *GI:* Nausea, vomiting, anorexia, abdominal pain. *CNS:* Fever, headache, dizziness, confusion, disorientation, malaise, hallucinations. *Allergic:* Pruritus, dermatitis, anaphylaxis.

Miscellaneous: Peripheral neuropathy (numbness, tingling), precipitation of gout, thrombocytopenia, joint pain, toxic epidermal necrolysis. Renal damage. Also anaphylactic shock, peripheral neuritis (rare), hyperuricemia, and decreased liver function. Adverse symptoms usually appear during the early months of therapy and disappear thereafter. Periodic renal and hepatic function tests as well as uric acid determinations are recommended.

Drug Interactions: Aluminum may delay and decrease the absorption of ethambutol.

Dosage: Tablets. Initial treatment: 15 mg/kg/day given once daily until maximal improvement noted; **for retreatment:** 25 mg/kg daily as a single dose with at least one other tuberculostatic drug; **after 60 days:** 15 mg/kg administered once daily.

NURSING CONSIDERATIONS

See also *General Nursing Considerations For All Anti-Infectives,* p. 83.

Administration/Storage: Ethambutol should only be used in conjunction with at least one other antituberculosis drug.

Assessment

1. Obtain baseline liver and renal function studies and monitor throughout therapy.
2. Ascertain that client has had visual acuity test before ethambutol therapy and that client does not have preexisting visual problems.

Client/Family Teaching

1. Stress importance of vision test every 2–4 weeks while on therapy.

2. Reassure client that adverse ocular side effects generally disappear within several weeks to several months after therapy has been discontinued.
3. Women of childbearing age should practice birth control during therapy. If she should become pregnant, discontinue use of the drug and report immediately to physician.
4. Avoid aluminum-based antacids because these may interfere with drug absorption.

Evaluation

1. Determine client knowledge and understanding of disease and assess compliance with prescribed drug therapy.
2. Assess lab culture data to determine response to drug therapy.
3. Assess client for freedom from adverse side effects of drug therapy.

Ethanolamine oleate injection 5%

(eth-an-**OH**-lah-meen)
Ethamolin (Rx)

Classification: Sclerosing agent.

Action/Kinetics: The oleic portion of the product induces an inflammatory reaction of the intimal endothelium of the vein, leading to fibrosis and occlusion. The drug may also diffuse through the venous wall, producing an extravascular inflammatory response. Ethanolamine oleate disappears within 5 min from the injection site via the portal vein.

Use: To prevent rebleeding in clients with esophageal varices who have had a recent bleeding episode. **Note:** The drug has no effect on portal hypertension, the cause of esophageal varices; thus, retreatment may be necessary.

Contraindications: Clients with esophageal varices who have not bled. Known sensitivity to ethanolamine, oleic acid, or ethanolamine oleate. Not recommended for use in treating varicosities of the leg.

Special Concerns: Use during pregnancy only when clearly needed (pregnancy category: C). Use with caution during lactation. Safety and efficacy in children have not been determined.

Side Effects: *At site of varices:* Pleural effusion or infiltration, esophageal ulcer, esophageal stricture, retrosternal pain. Less commonly, esophagitis, necrosis, periesophageal abscess, tearing of the esophagus, sloughing of the mucosa overlying the injected varix, perforation. *Miscellaneous:* Pyrexia, pneumonia, aspiration pneumonia, anaphylaxis, acute renal failure. *Symptom of Overdose:* Severe intramural necrosis of the esophagus.

Dosage: Local IV only: 1.5–5 ml/varix. **Maximum total dose/treatment:** 20 ml.

NURSING CONSIDERATIONS

Administration/Storage

1. Smaller doses should be used in clients with significant liver dysfunction (Child Class C) or accompanying cardiopulmonary disease.
2. Submucosal injections should not be used because they may result in ulceration at the site of injection.

3. The drug may be given at the time of acute bleeding and again after 1 week, 6 weeks, 3 months, and 6 months to obliterate the varix.
4. The drug should be stored at room temperature (15°C–30°C or 59°F–86°F) and protected from light.

Assessment

1. Note any client history of sensitivity to ethanolamine, oleic acid, or ethanolamine oleate and document.
2. Determine if the client has any history of liver or cardiovascular disease.
3. Obtain baseline CBC, liver and renal function studies.
4. Determine when last bleed from esophageal varices occurred and what, if any, treatment was administered.

Interventions

1. Monitor CBC, liver and renal function studies throughout drug therapy.
2. Anticipate reduced dose in clients with impaired liver, cardiac, and/or renal function.
3. Monitor vital signs, intake and output and record.
4. Observe client closely for any evidence of rebleeding from esophageal varices.
5. Observe client for any symptoms associated with pleural effusion and/or pneumonia such as chest pain, dyspnea, cough, and pyrexia. Document and report to the physician because these are side effects related to drug therapy.

Evaluation: Evaluate client for prevention of a recurrence of esophageal bleeding.

Ethchlorvynol
(eth-klor-**VYE**-nohl)
Placidyl (C-IV, Rx)

Classification: Nonbarbiturate, nonbenzodiazepine sedative-hypnotic.

Action/Kinetics: Manifests anticonvulsant and muscle relaxant properties, as well as sedative and hypnotic effects. Said to depress REM sleep. Chronic use produces psychologic and physical dependence. Produces less respiratory depression than occurs with barbiturates. **Onset:** 15–60 min. **Peak blood levels:** 1–1.5 hr. **Duration:** 5 hr. $t\frac{1}{2}$: initial, 1–3 hr; final, 10–25 hr. Approximately 90% metabolized in liver and excreted in urine.

Uses: Short-term treatment of insomnia (treatment not to exceed 1 week). Has generally been replaced by other sedative-hypnotic drugs. *Investigational:* Sedation.

Contraindications: Porphyria, hypersensitivity.

Special Concerns: Pregnancy category: C. Use during the third trimester may result in CNS depression and withdrawal symptoms in the neonate. Geriatric clients may be more sensitive to the effects of this drug; also, a decrease in dose may be necessary in these clients due to age-related decreases in both hepatic and renal function.

Side Effects: *CNS:* Initial excitement, giddiness, vertigo, mental confusion, headache, blurred vision, hangover, fatigue, ataxia. *GI:*

Bad aftertaste, nausea, vomiting, gastric upset. *CV:* Hypotension, fainting. *Miscellaneous:* Skin rash, thrombocytopenia, jaundice, pulmonary edema (following IV abuse). Overdose produces symptoms similar to those of barbiturate intoxication.

Drug Interactions

Anticoagulants, oral / ↓ Effect of anticoagulants due to ↑ breakdown by liver

Antidepressants, tricyclic / Combination may result in transient delirium

Laboratory Test Interference: ↓ Prothrombin time (clients on coumadin).

Dosage: Capsules. Adult, usual: 500 mg at bedtime; up to 1,000 mg may be required if insomnia is severe. If client awakens, a 100- to 200-mg supplemental dose can be given. Adjust dose carefully in geriatric or debilitated clients. *Sedation:* 100–200 mg b.i.d.–t.i.d.

NURSING CONSIDERATIONS

See also *Nursing Considerations* for *Barbiturates,* p. 104.

Interventions

1. Monitor liver and renal function studies and anticipate a decreased dose in clients with altered function.
2. Advise client to use caution in driving or operating machinery until daytime sedative effects are evaluated. Milk or food taken with the medication may reduce these symptoms.
3. Assess closely for tolerance and for psychologic and physical dependence.

Evaluation: Evaluate client for

reports of enhanced duration and quality of sleep and less frequent awakenings.

Ethosuximide
(eth-oh-**SUCKS**-ih-myd)
Zarontin (Rx)

See also *Anticonvulsants,* p. 61, and *Succinimides,* p. 212.

Classification: Anticonvulsant, succinimide type.

Action/Kinetics: Peak serum levels: 3–7 hr. **t½: adults,** 60 hr; **t½: children,** 30 hr. Steady serum levels reached in 7–10 days. **Therapeutic serum levels:** 40–100 mcg/ml. The drug is metabolized in the liver. Both inactive metabolites and unchanged drug are excreted in the urine.

Uses: To control absence (petit mal) seizures.

Additional Drug Interactions: Both isoniazid and valproic acid may ↑ the effects of ethosuximide.

Dosage: Capsules, Syru̲. Adults and children over 6 years, initial: 250 mg b.i.d.; the dose may be increased by 250 mg daily at 4–7-day intervals until seizures are controlled or until total daily dose reaches 1.5 g. **Children under 6 years, initial:** 250 mg once daily; dosage may be increased by 250 mg daily every 4–7 days until control is established or total daily dose reaches 1 g.

NURSING CONSIDERATIONS

See also *Nursing Considerations* for *Anticonvulsants,* p. 63, and *Succinimides,* p. 213.

Administration/Storage: The drug may be given with other anticonvulsants when other forms of epilepsy are present.

Client/Family Teaching

1. Instruct the client to take medication with meals to minimize GI upset.
2. Do not engage in hazardous activities while on drug therapy.
3. Do not stop drug abruptly because this may precipitate withdrawal seizures.
4. Stress the importance of labs every three months to assess CBC, liver and renal function.

Evaluation: Evaluate client for evidence of control of seizures.

Ethylnorepinephrine hydrochloride
(eth-ill-nor-ep-ih-**NEF**-rin)
Bronkephrine (Rx)

See also *Sympathomimetic Drugs,* p. 218.

Classification: Direct-acting adrenergic agent.

Action/Kinetics: Ethylnorepinephrine stimulates beta-1 and beta-2 receptors similarly to epinephrine with minor effects on alpha receptors. Has little effect on BP and may be safer than epinephrine. Especially suitable for children, for diabetic asthmatics, and for clients refractory to isoproterenol or epinephrine. **Onset, SC or IM:** 6–12 min. **Duration:** 1–2 hr.

Uses: Treatment of bronchial asthma, bronchospasms due to emphysema or bronchitis, bronchiectasis, obstructive pulmonary disease.

Special Concerns: Pregnancy category: C.

Dosage: IM, SC. Adults: 1–2 mg (0.5–1 ml of 0.2% solution); **pediatric:** 0.2–1 mg (0.1–0.5 ml of 0.2% solution).

NURSING CONSIDERATIONS

See *Nursing Considerations* for *Sympathomimetic Drugs,* p. 220.

Etidronate disodium (oral)
(eh-tih-**DROH**-nayt)
Didronel (Rx)

Etidronate disodium (parenteral)
(eh-tih-**DROH**-nayt)
Didronel IV (Rx)

Classification: Bone growth regulator, antihypercalcemic.

Action/Kinetics: Paget's disease is characterized by bone resorption, compensatory new bone formation, and increased vascularization of the bone. Etidronate disodium slows bone metabolism, thereby decreasing bone resorption, bone turnover, and new bone formation; it also reduces bone vascularization. Renal tubular reabsorption of calcium is not affected. **Absorption:** Dose-dependent; after 24 hr, one-half of absorbed drug is excreted unchanged. **Onset:** 1 month for Paget's disease and within 24 hr for hypercalcemia. The drug remaining in the body is adsorbed to bone, where therapeutic effects for Paget's disease persist 3–12 months after discontinuation of the drug. **Plasma t½:** 6 hr. Approximately 50% excreted unchanged in the urine; unabsorbed drug is excreted through the feces.

Uses: *Oral:* Paget's disease (osteitis deformans), especially of the polyostotic type accompanied by pain and increased urine levels of hydroxyproline and serum alkaline phosphatase. Heterotopic ossification due to spinal cord injury or total hip replacement. *Parenteral:* Hypercalcemia due to malignancy, which is not responsive to hydration or dietary control. *Investigational:* Prevention and treatment of osteoporosis in clients on total parenteral nutrition.

Contraindications: Enterocolitis, fracture of long bones, hypercalcemia of hyperparathyroidism.

Special Concerns: Pregnancy category: B for tablets and C for parenteral form. Use with caution in the presence of renal dysfunction and during lactation. Dosage has not been established in children.

Side Effects: *GI:* Nausea, diarrhea, loose bowel movements. *Bones:* Increased incidence of bone fractures and increased or recurrent bone pain. Drug should be discontinued if fracture occurs and not restarted until healing takes place. *Allergy:* Angioedema, rash, pruritus, urticaria. Symptoms of rachitic syndrome have been reported in children receiving 10 mg or more/kg daily for long periods (up to 1 year) to treat heterotopic ossification or soft tissue calcification.

Dosage: Tablets. *Paget's disease:* **Adults, initial:** 5–10 mg/kg/day for 6 months or less; 11 mg/kg up to a maximum of 20 mg/kg/day for clients when bone metabolism suppression is highly advisable; treatment at this dose level should not exceed 3 months. Another course of therapy may be instituted after rest period of 3 months. *Heterotopic ossification due to spinal cord injury:* **Adults:** 20 mg/kg/day for 2 weeks; **then** 10 mg/kg/day for 10

weeks. *Heterotopic ossification complicating total hip replacement:* 20 mg/kg/day for 30 days preoperatively; **then,** 20 mg/kg/day for 90 days postoperatively. *Hypercalcemia:* **Adults:** 20 mg/kg daily for 30 days (up to a maximum of 90 days). **IV infusion.** *Hypercalcemia due to malignancy:* 7.5 mg/kg daily for 3 successive days. If necessary, a second course of treatment may be instituted after a 3-day rest period. The safety and effectiveness of more than 2 courses of therapy has not been determined. Etidronate tablets may be started the day after the last infusion at a dose of 20 mg/kg daily for 30 days (treatment may be extended to 90 days if serum calcium levels are normal). Use for more than 90 days is not recommended.

NURSING CONSIDERATIONS

Administration/Storage

1. Administer as a single dose of medication with juice or water 2 hr before meals.
2. Urinary hydroxyproline excretion and/or serum alkaline phosphatase levels should be determined periodically when the drug is given for Paget's disease.
3. There are no indications to date that etidronate will affect mature heterotopic bone.
4. The IV dose must be diluted in at least 250 ml of sterile normal saline.
5. The IV dose, diluted, should be administered over a period of 2 hr.
6. A metallic taste may be experienced during IV administration.

Assessment

1. Note if the client has any evidence of renal dysfunction.

Obtain baseline renal function studies and monitor during drug therapy.

2. If the client is of childbearing age and is sexually active, determine the possibility of pregnancy.

Client/Family Teaching

1. Assist the client and family in understanding the importance of maintaining a well-balanced diet with adequate intake of calcium and vitamin D.

2. Advise clients not to eat for 2 hr after taking medication because foods particularly high in calcium may reduce the absorption of the drug.

3. Review signs and symptoms of hypercalcemia that require immediate reporting, i.e., lethargy, nausea, vomiting, anorexia, tremors, and bone pain.

Evaluation

1. During treatment of Paget's disease determine levels of urinary hydroxyproline excretion and serum alkaline phosphatase because reduction in these levels is the first indication of a beneficial therapeutic response. Levels usually decrease 1–3 months after initiation of therapy.

2. In clients with hypercalcemia, determine serum calcium levels to assess drug response.

Etodolac
(ee-toh-**DOH**-lack)
Lodine (Rx)

See also *Nonsteroidal Anti-Inflammatory Drugs,* p. 186.

Classification: Nonsteroidal anti-inflammatory drug.

Action/Kinetics: Etodolac is a nonsteroidal anti-inflammatory drug (NSAID) in a class called the pyranocarboxylic acids. **Time to peak levels:** 1–2 hr. **Onset of analgesic action:** 30 min; **duration:** 4–12 hr. **t½:** 7.3 hr. The drug is metabolized by the liver and metabolites are excreted through the kidneys.

Uses: Acute and chronic treatment of osteoarthritis, mild to moderate pain.

Contraindications: Clients in whom etodolac, aspirin, or other NSAIDs have caused asthma, rhinitis, urticaria, or other allergic reactions. Use during lactation, during labor and delivery, and in children.

Special Concerns: Pregnancy category: C. Use with caution in impaired renal or hepatic function, heart failure, those on diuretics, and in geriatric clients. Safety and effectiveness have not been determined in children.

Additional Side Effects: *GI:* Diarrhea, gastritis, thirst, ulcerative stomatitis, anorexia. *CNS:* Nervousness, depression. *CV:* Syncope. *Respiratory:* Asthma. *Dermatologic:* Angioedema, vesiculobullous rash, cutaneous vasculitis with purpura, hyperpigmentation. *Miscellaneous:* Jaundice, hepatitis.

Symptoms of Overdose: Nausea, vomiting, drowsiness, lethargy, epigastric pain, anaphylaxis. Rarely, hypertension, acute renal failure, respiratory depression.

Additional Drug Interactions

Cyclosporine / ↑ Serum levels of cyclosporine due to ↓ renal excretion; ↑ risk of cyclosporine-induced nephrotoxicity

Digoxin / ↑ Serum levels of digoxin due to ↓ renal excretion
Lithium / ↑ Serum levels of lithium due to ↓ renal excretion
Methotrexate / ↑ Serum levels of methotrexate due to ↓ renal excretion

Laboratory Test Interferences: False + reaction for urinary bilirubin and for urinary ketones (using the dip-stick method). ↑ Liver enzymes, serum creatinine. Increased bleeding time.

Dosage: Capsules. *Osteoarthritis:* **initial,** 800–1,200 mg daily in divided doses; **then,** adjust dose within the range of 600–1,200 mg daily in divided doses (400 mg b.i.d.–t.i.d.; 300 mg b.i.d., t.i.d., or q.i.d.; 200 mg t.i.d. or q.i.d.). Total daily dose should not exceed 1,200 mg. *Acute pain:* 200–400 mg q 6–8 hr as needed, not to exceed 1,200 mg daily. For clients weighing less than 60 kg, the dose should not exceed 20 mg/kg.

NURSING CONSIDERATIONS

See also *Nursing Considerations* for *Nonsteroidal Anti-Inflammatory Drugs,* p. 189.

Administration/Storage

1. The capsules should be protected from moisture.
2. *Treatment of Overdose:* Since there are no antidotes, treatment is supportive and symptomatic. If discovered within 4 hr, emesis followed by activated charcoal and an osmotic cathartic may be tried.

Assessment

1. Note any previous experience with NSAIDs or acetylsalicylic acid and the results.

2. Obtain baseline bleeding parameters, liver and renal function studies.
3. Determine any history of heart disease or cardiac failure.
4. Note age and weight of client and if currently prescribed diuretics.

Evaluation: Evaluate client for reports of effective control of pain with improved joint mobility.

Etomidate
(eh-**TOM**-ih-dayt)
Amidate (Rx)

Classification: General anesthetic and adjunct to general anesthesia.

Action/Kinetics: Etomidate is actually a hypnotic without any analgesic activity. The drug seems to act like gamma-aminobutryic acid (GABA) and is thought to exert its mechanism by depressing the activity of the brain stem reticular system. It has minimal cardiovascular and respiratory depressant effects. **Onset:** 1 min. **Duration:** 3–5 min. **t½:** 75 min. Rapidly metabolized in the liver with inactive metabolites excreted mainly through the urine.

Uses: Induction of general anesthesia. As a supplement to nitrous oxide during short surgical procedures.

Special Concerns: Pregnancy category: C. Use with caution during lactation. Safety and efficacy have not been established in children less than 10 years of age.

Side Effects: *Skeletal muscle:* Myoclonic skeletal muscle movements, tonic movements. *Respiratory:* Apnea, hyperventilation or hypoventilation, laryngospasm. *Cardio-*

vascular: Either hypertension or hypotension; tachycardia or bradycardia; arrhythmias. *GI:* Nausea, vomiting. *Miscellaneous:* Eye movements (common), hiccoughs, snoring.

Dosage: IV only. *Induction of anesthesia:* **Adults and children over 10 years of age,** 0.2–0.6 mg/kg (usual: 0.3 mg/kg) injected over 30–60 sec.

NURSING CONSIDERATIONS

Administration/Storage

1. Lower doses of etomidate may be used as adjuncts to supplement less potent general anesthetics such as nitrous oxide.
2. Etomidate may be used following preanesthetic medications.
3. The drug should be protected from extreme heat and freezing.

Interventions

1. Nausea and vomiting are likely to occur postoperatively. Have essential equipment available to counteract the problem.
2. Monitor during the immediate postoperative period, for both hypotension and hypertension, tachycardia and bradycardia. Document and report to the physician.

Etoposide (VP-16–213)
(eh-**TOH**-poh-syd)
VePesid (Rx)

See also *Antineoplastic Agents,* p. 85.

Classification: Antineoplastic, miscellaneous.

Action/Kinetics: Etoposide is a semisynthetic derivative of podophyllotoxin. Etoposide acts as a mitotic inhibitor at the G_2 portion of the cell cycle to inhibit DNA synthesis. At high doses, cells entering mitosis are lysed, whereas at low doses, cells will not enter prophase. **t½:** biphasic, initial, 1.5 hr; final, 4–11 hr. **Effective plasma levels:** 0.3–10 mcg/ml. Poor penetration to the CNS. The drug is eliminated through both the urine and bile unchanged and as liver metabolites.

Uses: With combination therapy to treat refractory testicular tumors and small cell lung cancer. *Investigational:* Alone or in combination to treat acute monocytic leukemia, non-Hodgkin's lymphoma, Hodgkin's disease, AIDS-associated Kaposi's sarcoma, Ewing's sarcoma. Also, choriocarcinoma; hepatocellular carcinoma; non-small cell lung, breast, endometrial, and gastric cancers; acute lymphocytic leukemia; soft tissue carcinoma; rhabdomyosarcoma.

Contraindications: Lactation.

Special Concerns: Pregnancy category: D. Safety and efficacy in children have not been established. Severe myelosuppression may occur.

Additional Side Effects: Anaphylactic-type reactions, hypotension, peripheral neuropathy, somnolence.

Dosage: IV. *Testicular carcinoma:* 50–100 mg/m²/day on days 1–5 or 100 mg/m²/day on days 1, 3, and 5 every 3–4 weeks (i.e., after recovery from toxic effects). Used in combination with other agents. *Small cell lung carcinoma:* 35 mg/m²/day for 4 days to 50 mg/m²/day for 5 days, repeated q 3–4 weeks.

Capsules. *Small cell lung carcinoma:* 70 mg/m^2 (rounded to the nearest 50 mg) daily for 4 days to 100 mg/m^2 (rounded to the nearest 50 mg) daily for 5 days; repeat q 3–4 weeks.

NURSING CONSIDERATIONS

See also *Nursing Considerations* for *Antineoplastic Agents,* p. 88.

Administration/Storage

1. A slow IV infusion over 30–60 min will decrease the chance of hypotension. The drug should not be given by rapid IV push.
2. For IV use, the drug should be diluted with either 5% dextrose or 0.9% sodium chloride injection for a final concentration of 0.2 or 0.4 mg/ml.
3. Medical personnel should wear gloves when preparing this medication; if the drug comes in contact with the skin or mucosa, the area should be washed immediately and thoroughly with soap and water.
4. Diluted solutions to give a final concentration of 0.2 mg/ml are stable for 96 hr at room temperature; final concentrations of 0.4 mg/ml are stable for 48 hr at room temperature.
5. Capsules must be stored at 2°C–8°C (36°F–46°F) but should not be frozen.
6. Be prepared to treat anaphylactic reactions. Have available corticosteroids, pressor agents, antihistamines, and plasma expanders.

Assessment

1. Obtain baseline hemoglobin level and white blood cell count with differential before drug is administered.
2. Determine pregnancy if female of childbearing years.

Interventions

1. Monitor for signs of infection and bleeding, which are more likely to occur with this drug than with most antineoplastic agents.
2. Record BP frequently during infusions and at least twice a day with oral therapy and note any significant decreases.
3. Report any tingling sensations, numbness, and other signs of peripheral neuropathy.
4. Be aware that client may feel fatigued and be sleepy during and after drug administration. Schedule nursing activities accordingly.
5. Anticipate pretreatment with an antiemetic as drug may cause nausea and vomiting.

Client/Family Teaching

1. Report any flu-like symptoms because drug may cause severe myelosuppression.
2. Advise client to practice barrier contraception during treatment.
3. Provide a printed list of side effects that require immediate reporting.

Evaluation: Evaluate client for evidence of a decrease in the size and spread of malignant process.

Etretinate

(eh-**TRET**-ih-nayt)
Tegison (Rx)

Classification: Systemic antipsoriatic.

Action/Kinetics: Etretinate is related to vitamin A; it acts to decrease the thickness, erythema, and scale of lesions in individuals with psoriasis. Significant first-pass metabolism occurs to the active acid form of the drug. The ingestion of milk or a high-lipid diet increases the absorption of etretinate. Has a long half-life due to storage in adipose tissue. The drug has been found in the blood of certain clients up to 3 years after therapy was terminated. Etretinate itself is bound more than 99% to plasma lipoproteins, whereas the active acid metabolite is bound to albumin.

Uses: Severe recalcitrant psoriasis unresponsive to psoralens plus UVA light, systemic corticosteroids, methotrexate, or topical tar plus UVB light. *Investigational:* Severe, intractable keratinization disorders; severe, intractable oral lichen planus.

Contraindications: Individuals who are pregnant, intend to become pregnant, or who are not using effective contraceptive measures while taking the drug (pregnancy category: X). Lactation. Use in children unless other alternatives have been exhausted.

Side Effects: The toxic effects of etretinate resemble those of hypervitaminosis A. They include benign intracranial hypertension (pseudotumor cerebri); the symptoms include headache, nausea, vomiting, papilledema, and visual disturbances. *CNS:* Fatigue, headache, fever, lethargy, pain, dizziness, rigors, amnesia, anxiety, abnormal thought processes, depression, emotional lability, flu-like symptoms, faint feeling. *CV:* Edema, thrombosis, fainting, postural hypotension, chest pain, atrial fibrillation, phlebitis. *GI:* GI pain, changes in appetite, nausea, constipation, flatulence, melena, diarrhea, alteration in taste, ulcers of mouth, tooth caries. *Hepatic:* Hepatitis. *Ophthalmic:* Decreased visual acuity, blurred vision, decrease in night vision, corneal erosion, irregular and punctate staining, abrasions, iritis, retinal hemorrhage, photophobia, eye irritation, eyeball pain, double vision, scotoma. *Dermatologic:* Peeling of soles, palms, fingertips; loss of hair, itching, rash, dry skin, skin fragility, red scaly face, bruising, sunburn, cold clammy skin, bullous eruptions, onycholysis, changes in perspiration, paronychia, pyogenic granuloma, impaired healing, herpes simplex, hirsutism, abnormal skin odor, urticaria, granulation tissue. Skin atrophy, infection, fissures, nodules or ulceration. *Musculoskeletal:* Joint and bone pain, myalgia, muscle cramps, gout, ossification of interosseous ligaments and tendons of extremities, hyperkinesia. *Hematologic:* Significant alterations of platelets, reticulocytes, hemoglobin, white blood cells, or prothrombin time. *Renal:* Kidney stones; white blood cells, proteins, glucose, acetone, blood, casts, or hemoglobin in the urine; dysuria, urinary retention, polyuria. *Other:* Dyspnea, coughing, changes in electrolytes (either increased or decreased potassium, sodium, chloride, calcium, phosphorus, carbon dioxide), abnormal menses, earache, otitis externa, changes in equilibrium, drainage or infection of ear.

Laboratory Test Interferences: ↑ Triglycerides, AST, ALT, globulin, cholesterol, alkaline phosphatase, bilirubin, BUN. ↑ or ↓ Total protein albumin.

Dosage: Capsules. Adults: initial, 0.75–1 mg/kg/day in divided doses, not to exceed 1.5 mg/kg/day. **Maintenance:** 0.5–0.75 mg/kg/day, usually after 8–16 weeks of therapy. *Erythrodermic psoriasis:* **initial,** 0.25 mg/kg/day; **then,** increase by 0.25 mg/kg/day each week until optimum response has been obtained.

NURSING CONSIDERATIONS

Administration/Storage

1. Individualization of dosage is required to achieve maximal therapeutic effects with a tolerable degree of side effects.
2. Lesions may require up to 9 months of therapy to be completely cleared.
3. The drug should be administered with food.
4. Most clients have relapses within 2 months after therapy is terminated. Subsequent courses of therapy, up to 9 months, result in a response similar to that achieved during the initial course of therapy.

Assessment

1. Determine if female clients are sexually active and likely to be pregnant, prior to initiating therapy.
2. Ensure that women of childbearing age, who are to receive this medication, are using reliable forms of birth control.
3. Obtain pretreatment blood lipids under fasting conditions.

Client/Family Teaching

1. Clients may experience a worsening of psoriasis at the beginning of therapy.
2. Take the medication with meals to avoid GI upset.
3. The ingestion of milk or a high-lipid diet increases the absorption of drug. Review dietary recommendations.
4. Discuss with clients who wear contact lenses the fact that they may experience a decreased tolerance to contact lenses during and following therapy.
5. Provide a printed list of drug side effects. Report any symptoms that may indicate toxicity, such as headaches, nausea and vomiting, dizziness, and visual disturbances to the physician.
6. Do not take vitamin A supplements during therapy since etretinate is similar to vitamin A.
7. Stress the importance of reporting for all laboratory tests.
8. Advise client not to donate blood during therapy and for several years thereafter due to the possible risks to a developing fetus if a pregnant client receives such blood.

Evaluation: Evaluate client for:
- A positive clinical response as evidenced by improvement in skin lesions in psoriasis
- Freedom from severe complications of side effects of drug therapy

F

Famotidine

(fah-**MOH**-tih-deen)
Pepcid, Pepcid IV (Rx)

Classification: Histamine H_2-receptor antagonist.

Action/Kinetics: Famotidine is a competitive inhibitor of histamine H_2-receptors, thus leading to inhibition of gastric acid secretion. Both basal and nocturnal gastric acid secretion, as well as secretion stimulated by food or pentagastrin, are inhibited. **Peak plasma levels:** 1–3 hr. **t½:** 2.5–3.5 hr. **Onset:** 1 hr. **Duration:** 10–12 hr. Famotidine does not inhibit the cytochrome P-450 system in the liver; thus, drug interactions, as a result of inhibition of liver metabolism, are not expected to occur. From 25%–30% of an oral dose is eliminated through the kidney unchanged.

Uses: Short-term treatment of active duodenal ulcer (up to 8 weeks). Maintenance therapy for duodenal ulcer, at reduced dosage, after active ulcer has healed. Pathologic hypersecretory conditions such as Zollinger-Ellison syndrome or multiple endocrine adenomas. Benign gastric ulcer. *Investigational:* Gastroesophageal reflux disease, prevent aspiration pneumonitis, prophylaxis of stress ulcers, acute upper GI bleeding.

Contraindications: Cirrhosis of the liver, impaired renal or hepatic function.

Special Concerns: Pregnancy category: B. Assess benefits versus risks during lactation. Safety and efficacy in children have not been established.

Side Effects: *GI:* Constipation, diarrhea, nausea, vomiting, anorexia, dry mouth, abdominal discomfort. *CNS:* Dizziness, headache, paresthesias, depression, anxiety, confusion, hallucinations, insomnia, fatigue, sleepiness. *Skin:* Rash, acne, pruritus, alopecia, urticaria, dry skin, flushing. *CV:* Palpitations. *Musculoskeletal:* Arthralgia, asthenia, musculoskeletal pain. *Other:* Fever, liver enzyme abnormalities, orbital edema, conjunctival injection, bronchospasm, tinnitus, taste disorders, thrombocytopenia, loss of libido, impotency, pain at injection site (transient).

Drug Interactions

Antacids / ↓ Absorption of famotidine from the GI tract
Diazepam / ↓ Absorption of diazepam from the GI tract

Dosage: Oral Suspension, Tablets. *Duodenal ulcer, acute therapy:* 40 mg once daily at bedtime or 20 mg b.i.d. for up to 8 weeks. *Duodenal ulcer, maintenance therapy:* 20 mg once daily at bedtime. *Benign gastric ulcers:* 40 mg at bedtime. *Hypersecretory conditions:* **Individualized. Initial, adults:** 20 mg q 6 hr; **then,** adjust dose to response, although doses of up to 160 mg q 6 hr may be required for severe cases.

IV, IV infusion. *Hospitalized clients with hypersecretory conditions, duodenal ulcers, gastric ulcers, clients unable to take PO medication:* 20 mg q 12 hr.

NURSING CONSIDERATIONS

Administration/Storage

1. Antacids may be used concomitantly if required.

2. In clients with a creatinine clearance less than 10 ml/min, the dose may be reduced to 20 mg at bedtime or the interval between doses may be increased to 36–48 hr.

3. For IV injection, dilute 2 ml with 0.9% sodium chloride injection to a total volume of 5–10 ml and give over at least a 2-min period.

4. For IV infusion, dilute 2 ml with 100 ml of 5% dextrose and infuse over 15–30 min.

5. Famotidine is stable when mixed with various total parenteral nutrition solutions.

Assessment

1. If the client is pregnant, discuss with the physician the advisability of using the drug.

2. Prior to administering the drug, determine if the client has a history of seizures, document and report to the physician.

3. Perform a baseline exam of the client's mental status.

4. Note location, extent, and intensity of abdominal pain.

5. Assess for occult blood in stools and gastric secretions.

Interventions

1. Observe the client for CNS effects such as dizziness, headaches, and anxiety.

2. Periodically assess the client for signs of depression. Report any changes in client attitude such as increasing lack of concern for personal appearance or sleeplessness.

3. Check the client's eyes routinely and report any complaints of eye problems.

4. Monitor for GI effects, such as diarrhea, constipation, or loss of appetite, document and report.

5. Check urinary output. If there is evidence of renal insufficiency, order a urinalysis, BUN, and serum creatinine and report the results to the physician because a reduction in dosage may be indicated.

Evaluation: Evaluate client for
- Reduction of abdominal pain
- Prevention of GI irritation and bleeding
- Evidence (x-ray or endoscopic) of duodenal ulcer healing

Felodipine
(feh-**LOHD**-ih-peen)
Plendil (Rx)

See also *Calcium Channel Blocking Agents,* p. 118.

Classification: Calcium channel blocking agent.

Action/Kinetics: Onset after PO: 120–300 min. **Peak plasma levels:** 2.5–5 hr. Over 99% bound to plasma protein. **t½, elimination:** 11–16 hr. Metabolized in the liver.

Uses: Treatment of mild to moderate hypertension.

Contraindications: Use during lactation.

Special Concerns: Pregnancy category: C. Safe use in clients with heart failure has not been determined; thus, use with caution in clients with heart failure or compromised ventricular function, especially in combination with a beta-adrenergic blocking agent. Felodipine may cause a greater hypotensive effect in geriatric clients. Safety and effectiveness have not been determined in children.

Side Effects: *CV:* Significant hypotension, syncope, angina pectoris, peripheral edema, palpitations, AV block, myocardial infarction, arrhythmias, tachycardia. *CNS:* Dizziness, lightheadedness, headache, nervousness, sleepiness, irritability, anxiety, insomnia, paresthesia, depression, amnesia, paranoia, psychosis, hallucinations. *Body as a whole:* Asthenia, flushing, muscle cramps, pain, inflammation, warm feeling, influenza. *GI:* Nausea, abdominal discomfort, cramps, dyspepsia, diarrhea, constipation, vomiting, dry mouth, flatulence. *Dermatologic:* Rash, dermatitis, urticaria, pruritus. *Respiratory:* Rhinitis, rhinorrhea, pharyngitis, sinusitis, nasal and chest congestion, shortness of breath, wheezing, dyspnea, cough, bronchitis, sneezing, respiratory infection. *Miscellaneous:* Anemia, gingival hyperplasia, sexual difficulties, epistaxis, back pain, facial edema, erythema, urinary frequency or urgency, dysuria.

Additional Drug Interactions

Digoxin / ↑ Peak plasma levels of digoxin
Fentanyl / Possible severe hypotension or ↑ fluid volume
Ranitidine / ↑ Bioavailability of felodipine

Dosage: Tablets. Initial, 5 mg once daily; **then:** adjust dose according to response, usually at 2-week intervals with the usual dosage range being 5–10 mg once daily, up to a maximum of 20 mg once daily.

NURSING CONSIDERATIONS

See also *Nursing Considerations* for *Calcium Channel Blocking Agents,* p. 119.

Administration/Storage

1. Tablets should be swallowed whole and not chewed or crushed.
2. The bioavailability is not affected by food although it is increased more than twofold when taken with doubly concentrated grapefruit juice when compared with water or orange juice.

Assessment

1. Note any history of heart failure or compromised ventricular function.
2. List drugs currently prescribed and note any potential interactions.

Interventions: Blood pressure should be closely monitored in geriatric clients over 65 years of age and in clients with impaired hepatic function during any adjustment of dosage.

Client/Family Teaching

1. Do not stop drug abruptly as abrupt withdrawal may cause an increased frequency and duration of chest pain.
2. Avoid activities that require mental alertness until drug effects are realized.
3. Rise slowly from a lying position and dangle feet before standing to minimize postural effects.
4. Advise client to practice frequent careful oral hygiene to minimize the incidence and

severity of drug-induced gingival hyperplasia.

Evaluation: Evaluate client for evidence of control of hypertension.

Fenfluramine

(fen-**FLUR**-ah-meen)

Ponderal ✱, Pondimin (C-IV) (Rx)

See also *Amphetamines and Derivatives,* p. 29.

Classification: Anorexiant

Action/Kinetics: This drug produces more CNS depression and less stimulation than does amphetamine. It may exert its activity by affecting turnover of serotonin in the brain or to increased use of glucose. The abuse potential of fenfluramine appears to be different from other anorexiants in that it produces euphoria, derealization, and perceptual changes with doses of 80–400 mg. **Onset:** 1–2 hr. **Maximum effect:** 2–4 hr. **Duration:** 4–6 hr. **t½:** 11–30 hr. Excretion is pH dependent and is through the urine (alkaline urine decreases excretion).

Uses: Short-term treatment (8–12 weeks) of exogenous obesity in conjunction with a weight reduction program including reduced caloric intake, exercise, and behavior modification. To treat autistic children with high serotonin levels.

Additional Contraindication: Alcoholism.

Special Concerns: Pregnancy category: C.

Additional Side Effects: Hypoglycemia, CNS depression, impotence, drowsiness. Following long-term use (1 month), withdrawal symptoms have been observed including: tremor, ataxia, loss of sense of reality, visual hallucinations, depression, disturbed concentration and memory, suicidal feelings.

Symptoms of overdose: CNS: Agitation, drowsiness, confusion, convulsions, coma. *Musculoskeletal:* Tremor, shivering, increased or decreased reflexes. *CV:* Tachycardia, ventricular extrasystoles, culminating in ventricular fibrillation and cardiac arrest (at high doses). *Miscellaneous:* Flushing, fever, sweating, abdominal pain, hyperventilation, rotary nystagmus, dilated nonreactive pupils. Treatment should be symptomatic and supportive; however, emesis should not be induced due to the depressant effects of the drug.

Additional Drug Interactions: Fenfluramine may ↑ effect of alcohol, CNS depressants, guanethidine, methyldopa, reserpine, thiazide diuretics, and tricyclic antidepressants.

Dosage: Tablets. Adults: 20 mg t.i.d. 30–60 min before meals. May be increased weekly to a maximum of 40 mg t.i.d. If initial dose is not well tolerated, reduce to 40 mg daily and increase gradually. Total daily dose should not exceed 120 mg.
Extended-release Capsules. Adults: 60 mg once daily; the dose may be increased to a maximum of 120 mg daily, if needed.

NURSING CONSIDERATIONS

See also *Nursing Considerations* for *Amphetamines and Derivatives,* p. 31.

Administration/Storage

1. Anticipate the drug will produce anorexiant effects within 1–2 hr after ingestion.
2. The effects of the drug should last approximately 4–6 hr.
3. The drug should not be abruptly withdrawn because depression may occur.

Evaluation

1. Assess client for ↓ in weight and evidence of compliance with weight reduction program.
2. In autistic children, assess for a ↓ in serotonin levels.

Fenoprofen calcium
(fen-oh-**PROH**-fen)
Nalfon (Rx)

See also *Nonsteroidal Anti-Inflammatory Drugs,* p. 186.

Classification: Nonsteroidal anti-inflammatory analgesic.

Action/Kinetics: Peak serum levels: 1–2 hr; **t½:** 2–3 hr. Ninety-nine percent protein bound. Food (but not antacids) delays absorption and decreases the total amount absorbed. When used for arthritis, onset of action is within 2 days but 2–3 weeks may be necessary to assess full therapeutic effects. Safety and efficacy in children have not been established.

Uses: Rheumatoid arthritis, osteoarthritis, mild to moderate pain. *Investigational:* Juvenile rheumatoid arthritis, prophylaxis of migraine, migraine due to menses, sunburn.

Additional Contraindications: Renal dysfunction.

Special Concerns: Pregnancy category: B. Dosage has not been determined in children.

Additional Side Effects: *GU:* Dysuria, hematuria, cystitis, interstitial nephritis, nephrotic syndrome. Overdosage has caused tachycardia and hypotension.

Dosage: Capsules, Tablets. *Rheumatoid and osteoarthritis:* 300–600 mg t.i.d.–q.i.d. Adjust dose according to response of client. *Mild to moderate pain:* 200 mg q 4–6 hr. Maximum daily dose for all uses: 3,200 mg.

NURSING CONSIDERATIONS

See also *Nursing Considerations* for *Nonsteroidal Anti-Inflammatory Drugs,* p. 189.

Administration/Storage

1. Give the drug 30 min before or 2 hr after meals. Food decreases the rate and extent of absorption of fenoprofen.
2. Expect the peak effect to be realized in 2–3 hr and to last for 4–6 hr.
3. Two to 3 weeks may be required before a beneficial effect is seen.
4. Elderly clients over 70 years of age usually require half the usual adult dose of fenoprofen.
5. The drug is not recommended for children under 12 years of age or for pregnant women.
6. For clients who have difficulty swallowing, the tablets can be crushed and the contents mixed with applesauce or other similar foods.
7. If fenoprofen is given chronically, auditory tests should be performed periodically.

Assessment

1. Note the drugs the client is currently taking to assure that there is no potential drug interactions.
2. Obtain a baseline ophthalmic and auditory examination against which to measure any auditory or visual changes once drug therapy begins.
3. Obtain baseline liver and renal function studies.

Interventions

1. Note client complaints of headache, sleepiness, dizziness, nervousness, weakness or fatigue. These may be drug side effects and should be documented and reported to the physician.
2. Monitor intake and output. If the client is vomiting or has diarrhea, also monitor client's weight.
3. Perform a routine urinalysis, serum electrolytes, BUN, and creatinine to detect evidence of renal failure and nephrotic syndrome.
4. Note evidence of easy bruising, prolonged bleeding times, or anemia. Inspect the client for petechiae, oozing of blood from the gums, nosebleeds, sore throat, and fever. Report these findings to the physician.
5. Monitor CBC with differential, platelet counts, and PT/PTT during therapy.
6. Assess clients for the development of jaundice, right upper quadrant abdominal pain, or a change in the color and consistency of stools. Document and report to the physician.

Client/Family Teaching

1. Take the medication only as prescribed.
2. Explain that it takes 2–3 weeks of therapy to realize improvement in arthritic conditions.
3. Do not take aspirin during therapy with fenoprofen.
4. Provide a printed list of drug side effects. Identify those that require immediate reporting.

Evaluation: Assess client for reports of symptomatic improvement in joint pain and mobility.

Fentanyl citrate
(FEN-tah-nil)
Sublimaze (C-II, Rx)

See also *Narcotic Analgesics,* p. 174.

Classification: Narcotic analgesic, morphine type.

Action/Kinetics: Similar to those of morphine and meperidine. **Onset:** 7–8 min. **Peak effect:** Approximately 30 min. **Duration:** 1–2 hr. $t^{1/2}$: 1.5–6 hr. The drug is faster-acting and of shorter duration than morphine or meperidine.

Uses: Preanesthetic medication, induction, and maintenance of anesthesia of short duration and immediate postoperative period. Supplement in general or regional anesthesia. Combined with droperidol for preanesthetic medication, induction of anesthesia, or as adjunct in maintenance of general or regional anesthesia. Combined with oxygen for anesthesia in high-risk clients undergoing open heart surgery, orthopedic procedures, or complicated neurologic procedures.

Additional Contraindications: Myasthenia gravis and other conditions in which muscle relaxants should not be used. Clients particularly sensitive to respiratory depression. Use during labor.

Special Concerns: Pregnancy category: C. Safety and effectiveness have not been determined in children less than 2 years of age. Use with caution and at reduced dosage in poor-risk clients, children, the elderly, and when other CNS depressants are used.

Additional Side Effects: Skeletal and thoracic muscle rigidity, especially after rapid IV administration. Bradycardia, seizures, diaphoresis.

Additional Drug Interaction: ↑ Risk of cardiovascular depression when high doses of fentanyl are combined with nitrous oxide or diazepam.

Dosage: *Preoperatively:* **IM,** 0.05–0.1 mg 30–60 min before surgery. *Adjunct to anesthesia: induction,* **IV,** 0.002–0.05 mg/kg, depending on length and depth of anesthesia desired; *maintenance:* **IV, IM,** 0.025–0.1 mg/kg when indicated. *Adjunct to regional anesthesia:* **IM, IV,** 0.05–0.1 mg over 1–2 min when indicated. *Postoperatively:* **IM,** 0.05–0.1 mg q 1–2 hr for control of pain. *As general anesthetic with oxygen and a muscle relaxant:* 0.05–0.1 mg/kg (up to 0.15 mg/kg may be required).
    Pediatric, 2–12 years: *Induction and maintenance:* 1.7–3.3 mcg/kg.

NURSING CONSIDERATIONS

See also *Nursing Considerations* for *Narcotic Analgesics,* p. 177.

Administration/Storage

1. Direct IV infusions may be given, undiluted, over a period of 2–3 min.

2. After an IV injection, anticipate that the client will feel the onset of action within a few minutes and it should last for 30–60 min.
3. Clients receiving an IM injection of drug can expect to have relief within 15 min and expect a duration of 1–2 hr.
4. Protect drug from light.

Fentanyl Transdermal System
(FEN-tah-nil)
Duragesic-25, -50, -75, and -100 (C-II, Rx)

See also *Narcotic Analgesics,* p. 174 and *Fentanyl citrate,* p. 636.

Classification: Narcotic analgesic.

Action/Kinetics: The system provides continuous delivery of fentanyl for up to 72 hr. The amount of fentanyl released from each system/hr depends on the surface area (25 mcg/hr is released from each 10 cm^2). Each system also contains 0.1 ml of alcohol/10 cm^2; the alcohol enhances the rate of drug flux through the copolymer membrane and also increases the permeability of the skin to fentanyl. Following application of the system, the skin under the system absorbs fentanyl resulting in a depot of the drug in the upper skin layers, which is then available to the general circulation. After the system is removed, the residual drug in the skin continues to be absorbed so that serum levels fall 50% in about 17 hr. The drug is metabolized in the liver and excreted mainly in the urine.

Uses: Chronic pain for clients requiring a narcotic analgesic.

Contraindications: Use for postoperative pain due to variability in absorption and disposition seen in such clients. Hypersensitivity to fentanyl or adhesives. Increased intracranial pressure, impaired consciousness, coma, medical conditions causing hypoventilation. Use during labor and delivery. Lactation.

Special Concerns: Doses higher than 25 mcg/hr are too high for initiation of therapy. Use with caution in clients with brain tumors and bradyarrhythmias, as well as in elderly, cachectic, or debilitated individuals. Safety and efficacy have not been determined in children. The systems should be kept out of the reach of children; used systems should be disposed of properly.

Additional Side Effects: Sustained hypoventilation.

Dosage: Transdermal system. Adults: *Individualized.* **Usual initial:** 25 mcg/hr unless the client is tolerant to opioids (Duragesic-50, -75, and -100 are intended for use only in clients tolerant to opioids). Initial dose should be based on (1) the daily dose, potency, and characteristics (i.e., pure agonist, mixed agonist-antagonist) of the drug the client has been taking; (2) the reliability of the relative potency estimates used to calculate the dose as estimates vary depending on the route of administration; (3) the degree, if any, of tolerance to narcotics; and, (4) the general condition and status of the client.

To convert clients from oral or parenteral opioids to the transdermal system, the following method should be used: (1) the previous 24-hr analgesic requirement should be calculated; (2) convert this amount to the equianalgesic oral morphine dose; (3) find the calcu-

lated 24-hr morphine dose and the corresponding transdermal fentanyl dose using the table provided with the product; and, (4) initiate treatment using the recommended fentanyl dose. The dose may be increased no more frequently than 3 days after the initial dose or than every 6 days thereafter. The ratio of 90 mg/24 hr of oral morphine to 25 mcg/hr increase in transdermal fentanyl dose should be used to base appropriate dosage increments on the daily dose of supplementary opioids.

If the dose of the fentanyl transdermal system exceeds 300 mcg/hr, it may be necessary to change clients to another narcotic analgesic. In such cases, the transdermal system should be removed and treatment initiated with one-half the equianalgesic dose of the new opioid 12–18 hr later. The dose of the new analgesic should be titrated based on the level of pain reported by the client.

NURSING CONSIDERATIONS

See also *Nursing Considerations* for *Narcotic Analgesics,* p. 177, and *Fentanyl citrate,* p. 637.

Administration/Storage

1. The system should be applied to a nonirritated and nonirradiated flat surface of the skin on the upper torso. If needed, hair should be clipped (not shaved) from the site prior to application.
2. Only clear water, if needed, should be used to cleanse the site prior to application. Soaps, oils, lotions, alcohol, or other agents that might irritate the skin should not be used. The skin should be allowed to dry completely prior to applying the system.

3. The system should be removed from the sealed package and applied immediately by pressing firmly in place (for 10–20 sec) with the palm of the hand. Ensure that contact of the system is complete, especially around the edges.

4. Each system should remain in place for 72 hr; if additional analgesia is required, a new system can be applied to a different skin site after removal of the previous system.

5. Systems removed from a skin site should be folded so that the adhesive side adheres to itself; it should then be flushed down the toilet immediately after removal.

6. Any unused systems should be disposed of as soon as they are no longer needed by removing them from their package and flushing down the toilet. During hospitalization, appropriate institutional guidelines for disposing of controlled substances should be addressed.

7. Multiple systems may be used if the delivery rate needs to exceed 100 mcg/hr.

8. The initial evaluation of the maximum analgesic effect should not be undertaken until 24 hr after the system is applied.

9. If required, clients can use a short-acting analgesic for the first 24 hr (i.e., until analgesic efficacy is reached with the transdermal system).

10. Clients may require periodic supplemental doses of a short-acting analgesic to treat breakthrough pain.

11. If opioid therapy is to be discontinued, a gradual decrease in dose is recommended to minimize signs and symptoms of abrupt narcotic withdrawal.

Client/Family Teaching

1. Review and demonstrate the appropriate method for fentanyl transdermal patch application.

2. Stress the importance of administering *only* as prescribed.

3. Review the safe, appropriate method for drug storage and disposal.

4. Provide a printed list of adverse drug effects that require immediate reporting to the physician.

5. Advise client not to stop drug system suddenly without physician knowledge.

6. Use a prescribed short-acting analgesic for breakthrough pain. Notify physician if use exceeds expected needs because transdermal dosage may require adjustment.

7. Assist client to develop a written record of drug administration for the transdermal system and for short-acting analgesics. Advise client to date the patches when they are applied to avoid any confusion.

Evaluation

1. Evaluate client for:
   - Control of pain as evidenced by improved appetite, increased activity, and socialization
   - Reports of effective control of pain

2. Assess client record of short-acting analgesic utilization (for breakthrough pain) to determine if transdermal dosage requires adjustment.

Ferrous fumarate

(FAIR-us FYOU-mar-ayt)
**Femiron, Feostat, Feostat Drops
and Suspension, Fumasorb,
Fumerin, Hemocyte, Ircon,
NeoFer✺, Nephro-Fer,
Novofumar✺, Palafer✺, Palafer
Pediatric Drops✺, Span-FF
(OTC)**

See also *Antianemic Drugs,* p. 42.

Classification: Antianemic, iron.

Action/Kinetics: Better tolerated than ferrous gluconate or ferrous sulfate. Contains 33% elemental iron.

Dosage: Extended-release Capsules: Adults: 325 mg daily (for prophylaxis) or 325 mg b.i.d. (to treat anemia). Capsules are not recommended for use in children. **Oral Solution, Oral Suspension, Tablets, Chewable Tablets: Adults:** 200 mg daily (for prophylaxis) or 200 mg t.i.d.–q.i.d. (to treat anemia). **Pediatric:** 3 mg/kg daily (prophylaxis) or 3 mg/kg t.i.d., up to 6 mg/kg daily, if needed (to treat anemia).

NURSING CONSIDERATIONS

See *Nursing Considerations* for *Antianemic Drugs,* p. 45.

Ferrous gluconate

(FAIR-us GLUE-kon-ayt)
**Apo-Ferrous Gluconate✺,
Fergon, Ferralet, Ferralet Slow
Release, Fertinic✺, Novo–
Ferrogluc✺, Simron (OTC)**

See also *Antianemic Drugs,* p. 42.

Classification: Antianemic, iron.

Use: Particularly indicated for clients who cannot tolerate ferrous sulfate because of gastric irritation.

Dosage: Preparation contains 11.6% elemental iron. **Capsules, Tablets. Adults:** 325 mg daily (prophylaxis) or 325 mg q.i.d. (for anemia). Can be increased to 650 mg q.i.d. if needed and tolerated. **Pediatric, 2 years and older:** 8 mg/kg daily (prophylaxis) or 16 mg/kg t.i.d. (for anemia). **Elixir, Syrup. Adults:** 300 mg daily (prophylaxis) or 300 mg q.i.d. (for anemia). Can be increased to 600 mg q.i.d. as needed and tolerated. **Pediatric, 2 years and older:** 8 mg/kg daily (prophylaxis) or 16 mg/kg t.i.d. (for anemia).

The physician must determine dosage for children less than 2 years of age.

NURSING CONSIDERATIONS

See *Nursing Considerations* for *Antianemic Drugs,* p. 45.

Ferrous sulfate

(FAIR-us SUL-fayt)
**Apo-Ferrous Sulfate✺, Feosol,
Fer-In-Sol, Fer-Iron, Fero-Grad✺,
Fero-Gradumet, Ferospace,
Feratab, Mol-Iron, Novo–
Ferrosulfa✺, PMS Ferrous
Sulfate✺ (OTC)**

Ferrous sulfate, dried

(FAIR-us SUL-fayt)
**Feosol, Fer-in-Sol, Ferralyn
Lanacaps, Ferra-TD, Slow-FE
(OTC)**

See also *Antianemic Drugs,* p. 42.

Classification: Antianemic, iron.

Action/Kinetics: Least expensive, most effective iron salt for oral therapy. Ferrous sulfate products contain 20% elemental iron, whereas ferrous sulfate dried products contain 30% elemental iron. The exsiccated form is more stable in air.

Dosage: *Ferrous Sulfate.* **Extended-release Capsules. Adults:** 150–250 mg 1–2 times daily. This dosage form is not recommended for children. **Elixir, Oral Solution, Tablets, Enteric-coated Tablets. Adults:** 300 mg daily (prophylaxis) or 300 mg b.i.d. increased to 300 mg q.i.d. as needed and tolerated (for anemia). **Pediatric:** 5 mg/kg daily (prophylaxis) or 10 mg/kg t.i.d. (for anemia). The enteric-coated tablets are not recommended for use in children. **Extended-Release Tablets. Adults:** 525 mg 1–2 times daily. This dosage form is not recommended for use in children.

Ferrous Sulfate, Dried. **Capsules. Adults:** 300 mg daily (prophylaxis) or 300 mg b.i.d. up to 300 mg q.i.d. as needed and tolerated (for anemia). **Pediatric:** 5 mg/kg daily (prophylaxis) or 10 mg/kg t.i.d. (for anemia). **Tablets. Adults:** 200 mg daily (prophylaxis) or 200 mg t.i.d. up to 200 mg q.i.d. as needed and tolerated (for anemia). **Pediatric:** Same dosage as ferrous sulfate, dried capsules. **Extended-release Tablets. Adults:** 160 mg 1–2 times daily. This dosage form is not recommended for use in children.

NURSING CONSIDERATIONS

See *Nursing Considerations* for *Antianemic Drugs,* p. 45.

Filgrastim
(fill-**GRASS**-tim)
Neupogen (Rx)

Classification: Human granulocyte colony-stimulating factor (G-CSF).

Action/Kinetics: Filgrastim is a human granulocyte colony-stimulating factor (G-CSF). It is produced by recombinant DNA technology by *Escherichia coli* that has been inserted with the human G-CSF gene. Endogenous G-CSF is a glycoprotein that is produced by monocytes, fibroblasts, and other endothelial cells and that regulates the production of neutrophils in the bone marrow. It has minimal effects, either in vivo or in vitro, on the production of other hematopoietic cell types. Filgrastim has an amino acid sequence that is identical to the natural sequence predicted from human DNA sequence analysis except there is an N-terminal methionine that is required for expression in *E. coli.* IV infusion of 20 mcg/kg over 24 hr resulted in a mean serum level of 48 ng/ml, whereas SC administration of 11.5 mcg/kg resulted in a maximum serum level of 49 ng/ml within 2–8 hr. **t½, elimination:** 3.5 hr.

Uses: To decrease the incidence of infection, as manifested by febrile neutropenia, in clients with non-myeloid malignancies who are receiving myelosuppressive anticancer drugs, which are associated with severe neutropenia with fever.

Contraindications: Hypersensitivity to proteins derived from *E. coli.* The safety and effectiveness of filgrastim given simultaneously with cytotoxic chemotherapy have not been determined; thus, filgrastim should not be given 24 hr before to 24 hr after cytotoxic chemotherapy.

Special Concerns: Pregnancy category: C. Use with caution during lactation. Use with caution in any malignancy with myeloid characteristics since the drug may act as a growth factor for any tumor type. Filgrastim does not cause any greater incidence of toxicity in children than in adults. The safety and effectiveness of chronic filgrastim therapy have not been determined.

Side Effects: *Musculoskeletal:* Medullary bone pain, skeletal pain. *GI:* Nausea, vomiting, diarrhea, anorexia, stomatitis, constipation. *Respiratory:* Dyspnea, cough, chest pain, sore throat. *Body as a whole:* Alopecia, neutropenic fever, fever, fatigue, headache, skin rash, mucositis, generalized weakness, unspecified pain. *CV:* Decreased blood pressure (transient), arrhythmias, myocardial infarction.

Laboratory Test Interferences: ↑ Uric acid, lactic dehydrogenase, alkaline phosphatase.

Dosage: SC, IV. Initial, 5 mcg/kg/day as a single injection. The dose may be increased in increments of 5 mcg/kg for each chemotherapy cycle depending on the duration and severity of the absolute neutrophil count (ANC) nadir.

NURSING CONSIDERATIONS

Administration/Storage

1. Filgrastim is given daily for up to 2 weeks until the ANC has reached $10,000/m^3$ following the expected chemotherapy-induced neutrophil nadir.
2. Therapy should be discontinued if the ANC is greater than $10,000/mm^3$ after the expected chemotherapy-induced neutrophil nadir.
3. Discontinuing therapy usually results in a 50% decrease in circulating neutrophils within 1–2 days with a return to pretreatment levels in 1–7 days.

4. The product should not be frozen but stored in the refrigerator at 2°–8°C (36°–46°F). Prior to use, filgrastim can be at room temperature for a maximum of 6 hr. Any product left at room temperature for more than 6 hr should be discarded.
5. The product should not be shaken.
6. Only one dose should be used for each vial; the vial should not be re-entered.

Assessment

1. Determine any client hypersensitivity to *E. coli*-derived products.
2. Obtain baseline CBC and platelet counts and perform twice weekly during therapy (to prevent leukocytosis).
3. Document last dose of cytotoxic agent and determine ANC nadir. Drug should not be administered 24 hr before to 24 hr after cytotoxic chemotherapy.

Client/Family Teaching

1. Review the appropriate technique for administration of prescribed drug therapy and have client return demonstrate. Provide written guidelines concerning dose, administration time, drug storage and the proper method for storing, handling, and discarding of syringes.
2. Ensure that the client has the appropriate materials for drug administration and for proper disposal of equipment.
3. Remind client not to shake the container and to only enter the vial once.
4. Advise that "flu-like" symptoms (nausea, vomiting, and aching)

may be side effects of drug therapy. Also, bone pain has occurred and advise client to take prescribed analgesics and to report if persistent.

5. Encourage client to maintain a record of daily temperatures.
6. Advise to report for scheduled laboratory follow-up to evaluate the effectiveness of drug therapy.

Evaluation: Evaluate client for:
- Evidence of the prevention of infection during therapy with myelosuppressive anticancer drugs
- Laboratory confirmation of improved neutrophil counts

—— *COMBINATION DRUG* ——

Fiorinal
(fee-**OR**-in-al)

(Rx)

Fiorinal with Codeine
(fee-**OR**-in-al, **KOH**-deen)

(C-III, Rx)

See also *Narcotic Analgesics,* p. 174, *Aspirin,* p. 260, and *Barbiturates,* p. 101.

Classification/Content: Each Fiorinal capsule or tablet contains:
Nonnarcotic analgesic: Aspirin, 325 mg.
Sedative barbiturate: Butalbital, 50 mg.
CNS stimulant: Caffeine, 40 mg.

In addition to the above, Fiorinal with Codeine capsules contain phosphate, 7.5 mg (No. 1), 15 mg (No. 2), or 30 mg (No. 3).

Uses: Fiorinal is indicated for tension headaches. Fiorinal with Codeine is indicated as an analgesic for all types of pain.

Special Concerns: Pregnancy category: C (Fiorinal with Codeine).

Dosage: Capsules, Tablets. *Fiorinal:* 1–2 tablets or capsules q 4 hr not to exceed 6 tablets or capsules daily. *Fiorinal with Codeine.* **Initial,** 1–2 capsules; **then,** dose may be repeated, if necessary, up to maximum of 6 capsules daily.

NURSING CONSIDERATIONS

See *Nursing Considerations* for *Aspirin,* p. 264, and *Narcotic Analgesics,* p. 177.

Flavoxate hydrochloride
(flay-**VOX**-ayt)

Urispas (Rx)

Classification: Urinary tract antispasmodic.

Action/Kinetics: Flavoxate relieves muscle spasms of the urinary tract by acting directly on the smooth muscle; it relaxes the detrusor muscle by cholinergic blockade. The drug has local anesthetic and analgesic effects also. It is well absorbed from GI tract; 10%–30% is excreted in urine.

Uses: Symptomatic relief of urinary tract irritation, dysuria, urgency, nocturia, suprapubic pain, incontinence associated with cystitis, prostatitis, urethritis, urethrocystitis, and other urinary tract disorders. Compatible for use with urinary tract germicides.

Contraindications: Obstructive disorders of urinary tract, including pyloric or duodenal obstructions, intestinal lesions, ileus, achalasia (absence of gastric acid), and GI hemorrhage.

Special Concerns: Use with caution in glaucoma. Safe use in pregnancy (category: B) not established. Use with caution during lactation. Confusion is more likely to occur in geriatric clients. Safety and effectiveness have not been determined in children less than 12 years of age.

Side Effects: *GI:* Nausea, vomiting, xerostomia. *CNS:* Drowsiness, headache, vertigo, nervousness, mental confusion (especially in the elderly). *CV:* Tachycardia, palpitations. *Hematologic:* Eosinophilia, leukopenia. *Ophthalmologic:* Blurred vision, increased ocular tension, accommodation disturbances. *Other:* Urticaria, skin rashes, fever, dysuria.

Dosage: Tablets. Adults and children over 12 years: 100 or 200 mg t.i.d.–q.i.d. Dose may be reduced when symptoms decrease.

NURSING CONSIDERATIONS

See also *Nursing Considerations* for *Cholinergic Blocking Agents,* p. 138.

Client/Family Teaching

1. Do not drive a car or operate hazardous machinery because drug may cause drowsiness and blurred vision.
2. Practice good oral hygiene. Relieve dryness of mouth with ice chips or hard candy.
3. Report any persistent, bothersome side effects.

Evaluation: Evaluate client for
- Reports of symptomatic improvement in urinary tract symptoms and discomfort
- Evidence of any adverse side effects that would necessitate discontinuation of drug therapy

Flecainide acetate
(fleh-**KAY**-nyd)
Tambocor (Rx)

See also *Antiarrhythmic Drugs,* p. 51.

Classification: Antiarrhythmic, type IC.

Action/Kinetics: Flecainide produces its antiarrhythmic effect by a local anesthetic action, especially on the His–Purkinje system in the ventricle. The drug decreases single and multiple premature ventricular contractions and reduces the incidence of ventricular tachycardia. **Peak plasma levels:** 3 hr.; **steady state levels:** 3–5 days. **Effective plasma levels:** 0.2–1 mcg/ml. **t½:** 20 hr. Approximately 30% is excreted in urine unchanged. Impaired renal function decreases rate of elimination of unchanged drug. Food or antacids do not affect absorption.

Uses: Life-threatening arrhythmias manifested as sustained ventricular tachycardia. Prevention of paroxysmal supraventricular tachycardias (PSVT) and paroxysmal atrial fibrillation or flutter (PAF) associated with disabling symptoms but not structural heart disease.

Contraindications: Cardiogenic shock, preexisting second- or third-degree AV block, right bundle branch block when associated with bifascicular block (unless pacemaker is present to maintain cardiac rhythm). Frequent premature ventricular complexes and symptomatic nonsustained ventricular arrhythmias.

Special Concerns: Safe use has not been established in pregnancy (category: C) and lactation. Use with caution in sick sinus syndrome, congestive heart failure, myocardial infarction, in disturbances of potassium levels, in clients with permanent pacemakers or temporary pacing electrodes, renal and liver impairment. Safety and efficacy in children less than 18 years of age are not established. The incidence of proarrhythmic effects may be increased in geriatric clients.

Side Effects: *CV:* New or worsening ventricular arrhythmias, new or worsened congestive heart failure, palpitations, chest pain, sinus bradycardia, sinus pause, sinus arrest, ventricular fibrillation, ventricular tachycardia that cannot be resuscitated, second- or third-degree AV block, tachycardia, hypertension, hypotension, angina pectoris. *CNS:* Dizziness, faintness, syncope, lightheadedness, unsteadiness, headache, fatigue, paresthesia, paresis, insomnia, anxiety, malaise, vertigo, depression, seizures, euphoria, confusion, depersonalization, apathy, morbid dreams, speech disorders, stupor, amnesia, weakness, speech disorders. *GI:* Nausea, constipation, abdominal pain, vomiting, anorexia, dyspepsia, dry mouth, diarrhea, flatulence, change in taste. *Ophthalmic:* Blurred vision, difficulty in focusing, spots before eyes, diplopia, eye irritation, photophobia, eye pain, nystagmus, eye irritation, photophobia. *Hematologic:* Leukopenia, thrombocytopenia. *Genitourinary:* Decreased libido, impotence, urinary retention, polyuria. *Musculoskeletal:* Asthenia, tremor, ataxia, arthralgia, myalgia. *Other:* Edema, skin rashes, urticaria, exfoliative dermatitis, pruritus, dyspnea, fever, bronchospasm, flushing, sweating, swollen mouth, lips, and tongue.

Symptoms of Overdose: Lengthening of PR interval; increase in QRS duration, QT interval, and amplitude of T wave; decrease in heart rate and contractility; conduction disturbances; hypotension; respiratory failure or asystole.

Drug Interactions

Acidifying agents / ↑ Renal excretion of flecainide
Alkalinizing agents / ↓ Renal excretion of flecainide
Digitalis / ↑ Digoxin plasma levels
Disopyramide / Additive negative inotropic effects
Propranolol / Additive negative inotropic effects; also, ↑ plasma levels of both drugs
Verapamil / Additive negative inotropic effects

Dosage: Tablets. *Sustained ventricular tachycardia:* **initial,** 100 mg q 12 hr; **then,** increase by 50 mg b.i.d. q 4 days until effective dose reached. **Usual effective dose:** 150 mg q 12 hr; dose should not exceed 400 mg daily. *PSVT, PAF:* 50 mg q 12 hr.

NURSING CONSIDERATIONS

See also *Nursing Considerations* for *Antiarrhythmic Drugs,* p. 52.

Administration/Storage

1. For most situations, therapy should be started in a hospital setting (especially in clients with symptomatic congestive heart failure, sustained ventricular arrhythmias, compensated clients with significant myocardial dysfunction, or sinus node dysfunction).
2. For clients with renal impairment, the dosage should be increased at intervals greater

than 4 days. The client should be monitored carefully for adverse toxic effects.

3. The chance of toxic effects increases if the trough plasma levels exceed 1 mcg/ml.

4. If client is being transferred to flecainide from another anti-arrhythmic, at least two to four plasma half-lives should elapse for the drug being discontinued before initiating flecainide therapy.

5. An occasional client may benefit from dosing at 8-hr intervals.

6. To minimize toxicity, the dose may be reduced once the arrhythmia is controlled.

7. *Treatment of Overdose:* Administration of dopamine, dobutamine, or isoproterenol. Artificial respiration. Intraaortic balloon pumping, transvenous pacing (to correct conduction block). Due to the long duration of action of the drug, treatment measures may have to be continued for a prolonged period of time.

Assessment

1. Obtain baseline ECG, electrolytes, and renal function studies prior to initiating therapy.

2. Review client history and ECGs for evidence of congestive heart failure, ventricular arrhythmias, sinus node dysfunction, or abnormal ejection fractions.

Interventions

1. Monitor ECG for increased arrhythmias or AV block and report immediately to the physician.

2. Check serum potassium levels. Preexisting hypokalemia or hy-

perkalemia may alter the effects of the drug and should be corrected before starting therapy with flecainide.

3. Assess the client for labile blood pressure and document.

4. Note adverse CNS effects, such as client complaints of dizziness, visual disturbances, headaches, nausea, or depression and report.

5. Obtain urinary pH to detect alkalinity or acidity. Alkalinity of the urine decreases renal excretion and acidity increases renal excretion which in turn affects the rate of drug elimination.

6. Observe for any evidence of congestive heart failure.

7. Concomitant administration of flecainide with disopyramide, propranolol, or verapamil will promote additive negative inotropic effects.

Client/Family Teaching

1. Report any bruising or increased bleeding tendencies.

2. Observe for and report changes in elimination patterns.

3. Stress the importance of taking the medication in the dose and frequency prescribed.

Evaluation: Evaluate client for
- Successful termination of lethal ventricular arrhythmias
- Laboratory evidence of therapeutic serum drug level (0.2–1.0 mcg/ml)

Floxuridine
(flox-YOUR-ih-deen)
FUDR (Rx)

See also *Antineoplastic Agents,* p. 85.

Classification: Antineoplastic, antimetabolite.

Action/Kinetics: Floxuridine is cell-cycle specific for the S phase of cell division. The drug is rapidly metabolized to fluorouracil (see below). The drug inhibits DNA and RNA synthesis. Crosses blood-brain barrier. $t^{1/2}$: 5–20 min. From 60%–80% of fluorouracil is excreted as respiratory CO_2 (8–12 hr); small amount (15%) excreted in urine (1–6 hr).

Uses: Intra-arterially as palliative treatment of GI adenocarcinoma metastatic to the liver (especially in clients incurable by surgery or other treatment). Used in clients with disease limited to an area capable of infusion by a single artery. *Investigational:* Cancer of the breast, ovaries, cervix, bladder, kidney, and prostate.

Contraindications: If client is at poor risk, including depressed bone marrow function, nutritionally poor, or potentially serious infections. Lactation. Should not be used during pregnancy unless benefits clearly outweigh risks.

Additional Side Effects: Esophagopharyngitis, myocardial ischemia, angina, acute cerebellar syndrome, photophobia, lacrimation, decreased vision. Complications of intra-arterial administration are arterial aneurysm, arterial ischemia, arterial thrombosis, bleeding at catheter site, occluded, displaced, or leaking catheters, embolism, fibromyositis, infection at catheter site, thrombophlebitis.

Laboratory Test Interferences: ↑ Excretion of 5-hydroxyindole-acetic acid. ↑ Serum transaminase and bilirubin, lactic dehydrogenase, alkaline phosphatase. ↓ Plasma albumin.

Dosage: Intra-arterial infusion: 0.1–0.6 mg/kg/day by continuous infusion over 24 hr. Infusion is continued until a response or toxicity occurs (usually for 14–21 days with a rest period of 2 weeks between courses of therapy).

NURSING CONSIDERATIONS

See also *Nursing Considerations* for *Antineoplastic Agents,* p. 88.

Administration/Storage

1. Higher doses (0.4–0.6 mg) are best given by hepatic artery infusion because the liver metabolizes the drug, reducing the possibility of systemic toxicity.
2. The drug should be given until adverse effects are manifested. Resume therapy after adverse effects have subsided.
3. An infusion pump should be used to overcome pressure in the large arteries and to assure a uniform rate of infusion.
4. The drug should be reconstituted with 5 ml sterile water.
5. Reconstituted vials should be stored in the refrigerator at 2°C–8°C (36°F–46°F) for no longer than 2 weeks.

Fluconazole
(flew-**KON**-ah-zohl)
Diflucan (Rx)

Classification: Antifungal agent.

Action/Kinetics: Fluconazole inhibits the enzyme cytochrome P-450, which is essential to survival of fungal cells. Inhibition of the enzyme results in a decrease in cell wall integrity and extrusion of intracellular material. Fluconazole apparently does not affect the cytochrome P-450 enzyme in animals or humans. **Peak plasma levels:** 1–2 hr. **t½:** 30 hr, which allows for once daily dosing. The drug penetrates all body fluids at steady state. Bioavailability is not affected by agents that increase gastric pH. Eighty percent of the drug is excreted unchanged by the kidneys.

Uses: Oropharyngeal and esophageal candidiasis. Serious systemic candidal infection (including urinary tract infections, peritonitis, and pneumonia). Cryptococcal meningitis. Maintenance therapy to prevent cryptococcal meningitis in AIDS clients.

Contraindications: Hypersensitivity to fluconazole.

Special Concerns: Use with caution if client shows hypersensitivity to other azoles. Use during pregnancy (category: C) only if the potential benefit justifies the potential risk to the fetus. Care should be used when fluconazole is prescribed during lactation. The effectiveness of the drug has not been adequately assessed in children.

Side Effects: Side effects are more frequently reported in HIV infected clients than in non-HIV infected clients. *GI:* Nausea, vomiting, abdominal pain, diarrhea. *Miscellaneous:* Headache, skin rash, hepatotoxicity, exfoliative skin disorders.

Laboratory Test Interferences: ↑ AST, serum transaminase (especially if used with isoniazid, oral hypoglycemic agents, phenytoin, rifampin, valproic acid).

Drug Interactions

Cimetidine / ↓ Plasma levels of fluconazole
Cyclosporine / Fluconazole may ↑ cyclosporine levels in renal transplant clients with or without impaired renal function
Hydrochlorothiazide / ↑ Plasma levels of fluconazole due to ↓ renal clearance
Glipizide / ↑ Plasma levels of glipizide due to ↓ breakdown by the liver
Glyburide / ↑ Plasma levels of glyburide due to ↓ breakdown by the liver
Phenytoin / Fluconazole ↑ plasma levels of phenytoin
Rifampin / ↓ Plasma levels of fluconazole due to ↑ breakdown by the liver
Tolbutamide / ↑ Plasma levels of tolbutamide due to ↓ breakdown by the liver
Warfarin / ↑ Prothrombin time

Dosage: Tablets, IV, Adults: *Oropharyngeal or esophageal candidiasis:* **first day,** 200 mg; **then,** 100 mg once daily for a minimum of 14 days (for oropharyngeal candidiasis) or 21 days (for esophageal candidiasis). Up to 400 mg daily may be required for esophageal candidiasis. *Systemic candidiasis:* **first day,** 400 mg; **then,** 200 mg daily for at least 28 days. *Acute cryptococcal meningitis:* **first day,** 400 mg; **then,** 200 mg daily (up to 400 mg may be required) for 10–12 weeks after CSF culture is negative. *Maintenance to prevent relapse of cryptococcal meningitis:* 200 mg daily. **Pediatric:** 3–6 mg/kg daily. In clients with renal impairment, an initial loading dose of 50–400 mg can be given; daily dose is based then on creatinine clearance.

NURSING CONSIDERATIONS

Administration/Storage

1. The IV solution should not be used if it is cloudy or precipitated or the seal is not intact.

2. The rate of IV infusion of fluconazole should not exceed 200 mg/hr as a continuous infusion.
3. Supplementary medication should not be added to the IV bag.

Assessment

1. Take a thorough nursing and drug history. Note any history of hypersensitivity to azoles or similar class of drugs.
2. Determine if client is HIV infected (if possible) because this may place client at an increased risk for possible side effects.

Interventions

1. Due to a long half-life, once daily dosing (either IV or PO) is possible.
2. Obtain baseline liver function studies. Clients who develop abnormal liver function tests should be closely monitored for the development of more serious liver toxicity.
3. Observe immunocompromised clients closely for evidence of a rash; if lesions progress, the drug should be discontinued.

Client/Family Teaching

1. Review goals of therapy and appropriate method and schedule for medication administration.
2. Stress the importance of reporting any rash or persistent side effects to the physician and to report for all scheduled lab studies.

Evaluation

1. Note status of pretreatment symptoms and laboratory culture results to assess response to therapy.
2. Assess reports of any adverse effects that would necessitate discontinuation of drug therapy.

Flucytosine
(flew-**SYE**-toe-seen)
Ancobon, Ancotil✹ (Rx)

Classification: Antibiotic, antifungal.

Action/Kinetics: Flucytosine is indicated only for serious systemic fungal infections. The drug is less toxic than amphotericin B. Liver, renal system, and hematopoietic system must be monitored closely.

Flucytosine appears to penetrate the fungal cell membrane and then, after metabolism, to act as an antimetabolite interfering with nucleic acid and protein synthesis. It is well absorbed from the GI tract and is distributed to the joints, aqueous humor, peritoneal and other body fluids and tissues. **Peak plasma concentration:** 2–6 hr. **Therapeutic serum concentration:** 20–25 mcg/ml. **t½:** 2–5 hr, higher in presence of impaired renal function. 80–90% of the drug is excreted unchanged in urine.

Uses: Serious systemic infections by susceptible strains of *Candida* (e.g., endocarditis, septicemia, urinary tract infections) or *Cryptococcus* (pulmonary or urinary tract infections, meningitis, septicemia).

Contraindications: Hypersensitivity to drug. Lactation.

Special Concerns: Pregnancy category: C. Safety and effectiveness have not been determined in children. Use with extreme caution in clients with kidney disease or history of bone marrow depression. Use during childbearing age only if benefits clearly outweigh risks. The bone marrow depressant effects may cause an increased incidence of microbial infection, gingival bleeding, and delayed healing.

Side Effects: *GI:* Nausea, vomiting, diarrhea, abdominal pain, dry mouth, anorexia, duodenal ulcer, GI hemorrhage, ulcerative colitis. *Hematologic:* Anemia, leukopenia, thrombocytopenia, aplastic anemia, agranulocytosis, pancytopenia, eosinophilia. *CNS:* Headache, vertigo, confusion, sedation, hallucinations, paresthesia, parkinsonism, psychosis, pyrexia. *Hepatic:* Hepatic dysfunction, jaundice, elevation of hepatic enzymes, increase in bilirubin. *GU:* Increase in BUN and creatinine, azotemia, crystalluria, renal failure. *Respiratory:* Chest pain, dyspnea, respiratory arrest. *Dermatologic:* Pruritus, rash, urticaria, photosensitivity. *Other:* Ataxia, hearing loss, peripheral neuropathy, weakness, hypoglycemia, fatigue, cardiac arrest, hypokalemia.

Symptoms of Overdose (serum levels greater than 100 mcg/ml): Nausea, vomiting, diarrhea, leukopenia, thrombocytopenia, hepatitis.

Drug Interactions

Amphotericin B / ↑ Effect and toxicity of flucytosine due to kidney impairment

Cytosine / Inactivates antifungal effect of flucytosine

Dosage: Capsules. Adult and children: 50–150 mg/kg daily in 4 divided doses. Clients with renal impairment receive lower dosages.

NURSING CONSIDERATIONS

See also *General Nursing Considerations For All Anti-Infectives,* p. 83.

Administration/Storage

1. Reduce or avoid nausea by administering capsules a few at a time over a 15-min period.
2. *Treatment of Overdose:* Prompt induction of vomiting or gastric lavage. Adequate fluid intake (by IV if necessary). Monitor blood, liver, and kidney parameters frequently. Hemodialysis will quickly decrease serum levels.

Assessment

1. Obtain baseline CBC and liver and renal function studies and monitor throughout therapy.
2. Before administering first dose, check that culture has been taken.

Interventions

1. Ascertain that weekly cultures are taken to determine that strains have not become resistant. A strain is considered resistant if the minimal inhibitory concentration (MIC) value is greater than 100.
2. Monitor intake and output. Report reduction in urine output as well as any blood, sediment, or cloudiness in the urine.
3. Anticipate reduced dose with impaired renal function.
4. Hepatic function should be monitored frequently during therapy.

Fludarabine phosphate
(floo-**DAIR**-ah-bean)
Fludara (Rx)

See also *Antineoplastic Agents,* p. 85.

Classification: Antineoplastic, antimetabolite.

Action/Kinetics: Fludarabine is rapidly dephosphorylated to 2-fluoro-ara-A and then phosphorylated within the cell by the enzyme deoxycytidine kinase to the active 2-fluoro-ara-ATP. This compound inhibits DNA polymerase alpha, ribonucleotide reductase, and DNA primase, resulting in inhibition of DNA synthesis. $t^{1/2}$, **2-fluoro-ara-A:** About 10 hr. Approximately 23% of a dose of fludarabine is excreted in the urine as unchanged 2-fluoro-ara-A.

Uses: Chronic lymphocytic leukemia in individuals who have not responded to at least one standard alkylating agent-containing regimen. *Investigational:* Non-Hodgkin's lymphoma, macroglobulinemic lymphoma, prolymphocytic leukemia or prolymphocytoid variant of chronic lymphocytic leukemia, mycosis fungoides, hairy-cell leukemia, Hodgkin's disease.

Contraindications: Lactation.

Special Concerns: Pregnancy category: D. Use with caution in clients with renal insufficiency. The safety and effectiveness of fludarabine in children and in previously untreated or nonrefractory chronic lymphocytic leukemia clients have not been established. Fludarabine produces dose-dependent toxic effects. An increased risk of toxicity is possible in geriatric clients, in renal insufficiency, and in bone marrow impairment.

Side Effects: *Hematologic:* Neutropenia, thrombocytopenia, anemia. *Tumor lysis syndrome:* Hyperuricemia, hyperphosphatemia, hypocalcemia, hyperkalemia, hematu-

ria, metabolic acidosis, urate crystalluria, renal failure. Flank pain and hematuria may signal the onset of the syndrome. *GI:* Nausea, vomiting, anorexia, stomatitis, diarrhea, GI bleeding. *CNS:* Malaise, fatigue, weakness, agitation, confusion, coma. *Neuromuscular:* Peripheral neuropathy, paresthesia, myalgia. *Respiratory:* Pneumonia, dyspnea, cough, interstitial pulmonary infiltrate. *GU:* Dysuria, urinary infection, hematuria. *Miscellaneous:* Edema (common), skin rashes, fever, chills, serious opportunistic infections, pain, visual disturbances, hearing loss.

Symptoms of Overdose: Irreversible CNS toxicity including delayed blindness, coma, and death. Severe thrombocytopenia and neutropenia.

Dosage: IV, Adults, usual: 25 mg/m^2 given over a period of 30 min for 5 consecutive days. A 5-day course of therapy should be initiated every 28 days.

NURSING CONSIDERATIONS

See also *Nursing Considerations* for *Antineoplastic Agents,* p. 88.

Administration/Storage

1. The dose may be decreased or delayed based on the presence of hematologic or neurotoxicity.
2. It is recommended that after a maximal response has been seen that three additional cycles be administered; the drug should then be discontinued.
3. The lyophilized product should be reconstituted with 2 ml of sterile water for injection, USP. Each ml of the resulting solution will contain 25 mg fludarabine phosphate with the

final pH ranging from 7.2–8.2. This may then be diluted in 100 or 125 ml of 5% dextrose injection, USP or 0.9% sodium chloride, USP.

4. Reconstituted fludarabine contains no preservatives; thus, it must be used within 8 hr.

5. If the solution comes in contact with the skin or mucous membranes, wash thoroughly with soap and water. Eyes should be rinsed thoroughly with plain water.

6. The product should be stored under refrigeration at a temperature of 2°–8°C (36°–46°F).

7. *Treatment of Overdose:* Discontinue administration of the drug and treat symptoms. The hematologic profile should be monitored.

Assessment

1. Perform a baseline CNS assessment and document.

2. Obtain baseline hematologic parameters and renal function studies and monitor throughout therapy.

Client/Family Teaching

1. Advise client to report any evidence of flank pain or hematuria as this may preclude a tumor lysis syndrome.

2. Practice barrier birth control during drug therapy.

3. Report any evidence of infection (sore throat, fever) and the development of any abnormal bruising or bleeding.

Evaluation: Evaluate client for hematologic evidence of control of the malignant process.

Fludrocortisone acetate

(flew-droh-**KOR**-tih-sohn)

Florinef (Rx)

See also *Adrenocorticosteroids and Analogs,* p. 8.

Classification: Adrenocorticosteroid, synthetic; mineralocorticoid type.

Action/Kinetics: Produces marked sodium retention and inhibits excess adrenocortical secretion. Should not be used systemically for its anti-inflammatory effects. Supplementary potassium may be indicated.

Uses: Addison's disease and adrenal hyperplasia.

Special Concerns: Pregnancy category: C.

Dosage: Tablets. *Addison's disease:* 0.1–0.2 mg daily to 0.1 mg 3 times/week, usually in conjunction with hydrocortisone or cortisone. *Salt-losing adrenogenital syndrome:* 0.1–0.2 mg/day.

NURSING CONSIDERATIONS

See *Nursing Considerations* for *Adrenocorticosteroids and Analogs,* p. 15.

Flunisolide

(flew-**NISS**-oh-lyd)

Inhalation: AeroBid, Bronalide Aerosol✤ (Rx). Intranasal: Nasalide, Rhinalar✤ (Rx)

See also *Adrenocorticosteroids and Analogs,* p. 8.

Classification: Intranasal and inhalation corticosteroid.

Action/Kinetics: Produces anti-inflammatory effects intranasally with minimal systemic effects. Several days may be required for full beneficial effects. After inhalation, there is a significant first-pass effect through the liver and the drug is rapidly metabolized. **t½:** 1.8 hr.

Uses: Inhalation: Bronchial asthma in combination with other therapy. Not used when asthma can be relieved by other drugs, in clients where systemic corticosteroid treatment is infrequent, and in nonasthmatic bronchitis. **Intranasal:** Seasonal or perennial rhinitis, especially if other treatment has proven unsatisfactory.

Contraindications: Active or quiescent tuberculosis, especially of the respiratory tract. Untreated fungal, bacterial, systemic viral infections. Ocular herpes simplex. Do not use until healing occurs following recent ulceration of nasal septum, nasal surgery, or trauma. Lactation.

Special Concerns: Pregnancy category: C. Safety and effectiveness in children less than 6 years of age have not been determined.

Additional Side Effects: *Respiratory:* Hoarseness, coughing, throat irritation; *Candida* infections of nose, larynx, and pharynx. *After intranasal use:* Nasopharyngeal irritation, stinging, burning, dryness, headache. *GI:* Dry mouth. Systemic corticosteroid effects, especially if recommended dose is exceeded.

Dosage: Inhalation. Adults: 2 inhalations (total of 500 mcg flunisolide) in A.M. and P.M., not to exceed 4 inhalations b.i.d. (i.e., total daily dose of 2 mg). **Pediatric, 6–15 years:** 2 inhalations b.i.d.

Intranasal. Adults: initial, 50 mcg (2 sprays) in each nostril b.i.d.; may be increased to 2 sprays t.i.d. up to maximum daily dose of 400 mcg (i.e., 8 sprays in each nostril). **Pediatric, 6–14 years: initial,** 25 mcg (1 spray) in each nostril t.i.d. or 50 mcg (2 sprays) in each nostril b.i.d. Up to maximum daily dose of 200 mcg (i.e., 4 sprays in each nostril). **Maintenance, adults, children:** Smallest dose necessary to control symptoms. Some clients (approximately 15%) are controlled on 1 spray in each nostril daily.

NURSING CONSIDERATIONS

See also *Nursing Considerations* for *Adrenocorticosteroids and Analogs,* p. 15.

Administration/Storage

1. When initiating the inhalant in clients receiving corticosteroids systemically, the aerosol should be used concomitantly with the systemic steroid for 1 week. Then, slowly withdraw the systemic corticosteroid over several weeks.
2. If nasal congestion is present, use a decongestant before administration to ensure the drug reaches the site of action.
3. If beneficial effects do not occur within 3 weeks, discontinue therapy.

Interventions: Assess the oral mucosa closely for any evidence of fungal infections.

Client/Family Teaching

1. Instruct client and family how to administer nasal spray.
2. Remind clients to rinse their mouth with water after inhala-

tion to prevent alterations in taste and to maintain adequate oral hygiene.
3. Provide a printed list of drug side effects. Identify those that require immediate reporting.

Evaluation: Evaluate client for
- Knowledge and understanding of illness as well as level of compliance with drug therapy
- Reports of symptomatic improvement in pretreatment symptoms

---

Fluorouracil (5-Fluorouracil, 5-FU)

(flew-roh-**YOUR**-ah-sill)
Adrucil, Efudex, Fluoroplex (Abbreviation: 5-FU) (Rx)

See also *Antineoplastic Agents,* p. 85.

Classification: Antineoplastic, antimetabolite.

Action/Kinetics: Pyrimidine antagonist that inhibits the methylation reaction of deoxyuridylic acid to thymidylic acid. Thus, the synthesis of DNA, and to a lesser extent, RNA, is inhibited. The drug is cell-cycle specific for the S phase of cell division. $t\frac{1}{2}$, **initial:** 5–20 min; **final:** 20 hr. From 60%–80% eliminated as respiratory CO_2 (8–12 hr); small amount (15%) excreted unchanged in urine (1–6 hr).

Highly toxic; initiate use in hospital. Initially, topical creams cause ulcers, which might heal only 1–2 months after cessation of therapy.

Uses: Systemic: Palliative management of certain cancers of the rectum, stomach, colon, pancreas, and breast. Relieves pain and reduces size of tumor. In combina-

tion with levamisole for Dukes' stage C colon cancer. In combination with leucovorin for metastatic colorectal cancer. **Topical (as solution or cream):** Actinic or solar keratosis, superficial basal cell carcinoma. *Investigational:* **Systemic:** Cancer of the bladder, ovaries, prostate, cervix, endometrium, lung, liver, head, and neck. Also, malignant pleural, peritoneal, and pericardial effusions. **Topical:** Actinic cheilitis, mucosal leukoplakia, Bowen's disease, radiodermatitis, erythroplasia of Queyrat.

Additional Contraindications: Systemic: Clients in poor nutritional state, with severe bone marrow depression, severe infection, or recent (4-week-old) surgical intervention. Lactation. To be used with caution in clients with hepatic or liver dysfunction.

Special Concerns: Use during pregnancy only if benefits clearly outweigh risks (pregnancy category: D).

Additional Side Effects: Esophagopharyngitis, myocardial ischemia, angina, acute cerebellar syndrome, photophobia, lacrimation, decreased vision. Also, arterial thrombosis, arterial ischemia, arterial aneurysm, bleeding or infection at site of catheter, thrombophlebitis, embolism, fibromyositis, abscesses.

Symptoms of Overdose: Nausea, vomiting, diarrhea, GI ulceration, GI bleeding, thrombocytopenia, agranulocytosis, leukopenia.

Drug Interactions: Leucovorin calcium ↑ toxicity of fluorouracil.

Laboratory Test Interferences: ↑ Alkaline phosphatase, lactic dehydrogenase, serum bilirubin, and serum transaminase.

Dosage: IV. Individualize dosage. Initial: 12 mg/kg/day for 4 days, not to exceed 800 mg/day. If no toxicity seen, administer 6 mg/kg on days 6, 8, 10, and 12. Discontinue therapy on day 12 even if there are no toxic symptoms. **Maintenance:** Repeat dose of first course every 30 days or when toxicity from initial course of therapy is gone; or, give 10–15 mg/kg/week as a single dose. Do not exceed 1 g/week. **If client is debilitated or is a poor risk:** 6 mg/kg/day for 3 days; if no toxicity, give 3 mg/kg on days 5, 7, and 9 (daily dose should not exceed 400 mg). *Metastatic colorectal cancer:* Leucovorin, **IV,** 200 mg/m²/day for 5 days followed by fluorouracil, **IV,** 370 mg/m²/day for 5 days. Repeat q 28 days to maximize response and to prolong survival. **Cream, Topical Solution:** *Actinic or solar keratoses:* Apply 1%–5% cream or solution to cover lesion 1–2 times daily for 2–6 weeks. *Superficial basal cell carcinoma:* Apply 5% cream or solution to cover lesion b.i.d. for 3–6 weeks (up to 10–12 weeks may be required).

NURSING CONSIDERATIONS

See also *Nursing Considerations* for *Antineoplastic Agents,* p. 88.

Administration/Storage

IV

1. Store in a cool place (50°F–80°F or 10°C–27°C). Do not freeze. Excessively low temperature causes precipitation.
2. Do not expose the solution to light.
3. Solution may discolor slightly during storage, but potency and safety are not affected.
4. If precipitate forms, resolubilize by heating to 140°F with vigorous shaking. Allow to return to room temperature and allow air to settle out before withdrawing and administering medication.
5. Further dilution is not needed, and solution may be injected directly into the vein with a 25-gauge needle.
6. Drug can be administered by IV infusion for periods of 30 min–8 hr. This method has been reported to produce less systemic toxicity than rapid injection.
7. The drug should not be mixed with other drugs or IV additives.
8. *Treatment of Overdose:* Monitor hematologically for at least 4 weeks.

TOPICAL

1. Apply with fingertips, nonmetallic applicator, or rubber gloves. Wash hands immediately thereafter.
2. Avoid contact with eyes, nose, and mouth.
3. Limit occlusive dressings to lesions, since they are responsible for an increased incidence of inflammatory reactions in normal skin.
4. Complete healing of keratoses may require 2 months.

Assessment

1. Observe for intractable vomiting, stomatitis, and diarrhea, all of which are early signs of toxicity and thus indicate immediate discontinuation of drug.
2. The drug also should be discontinued if WBC and platelet counts are depressed below 3,500/mm³ and 100,000/mm³, respectively.

Interventions

1. Practice reverse isolation techniques when WBC count is below 2,000/mm³.
2. Prevent exposure to strong sunlight and other ultraviolet rays because these rays intensify skin reaction to the drug.

Client/Family Teaching

1. Review and demonstrate appropriate method for topical administration.
2. Advise to drink plenty of fluids during therapy with fluorouracil.
3. Instruct both men and women to practice barrier contraception during drug therapy.
4. Avoid exposure to sunlight. If exposure is necessary, wear protective clothing and sunscreen.
5. Provide a printed list of drug side effects. Stress those that require immediate reporting.

Evaluation: Assess client for a positive tumor response as evidenced by a ↓ in tumor size and spread.

Fluoxetine hydrochloride
(flew-**OX**-eh-teen)
Prozac (Rx)

Classification: Antidepressant, miscellaneous

Action/Kinetics: Fluoxetine is not related chemically to tricyclic, tetracyclic, or other antidepressants. The antidepressant effect is thought to be due to inhibition of uptake of serotonin into CNS neurons. The drug also binds to musca-

rinic, histaminergic, and alpha-1-adrenergic receptors, accounting for many of the side effects. Fluoxetine is metabolized in the liver to norfluoxetine, a metabolite with equal potency to fluoxetine. Norfluoxetine is further metabolized by the liver to inactive metabolites that are excreted by the kidneys. **t½, fluoxetine:** 2–7 days; **t½, norfluoxetine:** 7–9 days. Steady-state plasma levels are achieved after 4–5 weeks. Active drug will be maintained in the body for weeks after withdrawal.

Uses: Depression manifested by outpatients. Use in hospitalized clients or for longer than 5–6 weeks has not been studied adequately. *Investigational:* Treatment of obesity and bulimia nervosa and obsessive-compulsive disorders.

Special Concerns: Use with caution during pregnancy (category: B) and lactation and in clients with impaired liver or kidney function. Safety and efficacy have not been determined in children. A lower initial dose may be necessary in geriatric clients.

Side Effects: A large number of side effects have been reported for this drug. Listed are those with a reported frequency of greater than 1%. *CNS:* Headache (most common), activation of mania or hypomania, insomnia, anxiety, nervousness, dizziness, fatigue, sedation, decreased libido, drowsiness, light-headedness, decreased ability to concentrate, tremor, disturbances in sensation, agitation, abnormal dreams. Although less frequent than 1%, some clients may experience seizures or attempt suicide. *GI:* Nausea (most common), diarrhea, vomiting, constipation, dry mouth, dyspepsia, anorexia, abdominal pain, flatulence, alteration in taste, gastroenteritis, increased appetite. *CV:* Hot flashes, palpitations. *GU:* Sexual dysfunction, frequent urination, infection of the urinary tract, dysmenorrhea. *Respiratory:* Upper respiratory tract infections, pharyngitis, cough, dyspnea, rhinitis, bronchitis, nasal congestion. *Skin:* Rash, pruritus, sweating. *Musculoskeletal:* Muscle, joint, or back pain. *Miscellaneous:* Flu-like symptoms, asthenia, fever, chest pain, allergy, visual disturbances, weight loss.

Drug Interactions

Diazepam / Fluoxetine ↑ half-life of diazepam → excessive sedation or impaired psychomotor skills

Digoxin / ↑ Effect of fluoxetine due to ↓ plasma protein binding

Lithium / ↑ Serum levels of lithium → possible neurotoxicity

MAO inhibitors / MAO inhibitors should be discontinued 14 days before initiation of fluoxetine therapy

Tricyclic antidepressants / ↑ Pharmacologic and toxicologic effects of tricyclics due to ↓ breakdown by liver

Tryptophan / Symptoms of agitation, GI distress, restlessness

Warfarin / ↑ Effect of fluoxetine due to ↓ plasma protein binding

Dosage: Capsules, Liquid. Adults, initial: 20 mg daily in the morning. If clinical improvement is not observed after several weeks, the dose may be increased to a maximum of 80 mg daily in two equally divided doses.

NURSING CONSIDERATIONS

Administration/Storage

1. Doses greater than 20 mg daily should be divided and given in the morning and at noon.
2. If doses lower than 20 mg are necessary, the drug may be emptied from the capsule into cranberry, orange, or apple juice; this should not be refrigerated (is stable for 2 weeks). Note: A liquid preparation (20 mg/5 ml) is also available.
3. The maximum therapeutic effect may not be observed until 4 weeks after beginning therapy.
4. Elderly clients or clients taking multiple medications should take lower or less frequent doses.
5. Lower doses should be used in clients with liver or kidney dysfunction.

Assessment

1. Obtain baseline liver and renal function studies prior to initiating therapy. Anticipate reduced dose in clients with hepatic and/or renal insufficiency.
2. In women of childbearing age, determine if pregnant or lactating.

Client/Family Teaching

1. Use caution when driving or performing tasks that require mental alertness because drug may cause drowsiness and/or dizziness.
2. Report any side effects, especially rashes, hives, increased anxiety, and loss of appetite.
3. Stress the importance of taking the medication at the specific times designated by the physician.

4. Remind client that it usually takes 1 month to note any significant benefits from therapy and not to become discouraged and discontinue the medication before benefits are attained and evaluated.
5. Do not take any OTC medications without first consulting with physician.
6. Avoid ingestion of alcohol.
7. Stress the importance of reporting for all scheduled lab and medical visits.
8. Any thoughts of suicide or evidence of increased suicide ideations should be reported immediately to the physician.

Evaluation: Evaluate client for:
- Reports of a reduction in level of depression
- Improved appetite and evidence of increased social involvement and activity
- Freedom from complications of adverse drug effects

Fluphenazine decanoate

(flew-**FEN**-ah-zeen)

Prolixin Decanoate, Modecate Decanoate ✹, Modecate Concentrate ✹ (Rx)

Fluphenazine enanthate

(flew-**FEN**-ah-zeen)

Prolixin Enanthate, Moditen Enanthate ✹ (Rx)

Fluphenazine hydrochloride

(flew-**FEN**-ah-zeen)

Apo-Fluphenazine ✹, Permitil, Prolixin, Moditen HCl ✹, Moditen HCl-H.P. ✹ (Rx)

See also *Phenothiazines,* p. 201.

Classification: Antipsychotic, piperazine-type phenothiazine.

Action/Kinetics: Fluphenazine is accompanied by a high incidence of extrapyramidal symptoms and a low incidence of sedation, anticholinergic effects, antiemetic effects, and orthostatic hypotension. The enanthate and decanoate esters dramatically increase the duration of action. *Decanoate:* **Onset,** 24–72 hr; **peak plasma levels,** 24–48 hr; **t½** (approximate), 14 days; **duration:** up to 4 weeks. *Enanthate:* **Onset,** 24–72 hr; **peak plasma levels,** 48–72 hr; **t½** (approximate): 3.6 days; **duration:** 1–3 weeks.

Fluphenazine hydrochloride can be cautiously administered to clients with known hypersensitivity to other phenothiazines.

Fluphenazine enanthate may replace fluphenazine hydrochloride if desired response occurs with hypersensitivity reaction to fluphenazine.

Uses: Psychotic disorders. Adjunct to tricyclic antidepressants for chronic pain states (e.g., diabetic neuropathy, and clients trying to withdraw from narcotics).

Dosage: Fluphenazine hydrochloride is administered **PO and IM.** Fluphenazine enanthate or decanoate are administered **SC and IM.**

Elixir, Oral Solution, Tablets. *Psychotic disorders:* **Adults and adolescents, initial:** 2.5–10 mg/day in divided doses q 6–8 hr; **then,** reduce gradually to maintenance dose of 1–5 mg/day (usually given as a single dose, not to exceed 20 mg/day). *Geriatric, emaciated, debilitated clients:* **Initial:** 1–2.5 mg/day; **then,** dosage determined by response. **Pediatric:** 0.25–0.75 mg 1–4 times daily.

IM, Hydrochloride. Adults and adolescents: 1.25–2.5 mg q 6–8 hr as needed. Maximum daily dose: 10 mg. Elderly, debilitated, or emaciated clients should start with 1–2.5 mg daily.

IM, SC. Decanoate. *Psychotic disorders:* **Adults, initial,** 12.5–25 mg; **then,** the dose may be repeated or increased q 1–3 weeks. The usual maintenance dose is 50 mg q 1–4 weeks. Maximum adult dose: 100 mg/dose. **Pediatric, 12 years and older:** 6.25–18.75 mg weekly; the dose can be increased to 12.5–25 mg given q 1–3 weeks. **Pediatric, 5–12 years:** 3.125–12.5 mg with this dose being repeated q 1–3 weeks.

IM, SC. Enanthate. *Psychotic disorders:* **Adults and adolescents:** 25 mg; dose can be repeated or increased q 1–3 weeks. For doses greater than 50 mg, increases should be made in increments of 12.5 mg. Maximum adult dose: 100 mg/dose.

NURSING CONSIDERATIONS

See also *Nursing Considerations* for *Phenothiazines,* p. 205.

Administration/Storage

1. Protect all forms of medication from light.
2. Store at room temperature and avoid freezing.
3. Color of parenteral solution may vary from colorless to light amber. Do not use solutions that are darker than light amber.
4. The hydrochloride concentrate should not be mixed with any beverage containing caffeine, tannates (e.g., tea), or pectins (e.g., apple juice) due to a physical incompatibility.
5. Clients beginning therapy with

phenothiazines should first receive a short-acting form of the drug; the decanoate and enanthate can be considered after the response to the drug has been evaluated.

Assessment: Note the age and condition of the client. Elderly and debilitated clients are particularly at risk for acute extrapyramidal symptoms.

Evaluation: Evaluate client for:
- Evidence of improved behavior patterns
- Reports of improved coping mechanisms
- Evidence of a reduction in paranoia and withdrawal behaviors

---

Flurazepam hydrochloride

(flur-**AYZ**-eh-pam)
Apo-Flurazepam ✿, Dalmane, Durapam, Novo–Flupam ✿, Somnol ✿,(C-IV, Rx)

See also *Benzodiazepines,* p. 108.

Classification: Benzodiazepine sedative-hypnotic.

Action/Kinetics: Flurazepam acts at benzodiazepine receptors, which are part of the benzodiazepine-GABA receptor-chloride ionophore complex. Interaction with the complex enhances the inhibitory action of GABA leading to interference of transmission of nerve impulses in the reticular activating system. **Onset:** 17 min. The major active metabolite, *N*-desalkyl-flurazepam, is active and has a $t\frac{1}{2}$ of 47–100 hr. **Time to peak plasma levels, flurazepam:** 0.5–1 hr; **active metabolite:** 1–3 hr. **Duration:** 7–

8 hr. **Maximum effectiveness:** 2–3 days (due to slow accumulation of active metabolite). Significantly bound to plasma protein. Elimination is slow because metabolites remain in the blood for several days. Exceeding the recommended dose may result in development of tolerance and dependence.

Use: Insomnia (all types). Flurazepam is increasingly effective on the second or third night of consecutive use and for one or two nights after the drug is discontinued.

Contraindications: Hypersensitivity. Pregnancy or in women wishing to become pregnant. Depression, renal or hepatic disease, chronic pulmonary insufficiency, children under 15 years.

Special Concerns: Use during the last few weeks of pregnancy may result in CNS depression of the neonate. Use during lactation may cause sedation and feeding problems in the infant. Geriatric clients may be more sensitive to the effects of flurazepam.

Side Effects: *CNS:* Ataxia, dizziness, drowsiness/sedation, headache, disorientation. Symptoms of stimulation including nervousness, apprehension, irritability, and talkativeness. *GI:* Nausea, vomiting, diarrhea, gastric upset or pain, heartburn, constipation. *Miscellaneous:* Arthralgia, chest pains, or palpitations. Rarely, symptoms of allergy, shortness of breath, jaundice, anorexia, blurred vision.

Drug Interactions

Cimetidine / ↑ Effect of flurazepam due to ↓ breakdown by liver

CNS depressants / Addition or potentiation of CNS depressant effects—drowsiness, lethargy, stupor, respiratory depression or collapse, coma, and possible death

Disulfiram / ↑ Effect of flurazepam due to ↓ breakdown by liver

Ethanol / Additive depressant effects up to the day following flurazepam administration

Isoniazid / ↑ Effect of flurazepam due to ↓ breakdown by liver

Oral contraceptives / Either ↑ or ↓ effect of benzodiazepines due to effect on breakdown by liver

Rifampin / ↓ Effect of benzodiazepines due to ↑ breakdown by liver

Laboratory Test Interference: ↑ Alkaline phosphatase, bilirubin, serum transaminases.

Dosage: Capsules. Adults: 15–30 mg at bedtime; 15 mg for geriatric and/or debilitated clients.

NURSING CONSIDERATIONS

See also *Nursing Considerations for Benzodiazepines,* p. 111.

Client/Family Teaching

1. Avoid the ingestion of alcohol during therapy with flurazepam.
2. Use caution in driving or operating machinery until daytime sedative effects are evaluated.
3. Report tolerance and any symptoms of psychologic and/or physical dependence.
4. Clients suffering from simple insomnia should be instructed to try warm baths, warm drinks, and other relaxation techniques to induce sleep.

Evaluation

1. Client reports improved sleeping patterns and less frequent awakenings.
2. Note any evidence of dependence, which would require discontinuation of drug therapy.

Flurbiprofen

(flur-**BIH**-proh-fen)
Ansaid, Froben✲ (Rx)

Flurbiprofen sodium

(flur-**BIH**-proh-fen)
Ocufen (Rx)

Classification: Nonsteroidal anti-inflammatory drug, ophthalmic and systemic use.

Action/Kinetics: By inhibiting prostaglandin synthesis, flurbiprofen reverses prostaglandin-induced vasodilation, leukocytosis, increased vascular permeability, and increased intraocular pressure. The drug also inhibits miosis, which occurs during cataract surgery. **PO form, time to peak levels:** 1.5 hr; **t½:** 5.7 hr.

Uses: *Ophthalmic:* Prevention of intraoperative miosis. *PO:* Rheumatoid arthritis, osteoarthritis. *Investigational:* Inflammation following cataract surgery, uveitis syndromes. Topically to treat cystoid macular edema. Primary dysmenorrhea, sunburn, mild to moderate pain.

Contraindications: Dendritic keratitis.

Special Concerns: Pregnancy category: B for flurbiprofen and C for flurbiprofen sodium. Use with caution in clients hypersensitive to aspirin or other NSAIDs. Use with caution during lactation. Safety and efficacy in children have not been established.

Additional Side Effects: *Ophthalmic:* Ocular irritation, transient stinging or burning following use, delay in wound healing.

Dosage: *Ophthalmic:* Beginning 2 hr before surgery, instill 1 drop every 30 min (i.e., total of 4 drops of 0.03% solution). **Tablets.** *Rheumatoid arthritis, osteoarthritis:* **initial,** 200–300 mg daily in divided doses b.i.d.–q.i.d.; **then,** adjust dose to client response. Doses greater than 300 mg daily are not recommended. *Dysmenorrhea:* 50 mg q.i.d.

NURSING CONSIDERATIONS

See also *Nursing Considerations* for *Nonsteroidal Anti-Inflammatory Drugs,* p. 189.

Administration/Storage: The maximum dose of 300 mg should be used only for initiating therapy or for treating acute exacerbations of the disease.

Interventions

1. Assess and report any delays in wound healing.
2. Prior to surgery, carefully follow the prescribed administration regimen.

Client/Family Teaching

1. Instruct client and family in the appropriate method of administering the eye medication.
2. Advise clients to avoid rubbing the eyes after the medication has been administered.
3. Instruct the client to report any stinging, burning, or irritation immediately to the physician.

Evaluation: Evaluate client for
- Reports of decreased pain and improved joint mobility
- A reduction of optic inflammation and ↓ intraocular pressure

Flutamide

(FLOO-tah-myd)

Euflex✹, Eulexin (Rx)

See also *Antineoplastic Agents,* p. 85.

Classification: Antineoplastic, hormonal agent.

Action/Kinetics: Flutamide acts either to inhibit uptake of androgen or to inhibit nuclear binding of androgen in target tissues. Thus, the effect of androgen is decreased in androgen-sensitive tissues. Flutamide is rapidly metabolized to active (alpha-hydroxylated derivative) and inactive metabolites in the liver and mainly excreted in the urine. **t½ of active metabolite:** 6 hr (8 hr in geriatric clients). 94%–96% is bound to plasma proteins.

Uses: In combination with leuprolide acetate (i.e., a LHRH-agonist) to treat stage D_2 metastatic prostatic carcinoma. Treatment must be initiated simultaneously with both drugs for maximum benefit.

Contraindications: Use during pregnancy (category: D).

Side Effects: Side effects are listed for treatment of flutamide with LHRH-agonist. *GU:* Loss of libido, impotence. *CV:* Hot flashes, hypertension. *GI:* Nausea, vomiting, diarrhea, GI disturbances, anorexia. *CNS:* Confusion, depression, drowsiness, anxiety, nervousness. *Hematologic:* Anemia, leukopenia, thrombocytopenia, hemolytic anemia, macrocytic anemia. *Hepatic:* Elevated transaminases, bilirubin, or creatinine; hepatitis, cholestatic jaundice, hepatic encephalopathy, hepatic necrosis. *Dermatologic:* Rash, photosensitivity, irritation at injection site. *Miscellaneous:* Gynecomastia, edema, neuromuscular symptoms, pulmonary symptoms.

Symptoms of Overdose: Breast tenderness, gynecomastia, increases in AST. Also possible are ataxia, anorexia, vomiting, decreased respiration, lacrimation, sedation, hypoactivity, and piloerection.

Laboratory Test Interferences: ↑ AST, ALT, creatinine, alpha-glutamyl transferase.

Dosage: Capsules: 250 mg (2 capsules) t.i.d. q 8 hr for a total daily dose of 750 mg.

NURSING CONSIDERATIONS

See also *Nursing Considerations for Antineoplastic Agents,* p. 88.

Administration/Storage: *Treatment of Overdose:* Induce vomiting if client is alert. Frequently monitor vital signs and observe client closely.

Interventions

1. Anticipate concomitant administration with an LHRH-agonist (such as leuprolide acetate).
2. Periodic CBC and liver function tests should be performed in clients on long-term flutamide therapy.

Client/Family Teaching

1. Clients should be informed to take flutamide and the LHRH-agonist (leuprolide) at the same time.

2. Drug therapy should not be interrupted or discontinued without consulting the physician.
3. Hot flashes, impotence, and diarrhea are all potential side effects of drug therapy and instruct client to report if persistent or bothersome.

Evaluation: Evaluate client for evidence of a ↓ in size and spread of tumor.

Fluticasone propionate
(flew-**TIH**-kah-sohn)
Cutivate (Rx)

See also *Adrenocorticosteroids and Analogs,* p. 8.

Classification: Adrenocorticosteroid, topical.

Action/Kinetics: Anti-inflammatory, antipruritic, and antiproliferative activity when used topically.

Uses: Dermatoses responsive to adrenocorticosteroid therapy including inflammation and itching of eczema, atopic dermatitis, and psoriasis.

Contraindications: Primary bacterial infections, *Candida,* dermatophytes, herpes simplex, herpes zoster.

Special Considerations: Pregnancy category: C. Use with caution during lactation. Safety and effectiveness have not been determined in children. Systemic absorption may result in suppression of the hypothalamic-pituitary axis. Use with caution around the eyes.

Side Effects: *Dermatologic:* Burning, itching, erythema, dryness, pruritus, irritation, folliculitis, hypertrichosis, acneiform eruptions, hypopigmentation, perioral dermatitis, allergic contact dermatitis, cracking of skin, maceration of skin, secondary infection, skin atrophy, striae, miliaria. *Miscellaneous:* Numbness of fingers. *Note:* In children, intracranial hypertension, Cushing's syndrome, and suppression of the hypothalamic-pituitary axis have been observed.

Dosage: Cream (0.05%), Ointment (0.005%): Apply a thin film to the affected area b.i.d.–q.i.d. and rub in gently.

NURSING CONSIDERATIONS

See *Nursing Considerations* for *Topical Corticosteroids* under *Adrenocorticosteroids and Analogs,* p. 15.

Folic acid
(**FOH**-lik **AH**-sid)
Apo-Folic✸, Folvite, Novo– Folacid✸ (Rx and OTC)

Classification: Vitamin B complex.

Action/Kinetics: Folic acid (which is converted to tetrahydrofolic acid) is necessary for normal production of red blood cells and for synthesis of nucleoproteins. Synthetic folic acid is absorbed from the GI tract even if the client suffers from malabsorption syndrome. Is stored in the liver.

Uses: Prophylaxis and treatment of folic acid deficiency (e.g., sprue, pregnancy, infancy or childhood, nutritional causes). Diagnosis of folate deficiency.

Contraindications: Use in aplastic, normocytic, or pernicious anemias (is ineffective). Folic acid injection that contains benzyl alcohol should not be used in neonates or immature infants.

Side Effects: Allergies.

Drug Interactions

Corticosteroids (chronic use) / ↑ Folic acid requirements
Methotrexate / Is a folic acid antagonist
Oral contraceptives / ↑ Risk of folate deficiency
Phenytoin / Folic acid ↑ seizure frequency; also, phenytoin ↓ serum folic acid levels.
Pyrimethamine / Folic acid ↓ effect of pyrimethamine in toxoplasmosis; also, pyrimethamine is a folic acid antagonist
Sulfonamides / ↓ Absorption of folic acid
Triamterene / ↓ Utilization of folic acid as it is a folic acid antagonist
Trimethoprim / ↓ Utilization of folic acid as it is a folic acid antagonist

Dosage: Tablets. *Dietary supplement:* **Adults and children:** 100 mcg daily (up to 1 mg in pregnancy); may be increased to 500–1,000 mcg if requirements increase. *Treatment of deficiency:* **Adults, initial:** 250–1,000 mcg daily until a hematologic response occurs; **maintenance:** 400 mcg daily (800 mcg during pregnancy and lactation). **Pediatric, initial:** 250–1,000 mcg daily until a hematologic response occurs. **Maintenance, infants:** 100 mcg daily; **children up to 4 years:** 300 mcg daily; **children 4 years and older:** 400 mcg daily.

IM, IV, Deep SC. *Treatment of deficiency:* **Adults and children:** 250–1,000 mcg daily until a hematologic response occurs. *Diagnosis of folate deficiency:* **Adults, IM:** 100–200 mcg daily for 10 days plus low dietary folic acid and vitamin B_{12}.

NURSING CONSIDERATIONS

Administration/Storage

1. Folic acid is given orally unless there is severe malabsorption in which case it can be given either IV or SC.
2. Regardless of age, the dosage should never be less than 0.1 mg daily.
3. Folic acid will remain stable in solution if the pH is kept above 5.
4. The drug may be administered IM or by direct IV push or added to infusions. However, if administered by IV, the rate should not exceed 5 mcg/min.
5. When parenteral forms are used, have drugs and equipment available to treat potential allergic drug reactions.

Evaluation: Evaluate client for:
- Laboratory evidence of a positive hematologic response
- Reports of improvement in symptoms of folate deficiency

Foscarnet sodium
(fos-**KAR**-net)
Foscavir (Rx)

Classification: Antiviral agent.

Action/Kinetics: Foscarnet inhibits replication of all known herpes viruses. The drug acts by selective inhibition at the pyrophosphate binding site on virus-specific DNA polymerases and reverse transcriptases at levels that do not affect cellular DNA polymerases. It is active against herpes simplex virus mutants deficient in thymidine kinase. Cytomegalovirus (CMV) strains resistant to ganciclovir may be sensitive to foscarnet; viral reactivation of CMV occurs after termination of foscarnet therapy. The latent state of any of the human herpes viruses is not sensitive to foscarnet. The drug is believed to accumulate in human bone and has variable penetration into the cerebrospinal fluid. Approximately 80%–90% of IV foscarnet is excreted unchanged through the urine.

Uses: Treatment of cytomegalovirus retinitis in clients with AIDS.

Special Concerns: Pregnancy category: C. Use with caution during lactation and in clients with impaired renal function (the effects of the drug have not been determined in clients with a creatinine clearance less than 50 ml/min or serum creatinine more than 2.8 mg/dl). Safety and effectiveness in children have not been determined. Transient changes in electrolytes may increase the risk of cardiac disturbances and seizures. Safety and effectiveness have not been determined for the treatment of other CMV infections such as pneumonitis or gastroenteritis, for congenital or neonatal CMV disease, and in non-immunocompromised clients. Use with caution with drugs that alter serum calcium levels as foscarnet decreases serum levels of ionized calcium. Side effects such as renal impairment, electrolyte abnormalities, and seizures may contribute to client death.

Side Effects: *GU:* Renal impairment (most common), albuminuria, dysuria, polyuria, urinary retention, urethral disorder, urinary tract infections, acute renal failure, nocturia, hematuria, glomerulonephritis, urinary frequency, toxic nephropathy, nephrosis, urinary incontinence, pyelonephritis, renal tubular disorders, urethral irritation, uremia, perineal pain in women, penile inflammation. *Metabolic/Electrolyte:* Hypocalcemia, hypokalemia, hypomagnesemia, hypophosphatemia, hyperphosphatemia, hyponatremia, hypercalcemia, acidosis, thirst, decreased weight, dehydration, glycosuria, diabetes mellitus, abnormal glucose tolerance, hypochloremia, hypervolemia, hypoproteinemia. *Hematologic:* Anemia (one-third of clients), granulocytopenia, neutropenia, leukopenia, thrombocytopenia, platelet abnormalities, thrombosis, white blood cell abnormalities, lymphadenopathy, coagulation disorders, decreased coagulation factors, decreased prothrombin, hypochromic anemia, pancytopenia, hemolysis, leukocytosis, cervical lymphadenopathy, lymphopenia. *Body as a whole:* Fever, fatigue, asthenia, pain, infection, rigors, malaise, sepsis, death, back or chest pain, cachexia, flu-like symptoms, edema, bacterial or fungal infections, abscess, moniliasis, leg edema, peripheral edema, hypothermia, syncope, substernal chest pain, ascites, malignant hyperpyrexia, herpes simplex, viral infections, toxoplasmosis. *CNS:* Headache, dizziness, seizures (including tonic-clonic), tremor, ataxia, dementia, stupor, meningitis, aphasia, abnormal coordination, EEG abnormalities, vertigo, coma, encephalopathy, dyskinesia, extrapyramidal disorders, hemiparesis, paraplegia, speech disorders, tetany, cerebral edema, depression, confusion, anxiety, insomnia, somnolence, amnesia, aggressive reaction, nervousness, agitation, hallucinations, impaired concentration, emotional liability, psychosis, suicide attempt, delirium, sleep disorders, personality disorders. *Peripheral nervous system:* Hypoesthesia, neuropathy, sensory disturbances, generalized spasms, abnormal gait, hyperesthesia, hypertonia, hyperkinesia, vocal cord paralysis, hyporeflexia, hyperreflexia, neuralgia, neuritis, peripheral neuropathy. *Musculoskeletal:* Arthralgia, myalgia, involuntary muscle contractions, leg cramps, arthrosis, synovitis, torticollis. *GI:* Nausea, vomiting, diarrhea, anorexia, abdominal pain, dry mouth, dysphagia, dyspepsia, rectal hemorrhage, constipation, melena, flatulence, pancreatitis, ulcerative stomatitis, enteritis, glossitis, enterocolitis, proctitis, stomatitis, tenesmus, pseudomembranous colitis, gastroenteritis, oral leukoplakia, oral hemorrhage, rectal disorders, colitis, duodenal ulcer, hematemesis, paralytic ileus, ulcerative proctitis, tongue ulceration, esophageal ulceration. *Hepatic:* Abnormal hepatic function, cholecystitis, cholelithiasis, hepatitis, hepatosplenomegaly, cholestatic hepatitis, jaundice. *CV:* Hypertension, palpitations, sinus tachycardia, first degree AV block, nonspecific ST-T segment changes, hypotension, flushing, cerebrovascular disorder, cardiomyopathy, cardiac failure, cardiac arrest, bradycardia, arrhythmias, extrasystole, atrial fibrillation, phlebitis, superficial thrombophlebitis of arm, mesenteric vein thrombophlebitis. *Respiratory:* Cough, dyspnea, pneumonia, sinusitis, rhinitis, pharyngitis, respiratory insufficiency, pulmonary infiltration, pulmonary embolism, pneumothorax, hemoptysis, stridor, bronchospasm, laryngitis, bronchitis, respiratory depression, pleural effusion, pulmonary hemorrhage, pneumonitis. *Ophthalmic:* Visual field defects, nystagmus, periorbital edema, eye pain, conjunctivitis, diplopia, blindness, retinal detachment, mydriasis, photophobia. *Ear:* Deafness, earache, tinnitus, otitis. *Dermatologic:* Increased sweating, rash, skin ulceration, pruritus, seborrhea, erythematous rash, maculopapular rash, facial edema, skin discoloration, acne, alopecia, dermatitis, anal pruritus, genital pruritus, aggravated psoriasis, psoriaform rash, skin disorders, dry skin, urticaria, skin hypertrophy, verruca. *Miscellaneous:* Epistaxis, taste perversions, pain or inflammation at injection site, lymphoma-like disorder, sarcoma, malignant lymphoma, antidiuretic hormone disorders, decreased gonadotropins, gynecomastia.

Symptoms of Overdose: Extensions of the above side effects. Of most concern are development of seizures, renal function impairment, paresthesias in limbs or periorally, and electrolyte disturbances especially involving calcium and phosphate.

Drug Interactions

Aminoglycosides / ↓ Elimination of foscarnet → ↑ risk of renal impairment

Amphotericin / ↓ Elimination of foscarnet → ↑ risk of renal impairment

Pentamidine, IV / ↓ Elimination of foscarnet → ↑ risk of renal impairment; also, pentamidine causes hypocalcemia

Zidovudine / ↑ Risk of anemia

Laboratory Test Interferences: ↑ Alkaline phosphatase, AST, ALT, LDH, BUN, creatine phosphokinase, serum creatinine. ↓ Creatinine clearance. Abnormal X-ray. Abnormal A-G ratio.

Dosage: IV infusion. Individualized. Induction: 60 mg/kg for clients with normal renal function given IV at a constant rate over a minimum of 1 hr q 8 hr for 2–3 weeks, depending on the response. **Maintenance:** 90–120 mg/kg daily (depending on renal function) given as an IV infusion over 2 hr. Most clients should be started on the 90 mg/kg daily dose.

NURSING CONSIDERATIONS

Administration/Storage

1. To avoid local irritation, foscarnet should be infused only into veins with adequate blood flow to allow rapid dilution and distribution.
2. The rate of infusion must be no more than 1 mg/kg/min using controlled IV infusion either by a central venous line or a peripheral vein.
3. If using a central venous catheter for infusion, the standard 24 mg/ml solution may be used without dilution. However, if a peripheral vein catheter is used, the 24 mg/ml solution should be diluted to 12 mg/ml with 5% dextrose in water or with normal saline to avoid vein irritation. Diluted solutions should be used within 24 hr of first entry into a sealed bottle.
4. The potential for renal impairment may be minimized by hydrating the client during administration of the drug to establish and maintain diuresis.
5. The dose must be adjusted in renal impairment using the dosing guide provided with the drug.
6. No other drug or supplement should be given through the same catheter as foscarnet. Foscarnet is incompatible with 30% dextrose, amphotericin B, and calcium-containing solutions (e.g., Ringer's lactate and TPN). Other incompatibilities include acyclovir sodium, diazepam, digoxin, ganciclovir, leucovorin, midazolam, pentamidine, phenytoin, prochlorperazine, trimethoprim/sulfamethoxazole, and vancomycin. A precipitate can result if foscarnet is given at the same time as divalent cations.
7. *Treatment of Overdose:* Monitor the client for signs and symptoms of electrolyte imbalance and renal impairment. Symptomatic treatment. Hemodialysis and hydration may be of some benefit.

Assessment

1. Note any history of cardiac or neurologic dysfunction.
2. Obtain baseline CBC, serum electrolytes, calcium, phosphorus, magnesium, liver, and renal function studies.
3. Determine confirmation of the diagnosis of CMV retinitis by indirect ophthalmoscopy.
4. Ensure that appropriate laboratory cultures have been performed before instituting therapy.

Interventions

1. Due to the possibility of decreased renal function, creatinine clearance should be de-

termined at baseline, 2–3 times weekly during induction therapy, and at least once every 1–2 weeks during maintenance therapy. This is especially true in geriatric clients who commonly have decreased glomerular filtration rates.

2. Monitor I&O and vital signs. Ensure that client is well hydrated.

3. Monitor appropriate labs and observe clients for the possibility of chelation of divalent metal ions, which will alter serum levels of electrolytes. Thus, levels of electrolytes, calcium, magnesium, and creatinine are especially important to determine.

4. Observe client closely for evidence of seizure activity and use seizure precautions.

5. Follow dilution and administration guidelines carefully. Ideally, product should be prepared daily, under a biologic hood, by the pharmacist.

Client/Family Teaching

1. Remind clients that foscarnet is not a cure for CMV retinitis and that they may continue to experience progression of the condition during or following treatment.

2. Stress the importance of reporting for regularly scheduled ophthalmic examinations.

3. Report any evidence of numbness of the extremities, paresthesias, or perioral tingling as these are symptoms of hypocalcemia and the infusion should be stopped, the physician notified, and appropriate steps taken to correct the imbalance before resuming the infusion.

Evaluation: Evaluate for ophthalmic evidence of successful treatment of CMV retinitis in clients with AIDS.

Fosinopril sodium
(foh-**SIN**-oh-prill)
Monopril (Rx)

See also *Angiotensin-Converting Enzyme (ACE) Inhibitors*, p. 33.

Classification: Angiotensin-converting enzyme (ACE) inhibitor.

Action/Kinetics: Onset: 1 hr. **Time to peak serum levels:** About 3 hr. Metabolized in the liver to the active fosinoprilat. Fosinoprilat is significantly bound to plasma proteins. **t½:** 12 hr (prolonged in impaired renal function) following IV administration. **Duration:** 24 hr. Approximately 50% excreted through the urine and 50% in the feces.

Uses: Alone or in combination with other antihypertensive agents (especially thiazide diuretics) for the treatment of hypertension.

Contraindications: Use during lactation.

Special Concerns: Pregnancy category: D.

Side Effects: *CV:* Orthostatic hypotension, chest pain, hypotension, palpitations, angina pectoris, cerebrovascular accident, myocardial infarction, rhythm disturbances, hypertensive crisis, claudication. *CNS:* Headache, dizziness, fatigue, confusion, anxiety, insomnia, sleep disturbances. *GI:* Nausea, vomiting, diarrhea, abdominal pain, constipation, dry mouth, dysphagia, abdominal distention, flatulence, heartburn, taste disturbances, appetite changes, weight changes. *Respiratory:* Cough, sinusitis, bronchospasm, pharyngitis, laryngitis. *Hematologic:* Leukopenia, eosinophilia, neutropenia. *Dermatologic:* Diaphoresis, photosensitivity, flushing, pruritus, rash, urticaria. *Body as a whole:* Angioedema, muscle cramps, syncope, myalgia, arthralgia, edema, weakness, musculoskeletal pain. *Miscellaneous:* Paresthesias, hepatitis, pancreatitis, tinnitus, decreased libido, sexual dysfunction, gout, lymphadenopathy, rhinitis, epistaxis, vision disturbances, eye irritation, renal insufficiency, urinary frequency.

Laboratory Test Interferences: Transient ↓ hemoglobin and hematocrit.

Dosage: Tablets. Initial: 10 mg once daily; **then,** adjust depending on blood pressure response at peak (2–6 hr after dosing) and trough (24 hr after dosing) blood levels. **Maintenance:** Usually 20–40 mg daily, although some clients manifest beneficial effects at doses up to 80 mg.

NURSING CONSIDERATIONS

See also *Nursing Considerations* for *Angiotensin-Converting Enzyme Inhibitors,* p. 35.

Administration/Storage

1. If the antihypertensive effect decreases at the end of the dosing interval in clients taking the medication once daily, twice daily administration should be considered.
2. If the client is taking a diuretic, the diuretic should be discontinued 2–3 days prior to beginning fosinopril therapy. If the blood pressure is not controlled, the diuretic should be

reinstituted. If the diuretic cannot be discontinued, an initial dose of fosinopril should be 10 mg.
3. The dose of fosinopril does not have to be adjusted in clients with renal insufficiency.

Evaluation: Evaluate client for evidence of effective control of hypertension.

Furosemide
(fur-**OH**-seh-myd)
Apo-Furosemide✸, **Furoside**✸, **Lasix, Lasix Special**✸, **Myrosemide, Novo–Semide**✸, **Uritol**✸ **(Rx)**

See also *Diuretics,* p. 140.

Classification: Loop diuretic.

Action/Kinetics: Furosemide inhibits the reabsorption of sodium and chloride in the ascending loop of Henle, resulting in the excretion of sodium, chloride, and, to a lesser degree, potassium and bicarbonate ions. The drug also decreases reabsorption of sodium and chloride and increases the excretion of potassium in the distal tubule. The resulting urine is more acid. Diuretic action is independent of changes in clients' acid-base balance. Furosemide has a slight antihypertensive effect. **Onset: PO, IM:** 30–60 min; **IV:** 5 min. **Peak: PO, IM:** 1–2 hr; **IV:** 20–60 min. **Duration: PO, IM:** 6–8 hr; **IV:** 2 hr. Metabolized in the liver and excreted through the urine.

The drug may be effective for clients resistant to thiazides and for those with reduced glomerular filtration rates.

Uses: Edema associated with congestive heart failure, nephrotic syndrome, hepatic cirrhosis, and ascites. Hypertension alone or as an adjunct. IV for acute pulmonary edema. Furosemide can be used in conjunction with spironolactone, triamterene, and other diuretics *except* ethacrynic acid. *Investigational:* Hypercalcemia.

Contraindications: Never use with ethacrynic acid. Anuria, hypersensitivity to drug, severe renal disease associated with azotemia and oliguria, hepatic coma associated with electrolyte depletion. Lactation.

Special Concerns: Use during pregnancy (category: C) only when benefits clearly outweigh risks. Use with caution in premature infants and neonates due to prolonged half-life in these clients (dosing interval must be extended). Geriatric clients may be more sensitive to the usual adult dose.

Side Effects: *Electrolyte and fluid effects:* Fluid and electrolyte depletion leading to dehydration, hypovolemia, thromboembolism. Hypokalemia and hypochloremia may cause metabolic alkalosis. Hyperuricemia, azotemia, hyponatremia. *GI:* Nausea, GI irritation, vomiting, anorexia, diarrhea (especially in children) or constipation, cramps. *Otic:* Tinnitus, hearing impairment (may be reversible or permanent), reversible deafness. Usually following rapid IV or IM administration of high doses. *CNS:* Vertigo, headache, dizziness, lightheadedness, blurred vision, weakness, restlessness, paresthesias, xanthopsia. *CV:* Orthostatic hypotension, thrombophlebitis, chronic aortitis. *Hematologic:* Anemia, thrombocytopenia, neutropenia, leukopenia, agranulocytosis,

purpura. Rarely, aplastic anemia. *Allergic:* Rashes, pruritus, urticaria, photosensitivity, exfoliative dermatitis, vasculitis, erythema multiforme. *Miscellaneous:* Hyperglycemia, glycosuria, exacerbation of, aggravation of or worsening of systemic lupus erythematosus, increased perspiration, muscle spasms, urinary bladder spasm, urinary frequency.

Following IV use: Thrombophlebitis, cardiac arrest. *Following IM use:* Pain at injection site, cardiac arrest.

Because this drug is resistant to the effects of pressor amines and potentiates the effects of muscle relaxants, it is recommended that the oral drug be discontinued 1 week before surgery and the IV drug 2 days before surgery.

Symptoms of Overdose: Profound water loss, electrolyte depletion (manifested by weakness, anorexia, vomiting, lethargy, cramps, mental confusion, dizziness), decreased blood volume, circulatory collapse (possibly vascular thrombosis and embolism).

Drug Interactions

Adrenergic blocking agents /
    Potentiation of effects
Alcohol / ↑ Orthostatic
    hypotension
Aminoglycoside antibiotics /
    Additive ototoxicity and
    nephrotoxicity
Anticoagulants / ↑ Effect of
    anticoagulant due to ↓ plasma
    protein binding
Antidiabetic agents / Furosemide
    antagonizes hypoglycemic effect
    of antidiabetics
Antihypertensive agents /
    Potentiation of antihypertensive
    effect

Barbiturates / ↑ Orthostatic hypotension

Cephalosporins / ↑ Renal toxicity of cephalosporins

Cisplatin / ↑ Risk of ototoxicty

Corticosteroids / Enhanced K loss due to K-depleting properties of both drugs

Digitalis glycosides / Furosemide produces excess K and Mg loss with ↑ chance of cardiac arrhythmias

Ethacrynic acid / Combination may result in hypokalemia, tachycardia, deafness, hypotension—**do not use together**

Ganglionic blocking agents / Potentiation of effects

Indomethacin / ↓ Diuretic and antihypertensive effects of furosemide

Lithium / ↓ Renal clearance of lithium leading to ↑ risk of toxicity

Narcotics / ↑ Orthostatic hypotension

Phenytoin / ↓ Diuretic effect of furosemide due to ↓ absorption

Salicylates / ↑ Risk of salicylate toxicity due to ↓ renal excretion

Succinylcholine / Effect of succinylcholine is ↑ by low doses and ↓ by high doses of furosemide.

Theophylline / Furosemide may ↑ or ↓ the effect of theophyllines

d-Tubocurarine / Effect of tubocurarine is ↑ by low doses and ↓ by high doses of furosemide

Dosage: Oral Solution, Tablets. *Diuretic.* **Adults, initial:** 20–80 mg daily as a single dose. For resistant cases, dosage can be increased by 20–40 mg q 6–8 hr until desired diuretic response is attained. Max-

imum daily dose should not exceed 600 mg. **Pediatric, initial:** 2 mg/kg as a single dose; **then,** dose can be increased by 1–2 mg/kg q 6–8 hr until desired response is attained (up to 5 mg/kg may be required in children with nephrotic syndrome; maximum dose should not exceed 6 mg/kg). *Hypertension:* **Adults, initial:** 40 mg b.i.d. Adjust dosage depending on response. *Antihypercalcemic:* **Adults:** 120 mg daily in 1–3 doses.

IV, IM. *Diuretic:* **Adults, initial:** 20–40 mg; if response inadequate after 2 hr, increase dose in 20 mg increments. **Pediatric, initial:** 1 mg/kg given slowly; if response inadequate after 2 hr, increase dose by 1 mg/kg. Doses greater than 6 mg/kg should not be given. **IV.** *Acute pulmonary edema:* **Adults:** 40 mg slowly over 1–2 min; if response inadequate after 1 hr, give 80 mg slowly over 1–2 min. Concomitant oxygen and digitalis may be used. *Hypertensive crisis, normal renal function:* **Adults, IV:** 40–80 mg. *Hypertensive crisis with pulmonary edema or acute renal failure:* **Adults, IV:** 100–200 mg. *Antihypercalcemic:* **Adults, IM, IV:** 80–100 mg for severe cases; dose may be repeated q 1–2 hr if needed.

NURSING CONSIDERATIONS

See also *Nursing Considerations* for *Diuretics,* p. 141.

Administration/Storage

1. The drug should be given 2–4 days/week.
2. If used IV, furosemide should not be mixed with solutions with a pH below 5.5.
3. When high doses of the medication are required parenteral-

ly, administer by infusion at a rate not to exceed 4 mg/min.

4. Food decreases the bioavailability of furosemide and ultimately the degree of diuresis.

5. Discoloration resulting from light does not affect potency.

6. Store in light-resistant containers.

7. *Treatment of Overdose:* Replace fluid and electrolytes. Monitor urine electrolyte output and serum electrolytes. Induce emesis or perform gastric lavage. Oxygen or artificial respiration may be needed. Treat symptoms.

Interventions

1. Monitor serum electrolytes and observe client for signs and symptoms of hypokalemia.

2. In clients with rapid diuresis, observe for dehydration and circulatory collapse. Monitor BP and pulse and document.

3. When the client has renal impairment or is receiving other ototoxic drugs, observe for ototoxicity.

4. Assess closely for signs of vascular thrombosis and embolism, particularly in the elderly.

Client/Family Teaching

1. Assure the client that any pain after IM injection will be transitory.

2. Take medication in the morning to avoid interruption of sleep.

3. Provide a printed list of adverse side effects of drug therapy. Stress those that require immediate reporting.

4. Assist clients to establish the timing of the diuretic so that they can participate in social activities.

5. Advise client that before taking aspirin for any reason, to consult with the physician. Salicylate intoxication occurs at lower levels than normal because of competition at the renal excretory sites.

6. Use sunscreens and protective clothing when exposed to the sun to minimize the effects of drug-induced photosensitivity.

7. Discuss the need for a diet high in potassium. Supplement diet with vegetables and fruits high in potassium.

Evaluation: Evaluate client for:

- Evidence of an increased urinary output, a decrease in dependent edema, a decrease in BP, and a decrease or stabilization of weight
- Freedom from complications of adverse drug effects that may require discontinuation of therapy

G

Gallium nitrate
(Gal-ee-um NIGH-trayt)
Ganite (Rx)

Classification: Antihypercalcemic agent.

Action/Kinetics: Gallium nitrate produces a hypocalcemic effect by inhibiting calcium resorption from bone; it may reduce increased bone turnover. After infusion, steady state is reached in 24–48 hr. **Plasma levels:** 1134–2399 ng/ml. The drug is not metabolized by the liver or kidney and is excreted through the kidneys.

Uses: Cancer-related hypercalcemia that is not responsive to adequate hydration and where there are symptoms of hypercalcemia.

Contraindications: Severe renal impairment (serum creatinine>2.5 mg/dl). Lactation.

Special Concerns: Pregnancy category: C. Safety and effectiveness have not been determined in children.

Side Effects: *Metabolic:* Hypocalcemia, transient hypophosphatemia, decreased serum bicarbonate (possibly secondary to mild respiratory alkalosis). *GU:* Increased BUN and creatinine. *Hematologic:* Anemia (relationship to drug itself not certain), leukopenia. *GI:* Nausea, vomiting, diarrhea, constipation. *CV:* Tachycardia, edema of lower extremities, decrease in mean systolic and diastolic blood pressure. *Respiratory:* Dyspnea, rales and rhonchi, pulmonary infiltrates, pleural effusion. *Miscellaneous:* Acute optic neuritis, visual impairment, decreased hearing, hypothermia, fever, skin rash, lethargy, confusion.

Symptoms of Overdose: Nausea, vomiting, increased risk of renal insufficiency.

Drug Interactions: Use of gallium nitrate with nephrotoxic drugs (e.g., aminoglycosides, amphotericin B) may increase the incidence of renal insufficiency in clients with hypercalcemia due to cancer.

Dosage: IV infusion, Adults: 200 mg/m² daily for 5 consecutive days. *Mild hypercalcemia:* 100 mg/m² for 5 consecutive days.

NURSING CONSIDERATIONS
Administration/Storage

1. The daily dose must be given as an IV infusion over 24 hr.
2. If serum calcium levels are brought into the normal range in less than 5 days, treatment may be discontinued early.
3. The daily dose should be diluted in 1 L of 0.9% sodium chloride injection or 5% dextrose injection. When diluted as such, it is stable for 48 hr at room temperature and for 7 days if refrigerated.
4. Since the product contains no preservative, any unused portion should be discarded.
5. *Treatment of Overdose:* Discontinue administration of the drug and monitor serum calcium. Give fluids IV, with or without diuretics, for 2–3 days. Carefully monitor renal function and urinary output.

Assessment

1. Determine that cancer-related hypercalcemia was previously unresponsive to saline hydration. In treating hypercalcemia due to carcinoma, it is important to first establish adequate hydration to increase renal excretion of calcium and to correct for dehydration caused by hypercalcemia.
2. Obtain baseline CBC, serum calcium, phosphorus, and renal function studies and monitor throughout therapy.

Interventions

1. Monitor serum calcium levels closely and observe client for symptoms of hypocalcemia. If hypocalcemia occurs, stop gallium infusion and notify physician.
2. Monitor I&O. Hypercalcemia is frequently associated with impaired renal function; thus, serum creatinine and BUN should also be monitored during therapy. Therapy should be discontinued if serum creatinine levels exceed 2.5 mg/dl.
3. A satisfactory urine output (2 L/day) should be established before gallium nitrate therapy is initiated. Adequate hydration should be maintained throughout therapy with care taken to avoid overhydration in clients with compromised cardiovascular function.
4. Diuretic therapy should *not* be used prior to correction of hypovolemia.
5. Encourage client to immediately report any visual or hearing disturbances as these may be drug related.

Evaluation: Evaluate client for laboratory evidence that serum calcium levels are within desired range (8.8–10.4 mg/dl).

Ganciclovir sodium (DHPG)
(gan-**SYE**-kloh-veer)
Cytovene (Rx)

Classification: Antiviral.

Action/Kinetics: Upon entry into viral cells infected by cytomegalovirus (CMV), ganciclovir is converted to ganciclovir triphosphate by the CMV. Ganciclovir triphosphate inhibits viral DNA synthesis by competitive inhibition of viral DNA polymerases and direct incorporation into viral DNA; this results in eventual termination of viral DNA elongation. Ganciclovir is active against CMV, herpes simplex virus-1 and -2, Epstein-Barr virus, and varicella zoster virus. $t^{1/2}$: Approximately 2.9 hr. The drug is believed to cross the blood-brain barrier. Most of the drug is excreted unchanged through the urine. Renal impairment increases the $t^{1/2}$ of the drug.

Uses: At the present time, ganciclovir is indicated only in immunocompromised clients with CMV retinitis, including AIDS clients. Diagnosis may be confirmed by culture of CMV from the blood, urine, or throat; note that a negative CMV culture does not rule out CMV retinitis.

Contraindications: Hypersensitivity to acyclovir or ganciclovir. Lactation.

Special Concerns: Safety and effectiveness of ganciclovir have not been established for nonimmuno-compromised clients, treatment of other CMV infections such as pneumonitis or colitis, or for congenital or neonatal CMV disease. Use with caution in impaired renal function and in elderly clients. Use during pregnancy (category: C) and in children only if potential benefits outweigh potential risks.

Side Effects: *Hematologic:* Granulocytopenia, thrombocytopenia, neutropenia (may be irreversible), eosinophilia, anemia. *CNS:* Ataxia, coma, confusion, abnormal dreams or thoughts, dizziness, headache, paresthesia, psychosis, nervousness, somnolence, tremor. *GI:* Nausea, vomiting, diarrhea, anorexia, hemorrhage, abdominal pain. *CV:* Hypertension or hypotension, arrhythmias. *Body as a whole:* Fever (most common), chills, edema, infections, malaise. *Dermatologic:* Rash (most common), alopecia, pruritus, urticaria. *Miscellaneous:* Abnormal liver function values; inflammation, pain, or phlebitis at injection site; hematuria, dyspnea, retinal detachment in CMV retinitis patients.

Symptoms of Overdose: Neutropenia. Possibility of hypersalivation, anorexia, vomiting, bloody diarrhea, inactivity, cytopenia, testicular atrophy, increased BUN and liver function test results.

Laboratory Test Interferences: ↑ Serum creatinine, BUN. ↓ Blood glucose.

Drug Interactions

Adriamycin / Additive cytotoxicity
Amphotericin B / Additive cytotoxicity
Dapsone / Additive cytotoxicity
Flucytosine / Additive cytotoxicity

Imipenem/Cilastatin combination / Possibility of seizures
Pentamidine / Additive cytotoxicity
Probenecid / ↑ Effect of ganciclovir due to ↓ renal excretion
Sulfamethoxazole/Trimethoprim combinations / Additive cytotoxicity
Vinblastine / Additive cytotoxicity
Vincristine / Additive cytotoxicity
Zidovudine / ↑ Risk of granulocytopenia

Dosage: IV infusion, induction: 5 mg/kg over 1 hr q 12 hr for 14–21 days in clients with normal renal function. **Maintenance:** 5 mg/kg over 1 hr by IV infusion daily for 7 days or 6 mg/kg daily for 5 days each week. Dosage must be reduced in clients with renal impairment.

NURSING CONSIDERATIONS

Administration/Storage

1. Doses greater than 6 mg/kg infused over 1 hr may result in increased toxicity.

2. Due to the high pH (9–11) of reconstituted ganciclovir, the drug should not be given by IM or SC injection. The drug should not be given by IV bolus or rapid IV injection.

3. To minimize phlebitis or pain at the injection site, ganciclovir should be given into veins with an adequate blood flow to allow rapid dilution and distribution.

4. The dose should not exceed 1.25 mg/kg daily in clients undergoing hemodialysis.

5. The drug should be reconstituted by injecting 10 ml sterile water for injection followed by

shaking. The vial should be discarded if particulate matter or discoloration is noted. Since parabens is incompatible with ganciclovir, bacteriostatic water for injection should not be used for reconstitution.

6. The reconstituted solution is stable for 12 hr at room temperature.

7. IV infusion concentrations greater than 10 mg/ml are not recommended.

8. Reconstituted ganciclovir is compatible with the following infusion solutions: 5% dextrose, lactated Ringer's injection, Ringer's injection, 0.9% sodium chloride.

9. *Treatment of Overdose:* Hydration, hemodialysis.

Assessment: Note lab reports for evidence of hematologic disorders that could preclude use of the drug.

Interventions

1. Monitor CBC frequently because granulocytopenia and thrombocytopenia are side effects of drug therapy. Ganciclovir should not be administered if neutrophil count drops below 500 cells/mm^3 or the platelet count falls below 25,000/mm^3.

2. Anticipate reduced dose in clients with impaired renal function; monitor renal function studies throughout therapy.

3. Assess intake and output. Ensure that client is adequately hydrated before and during therapy with ganciclovir because drug is excreted through the kidneys.

4. Concomitant therapy with zido-

vudine may increase neutropenia.

5. Client may experience pain and/or phlebitis at infusion site because pH of *diluted* solution is high (pH 9–11). Follow administration guidelines carefully.

6. Review list of drug interactions as some may induce renal failure and have additive toxicity if given during ganciclovir therapy.

7. Follow guidelines for handling cytotoxic drugs during handling and disposal of drug. Avoid inhalation and contact with skin. Latex gloves and safety glasses should be used when handling drug. Ideally, ganciclovir should be mixed under a laminar flow hood.

8. Hemodialysis and hydration may reduce plasma levels in cases of overdosage.

Client/Family Teaching

1. Drug therapy should not be interrupted unless deemed necessary by physician because a relapse may occur.

2. Report any dizziness, confusion, and/or seizures immediately.

3. Stress the importance of reporting for scheduled lab studies because results may require adjustment of dose or even discontinuation of therapy.

4. Stress the importance of regular ophthalmologic examinations because retinitis may progress to blindness.

5. Ganciclovir may impair fertility.

6. During and for 90 days following drug therapy, women of childbearing age should use

safe contraception and men should practice barrier contraception.

Evaluation

1. Assess client/family knowledge and understanding of illness, response to therapy and to teaching.
2. Review hematologic studies carefully because drug may need to be discontinued.
3. Follow ophthalmologic exams closely to evaluate progression of CMV retinitis and response to therapy.

——— COMBINATION DRUG ———

Gelusil and Gelusil-II
(**JELL**-you-sill)
(OTC)

See also *Antacids,* p. 37.

Classification/Content: Gelusil contains the following in each tablet or 5 ml:

Antacid: Aluminum hydroxide, 200 mg.
Antacid: Magnesium hydroxide, 200 mg.
Antiflatulent: Simethicone, 25 mg.

Gelusil-II contains aluminum hydroxide and magnesium hydroxide, each 400 mg, and simethicone, 30 mg. See also information on individual components.

Action/Kinetics: Gelusil has a high capacity to neutralize acid and has a low sodium content.

Uses: To treat acid indigestion, heartburn, sour stomach; relieve symptoms of gas. Also as an adjunct in the treatment of peptic ulcer.

Additional Contraindication: Kidney disease.

Dosage: Oral Suspension, Chewable Tablets. *Gelusil, Gelusil-II:* Two or more tablets or teaspoonfuls 1 hr after meals and at bedtime.

NURSING CONSIDERATIONS

See also *Nursing Considerations* for *Antacids,* p. 38.

Administration/Storage

1. Tablets should be chewed before being swallowed.
2. The maximum daily dosage of Gelusil should be 12 tablets or teaspoons, and the maximum daily dosage for Gelusil-II should be 8 tablets or teaspoonsful. Maximum dosage should not be taken for more than 2 weeks.

Evaluation: Evaluate client for reports of symptomatic improvement in GI upset and gas.

Gemfibrozil
(jem-**FIH**-broh-zill)
Lopid (Rx)

Classification: Antihyperlipidemic.

Action/Kinetics: Gemfibrozil, which resembles clofibrate, decreases triglycerides, cholesterol, and VLDL and increases HDL; LDL levels either decrease or do not change. In addition, the drug decreases hepatic triglyceride production by inhibiting peripheral lipolysis and decreasing extraction of free fatty acids by the liver. Also, gemfibrozil decreases VLDL synthesis by inhibiting synthesis of VLDL carrier apolipoprotein B as well as inhibits peripheral lipolysis and decreases hepatic extraction of free fatty acids (thus decreasing hepatic triglyceride production). The drug may be beneficial in inhibiting development of atherosclerosis. **Onset:** 2–5 days. **Peak plasma levels:** 1–2 hr; **t½:** 1.5 hr. Nearly 70% is excreted unchanged.

Uses: Hypertriglyceridemia (type IV and type V hyperlipidemia) unresponsive to dietary control or in clients who are at risk of pancreatitis and abdominal pain. (Response variable; discontinue if significant improvement not observed within 3 months.) Reduce risk of coronary heart disease in clients with type IIb hyperlipidemia who have not responded to diet, weight loss, exercise, and other drug therapy.

Contraindications: Gallbladder disease, primary biliary cirrhosis, hepatic or renal dysfunction.

Special Concerns: Pregnancy category: B. Use with caution during lactation. Safety and efficacy have not been established in children. The dose may have to be reduced in geriatric clients due to age-related decreases in renal function.

Side Effects: Cholelithiasis; increased chance of viral and bacterial infections. *GI:* Abdominal or epigastric pain, nausea, vomiting, diarrhea, dyspepsia, constipation, acute appendicitis, colitis, pancreatitis, cholestatic jaundice, hepatoma. *CNS:* Dizziness, headache, fatigue, vertigo, somnolence, paresthesia, hypesthesia, depression, confusion, syncope, seizures. *CV:* Atrial fibrillation, extrasystole, peripheral vascular disease, intracerebral hemorrhage. *Hematopoietic:* Anemia, leukopenia, eosinophilia, thrombocytopenia, bone narrow hypoplasia. *Musculoskele-*

tal: Painful extremities; possibly arthralgia, muscle cramps, swollen joints, back pain, myalgia, myopathy, myasthenia, rhabdomyolysis. *Allergic:* Urticaria, lupus-like syndrome, angioedema, laryngeal edema, vasculitis, anaphylaxis. *Dermatologic:* Eczema, dermatitis, pruritus, skin rashes, exfoliative dermatitis, alopecia. *Miscellaneous:* Increased chance of viral and bacterial infections, taste perversion, impotence, decreased male fertility, weight loss.

Drug Interaction

Anticoagulants, oral /
   Gemfibrozil may ↑ effect of
   anticoagulants; dosage
   adjustment necessary
Lovastatin / Rhabdomyolysis
   when combined with
   gemfibrozil

Laboratory Test Interference: ↑ AST, ALT, LDH, CPK, alkaline phosphatase, bilirubin. Hypokalemia. Positive antinuclear antibody. ↓ Hemoglobin, white blood cells, hematocrit.

Dosage: **Capsules / Tablets. Adults:** 600 mg 30 min before the morning and evening meal (range: 900–1,500 mg/day). Dosage has not been established in children.

NURSING CONSIDERATIONS

See also *Nursing Considerations for Clofibrate,* p. 463.

Client / Family Teaching

1. Limit the intake of alcohol.
2. Take only as directed and follow prescribed dietary guidelines.
3. Observe for bruising or bleeding and report, especially if client is also on anticoagulant

therapy. A reduction in anticoagulant drug dosage is indicated if gemfibrozil therapy is instituted.

4. Be alert for signs and symptoms associated with gallstones, such as abdominal pain and vomiting. Report any persistent GI symptoms to the physician.
5. Report any right upper quadrant abdominal pain or change in color and consistency of the stools.
6. Use caution when driving or performing other dangerous tasks because drug may cause dizziness or blurred vision.

Evaluation: Evaluate client for laboratory evidence of a ↓ in serum cholesterol and triglyceride levels after 3 months of therapy.

—— COMBINATION DRUG ——
Genora 0.5/35 21 Day and Genora 0.5/35 28 Day
(jen-OR-ah)
(Rx)

Genora 1/35 21 Day and Genora 1/35 28 Day
(jen-OR-ah)
(Rx)

Genora 1/50 21 Day and Genora 1/50 28 Day
(jen-OR-ah)
(Rx)

See also *Oral Contraceptives,* p. 192.

Classification: Monophasic combination oral contraceptive.

Components: Genora 0.5/35: Each tablet of the 21 day and the first 21 tablets of the 28 day contains ethinyl estradiol, 35 mcg, and norethindrone, 0.5 mg (white tablets); the 28s also contain 7 inert peach tablets.

Genora 1/35: Each tablet of the 21 day and the first 21 tablets of the 28 day contains ethinyl estradiol, 35 mcg, and norethindrone, 1 mg (blue tablets); the 28s also contain 7 inert peach tablets.

Genora 1/50: Each tablet of the 21 day and the first 21 tablets of the 28 day contains mestranol, 50 mcg, and norethindrone, 1 mg (white or pale blue tablets); the 28s also contain 7 inert peach tablets.

Special Concerns: Pregnancy category: X.

NURSING CONSIDERATIONS
See *Oral Contraceptives,* p. 192.

Gentamicin sulfate
(jen-tah-MY-sin)
Alcomicin ✹, Cidomycin ✹, Garamycin, Garamycin Intrathecal, Garamycin IV Piggyback, Garamycin Ophthalmic Ointment, Garamycin Ophthalmic Solution, Garamycin Pediatric, Genoptic Ophthalmic Liquifilm, Genoptic S.O.P. Ophthalmic, Gentacidin Ophthalmic, Gentafair, Gent-AK Ophthalmic, Gentamicin, Gentamicin Ophthalmic, Gentamicin Sulfate IV Piggyback, Gentrasul Ophthalmic, G-myticin Topical, Jenamicin, Pediatric Gentamicin Sulfate, PMS Gentamicin Sulfate ✹ (Rx)

See also *Aminoglycosides,* p. 23.

Classification: Antibiotic, amino-glycoside.

Action/Kinetics: Therapeutic serum levels: IM, 4–8 mcg/ml. Prolonged serum levels above 12 mcg/ml should be avoided. **t½:** 2 hr.

The drug can be used concurrently with carbenicillin for the treatment of serious *Pseudomonas* infections. However, the drugs should not be mixed in the same flask because carbenicillin will inactivate gentamicin.

Uses: *Systemic:* Gentamicin is the drug of choice for hospital-acquired gram-negative sepsis (including neonatal sepsis). In combination with carbenicillin for life-threatening infections caused by *Pseudomonas aeruginosa.* Serious staphylococcal infections.

Ophthalmic: Ophthalmic infections due to *Staphylococcus, Streptococcus pneumoniae,* beta-hemolytic streptococci, *Escherichia coli, Hemophilus influenzae, H. aegyptius, Klebsiella pneumoniae, Neisseria gonorrhoeae, Proteus* species, *Enterobacter aerogenes, Pseudomonas aeruginosa, Moraxella lacunata.*

Topical: Prevention of infections following minor cuts, wounds, burns, and skin abrasions. Treatment of superficial infections of the skin.

Special Concerns: Pregnancy category: C. Use with caution in premature infants and neonates.

Additional Side Effects: Muscle twitching, numbness, seizures, increased blood pressure, alopecia, purpura, pseudotumor cerebri. Photosensitivity when used topically.

Additional Drug Interaction: With carbenicillin or ticarcillin, gentamicin may result in increased effect when used for *Pseudomonas* infections.

Dosage: IM (usual), IV. Adults with normal renal function: 1 mg/kg q 8 hr, up to 5 mg/kg daily in life-threatening infections; **children:** 2–2.5 mg/kg q 8 hr; **infants and neonates:** 2.5 mg/kg q 8 hr; **premature infants or neonates less than 1 week of age:** 2.5 mg/kg q 12 hr. *Prevention of bacterial endocarditis, dental or respiratory tract procedures:* **Adults:** 1.5 mg/kg gentamicin (not to exceed 80 mg) plus 1 g ampicillin, each IM or IV, 30–60 min before the procedure; one additional dose of each can be given 8 hr later (alternative: penicillin V, 1 g PO, 6 hr after initial dose). *Prophylaxis of bacterial endocarditis in GI or GU tract procedures or surgery:* **Adults,** 1.5 mg/kg gentamicin (not to exceed 80 mg) plus 2 g ampicillin, each IM or IV, 30–60 min before procedure; dose should be repeated 8 hr later. **Children:** 2 mg/kg gentamicin plus penicillin G, 30,000 units/kg, or ampicillin, 50 mg/kg in same dosage interval as for adults. Pediatric dosage should not exceed single or 24-hr adult doses. **Note:** In clients allergic to penicillin, vancomycin, 1 g IV given slowly over 1 hr, may be substituted; the dose of vancomycin should be repeated 8–12 hr later. **Adults with impaired renal function:** To calculate interval (hr) between doses, multiply serum creatinine level (mg/100 ml) by 8. **IV:** *Septicemia,* **initially,** 1–2 mg/kg infused over 30–60 min; **then,** maintenance doses may be administered. **Intrathecal** (*for men-*

ingitis): **Use only the intrathecal preparation. Adults, usual:** 4–8 mg once daily; **children and infants 3 months and older:** 1–2 mg once daily.

Ophthalmic solution (0.3%): *Acute infections:* **initially,** 1–2 drops in conjunctival sac q 15–30 min; **then,** as infection improves, reduce frequency. *Moderate infections:* 1–2 drops in conjunctival sac 4–6 times daily. *Trachoma:* 2 drops in each eye b.i.d.–q.i.d.; treatment should be continued for up to 1–2 months. **Ophthalmic ointment (0.3%):** Depending on the severity of infection, ½ inch ribbon from q 3–4 hr to 2–3 times daily.

Topical Cream/Ointment (0.1%): Apply 1–5 times daily to affected area. The area may be covered with a sterile bandage.

NURSING CONSIDERATIONS

See also *Nursing Considerations* for *Aminoglycosides*, p. 25.

Administration/Storage

1. For intermittent IV administration, the adult dose should be diluted in 50–200 ml of sterile 5% dextrose in water or isotonic saline and administered over a 30–120 min period. The volume should be less for infants and children.
2. Gentamicin should not be mixed with other drugs for parenteral use.
3. For parenteral use, the duration of treatment is 7–10 days, although a longer course of therapy may be required for severe or complicated infections.
4. When used intrathecally, the usual site is the lumbar area.
5. With topical administration:
   * Remove the crusts of impe-

tigo contagiosa before applying ointment to permit maximum contact between antibiotic and infection.
* Apply ointment gently and cover with gauze dressing if desirable or as ordered.
* Avoid direct exposure to sunlight as photosensitivity reaction may occur.
* Avoid further contamination of infected skin.

Evaluation

1. Assess lab culture data to determine effectiveness of drug therapy.
2. During systemic administration, evaluate for laboratory evidence of therapeutic drug levels (4–8 mcg/ml).

Gentian Violet
(**JEN**-shun **VYE**-oh-let)
Genapax (Rx)

Classification: Topical and vaginal anti-infective.

Action/Kinetics: This traditional rosaniline dye is effective against some gram-positive bacteria, many fungi (yeasts and dermatophytes), and many strains of *Candida*. Treatment should continue until symptoms subside and cultures are negative.

Uses: Topically for treatment of cutaneous and mucocutaneous *Candida albicans* infections such as thrush, intertriginous and paronychial candidiasis. Vulvovaginal candidiasis.

Contraindications: Hypersensitivity to gentian violet, presence of other vaginal infections, extensive vaginal excoriation, and ulceration. Ulcerative lesions of the face.

Special Concerns: Safe use during pregnancy (category: C) has not been determined. Use with caution in clients suspected of having diabetes mellitus because vaginal infections often are the first symptoms of this disease.

Side Effects: *Topical:* Irritation, hypersensitivity, ulceration of mucous membranes, permanent staining if applied to granulation tissue. *GI:* Following use for oral candidiasis, esophagitis, laryngitis, tracheitis, laryngeal obstruction. *Vaginal:* Vaginal burning, pain, itching, or other signs of irritation.

Dosage: Vaginal: One tampon (5 mg) inserted for 3–4 hr once or twice daily for 12 consecutive days. An additional tampon may be used overnight in resistant cases. **Topical solution:** Apply 1% or 2% solution to affected areas b.i.d.– t.i.d. for 3 days.

NURSING CONSIDERATIONS

Administration/Storage

1. Tampon should be inserted high into vagina. During last trimester of pregnancy, the suppository should be inserted partially into vagina, preferably by hand.
2. The solution should not be used in or around the eyes.

Client/Family Teaching

1. Review the appropriate method for administration.
2. Stress the importance of good skin care and proper hygiene to prevent further infection.
3. Keep exposed areas as dry as possible.
4. Wear clean panties with a cotton crotch.
5. Protect skin and clothing from dye as it will stain.

6. Male partner should wear a condom to prevent reinfection.

Evaluation

1. Review lab culture data to determine effectiveness of drug therapy.
2. Evaluate client for reports of symptomatic improvement.

Glipizide

(**GLIP**-ih-zyd)
Glucotrol (Rx)

See also *Antidiabetic Agents, Oral,* p. 65.

Classification: Second-generation sulfonylurea.

Action/Kinetics: Glipizide also has mild diuretic effects. **Onset:** 1–1.5 hr. **t½:** 2–4 hr. **Time to peak levels:** 1–3 hr. **Duration:** 12–24 hr. Metabolized in liver to inactive metabolites, which are excreted through the kidneys.

Special Concerns: Pregnancy category: C.

Additional Drug Interaction: Cimetidine may ↑ effect of glipizide due to ↓ breakdown by liver.

Dosage: PO. Adults, initial: 5 mg before breakfast; **then,** adjust dosage by 2.5–5 mg q few days until adequate control is achieved. **Maintenance:** 15–40 mg daily. Older clients should begin with 2.5 mg.

NURSING CONSIDERATIONS

See also *Nursing Considerations* for *Antidiabetic Agents, Oral,* p. 68.

Administration/Storage

1. Maintenance doses greater than 15 mg daily should be

divided and given before the morning and evening meals.

2. For greatest effect, give 30 min before meals.

Client/Family Teaching

1. Advise client that complaints of CNS side effects such as drowsiness or headache should be reported to the physician.

2. Some clients may suffer from anorexia, constipation or diarrhea, vomiting, and gastralgia. If the symptoms are severe, advise client to record weight and intake and output.

3. Skin reactions may occur and skin changes should be reported. Advise clients to avoid exposure to the sun, to use a sunscreen when in the sun, and to keep their arms and extremities covered.

4. Avoid alcohol in any form.

5. Practice barrier form of contraception.

Evaluation: Evaluate client for laboratory evidence that serum glucose levels are within desired range.

Glucagon
(**GLOO**-kah-gon)
(Rx)

Classification: Insulin antagonist.

Action/Kinetics: Glucagon is a hormone produced by the alpha islet cells of the pancreas. The hormone increases blood glucose by increasing breakdown of glycogen to glucose, stimulating gluconeogenesis from amino acids and fatty acids, and inhibiting conversion of glucose to glycogen. Also, lipolysis is increased, resulting in free fatty acids and glycerol for gluconeogenesis. The drug is effective in overcoming hypoglycemia only if the liver has a glycogen reserve. **Onset, hypoglycemia:** 5–20 min. **Maximum effect:** 30 min. **Duration:** 1–2 hr. **t½:** 3–6 min. Metabolized in the liver, kidney, plasma membrane receptor sites, and plasma.

Uses: Used to terminate insulin-induced shock in diabetic or psychiatric clients. Client usually regains consciousness 5–20 min after the parenteral administration of glucagon. The drug should only be used under medical supervision or in accordance with strict instructions received from the physician. Failure to respond may be an indication for IV administration of glucose—especially true in the juvenile diabetics. As a diagnostic aid in radiologic examination of the GI tract when a hypotonic state is desirable. *Investigational:* Inhibit bowel peristalsis in abdominal digital vascular imaging and in abdominal CT scanning to prevent misregistration artifact. Adjunct in diagnosis of GI bleeding. Treatment of toxicity due to beta-adrenergic blocking agents, quinidine, or tricyclic antidepressants.

Special Concerns: Pregnancy category: B. Use with caution in clients with renal or hepatic disease, in those who are undernourished and emaciated, and in clients with a history of pheochromocytoma or insulinoma.

Side Effects: *GI:* Nausea, vomiting. *Allergy:* Respiratory distress, urticaria, hypotension. Stevens-Johnson syndrome when used as diagnostic aid. *Symptoms of Overdose:* Nausea, vomiting, hypokalemia.

G

Drug Interactions

Anticoagulants,, oral / ↑ Effect of anticoagulants by ↑ hypoprothrombinemia

Antidiabetic agents / Hyperglycemic effect of glucagon antagonizes hypoglycemic effect of antidiabetics

Corticosteroids, Epinephrine, Estrogens, Phenytoin / Additive hyperglycemic effect of drugs listed

Dosage: IM, IV, SC. *Hypoglycemia:* **Adults:** 0.5–1 mg; 1–2 additional doses may be given at 20 min intervals, if necessary. **Pediatric:** 0.025 mg/kg, up to a maximum of 1 mg; may be repeated in 20 min if needed. *Insulin shock therapy:* **IM, IV, SC,** 0.5–1 mg after 1 hr of coma; if no response, dose may be repeated. *Diagnostic aid for GI tract:* dose dependent on desired onset of action and duration of effect necessary for the examination: **IV,** 0.25–0.5 mg (onset: 1 min; duration: 9–17 min); 2 mg (onset: 1 min; duration 22–25 min). **IM,** 1 mg (onset: 8–10 min; duration: 12–27 min); 2 mg (onset: 4–7 min; duration: 21–32 min). *For colon examination:* **IM,** 2 mg 10 min prior to procedure. *Treatment of toxicity of beta-adrenergic blocking agents:* **Adults, IV, initial:** 2–3 mg given over 30 sec; may be repeated at the rate of 5 mg/hr until client is stabilized.

NURSING CONSIDERATIONS

Administration/Storage

1. Once the client with hypoglycemia responds, supplemental carbohydrates should be given to prevent secondary hypoglycemia.

2. Before reconstituting, the powder should be stored at room temperature.

3. Following reconstitution, the solution should be used immediately. However, if necessary, the solution may be stored at 5°C (41°F) for up to 2 days.

4. Doses higher than 2 mg should be reconstituted with sterile water for injection and used immediately.

5. Administer with dextrose solutions. A precipitate may form if saline solutions are used.

6. *Treatment of Overdose:* Symptomatic.

Interventions

1. Following the administration of glucagon, administer a carbohydrate after the client awakens.

2. Have rapidly available sugar, such as orange juice and Karo syrup in water, to administer. If the shock was caused by a long-acting medication, administer slowly digestible carbohydrates, such as bread with honey.

Client/Family Teaching

1. Instruct the family in the administration of glucagon SC or IM in the event the client has a hypoglycemic reaction and loses consciousness.

2. Discuss the need to keep the physician informed of hypoglycemic reactions so that the dosage of insulin can be properly adjusted.

3. Advise the family not to try to administer fluids by mouth if the client has a reaction and is not fully conscious. The client

could easily aspirate these fluids into the lungs.

Evaluation: Evaluate for a positive clinical response as evidenced by an increased serum glucose level and an improvement in the client's level of consciousness during treatment for hypoglycemia.

Glutethimide
(gloo-**TETH**-ih-myd)
Doriden, Doriglute (C-II, Rx)

Classification: Nonbarbiturate, nonbenzodiazepine sedative-hypnotic.

Action/Kinetics: Glutethimide produces CNS depressant effects comparable to barbiturates, including suppression of REM sleep and REM rebound. Other effects include anticholinergic with mydriasis, inhibition of salivary secretion, and decreased GI motility. At comparable doses, glutethimide produces less respiratory depression but greater hypotension than occurs with barbiturates. Psychologic and physical dependence may develop. **Onset:** 30 min. **Peak plasma concentration:** 1–6 hr (erratically absorbed from GI tract). **t½:** 10–12 hr. **Duration:** 4–8 hr. About 50% is bound to plasma protein. Metabolized in liver and excreted in urine.

Uses: Short-term treatment of insomnia (use should not exceed 1 week). Has generally been replaced by other sedative-hypnotics.

Contraindications: Hypersensitivity to drug. Porphyria. Clients with a history of drug dependence, alcoholism, or emotional disorders. Use not recommended during pregnancy, during lactation, and in children. **Do not give to client with glaucoma or to clients with a history of drug dependence, alcoholism, or emotional disorders.**

Special Concerns: Pregnancy category: C. Use during lactation may cause sedation in the infant. Dosage adjustment may be necessary in geriatric clients due to age-related prostatic hypertrophy and impairment of renal function.

Side Effects: *GI:* Nausea, vomiting, anorexia, xerostomia. *CNS:* Headache, hangover, dizziness, confusion, drowsiness. *Dermatologic:* Skin rash (cause for discontinuing drug), urticaria, purpura. *Miscellaneous:* Osteomalacia following long-term use. *Rarely:* Excitation, blurred vision, acute hypersensitivity, exfoliative dermatitis, intermittent porphyria, and blood dyscrasias including thrombocytopenia, aplastic anemia, and leukopenia. Abrupt withdrawal of large doses may be dangerous—withdrawal symptoms are similar to those of barbiturates. Occasionally, symptoms similar to withdrawal occur in clients who have been taking only moderate doses, even when there is no abstention (tremulousness, nausea, tachycardia, fever, tonic muscle spasms, generalized convulsions).

Chronic Toxicity: Characterized by psychosis, confusion, delirium, hallucinations, ataxia, tremor, hyporeflexia, slurred speech, memory loss, irritability, fever, weight loss, mydriasis, xerostomia, nystagmus, headache, and convulsions. Treatment consists of careful, cautious withdrawal of drug over a period of several days or weeks.

Acute Toxicity: Characterized by

coma, hypotension, hypothermia, followed by fever, tachycardia, depression or absence of reflexes (including pupillary response), sudden apnea, cyanosis, tonic muscle spasms, convulsions, and hyperreflexia. Treatment of acute toxicity is supportive, starting with gastric lavage, CNS stimulants (used with caution), vasopressors, and maintenance of pulmonary ventilation. Parenteral fluids are administered cautiously, and hemodialysis may be necessary. Endotracheal intubation or tracheotomy may be indicated.

Drug Interactions

Anticoagulants, oral / ↓ Effect of anticoagulants due to ↑ breakdown by liver
Antidepressants, tricyclic / Additive anticholinergic side effects
CNS depressants / Additive CNS depression

Laboratory Test Interference: ↑ or ↓ 17-ketogenic steroids, 17-hydroxycorticosteroids.

Dosage: Tablets. Adults: Individualize to minimize chance of overdosage. **Usual:** 500 mg at bedtime. Dose may be repeated but not less than 4 hr before client arises. **Geriatric or debilitated clients:** Initial daily dose should not exceed 500 mg. **Not recommended for children.**

NURSING CONSIDERATIONS

Administration/Storage: *Treatment of Overdose*
- Assist with gastric lavage for treatment of acute toxicity.
- Monitor vital signs.
- Have emergency drugs and equipment available.

- Anticipate hemodialysis in severe cases.

Interventions

1. Incorporate safety measures such as side rails and assisted ambulation.
2. Provide special mouth care for clients to avoid or minimize xerostomia.
3. Check clients for bowel regularity. Provide extra fluids and increased dietary roughage. Consult with the physician regarding the need for a stool softener or laxative.
4. If the client seems to be depressed or have suicidal tendencies, withhold the drug, document, and report to the physician.
5. Withdraw the drug gradually to minimize withdrawal symptoms.
6. The drug suppresses REM sleep. Therefore, try alternative methods to induce sleep, such as relaxation methods, having the client drink warm milk, or give client a backrub.

Client/Family Teaching

1. Warn clients receiving glutethimide not to drive a car or operate other machinery after taking medication because drug may cause drowsiness.
2. Advise to avoid alcohol in any form and any other CNS depressants.
3. Provide a printed list of drug side effects. Stress those that require immediate reporting.

Evaluation: Evaluate client for:
- Reports of improved sleeping patterns with less frequent awakenings

- Freedom from complications of drug therapy and associated psychological dependence

Glyburide

(GLYE-byou-ryd)

Diabeta, Euglucon✦, Micronase (Rx)

See also *Antidiabetic Agents, Oral,* p. 65.

Classification: Second-generation sulfonylurea.

Action/Kinetics: Glyburide has a mild diuretic effect. **Onset:** 2–4 hr. **t½:** 10 hr. **Time to peak levels:** 4 hr. **Duration:** 24 hr. Metabolized in liver to weakly active metabolites. Excreted in bile (50%) and through the kidneys (50%).

Special Concerns: Pregnancy category: B.

Dosage: PO. Adults, initial: 2.5–5 mg daily given with breakfast (or the first main meal); **then,** increase by 2.5 mg at weekly intervals to achieve the desired response. **Maintenance:** 1.25–20 mg daily. Clients sensitive to sulfonylureas should start with 1.25 mg/day.

NURSING CONSIDERATIONS

See *Nursing Considerations* for *Antidiabetic Agents, Oral,* p. 68.

Administration/Storage

1. For best results, administer prior to meals.
2. If daily dosage exceeds 15 mg, the dose should be divided and given before the morning and evening meals.

Evaluation: Assess client for laboratory evidence that serum glucose levels are within desired range.

Glycerin suppositories

(GLIH-sir-in)

Fleet Babylax, Sani-Supp (OTC)

Classification: Miscellaneous laxative.

Action/Kinetics: Glycerin suppositories promote defecation by irritating the rectal mucosa as well as by a hyperosmotic action. Glycerin may also soften and lubricate fecal material. The suppository does not have to melt to be effective. **Onset:** 15–60 min.

Use: To establish normal bowel function in clients dependent on laxatives. To evacuate the colon prior to rectal and bowel examinations as well as colon surgery.

Contraindications: Should not be used in the presence of anal fissures, fistulas, ulcerative hemorrhoids, or proctitis.

Side Effects: Mucous membrane irritation.

Dosage: Suppository: Insert one adult or pediatric suppository high in the rectum and hold for 15 min. **Liquid:** The contents of one unit (4 ml) inserted gently with the tip of the applicator pointed toward the navel.

NURSING CONSIDERATIONS

See also *Nursing Considerations* for *Laxatives,* p. 172.

Administration/Storage

1. Store in a tight container in the refrigerator below 25°C (77°F).

2. A small amount of liquid glycerin will remain in the applicator unit.
3. Anticipate onset of action within 1 hr.
4. The suppository does not need to melt in order to produce a laxative effect.

Evaluation: Evaluate client for reports of successful evacuation of a soft, formed stool.

G

Glycopyrrolate

(glye-koh-**PYE**-roh-layt)
Robinul, Robinul Forte (Rx)

See also *Cholinergic Blocking Agents,* p. 136.

Classification: Cholinergic blocking agent.

Action/Kinetics: Onset: PO, 1 hr; **IV,** 1 min; **IM, SC:** 15–30 min. **Duration: decrease salivation,** Up to 7 hr; **block vagal activity:** 2–3 hr. **t½:** 0.6–4.6 hr.

Uses: PO. Adjunct in treatment of peptic ulcer. Antidiarrheal. **IM, IV.** To reduce salivation, tracheobronchial and pharyngeal secretions during surgery. To decrease acidity and volume of gastric secretions; to block cardiac vagal inhibitory reflexes during induction of anesthesia and intubation. Prophylaxis of aspiration of gastric contents during anesthesia. Adjunct with neostigmine or pyridostigmine to reverse neuromuscular blockade due to nondepolarizing muscle relaxants.

Additional Contraindication: Peptic ulcer in children under 12 years of age.

Special Concerns: Pregnancy category: B. Dosage has not been determined for the injection in children with peptic ulcer.

Laboratory Test Interferences: ↓ Serum uric acid in clients with gout or hyperuricemia.

Dosage: Tablets. *Peptic ulcer:* **Adults, initial:** 1–2 mg t.i.d. or 2 mg b.i.d.–t.i.d. (may also give 2 mg at bedtime); **maintenance:** 1 mg b.i.d. with dose adjusted as needed up to a maximum of 8 mg. **IM, IV.** *Peptic ulcer:* **Adults, IM, IV,** 0.1–0.2 mg t.i.d.–q.i.d. *Prophylaxis of excessive salivation, respiratory tract secretions, gastric hypersecretion during anesthesia:* **Adults, IM,** 0.0044 mg/kg 30–60 min prior to anesthesia or at the time the preanesthetic sedative and/or narcotic are given; **pediatric, less than 12 years:** 0.0044–0.0088 mg/kg 30–60 min before anesthetic or at the time preanesthetic medication is given. *Prophylaxis of arrhythmias during anesthesia and surgery:* **Adults, IV,** 0.1 mg repeated, as needed, q 2–3 min; **pediatric, IV,** 0.0044 mg/kg not to exceed 0.1 mg/dose, repeated, as needed, q 2–3 min. *Reversal of neuromuscular blockade.* **IV: Adults and children:** 0.2 mg for each 1 mg neostigmine or 5 mg pyridostigmine. Give IV at the same time and in the same syringe.

NURSING CONSIDERATIONS

See also *Nursing Considerations for Cholinergic Blocking Agents,* p. 138.

Administration/Storage

1. Do not add to IV solution containing sodium chloride or bicarbonate.
2. Parenteral use may slow stomach emptying and cause pain at the injection site.

Assessment: Note the age of the client. Elderly clients are more sensitive to the side effects of drug therapy than younger clients.

Evaluation: Evaluate client for:
- ↓ frequency of diarrheal stools
- ↓ salivation preop
- ↓ acidity and volume of gastric secretions

Gold sodium thiomalate

(gold **SO**-dee-um thigh-oh-**MAH**-layt)
Myochrysine (Rx)

Classification: Antirheumatic.

Action/Kinetics: Although the exact mechanism is not known, gold salts may inhibit lysosomal enzyme activity in macrophages and decrease macrophage phagocytic activity. Other mechanisms may include alteration of the immune response and alteration of biosynthesis of collagen. Gold salts suppress, but do not cure, arthritis and synovitis. The beneficial effects may not be seen for 3–12 months. Most clients experience transient side effects, although serious effects may be manifested in some. **Peak blood levels (IM):** 4–6 hr. **t½:** increases with continued therapy. Gold may accumulate in tissues and persist for years. Significantly bound to plasma proteins. The drug is eliminated slowly through both the urine (60%–90%) and feces (10%–40%). This preparation contains 50% gold.

Uses: Adjunct to the treatment of rheumatoid arthritis (active and progressive stages) in children and adults. It is most effective in the early stages of the disease.

Contraindications: Hepatic disease, cardiovascular problems such as hypertension or congestive heart failure, severe diabetes, debilitated clients, renal disease, blood dyscrasias, agranulocytosis, hemorrhagic diathesis, clients receiving radiation treatments, colitis, lupus erythematosus, pregnancy, lactation, children under 6 years of age. Clients with eczema or urticaria.

Special Concerns: Pregnancy category: C.

G

Side Effects: *Skin:* Dermatitis (most common), pruritus, erythema, dermatoses, gray to blue pigmentation of tissues, alopecia, loss of nails. *GI:* Stomatitis (second most common), metallic taste, gastritis, colitis, gingivitis, glossitis, nausea, vomiting, diarrhea (may be persistent), colic, anorexia, cramps, enterocolitis. *Hematologic:* Anemia, thrombocytopenia, granulocytopenia, leukopenia, eosinophilia, hemorrhagic diathesis. *Allergic:* Flushing, fainting, sweating, dizziness, anaphylaxis, syncope, bradycardia, angioneurotic edema, respiratory difficulties. *Other:* Interstitial pneumonitis, pulmonary fibrosis, nephrotic syndrome, glomerulitis (with hematuria), proteinuria, hepatitis, fever, headache, arthralgia, ophthalmologic problems including corneal ulcers, iritis, gold deposits, EEG abnormalities, peripheral neuritis. Corticosteroids may be used to treat symptoms such as stomatitis, dermatitis, GI, renal, hematologic, or pulmonary problems. Also, if symptoms are severe and do not respond to corticosteroids, a chelating agent such as dimercaprol may be used. Clients should be monitored carefully. *Symptoms of Overdose:* Hematuria, proteinuria, thrombocytopenia, granulocytopenia, nausea, vomiting, diarrhea, fever, papulovesicular lesions, urticaria, exfoliative dermatitis, severe pruritus.

Drug Interactions: Concomitant use contraindicated with drugs known to cause blood dyscrasias (e.g., antimalarials, cytotoxic drugs, pyrazolone derivatives, immunosuppressive drugs).

Laboratory Test Interference: Alters liver function tests. Urinary protein and RBCs, altered blood counts (indicative of toxic effect of drug).

Dosage: IM. *Rheumatoid arthritis.* **Adults,** *week 1:* 10 mg as a single injection; *week 2:* 25 mg as a single dose. Thereafter, 25–50 mg/week until 0.8–1 g total has been given. Thereafter according to individual response. *Usual maintenance:* 25–50 mg every other week for up to 20 weeks. If condition remains stable, the dose can be given every third or fourth week indefinitely. **Pediatric: initial,** *week 1:* 10 mg; **then,** usual dose is 1 mg/kg, not to exceed 50 mg/injection using the same spacing of doses as for adults.

NURSING CONSIDERATIONS

Administration/Storage

1. Shake vial well to ensure uniformity of suspension before withdrawing medication.
2. Inject into gluteus maximus.
3. Gold therapy may be reinstituted following mild toxic symptoms but not after severe symptoms.
4. Geriatric clients manifest a lower tolerance to gold.
5. *Treatment of Overdose:* Discontinue use of the drug immediately. Give dimercaprol. Give supportive treatment for hematologic or renal complications.

Interventions

1. Have the client remain in a recumbent position for at least 20 min after the injection to prevent falls resulting from transient vertigo or giddiness.
2. Have dimercaprol (BAL) readily available to use as an antidote in case of severe toxicity.

Client/Family Teaching

1. Explain that close medical supervision is required during gold therapy.
2. Advise client not to become discouraged. Stress that beneficial effects are slow to appear but that therapy may be continued for up to 12 months in anticipation of relief.
3. Provide a printed list of adverse drug effects. Identify those that require immediate reporting.
4. Practice contraception during therapy.
5. Avoid direct sun exposure as a photosensitivity reaction may occur. Wear sunscreen, protective clothing, and a hat if exposure is necessary.

Evaluation: Evaluate client for:
- Reports of symptomatic improvement in joint pain and mobility
- Freedom from complications of drug therapy

Gonadorelin acetate
(go-nad-oh-**RELL**-in)
Factrel ✹, Lutrepulse (Rx)

Classification: Gonadotropin-releasing hormone.

Action/Kinetics: Gonadorelin is a synthetic hormone identical in amino acid sequence to the naturally occurring gonadotropin-releasing hormone. Thus, gonadorelin stimulates the synthesis, and release of FSH and LH from the adenohypophysis. FSH and LH then stimulate the ovaries to synthesize estrogen and progesterone, which are necessary for development and release of an ovum. **t½, initial:** 2–10 min; **final:** 10–40 min. Gonadorelin is metabolized to inactive peptide fragments, which are excreted in the urine.

Uses: Primary hypothalamic amenorrhea.

Contraindications: Sensitivity to gonadorelin acetate or gonadorelin HCl (used for determining gonadotropic function of the pituitary). Pituitary prolactinoma, causes of anovulation other than those of hypothalamic origin (e.g., ovarian cysts), hormone-dependent tumors.

Special Concerns: Pregnancy category: B. There is no indication for use of gonadorelin acetate during lactation. Safety and efficacy have not been determined in children less than 18 years of age.

Side Effects: *Ovarian hyperstimulation:* Ovarian enlargement, ascites with or without pain, pleural effusion. *Local, due to use of infusion pump:* Inflammation, infection, mild phlebitis, hematoma at site of catheter. *Anaphylaxis:* Bronchospasm, flushing, tachycardia, urticaria, induration at injection site. *Miscellaneous:* Multiple pregnancy.

Drug Interactions: Gonadorelin should not be used with ovarian stimulators.

Dosage: IV: 5 mcg q 90 min (range: 1–20 mcg) delivered by Lutrepulse pump using the 0.8 mg solution at 50 mcl/pulse. The recommended treatment interval is 21 days. If there is no response after three treatment intervals, the dose should be increased cautiously and in step wise fashion.

NURSING CONSIDERATIONS

Administration/Storage

1. The kit contains the lyophilized powder for injection, diluent, catheter and tubing, alcohol swabs, IV cannula units, syringe and needle, elastic belt, batteries, the Lutrepulse pump, physician pump manual, and package insert.
2. Gonadorelin is reconstituted with 8 ml of diluent immediately prior to use and then transferred to the plastic reservoir.
3. The presterilized bag with the supplied infusion catheter set is filled with the reconstituted solution for IV administration.
4. The drug is then administered IV using the "Lutrepulse" pump which can deliver 25 or 50 mcl of solution over a period of 1 min and at a pulse frequency of 90 min. Depending on the concentration of the solution and the volume/pulse, the pump can deliver 2.5, 5, 10, or 20 mcg of gonadorelin.
5. The 8 ml of solution will last for approximately 7 consecutive days.
6. The cannula and IV site should be changed every 48 hr.
7. Have emergency drugs and equipment available in the event of an anaphylactic reaction.

Assessment

1. Perform a thorough nursing history. Proper diagnosis is

critical for treatment to be successful.

2. Determine that hypothalamic amenorrhea or hypogonadism is due to a deficiency in quantity or pulsing of endogenous gonadotropin-releasing hormone.

3. Note any history of ovarian cysts or pituitary tumors because drug is contraindicated under these circumstances.

4. Obtain baseline ovarian ultrasound, pelvic exam, and midluteal phase serum progesterone level prior to initiating therapy.

Client/Family Teaching

1. Demonstrate the appropriate method for drug administration. Provide detailed instructions both orally and in writing regarding the proper use and care of the Lutrepulse infusion pump.

2. Stress the importance of using aseptic technique.

3. Have client return demonstrate so that any problems or questions may be identified prior to leaving the office. Provide client with a phone number where assistance may be found 24 hr a day.

4. Instruct the client in how to assess the infusion site for evidence of inflammation, phlebitis, erythema, infection, or hematoma and to report these findings to the physician because the site will need to be changed.

5. Provide a list of symptoms of hyperstimulation of the ovaries and advise the client to avoid having intercourse if these symptoms occur. A rupture of an ovarian cyst could occur, resulting in hemoperitoneum.

6. Explain the importance of careful record-keeping in relation to menses, basal temperatures and graph recordings, medication administration, and any side effects that may be noted. All side effects should always be reported to the physician.

7. Explain to the client that if ovulation occurs with the pump in place, notify the physician because the therapy should be continued for 2 more weeks to maintain the corpus luteum.

8. Explain that clinical response to gonadorelin acetate therapy is generally monitored by ovarian ultrasound, mid-luteal phase serum progesterone levels, and regularly scheduled physical exams including a pelvic. Additionally, the infusion site will be examined and changed every 48 hr. Stress the importance of complying with these frequently scheduled tests. This therapy may require a relatively long-term commitment by the client.

Evaluation: Evaluate client for:
- Restoration of menstrual cycle with evidence of ovum production (response to gonadorelin usually occurs within 2–3 weeks after initiation of therapy)
- Freedom from complications of drug therapy

Goserelin acetate
(GO-seh-rel-in)
Zoladex (Rx)

Classification: Antineoplastic, hormonal agent.

Action/Kinetics: Goserelin acetate is a synthetic decapeptide analog of luteinizing hormone-releasing hormone (LHRH or GnRH). The drug is a potent inhibitor of gonadotropin secretion from the pituitary gland. Initially, there is actually an increase in serum LH and FSH. This is followed by a long-term suppression of pituitary gonadotropins with serum levels of testosterone decreasing to those seen in surgically castrated males. **Peak serum levels after SC implantation:** 12–15 days. **Mean peak serum levels:** Approximately 2.5 ng/ml. The drug is available as an implant in a preloaded syringe. For the first 8 days of the treatment cycle, the rate of absorption is slower than for the remainder of the period.

Uses: Palliative treatment of advanced prostatic carcinoma as an alternative to orchiectomy or estrogen administration when these are either unacceptable to the client or not indicated.

Contraindications: Pregnancy category: X. Lactation.

Special Concerns: Safety and effectiveness have not been determined in clients less than 18 years of age. There may be transient worsening of symptoms during the first few weeks of therapy.

Side Effects: *GU:* Sexual dysfunction, decreased erections, lower urinary tract symptoms, renal insufficiency, urinary obstruction, urinary tract infection. Impairment of fertility. *CNS:* Lethargy, dizziness, insomnia, anxiety, depression, headache. *GI:* Anorexia, nausea, constipation, diarrhea, vomiting, ulcer formation. *CV:* Edema, congestive heart failure, arrhythmias, cerebrovascular accident, myocardial infarction, peripheral vascular disorder, hypertension, chest pain. *Miscellaneous:* Hot flashes (common), upper respiratory tract infection, rash, sweating, chronic obstructive pulmonary disease, worsened pain for the first 30 days, breast swelling/tenderness, fever, chills, anemia, gout, hyperglycemia, weight increase.

Dosage: SC Implant: 3.6 mg q 28 days into the upper abdominal wall using sterile technique under the direction of a physician.

NURSING CONSIDERATIONS

See also *Nursing Considerations* for *Antineoplastic Agents,* p. 88.

Administration/Storage

1. The sterile syringe, in which the drug is contained, should not be removed until immediately before use. The syringe should be examined for damage and to ensure the drug is visible in the translucent chamber.
2. The area should be cleaned with an alcohol swab; a topical (i.e., ethyl chloride) or a local anesthetic may be used prior to the injection.
3. To administer the drug, the client's skin should be stretched with one hand and the needle gripped with the fingers around the barrel of the syringe. The needle is inserted into the SC fat and should not be aspirated. If a large vessel is penetrated, blood will be seen immediately in the syringe; the needle should be withdrawn and the injection made elsewhere with a new syringe.
4. The direction of the needle is

changed so it parallels the abdominal wall. The needle is then pushed in until the barrel hub touches the client's skin and then withdrawn approximately 1 cm to create a space to inject the drug. The plunger is depressed to deliver the drug.
5. The needle is then withdrawn and the area bandaged.
6. To confirm the drug has been delivered, ensure that the tip of the plunger is visible within the tip of the needle.
7. The drug should be stored at room temperature not exceeding 25°C (77°F).
8. There is no evidence the drug accumulates in clients with either hepatic and/or renal dysfunction.

Interventions

1. Goserelin should not be used in women who are likely to become pregnant or who are pregnant. Clients must be appraised of potential hazards to the fetus in the event of pregnancy.
2. Administration of the drug should be under the supervision of a physician.
3. The 28-day schedule should be adhered to as closely as possible.
4. If there is need to remove goserelin surgically, it can be located by ultrasound.
5. Be prepared to provide emotional support to clients and families.

Client/Family Teaching

1. Remind client that the most common adverse side effects (especially hot flashes, decreased erections, and sexual

dysfunction) are due to decreased testosterone levels.
2. Drug may impair fertility.
3. Advise that there may be initial worsening of symptoms or the occurrence of new symptoms of prostatic cancer. This is the result of transient increases of testosterone.
4. Clients may complain of an increase in bone pain and develop spinal cord compression or ureteral obstruction. Client and family should be reassured that these symptoms are usually only temporary.

Evaluation: Evaluate client for evidence of a decrease in tumor size and spread.

Griseofulvin microsize
(griz-ee-oh-**FULL**-vin)
Fulvicin-U/F, Grifulvin V, Grisactin, Grisactin 500, Grisovin-FP ✹ (Rx)

Griseofulvin ultramicrosize
(grih-see-oh-**FULL**-vin)
Fulvicin-P/G, Grisactin Ultra, Gris-PEG (Rx)

See also *Anti-Infectives,* p. 80.

Classification: Antibiotic, antifungal.

Action/Kinetics: Griseofulvin is a natural antibiotic derived from a species of *Penicillium.* It is believed to interfere with cell division (metaphase) or DNA replication. When taken systemically, the drug is deposited in the newly formed skin and nails, which are then resistant to reinfection by the tinea. Griseofulvin is absorbed from the duodenum. **Peak plasma concentration:** 0.37–2 mcg/ml after 4 hr.

$t\frac{1}{2}$: 9–24 hr. Levels may be increased by giving the drug with a high-fat diet. The GI absorption of the ultramicrosize products is about 1.5 times that of the microsize products.

Uses: Tinea (ringworm) infections of skin (including athlete's foot), scalp, groin, and nails. The drug is effective against tinea corporis, tinea pedis, tinea barbae, tinea unguium, tinea cruris, tinea capitis due to *Trichophyton* species, *Microsporum audouinii, M. canis, M. gypseum,* and *Epidermophyton floccosum*. It is the only oral drug effective against dermatophytic (tinea ringworm) infections. The drug is not effective against *Candida*. Susceptibility of the infectious agent should be established before treatment is begun.

Contraindications: Pregnancy. Porphyria or history thereof, hepatocellular failure, and hypersensitivity to drug. Exposure to artificial light or sunlight. Use for infections due to bacteria, candidiasis, actinomycosis, sporotrichosis, tinea versicolor, histoplasmosis, chromoblastomycosis, coccidioidomycosis, cryptococcosis, and North American blastomycosis.

Special Concerns: Pregnancy category: C. Cross sensitivity with penicillin is possible.

Side Effects: *Hypersensitivity:* Rashes, urticaria, angioneurotic edema, allergic reactions. *GI:* Nausea, vomiting, diarrhea, epigastric pain. *CNS:* Dizziness, headache, tiredness, confusion, fatigue, insomnia. *Miscellaneous:* Oral thrush, acute intermittent porphyria, paresthesias of extremities, proteinuria, leukopenia, photosensitivity, worsening of lupus erythematosus.

Drug Interactions

Alcohol, ethyl / Tachycardia and flushing

Anticoagulants, oral / ↓ Effect of anticoagulants due to ↑ breakdown in liver

Barbiturates / ↓ Effect of griseofulvin due to ↓ absorption from GI tract

Oral contraceptives / ↓ Effect of contraceptives → breakthrough bleeding, pregnancy, or amenorrhea

Laboratory Test Interferences: ↑ ALT, AST, alkaline phosphatase, BUN, and creatinine level values.

Dosage: Capsules, Oral Suspension, Tablets. Adults: *Tinea corporis, cruris, or capitis:* 0.5 g griseofulvin microsize daily in a single dose or divided dose (or 330–375 mg ultramicrosize). *Tinea pedis or unguium:* 0.75–1 g daily of griseofulvin microsize (or 660–750 mg ultramicrosize). After response, decrease dose of microsize to 0.5 g daily. **PO. Pediatric, 13.6–22.7 kg:** 125–250 mg griseofulvin microsize daily (or 82.5–165 mg ultramicrosize); **pediatric, over 22.7 kg:** 250–500 mg microsize daily (or 165–330 mg ultramicrosize). **Note:** Dose has not been determined in children less than 2 years of age.

NURSING CONSIDERATIONS

See also *General Nursing Considerations For All Anti-Infectives,* p. 83.

Administration/Storage: Treatment must be of sufficient duration to eradicate the infecting organism. For example, treatment for tinea capitis should be from 4–6 weeks; 2–4 weeks for tinea corporis, 4–8 weeks for tinea pedis, and tinea unguium for 4 months (fingernails) to 6 months (toe nails).

Client/Family Teaching

1. Eat a high-fat diet because fat enhances the absorption of griseofulvin from the intestines. Refer to dietician as necessary for assistance with diet and meal planning.
2. Take all medication as prescribed to prevent any recurrence of infection.
3. Practice appropriate hygiene to prevent reinfection.
4. Avoid exposure to intense natural and artificial light because photosensitivity reactions may occur.
5. Report fever, sore throat, and malaise, (all symptoms of leukopenia) to the physician.
6. Advise client that to be considered cured, repeated cultures and scrapings of affected sites must be negative.
7. Advise client to practice a nonhormonal form of birth control.

Evaluation: Evaluate client for:

- Status of pretreatment symptoms and culture and scraping results
- Client/family knowledge and understanding of illness and their response to therapy and level of compliance with the prescribed drug therapy

---

Guaifenesin (Glyceryl guaiacolate)

(gwye-FEN-eh-sin)

Amonidrin, Anti-Tuss, Balminil Expectorant✿, Benylin-E✿, Breonesin, Fenesin, Gee-Gee, Genatuss, GG-Cen, Glyate, Glycotuss, Glytuss, Guiatuss, Halotussin, Humibid L.A., Humibid Sprinkle, Hytuss, Hytuss-2X, Malotuss, Mytussin, Naldecon Senior EX, Resyl✿, Robitussin, Scot-tussin, Sinumist-SR Capsules, Uni-tussin (OTC)

Classification: Expectorant.

Action/Kinetics: Guaifenesin increases the output of fluid of the respiratory tract by reducing the viscosity and surface tension of respiratory secretions, thereby facilitating their expectoration. Data on efficacy are lacking; however, guaifenesin is an ingredient of many nonprescription cough preparations.

Uses: Dry, nonproductive cough due to colds and minor upper respiratory tract infections.

Contraindications: Chronic cough, cough accompanied by excess secretions.

Side Effects: *GI:* Nausea, vomiting, GI upset. *CNS:* Dizziness, headache. *Dermatologic:* Rash, urticaria. *Symptoms of Overdose:* Nausea, vomiting.

Drug Interaction: Inhibition of platelet adhesiveness by guaifenesin may result in bleeding tendencies.

Laboratory Test Interferences: False + urinary 5-hydroxyindole-acetic acid. Color interference with determination of urinary vanillylmandelic acid.

Dosage: Capsules, Oral Solution, Syrup, Tablets. Adults and children over 12 years: 200–400 mg q 4 hr, not to exceed 2.4 g/day; **pediatric, 6–12 years:** 100–200 mg q 4 hr, not to exceed 600 mg/day; **pediatric, 2–6 years:** 50–100 mg q 4 hr, not to exceed

300 mg/day. If less than 2 years of age, the dosage must be individualized by the physician. **Extended-release Capsules, Extended-release Tablets. Adults and children over 12 years:** 600–1,200 mg q 12 hr, not to exceed 2.4 g/day; **pediatric, 6–12 years:** 600 mg q 12 hr, not to exceed 1.2 g/day; **pediatric, 2–6 years:** 300 mg q 12 hr, not to exceed 600 mg/day. **Note:** The liquid dosage forms may be more suitable for children less than 6 years of age.

NURSING CONSIDERATIONS

Client/Family Teaching

1. Take only as directed and do not exceed prescribed dosing guidelines.
2. If symptoms persist more than one week, medical intervention should be sought as cough may indicate a serious condition.
3. Any evidence of increased bleeding tendencies or increased bruising should be reported to the physician.
4. Advise client not to perform activities that require mental alertness because drug may cause drowsiness.

Evaluation: Evaluate client for:
- Reports of improvement in the frequency and duration of coughing episodes
- Improved mobilization and expectoration of mucus

Guanabenz acetate
(GWON-ah-benz)
Wytensin (Rx)

Classification: Antihypertensive, centrally acting antiadrenergic.

Action/Kinetics: Guanabenz stimulates alpha-adrenergic receptors in the CNS, resulting in a decrease in sympathetic impulses and in sympathetic tone. It also decreases the pulse rate, but postural hypotension has not been manifested. **Onset:** 60 min. **Peak effect:** 2–4 hr. **Peak plasma levels:** 2–5 hr. **t½:** 6 hr. **Duration:** 8–12 hr.

Uses: Hypertension, alone or as adjunct with thiazide diuretics.

Contraindications: Lactation, children under 12 years of age.

Special Concerns: Pregnancy category: C. Use with caution in severe coronary insufficiency, cerebrovascular disease, recent myocardial infarction, hepatic or renal disease. Geriatric clients may be more sensitive to the hypotensive and sedative effects of guanabenz; also, it may be necessary to decrease the dose in these clients due to age-related decreases in renal function.

Side Effects: *CNS:* Drowsiness and sedation (common), dizziness, weakness, headache, ataxia, depression, disturbances in sleep, excitement. *GI:* Dry mouth (common), nausea, vomiting, diarrhea, constipation, abdominal pain or discomfort. *CV:* Palpitations, chest pain, arrhythmias. *Miscellaneous:* Edema, blurred vision, muscle aches, dyspnea, rash, pruritus, nasal congestion, urinary frequency, gynecomastia, alterations in taste, disturbances of sexual function, taste disorders, aches in extremities. *Symptoms of Overdose:* Hypotension, sleepiness, irritability, miosis, lethargy, bradycardia.

Drug Interaction: Use with CNS depressants may result in significant sedation.

Dosage: Tablets. Adults: initial, 4 mg b.i.d. alone or with a diuretic; **then,** increase by 4–8 mg q 1–2 weeks until control achieved. Maximum recommended dose: 32 mg b.i.d.

NURSING CONSIDERATIONS

See also *Nursing Considerations* for *Antihypertensive Agents,* p. 78.

Administration/Storage

1. The drug should be kept tightly closed and protected from light.
2. *Treatment of Overdose:* Supportive treatment. Vital signs and fluid balance should be monitored. Syrup of ipecac or gastric lavage followed by activated charcoal; administration of fluids, pressor agents, and atropine. Adequate airway should be maintained; artificial respiration may be required.

Client/Family Teaching

1. Do not drive an automobile or operate machinery until the sedative effect of this drug has been assessed.
2. Be alert to disturbances in sleep that may indicate a depressive episode. Report these symptoms to the health care provider.

Evaluation: Evaluate client for:
- Control of hypertension
- Freedom from complications of adverse drug effects

Guanadrel sulfate

(GWON-ah-drell)

Hylorel (Rx)

Classification: Antihypertensive, peripherally acting antiadrenergic

Action/Kinetics: Similar to that of guanethidine. Inhibits vasoconstriction by blocking efferent, peripheral sympathetic pathways by depleting norepinephrine reserves and inhibiting norepinephrine release. Causes increased sensitivity to norepinephrine. **Onset:** 2 hr. **Peak plasma levels:** 1.5–2 hr. **Peak effect:** 4–6 hr. **$t\frac{1}{2}$:** Approximately 10 hr. **Duration:** 4–14 hr. Excreted through the urine as unchanged drug (40%) and metabolites.

Uses: Hypertension (usually Step 2 therapy).

Contraindications: Pheochromocytoma, congestive heart failure, within 1 week of MAO drug use, within 2–3 days of elective surgery.

Special Concerns: Use with caution in bronchial asthma and peptic ulcer. Safety not established during pregnancy (category: B), lactation and in children. Geriatric clients may be more sensitive to the hypotensive effects.

Side Effects: *CNS:* Fainting, fatigue, headache, drowsiness, paresthesias, confusion, depression, sleep disorders, visual disturbances. *CV:* Exertional or resting shortness of breath, chest pain, orthostatic hypotension, palpitations, peripheral edema. *GI:* Increase in number of bowel movements, constipation, anorexia, indigestion, flatus, glossitis, nausea and vomiting, dry mouth and throat. *GU:* Difficulty in ejaculation, impotence, nocturia, hematuria, urinary urgency or frequency. *Miscellaneous:* Cough, leg cramps, changes in weight (gain or loss), backache, neckache, joint pain. *Symptoms of Overdose:* Postural hypotension, syncope, dizziness, blurred vision.

Drug Interactions

Beta-adrenergic blocking agents / Excessive hypotension, bradycardia

Ephedrine / Reverses effect of guanadrel

Norepinephrine / Guanadrel ↑ effect of norepinephrine

Phenothiazines / Reverses effect of guanadrel

Phenylpropanolamine / ↓ Effect of guanadrel

Reserpine / Excessive hypotension, bradycardia

Tricyclic antidepressants / Reverses effect of guanadrel

Vasodilators / ↑ Risk of orthostatic hypotension

Dosage: Tablets. Individualized. Initial: 5 mg b.i.d.; **then,** increase dosage to maintenance level of 20–75 mg/day in 2–4 divided doses.

NURSING CONSIDERATIONS

See also *Nursing Considerations* for *Antihypertensive Agents,* p. 78

Administration/Storage

1. Tolerance may occur with long-term therapy, necessitating a dosage increase.
2. While adjusting dosage, both supine and standing blood pressure should be monitored.
3. *Treatment of Overdose:* Administration of a vasoconstrictor (e.g., phenylephrine) if hypotension persists. If used, monitor carefully as client may be hypersensitive.

Client/Family Teaching

1. Warn clients that they may develop a dry mouth and become drowsy. Therefore, care should be taken not to perform any tasks that require mental alertness, such as driving a car.

2. Clients may develop diarrhea. If this is persistent the condition should be called to the physician's attention. The client could develop a severe electrolyte imbalance. This is particularly true with elderly clients.

Evaluation: Evaluate client for control of hypertension.

Guanethidine sulfate

(gwon-**ETH**-ih-deen)

Apo-Guanethidine✦, Ismelin Sulfate (Rx)

Classification: Antihypertensive, peripherally acting antiadrenergic.

Action/Kinetics: Guanethidine produces selective adrenergic blockade of efferent, peripheral sympathetic pathways by depleting norepinephrine reserve and inhibiting norepinephrine release. It induces a gradual, prolonged drop in both systolic and diastolic blood pressure, usually associated with bradycardia, decreased pulse pressure, a decrease in peripheral resistance, and small changes in cardiac output. The drug is not a ganglionic blocking agent and does not produce central or parasympathetic blockade. In clients with depleted catecholamines, guanethidine can directly depress the myocardium and can cause an increase in the sensitivity of tissues to catecholamines. Incompletely and variably absorbed from the GI tract (3%–30%) but is relatively constant for any given client. **Peak effect:** 6–8 hr. **Duration:** 24–48 hr. **Maximum effect:** 1–3 weeks. **Duration:** 7–10 days after discontinuation. **t½:** approximately 5 days. From 25%–50% excreted through the kidneys unchanged.

Uses: Moderate to severe hypertension—used alone or in combination. Renal hypertension.

Contraindications: Mild, labile hypertension; pheochromocytoma, CHF not due to hypertension, use of MAO inhibitors.

Special Concerns: Use during pregnancy (category: C) only when benefits clearly outweigh risks. Administer with caution and at a reduced rate to clients with impaired renal function, coronary disease, cardiovascular disease, especially when associated with encephalopathy, or to those who have suffered a recent myocardial infarction. During prolonged therapy, cardiac, renal, and blood tests should be performed. Used with caution in peptic ulcer. Geriatric clients may be more sensitive to the hypotensive effects of guanethidine; also, it may be necessary to decrease the dose in these clients due to age-related decreases in renal function.

Side Effects: *CNS:* Dizziness, weakness, lassitude. Rarely, dyspnea, fatigue, psychic depression. *CV:* Syncope due to exertional or postural hypotension, bradycardia, fluid retention and edema with possible congestive heart failure. Less commonly, angina. *GI:* Persistent diarrhea, increased frequency of bowel movements. Nausea, vomiting, dry mouth, and parotid tenderness are less common. *Miscellaneous:* Inhibition of ejaculation. Less commonly, dyspnea, nocturia, urinary incontinence, dermatitis, alopecia, increased blood urea nitrogen, drooping of upper eyelid, blurred vision, myalgia, muscle tremors, chest paresthesia, nasal congestion, asthma in susceptible individuals, weight gain, blurred vision, ptosis of the lids. Rarely, impotence, anemia, thrombocytopenia, priapism, impotence. *Symptoms of Overdose:* Bradycardia, postural hypotension, diarrhea (may be severe).

Drug Interactions

Alcohol, ethyl / Additive orthostatic hypotension
Amphetamines / ↓ Effect of guanethidine by ↓ uptake of the drug to its site of action
Anesthetics, general / Additive hypotension
Antidepressants, tricyclic / ↓ Effect of guanethidine by ↓ uptake of the drug to its site of action
Antidiabetic drugs / Additive effect ↓ in blood glucose
Cocaine / ↓ Effect of guanethidine by ↓ uptake of the drug at its site of action
Digitalis / Additive slowing of heart rate
Ephedrine / ↓ Effect of guanethidine by ↓ uptake of the drug at its site of action
Epinephrine / Guanethidine ↑ effect of epinephrine
Haloperidol / ↓ Effect of guanethidine by ↓ uptake of the drug at its site of action
Levarterenol / See norepinephrine
MAO inhibitors / Reverse effect of guanethidine
Metaraminol / Guanethidine ↑ effect of metaraminol
Methotrimeprazine / Additive hypotensive effect
Methoxamine / Guanethidine ↑ effect of methoxamine
Minoxidil / Profound drop in blood pressure
Norepinephrine / ↑ Effect of norepinephrine probably due to ↑ sensitivity of

norepinephrine receptor and ↓ uptake of norepinephrine by the neuron

Oral contraceptives / ↓ Effect of guanethidine by ↓ uptake of the drug to its site of action

Phenothiazines / ↓ Effect of guanethidine by ↓ uptake of the drug to its site of action

Phenylephrine / ↑ Response to phenylephrine in guanethidine-treated patients

Phenylpropanolamine / ↓ Effect of guanethidine by ↓ uptake of the drug to its site of action

Procainamide / Additive hypotensive effect

Procarbazine / Additive hypotensive effect

Propranolol / Additive hypotensive effect

Pseudoephedrine / ↓ Effect of guanethidine by ↓ uptake of the drug at its site of action

Quinidine / Additive hypotensive effect

Reserpine / Excessive bradycardia, postural hypotension, and mental depression

Thiazide diuretics / Additive hypotensive effect

Thioxanthines / ↓ Effect of guanethidine by ↓ uptake of the drug at its site of action

Vasodilator drugs, peripheral / Additive hypotensive effect

Vasopressor drugs / ↑ Effect of vasopressor agents probably due to ↑ sensitivity of norepinephrine receptor and ↓ uptake of vasopressor agent by the neuron

Laboratory Test Interference: ↑ BUN, AST, and ALT. ↓ Prothrombin time, serum glucose, and urine catecholamines. Alteration of electrolyte balance.

Dosage: Tablets. *Ambulatory clients:* **initial:** 10–12.5 mg once daily; increase in 10–12.5 mg increments q 5–7 days; **maintenance:** 25–50 mg once daily. *Hospitalized clients:* **initial:** 25–50 mg; increase by 25 or 50 mg daily or every other day; **maintenance:** estimated to be approximately one-seventh of loading dose. **Pediatric, initial:** 0.2 mg/kg/day (6 mg/m²) given in one dose; **then,** dose may be increased by 0.2 mg/kg/day q 7–10 days to maximum of 3 mg/kg/day.

NURSING CONSIDERATIONS

See also *Nursing Considerations* for *Antihypertensive Agents,* p. 78

Administration/Storage

1. The loading dose for severe hypertension is given t.i.d. at 6-hr intervals with no nighttime dose.
2. Drug should be given daily or every other day.
3. Often used concomitantly with thiazide diuretics to reduce severity of sodium and water retention caused by guanethidine. When used together, the dose of guanethidine should be reduced.
4. When control is achieved, dosage should be reduced to the minimal dose required to maintain lowest possible BP.
5. Guanethidine sulfate should be discontinued or dosage decreased at least 2 weeks before surgery.
6. *Treatment of Overdose:* If the client was previously normotensive, keep in a supine position (symptoms usually subside within 72 hr). If the client was previously hypertensive (especially with impaired cardiac reserve or other cardiovascular problems or renal disease), intensive treatment

may be needed. Vasopressors may be required. Severe diarrhea should be treated.

Interventions

1. Ascertain that hepatic and renal function studies are completed before therapy is initiated.
2. Note the presence of bradycardia and report to the physician. An anticholinergic drug, such as atropine, may be indicated for severe bradycardia.
3. Note client complaints of persistent diarrhea. Severe electrolyte imbalance could occur. Document and report such incidents to the physician.
4. Weigh the client daily and record. Note any sudden increases in weight because this could indicate the presence of edema.
5. Monitor intake and output; observe for any reduction in urine volume.
6. Assess client for any undue stress, which could precipitate cardiovascular collapse. Assist to reduce such stress whenever possible.
7. Observe client closely for drug interactions. Since guanethidine interacts with many drugs the dosage may need to be adjusted.

Client/Family Teaching

1. Limit alcohol intake; otherwise, orthostatic hypotension may be further precipitated.
2. Avoid any sudden or prolonged standing or exercise.
3. Report any nausea, vomiting or diarrhea.

Evaluation: Evaluate client for control of hypertension with a minimum of side effects.

Guanfacine hydrochloride
(**GWON**-fah-seen)
Tenex (Rx)

Classification: Antihypertensive, centrally acting.

Action/Kinetics: Guanfacine is thought to act by central stimulation of alpha-2 receptors resulting in a decrease in peripheral sympathetic output and heart rate resulting in a decrease in blood pressure. The drug may also manifest a direct peripheral alpha-2 receptor stimulant action. **Onset:** 2 hr. **Peak plasma levels:** 1–4 hr. **Peak effect:** 6–12 hr. **t½:** 12–23 hr. **Duration:** 24 hr. Approximately 50% is excreted through the kidneys unchanged.

Uses: Hypertension concomitantly with a thiazide diuretic. *Investigational:* Withdrawal from heroin use.

Contraindications: Hypersensitivity to guanfacine. Acute hypertension associated with toxemia. Children less than 12 years of age.

Special Concerns: Use with caution during pregnancy (category: B) and lactation. Use with caution in clients with recent myocardial infarction, cerebrovascular disease, chronic renal or hepatic failure, or severe coronary insufficiency. Geriatric clients may be more sensitive to the hypotensive and sedative effects.

Side Effects: *GI:* Dry mouth, constipation, nausea, abdominal pain, diarrhea, dyspepsia, dysphagia. *CNS:* Sedation, weakness, dizziness, headache, fatigue, insomnia, amnesia, confusion, depression. *CV:* Bradycardia, substernal pain, palpitations. *Ophthalmic:* Visual disturbances, conjunctivitis, iritis. *Dermatologic:* Pruritus, dermatitis, purpura, sweating. *Other:* Decreased libido, impotence, rhinitis, tinnitus, alterations in taste, leg cramps, dyspnea, urinary incontinence, paresthesia, paresis, asthenia, hypokinesia, malaise, testicular disorder. **Note:** If therapy is abruptly discontinued, a rebound reaction may occur within 2–4 days, which is manifested by nervousness, anxiety, and increased blood pressure.

Drug Interactions: Additive sedative effects when used concomitantly with CNS depressants.

Dosage: Tablets. *Hypertension:* **initial:** 1 mg daily at bedtime; if satisfactory results are not obtained in 3–4 weeks, dosage may be increased by 1 mg at 1- to 2-week intervals up to a maximum of 3 mg daily in 1–2 divided doses. *Heroin withdrawal:* 0.03–1.5 mg daily.

NURSING CONSIDERATIONS

See also *Nursing Considerations* for *Antihypertensive Agents,* p. 78

Administration/Storage

1. If a decrease in blood pressure is not maintained for over 24 hr, the daily dose may be more effective if divided, although the incidence of side effects increases.
2. Adverse effects increase significantly when the daily dose exceeds 3 mg.
3. Therapy should be initiated in clients already taking a thiazide diuretic.

Client/Family Teaching: Stress the importance of not discontinuing the drug abruptly.

Evaluation: Assess client for control of hypertension with a minimum of side effects.

Guanidine hydrochloride
(**GWON**-ih-deen)
(Rx)

Classification: Cholinergic muscle stimulant.

Action/Kinetics: Guanidine hydrochloride increases the release of acetylcholine at the synapses following nerve impulse transmission; it slows the rate of depolarization and repolarization of the muscle cell membrane, therefore acting as a cholinergic muscle stimulant. It is ineffective in the treatment of myasthenia gravis.

Uses: Reduction of muscle weakness and relief of fatigue associated with Eaton-Lambert syndrome.

Contraindications: Hypersensitivity to and intolerance of drug. Lactation. Use in myasthenia gravis.

Special Concerns: Use during pregnancy only if benefits clearly outweigh risks. Safety for use in children not established.

Side Effects: *CNS:* Nervousness, tremors, irritability, lightheadedness, ataxia, jitteriness, psychoses, confusion, changes in mood and emotions, hallucinations. *Neurologic:* Paresthesia of face, feet, hands, and lips; hands and feet feel cold. *GI:* Nausea, cramps, diarrhea, anorexia, dry mouth, gastric irritation. *Dermatologic:* Rashes, petechiae, ecchymoses, sweating, dry skin, scaling of skin, folliculitis, purpura, flushing. *CV:* Hypotension, atrial fibrillation, tachycardia, palpitations. *Hematologic:* Anemia, leukopenia, thrombocytopenia. *Renal:* Uremia, renal tubular necrosis, chronic interstitial nephritis. *Other:* Sore throat, fever. *Symptoms of Overdose:* Anorexia, diarrhea. If intoxication is severe, symptoms include salivation, vomiting, diarrhea, hypoglycemia, nervous hyperirritability, fibrillary tremors and convulsive contractions of muscle, circulatory disturbances.

Laboratory Test Interferences: Increase in blood creatinine, uremia, abnormal liver function tests.

Dosage: Tablets. *Individualized,* **Adults: initial,** 10–15 mg/kg/day in 3–4 divided doses; **then,** increase dose gradually to 35 mg/kg/day or up to the development of side effects.

NURSING CONSIDERATIONS

Administration/Storage: *Treatment of Overdose:* Calcium gluconate given IV to control neuromuscular and convulsive symptoms. Atropine will help the GI symptoms, hypoglycemia, and circulatory disturbances.

Assessment

1. Take a complete nursing history.

2. Note any history of myasthenia gravis as the drug is contraindicated.
3. Obtain baseline CBC, liver and renal function studies prior to initiating therapy.

Interventions

1. Monitor CBC, liver and renal function tests periodically while client is receiving the drug because damage may be dose-related.
2. If client experiences anorexia, increased peristalsis, or diarrhea, notify the physician. These are early warnings that suggest the drug should be discontinued.
3. Symptoms of hyperirritability, tremors, convulsive contractions of muscles, increased salivation, vomiting, diarrhea, and hypoglycemia are usually toxic manifestations of drug therapy.
4. The drug is highly toxic and treatment should continue only as long as necessary.

Evaluation: Evaluate for decreased complaints of muscle weakness and fatigue in clients with Eaton-Lambert syndrome.

H

Halazepam
(hal-**AYZ**-eh-pam)
Paxipam (C-IV, Rx)

See also *Benzodiazepines,* p. 108.

Classification: Antianxiety agent, benzodiazepine type.

Action/Kinetics: $t\frac{1}{2}$: 14 hr. Metabolized in liver to *N*-desmethyldiazepam (active with a $t\frac{1}{2}$ of 30–

100 hr) and to inactive conjugates. **Maximum plasma levels of active metabolite:** 3–6 hr. Excreted through the kidneys.

Use: Short-term relief of anxiety.

Additional Contraindication: Acute narrow-angle glaucoma.

Special Concerns: Pregnancy category: D. Dose has not been established in children less than 18 years of age.

Dosage: Tablets. Adults: 20–40 mg t.i.d.–q.i.d. In elderly or debilitated clients: **initial,** 20 mg 1–2 times daily.

NURSING CONSIDERATIONS

See *Nursing Considerations* for *Benzodiazepines,* p. 111.

Evaluation: Evaluate client for reports of improvement in anxiety levels and coping ability.

Halobetasol propionate
(hay-loh-**BET**-ah-sohl)
Ultravate (Rx)

See also *Adrenocorticosteroids and Analogs,* p. 8.

Classification: Adrenocorticosteroid, topical.

Action/Kinetics: Anti-inflammatory, antipruritic, and antiproliferative activity when used topically.

Uses: Dermatoses responsive to adrenocorticosteroid therapy.

Contraindications: Primary bacterial infections, *Candida,* dermatophytes, herpes simplex, herpes zoster.

Special Considerations: Pregnancy category: C. Use with caution during lactation and in children. Systemic absorption may result in suppression of the hypothalamic-pituitary axis. Use with caution around the eyes.

Side Effects: *Dermatologic:* Burning, itching, erythema, dryness, irritation, folliculitis, hypertrichosis, acneiform eruptions, hypopigmentation, perioral dermatitis, allergic contact dermatitis, cracking of skin, maceration of skin, secondary infection, skin atrophy, striae, miliaria.

Dosage: Cream (0.05%), Ointment (0.05%): Apply sparingly b.i.d.–q.i.d.

NURSING CONSIDERATIONS

See *Nursing Considerations* for *Topical Corticosteroids* under *Adrenocorticosteroids and Analogs,* p. 15.

Haloperidol
(hah-low-**PAIR**-ih-dohl)
Apo-Haloperidol ✹, Haldol, Halperon, Novo–Peridol ✹, Peridol ✹, PMS Haloperidol ✹ (Rx)

Haloperidol decanoate
(hah-low-**PAIR**-ih-dohl)
Haldol Decanoate 50 and 100, Haldol LA ✹ (Rx)

Haloperidol lactate
(hah-low-**PAIR**-ih-dohl)
Haldol Lactate (Rx)

Classification: Antipsychotic, butyrophenone.

Action/Kinetics: Although the precise mechanism is not known, haloperidol does competitively block dopamine receptors in the tuberoinfundibular system to cause sedation. The drug also causes alpha-adrenergic blockade, decreases release of growth hormone, and increases prolactin release by the pituitary. Haloperidol causes significant extrapyramidal effects, as well as a low incidence of sedation, anticholinergic effects, and orthostatic hypotension. The margin between the therapeutically effective dose and that causing extrapyramidal symptoms is narrow. The drug also has antiemetic effects. **Peak plasma levels: PO,** 2–6 hr; **IM,** 20 min; **IM, decanoate:** approximately 6 days. **Therapeutic serum levels:** 3–10 ng/ml. **t½, PO:** 12–38 hr; **IM:** 13–36 hr; **IM, decanoate:** 3 weeks; **IV:** approximately 14 hr. **Plasma protein binding:** 90%. Metabolized in liver, slowly excreted in urine and bile.

Uses: Psychotic disorders including manic states, drug-induced psychoses, and schizophrenia. Aggressive and agitated clients, including chronic brain syndrome or mental retardation. Severe behavior problems in children. Short-term treatment of hyperactive children. Control of tics and vocal utterances associated with Gilles de la Tourette's syndrome.

Investigational: Antiemetic for cancer chemotherapy, infantile autism, Huntington's chorea.

Contraindications: Use with extreme caution, or not at all, in clients with parkinsonism. Lactation.

Special Concerns: Pregnancy category: C (decanoate form). Oral dosage has not been determined in children less than 3 years of age; IM dosage is not recommended in children. Geriatric clients are more likely to exhibit orthostatic hypotension, anticholinergic effects, sedation, and extrapyramidal side effects (such as parkinsonism and tardive dyskinesia).

Side Effects: Extrapyramidal symptoms, especially akathisia and dystonias, occur more frequently than with the phenothiazines. Overdosage is characterized by severe extrapyramidal reactions, hypotension, or sedation. The drug does not elicit photosensitivity reactions like those of the phenothiazines.

Symptoms of Overdose: CNS depression, hypertension or hypotension, extrapyramidal symptoms, agitation, restlessness, fever, hypothermia, hyperthermia, seizures, cardiac arrhythmias, changes in the ECG, autonomic reactions, coma.

Drug Interactions

Amphetamine / ↓ Effect of amphetamine by ↓ uptake of drug at its site of action

Anticholinergics / ↓ Effect of haloperidol

Antidepressants, tricyclic / ↑ Effect of antidepressants due to ↓ breakdown by liver

Barbiturates / ↓ Effect of haloperidol due to ↑ breakdown by liver

Guanethidine / ↓ Effect of guanethidine by ↓ uptake of drug at site of action

Lithium / ↑ Toxicity of haloperidol

Methyldopa / ↑ Toxicity of haloperidol

Phenytoin / ↓ Effect of haloperidol due to ↑ breakdown by liver

Laboratory Test Interferences: ↑ Alkaline phosphatase, bilirubin, serum transaminase; ↓ prothrombin time (clients on coumarin), serum cholesterol.

Dosage: Oral Solution, Tablets. Adults: 0.5–2 mg b.i.d.–t.i.d. up to 3–5 mg b.i.d.–t.i.d. for severe symptoms; **maintenance:** reduce dosage to lowest effective level. Up to 100 mg/day may be required in some. **Geriatric or debilitated clients:** 0.5–2 mg b.i.d.–t.i.d. **Pediatric, 3–12 years:** 0.05 mg/kg daily in 2–3 divided doses; if necessary the daily dose may be increased by 0.5-mg increments q 5–7 days for a total of 0.15 mg/kg daily for psychotic disorders and 0.075 mg/kg for nonpsychotic behavior disorders and Tourette's syndrome.

IM. *Acute psychoses:* **Adults and adolescents, initial:** 2–5 mg; may be repeated if necessary q 4–8 hr to a total of 100 mg daily. Switch to **PO** therapy as soon as possible. **IM, Decanoate:** *Chronic therapy,* **initial dose:** 10–15 times the daily oral dose; **then,** repeat q 4 weeks (decanoate is not to be given IV).

NURSING CONSIDERATIONS

See also *Nursing Considerations* for *Phenothiazines,* p. 205.

Administration/Storage: *Treatment of Overdose:* Treat symptomatically. Antiparkinson drugs, diphenhydramine, or barbiturates can be used to treat extrapyramidal symptoms. Fluid replacement and vasoconstrictors (either norepinephrine or phenylephrine) can be used to treat hypotension. Ventricular arrhythmias can be treated with phenytoin. To treat seizures, use pentobarbital or diazepam. A saline cathartic can be used to hasten the excretion of sustained-release products.

Interventions

1. Use with caution in the elderly as they tend to exhibit toxicity more frequently and may benefit from a periodic drug "holiday."
2. Document any evidence of new onset of Parkinson's symptoms because drug has been reported to induce this disorder with some clients.

Evaluation: Evaluate client for:
- Improved patterns of behavior with a decrease in reported hallucinations, delusions, agitation, hostility and aggressiveness
- ↓ tics and vocal utterances in Tourette's syndrome
- Evidence of a reduction in hyperacitivy or hyperactive behaviors

Heparin calcium
(HEP-ah-rin)
Calcilean✿, Calciparine (Rx)

Heparin sodium injection
(HEP-ah-rin)
Hepalean✿, Heparin Leo✿, Liquaemin Sodium, Liquaemin Sodium Preservative Free (Rx)

Heparin sodium in dextrose injection
(HEP-ah-rin)
(Rx)

Heparin sodium in sodium chloride injection
(HEP-ah-rin)
(Rx)

See also *Anticoagulants,* p. 54.

Classification: Anticoagulant.

General Statement: Heparin is a naturally occurring substance isolated from porcine intestinal mucosa or bovine lung tissue. Must be given parenterally. Heparin does not interfere with wound healing. Leukocyte counts should be performed in heparinized blood within 2 hr after adding heparin. Heparinized blood should not be used for complement, isoagglutin, erythrocyte fragility test, or platelet counts.

Action/Kinetics: Heparin potentiates the inhibitory action of antithrombin III on various coagulation factors including factor IIa, IXa, Xa, XIa, and XIIa. This occurs due to the formation of a complex with and causing a conformational change in the antithrombin III molecule. Inhibition of factor Xa results in interference with thrombin generation; thus, the action of thrombin in coagulation is inhibited. Heparin also increases the rate of formation of antithrombin III-thrombin complex causing inactivation of thrombin and preventing the conversion of fibrinogen to fibrin. By inhibiting the activation of fibrin-stabilizing factor by thrombin, heparin also prevents formation of a stable fibrin clot. Therapeutic doses of heparin prolong thrombin time, whole blood clotting time, activated clotting time, and partial thromboplastin time. Heparin also decreases the levels of triglycerides by releasing lipoprotein lipase from tissues; the resultant hydrolysis of triglycerides causes increased blood levels of free fatty acids. **Onset: IV,** immediate; **deep SC:** 20–60 min. **t½:** 60–90 min in healthy persons. **t½** increases with dose, severe renal disease, cirrhosis, and in anephric clients and decreases with pulmonary embolism and liver impair-

ment other than cirrhosis. *Metabolism:* Probably by reticuloendothelial system. Clotting time returns to normal within 2–6 hr.

Uses: As an anticoagulant, heparin is used to prevent the extension of clots or to prevent thrombi and emboli from recurring. It is also used prophylactically in the management of thromboembolic disease and to prevent complications after many kinds of surgery, including cardiac and vascular surgery. To treat hyperlipemia and to prevent clotting in renal dialysis and blood transfusions. Diagnosis and treatment of disseminated intravascular coagulation (DIC). Prophylaxis of cerebral thrombosis in stroke. Coronary occlusion following myocardial infarction. Atrial fibrillation with embolization.

Contraindications: Active bleeding, blood dyscrasias (or other disorders characterized by bleeding tendencies such as hemophilia), purpura, thrombocytopenia, liver disease with hypoprothrombinemia, suspected intracranial hemorrhage, suppurative thrombophlebitis, inaccessible ulcerative lesions (especially of the GI tract), open wounds, extensive denudation of the skin, and increased capillary permeability (as in ascorbic acid deficiency).

The drug should not be administered during surgery of the eye, brain, or spinal cord or during continuous tube drainage of the stomach or small intestine. Use is also contraindicated in subacute endocarditis, shock, advanced kidney disease, threatened abortion, severe hypertension, or hypersensitivity to drug.

Use with caution during menstruation and in the postpartum period, as well as in clients with a history of asthma, allergies, mild liver or kidney disease, or in alcoholics. Should not be used in premature neonates due to the possibility of a fatal "gasping syndrome."

Special Concerns: Pregnancy category: C. Women over aged 60 may be more susceptible to hemorrhage during heparin therapy.

Side Effects: Hemorrhage ranging from minor local ecchymoses to major hemorrhagic complications. Such reactions are more likely to occur in prophylactic administration during surgery than in the treatment of thromboembolic disease. Thrombocytopenia.

Rare allergic reactions characterized by chills, fever, pruritus, urticaria, burning feet, rhinitis, conjunctivitis, lacrimation, asthma-like reactions, hyperemia, arthralgia, and anaphylactoid reactions have been noted. Use a test dose of 1,000 units in clients with a history of asthma or allergic disease. Long-term therapy may cause osteoporosis and/or spontaneous fractures and hypoaldosteronism.

Discontinuance of heparin has resulted in rebound hyperlipemia, priapism, transient alopecia, and decreased aldosterone synthesis. Heparin resistance has been observed in some elderly clients. In these cases, large doses may be required.

IM injections of heparin may produce local irritation, hematoma, and tissue sloughing.

Symptoms of Overdose: Nosebleeds, hematuria, tarry stools, petechiae, and easy bruising may be the first signs.

Drug Interactions

ACTH / Heparin antagonizes effect of ACTH

Alteplase, recombinant / ↑ Risk of bleeding, especially at arterial puncture sites

Anticoagulants, oral / Additive ↑ prothrombin time

Antihistamines / ↓ Effect of heparin

Aspirin / Additive ↑ prothrombin time

Corticosteroids / Heparin antagonizes effect of corticosteroids

Dextran / Additive ↑ prothrombin time

Diazepam / Heparin ↑ plasma levels of diazepam

Digitalis / ↓ Effect of heparin

Dipyridamole / Additive ↑ prothrombin time

Hydroxychloroquine / Additive ↑ prothrombin time

Ibuprofen / Additive ↑ prothrombin time

Indomethacin / Additive ↑ prothrombin time

Insulin / Heparin antagonizes effect of insulin

Phenylbutazone / Additive ↑ prothrombin time

Quinine / Additive ↑ prothrombin time

Tetracyclines / ↓ Effect of heparin

Laboratory Test Interferences: ↑ AST and ALT.

Dosage: Adjusted for each client on the basis of laboratory tests. **Deep SC: initial loading dose,** 10,000–20,000 units (preceded by 5,000 units IV); **maintenance:** 8,000–10,000 units q 8 hr or 15,000–20,000 units q 12 hr. *Use concentrated solution.* **Intermittent IV: initially,** 10,000 units undiluted or in 50–100 ml saline; **then,** 5,000–10,000 units q 4–6 hr undiluted or in 50–100 ml saline. **Continuous IV infusion:** 20,000–40,000 units/day in 1,000 ml saline (preceded initially by 5,000 units IV).

Prophylaxis of postoperative thromboembolism: **Deep SC:** 5,000 units of concentrated solution 2 hr before surgery and 5,000 units q 8–12 hr thereafter for 7 days or until client is ambulatory. *Surgery of heart and blood vessels:* **initial,** 150–400 units/kg (dose depends on estimated length of surgery); to prevent clotting in the tube system, add heparin to fluids in pump oxygenator. *Extracorporeal renal dialysis:* See instructions on equipment. *Blood transfusion:* 400–600 units/100 ml whole blood. *Laboratory samples:* 70–150 units/10- to 20-ml sample to prevent coagulation.

NURSING CONSIDERATIONS

See also *Nursing Considerations* for *Anticoagulants,* p. 55.

Administration/Storage

1. Client should be hospitalized for IV heparin therapy.
2. Protect solutions from freezing.
3. Heparin should not be administered IM.
4. Administer by deep SC injection to minimize local irritation, hematoma, and tissue sloughing and to prolong action of drug.
   - Z-track method: Use any fat roll, but abdominal fat rolls are preferred. Use a ½-inch or ⅝-inch needle. Grasp the skin layer of the fat roll and lift it up. Insert the needle at about a 45° angle to the skin surface and then administer the medication. With this medication, it is not necessary to aspirate to check whether or not the needle is in a blood vessel. Rapidly withdraw the needle while releasing the skin.
   - "Bunch technique" method: Grasp the tissue around the injection site, creating a tissue roll of about ½ inch in diameter. Insert the needle into the tissue roll at a 90° angle to the skin surface and inject the medication. Again, it is not necessary to aspirate to check whether or not the needle is in a blood vessel. Withdraw the needle rapidly when the skin is released.
   - Do not administer within 2 inches of the umbilicus because of increased vascularity of area.
5. Do not massage before or after injection.
6. Change sites of administration.
7. Caution should be used to prevent negative pressure (with a roller pump), which would increase the rate at which heparin is injected into the system. Administer with a constant rate infusion pump.
8. Have protamine sulfate, a heparin antagonist, available should the client develop excessive bleeding and anticoagulant effects.
9. *Treatment of Overdose:* Drug withdrawal is usually sufficient to correct heparin overdosage. In some cases, blood transfusion or the administration of protamine sulfate may be necessary.

Assessment

1. Inquire about any bleeding incidents a client may have had, i.e., bleeding tendencies, family history of bleeding tendencies, or any incidents of active bleeding.
2. Determine any history of pep-

tic ulcer disease. This may be an indication for a potential site of bleeding.
3. Note any evidence of possible intracranial hemorrhage.
4. If the client is receiving one of the many drugs that interact with anticoagulants, document and anticipate an adjustment in the dosage of heparin.

Interventions

1. Assure that all appropriate blood work has been completed prior to initiating therapy (Lee-White whole blood clotting time tests and activated partial thromboplastin times-APTT) and that the results are reported promptly to the physician.
2. With full-dose heparin administered by continuous IV, the APTT should be done before onset of therapy, q 4 hr during the early stages, and then daily.
3. During full-dose therapy, the accepted therapeutic range for the APTT is 1.5–2.5 times the control value in seconds. The activated coagulation time (ACT) may also be used.
   • ACT can be done at the bedside, (although it is time consuming), thus it is convenient for monitoring the degree of anticoagulation in clients with extracorporeal circulation.
   • The accepted therapeutic range for the ACT is two to three times the control value.
4. With full-dose intermittent IV heparin therapy, the APTT should be done before the start of therapy. In the early stages it may be repeated before each dose of drug, and then daily.

5. Anticipate that heparin therapy will be ordered on an individual basis after the coagulation time has been evaluated by the physician. Exceptions are when small doses are administered for prophylaxis.

Client/Family Teaching

1. Instruct and stress the importance of reporting any signs of active bleeding.
2. In women of childbearing age, any excessive menstrual flow should be reported because increased flow may be caused by the drug, necessitating a reduction in dosage.
3. Reassure client that alopecia, if it occurs, is generally only temporary.
4. Alterations in GU function and any injury should be immediately reported to the physician prescribing heparin.
5. Use an electric razor for shaving.
6. Use a soft-bristle toothbrush to decrease gum irritation.
7. Arrange furniture in the home to allow open space for unimpeded ambulation and to diminish chances of bumping into objects that may cause bruising and bleeding.
8. Use a night light to provide illumination during trips to the bathroom at night.
9. Encourage clients to eat potassium-rich foods (e.g., baked potato, orange juice, bananas, beef, flounder, haddock, sweet potato, turkey, raw tomato).
10. Advise clients against eating large amounts of vitamin K foods. These are mostly yellow and dark green vegetables.
11. Advise client to report any

evidence of increased bruising, bleeding of nose, mouth, gums, tarry stools, or GI upset.

12. Avoid using alcohol as this creates an increased anticoagulant response.

Evaluation

1. Prothrombin time and/or partial thromboplastin time should be within desired range.
2. Assess client for freedom from evidence of abnormal bleeding and/or hemorrhage.

Heparin lock flush solution

(HEP-ah-rin)

Hepalean-Lok✦. Hep-Lock (Rx)

See also *Anticoagulants,* p. 54.

Classification: Anticoagulant flushing agent.

Use: Dilute solutions of heparin sodium (100 USP units/ml) are used to maintain patency of indwelling catheters used for IV therapy or blood sampling. Not to be used therapeutically. See *Heparin,* for all other information.

NURSING CONSIDERATIONS

See also *Nursing Considerations* for *Anticoagulants,* p. 55.

Interventions

1. Aspirate lock to determine patency. Maintain patency by injecting 1 ml of heparin lock flush solution into the diaphragm of the device after each use. This dose should maintain patency for up to 8 hr for a converted (capped) catheter.
2. When a drug incompatible with

heparin is to be administered, flush the device with 0.9% sodium chloride injection or sterile water for injection before and immediately after the incompatible drug is administered. After the final flush, inject another dose of heparin lock flush solution.

3. Clients with underlying coagulation disorders may be at a risk for bleeding; observe coagulation times carefully.

4. When repeated blood samples are drawn from the venipuncture device, the presence of heparin or normal saline may cause interference with laboratory tests.

   • Clear the heparin lock flush solution by aspirating and discarding 1 ml of fluid from the device before withdrawing the blood sample.

   • Inject another 1 ml of heparin lock flush solution into the device after blood samples are drawn.

   • Because this is not the most reliable method of acquiring serum levels, if there are any excessively abnormal results, obtain a repeat sample from another site before initiating treatment.

Evaluation: Evaluate client for:

   • Determining patency of indwelling catheter

   • Any allergic reactions to heparin due to various biological sources of the product

   • Evidence of thrombocytopenia, a possible side effect of heparin therapy

Special Concerns: Recent studies have shown that 0.9% NaCl is effective in maintaining patency of peripheral (noncentral) intermittent infusion devices. The following procedure has been recommended:

- Determine patency by aspirating lock.
- Flush with 2 ml NSS.
- Administer medication therapy. (Flush between drugs.)
- Flush with 2 ml NSS.
- This does *NOT* apply to any central venous access devices.

Human insulin

Buffered Human Insulin: Humulin BR. Insulin Injection: Humulin R, Novolin R, Novolin R PenFill, Velosulin. Insulin Zinc Suspension: Humulin L, Novolin L. Insulin Zinc Suspension and Insulin Injection: Humulin 70/30, Mixtard Human 70/30, Novolin 70/30, Novolin 70/30 PenFill. Insulin Zinc Suspension Extended: Humulin U Ultralente. Isophane Insulin Suspension: Humulin N, Insulatard NPH, Novolin N, Novolin N PenFill.

See also *Insulins,* p. 156.

Classification: Human insulin from semisynthetic or recombinant DNA sources.

Action/Kinetics: Human insulin derived from recombinant DNA technology utilizes genetically modified *Escherichia coli.* These organisms synthesize each chain of insulin into the same amino acid sequence as human insulin. The chains are then combined and purified to produce human insulin. Human insulin prepared semisynthetically undergoes a process whereby the terminal amino acid of porcine insulin is enzymatically substituted for an amino acid, making the product identical to human insulin. This product is then purified. **Note:** Human insulins are available as regular, insulin zinc, extended, and isophane; for the kinetics of these products, please refer to the appropriate products described elsewhere. Human insulins cause fewer allergic reactions and less insulin-induced antibody formation than insulins from animal sources.

Uses: Management of type I diabetes mellitus. At this time, as long as the client is well controlled on insulin from porcine or beef sources, transfer to human insulin may not be recommended. Human insulin may be preferred in the following situations: local or systemic allergic reactions to products from animal sources, lipoatrophy at injection site, type II diabetes that requires short-term insulin treatment, in clients resistant to insulin from animal sources, in pregnancy, and in newly diagnosed diabetics.

Dosage: Dosage and routes of administration are similar to products from animal sources.

NURSING CONSIDERATIONS

See also *Nursing Considerations* for *Insulins,* p. 160.

Client/Family Teaching: Remind clients that dose may have to be reduced, so it is particularly important to watch for and report signs and symptoms of hypoglycemia.

Evaluation: Evaluate client for laboratory evidence that serum glucose levels are within desired range.

H

Hyaluronidase

(hy-al-your-**ON**-ih-days)
Hyalase ✹, Wydase (Rx)

Classification: Enzyme, miscellaneous.

Action/Kinetics: Hyaluronidase, an enzyme that hydrolyzes hyaluronic acid, a constituent of connective tissue, acts to promote the diffusion of injected liquids. The purified enzyme has no effect on blood pressure, respiration, temperature, and kidney function. However, it is antigenic and repeated use may induce the formation of antibodies which neutralize the effect. It will not result in spread of localized infection as long as it is not injected into the infected area. The effects last 24–48 hr.

Uses: Adjunct to promote absorption and dispersion of liquids and drugs, for hypodermoclysis, adjunct in urography to improve resorption of radiopaque agents, administration of local anesthetics. (Hyaluronidase can be added to primary drug solution or injected prior to administration of primary drug solution.)

Contraindications: Do not inject into acutely infected or cancerous areas.

Special Concerns: Pregnancy category: C. Use with caution during lactation.

Side Effects: Rarely, sensitivity reactions, including urticaria and anaphylaxis. *Symptoms of Overdose:* Local edema or urticaria, chills, erythema, dizziness, nausea, vomiting, tachycardia, hypotension.

Dosage: *Drug and fluid dispersion:* **Adults and older children, usual:** 150 units added to the injection solution. *Subcutaneous urography:* (when IV injection cannot be used) *with client in prone position:* 75 units **SC** over each scapula, followed by contrast medium in same site. *Hypodermoclysis:* 150 units which facilitates absorption of 1,000 ml fluid (give at a rate no faster than would be used for IV infusion); **pediatric, less than 3 years:** volume of single clysis should be limited to 200 ml; **premature infants, neonates:** volume should not exceed 25 ml/kg/day given at a rate no greater than 2 ml/min.

NURSING CONSIDERATIONS

Administration/Storage

1. Conduct a preliminary skin test for sensitivity by injecting 0.02 ml of the solution intradermally. A positive reaction occurs within 5 min when a wheal with pseudopods appears and persists for 20–30 min and is accompanied by localized itching. The appearance of erythema alone is not a positive reaction.
2. Methods for administering hyaluronidase during clysis therapy:
   • Inject hyaluronidase under the skin before clysis is started.
   • After the clysis has been started, inject solution of hyaluronidase into tubing close to the needle.
3. Control rate and volume of fluid for the older client so that it will not exceed those used for IV administration.
4. Do not inject hyaluronidase into a malignant area.
5. Check the physician's orders for dosage of hyaluronidase, type and amount of parenteral

solution, the rate of flow, and the site of injection.

6. Hyaluronidase is incompatible with heparin and epinephrine.
7. Hyaluronidase solution must be refrigerated. The reconstituted sterile solution maintains potency for 2 weeks if stored below 30°C (86°F).
8. *Treatment of Overdose:* Discontinue and begin supportive treatment immediately. Epinephrine, corticosteroids, and antihistamines may be required to treat symptoms.

Interventions

1. Monitor the client's PT/PTT during parenteral infusion therapy.
2. Monitor liver and renal function studies and compare with premedication studies.
3. Observe the area receiving clysis for pale color, coldness, hardness, and pain. If these signs occur, reduce the rate of flow and notify the physician.

———— *COMBINATION DRUG* ————
Hycodan syrup and tablets
(**HY**-koh-dan)
(Rx) (C-III)

Classification/Content: Each tablet or 5 ml contains: *Antitussive, narcotic:* hydrocodone bitartrate, 5 mg; *anticholinergic:* homatropine methylbromide, 1.5 mg.

See also information on narcotic analgesics and cholinergic blocking drugs.

Uses: Relief of symptoms of cough.

Special Concerns: Pregnancy category: C. May be habit-forming. Use with caution in children with croup,

in geriatric or debilitated clients, impaired renal or hepatic function, hyperthyroidism, asthma, narrow-angle glaucoma, prostatic hypertrophy, urethral stricture, Addison's disease. Safety and effectiveness in children less than 6 years of age have not been determined.

Dosage: Syrup, Tablets. Adults and children over 12 years: 1 tablet or 5 ml q 4–6 hr as needed, not to exceed 6 tablets or 30 ml in 24 hr. **Pediatric, 6–12 years:** ½ tablet or 2.5 ml q 4–6 hr as needed, not to exceed 3 tablets or 15 ml in 24 hr.

NURSING CONSIDERATIONS

See also *Nursing Considerations* for *Cholinergic Blocking Agents,* p. 138, and *Narcotic Analgesics,* p. 177.

Administration/Storage

1. The single maximum dose of medication for adults is 3 tablets or 15 ml of syrup after meals and at bedtime.
2. For children over 12 years of age, the maximum dosage is 2 tablets or 10 ml of syrup after meals and at bedtime.
3. For children 2–12 years of age, the maximum dosage is 1 tablet or 5 ml of syrup after meals and at bedtime.
4. For children less than 2 years old, the maximum dosage is ¼ tablet or 1.25 ml of syrup after meals and at bedtime.
5. Doses should be taken at least 4 hr apart.

Client/Family Teaching

1. Caution that the drug may cause drowsiness and/or dizziness. Advise client to avoid tasks that require mental alert-

ness, such as operating machinery or driving a car.

2. Notify the physician if symptoms persist or intensify as medical intervention may be necessary.

3. Explain that the drug may be habit-forming if used over a prolonged period of time.

Evaluation: Evaluate client for reports of control of cough and uninterrupted periods of sleep.

Hydralazine hydrochloride

(hy-**DRAL**-ah-zeen)

Apo-Hydralazine✽, Apresoline, Novo-Hylazin✽ (Rx)

Classification: Antihypertensive, direct action on vascular smooth muscle.

Action/Kinetics: Exerts a direct vasodilating effect on vascular smooth muscle. It also increases blood flow to the kidneys and brain and increases cardiac output by a reflex action. To minimize the cardiac effects, hydralazine is often given with drugs that decrease activity of sympathetic nerves. For example, it is found in Apresazide and Ser-Ap-Es. Food increases bioavailability of the drug. **PO: Onset,** 45 min; **peak plasma level:** 2 hr; **duration:** 3–8 hr. **$t^{1/2}$:** 3–7 hr. **IM: Onset,** 10–30 min; **peak plasma level:** 1 hr; **duration:** 2–6 hr. **IV: Onset,** 10–20 min; **maximum effect:** 10–80 min; **duration:** 2–6 hr. Metabolized in the liver and excreted through the kidney (2%–5% unchanged after PO use and 11%–14% unchanged after IV administration).

Uses: *PO:* In combination with other drugs for essential hypertension. *Parenteral:* Hypertensive emergencies. *Investigational:* To reduce afterload in congestive heart failure, severe aortic insufficiency after valve replacement.

Contraindications: Coronary artery disease, angina pectoris, advanced renal disease (as in chronic renal hypertension), rheumatic heart disease (e.g., mitral valvular) and chronic glomerulonephritis.

Special Concerns: Pregnancy category: C. Use with caution in stroke clients. Use with caution during lactation, in clients with advanced renal disease, and in clients with tartrazine sensitivity. Safety and efficacy have not been established in children. Geriatric clients may be more sensitive to the hypotensive and hypothermic effects of hydralazine; also, a decrease in dose may be necessary in these clients due to age-related decreases in renal function.

Side Effects: *CV:* Orthostatic hypotension, myocardial infarction, angina pectoris, palpitations, tachycardia. *CNS:* Headache, dizziness, psychoses, tremors, depression, anxiety, disorientation. *GI:* Nausea, vomiting, diarrhea, anorexia, constipation, paralytic ileus. *Allergic:* Rash, urticaria, fever, chills, arthralgia, pruritus, eosinophilia. Rarely, hepatitis, obstructive jaundice. *Hematologic:* Decrease in hemoglobin and red blood cells, purpura, agranulocytosis, leukopenia. *Other:* Peripheral neuritis, impotence, nasal congestion, edema, muscle cramps, lacrimation, conjunctivitis, difficulty in urination, lupus-like syndrome, lymphadenopathy, splenomegaly. Side effects are less severe when dosage is increased slowly.

Symptoms of Overdose: Hypotension, tachycardia, skin flushing, headache. Also, myocardial ischemia, cardiac arrhythmias, myocardial infarction, and severe shock can occur.

Drug Interactions

Beta-adrenergic blocking agents / ↑ Effect of both drugs
Methotrimeprazine / Additive hypotensive effect
Procainamide / Additive hypotensive effect
Quinidine / Additive hypotensive effect
Sympathomimetics / ↑ Risk of tachycardia and angina

Dosage: Tablets. Adult, initial: 10 mg q.i.d for 2–4 days; **then,** increase to 25 mg q.i.d. for rest of first week. For second and following weeks, increase to 50 mg q.i.d. **Maintenance:** individualized to lowest effective dose; maximum daily dose should not exceed 300 mg. **Pediatric, initial:** 0.75 mg/kg/day (25 mg/m²/day) in 2–4 divided doses; dosage may be increased gradually up to 7.5 mg/kg/day (or 300 mg daily). Food increases the bioavailability of the drug.

IV, IM. *Hypertensive crisis:* **adults, usual:** 20–40 mg, repeated as necessary. Blood pressure may fall within 5–10 min, with maximum response in 10–80 min. Usually switch to PO medication in 1–2 days. Dosage should be decreased in clients with renal damage. **Pediatric:** 1.7–3.5 mg/kg/day (50–100 mg/m²/day) divided into 4–6 divided doses.

NURSING CONSIDERATIONS

See also *Nursing Considerations* for *Antihypertensive Agents,* p. 78

Administration/Storage

1. Parenteral injections should be made as quickly as possible after being drawn into the syringe.
2. To enhance bioavailability, the tablets should be taken with food.
3. The presence of a metal filter will cause a change in color of hydralazine.
4. *Treatment of Overdose:* If the cardiovascular status is stable, induce vomiting or perform gastric lavage followed by activated charcoal. Treat shock with volume expanders, without vasopressors; if a vasopressor is necessary, one should be used that is least likely to cause or aggravate tachycardia and cardiac arrhythmias. Renal function should be monitored.

Assessment

1. Note any client history of hypersensitivity to the drug.
2. Document other drugs the client may be taking that would interact unfavorably with hydralazine.
3. Determine baseline BP and weight
4. Note any history of coronary or renal disease.

Interventions

1. Record daily weights and compare to baseline; observe for any evidence of edema.
2. Place the client on intake and output. Note especially any reduction in urine output.

3. If the client is to receive the drug by parenteral injection, take the BP within 5 min and p.r.n. following the injection.
4. Monitor serum electrolytes.
5. The BP should be taken several times a day under standardized conditions, either sitting or standing, as ordered by the physician.
6. Anticipate that client's cardiac condition may require monitoring during drug therapy.

Client/Family Teaching

1. Take oral prescribed drugs with meals to avoid gastric irritation.
2. Explain the possible side effects of the drug, which the client may experience after taking the first dose. These may include headaches, palpitations, and possibly mild postural hypotension and may persist for 7–10 days with continued treatment.
3. Report tingling sensations or discomfort in the hands or feet. These generally are signs of peripheral neuropathies and need to be reported. The problem may be reversed with the use of other drugs, usually pyridoxine.
4. Avoid the use of alcohol or other drugs that could also lower blood pressure.

Evaluation: Evaluate client for:
- Control of hypertension
- Development of arthralgia, dermatoses, fever, anemia, or splenomegaly since these may require discontinuation of drug therapy
- Development of a rheumatoid-like or influenza-like

syndrome as this would necessitate discontinuing hydralazine therapy

Hydrochlorothiazide

(hy-droh-klor-oh-**THIGH**-ah-zyd)
Apo-Hydro❋, Esidrex, Hydro-DIURIL, Neo-Codema❋, Novo-Hyrazide❋, Oretic (Rx)

See also *Diuretics*, p. 140, and *Thiazide and Related Diuretics*, p. 231.

Classification: Diuretic, thiazide type.

Action/Kinetics: Onset: 2 hr. **Peak effect:** 4–6 hr. **Duration:** 6–12 hr. **t½:** Approximately 15 hr. Hydrochlorothiazide is also found in Aldactazide, Aldoril, Apresazide, Dyazide, Hydropres, and Ser-Ap-Es.

Special Concerns: Pregnancy category: B. Geriatric clients may be more sensitive to the usual adult dose.

Dosage: Oral Solution, Tablets. *Antidiuretic, diabetes insipidus:* **Adults:** 25–100 mg once or twice daily, once every other day, or once a day for 3–5 days a week. *Antihypertensive:* **Adults:** 25–100 mg/day as a single dose or in two divided doses. **Pediatric, all uses:** 1–2 mg/kg (30–60 mg/m²) daily as a single dose or two divided doses. Infants up to 6 months of age may require up to 3 mg/kg daily.

NURSING CONSIDERATIONS

See also *Nursing Considerations* for *Diuretics,* p. 141, and *Thiazide and Related Diuretics,* p. 233.

Administration/Storage

1. Divide daily doses in excess of 100 mg.
2. Give b.i.d. at 6- to 12-hr intervals.

Evaluation: Evaluate client for evidence of ↓ blood pressure, as well as ↓ edema, ↓ weight, and/or ↑ in urine output.

——— *COMBINATION DRUG* ———
Hydrochlorothiazide and Lisinopril
(hy-droh-**KLOR**-roh-**THIGH**-ah-zyd, lyes-**IN**-oh-prill)
Prinzide, Zestoretic (Rx)

See also *Lisinopril*, p. 805, and *Hydrochlorothiazide*, p. 718.

Classification/Contents: Lisinopril is an angiotensin-converting enzyme inhibitor and hydrochlorothiazide is a diuretic. Prinzide 12.5 and Zestoretic 20–12.5: Lisinopril, 20 mg and hydrochlorothiazide, 12.5 mg. Prinzide 25 and Zestoretic 20–25: Lisinopril, 20 mg and hydrochlorothiazide, 25 mg.

Uses: Hypertension in clients in whom combination therapy is appropriate. Not for initial therapy.

Special Concerns: Pregnancy category: C.

Dosage: Individualized. PO, usual: 1 or 2 tablets once daily of Prinzide 12.5, Prinzide 25, Zestoretic 20–12.5, or Zestoretic 20–25.

NURSING CONSIDERATIONS

See also *Nursing Considerations for Lisinopril*, p. 806, and *Thiazide Diuretics*, p. 233.

Administration/Storage

1. Clients whose blood pressure is controlled with lisinopril, 20 mg plus hydrochlorothiazide, 25 mg given separately should be given a trial of Prinzide 12.5 or Zestoretic 20–12.5 before Prinzide 25 or Zestoretic 20–25 mg is used.

2. The maximum recommended daily dose of lisinopril is 80 mg in a single daily dose. However, clients usually do not require hydrochlorothiazide in doses exceeding 50 mg daily, especially if combined with other antihypertensives.

3. Use of potassium supplements, potassium-sparing diuretics, or potassium salt substitutes with Prinzide or Zestoretic may lead to increases in serum potassium.

4. Prinzide or Zestoretic is recommended for those clients with a creatinine clearance greater than 30 ml/min.

Client/Family Teaching

1. Stress the importance of reporting for scheduled laboratory studies.
2. Avoid all potassium supplements as well as foods high in potassium.
3. Instruct how to take blood pressure and maintain written record for physician review.

Evaluation: Evaluate client for evidence of a ↓ blood pressure, as well as a ↑ urine output, ↓ weight, and/or ↓ edema.

Hydrocortisone (Cortisol)
(hy-droh-**KOR**-tih-zohn)
**Parenteral: Sterile Hydrocortisone Suspension.
Rectal: Dermolate Anal-Itch,
Proctocort, Rectocort✽.
Retention Enema: Cortenema,
Hycort✽, Rectocort✽. Tablets:
Cortef, Hydrocortone. Topical
Aerosol Solution: Aeroseb-HC,
CaldeCORT Anti-Itch. Topical**

Cream: Ala-Cort, Allercort, Alphaderm, Bactine, Cortate✿, Cort-Dome, Cortifair, Dermacort, DermiCort, Dermolate Anti-Itch, Dermtex HC, Emo-Cort✿, H₂Cort, Hi-Cor 1.0 and 2.5, Hydro-Tex, Hytone Lemoderm, Nutracort, Penecort, Prevex HC✿, Synacort,Unicort✿. Topical Lotion: Acticort 100, Ala-Cort, Ala-Scalp HP, Allercort, Cetacort, Cortate✿, Cort-Dome, Delacort, Dermacort, Dermolate Scalp-Itch, Emo-Cort✿, Gly-Cort, Hytone, LactiCare-HC, Lemoderm, Lexocort Forte, My Cort, Nutracort, Pentacort, Rederm, Sarna HC 1.0%✿, S-T Cort. Suppository: Cortiment✿. Topical Ointment: Allercort, Cortril, Dermolate Anal-Itch, Hytone, Lemoderm, Penecort. Topical Solution: Penecort, Emo-Cort Scalp Solution, Texacort Scalp Solution. Topical Spray: Cortaid, Dermolate Anti-Itch. (OTC, Rx)

Hydrocortisone acetate

(hy-droh-**KOR**-tih-zohn)
Dental Paste: Orabase-HCA. Intrarectal Foam: Cortifoam. Ophthalmic/Otic: Cortamed✿. Parenteral: Hydrocortone Acetate. Rectal: Anusol HC, Cort-Dome High Potency, Cortenema, Corticaine, Cortifoam,Cortiment-10 and -40✿. Suppository: Cortiment✿. Topical Aerosol Foam: Epifoam. Topical Cream: Allocort✿, Anusol-HC, CaldeCORT Anti-Itch, CaldeCORT Light, Carmol-HC, Cortacet✿, Cortaid, Cortef Feminine Itch, Corticaine, Corticreme✿, FoilleCort, Gynecort, Hyderm✿, Lanacort, Novo-Hydrocort✿, Pharma-Cort, Rhulicort. Topical Lotion:

Cortaid, Rhulicort. Topical Ointment: Cortaid, Cortef Acetate, Cortoderm✿, Dermaflex HC 1%✿, Lanacort, Nov-Hydrocort. (OTC, Rx)

Hydrocortisone butyrate

(hy-droh-**KOR**-tih-zohn)
Topical Cream: Locoid (Rx)

Hydrocortisone cypionate

(hy-droh-**KOR**-tih-zohn)
Oral Suspension: Cortef (Rx)

Hydrocortisone sodium phosphate

(hy-droh-**KOR**-tih-zohn)
Parenteral: Hydrocortone Phosphate (Rx)

Hydrocortisone sodium succinate

(hy-droh-**KOR**-tih-zohn)
Parenteral: A-hydroCort, Solu-Cortef (Rx)

Hydrocortisone valerate

(hy-droh-**KOR**-tih-zohn)
Topical Cream/Ointment: Westcort (Rx)

See also *Adrenocorticosteroids and Analogs,* p. 8.

Classification: Adrenocorticosteroid, naturally occurring; glucocorticoid-type.

Action/Kinetics: Short-acting. $t^{1/2}$: 80–118 min. Topical products are available without a prescription in strengths of 0.5% and 1%.

Dosage: *Hydrocortisone.* **PO:** 20–240 mg/day, depending on disease. **IM only:** one-third to one-half the oral dose q 12 hr. **Rectal:** 100 mg in retention enema nightly for 21 days (up to 2 months of therapy may be needed; discontinue gradually if therapy exceeds 3 weeks). **Topical (ointment, cream, gel, lotion, solution, spray):** Apply sparingly to affected area and rub in lightly t.i.d.–q.i.d.

Hydrocortisone acetate. **Intralesional, intra-articular, soft tissue:** 5–50 mg, depending on condition. **Intrarectal Foam:** 1 applicatorful (90 mg) 1–2 times/day for 2–3 weeks; **then** every second day. **Topical:** See *Hydrocortisone.*

Hydrocortisone butyrate. **Topical:** See *Hydrocortisone.*

Hydrocortisone cypionate (as suspension). 20–240 mg/day, depending on the severity of the disease.

Hydrocortisone sodium phosphate. **IV, IM, SC: initial,** 15–240 mg/day depending on use and on severity of the disease. Usually, one-half to one-third of the oral dose is given q 12 hr. *Adrenal insufficiency, acute.* **IV, adults: initial,** 100 mg; **then,** 100 mg q 8 hr in an IV fluid; **older children: initial, IV bolus,** 1–2 mg/kg; **then,** 150–250 mg/kg daily **IV** in divided doses; **infants: initial, IV bolus,** 1–2 mg/kg; **then,** 25–150 mg/kg daily in divided doses.

Hydrocortisone sodium succinate. **IM, IV, initial:** 100–500 mg; **then,** may be repeated at 2-, 4-, and 6-hr intervals depending on response and severity of condition.

Hydrocortisone valerate. **Topical (cream):** See *Hydrocortisone.*

NURSING CONSIDERATIONS

See also *Nursing Considerations* for *Adrenocorticosteroids and Analogs,* p. 15.

Administration/Storage

1. Check label of parenteral hydrocortisone to verify route that can be used for a particular preparation, because IM and IV routes are not necessarily interchangeable.

2. No part of the hydrocortisone acetate intrarectal foam aerosol container should be inserted into the anus.

3. When using topical products, washing the area prior to application may increase the penetration of the drug.

4. Topical products should not come in contact with the eyes.

5. Prolonged use of topical products should be avoided near the genital/rectal areas, eyes, on the face, and in creases of the skin.

Hydromorphone hydrochloride

(hy-droh-**MOR**-fohn)

Dilaudid, Dilaudid-HP (C-II, Rx)

See also *Narcotic Analgesics,* p. 174.

Classification: Narcotic analgesic, morphine type.

Action/Kinetics: Hydromorphone is 7–10 times more analgesic than morphine, with a shorter duration of action. It manifests less sedation, less vomiting, and less nausea than morphine, although it induces pronounced respiratory depression. **Onset:** 15–30 min. **Peak effect:** 30–60 min. **Duration:** 4–5 hr. **t½:** 2–3 hr. The drug can be given rectally for prolonged activity.

Uses: Analgesia for moderate to severe pain (e.g., surgery, cancer, biliary colic, burns, renal colic, myocardial infarction, bone trauma).

Additional Contraindications: Migraine headaches. Use in children. Status asthmaticus, obstetrics, respiratory depression in absence of resuscitative equipment.

Special Concerns: Pregnancy category: C.

Additional Side Effect: Nystagmus.

Dosage: Tablets. Adults: 2 mg q 4–6 hr as necessary. For severe pain, 4 or more mg q 4–6 hr. **Suppositories:** 3 mg q 6–8 hr. **SC, IM, IV:** 1–2 mg q 4–6 hr. For severe pain, 3–4 mg q 4–6 hr.

NURSING CONSIDERATIONS

See also *Nursing Considerations* for *Narcotic Analgesics,* p. 177.

Administration/Storage

1. May be administered by slow IV injection. When using this route, administer the drug slowly to minimize hypotensive effects and respiratory depression. Dilute with 5 ml of sterile water or normal saline.
2. Suppositories should be refrigerated.
3. Drug may be administered as Dilaudid brand cough syrup. Be alert to the possibility of an allergic response in people sensitive to yellow dye #5.

Assessment: Take a complete history of client response to narcotic agents. If the drug is to be administered as a cough syrup determine and record any allergies to dyes.

Interventions: Observe client closely for respiratory depression, as it is more profound with hydromorphone than with other narcotic analgesics.

Evaluation: Evaluate client for:
- Reports of effective control of pain
- Evidence of control of cough permitting uninterrupted periods of sleep

Hydroxychloroquine sulfate

(hy-drox-ee-**KLOR**-oh-kwin)
Plaquenil Sulfate (Rx)

See also *4-Aminoquinolines,* p. 27.

Classification: 4-Aminoquinoline, antimalarial, and antirheumatic.

Action/Kinetics: Hydroxychloroquine is not a drug of choice for rheumatoid arthritis and should be discontinued after 6 months if no beneficial effects are noted. **Peak plasma levels:** 1–3 hr. Unchanged drug is excreted in the urine. Excretion may be enhanced by acidifying the urine and decreased by alkalizing the urine.

Uses: Antimalarial, antirheumatic, discoid and lupus erythematosus. Not used as a first line of therapy.

Additional Contraindications: Long-term therapy in children, ophthalmologic changes due to 4–aminoquinolines.

Special Concerns: Use with caution in alcoholism or liver disease.

Additional Side Effects: The appearances of skin eruptions or of misty vision and visual halos are indications for withdrawal. Clients on long-term therapy should be examined thoroughly at regular intervals for knee and ankle reflexes and hematopoietic studies.

Drug Interactions

Digoxin / Hydroxychloroquine ↑ serum digoxin levels

Gold salts / Dermatitis and ↑ risk of severe skin reactions

Phenylbutazone / Dermatitis and ↑ risk of severe skin reactions

Dosage: Tablets. *Acute malarial attack:* **Adults, initial,** 800 mg; **then,** 400 mg after 6–8 hr and 400 mg/day for next 2 days. **Children:** A total of 32 mg/kg given over a 3-day period as follows: **initial,** 12.9 mg/kg (not to exceed a single dose of 800 mg); **then,** 6.4 mg/kg (not to exceed a single dose of 400 mg) 6, 24, and 48 hr after the first dose. *Suppression of malaria:* **Adults,** 400 mg q 7 days. If therapy has not been initiated 14 days prior to exposure, an initial loading dose of 800 mg may be given in 2 divided doses 6 hr apart. **Children:** 6.4 mg/kg (not to exceed the adult dose) q 7 days. If therapy has not been initiated 14 days prior to exposure, an initial loading dose of 12.9 mg/kg may be given in 2 doses 6 hr apart.

Rheumatoid arthritis: **Adults,** 400–600 mg daily taken with milk or meals; **maintenance** (usually after 4–12 weeks): 200–400 mg daily. (**Note:** Several months may be required for a beneficial effect to be seen). *Lupus erythematosus:* **Adults, usual,** 400 mg once or twice daily; **prolonged maintenance:** 200–400 mg daily.

NURSING CONSIDERATIONS

See also *Nursing Considerations for 4-Aminoquinolines,* p. 28, and *General Nursing Considerations for All Anti-Infectives,* p. 83.

Assessment

1. Determine if client has any history of liver disease or alcohol abuse.
2. Ensure that baseline CBC and ophthalmic exams are completed.
3. Note condition of skin and record strength of ankle and knee reflexes.

Interventions

1. When the drug is given for rheumatoid arthritis:
   - Reassure client and indicate that benefits may not occur until 6–12 months after therapy has been initiated.
   - Anticipate that side effects may necessitate a reduction of therapy. After 5–10 days of reduced dosage, it may gradually be increased again to the desired level.
   - Anticipate that dosage will be reduced when the desired response is attained. Drug will again be effective in case of flare-up.
   - Reduce GI irritation by administering drug with meal or glass of milk.
   - Corticosteroids and salicylates may be used concomitantly.
2. When the drug is given for lupus erythematosus, administer dose with the evening meal.
3. Suppressive antimalarial therapy should be initiated 2 weeks prior to exposure and should be continued for 6–8 weeks after leaving the endemic area. If therapy is not started prior to exposure, the initial loading dose should be doubled (i.e., adults, 620 mg as the base and children 10 mg/kg as the base) and given in two doses 6 hr apart.

Client/Family Teaching

1. Any skin eruptions should be reported because this is an indication to stop drug therapy.

2. Stress the importance of reporting for regular ophthalmic exams and of reporting any visual disturbances because the drug may need to be discontinued.

Evaluation: Evaluate client for:

- Evidence of termination of acute malarial attack and suppression of malarial symptoms
- Reports of improvement in joint pain and mobility

Hydroxypropyl cellulose ophthalmic insert

(hy-**DROX**-ee-proh-pill **SELL**-you-lohs)

Lacrisert (Rx)

Classification: Wetting agent, hydrophilic.

Action/Kinetics: Lacrisert contains 5 mg of hydroxypropyl cellulose in a rod-shaped (1.27 mm diameter; 3.5 mm long), water-soluble preparation. It contains no preservatives or other ingredients. This preparation stabilizes and thickens precorneal tear film and prolongs the breakup time for tear film. It also lubricates and protects the eye.

Use: Moderate to severe dry eye syndrome including keratoconjunctivitis sicca. Also exposure keratitis, decreased corneal sensitivity, and recurrent corneal lesions. *Investigational:* Ocular lubricant, neuroparalytic keratitis.

Contraindications: Hypersensitivity to hydroxypropyl cellulose.

Side Effects: Transient blurring of vision, ocular discomfort or irritation, photophobia, hypersensitivity, edema of eyelids, eyelids mat or become sticky, hyperemia.

Dosage: Ocular system. Adults and children: One 5-mg insert daily placed into the conjunctival sac of the eye. Some clients may require two inserts daily.

NURSING CONSIDERATIONS

Interventions

1. Review instructions in the package insert on how to insert and remove Lacrisert. Follow the instructions carefully.
2. Assess closely for signs and symptoms of drug side effects. These may include conjunctival hyperemia, exudation, itching, burning, a sensation of the presence of a foreign body, smarting, photophobia, and blurred or cloudy vision. Document and determine client's ability to tolerate these side effects.

Client/Family Teaching

1. Instruct the client in how to insert and remove Lacrisert. Review the package insert with the client and advise to follow the instructions provided.
2. Avoid rubbing the eyes, thereby preventing a dislodgement of Lacrisert.
3. If Lacrisert is accidentally expelled, client may insert another Lacrisert as needed.
4. Report for regular ophthalmic examinations as scheduled.
5. Discuss the need to report any adverse reactions to the ophthalmologist.
6. Explain that the medication may retard, stop, or reverse progressive visual deterioration.

7. Avoid operating a car or other hazardous machinery because the drug may cause transitory blurring of vision.

Evaluation: Evaluate client for reports of symptomatic improvement in corneal lubrication, pain, and sensitivity.

Hydroxyurea
(hy-**DROX**-ee-you-**ree**-ah)
Hydrea (Abbreviation: HYD)

See also *Antineoplastic Agents,* p. 85.

Classification: Antineoplastic, antimetabolite.

Action/Kinetics: Thought to be cell-cycle specific for the S phase of cell division. Believed to interfere with DNA but not synthesis of RNA or protein. Most active in inhibiting incorporation of thymidine into DNA. Rapidly absorbed from GI tract. **Peak serum concentration:** 2 hr. **t½:** 3–4 hr. The drug crosses the blood-brain barrier. Degraded in liver; 80% excreted through the urine with 50% unchanged; also excreted as respiratory CO_2.

Uses: Chronic, resistant, myelocytic leukemia. Carcinoma of the ovary (recurrent, inoperable, or metastatic). Melanoma. With irradiation to treat primary squamous cell carcinoma of the head and neck (but not the lip).

Contraindications: Leukocyte count less than 2,500/mm³ or thrombocyte count less than 100,000/mm³. Severe anemia.

Special Concerns: Use during pregnancy only if benefits clearly outweigh risks. Give with caution to clients with marked renal dysfunction. Dosage has not been established in children.

Additional Side Effects: Erythrocyte abnormalities including megaloblastic erythropoiesis. Constipation, redness of the face, maculopapular rash.

Laboratory Test Interference: ↑ Uric acid in serum; ↑ BUN and creatinine.

Dosage: Capsules. Dose individualized. *Solid tumors, intermittent therapy or when used together with irradiation:* 60–80 mg/kg as a single dose q third day; *solid tumors, continuous therapy:* 20–30 mg/kg daily as a single dose. Intermittent dosage offers advantage of reduced toxicity. If effective, maintain client on drug indefinitely unless toxic effects preclude such a regimen. *Resistant chronic myelocytic leukemia:* 20–30 mg/kg/day in a single dose or two divided daily doses.

NURSING CONSIDERATIONS

See also *Nursing Considerations* for *Antineoplastic Agents,* p. 88.

Administration/Storage

1. Dosage should be calculated on the basis of actual or ideal weight (whichever is less).
2. Therapy should be continued for at least 6 weeks before efficacy is assessed.
3. If the client cannot swallow a capsule, contents may be given in glass of water that should be drunk immediately, even though some material may not dissolve and may float on top of glass.
4. Hydroxyurea should be started 7 days before irradiation.

Interventions

1. Observe for exacerbation of postirradiation erythema.
2. Monitor liver and renal function studies during therapy.

Evaluation: Evaluate client for:
- Laboratory evidence of improved hematologic parameters
- Evidence of a decrease in tumor size and spread

Hydroxyzine hydrochloride
(hy-DROX-ih-zeen)
Anxanil, Apo-Hydroxyzine✱, Atarax, Atozine, E-Vista, Hydroxacen, Hyzine-50, Multipax✱, Novo–Hydroxyzin✱, PMS Hydroxyzine✱, Quiess, Vistaject-25 and -50, Vistaquel 50, Vistaril, Vistazine 50 (Rx)

Hydroxyzine pamoate
(hy-DROX-ih-zeen)
Vamate, Vistaril (Rx)

Classification: Antianxiety agent, miscellaneous.

Action/Kinetics: The action of hydroxyzine may be due to a depression of activity in selected important regions of the subcortical areas of the CNS. Hydroxyzine manifests anticholinergic, antiemetic, antispasmodic, local anesthetic, antihistaminic, and skeletal relaxant effects. The drug also has mild antiarrhythmic activity and mild analgesic effects. **Onset:** 15–30 min. **t½:** 3 hr. **Duration:** 4–6 hr. Metabolized by the liver and excreted through the urine. The pamoate salt is believed to be converted to the hydrochloride in the stomach.

Uses: PO use: Psychoneurosis and tension states, anxiety, and agitation. Anxiety observed in organic disease. Adjunct in the treatment of chronic urticaria. Control of nausea and vomiting accompanying various diseases. Preanesthetic medication. **IM use:** Acute hysteria or agitation, withdrawal symptoms (including delirium tremens) in the acute or chronic alcoholic, asthma, nausea and vomiting (except that due to pregnancy), pre- or postoperative and pre- or postpartum to allow decrease in dosage of narcotics.

Contraindications: Pregnancy (especially early) or lactation; not recommended for the treatment of morning sickness during pregnancy or as sole agent for treatment of psychoses or depression. Hypersensitivity to drug. Not to be used IV, SC, or intra-arterially.

Special Concerns: Geriatric clients may manifest increased anticholinergic and sedative effects.

Side Effects: Low incidence at recommended dosages. Drowsiness, dryness of mouth, involuntary motor activity, dizziness, urticaria, or skin reactions. Marked discomfort, induration, and even gangrene have been reported at site of IM injection.

Symptom of Overdose: Oversedation.

Drug Interactions: Additive effects when used with other CNS depressants. See *Drug Interactions* for *Benzodiazepines,* p. 108.

Laboratory Test Interference: Hydroxycorticosteroids.

Dosage: Capsules, Oral Suspension, Syrup. Hydroxyzine hydrochloride and **hydroxyzine**

pamoate. *Antianxiety:* **Adults,** 50–100 mg q.i.d.; **pediatric under 6 years:** 50 mg daily; **over 6 years:** 50–100 mg daily in divided doses. *Pruritus:* **Adults,** 25 mg t.i.d.–q.i.d.; **children under 6 years:** 50 mg daily in divided doses; **children over 6 years:** 50–100 mg/day in divided doses. *Preoperatively:* **Adults,** 50–100 mg; **children:** 0.6 mg/kg.

IM. Hydroxyzine hydrochloride. *Acute anxiety, including alcohol withdrawal:* **Initial,** 50–100 mg repeated q 4–6 hr as needed. *Nausea, vomiting, pre- and post operative, pre- and postpartum:* **Adults,** 25–100 mg; **pediatric,** 1.1 mg/kg. Switch to **PO** as soon as possible.

NURSING CONSIDERATIONS

See also *Nursing Considerations* for *Benzodiazepines,* p. 111.

Administration/Storage

1. Inject IM only. Injection should be made into the upper, outer quadrant of the buttocks or the midlateral muscles of the thigh.

In children the drug should be injected into the midlateral muscles of the thigh.

2. *Treatment of Overdose:* Immediate induction of vomiting or performance of gastric lavage. General supportive care with monitoring of vital signs. Control hypotension with IV fluids and either norepinephrine or metaraminol (epinephrine should not be used).

Client/Family Teaching

1. Frequent rinsing of the mouth and increased fluid intake may relieve dryness of the mouth.
2. Wait and evaluate the sedative effects of hydroxyzine before performing any tasks that require mental alertness.
3. Avoid ingestion of alcohol.

Evaluation: Evaluate client for:
- Evidence of a ↓ in anxiety levels, itching, and allergic symptoms
- Reports of effective control of nausea and vomiting

Ibuprofen

(eye-byou-**PROH**-fen)

Rx: Apo-Ibuprofen✶, Amersol✶, Children's Advil, Ibuprohm, Ibu-Tab, Motrin, Novo–Profen✶, PediaProfen, Rufen, Saleto-400, -600, and -800. OTC: Aches-N-Pain, Advil Caplets and Tablets, Genpril Caplets and Tablets, Haltran, Ibuprin, Ibuprohm Caplets and Tablets, Ibu-Tab,

Medipren, Midol 200, Motrin-IB Caplets and Tablets, Nuprin Caplets and Tablets, Pamprin-IB, Saleto-200, Trendar

See also *Nonsteroidal Anti-Inflammatory Drugs,* p. 186.

Classification: Anti-inflammatory, nonsteroidal analgesic.

Action/Kinetics: Time to peak levels: 1–2 hr. **Onset:** 30 min for analgesia and approximately 1 week for anti-inflammatory effect. **Peak serum levels:** 1–2 hr. **t½:** 2 hr. **Duration:** 4–6 hr for analgesia and 1–2 weeks for anti-inflammatory effect. Food delays absorption rate but not total amount of drug absorbed.

The OTC products each contain 200 mg of ibuprofen; tablets containing 300 mg, 400 mg, 600 mg, 800 mg or the oral suspension containing 100 mg/5 ml are all available by prescription only.

Uses: Analgesic for mild to moderate pain. Primary dysmenorrhea, rheumatoid arthritis, osteoarthritis, antipyretic. *Investigational:* Resistant acne vulgaris (with tetracyclines); inflammation due to ultraviolet-B exposure (sunburn); juvenile rheumatoid arthritis.

Contraindications: Use of ibuprofen is not recommended during pregnancy, especially during the last trimester.

Special Concerns: The dosage must be individually determined for children less than 12 years of age as safety and effectiveness have not been established.

Additional Side Effects: Dermatitis (maculopapular type), rash. Hypersensitivity reaction consisting of abdominal pain, fever, headache, meningitis, nausea, signs of liver damage, and vomiting; especially seen in clients with systemic lupus erythematosus.

Additional Drug Interactions

Furosemide / Ibuprofen ↓ diuretic effect of furosemide due to ↓ renal prostaglandin synthesis
Lithium / Ibuprofen ↑ plasma levels of lithium

Thiazide diuretics / Ibuprofen ↓ diuretic effect of furosemide due to ↓ renal prostaglandin synthesis

Dosage: Tablets. *Rheumatoid arthritis, osteoarthritis:* Either 300 mg q.i.d. or 400, 600, or 800 mg t.i.d.–q.i.d.; adjust dosage according to client response. Full therapeutic response may not be noted for 2 or more weeks. *Juvenile arthritis:* 30–40 mg/kg daily in 3–4 divided doses. *Mild to moderate pain:* 400 mg q 4–6 hr. *Antipyretic:* **Pediatric:** 5 mg/kg if baseline temperature is 102.5°F or below or 10 mg/kg if baseline temperature is greater than 102.5°F. *Dysmenorrhea:* 400 mg q 4 hr. **OTC use:** *Mild to moderate pain, antipyretic, dysmenorrhea:* 200 mg q 4–6 hr, not to exceed 1,200 mg daily.

NURSING CONSIDERATIONS

See also *Nursing Considerations* for *Nonsteroidal Anti-Inflammatory Drugs,* p. 189.

Administration/Storage

1. Ibuprofen purchased OTC should not be used as an antipyretic for more than 3 days.
2. This drug should not be used as an analgesic for more than 10 days unless approved by a physician.
3. Anticipate an onset of action in 30 min and that the effect will last 2–4 hr.
4. No more than 3.2 g/day should be taken of prescription products and no more than 1.2 g/day should be taken of OTC products.
5. Can be taken with meals or milk if GI upset occurs.

Assessment

1. Take a complete drug history, noting if the client is currently taking any of the drugs with which ibuprofen interacts unfavorably. Document any evidence of lupus.
2. Note the age of the client, and if female determine if sexually active and potentially pregnant. The drug is contraindicated in pregnancy.
3. Obtain a baseline eye examination prior to initiating drug therapy.

Client/Family Teaching

1. Take the medication only as prescribed.
2. Provide a printed list of adverse side effects. Stress those that should be reported to the physician immediately.
3. Take the medication with a snack, milk, antacid, or meals to decrease GI upset. If nausea, vomiting, diarrhea, or constipation persist, report to the physician because the drug may need to be discontinued.
4. Clients with a history of congestive heart failure or compromised cardiac function should keep careful records of weight and report any evidence of edema. Records of BP and intake and output may additionally be requested with some individuals.
5. Report any evidence of blurred vision. Periodic eye examinations should be performed on clients undergoing long-term therapy.
6. Remind the client that it may take 2–3 weeks of therapy to realize an improvement in arthritic pain. Therefore, the

client should remain on the drug unless side effects occur.
7. Stress the importance of reporting for scheduled lab tests including BUN, serum electrolytes, creatinine, and urinalysis.

Evaluation: Evaluate client for:
- Reports of effective relief of pain
- Relief of joint pain and improved joint mobility
- Reduction of fever

Idarubicin hydrochloride
(eye-dah-**ROOB**-ih-sin)
Idamycin For Injection (Rx)

Classification: Antineoplastic agent.

Action/Kinetics: Idarubicin is an anthracycline that inhibits nucleic acid synthesis and interacts with the enzyme topoisomerase II. It is rapidly taken up into cells due to its significant lipid solubility. **t½ (terminal):** 22 hr when used alone and 20 hr when used with cytarabine. The drug is metabolized in the liver to the active idarubicinol, which is excreted through both the bile and urine. Both idarubicin and idarubicinol are significantly bound (97% and 94%, respectively) to plasma proteins.

Uses: In combination with other drugs (often cytarabine) to treat acute myeloid leukemia (AML) in adults, including French-American-British classifications M1 through M7. Comparison with daunorubicin indicates that idarubicin is more effective in inducing complete remissions in clients with AML.

Contraindications: Lactation. Pre-existing bone marrow suppression induced by previous drug therapy or radiotherapy (unless benefit outweighs risk). Administration by the IM or SC routes.

Special Concerns: Pregnancy category: D. Safety and effectiveness have not been demonstrated in children. Skin reactions may occur if the powder is not handled properly.

Side Effects: *GI:* Nausea, vomiting, mucositis, diarrhea, abdominal pain, abdominal cramps, hemorrhage. *Hematologic:* Severe myelosuppression. *Dermatologic:* Alopecia, generalized rash, urticaria, bullous erythrodermatous rash of the palms and soles, hives at injection site. *CNS:* Headache, seizures, altered mental status. *CV:* Congestive heart failure, serious arrhythmias including atrial fibrillation, chest pain, myocardial infarction, cardiomyopathies, decrease in left ventricular ejection fraction. **Note:** Cardiac toxicity is more common in clients who have received anthracycline drugs previously or who have preexisting cardiac disease. *Miscellaneous:* Altered hepatic and renal function tests, infection (95% of clients), fever, pulmonary allergy, neurologic changes in peripheral nerves.
Symptoms of Overdose: Severe GI toxicity, myelosuppression.

Dosage: **IV.** *Induction therapy in adults:* 12 mg/m² daily for 3 days by slow (10–15 min) IV injection in combination with cytarabine, 100 mg/m² daily given by continuous infusion for 7 days or as a 25 mg/m² IV bolus followed by 200 mg/m² daily for 5 days by continuous infusion. A second course may be given if there is evidence of leukemia after the first course.

NURSING CONSIDERATIONS

Administration/Storage

1. The 5-mg and 10-mg vials should be reconstituted with 5 ml and 10 ml, respectively, of 0.9% sodium chloride injection to give a final concentration of 1 mg/ml. Diluents containing bacteriostatic agents should not be used.
2. To minimize aerosol formation during reconstitution, the contents of the vial are under negative pressure. Care should be taken to avoid inhalation of any aerosol formed.
3. The drug should be given slowly into a freely flowing IV infusion.
4. The IV solution of idarubicin should not be mixed with any other drugs.
5. Reconstituted solutions are stable for 7 days if refrigerated and 3 days at room temperature. Unused solution should be discarded.
6. If the drug comes in contact with the skin, the area should be washed thoroughly with soap and water. Goggles, gloves, and protective gowns should be used during preparation and administration of idarubicin.
7. *Treatment of Overdose:* Supportive treatment including antibiotics and platelet transfusions. Treat mucositis.

Assessment

1. Document any preexisting cardiac disease.
2. Note any history of previous radiation treatments or therapy with anthracyclines.

3. Obtain baseline CBC, platelets, liver and renal function studies and monitor throughout therapy.

Interventions

1. Anticipate that the dose should be reduced in clients with impaired hepatic or renal function or if bilirubin levels are greater than 5 mg/dl.
2. Severe myelosuppression is a side effect of drug therapy. Observe closely for early evidence of hemorrhaging and infection.
3. Medicate as needed for nausea and diarrhea; frequent side effects of drug therapy.
4. Evaluate complaints of severe abdominal pain and perform careful abdominal assessments.
5. Document any evidence of SOB or chest pain as drug may cause myocardial toxicity.
6. Monitor I&O, encourage a high fluid intake and keep the urine slightly alkaline to prevent the formation of uric acid stones.
7. If extravasation is suspected or has occurred, elevate the extremity and apply intermittent ice packs (immediately for 1/2 hr, then four times a day at 1/2-hr intervals for 3 days) over the affected area.

Evaluation

1. Determine client's response to treatment and note the presence of leukemia cells because a second course of therapy may be indicated after hematologic recovery.
2. Assess client for evidence of a complete remission and improved hematologic parameters.

Idoxuridine (IDU)
(eye-dox-**YOUR**-ih-deen)
Herplex Liquifilm, Herplex-D Liquifilm✦, Stoxil (Rx)

Classification: Antiviral agent, ophthalmic.

Action/Kinetics: Idoxuridine, which resembles thymidine, inhibits thymidylic phosphorylase and specific DNA polymerases required for incorporation of thymidine into viral DNA. Idoxuridine, instead of thymidine, is incorporated into viral DNA, resulting in faulty DNA and the inability of the virus to infect tissue or reproduce. Idoxuridine may also be incorporated into mammalian cells. The drug does not penetrate the cornea well. It is rapidly inactivated by nucleotidases or deaminases.

Uses: Herpes simplex keratitis, especially for initial epithelial infections characterized by the presence of thread-like extensions. **Note:** Idoxuridine will control infection but will not prevent scarring, loss of vision, or vascularization. Alternative form of treatment must be instituted if no improvement is noted after 7 days or if complete reepithelialization fails to occur after 21 days of therapy.

Contraindications: Hypersensitivity; deep ulcerations involving stromal layers of cornea. Lactation. Concomitant use of corticosteroids in herpes simplex keratitis.

Special Concerns: Use with caution during pregnancy.

Side Effects: Localized to eye. Temporary visual haze, irritation, pain, pruritus, inflammation, follicular conjunctivitis with preauricular adenopathy, mild edema of eyelids and cornea, allergic reactions (rare), photosensitivity, corneal clouding and stippling, small punctate defects. **Note:** Squamous cell carcinoma has been reported at the site of application.

Symptom of Overdose (frequent administration: Defects on corneal epithelium.

Drug Interaction: Concurrent use of boric acid may cause irritation.

Dosage: Ophthalmic (0.1%) solution: initially, 1 drop q hr during day and q 2 hr during night; **following improvement:** 1 drop q 2 hr during day and q 4 hr at night. Continue for 3–5 days after healing is complete. **Ophthalmic (0.5%) ointment:** Insert in conjunctival sac 5 times/day q 4 hr, with last dose at bedtime; continue for 3–5 days after healing is complete.

NURSING CONSIDERATIONS

See also *General Nursing Considerations For All Anti-Infectives,* p. 83.

Administration/Storage

1. Store idoxuridine solution at 2°C–8°C (36°F–46°F) and protect from light.
2. Do not mix with other medications.
3. Store idoxuridine ointment at 2°C–15°C (36°F–59°F).
4. Administer ophthalmic medication as scheduled, even during the night.
5. Do not use drug that was improperly stored because of loss of activity and increased toxic effects.
6. Topical corticosteroids may be used with idoxuridine in the treatment of herpes simplex with corneal edema, stromal lesions, or iritis.
7. To control secondary infec-

tions, antibiotics may be used with idoxuridine.
8. Atropine may be used concomitantly with idoxuridine, if appropriate.

Interventions

1. *Assess* client for symptoms of vision loss.
2. *Do not* apply boric acid to the eye when client is on idoxuridine therapy because boric acid may cause irritation.
3. Reassure client that hazy vision following instillation of medication will be of short duration.
4. Encourage clients to wear dark glasses if photophobia occurs.
5. Anticipate that if idoxuridine has been used concurrently with corticosteroids, the idoxuridine will be continued longer than the steroid, to prevent reinfection.

Evaluation: Evaluate client for clinical evidence of control of infection and re-epitheliazation of herpetic eye lesions.

Ifosfamide
(eye-**FOS**-fah-myd)
Ifex (Rx)

See also *Antineoplastic Agents,* p. 85, and *Alkylating Agents,* p. 20.

Classification: Antineoplastic, alkylating agent.

Action/Kinetics: Ifosfamide, a synthetic analog of cyclophosphamide, must be converted in the liver to active metabolites. The alkylated metabolites of ifosfamide then interact with DNA. **t½:** 7 hr. Excreted in the urine both as unchanged drug and metabolites.

Uses: As third-line therapy, in combination with other antineoplastic drugs, for germ cell testicular cancer. Ifosfamide should always be given with mesna (p. 845) to prevent ifosfamide-induced hemorrhagic cystitis. *Investigational:* Cancer of the breast, lung, pancreas, ovary, and stomach. Also for sarcomas, acute leukemias (except AML), malignant lymphomas.

Contraindications: Severe bone marrow depression. Lactation.

Special Concerns: Pregnancy category: D. Use with caution in clients with compromised bone marrow reserve, impaired renal function, and during lactation. Safety and efficacy have not been established in children. May interfere with wound healing.

Additional Side Effects: *GU:* Hemorrhagic cystitis, hematuria, dysuria, urinary frequency. *CNS:* Confusion, depressive psychosis, somnolence, hallucinations. Less frequently: dizziness, disorientation, cranial nerve dysfunction, seizures, coma. *GI:* Salivation, stomatitis. *Miscellaneous:* Alopecia, infection, liver dysfunction, phlebitis, fever of unknown origin, dermatitis, fatigue, hypertension, hypotension, polyneuropathy, pulmonary symptoms, cardiotoxicity, interference with normal wound healing.

Laboratory Test Interferences: ↑ Liver enzymes, bilirubin.

Dosage: IV: 1.2 g/m²/day for 5 consecutive days. Treatment may be repeated q 3 wks or if platelet counts are at least 100,000/μl and white blood cells are at least 4,000/μl.

NURSING CONSIDERATIONS

See also *Nursing Considerations* for *Antineoplastic Agents,* p. 88.

Administration/Storage

1. To prevent bladder toxicity, ifosfamide should be given with at least 2 L of oral or IV fluid per day as well as with mesna.
2. Dosage should be administered slowly over 30 min.
3. The drug is reconstituted by adding either sterile water for injection or bacteriostatic water for injection for a final concentration of 50 mg/ml. Solutions may be further diluted to achieve concentrations from 0.6–20 mg/ml by adding 5% dextrose injection, 0.9% sodium chloride injection, sterile water for injection, or lactated Ringer's injection.
4. Reconstituted solutions (50 mg/ml) are stable for 1 week at 30°C (86°F) or 3 weeks at 5°C (41°F).
5. Dilutions of ifosfamide not prepared with bacteriostatic water for injection should be refrigerated and used within 6 hr.

Interventions

1. Anticipate concomitant administration with mesna to minimize occurrence of hemorrhagic cystitis.
2. Monitor input and output; promote high fluid intake during therapy.
3. Obtain and send urine for analysis prior to each dose of ifosfamide.
4. Monitor CBC and platelets closely; obtain WBC and platelet parameters for drug administration.
5. Note the presence of marked leukopenia and protect the client from possible infection.

Immunosuppression may activate latent infections such as herpes.
6. Check client's mouth for furry patches on the tongue or oral membranes. Document and report to the physician.

Client/Family Teaching

1. Reinforce that hair loss, nausea, and vomiting are frequent side effects of drug therapy.
2. Stress that normal wound healing may be impaired during drug therapy. Report any injury or interference with normal wound healing.
3. Report any confusion, hallucinations, or marked drowsiness because these symptoms may necessitate discontinuation of drug therapy.
4. Warn clients that there may be hyperpigmentation of their skin and mucous membranes.
5. Advise female clients to practice contraceptive measures during the treatment and for at least 4 months after treatments have ceased.
6. If the treatment is to last 6 months, the client should be told that infertility may result.
7. Report the presence of frothy dark urine, jaundice, or light colored stools. These are signs of hepatotoxicity and adjustments may be needed in the dosage of drug or therapy may need to be changed.
8. Review symptoms of neurotoxicity and advise client to report these to the physician if evident. During outpatient treatment it is particularly important to elicit the support of the family in making observations and evaluations and encouraging them to keep a record of events and the times of their occurrence.

Evaluation: Evaluate client for:
- Evidence of a ↓ in tumor size and spread
- Designated hematologic parameters (platelet counts at least 100,000/µl and white blood cells at least 4,000/µl in order to continue the therapy)
- Complaints of joint or flank pain that may be caused by the increase in uric acid that results from the rapid cytolysis of tumor and red blood cells.

------ *COMBINATION DRUG* ------
Imipenem-Cilastatin sodium
(em-ee-**PEN**-em, sigh-lah-**STAT**-in)
Primaxin I.M., Primaxin I.V., Zienam✿ (Rx)

See also *Anti-Infectives*, p. 80.

Classification: Antibiotic combined with inhibitor of dehydropeptidase I.

Action/Kinetics: Imipenem inhibits cell wall synthesis and is thus bactericidal against a wide range of gram-positive and gram-negative organisms. It is stable in the presence of beta-lactamases. Addition of cilastatin prevents the metabolism of imipenem in the kidneys by dehydropeptidase I, thus ensuring high levels of the imipenem in the urinary tract. $t^{1/2}$, **after IV:** 1 hr for each component. **Peak plasma levels, after IM:** 10–12 mcg/ml within 2 hr. Compared with IV administration, imipenem is approximately 75% bioavailable after IM use with cilastatin being 95%

bioavailable. **t½, imipenem:** 2–3 hr.

Uses: IV. Serious infections of the lower respiratory tract and urinary tract. Also, serious gynecologic infections, skin and skin structure infections, bacterial septicemia, bone and joint infections, endocarditis, intra-abdominal infections, and infections caused by more than one agent. Infections resistant to aminoglycosides, cephalosporins, or penicillins have responded to imipenem.

IM. Lower respiratory tract infections, intra-abdominal infections, skin and skin structure infections, gynecologic infections.

Contraindications: IM use for severe or life-threatening infections or in clients allergic to local anesthetics of the amide type. IM use in clients with heart block (due to the use of lidocaine HCl diluent) or severe shock.

Special Concerns: Pregnancy category: C. Use with caution in pregnancy and lactation. Safety and effectiveness have not been determined in children less than 12 years of age.

Side Effects: *GI:* Pseudomembranous colitis, nausea, diarrhea, vomiting, abdominal pain, heartburn, increased salivation, hemorrhagic colitis, gastroenteritis, glossitis, pharyngeal pain, tongue papillar hypertrophy. *CNS:* Fever, confusion, seizures, dizziness, sleepiness, myoclonus, headache, vertigo, paresthesia, encephalopathy, tremor, psychic disturbances. *CV:* Hypotension, tachycardia, palpitations. *Dermatologic:* Rash, urticaria, pruritus, flushing, cyanosis, facial edema, erythema multiforme, toxic epidermal necrolysis. *Miscellaneous:* Candidiasis, pruritus vulvae, tinnitus, polyuria, increased sweating, joint pain, muscle weakness, anuria/oliguria, chest discomfort, dyspnea, hyperventilation, transient hearing loss in clients with existing hearing impairment, taste perversion, thrombocytopenia, leukopenia, thoracic spine pain, acute renal failure.

The following side effects may occur at the injection site: Thrombophlebitis, phlebitis, pain, erythema, induration, infection.

Drug Interactions: Use of ganciclovir with imipenem-cilastatin may result in generalized seizures.

Laboratory Test Interferences: ↑ AST, ALT, alkaline phosphatase, LDH, bilirubin, potassium, chloride, BUN, creatinine. ↓ Sodium. Positive Coombs' test and abnormal prothrombin time. Presence of red blood cells, white blood cells, casts, bilirubin, or urobilinogen in the urine.

Dosage: IV. *Gram-positive organisms, highly susceptible gram-negative organisms, anaerobes: Mild,* 250 mg q 6 hr; *moderate,* 500 mg q 6–8 hr; *severe/life-threatening,* 500 mg q 6 hr. *Urinary tract infections:* 250–500 mg q 6 hr, depending on severity.

Gram-negative organisms: Mild, 500 mg q 6 hr; *moderate,* 500–1,000 mg q 6–8 hr; *severe/life-threatening,* 1 g q 6–8 hr. *Urinary tract infections:* 250–500 mg q 6 hr, depending on severity.

The total daily dose should not exceed 50 mg/kg or 4 g, whichever is lower.

IM. *Lower respiratory tract, skin and skin structure, or gynecologic infections: mild to moderate,* 500 or 750 mg q 12 hr depending on severity. *Intra-abdominal: mild to moderate,* 750 mg q 12 hr. The total daily dose should not exceed 1.5 g.

NURSING CONSIDERATIONS

See also *General Nursing Considerations for All Anti-Infectives,* p. 83.

Administration/Storage

1. Doses between 250 and 500 mg should be given by IV infusion over 20–30 min; doses of 1 g should be given by IV infusion over 40–60 min. If nausea develops, the infusion rate should be decreased.
2. The package insert should be consulted for calculation of doses in adults with impaired renal function.
3. Reconstituted solutions vary from colorless to yellow.
4. Imipenem-cilastatin should not be physically mixed with other antibiotics; however, the drug may be administered with other antibiotics, if necessary.
5. Most reconstituted solutions can be stored at room temperature for 4 hr and, if refrigerated, for 24 hr. The exception is imipenem-cilastatin reconstituted with 0.9% sodium chloride solution, which is stable at room temperature for 10 hr and, if refrigerated, for 48 hr.
6. When used IM, the dose should be given in a large muscle mass with a 21-gauge 2-inch needle.
7. IM use should be continued for at least 2 days after signs and symptoms of infection are absent. Safety and effectiveness have not been established for use for more than 14 days.
8. Dosage should be reduced in clients with impaired renal function.

Imipramine hydrochloride
(im-**IHP**-rah-meen)
Apo-Imipramine✿, Impril✿, Janimine, Novo-Pramine✿, PMS Imipramine✿, Tofranil (Rx)

Imipramine pamoate
(im-**IHP**-rah-meen)
Tofranil-PM (Rx)

See also *Tricyclic Antidepressants,* p. 239.

Action/Kinetics: Imipramine is biotransformed into its active metabolite, desmethylimipramine (desipramine). **Effective plasma level of imipramine and desmethylimipramine:** 200–350 ng/ml. **$t\frac{1}{2}$:** 11–25 hr.

Uses: Symptoms of depression. Enuresis in children. Chronic, severe neurogenic pain. Bulimia nervosa.

Special Concerns: Pregnancy category: B.

Additional Side Effects: High therapeutic dosage may increase frequency of seizures in epileptic clients and cause seizures in nonepileptic clients. Elderly and adolescent clients may have low tolerance to the drug.

Laboratory Test Interferences: ↑ Metanephrine (Pisano test); ↓ Urinary 5-HIAA.

Dosage: Tablets, Capsules. *Depression:* **Hospitalized clients:** 50 mg b.i.d.–t.i.d. Can be increased by 25 mg every few days up to 200 mg daily. After 2 weeks, dosage may be increased gradually to maximum of 250–300 mg once daily at bedtime. **Outpatients:** 75–150 mg daily. Maximum dose for outpatients is

200 mg. Decrease when feasible to maintenance dosage: 50–150 mg once daily at bedtime. **Adolescent and geriatric clients:** 30–40 mg/day up to maximum of 100 mg/day. **Pediatric:** 1.5 mg/kg daily in 3 divided doses; can be increased 1–1.5 mg/kg daily q 3–5 days to a maximum of 5 mg/kg daily. *Childhood enuresis:* **age 6 years and over:** 25 mg/day 1 hr before bedtime. Dose can be increased to 50 mg/day up to 12 years of age and to 75 mg/day in children over 12 years of age.

   IM. Adults: *Antidepressant:* up to 100 mg daily in divided doses. IM route not recommended for use in children less than 12 years of age.

NURSING CONSIDERATIONS

See also *Nursing Considerations* for *Tricyclic Antidepressants,* p. 242.

Administration/Storage

1. Crystals, which may be present in the injectable form, can be dissolved by immersing closed ampules into hot water for 1 min.
2. Total daily dose can be given once daily at bedtime.
3. Protect from direct sunlight and strong artificial light.
4. Parenteral therapy should be used only in clients unwilling or unable to take oral medication. Switch to oral medication as soon as possible.
5. Imipramine injection should not be given IV.
6. When used for the treatment of enuresis, the drug can be given in doses of 25 mg in midafternoon and 25 mg at bedtime (this regimen may increase effectiveness).
7. When used as an enuretic in

children, the dose should not exceed 2.5 mg/kg daily.

Client/Family Teaching

1. Report increase in frequency of seizures in epileptics and any occurrence of seizures in nonepileptics.
2. Advise parents that children may experience mild nausea and vomiting, unusual tiredness, nervousness, or insomnia. If pronounced, these symptoms should be reported.

Evaluation: Evaluate client for:

- Evidence of improvement in symptoms of depression
- Reports of improved appetite, ↑ sense of well being, and evidence of socialization
- Prevention of bed wetting
- Reports of control of severe neurogenic pain
- Laboratory evidence of therapeutic serum drug levels (200–350 ng/ml)

Immune Globulin IV (Human)

(im-MYOUN GLOH-byou-lin)

Gamastan✿, Gamimune N, Gammagard, Immune Serum Globulin✿, Sandoglobulin, Venoglobulin-I (Rx)

Classification: IgG antibody product. **Note:** The available products differ significantly with respect to the process by which they are made (e.g., donor pool and fractionation/purification) as well as isotonicity. Thus, information on each product should be carefully read before use.

Action/Kinetics: Immune globulin IV is a polyvalent antibody product derived from a human volunteer pool. It contains the various IgG antibodies normally occurring in humans. The products may also contain traces of IgA and IgM. Plasma in the manufacturing pool has been found nonreactive for hepatitis B antigen. Also, there have been no documented cases of viral transmission. The antibodies present in the products will cause both opsonization and neutralization of microbes and toxins. The reconstituted products may contain sucrose, maltose, protein, and/or small amounts of sodium chloride. Doses of immune globulin IV will restore abnormally low IgG levels to within the normal range with equilibrium reached between the intra- and extravascular compartments within 6 days. The percentage of IgG in the products is over 90%. $t\frac{1}{2}$: Gamimune N and Sandoglobulin, 3 weeks; Venoglobulin-I, 29 days.

Use: Severe combined immunodeficiency and primary immunoglobulin deficiency syndromes, including congenital agammaglobulinemia, X-linked agammaglobulinemia, and Wiskott-Aldrich syndrome. Acute and chronic idiopathic thrombocytopenic purpura in both children and adults. B-cell chronic lymphocytic leukemia (Gammagard).

Contraindications: Clients with selective IgA deficiency who have antibodies to IgA (the products contain IgA). Sensitivity to human immune globulin.

Special Concerns: Pregnancy category: C. The various products are used for different conditions and at different doses; thus, check information carefully.

Side Effects: Headache. Hypersensitivity or anaphylactic reactions. Agammaglobulinemic and hypogammaglobulinemic clients never having received immunoglobulin therapy or where the time from the last treatment is more than 8 weeks may manifest side effects if the infusion rate exceeds 1 ml/min. Symptoms include flushing of the face, hypotension, tightness in chest, chills, fever, dizziness, diaphoresis, and nausea.

Dosage: IV only for all products.

Gamimune N. *Immunodeficiency syndrome:* 100–200 mg/kg given once a month; if response is satisfactory, dose can be increased to 400 mg/kg or infusion may be repeated more frequently than once a month. Rate of infusion: 0.01–0.02 ml/kg/min for 30 min; if no discomfort is experienced, the rate can be increased up to 0.08 ml/kg/min. *Idiopathic thrombocytopenic purpura:* 400 mg/kg for 5 consecutive days.

Gammagard. *Immunodeficiency syndrome:* 200–400 mg/kg (minimum of 100 mg/kg monthly). *B-cell lymphocytic leukemia:* 400 mg/kg q 3–4 weeks. *Idiopathic thrombocytopenic purpura:* 1,000 mg/kg; additional doses depend on platelet count (up to 3 doses can be given on alternate days). Rate of infusion: 0.5 ml/kg initially; may be increased gradually to 4 ml/kg/hr if there is no patient distress.

Sandoglobulin. *Immunodeficiency syndrome:* 200 mg/kg once monthly; increase to 300 mg/kg if client response satisfactory (i.e., IgG serum level of 300 mg/dl). Rate of administration: 3% solution at an initial rate of 0.5–1 ml/min; after 15–30 min can increase to 1.5–2.5 ml/min (subsequent infusions at a rate of 2–2.5 ml/min). If the 6%

solution is used, the initial infusion rate should be 1–1.5 ml/min and increased after 15–30 min to a maximum of 2.5 ml/min. *Idiopathic thrombocytopenic purpura:* 400 mg/kg for 2–5 consecutive days.

Venoglobulin-I. *Immunodeficiency disease:* 200 mg/kg monthly; can increase to 300–400 mg/kg if response is insufficient or can repeat infusion more frequently than once monthly. *Idiopathic thrombocytopenic purpura:* **Induction:** 500 mg/kg for 2–7 consecutive days; **maintenance:** 500–2,000 mg/kg as a single infusion q 2 weeks or less if platelet count falls to <30,000/μl.

NURSING CONSIDERATIONS

Administration/Storage

1. Follow the administration guidelines explicitly and follow the manufacturer's directions carefully for reconstitution of either the 3% or 6% solution.
2. In agamma- or hypogammaglobulinemic clients, the 3% solution should be used. Initially, administer at a rate of 10–20 drops/min (0.5–1 ml/min). After 15–30 min the rate may be increased to 30–50 drops/min (1.5–2.5 ml/min). Subsequent infusions may be given at a rate of 40–50 drops/min (2–2.5 ml/min). If the first bottle of the 3% solution is given in these clients with good tolerance, subsequent infusions may be given using the 6% solution.
3. The solutions should not be shaken because excessive foaming will occur.
4. The solution should be infused only if it is clear and at room temperature.
5. These products should be given only IV because the IM or SC routes have not been evaluated.
6. These products should be given by a separate IV line without mixing with other IV fluids or medications.
7. A rapid decrease in serum IgG level in the first week postinfusion will be observed; this is expected and is due to the equilibration of IgG between the plasma and extravascular space.
8. Utilize an electronic infusion device for administration.
9. Epinephrine should be readily available in the event of an acute anaphylactic reaction.

Interventions

1. Monitor vital signs throughout the infusion.
2. If the client develops hypotension, decrease or interrupt the rate of infusion until the hypotension subsides.
3. Administer drug therapy in a closely monitored environment.
4. Monitor liver function studies, hematologic values, IgG levels, and appropriate blood and urine chemistries.

Client/Family Teaching

1. Explain that drug may cause nausea, vomiting, fever, chills, flushing, lightheadedness, and tightness in the chest. These symptoms should be reported to the physician immediately because they may be related to the dosage and rate of drug administration.
2. Discuss the need to have drug therapy once a month to maintain appropriate IgG serum levels.

3. Explain that the drug is derived from human plasma and discuss the associated potential risks.

Evaluation: Evaluate client for:

- Laboratory evidence that IgG serum levels are within normal range following treatment
- Clinical evidence of passive immunity and ↑ platelet counts
- Freedom from complications of drug therapy

Indapamide
(in-**DAP**-ah-myd)
Lozide ❋, Lozol (Rx)

See also *Diuretics,* p. 140, and *Thiazide Diuretics,* p. 231.

Classification: Diuretic, thiazide type.

Action/Kinetics: Onset: 1–2 weeks after multiple doses. **Peak levels:** 2 hr. **Duration:** Up to 8 weeks with multiple doses. **t½:** 14 hr. Nearly 100% is absorbed from the GI tract. Excreted through the kidneys (70% with 7% unchanged) and the GI tract (23%).

Uses: Alone or in combination with other drugs for treatment of hypertension. Edema in congestive heart failure.

Special Concerns: Pregnancy category: B. Dosage has not been established in children. Geriatric clients may be more sensitive to the hypotensive and electrolyte effects.

Dosage: Tablets. *Edema, hypertension,* **adults:** 2.5 mg in the morning. If necessary, may be increased to 5 mg daily after 1 week if treating edema and 4 weeks if treating hypertension.

NURSING CONSIDERATIONS

See also *Nursing Considerations* for *Diuretics,* p. 141 and *Antihypertensive Agents,* p. 78.

Administration/Storage

1. May be combined with other antihypertensive agents if the response is inadequate. Initially, the dose of other agents should be reduced by 50%.
2. Doses greater than 5 mg daily do not increase effectiveness but may increase hypokalemia.

Evaluation: Evaluate client for:

- ↓ blood pressure
- ↑ urinary output, ↓ edema and rales with improvement in signs and symptoms of CHF

Indecainide hydrochloride
(in-deh-**KANE**-eyed)
Decabid (Rx)

Classification: Antiarrhythmic drug, Class IC.

Action/Kinetics: Although the mechanism of action is not known with certainty, indecainide is thought to block sodium movement into Purkinje and myocardial cells resulting in stabilization of the cell membrane and a slowing of conduction of cardiac impulses. Both AV and intraventricular conduction velocities are slowed with an increase in the AV nodal effective refractory period. At doses of 200 mg daily, the drug significantly reduces left ventricular ejection fraction both at rest and during exercise. Food has no effect on absorption and there is no first-pass effect. **Peak serum levels:** 4 hr. **t½:** Approximately 8 hr in normal clients. Indecainide is metabolized in the liver to inactive and one active (desisopropylindecainide) metabolite. Approximately 80% excreted in the urine (65% unchanged) and 17% in the feces.

Uses: Treatment of life-threatening ventricular arrhythmias (such as sustained ventricular tachycardia). Use should be reserved for those clients in whom benefits outweigh the risks of using the drug.

Contraindications: Use for less severe ventricular arrhythmias. Pre-existing second-or third-degree AV block or right bundle branch block associated with a left hemiblock (unless client has a pacemaker to sustain cardiac rhythm). Cardiogenic shock. Use during lactation.

Special Concerns: Pregnancy category: B. Safety and effectiveness have not been determined in children less than 18 years of age. Use with caution in clients with impaired renal function. Use with extreme caution in clients with sick sinus syndrome (drug may cause sinus bradycardia, sinus pause, or sinus arrest).

Side Effects: *CV:* Possibly increased mortality or nonfatal cardiac arrest in clients with asymptomatic non-life–threatening ventricular arrhythmias who experienced a myocardial infarction between 6 days and 2 years before use of the drug (this effect noted with use of encainide or flecainide). Proarrhythmic effects including new or worsening of arrhythmias; causing or worsening of congestive heart failure. Possibility of increased pacemaker thresholds. First- and third-degree AV block, syncope, sinus bradycardia, sinus pause, sinus arrest, angina pectoris, hypertension, hypotension, bundle branch block, palpitations. *GI:* Nausea, abdominal pain, constipation, diarrhea, dry mouth, dyspepsia, alteration in taste, vomiting. *CNS:* Dizziness, headache, circumoral paresthesia, insomnia, anxiety, emotional lability, vertigo, abnormal dreams, agitation, ataxia, confusion, nervousness, paresthesia, hypesthesia, seizures. *Respiratory:* Dyspnea, rhinitis, increased cough, chest pain. *Whole body:* Asthenia, back pain, general pain, fever, malaise. *Dermatologic:* Rash (including maculopapular or petechial), urticaria. *Hematologic:* Eosinophilia, anemia, leukopenia, thrombocytopenia. *Miscellaneous:* Hyperglycemia, tinnitus, diplopia, abnormal accommodation, arthralgia.

Drug Interactions

Antiarrhythmic drugs / Additive pharmacologic effects
Cimetidine / Significant ↑ in serum levels of indecainide

Laboratory Test Interfernces: ↑ BUN, creatinine clearance, AST, ALT.

Dosage: Extended-release Tablets. Adults, initial: 50 mg b.i.d. at 12-hr intervals. After a minimum of 4 days, dose can be increased to 75 mg b.i.d. if necessary. If the desired effect is not observed after 4 more days, the dosage may be increased to 100 mg b.i.d. Some clients may require as much as 300 mg daily and should be hospitalized for initial dosing at this level. In clients with a creatinine clearance of 30 ml/min or less, therapy should be initiated with a single daily dose of 50 mg; the dose may be increased to 75 mg once daily after 7 days. Thereafter, increase dose slowly (no more frequently than q 7 days) up to a maximum of 150 mg daily if necessary.

NURSING CONSIDERATIONS

See also *Nursing Considerations* for *Antiarrhythmic Drugs,* p. 52.

Administration/Storage

1. Therapy should be initiated in a hospital with facilities for monitoring cardiac rhythm because many of the serious proarrhythmic effects are observed within the first 1–2 weeks of therapy.
2. Extended-release tablets should be swallowed whole and not crushed or chewed.
3. Increments in dosage should not be undertaken more often than every 4 days.
4. When transferring clients from other antiarrhythmic drugs, the drug should be withdrawn for 2–5 plasma half-lives before beginning indecainide therapy. If withdrawal is potentially life-threatening, the client should be hospitalized and closely monitored.

Assessment

1. Obtain baseline ECG to determine if client has any evidence of advanced AV block because drug is contraindicated under these circumstances.
2. Note any client history of congestive heart failure.

Interventions

1. Indecainide is recommended only for the treatment of life-threatening ventricular arrhythmias. Client should be in a closely monitored environment and have rhythm strips to document these arrhythmias before, during, and throughout initial dosing adjustments.
2. Review serum electrolytes. Preexisting hypokalemia or hyperkalemia should be corrected before administration of indecainide.
3. Note renal function studies to determine if there is any evidence of impairment. Anticipate reduced dose and dosing intervals of 7 days when adjusting the dosage for clients with renal dysfunction.
4. Observe clients for complaints of dizziness, weakness, chest pain, or dyspnea because these are frequent side effects of drug therapy and should be documented and reported to the physician.

Evaluation

1. Evaluate client for successful termination of lethal ventricular arrhythmias.
2. Clients treated successfully with indecainide usually manifest trough serum levels between 300–600 mcg/L.

Indomethacin

(in-doh-**METH**-ah-sin)

Aspo-Indomethacin✷, Indocid✷, Indocid Ophthalmic Suspension✷, Indocid PDA✷, Indocin, Indocin SR, Novo–Methacin✷, Nu-Indo✷ (Rx)

Indomethacin sodium trihydrate

(in-doh-**METH**-ah-sin)

Indocin I.V. (Rx)

See also *Nonsteroidal Anti-Inflammatory Drugs,* p. 186.

Classification: Anti-inflammatory, analgesic, antipyretic.

Action/Kinetics: Indomethacin is not considered to be a simple analgesic and should only be used for the conditions listed. **PO. Onset:** 30 min for analgesia and up to 1 week for anti-inflammatory effect. **Peak plasma levels:** 1–2 hr (2–4 hr for sustained-release). **Duration:** 4–6 hr for analgesia and 1–2 weeks for anti-inflammatory effect. **Therapeutic plasma levels:** 10–18 mcg/ml. **t½:** Approximately 5 hr (up to 6 hr for sustained-release). **Plasma t½ following IV in infants:** 12–20 hr, depending on age and dose. Approximately 90% plasma protein bound. The drug is metabolized in the liver and excreted in both the urine and feces.

Uses: Moderate to severe rheumatoid arthritis, osteoarthritis, ankylosing spondylitis (drug of choice). Acute gouty arthritis, tendinitis, bursitis, acute painful shoulder. *IV:* Pharmacologic closure of persistent patent ductus arteriosus in premature infants. *Investigational:* Topically to treat cystoid macular edema (0.5% and 1% drops), sunburn, primary dysmenorrhea, prophylaxis of migraine, cluster headache, polyhydramnios.

Additional Contraindications: Pregnancy. Oral indomethacin in children under 14 years of age. GI lesions or history of recurrent GI lesions. *IV use:* GI or intracranial bleeding, thrombocytopenia, renal disease, defects of coagulation, necrotizing enterocolitis. *Suppositories:* Recent rectal bleeding, history of proctitis.

Special Concerns: Use in children should be restricted to those unresponsive to or intolerant of other anti-inflammatory agents. Geriatric clients are at greater risk of developing CNS side effects, especially confusion. To be used with caution in clients with history of epilepsy, psychiatric illness, parkinsonism, and in the elderly. Indomethacin should be used with extreme caution in the presence of existing, controlled infections.

Additional Side Effects: Reactivation of latent infections may mask signs of infection. More marked CNS manifestations than for other drugs of this group. Aggravation of depression or other psychiatric problems, epilepsy, and parkinsonism.

Additional Drug Interactions

Captopril / Indomethacin ↓ effect of captopril, probably due to inhibition of prostaglandin synthesis
Diflunisal / ↑ Plasma levels of indomethacin; also, possible fatal GI hemorrhage
Diuretics (loop, potassium-sparing, thiazide) / Indomethacin may reduce the antihypertensive and natriuretic action of diuretics
Lisinopril / Possible ↓ effect of lisinopril
Prazosin / Indomethacin ↓ antihypertensive effects of prazosin

Dosage: Capsules, Oral Suspension. *Moderate to severe arthritis, osteoarthritis, ankylosing spondylitis:* **Initial:** 25 mg b.i.d.–t.i.d.; may be increased by 25–50 mg at weekly intervals, according to condition, until satisfactory response is obtained. **Maximum daily dosage:** 150–200 mg. In acute flares of chronic rheumatoid arthritis, the dose may need to be increased by 25–50 mg daily until the acute phase is under control. *Gouty arthritis:* **Initial:** 50 mg t.i.d. until pain is tolerable; **then,** reduce dosage rapidly until drug is withdrawn. *Bursitis/tendinitis:* 75–150 mg/day in 3–4 divided doses for 1–2 weeks. **Extended-release Capsules.** *Antirheumatic, anti-inflammatory:* **Adults:** 75 mg, of which 25 mg is released immediately, 1–2 times daily.

Suppositories. *Anti-inflammatory, antirheumatic, antigout:* **Adults:** 50 mg up to q.i.d. **Pediatric:** 1.5–2.5 mg/kg daily in 3–4 divided doses (up to a maximum of 4 mg/kg or 250–200 mg daily, whichever is less).

IV only. *Patent ductus arteriosus:* 3 IV doses, depending on age of the infant, are given at 12- to 24-hr intervals. **Infants less than 2 days:** first dose, 0.2 mg/kg, followed by 2 doses of 0.1 mg/kg each; **infants 2–7 days:** 3 doses of 0.2 mg/kg each; **infants more than 7 days:** first dose, 0.2 mg/kg, followed by 2 doses of 0.25 mg/kg each. If patent ductus arteriosus reopens, a second course of 1–3 doses may be given. Surgery may be required if there is no response after 2 courses of therapy.

NURSING CONSIDERATIONS

See also *Nursing Considerations for Nonsteroidal Anti-Inflammatory Drugs,* p. 189.

Administration/Storage

1. Store in amber-colored containers.
2. The IV solution should be prepared with sodium chloride injection or water for injection. Diluent should not contain preservatives.
3. IV solutions should be freshly prepared prior to use.
4. The IV solution should be given over 5–10 sec.
5. Up to 100 mg of the total daily dose can be given at bedtime for clients with night pain or morning stiffness.
6. The sustained-release form should not be crushed and should not be used in clients with acute gouty arthritis.
7. If the client has difficulty swallowing capsules, the contents may be emptied into applesauce, food, or liquid to assure that the client receives the prescribed dose.
8. Suppositories (50 mg) may be used in clients unable to take oral medication. They should be stored below 30°C (86°F).
9. Anticipate a peak action of drug to occur in 24–36 hr in clients taking the medication for gout.
10. Peak drug activity in clients taking the medication for antirheumatic effect will occur in about 4 weeks.
11. The smallest effective dose of the drug should be administered, based on individual need. Adverse reactions are dose related.

Interventions

1. Monitor intake and output. If clients are experiencing nausea or vomiting, additionally monitor and record their weights.
2. Inspect the urine for signs of hematuria. Also monitor for signs and symptoms of anemia and report these to the physician.
3. If any adverse side effects occur, withhold the drug and report to the physician. Many of the adverse responses may be serious enough to discontinue the medication.

4. Indomethacin masks infections. Therefore, assess clients carefully, reporting any incidence of fever.

Client/Family Teaching

1. Report for scheduled ophthalmologic examinations and lab studies, especially if receiving long-term therapy.
2. Use caution when operating potentially hazardous equipment because of possible lightheadedness and decreased alertness.
3. Take the medication with food or milk to decrease GI upset.
4. Remind clients that it will take from 2–4 weeks of therapy before they will see significant improvement in arthritic conditions. Therefore, they should follow the prescribed drug regimen carefully and refrain from becoming discouraged.
5. Stress the importance of reporting any side effects from drug therapy immediately to the physician.

Evaluation

1. Evaluate client for reports of control of pain and improved joint mobility.
2. Assess for evidence of closure of patent ductus arteriosus in premature infants following IV administration.

Insulin injection (crystalline zinc insulin, unmodified insulin, regular insulin)

(IN-sue-lin)

Single peak: Regular Iletin I (beef and pork), Regular Insulin (pork). Purified: Regular Iletin II (beef), Regular Iletin II (pork), Regular Purified Pork Insulin, Velosulin (pork). Human: Humulin R, Humulin BR, Novolin R, Novolin R, PenFill, Velosulin. (OTC)

See also *Insulins,* p. 156, and *Human Insulin,* p. 713.

Classification: Rapid-acting insulin.

Action/Kinetics: This product is rarely administered as the sole agent due to its short duration of action. Injections of 100 units/ml are clear; cloudy, colored solutions should not be used. Regular insulin is the only preparation suitable for IV administration. Is available only as 100 units/ml. **Onset, SC:** 30–60 min; **IV:** 10–30 min. **Peak, SC:** 2–4 hr; **IV:** 15–30 min. **Duration, SC:** 6–8 hr; **IV:** 30–60 min.

Uses: Suitable for treatment of diabetic coma, diabetic acidosis, or other emergency situations. Especially suitable for the client suffering from labile diabetes.

During acute phase of diabetic acidosis or for the client in diabetic crisis, client is monitored by serum glucose and serum ketone levels.

Dosage: SC, Individualized. Adults: usual, initial: 5–10 units; **pediatric:** 2–4 units. Injection is given 15–30 min before meals and at bedtime. *Diabetic ketoacidosis:* **Adults:** 0.1 unit/kg/hr given by continuous IV infusion.

NURSING CONSIDERATIONS

See also *Nursing Considerations* for *Insulins,* p. 160.

Administration/Storage

1. When used IV, the rate of insulin infusion should be de-

creased when plasma glucose levels reach 250 mg/dl.

2. Due to the short half-life of regular insulin, large single IV doses should not be administered.

Insulin injection, concentrated

(IN-sue-lin)
Regular (Concentrated) Iletin II U-500 (Rx)

See also *Insulins,* p. 156.

Classification: Insulin, concentrated.

Action/Kinetics: This concentrated preparation (500 units/ml) of insulin injection (see above) is indicated for clients with a marked resistance to insulin who require more than 200 units/day. Clients must be kept under close observation until dosage is established. Depending on response, dosage may be given SC or IM as a single or as two or three divided doses.

Not suitable for IV administration because of possible allergic or anaphylactoid reactions.

Uses: Diabetic clients requiring more than 200 units insulin/day.

Contraindications: Allergy to pork or mixed pork/beef insulin (unless client has been desensitized).

Additional Side Effects: Deep secondary hypoglycemia 18–24 hr after administration.

Dosage: SC, IM: *Individualized.*

NURSING CONSIDERATIONS

See also *Nursing Considerations* for *Insulins,* p. 160.

Administration/Storage

1. Administer only water clear solutions (concentrated insulin may appear straw-colored).
2. Use a tuberculin type or insulin syringe for accuracy of measurement.
3. Deep secondary hypoglycemia may occur 18–24 hr after administration. Therefore, have 10%–20% dextrose solution or dextrose 50% bristojets available.
4. Keep insulin cool or refrigerated.

Interventions

1. Observe the client closely for signs and symptoms of hyper- or hypoglycemia during the period when the dosage is being established.
2. Monitor blood glucose levels frequently.

Client/Family Teaching: Teach the client to be alert for signs of hypoglycemia, which may indicate that responsiveness to insulin has been regained, and that a reduction in dosage is warranted.

Evaluation: Evaluate client for laboratory evidence that serum glucose is within desired range.

Insulin zinc suspension (Lente)

(IN-sue-lin)
Single Peak: Lente Iletin I (beef and pork), Lente Insulin (beef). Purified: Lente Iletin II (beef), Lente Iletin II (pork), Lente Purified Pork Insulin. Human: Humulin L, Novolin L. (OTC)

See also *Insulins,* p. 156.

Classification: Intermediate-acting insulin.

Action/Kinetics: Principal advantage is the absence of a sensitizing agent such as protamine. **Onset:** 1–2.5 hr. **Peak:** 7–15 hr. **Duration:** 18–28 hr.

Uses: Useful in clients allergic to other types of insulin and in clients disposed to thrombotic phenomena in which protamine may be a factor. Zinc insulin is not a replacement for regular insulin and is not suitable for emergency use.

Dosage: SC. Adults, initial: 7–26 units 30–60 min before breakfast. Dosage is then increased by daily or weekly increments of 2–10 units until satisfactory readjustment is established. A second smaller dose may be given prior to the evening meal or at bedtime.

Clients on NPH can be transferred to insulin zinc suspension on a unit-for-unit basis. Clients being transferred from regular insulin should begin zinc insulin at two-thirds to three-fourths the regular insulin dosage. If the client is being transferred from protamine zinc insulin, the dose of zinc insulin should be about 50% of that required for protamine zinc insulin.

NURSING CONSIDERATIONS

See *Nursing Considerations* for *Insulins,* p. 160.

Insulin zinc suspension, extended
Single Peak: Ultralente Iletin I (beef and pork), Ultralente Insulin (beef). Human: Humulin U Ultralente.

See also *Insulins,* p. 156.

Classification: Long-acting insulin.

Action/Kinetics: Large crystals of insulin and a high content of zinc are responsible for the slow-acting properties of this preparation. Products containing both 40 units/ml and 100 units/ml are available. **Onset:** 4–8 hr. **Peak:** 10–30 hr. **Duration:** 36 hr or longer.

Uses: Mild to moderate hyperglycemia in stabilized diabetics. Not suitable for the treatment of diabetic coma or emergency situations.

Dosage: SC. *Individualized.* **Usual, initial:** 7–26 units as a single dose 30–60 min before breakfast. **Do not administer IV.**

NURSING CONSIDERATIONS

See *Nursing Considerations* for *Insulins,* p. 160.

Insulin zinc suspension prompt (Semilente)
(IN-sue-lin)
Single Peak: Semilente Iletin I (beef and pork), Semilente Insulin (beef). (OTC)

See also *Insulins,* p. 156.

Classification: Fast-acting insulin.

Action/Kinetics: Contains small particles of zinc insulin in a nearly colorless suspension. Not suitable for emergency use. Cannot be injected IV. **Onset:** 1–1.5 hr. **Peak:** 5–10 hr. **Duration:** 12–16 hr.

Uses: In combination with insulin zinc or extended insulin zinc suspensions to control diabetes. May also be used alone for rapid control when initiating therapy.

**Dosage: SC. Individualized.
Adults, initial:** 10–20 units 30 min
before breakfast. A second daily
dose is usually required.

NURSING CONSIDERATIONS

See *Nursing Considerations* for
Insulins, p. 160.

Interferon alfa-2a recombinant (rI FN-A; IFLrA)

(in-ter-**FEER**-on **AL**-fah)
Roferon-A (Rx)

Classification: Antineoplastic, miscellaneous agent.

Action/Kinetics: Interferon alfa-
2a is the product of recombinant
DNA technology using strains of
genetically engineered *Escherichia
coli.* The activity of these drugs is
expressed as International Units,
which are determined by comparing the antiviral activity of recombinant interferons with the activity
of the international reference standard of human leukocyte interferon. Interferons bind to specific
receptors on the cell surface, resulting in inhibition of virus replication
in virus-infected cells, suppression
of cell proliferation, increase in the
phagocytic activity of macrophages,
and enhancement of the toxic effects of leukocytes for target cells.
Interferon A-2a. **Peak serum levels:** 3.8–7.3 hr. **t½:** 3.7–8.5 hr. The
drug is metabolized by the kidney.

Use: Hairy cell leukemia in clients
older than 18 years of age. Can be
used in splenectomized and nonsplenectomized clients. AIDS-related Kaposi's sarcoma in clients older
than 18 years of age. *Investigational:* The drug has been used for a
large number of other conditions.
Significant activity has been noted
against the following neoplastic
diseases: locally for superficial bladder tumors, carcinoid tumor,
chronic myelogenous leukemia,
cutaneous T-cell lymphoma, essential thrombocythemia, low-grade
non-Hodgkin's lymphoma. Limited
activity has been noted in acute
leukemias, cervical carcinoma,
chronic lymphocytic leukemia,
Hodgkin's disease, malignant
gliomas, melanoma, multiple myeloma, nasopharyngeal carcinoma,
osteosarcoma, ovarian carcinoma,
renal carcinoma. Interferon alfa-2a
has also been used to treat the
following viral infections: chronic
non-A, non-B hepatitis, condylomata acuminata, cutaneous
warts, cytomegaloviruses, herpes
keratoconjunctivitis, herpes simplex, papillomaviruses, rhinoviruses, vaccinia virus, varicella
zoster, and viral hepatitis B.

Contraindications: Lactation.

Special Concerns: Pregnancy category: C (use during pregnancy
only if clearly required). Use with
caution in clients with a history of
unstable angina, uncontrolled congestive heart failure, chronic obstructive pulmonary disease, diabetes mellitus prone to ketoacidosis,
thrombophlebitis, pulmonary embolism, seizure disorders, severe
renal and hepatic disease, compromised CNS function, and severe
myelosuppression. Safety and efficacy in individuals less than 18
years of age have not been established.

Side Effects: *Flu-like symptoms:*
Fever, headache, fatigue, arthralgia,
myalgias, chills. *CV:* Hypotension,
arrhythmias, syncope, hyperten-

sion, edema, chest pain, palpitations, transient ischemic attacks, pulmonary edema, myocardial infarction, congestive heart failure, stroke, hot flashes, Raynaud's phenomenon. *Respiratory:* Coughing, dyspnea, chest congestion, bronchospasm, tachypnea, rhinitis, rhinorrhea, sinusitis. *CNS:* Depression, confusion, dizziness, paresthesia, anxiety, nervousness, numbness, lethargy, sleep disturbances, visual disturbances, vertigo, decreased mental status, forgetfulness. *GI:* Anorexia, nausea, vomiting, diarrhea, hypermotility, abdominal fullness, abdominal pain, flatulence, constipation, gastric distress. *Hematologic:* Thrombocytopenia, neutropenia, leukopenia, decreased hemoglobin. *Musculoskeletal:* Myalgia, arthralgia, muscle contractions. *Dermatologic:* Rash, inflammation or dryness of the oropharynx, pruritus, dry skin, skin flushing, alopecia, urticaria. *Other:* Taste alteration, hepatitis, weight loss, diaphoresis, transient impotence, conjunctivitis, night sweats, excessive salivation, reactivation of herpes labialis, muscle contractions, cyanosis, eye irritation, earache.

Laboratory Test Interferences: ↑ AST, ALT, LDH, BUN, serum creatinine, alkaline phosphatase, bilirubin, uric acid, serum glucose, serum phosphorus. ↓ Hematocrit, hemoglobin. Hypocalcemia, proteinuria.

Dosage: IM, SC: *Hairy cell leukemia:* **induction,** 3 million IU/day for 16–24 weeks; **maintenance,** 3 million IU 3 times weekly. Doses higher than 3 million IU are not recommended. *AIDS-related Kaposi's sarcoma:* **IM, SC: induction,** 36 million IU/day for 10–12 weeks; or, 3 million IU/day on days 1–3; 9 million IU/day on days 4–6;

and 18 million IU/day on days 7–9 followed by 36 million IU/day for the remainder of the 10–12 week induction period. **Maintenance:** 36 million IU 3 times weekly. If severe side effects occur, the dose can be withheld or reduced by one-half.

NURSING CONSIDERATIONS

Administration/Storage

1. Treatment should be discontinued if the hairy cell leukemia does not respond within 6 months.
2. If severe reactions occur, the dose of the drug can be reduced by one-half or individual doses may be withheld. Also, assess the effect on bone marrow of previous x-ray therapy or chemotherapy.
3. Although the optimal duration of treatment has not been established, clients have been treated for up to 20 consecutive months.
4. The SC route of administration should be considered for clients who have a platelet count less than 50,000/mm³.

Interventions

1. Acetaminophen may be used to treat side effects of fever and headache.
2. Flu-like symptoms may be minimized by administering the drug at bedtime.
3. Clients should be well hydrated, especially when therapy is initiated.
4. Anticipate that hypotension may occur up to 2 days following drug therapy.

Client/Family Teaching

1. The most common side effects are flu-like symptoms, such as

fever, fatigue, headache, chills, nausea, and loss of appetite, and these symptoms may be minimized by taking the drug at bedtime. Notify physician if pronounced.

2. Flu-like symptoms usually diminish in severity as treatment continues.

3. Drink plenty of fluids during therapy.

4. Do not change brands of interferon without consulting physician because changes in dosage may occur with a different brand.

5. Stress the importance of reporting for laboratory tests, including CBC, electrolyte levels, and liver function studies as scheduled.

6. Report any evidence of neurologic or psychological disturbances.

7. Advise that hair loss may occur.

8. Practice contraception.

Evaluation: Evaluate client for:
- Evidence of a ↓ in tumor size and spread
- Laboratory findings of improved hematologic parameters in clients with hairy cell leukemia
- Reports and evidence of a reduction in lesions with Kaposi's sarcoma

---

Interferon alfa-2b recombinant (rI FN-α2; α-2-interferon)

(in-ter-**FEER**-on **AL**-fah)
Intron A, Wellferon ✲ (Rx)

Classification: Antineoplastic, miscellaneous agent.

Action/Kinetics: Interferon alpha-2b is a product of recombinant DNA technology using strains of genetically engineered *Escherichia coli.* The activity is expressed as International Units, which are determined by comparing the antiviral activity of the recombinant interferon with the activity of the international reference standard of human leukocyte interferon. Interferons bind to specific receptors on the cell surface, resulting in inhibition of virus replication in virus-infected cells, suppression of cell proliferation, increase in the phagocytic activity of macrophages, and enhancement of the toxic effects of leukocytes for target cells. *Interferon alpha-2b.* **Peak serum levels after IM, SC:** up to 116 IU/ml after 3–12 hr. $t^{1/2}$, **IM, SC:** 6–7 hr. **Peak serum levels after IV infusion:** up to 270 IU/ml at the end of the infusion. $t^{1/2}$, **IV:** 2 hr. The main site of metabolism may be the kidney.

Use: Hairy cell leukemia in clients older than 18 years of age. Can be used in splenectomized and nonsplenectomized clients. Intralesional use for genital or venereal warts (*Condylomata acuminata.*) AIDS-related Kaposi's sarcoma. Chronic hepatitis non-A, non-B/C in clients at least 18 years of age with compensated liver disease and a history of blood or blood product exposure or who are HIV antibody positive. *Investigational:* The drug has been used for a large number of conditions. Significant activity has been noted against the following neoplastic diseases: locally for superficial bladder tumors, carcinoid tumor, chronic myelogenous leukemia, cutaneous T-cell lymphoma, essential thrombocythemia, and low-grade non-Hodgkin's lymphoma. Limited activity has been noted in acute leukemias, cervical carcinoma, chronic lymphocytic leukemia, Hodgkin's disease, malignant gliomas, melanoma, multiple myeloma, nasopharyngeal carcinoma, osteosarcoma, ovarian carcinoma, renal carcinoma. Interferon alfa-2b has also been used to treat the following viral infections: cutaneous warts, cytomegaloviruses, herpes keratoconjunctivitis, herpes simplex, papillomaviruses, rhinoviruses, vaccinia virus, varicella zoster, and viral hepatitis B.

Contraindications: Lactation.

Special Concerns: Pregnancy category: C (use only if clearly required). Use with caution in clients with a history of unstable angina, uncontrolled congestive heart failure, chronic obstructive pulmonary disease, diabetes mellitus prone to ketoacidosis, thrombophlebitis, pulmonary embolism, seizure disorders, severe renal and hepatic disease, compromised CNS function, and severe myelosuppression. Safety and efficacy in individuals less than 18 years of age have not been established.

Side Effects: *Flu-like symptoms:* Fever, headache, fatigue, myalgia, chills. *CV:* Hypotension, arrhythmias, tachycardia, syncope, hypertension, coagulation disorders, chest pain, palpitations, flushing. *CNS:* Depression, confusion, somnolence, migraine, dizziness, ataxia, paresthesia, vertigo, anxiety, nervousness, insomnia, emotional lability, amnesia, impaired concentration, weakness, tremor, impotence, syncope, abnormal coordination, hypoesthesia. *GI:* Nausea, vomiting, diarrhea, stomatitis, paralytic ileus, alteration of taste, weight loss, anorexia, dyspepsia, flatulence, dry mouth, thirst, dehydration, constipation, eructation, abdominal pain. *Hematologic:* Thrombocytopenia, transient granulocytopenia. *Musculoskeletal:* Arthralgia, leg cramps, asthenia, arthrosis, back pain, bone disorders, rigors. *Respiratory:* Pharyngitis, coughing, dyspnea, sinusitis, rhinitis, epistaxis, nasal congestion. *EENT:* Alteration of taste, tinnitus, hearing disorders, conjunctivitis, photophobia, vision disorders, eye pain. *Dermatologic:* Rash, pruritus, alopecia, urticaria, dry skin, dermatitis, purpura, photosensitivity, acne, nail disorder, facial edema. *Other:* Pain, increased sweating, malaise, decreased libido, urinary frequency, menorrhagia, herpes simplex, lymphadenopathy, chest pain.

Drug Interactions

Aminophylline / ↓ Clearance of aminophylline due to ↓ breakdown by the liver
Zidovudine / ↑ Risk of neutropenia

Laboratory Test Interferences: ↑ AST, ALT, LDH, BUN, serum creatinine, alkaline phosphatase. ↓ Hematocrit, hemoglobin.

Dosage: IM, SC. *Hairy cell leukemia:* 2 million IU/m^2 3 times a week. Higher doses are not recommended. *AIDS-related Kaposi's sarcoma:* **IM, SC,** 30 million IU/m^2 3 times a week using only the 50 million IU vial. Using this dose, clients should tolerate an average dose of 110 million IU/week at the end of 12 weeks of therapy and 75 million IU/week at the end of 24 weeks of therapy. *Chronic hepatitis non-A, non-B/C:* 3 million IU 3 times weekly for up to 6 months.

Therapy should be discontinued if there is no response after 16 weeks.

Intralesional. *Genital or venereal warts:* 1 million IU/lesion 3 times weekly for 3 weeks. For this purpose, use only the vial containing 10 million units and reconstitute using no more than 1 ml diluent.

NURSING CONSIDERATIONS

See also *Nursing Considerations* for *Interferon alfa-2a Recombinant*, p. 749, and *Interferon alfa-n3*, p. 753.

Administration/Storage

1. Prior to administration, the drug must be reconstituted with bacteriostatic water for injection, which is provided. After reconstitution, the solution is stable for 1 month at 2°C–8°C (36°F–46°F).
2. If severe side effects occur, the dose can be reduced as much as 50% or therapy can be discontinued until side effects improve.
3. Treatment for hairy cell leukemia should be discontinued if the client does not respond within 6 months.
4. When used for venereal or genital warts, maximum response usually occurs 4–8 weeks after therapy is initiated. If results are not satisfactory after 12–16 weeks, a second course of therapy may be undertaken.
5. Although the optimal duration of treatment has not been established, clients have been treated for up to 20 consecutive months.
6. If the platelet count is less than 50,000/mm³, the drug should be given SC rather than IM.

Interventions

1. Prior to and periodically during therapy, the levels of hemoglobin, platelets, granulocytes and hairy cells, and bone marrow hairy cells should be determined.
2. Acetaminophen may be used to treat side effects of fever and headache.
3. Flu-like symptoms may be minimized by administering the drug at bedtime.
4. Clients should be well hydrated, especially when therapy is initiated.

Evaluation

1. If a positive response to the drug is manifested, treatment should be continued until no further beneficial effects are observed and laboratory values have been stable for 3 months.
2. Assess for a decrease in the size and number of genital and/or venereal warts; re-evaluate need for continued treatment if warts persist.

Interferon alfa-n3
(in-ter-FEER-on AL-fah)
Alferon N (Rx)

Classification: Antineoplastic.

Action/Kinetics: Interferon alfa-n3 is made from pooled human leukocytes induced by incomplete infection with Sendai (avian) virus. The product is a sterile, aqueous formulation of purified, natural, human interferon alpha proteins. The drug binds to receptors on cell surfaces leading to a sequence of events including inhibition of virus replication and suppression of cell proliferation. Also, interferon alfa-n3 causes immunomodulation characterized by enhanced phagocytosis by macrophages, augmentation of the cytotoxicity of lymphocytes, and enhancement of human leukocyte antigen expression. Intralesional use of interferon alfa-n3 does not result in detectable plasma levels of the drug.

Uses: Intralesional treatment of refractory or recurring external condylomata acuminata (genital or venereal warts) in clients 18 years of age or older. *Investigational:* Alpha interferons are being tested for use in a large number of neoplastic diseases and viral infections.

Contraindications: Hypersensitivity to human interferon alpha; clients who are allergic to mouse immunoglobulin (IgG), egg protein, or neomycin (the production process involves a nutrient medium containing neomycin although it has not been detected in the final product). Lactation.

Special Concerns: Pregnancy category: C (use only if clearly needed). Due to the manifestation of fever and flu-like symptoms with interferon alfa-n3 use, the drug should be used with caution in clients with debilitating diseases including unstable angina, uncontrolled congestive heart failure, chronic obstructive pulmonary disease, diabetes mellitus with ketoacidosis, thrombophlebitis, pulmonary embolism, hemophilia, severe myelosuppression, or seizure disorders. Safety and effectiveness have not been determined in children less than 18 years of age.

Side Effects: *Flu-like symptoms:* Commonly, fever, headache, myalgias which decrease with repeated doses. Also, chills, fatigue, malaise. *CNS:* Dizziness, lightheadedness, insomnia, depression, nervousness, decreased ability to concentrate. *GI:* Nausea, vomiting, heartburn, diarrhea, tongue hyperesthesia, thirst, altered taste, increased salivation. *Musculoskeletal/Skin:* Arthralgia, back pain, hot sensation at bottom of feet, tingling of legs/feet, muscle cramps. *Respiratory:* Nose or sinus drainage, nose bleed, throat tightness, pharyngitis. *Miscellaneous:* Pruritus, swollen lymph nodes, heat intolerance, visual disturbances, sensitivity to allergens, papular rash on neck, hot flashes, herpes labialis, dysuria, photosensitivity, decreased white blood count.

Note: When used for treatment of cancer, the incidence of many of the above side effects was increased. Additional side effects were noted including: *GI:* Constipation, anorexia, stomatitis, dry mouth, mucositis, sore mouth. *Laboratory Test Values:* Abnormal hemoglobin, white blood count, alkaline phosphatase, total bilirubin, platelet count, AST, and GGT. *Miscellaneous:* Insomnia, blurred vision, ocular rotation pain, sore injection site, chest pains, low blood pressure.

Dosage: Intralesional injection. *Condylomata acuminata:* 0.05 ml (250,000 IU)/wart twice a week for up to 8 weeks. The maximum recommended dose per treatment session is 0.5 ml (2.5 million IU). The safety and effectiveness of a second course of treatment have not been determined.

NURSING CONSIDERATIONS

See also *Nursing Considerations* for *Interferon alfa-2a Recombinant,* p. 749.

Administration/Storage

1. The drug should be injected into the base of the wart using a 30-gauge needle.
2. For large warts, the drug can be injected at several points around the periphery of the wart using a total dose of 0.05 ml/wart.
3. The drug should be stored at 2°C–8°C (36°F–46°F). It should not be frozen or shaken.

Assessment

1. Take client history, especially noting any history of allergic reactions to egg protein or neomycin. These could indicate an increased sensitivity to interferon alfa-n3.
2. Note any client history of pre-existing debilitating diseases.
3. For condylomata therapy, note the size of the wart. Measure it and document prior to initiating therapy.

Client/Family Teaching

1. Intralesional treatment should be continued for 8 weeks.
2. Genital warts may disappear both during treatment and after treatment has been discontinued. When this occurs, unless new warts appear or warts become enlarged, there should be a 3-month waiting period after the first 8-week course of therapy.
3. Do not change brands of interferon without consultation with the physician because the manufacturing process, strength, and type of interferon may vary.
4. Women should use contraceptive practices if fertile.
5. Review the early signs of hypersensitivity reactions (e.g., hives, chest tightness, generalized urticaria, hypotension, wheezing, anaphylaxis) and instruct client to contact their physician should these symptoms occur.

Evaluation

1. During therapy for condylomata, measure the warts to determine the extent to which they are decreasing in size at each treatment session.
2. Document the need for further therapy after a 3-month waiting period.

Interferon gamma-1b
(in-ter-**FEER**-on **GAM**-uh)
Actimmune (Rx)

Classification: Interferon.

Action/Kinetics: Interferon gamma-1b consists of a single-chain polypeptide of 140 amino acids. It is produced by fermentation of a genetically engineered *Escherichia coli* bacterium containing the DNA that encodes for the human protein. Interferon gamma manifests potent phagocyte-activating effects including generation of toxic oxygen metabolites within phagocytes. Such metabolites result in the death of microorganisms such as *Staphyloocccus aureus, Toxoplasma gondii, Leishmania donovani, Listeria monocytogenes,* and *Mycobacterium avium intracellulare.* Since interferon gamma regulates activity of immune cells, it is characterized as a lymphokine of the interleukin type. Data indicate that interferon gamma interacts functionally with other interleukin molecules (e.g., interleukin-2) and that all interleukins form part of a complex, lymphokine regulatory network. As an example, interferon gamma and interleukin-4 may interact reciprocally to regulate murine IgE levels; interferon gamma can suppress IgE levels and inhibit the production of collagen at the transcription level in humans.

Interferon gamma is rapidly cleared from the plasma after IV administration and is slowly absorbed after either IM or SC injection. **t½, elimination: IV,** 38 min; **IM,** 2.9 hr; **SC,** 5.9 hr. **Peak plasma levels:** 4 hr after IM and 7 hr after SC dosing.

Uses: Decrease the frequency and severity of serious infections associated with chronic granulomatous disease.

Contraindications: Hypersensitivity to interferon gamma or *E. coli*-derived products. Use during lactation.

Special Concerns: Pregnancy category: C. Safety and effectiveness have not been determined in children less than one year of age. Use with caution in clients with preexisting cardiac disease, including symptoms of ischemia, arrhythmia, or congestive heart failure, and in clients with myelosuppression, seizure disorders, or compromised CNS function.

Side Effects: The following side effects were noted in clients with chronic granulomatous disease receiving the drug SC. *GI:* Diarrhea, vomiting, nausea, abdominal pain, anorexia. *CNS:* Fever (over 50%), headache, fatigue, depression. *Miscellaneous:* Rash, chills, erythema or tenderness at injection site, pain at injection site, weight loss, myalgia, arthralgia, back pain.

When used in clients other than those with chronic granulomatous disease, in addition to above, the following side effects were reported. *GI:* GI bleeding, pancreatitis, hepatic insufficiency. *CV:* Hypotension, heart block, heart failure, syncope, tachyarrhythmia, myocardial infarction. *CNS:* Confusion, disorientation, symptoms of parkinsonism, gait disturbance, seizures, hallucinations, transient ischemic attacks. *Hematologic:* Deep venous thrombosis, pulmonary embolism. *Respiratory:* Bronchospasm, tachypnea, interstitial pneumonitis. *Metabolic:* Hyperglycemia, hyponatremia. *Miscellaneous:* Reversible renal insufficiency, worsening of dermatomyositis.

Dosage: SC. *Chronic granulomatous disease:* 50 mcg/m² (1.5 million U/m²) for clients whose body surface is greater than 0.5 m². If the body surface is less than 0.5 m², the dose of interferon gamma should be 1.5 mcg/kg/dose. The drug is given three times weekly (e.g., Monday, Wednesday, Friday).

NURSING CONSIDERATIONS

Administration/Storage

1. The preferred sites of injection are the right and left deltoid and anterior thigh.
2. The product does not contain a preservative. Thus, the vial is to be used only for a single dose with any unused portion discarded.
3. Safety and effectiveness have not been determined for doses greater or less than 50 mcg/m².
4. If severe side effects occur, the dose can be reduced by 50% or therapy can be discontinued until the side effects subside.
5. The drug may be administered using either sterilized glass or plastic disposable syringes.

6. Vials must be stored at 2°C–8°C (36°F–46°F) to assure optimal retention of activity. The vial should not be frozen.
7. The vial should not be shaken and vigorous agitation should be avoided.
8. Vials stored at room temperature for more than 12 hr should be discarded.

Assessment

1. Note any history or evidence of CAD.
2. Document any history of CNS disorders.
3. Obtain baseline urinalysis, CBC with differential and platelets, liver and renal function studies, and monitor every 3 months during drug therapy.
4. Determine client age of symptom (onset of chronic granulomatous disease) and what if any treatments in the past were used to reduce the frequency and severity of infections.

Client/Family Teaching

1. Review the appropriate method for medication administration and observe the client in self-administration.
2. Stress the importance of keeping the drug in the refrigerator and **not** to shake the container.
3. Advise client to take medication at bedtime with acetaminophen, unless contraindicated, to minimize fever and headaches associated with this drug therapy.
4. Provide a printed list of drug side effects stressing those that should be reported to the physician immediately.
5. Remind client that close medical supervision is imperative

with this disease and genetically engineered medication therapy as the dosage may require frequent adjustments. All concerns and any adverse effects should be reported immediately.

Intravenous Fat Emulsion
Intralipid 10% and 20%, Liposyn 10% and 20%, Liposyn II 10% and 20%, Soyacal 10% and 20%, Travamulsion 10% and 20% (Rx)

Classification: Nutritional agent.

Action/Kinetics: These products contain either soybean oil or safflower oil in a concentration of 10% or 20%, egg yolk phospholipids (1.2%), glycerin (2.21%–2.5%), and water for injection. The fatty acids present in these preparations (linoleic, linolenic, oleic, palmitic, and stearic) provide essential fatty acids to maintain normal cellular membrane function. The products provide from 1.1 cal/ml (10% oil) to 2.0 cal/ml (20% oil). Since it is isotonic, it can be administered into a peripheral vein. The preparations increase heat production, oxygen consumption, and decrease the respiratory quotient (ratio of CO_2/O_2; normal: 0.77–0.90).

Uses: Source of calories and essential fatty acids for prolonged parenteral nutrition (longer than 5 days). Fatty acid deficiency.

Contraindications: Disturbances of fat metabolism (e.g., lipoid nephrosis, pathologic hyperlipidemia, acute pancreatitis with hyperlipemia). Sensitivity to egg yolk.

Special Concerns: Safe use in pregnancy not established (pregnancy category: B for Soyacal 10%; pregnancy category: C for all others). Caution should be exercised when used in premature or jaundiced premature infants. Use with caution in clients with hepatic damage, anemia, respiratory disease, coagulation problems, or possibility of fat embolism.

Side Effects: *Premature infants:* Deaths due to intravascular fat accumulation in the lungs. **Acute side effects.** *GI:* Nausea, vomiting. *CNS:* Headache, fever, drowsiness, dizziness. *Other:* Hyperlipemia, dyspnea, increased coagulation, flushing, sweating, cyanosis, back and chest pain, pressure over eyes, hypersensitivity reactions with urticaria, increases in liver enzymes (transient). Neonates may manifest thrombocytopenia. **Long-term side effects.** *Hepatic:* Jaundice, hepatomegaly, alterations in liver function tests. *Overloading syndrome:* Splenomegaly, focal seizures, fever, leukocytosis, shock. *Other:* Deposition of pigment (brown) in reticuloendothelial system.

Sepsis and thrombophlebitis due to contamination or procedure.

Dosage: IV. *Total parenteral nutrition,* **Maximum:** 3 g/kg/day. **Pediatric maximum:** 4 g/kg/day. The product should not exceed 60% of daily caloric intake. *Fatty acid deficiency:* Approximately 8%–10% of caloric intake.

NURSING CONSIDERATIONS

See also *Nursing Considerations* for *Intravenous Nutritional Therapy,* p. 170.

Administration/Storage

1. Discard if oiling out occurs before administration.

2. May be given parenterally or centrally using a separate line, though it can be administered into same peripheral vein as carbohydrate-amino acid solutions using a Y-connection located near the infusion site. Flow rate of each solution should be controlled separately by an infusion pump. Do not use filters.

3. May be mixed with certain nutrient solutions (check package insert).

4. The rate of infusion should be: **Adults: 10% products, initial,** 1 ml/min for first 15–30 min; **then,** if no adverse effects, increase to 83–125 ml/hr up to 500 ml the first day. Amount may be increased the second day. **Adults: 20% products, initial,** 0.5 ml/min for first 15–30 min; **then,** if no adverse side effects, increase to 62.5 ml/hr up to 250–500 ml (depending on product) the first day. Amount may be increased the second day. Total daily dose should not exceed 3 g/kg. **Pediatric: 10% products, initial,** 0.1 ml/min for first 10–15 min; **then,** if no adverse effects, increase to maximum of 1 g/kg/4 hr (100 ml/hr). **Pediatric: 20% products, initial,** 0.05 ml/min over the first 10–15 min; **then,** if no adverse effects, increase to maximum of 1 g/4 hr (50 ml/hr). Total daily dose should not exceed 4 g/kg.

5. Carefully review and follow institutional guidelines for administration of IV fats.

6. Store in refrigerator at 4°C–8°C (39.2°F–46.4°F) if so designated on product literature.

Assessment

1. Perform baseline nutritional assessment and document weight.
2. Note any allergy to eggs.
3. Observe the client closely for the first 10–15 min of administration for signs of allergic reaction to the parenteral product. Stop the infusion, document, and report to the physician immediately.

Evaluation: Evaluate client for:

- Laboratory evidence that serum triglyceride and fatty acid levels within desired range
- Evidence of weight gain

Iodine Sources:
(**EYE**-oh-dyn)

Potassium Iodide
Pima, Thyro-Block✲ (Rx)

Sodium Iodide
(Rx)

Strong Iodine Solution
Lugol's Solution (Rx)

Classification: Source of iodine.

Action/Kinetics: Small doses of iodine are concentrated by the thyroid gland, resulting in an increased synthesis of thyroid hormones. However, large doses are capable of inhibiting thyroid hormone synthesis and release. This is the basis for the use of these drugs in treating hyperthyroidism. Iodine specifically produces involution of a hyperplastic thyroid gland, making it less friable and less vascular prior to surgery. Iodine also shortens the time required by other antithyroid drugs to reduce the

output of natural hormone. **Onset:** 1–2 days. **Peak effects:** 10–15 days. **Duration:** Up to 6 weeks. Strong Iodine Solution contains 5% iodine and 10% sodium iodide.

Uses: Prophylaxis of simple and colloid goiters, exophthalmic goiter. As adjunct with antithyroid drugs to prepare thyrotoxic clients for thyroidectomy, to treat thyrotoxic crisis, or neonatal thyrotoxicosis. Also, for thyroid blocking in radiation emergency. *Investigational, Potassium Iodide:* Erythema nodosum, iodine deficiency.

Contraindications: Iodine is contraindicated in tuberculosis because it may cause breakdown of healing of lesions. Pulmonary edema. In clients hypersensitive to iodine.

Special Concerns: Pregnancy category: C.

Side Effects: *Acute poisoning:* Vomiting, abdominal pain, diarrhea, gastritis, swelling of glottis or larynx, shock syndrome. May be treated by soluble starch gastric lavage followed by milk to relieve irritation. *Chronic toxicity (iodism):* *Dermatologic:* Skin reactions including acneiform, vesicular, bullous, or maculopapular eruptions. *Mucous membranes:* Swelling and inflammation, conjunctivitis, bronchial irritation, coryza. *CV:* Edema, erythema, purpura. *Miscellaneous:* Fever, irritability.

Symptoms of Overdose/Poisoning: GI tract irritation including symptoms of vomiting, diarrhea, abdominal pain. Death may result due to shock, corrosive gastritis, or asphyxiation due to swelling of the glottis or larynx.

Dosage: Sodium Iodide. IV. Thyroid crisis: 1–3 g/day.

Potassium Iodide. Oral Solution, Syrup, Tablets. *Thyroid blocking in radiation emergency:* **Adults,** 100–150 mg daily 24 before and for 3–10 days after administration of or exposure to radiation. **Pediatric, 1 year and older:** 130 mg once daily for 10 days following administration of or exposure to radiation; **less than 1 year of age:** 65 mg once daily for 10 days following administration of or exposure to radiation. *To prepare clients for thyroidectomy:* **Adults,** 5 drops of the 1 g/ml oral solution (about 250 mg), 4 ml of the syrup (about 260 mg), or 2 tablets dissolved in a glass of water (about 260 mg) daily for 10 days before surgery usually with an antithyroid drug.

Strong Iodine Solution. *Prior to thyroidectomy:* 2–6 drops t.i.d. for 10 days prior to surgery.

NURSING CONSIDERATIONS

See also *Nursing Considerations* for *Antithyroid Drugs,* p. 100.

Administration/Storage

1. Measure iodine solutions carefully, using a calibrated dropper. This medication is potent and the dosing volume tends to be small.
2. Dilute iodine in 60 ml of chocolate milk, plain milk, or orange juice. The medication has a bitter taste.
3. To decrease the burning sensation in the mouth and to prevent discoloration of the teeth, use drinking straws when administering iodine solutions.
4. Do not store other than in the original brown, light-resistant container.
5. *Treatment of Overdose/Poisoning:* Gastric lavage with either 15 g cornstarch or flour in 500 ml water. Sodium thiosulfate, 5% oral solution, will reduce iodine to iodide. To reduce gastric irritation, give milk. Correct fluid and electrolyte balance. Treat shock, if present.

Assessment

1. Note if the client has any allergy to iodine preparations.
2. Ask clients if they have had any side effects from medications or diagnostic tests where iodine has been used.
3. Obtain baseline data concerning the extent of the client's anxiety, nervousness, agitation, mood swings, and irritability.
4. Note if the client has exophthalmos, tremors, or increased tendon reflexes.
5. Obtain a baseline ECG, and measurement of blood pressure, pulse, and respirations.
6. Check the client's medication history for the use of oral anticoagulants, insulin, or anion exchange resins and document if in use.

Interventions

1. Monitor the client's blood pressure, temperature, respirations, weight. Determine glucose levels in the blood and urine as ordered during drug therapy.
2. Note if the client has a reduction in stress and changes in mood swings. Compare the client's responses with the baseline data obtained prior to initiating therapy.
3. If the client is receiving anticoagulants, monitor for increased bleeding tendencies.

Client/Family Teaching

1. Review with the client and family the purposes of drug therapy.
2. Describe the symptoms of acute iodine poisoning. Provide printed information listing these symptoms.
3. Withhold the drug and report any evidence of toxicity to the physician immediately.
4. Check with the physician before using iodized salt.
5. Sip the medication through a straw to avoid staining tooth enamel.
6. Dilute medication with water, juice, or milk to decrease gastric irritation
7. Review dietary intake for excessive ingestion of goitrogenic foods that could cause symptoms of hypothyroidism.
8. Stress the importance of reporting for medical visits and follow-up laboratory tests.

Evaluation: Evaluate client for:

- Evidence of improvement in psychological symptoms and sociability
- A ↓ pulse rate, a reduction in appetite, and ↓ in weight gain
- Evidence of a decrease in tremors, a lessening of exophthalmos, and a reduced diaphoresis within 3–8 weeks of therapy
- Reports of elimination of cold sensitivity

Ipecac Syrup
(IP-eh-kak)
PMS Ipecac Syrup ✤ (OTC)

Classification: Emetic.

Action/Kinetics: The active principle of ipecac, an alkaloid extracted from Brazil root, acts both locally on the gastric mucosa and centrally on the chemoreceptor trigger zone. **Onset:** 20 min. **Duration:** 20–25 min. In contrast to apomorphine, a second dose may be given if necessary. **Ipecac syrup must not be confused with ipecac fluid extract, which is 14 times as potent.** Syrup of ipecac can be purchased without a prescription. It has been abused by clients suffering from bulimia.

Uses: To empty the stomach promptly and completely after oral poisoning or drug overdose.

Contraindications: With corrosives or petroleum distillates, in individuals who are unconscious or semicomatose, severely inebriated, or in shock. Infants under 6 months of age.

Special Concerns: Pregnancy category: C. If used in children less than 12 months of age, there is an increased risk of aspiration of vomitus.

Drug Interactions: Activated charcoal adsorbs ipecac syrup, thus decreasing its effect.

Dosage: Syrup. Adults and children over 12 years: 15–30 ml followed by 240 ml of water; **pediatric up to 1 year:** 5–10 ml preceded or followed by 120–240 ml of water; **pediatric, 1–12 years:** 15 ml preceded or followed by 120–240 ml water.

NURSING CONSIDERATIONS

Administration/Storage

1. Check label of medication closely so that the syrup and the fluid extract are not confused.

2. Dosage may be repeated once if vomiting does not occur within 30 min. Gastric lavage should be considered if vomiting does not occur within 15 min after the second dose.
3. Administer ipecac syrup with 200–300 ml of water.

Client/Family Teaching

1. Provide with the name and telephone number of the local poison control center or hospital and advise the client/parent to contact before administering ipecac syrup.
2. Always have ipecac syrup available in the event of accidental poisoning.
3. Be sure that ipecac syrup is kept in a locked closet, out of the reach of children. Check expiration date periodically and before administering.
4. If the drug is to be used as an expectorant, instruct the client as to the correct dosage and the appropriate method of administration. Explain the difference between the dosage and methods used for expectorant purposes and emetic purposes.
5. Explain the potential for abuse, such as to induce vomiting after meals for weight reduction. (Some states have banned over-the-counter sales for this reason).

Evaluation

1. Assess for inducement of vomiting following drug overdose.
2. Consult with poison control center (See Appendix Five) and based on client response, determine if additional drug therapy and/or medical intervention is necessary.

Isoetharine hydrochloride

(eye-so-**ETH**-ah-reen)

Arm-a-Med Isoetharine HCl, Bronkosol, Dey-Dose Isoetharine HCl, Dey-Dose Isoetharine S/F, Dey-Lute Isoetharine, Dey-Lute Isoetharine S/F, Dispos-a-Med Isoetharine (Rx)

Isoetharine mesylate

(eye-so-**ETH**-ah-reen)

Bronkometer (Rx)

See also *Sympathomimetic Drugs,* p. 218.

Classification: Adrenergic agent, bronchodilator.

Action/Kinetics: Isoetharine has a greater stimulating activity on beta-2 receptors of the bronchi than on beta-1 receptors of the heart. Causes relief of bronchospasms. **Inhalation: Onset,** 1–6 min; **peak effect:** 15–60 min; **duration:** 1–4 hr. Partially metabolized; excreted in urine.

Special Concerns: Pregnancy category: C.

Uses: Bronchial asthma, bronchospasms due to chronic bronchitis or emphysema, bronchiectasis, pulmonary obstructive disease.

Special Concerns: Dosage has not been established in children.

Dosage: Inhalation Solution. Adults: *Hand nebulizer:* 3–7 inhalations (use undiluted) of the 0.5% or 1% solution. *Oxygen aerosolization or IPPB:* Dose depends on strength of solution used (range: 0.062%–1%) and whether the solution is used undiluted or diluted 1:3 according to the following: **0.5%– 1%:** 0.5–1 ml of 1:3 solution; **0.2%:**

2–2.5 ml used undiluted; **0.1%– 0.167%**: 2.5–4 ml used undiluted; **0.062% or 0.08%**: 3–4 ml used undiluted.

Mesylate Inhalation Aerosol. Adults: 0.34 mg (1 inhalation) repeated after 1–2 min if needed; **then,** dose may be repeated q 4 hr.

NURSING CONSIDERATIONS

See *Special Nursing Considerations For Adrenergic Bronchodilators* under *Sympathomimetics,* p. 221.

Administration/Storage

1. One or two inhalations are usually sufficient. Wait 1 min after giving initial dose to ensure necessity of another dose.
2. Treatment usually does not need to be repeated more than q 4 hr.
3. Do not use if solution contains a precipitate or is brown.

Assessment: Note any allergy to sulfites.

Evaluation: Evaluate client for evidence of improved airway exchange with ↓ in bronchospasm and/or bronchoconstriction.

Isoniazid
(eye-so-**NYE**-ah-zid)
INH, Isonicotinic Acid Hydrazide, Isotamine✿, Laniazid, Nydrazid, PMS Isoniazid✿, Teebaconin (Rx)

Classification: First-line antitubercular agent.

General Statement: Isoniazid is the most effective tuberculostatic agent. The metabolism of isoniazid is genetically determined and involves the level of a hepatic enzyme. Clients on isoniazid fall into two groups, depending on the manner in which they metabolize isoniazid. As a rule, 50% of whites and blacks inactivate the drug slowly, whereas the majority of American Indians, Eskimos, Japanese, and Chinese are rapid inactivators.

1. **Slow inactivators:** These clients show earlier, favorable response but have more toxic reactions (e.g., neuropathies because of higher blood levels of drug).
2. **Rapid inactivators:** These clients have possible poor clinical response due to rapid inactivation. This group requires an increased daily dose of the drug. They are more likely to develop hepatitis.

Action/Kinetics: Isoniazid probably interferes with lipid and nucleic acid metabolism of growing bacteria, resulting in alteration of the bacterial wall. The drug is tuberculostatic. It is readily absorbed after oral and parenteral (IM) administration and is widely distributed in body tissues. **Peak plasma concentration:** PO, 1–2 hr. $t^{1/2}$, **fast acetylators:** 0.5–6 hr; $t^{1/2}$, **slow acetylators:** 2–5 hr. These values are increased in association with liver and kidney impairment. Drug is metabolized in liver and excreted primarily in urine.

Uses: Tuberculosis caused by human, bovine, and BCG strains of *Mycobacterium tuberculosis.* The drug should not be used as the sole tuberculostatic agent. Prophylaxis of tuberculosis.

Contraindications: Severe hypersensitivity to isoniazid.

Special Concerns: Extreme caution should be exercised in clients with convulsive disorders, in whom the drug should be administered only when the client is adequately controlled by anticonvulsant medication. Also, use with caution for the treatment of renal tuberculosis and, in the lowest dose possible, in clients with impaired renal function and in alcoholics. Use during pregnancy only if benefits outweigh risks.

Side Effects: Peripheral neuritis, muscle twitches. *CNS:* Ataxia, stupor, seizures, toxic encephalopathy, euphoria, impaired memory, dizziness, toxic psychoses. *GI:* Nausea, vomiting, epigastric distress, xerostomia. *Hypersensitivity:* Fever, skin rashes, vasculitis, lymphadenopathy. *Hepatic:* Liver dysfunction, jaundice, bilirubinemia, hepatitis (especially in clients over 50 years of age). Increases in serum AST and ALT. *Hematologic:* Agranulocytosis, eosinophilia, thrombocytopenia, methemoglobinemia, anemias. *Miscellaneous:* Tinnitus, optic neuritis, optic atrophy, hyperglycemia, metabolic acidosis, urinary retention, gynecomastia in males, lupus-like syndrome, arthralgia.
   Note: Pyridoxine, 10–50 mg/day, may be given concomitantly with isoniazid to decrease CNS side effects. Ophthalmologic and liver function tests are recommended periodically.
   Symptoms of Overdose: Nausea, vomiting, dizziness, blurred vision, slurred speech, visual hallucinations within 30–180 min. Severe overdosage may cause respiratory distress, CNS depression (coma can occur), severe seizures, metabolic acidosis, acetonuria, hyperglycemia.

Drug Interactions

Aminosalicylic acid / ↑ Effect of isoniazid by ↑ blood levels
Atropine / ↑ Side effects of isoniazid
Disulfiram / ↑ Side effects of isoniazid (especially CNS)
Ethanol / ↑ Chance of isoniazid-induced hepatitis
Meperidine / ↑ Side effects of isoniazid
Phenytoin / ↑ Effect of phenytoin due to ↓ breakdown in liver
Rifampin / Additive liver toxicity

Laboratory Test Interferences: Altered liver function tests. False + or ↑ K, AST, ALT, urine glucose (Benedict's test, Clinitest).

Dosage: Syrup, Tablets. *Active tuberculosis:* **Adults,** 300 mg daily as a single dose; **children and infants:** 10–20 mg/kg/day (up to 300–500 mg total) in a single dose. *Prophylaxis:* **Adults,** 300 mg/day in a single dose; **children and infants:** 10 mg/kg/day (up to 300 mg total) in a single dose. **IM. Adults/adolescents:** *Prophylaxis,* 300 mg daily. *Treatment of tuberculosis:* 5 mg/kg (up to 300 mg) once daily. **Pediatric:** *Prophylaxis,* 10 mg/kg once daily. *Treatment of tuberculosis:* 10–20 mg/kg (up to 300 mg) once daily.

NURSING CONSIDERATIONS

See also *General Nursing Considerations For All Anti-Infectives*, p. 83.

Administration/Storage

1. Store in dark, tightly closed containers.
2. Solutions for IM injection may crystallize at low temperature and should be allowed to warm to room temperature if precipitation is evident.

3. Isoniazid should be administered with pyridoxine, 6–50 mg/day, in malnourished, alcoholic, or diabetic clients.
4. *Treatment of Overdose:* Maintain respiration and undertake gastric lavage (within first 2–3 hr providing seizures are not present). To control seizures, give diazepam or a short-acting IV barbiturate followed by pyridoxine (1 mg IV/1 mg isoniazid ingested). Sodium bicarbonate, IV, to correct metabolic acidosis. Forced osmotic diuresis; monitor fluid intake and output. For severe cases, hemodialysis or peritoneal dialysis should be considered.

Interventions

1. Obtain baseline liver and renal function studies and monitor throughout therapy.
2. Parenteral sodium phenobarbital is generally used for the control of isoniazid-induced neurotoxic symptoms, particularly convulsions; have readily available.
3. Anticipate that cholinergic drugs, atropine, and certain narcotic analgesics (e.g., meperidine) may aggravate adverse side effects.
4. If CNS stimulation is marked, withhold the drug and consult with physician.
5. Closely assess clients with diabetes because it is more difficult to control when isoniazid is administered.
6. Anticipate reduced dose with renal dysfunction. Monitor intake and output to ascertain that renal output is adequate to prevent systemic accumulation of the drug.

7. Provide client with only a 1-month supply of the drug because client should be examined and evaluated monthly while on isoniazid.
8. Anticipate a slight local irritation at the site of injection. Rotate and document injection sites.

Client/Family Teaching

1. Take drug on an empty stomach 1 hr before or 2 hr after meals.
2. Withhold drug and report fatigue, weakness, malaise, and anorexia immediately because these may be signs of hepatitis.
3. Stress the importance of taking drugs as ordered and of reporting for monthly follow-up and laboratory studies.
4. Explain that pyridoxine is given to prevent neurotoxic effects of isoniazid.
5. Do not use alcohol while on drug therapy.

Evaluation: Assess client for evidence of a positive clinical response as evidenced by negative lab culture results and a lack of toxic drug side effects.

Isophane insulin suspension (NPH)

(EYE-so-fayn IN-sue-lin)
Single peak: NPH Iletin I (beef and pork), NPH Insulin (beef). Purified: Beef NPH Iletin I, Insulatard NPH (pork), NPH Purified (pork), Pork NPH Iletin II. Human: Humulin N, Insulatard NPH, Novolin N, Novolin N PenFill (OTC)

See also *Insulins,* p. 156.

Classification: Intermediate-acting insulin.

Action/Kinetics: Contains zinc insulin crystals modified by protamine, appearing as a cloudy or milky suspension. Not recommended for emergency use. Not suitable for IV administration. Not useful in the presence of ketosis. **Onset:** 1–1.5 hr. **Peak:** 4–12 hr. **Duration:** 18–28 hr.

Dosage: SC, individualized. Adult, usual, initial: 7–26 units as a single dose 30–60 min before breakfast. A second smaller dose may be given, if needed, prior to the evening meal or at bedtime. If necessary, the daily dose may be increased in increments of 2–10 units at daily or weekly intervals until desired control is achieved.

Clients on insulin zinc may be transferred directly to isophane insulin on a unit-for-unit basis. If client is being transferred from regular insulin, the initial dose of isophane should be from two-thirds to three-fourths the dose of regular insulin.

NURSING CONSIDERATIONS

See *Nursing Considerations* for *Insulins,* p. 160.

——— COMBINATION DRUG ———
Isophane insulin suspension and insulin injection
(**EYE**-so-fayn **IN**-sue-lin)
Purified: Mixtard (pork). Human: Humulin 70/30, Mixtard Human 70/30, Novolin 70/30, Novolin 70/30 PenFill. (OTC)

See also *Insulins,* p. 156.

Classification: Mixture of insulins to achieve variable duration of action.

Action/Kinetics: Contains 30% insulin injection and 70% isophane insulin. This combination allows for a rapid onset (30–60 min) due to insulin injection and a long duration (24 hr) due to isophane insulin. **Peak effect:** 4–8 hr.

NURSING CONSIDERATIONS

See *Nursing Considerations* for *Insulins,* p. 160.

Isoproterenol hydrochloride
(eye-so-proh-**TER**-ih-nohl)
Dey-Dose Isoproterenol HCl, Dispos-a-Med Isoproterenol HCl, Isuprel, Isuprel Mistometer, Medihaler-Iso, Norisodrine Aerotrol (Rx)

Isoproterenol sulfate
(eye-so-proh-**TER**-ih-nohl)
Medihaler-Iso (Rx)

See also *Sympathomimetic Drugs,* p. 218.

Classification: Direct-acting sympathomimetic agent.

Action/Kinetics: Isoproterenol produces pronounced stimulation of both beta-1- and beta-2 receptors of the heart, bronchi, skeletal muscle vasculature, and the GI tract. In contrast to other sympathomimetics, isoproterenol produces a drop in BP. It also causes less hyperglycemia than epinephrine, but produces bronchodilation and the same degree of CNS excitation. **Inhalation: Onset,** 2–5 min; **peak effect:** 3–5 min; **duration:** 30–120 min. **IV: Onset,** immediate; **duration:** less than 1 hr. **Sublingual: Onset,** 15–30 min; **duration:** 1–2 hr. **Rectal: Onset,** 30 min; **duration:** 2–4 hr. Partially metabolized; excreted in urine.

Uses: Bronchodilator in asthma, chronic pulmonary emphysema, bronchiectasis, bronchitis, and other conditions involving bronchospasms. Treat bronchospasms during anesthesia. Cardiac arrest, heart block, syncope due to complete heart block, Adams-Stokes syndrome. Certain cardiac arrhythmias including ventricular tachycardia, ventricular arrhythmias; syncope due to carotid sinus hypersensitivity. Hypoperfusion shock syndrome.

Special Concerns: Pregnancy category: C. Use with caution in the presence of tuberculosis.

Additional Side Effects: Flushing, sweating, swelling of the parotid gland. Excessive inhalation causes refractory bronchial obstruction. Sublingual administration may cause buccal ulceration. Side effects of drug are less severe after inhalation.

Drug Interaction: Beta-adrenergic blocking agents reverse the effects of isoproterenol.

Dosage: *Isoproterenol hydrochloride. Shock:* **IV Infusion,** 0.5–5 mcg/min (0.25–2.5 ml of 1:500,000 diluted solution). *Cardiac standstill and cardiac arrhythmias:* **Adults, IM, SC:** 1 ml (0.2 mg) of 1:5,000 solution (range: 0.02–1 mg); **IV:** 1–3 ml (0.02–0.06 mg) of 1:50,000 solution (range: 0.01–0.2 mg); **IV infusion:** 5 mcg/min (1.25 ml of 1:250,000 solution/min); **Intracardiac (in extreme emergencies):** 0.1 ml of 1:5,000 solution. *Heart block:* **IV, SC, IM:** as above.
Acute bronchial asthma: **Hand bulb nebulizer:** 5–15 deep inhalations of 1:200 solution (or, in adults, 3–7 inhalations of the 1:100 solution); repeat once more if relief

not obtained after 5–10 min. **Metered-dose inhaler: Usual,** one inhalation; if relief not obtained after 2–5 min, administer again. **Maintenance:** 1–2 inhalations 4–6 times/day (**Note:** No more than 2 inhalations should be taken at once and no more than 6 in one hr.) *Chronic obstructive lung disease (bronchospasm):* **Hand bulb nebulizer:** 5–15 deep inhalations of 1:200 solution (or 3–7 inhalations of 1:100 solution) q 3–4 hr. **Nebulization by IPPE:** Dilute 0.5 ml of 1:200 solution in 2–2.5 ml diluent (to achieve concentration of 1:800–1:1,000) and deliver over 10–20 min. Can be repeated 5 times/day. **Metered-dose inhaler:** 1–2 inhalations q 3–4 hr. **Sublingual: Adults,** 10–20 mg depending on response (not to exceed 60 mg daily). **Pediatric:** 5–10 mg up to a maximum of 30 mg daily. Should not be given more than t.i.d. *Bronchospasms during anesthesia:* **IV,** 0.01–0.02 mg as required (1 ml of a 1:5,000 solution diluted to 10 ml with sodium chloride or dextrose injection).
Isoproterenol sulfate. Dispensed from metered aerosol inhaler for bronchospasms. See dosage above for *Hydrochloride.*

NURSING CONSIDERATIONS

See also *Special Nursing Considerations* for *Adrenergic Bronchodilators* under *Sympathomimetics,* p. 221.

Administration/Storage

1. Administration to children, except where noted, is the same as that for adults, because a child's smaller ventilatory exchange capacity will permit a proportionally smaller aerosol intake. For acute broncho-

spasms in children, use 1:200 solution.

2. In children, no more than 0.25 ml of the 1:200 solution should be used for each 10–15 min of programmed treatment.
3. Elderly clients usually receive a lower dose.

Interventions: Observe and report respiratory problems that seem to worsen after the administration of isoproterenol. Refractory reactions may necessitate withdrawal of the drug.

Client/Family Teaching

1. Rinse mouth with water to remove any drug residue and to minimize dryness, after inhalation therapy.
2. Maintain an adequate fluid intake of 2-3 L/day in order to help liquefy secretions.
3. The sputum and saliva may appear pink after inhalation therapy. This is due to the drug and the client should not become alarmed.
4. When also taking inhalant glucocorticoids advise to take isoproterenol first and to wait 15 min before using the second inhaler.
5. Do not use inhaler therapy more frequently than prescribed by the physician. Excessive use can cause severe cardiac and respiratory problems.
6. Show the client where the parotid gland is located. Instruct client to withhold the drug if parotid gland becomes enlarged. Advise to report this finding immediately to the physician and anticipate that the drug will be discontinued.

Evaluation: Evaluate client for:

- Clinical evidence and reports of improvement in airway exchange and breathing patterns
- ↑ in heart rate
- Evidence of improved cardiac output
- Effective termination of lethal ventricular arrhythmias

Isosorbide dinitrate chewable tablets
(eye-so-**SOR**-byd)

Isosorbide dinitrate extended-release capsules
(eye-so-**SOR**-byd)
Dilatrate-SR, Iso-Bid, Isordil Tembids, Isotrate Timecelles, Sorbitrate (Rx)

Isosorbide dinitrate extended-release tablets
(eye-so-**SOR**-byd)
Cedocard-SR✿, Coradur✿, Isordil Tembids, Sorbitrate SA (Rx)

Isosorbide dinitrate sublingual tablets
(eye-so-**SOR**-byd)
Apo-ISDN✿, Coronex✿, Isordil, Sorbitrate (Rx)

Isosorbide dinitrate tablets
(eye-so-**SOR**-byd)
Apo-ISDN✿, Coronex✿, Isordil Titradose, Novo–Sorbide✿, Sorbitrate (Rx)

See also *Antianginal Drugs,* p. 47.

Classification: Coronary vasodilator.

Action/Kinetics: Sublingual, chewable. Onset: 2–5 min; **duration:** 1–3 hr. **Oral Capsules/Tablets. Onset:** 15–40 min; **duration:** 4–6 hr. **Extended-release. Onset:** up to 4 hr; **duration:** 6–8 hr.

Additional Uses: Diffuse esophageal spasm. Oral tablets are only for prophylaxis while sublingual and chewable forms may be used to terminate acute attacks of angina.

Special Concerns: Pregnancy category: C. Dosage has not been established in children.

Additional Side Effects: Vascular headaches occur especially frequently.

Additional Drug Interactions

Acetylcholine / Isosorbide antagonizes the effect of acetylcholine
Norepinephrine / Isosorbide antagonizes the effect of norepinephrine

Dosage: Sublingual: *Acute attack:* 2.5–5 mg q 2–3 hr as required. *Prophylaxis:* 5–10 mg q 2–3 hr. **Chewable tablets:** *Acute attack:* **initial,** 5 mg q 2–3 hr. *Prophylaxis:* 5–10 mg q 2–3 hr. **Oral Capsules/Tablets, initial:** 5–20 mg; **maintenance:** 10–40 mg q 6 hr. **Sustained-release Tablets, initial:** 40 mg; **maintenance:** 40–80 mg q 8–12 hr.

NURSING CONSIDERATIONS

See also *Nursing Considerations for Antianginal Drugs,* p. 49.

Client/Family Teaching

1. Administer with meals to eliminate or reduce headaches; otherwise, take on an empty stomach.

2. None of the products should be crushed or chewed, unless specifically ordered by the physician.
3. Review appropriate method for administration. Remind client not to chew sublingual tablets.
4. Stress that chewable tablets should be held in the mouth for 1–2 min to allow for absorption through the buccal membranes.
5. Avoid alcohol or alcohol-containing products.
6. Acetaminophen (Tylenol) may assist to relieve headaches.

Evaluation: Evaluate client for:
- Reports of improvement in the frequency and severity of anginal attacks
- Effective resolution of esophageal spasm

Isotretinoin

(eye-so-**TRET**-ih-noyn)
Accutane, Accutane Roche ✦ (Rx)

Classification: Vitamin A metabolite (antiacne, keratinization stabilizer).

Action/Kinetics: Isotretinoin reduces sebaceous gland size, decreases sebum secretion, and inhibits abnormal keratinization. Approximately 25% of the oral dosage form is bioavailable. **Peak plasma levels:** 3 hr. **Steady-state blood levels following 80 mg daily:** 160 ng/ml. The drug is nearly 100% bound to plasma protein. **t½:** 10–20 hr. **Time to peak levels:** 3 hr. Metabolized in the liver to 4-oxo-isotretinoin which is also active. Approximately equal amounts are excreted through the urine and in the feces.

Uses: Severe recalcitrant cystic acne unresponsive to other therapy. *Investigational:* Cutaneous disorders of keratinization, leukoplakia, mycosis fungoides.

Contraindications: Due to the possibility of fetal abnormalities or spontaneous abortion, women who are pregnant or intend to become pregnant should not use the drug (pregnancy category: X). Certain conditions for use should be met in women with childbearing potential (see package insert). Use during lactation and in children.

Side Effects: *Skin:* Cheilitis, skin fragility, pruritus, dry skin, desquamation of facial skin, drying of mucous membranes, brittle nails, photosensitivity, rash, hypo- or hyperpigmentation, urticaria, erythema nodosum, hirsutism, excess granulation of tissues as a result of healing. *CNS:* Headache, fatigue, pseudotumor cerebri (i.e., headaches, papilledema, disturbances in vision), depression. *Ocular:* Conjunctivitis, optic neuritis, corneal opacities, dry eyes, decrease in acuity of night vision. *GI:* Dry mouth, nausea, vomiting, abdominal pain, inflammatory bowel disease, anorexia, weight loss, inflammation and bleeding of gums. *Neuromuscular:* Arthralgia, muscle pain, bone and joint pain and stiffness, skeletal hyperostosis. *Other:* Epistaxis, dry nose and mouth, respiratory infections, bruising, petechiae, disseminated herpes simplex, edema, transient chest pain, development of diabetes.

Symptoms of Overdose: Abdominal pain, ataxia, cheilosis, dizziness, facial flushing, headache, vomiting. Symptoms are transient.

Drug Interactions

Alcohol / Potentiation of ↑ in serum triglycerides
Benzoyl peroxide / ↑ Drying effects of isotretinoin
Minocycline / ↑ Risk of development of pseudotumor cerebri or papilledema
Tetracycline / ↑ Risk of development of pseudotumor cerebri or papilledema
Tretinoin / ↑ Drying effects of isotretinoin
Vitamin A / ↑ Risk of toxicity

Laboratory Test Interferences: ↑ Plasma triglycerides, sedimentation rate, platelet counts, alkaline phosphatase, AST, ALT, GGTP, LDH, fasting serum glucose, uric acid in blood, cholesterol, creatinine phosphokinase levels in clients who exercise vigorously. ↓ HDL, red blood cell parameters, white blood cell counts.

Dosage: Capsules. Adults, individualized, initial: 0.5–1 mg/kg daily (range: 0.5–2 mg/kg daily) divided in 2 doses for 15–20 weeks. Dose should be adjusted based on toxicity and clinical response; if cyst count decreases by 70% or more, drug may be discontinued. If necessary, a second course of therapy may be instituted after a rest period of 2 months. Doses of 0.05–0.5 mg/kg daily are effective but result in higher frequency of relapses. For keratinization disorders, doses up to 4 mg/kg daily have been used.

NURSING CONSIDERATIONS

Administration/Storage

1. Do not crush the drug.
2. Administer the drug with meals.
3. Before using the drug, the client should complete a client consent form included with the

package insert. Follow appropriate institutional guidelines for obtaining client consent.

4. If a second course of drug therapy is needed, the client should have a rest period of 2 months before it begins.

Assessment

1. Note if the client is female and of childbearing age. Perform a pregnancy test on all sexually active women of childbearing age.

2. Take a complete drug history, noting those medications with which the drug interacts unfavorably.

3. Obtain baseline blood glucose levels and liver function studies, especially lipoprotein, cholesterol and triglycerides.

Interventions

1. Once a month perform pregnancy tests on sexually active women of childbearing age. The drug is teratogenic. Advise the client to practice contraception.

2. Monitor the client's cholesterol, triglycerides, and blood glucose levels throughout the drug therapy.

3. To ensure compliance, give the client only a 30-day prescription.

Client/Family Teaching

1. Advise clients who receive isotretinoin to avoid donating blood for 30 days after the drug therapy has been discontinued.

2. Instruct females of childbearing age to practice some reliable form of birth control one month before, during, and for one month following this drug therapy because severe fetal damage may occur.

3. Report to the physician immediately if a persistent headache, nausea and vomiting, or visual disturbances develop.

4. Instruct clients who wear contact lenses that they may develop sensitivity to contacts during and after therapy. Excessively dry eyes may require an eye lubricant.

5. Explain that the condition may become worse before healing starts.

6. Avoid taking OTC medications, especially vitamin A, without physician knowledge and approval.

7. Eliminate or markedly reduce consumption of alcohol as it may ↑ triglyceride levels.

8. Avoid prolonged exposure to sunlight as the drug may cause photosensitivity. Wear protective clothing when exposure is necessary.

9. Lubricants may assist to diminish symptoms of dry, chapped skin and lips.

Evaluation: Evaluate client for evidence of a ↓ in the number and severity of cystic acne lesions.

Isoxsuprine
(eye-**SOX**-you-preen)
Vasodilan, Vasoprine (Rx)

Classification: Peripheral vasodilator.

Action/Kinetics: Direct relaxation of vascular smooth muscle in skeletal muscle, increasing peripheral blood flow. The drug has alpha-adrenergic receptor blocking activity and beta-adrenergic receptor stimulant properties. Isoxuprine also causes cardiac stimulation and uterine relaxation. Drug crosses placenta. In high doses it lowers blood viscosity and inhibits platelet aggregation. **Onset, PO:** 1 hr; **IV,** 10 min. **Peak serum levels:** 1 hr, persisting for approximately 3 hr. **t½:** 75 min. Mostly excreted in urine.

Uses: Symptomatic treatment of cerebrovascular insufficiency. Improves peripheral blood circulation in arteriosclerosis obliterans, Buerger's disease, and Raynaud's disease. *Investigational:* Dysmenorrhea, threatened premature labor.

Contraindications: Postpartum period, arterial bleeding.

Special Concerns: Use with caution parenterally in clients with hypotension and tachycardia. Safety for use during pregnancy has not been determined. Risk of drug-induced hypothermia may be increased in geriatric clients.

Side Effects: *CV:* Tachycardia, hypotension, chest pain. *GI:* Abdominal distress, nausea, vomiting. *CNS:* Lightheadedness, dizziness, nervousness, weakness. *Miscellaneous:* Severe rash.

Dosage: Tablets: 10–20 mg t.i.d.–q.i.d. **IM.** *Premature labor:* 5–10 mg b.i.d.–t.i.d. (Injection not available in the US).

NURSING CONSIDERATIONS
Assessment
1. Note if the client is taking a beta-blocking agent because this may diminish the response to isoxsuprine.
2. If administering the drug to a pregnant woman, determine if there is evidence of uterine relaxation.

3. Note any other drugs such as diuretics or hypotensive agents, that the client may be taking and document.

Interventions
1. If the client is postpartum, be aware that arterial bleeding may occur. Have emergency drugs available.
2. When the drug is used to control premature labor, monitor the intensity, frequency and duration of uterine contractions.
3. If the drug is used to counteract a threatened spontaneous abortion, monitor the fetal heart rate at regular intervals.

Client/Family Teaching
1. Review the goals of drug therapy.
2. Discuss the potential of the drug to cause hypotension, lightheadedness, and dizziness.
3. Avoid the use of alcoholic beverages.

Evaluation: Evaluate client for:
- Reports of symptomatic improvement
- Termination of premature labor

Isradipine
(iss-**RAD**-ih-peen)
DynaCirc (Rx)

See also *Calcium Channel Blocking Agents,* p. 118.

Classification: Calcium channel blocking agent.

Action/Kinetics: Isradipine binds to calcium channels resulting in the inhibition of calcium influx into cardiac and smooth muscle and subsequent arteriolar vasodilation. The reduced systemic resistance leads to a decrease in blood pressure with a small increase in resting heart rate. In clients with normal ventricular function, the drug reduces afterload leading to some increase in cardiac output. Isradipine is well absorbed from the GI tract although it undergoes significant first-pass metabolism. **Peak plasma levels:** 1 ng/ml after 1.5 hr. **Onset:** 2 hr. When taken with food, the time to peak effect is increased by approximately 1 hr, although the total bioavailability does not change. $t^{1/2}$, **initial:** 1.5–2 hr; **terminal,** 8 hr. The drug is completely metabolized in the liver with 60%–65% excreted through the kidneys and 25%–30% through the feces. The maximum effect may not be observed for 2–4 wk.

Uses: Alone or with thiazide diuretics in the management of essential hypertension.

Contraindications: Lactation.

Special Concerns: Pregnancy category: C. Safety and effectiveness have not been determined in children. Use with caution in clients with congestive heart failure, especially those taking a beta-adrenergic blocking agent. The bioavailability of isradipine increases in geriatric clients over 65 years of age, clients with impaired hepatic function, and those with mild renal impairment.

Side Effects: *CV:* Palpitations, edema, flushing, tachycardia, shortness of breath, hypotension, transient ischemic attack, stroke, atrial fibrillation, ventricular fibrillation, myocardial infarction, congestive

heart failure, angina. *CNS:* Headache, dizziness, fatigue, drowsiness, insomnia, lethargy, nervousness, depression, syncope, amnesia, psychosis, hallucinations, weakness, jitteriness, paresthesia. *GI:* Nausea, abdominal discomfort, diarrhea, vomiting, constipation, dry mouth. *Respiratory:* Dyspnea, cough. *Dermatologic:* Pruritus, urticaria. *Miscellaneous:* Chest pain, rash, pollakiuria, cramps of the legs and feet, nocturia, polyuria, hyperhidrosis, visual disturbances, numbness, throat discomfort, leukopenia, sexual difficulties.

Drug Interactions: Severe hypotension has been observed during fentanyl anesthesia with concomitant use of a beta blocker and a calcium channel blocking agent.

Laboratory Test Interferences: ↑ Liver function tests.

Dosage: Capsules. Adults, initial: 2.5 mg b.i.d. alone or in combination with a thiazide diuretic. If blood pressure is not decreased satisfactorily after 2–4 wk, the dose may be increased in increments of 5 mg/day at 2–4 wk intervals up to a maximum of 20 mg daily. Adverse effects increase, however, above doses of 10 mg/day.

Administration/Storage: The drug should be stored in a tight container protected from light.

NURSING CONSIDERATIONS

See *Nursing Considerations* for *Calcium Channel Blocking Agents,* p. 119.

Evaluation: Evaluate client for control of hypertension with a minimum of side effects.

K

Kanamycin sulfate

(kan-ah-**MY**-sin)
Anamid✿, Kantrex, Klebcil (Rx)

See also *Anti-Infectives,* p. 80, and *Aminoglycosides,* p. 23.

Classification: Antibiotic, aminoglycoside, and antitubercular agent (tertiary).

Action/Kinetics: The activity of kanamycin resembles that of neomycin and streptomycin. **Therapeutic serum levels: IM,** 8–16 mcg/ml. **t½:** 2–3 hr.

Uses: Adjunct in treatment of tuberculosis. Orally for hepatic encephalopathy to inhibit ammonia-forming bacteria in the GI tract. Orally to prepare the intestine prior to surgery. Peritoneally to irrigate infected wounds, cavities, surgical sites. As an aerosol for respiratory tract infections.

Special Concerns: Pregnancy category: D. Use with caution in premature infants and neonates.

Additional Side Effects: Sprue-like syndrome with steatorrhea, malabsorption, and electrolyte imbalance.

Additional Drug Interaction: Procainamide ↑ muscle relaxation.

Dosage: Capsules. *Intestinal bacteria suppression:* 1 g q hr for 4 hr; **then,** 1 g q 6 hr for 36–72 hr. *Hepatic coma:* 8–12 g/day in divided doses. **IM, IV. Adults and children:** 15 mg/kg/day in 2–3 equal doses. Maximum daily dose should not exceed 1.5 g regardless of route of administration. For calculating dosage interval (in hours) in clients with impaired renal function, multiply serum creatinine (mg/100 ml) by 9. **Intraperitoneal:** 500 mg diluted in 20 ml sterile distilled water. **Inhalation:** 250 mg in saline—nebulize b.i.d.–q.i.d. **Irrigation of abscess cavities, pleural space, ventricular cavities:** 0.25% solution.

Tuberculosis. **IM. Adults:** 15 mg/kg once daily. Not recommended for use in children.

NURSING CONSIDERATIONS

See also *Nursing Considerations* for *Aminoglycosides,* p. 25.

Administration

1. Do not mix with any other medication in IV bottle/bag. Administer IV slowly and at concentrations not exceeding 2.5 mg/ml.
2. Unopened vials may change color, but this does not affect potency of drug. Consult pharmacist if unsure of altered vials.
3. Do not mix with other drugs in same syringe for IM injection.
4. Inject deep into large muscle mass to minimize pain and local irritation. Rotate sites of injection. Local irritation may occur with large doses.
5. IV administration is rarely used and must not be used for clients with renal impairment.
6. Drug should not be administered for more than 12–14 days.

Ketamine hydrochloride

(**KEET**-ah-meen)
Ketalar (Rx)

Classification: General anesthetic.

Action/Kinetics: Ketamine is rapid-acting and produces good analgesia. The drug blocks afferent impulses associated with pain perception, depresses spinal cord activity, and affects transmitter systems in the CNS. There is no effect on the pharyngeal-laryngeal reflexes. There is, however, slightly enhanced skeletal muscle tone and cardiovascular and respiratory stimulation. **Onset, IV:** 30 sec following a dose of 2 mg/kg; **onset, IM:** 3–4 min. **Duration, IV:** 5–10 min following a dose of 2 mg/kg; **duration, IM:** 12–25 min following a dose of 10 mg/kg. **t½:** 7–11 min (distribution) and 2–3 hr (elimination). The anesthetic effect is terminated by redistribution to other tissues from the brain and by liver metabolism (the major metabolite is ⅓ as active as ketamine).

Uses: For procedures in which skeletal muscle relaxation is not required. Induction of anesthesia before use of other general anesthetics. As a supplement to nitrous oxide anesthesia. *Investigational:* Adjunct to local anesthesia to produce sedation and analgesia.

Contraindications: Schizophrenia, acute psychoses, hypertension (or in clients in whom a rise in blood pressure would be dangerous).

Special Concerns: Safe use during pregnancy has not been determined. Use with caution in the chronic alcoholic or if an individual is intoxicated with alcohol.

Side Effects: *Respiratory:* Apnea or severe respiratory depression following rapid IV administration, laryngospasm. *GI:* Nausea, vomiting, anorexia, increased salivation. *CV:* Increased blood pressure and pulse rate, bradycardia, hypotension, arrhythmias. *Skeletal muscle:* Tonic and clonic movements resembling seizures. *CNS:* Emergence reactions including dream-like states, hallucinations, delirium, vivid imagery, confusion, irrational behavior, excitement. *Ophthalmologic:* Increased intraocular pressure (slight), double vision, nystagmus. *Miscellaneous:* Morbilliform rash, transient erythema.

Symptom of Overdose: Respiratory depression.

Drug Interactions

Barbiturates / ↑ Recovery time from ketamine
Halothane / ↓ Pulse rate, blood pressure and cardiac output
Muscle relaxants, nondepolarizing / ↑ Neuromuscular effects → respiratory depression
Narcotic analgesics / ↑ Recovery time from ketamine
Thyroid hormones / Tachycardia and hypertension
Tubocurarine / ↑ Neuromuscular effects → respiratory depression

Dosage: IV. Individualized. *Induction,* **initial:** 1–2 mg/kg (of the base) at a rate of 0.5 mg/kg/min. **Maintenance:** 0.01–0.05 mg/kg by continuous infusion at a rate of 1–2 mg/min. *Adjunct to local anesthesia:* 5–30 mg (of the base) before giving the local anesthetic. *Sedation and analgesia:* 0.2–0.75 mg/kg (of the base) given over 2–3 min; **then,** 0.005–0.02 mg/kg (of the base)/min as a continuous IV infusion.

IM. *Induction,* **initial:** 5–10 mg/kg (of the base). Doses from one-half to the full amount of the induction dose may be used to maintain anesthesia. *Maintenance* *of ketamine used with diazepam:* 0.1–0.5 mg/min ketamine with 2–5 mg diazepam IV as required. *Sedation and analgesia:* 2–4 mg/kg (of the base); **then,** 0.005–0.2 mg/kg (of the base)/min by continuous IV infusion.

NURSING CONSIDERATIONS

Administration/Storage

1. The dose should be administered slowly over a 60-sec period to reduce respiratory depression and hypertension.
2. Vials containing 100 mg/ml should always be diluted first with an equal volume of sterile water for injection, normal saline, or 5% dextrose in water.
3. A precipitate will form if ketamine is combined with a barbiturate; thus, they should not be mixed in the same syringe.
4. Diazepam and ketamine should not be mixed in the same syringe or infusion flask.
5. Maintenance doses must be determined individually and are dependent, in part, on which additional anesthetic is used.
6. Tonic-clonic movements may occur during anesthesia; if manifested, they are not an indication for additional ketamine.
7. *Treatment of Overdose:* Artificial respiration.

Interventions

1. To prevent dreams that are likely to occur with ketamine, place client in a quiet area after anesthesia.
2. Take vital signs gently. Avoid making noises, bumping bed, and vigorously rousing or stimulating the client. Keep side rails up.

3. If the client is excessively active during the recovery phase, anticipate that a low dose of a barbiturate sedative may be required. This may also prolong recovery time.

Client/Family

1. Avoid alcohol and CNS depressants for at least 24 hr following anesthesia.
2. Do not perform tasks that require mental alertness until drug effects are realized.

Ketoconazole

(kee-toe-**KON**-ah-zohl)

Nizoral (Rx)

K

Classification: Broad-spectrum antifungal.

Action/Kinetics: Ketoconazole inhibits synthesis of sterols (e.g., ergosterol), damaging the cell membrane and resulting in loss of essential intracellular material. It also inhibits biosynthesis of triglycerides and phospholipids and inhibits oxidative and peroxidative enzyme activity. When used to treat *Candida albicans,* it inhibits transformation of blasto spores into the invasive mycelial form. Use in Cushing's syndrome is due to its ability to inhibit adrenal steroidogenesis. **Peak plasma levels:** 3.5 mcg/ml after 1–2 hr. **t½** [biphasic]: first, 2 hr; second, 8 hr. Requires acidity for dissolution. Metabolized in liver and most excreted through feces.

Uses: PO, Topical. Candidiasis, chronic mucocutaneous candidiasis, candiduria, histoplasmosis, chromomycosis, oral thrush, coccidioidomycosis, paracoccidioidomycosis. Recalcitrant cutaneous dermatophyte in fections. **Shampoo.** To reduce scaling due to dandruff. *Investigational:* Onychomycosis due to *Candida* and *Trichophyton*. Tinea versicolor; tinea pedis, corporis, and cruris; vaginal candidiasis. High doses to treat CNS fungal infections. Advanced prostate cancer, Cushing's syndrome. *Topical:* Tinea corporis, tinea cruris, and tinea versicolor. Cutaneous candidiasis, seborrheic dermatitis.

Contraindications: Hypersensitivity, fungal meningitis. Topical product not for ophthalmic use. Use during lactation.

Special Concerns: Pregnancy category: C. Use with caution in children less than 2 years of age.

Side Effects: *GI:* Nausea, vomiting, abdominal pain, diarrhea. *CNS:* Headache, dizziness, somnolence, fever, chills. *Hematologic:* Thrombocytopenia, leukopenia, hemolytic anemia. *Miscellaneous:* Hepatotoxicity, photophobia, pruritus, gynecomastia, impotence, bulging fontanelles, urticaria, anaphylaxis (rare). *Topical cream:* Stinging, irritation, pruritus. *Shampoo:* Increased hair loss, irritation, abnormal hair texture, itching, oiliness or dryness of the scalp and hair, scalp pustules.

Drug Interactions

Antacids / ↓ Absorption of ketoconazole due to ↑ pH induced by these drugs
Anticoagulants / ↓ Effect of anticoagulants
Anticholinergics / ↓ Absorption of ketoconazole due to ↑ pH induced by these drugs
Corticosteroids / ↑ Risk of corticosteroid toxicity due to ↑ bioavailability
Cyclosporine / ↑ Levels of cyclosporine (may be used therapeutically to decrease the dose of cyclosporine)
Histamine H$_2$-antagonists / ↓ Absorption of ketoconazole due to ↑ pH induced by these drugs
Isoniazid / ↓ Bioavailability of ketoconazole
Rifampin / ↓ Serum levels of both drugs
Theophyllines / ↓ Serum levels of theophylline

Laboratory Test Interference: Transient ↑ serum liver enzymes. ↓ Serum testosterone.

Dosage: Tablets. Adults: 200–400 mg as single dose/day. **Pediatric, over 2 years:** 3.3–6.6 mg/kg daily as a single dose. Dosage in children less than 2 years of age not established. *CNS fungal infections:* **PO,** 800–1,200 mg daily. *Advanced prostate cancer:* 400 mg q 8 hr. *Cushing's syndrome:* 800–1,200 mg daily. **Topical cream (2%).** *Tinea corporis, tinea cruris, tinea versicolor, cutaneous candidiasis:* Cover the affected and immediate surrounding areas once daily (twice daily for more resistant cases). Duration of treatment is usually 2 weeks. *Seborrheic dermatitis:* Apply to affected area b.i.d. for 4 weeks or until symptoms clear. **Shampoo (2%):** Use twice a week for 4 weeks with at least 3 days between each shampooing. **Then,** use as required to maintain control.

NURSING CONSIDERATIONS

See also *General Nursing Considerations For All Anti-Infectives,* p. 83.

Administration/Storage

1. Ketoconazole should be given a minimum of 2 hr before administration of drugs that

increase gastric pH (such as antacids, anticholinergics, or H_2 blockers). If antacids are needed, delay administration by 2 hr.

2. To decrease GI upset, take tablets with food.
3. The shampoo should be applied in sufficient quantities to cover the entire scalp for 1 min. Rinse with warm water and repeat, leaving the shampoo on the scalp for 3 min.
4. The minimum treatment for candidiasis (using tablets) is 1–2 weeks and for other systemic mycoses is 6 months.

Client/Family Teaching

1. Review the appropriate method for drug administration.
2. Report persistent fever, pain, or diarrhea.
3. If clients have achlorhydria, instruct them to dissolve each tablet in 4 ml aqueous solution of 0.2 N HCl and to use a straw (glass or plastic) to take this solution to avoid contact with their teeth. This is followed by drinking a glass of tap water.
4. Use caution when driving or when performing hazardous tasks because drug can cause headaches, dizziness, and drowsiness.
5. Avoid alcohol or alcohol-containing products.
6. Wear sunglasses and avoid sun exposure to prevent a photosensitivity reaction.

Evaluation: Evaluate client for:

- Improvement in pretreatment symptoms of fungal infections
- Knowledge and understanding of illness and compliance with drug therapy

Ketoprofen

(kee-toe-**PROH**-fen)

Apo-Keto ✱, Apo-Keto-E ✱, Orudis, Orudis-E ✱ Orudis-SR ✱, Rhodis ✱, Rhodis E ✱ (Rx)

See also *Nonsteroidal Anti-Inflammatory Drugs,* p. 186.

Classification: Nonsteroidal anti-inflammatory drug.

Action/Kinetics: The drug possesses anti-inflammatory, antipyretic, and analgesic properties. It is known to inhibit both prostaglandin and leukotriene synthesis, to have antibradykinin activity, and to stabilize lysosomal membranes. **Peak plasma levels:** 0.5–2 hr. **t½:** 2–4 hr. The **t½** is increased to approximately 5 hr in geriatric patients. Ketoprofen is 99% bound to plasma proteins. Food does not alter the bioavailability; however, the rate of absorption is reduced.

Uses: Acute or chronic rheumatoid arthritis and osteoarthritis. Primary dysmenorrhea. Analgesic for mild to moderate pain. *Investigational:* Juvenile rheumatoid arthritis, sunburn, prophylaxis of migraine, migraine due to menses.

Contraindications: Should not be used during late pregnancy. Use should be avoided during lactation and in children.

Special Concerns: Pregnancy category: B (use only if benefits outweigh risks). Safety and effectiveness have not been established in children. Geriatric clients may manifest increased and prolonged serum levels due to decreased protein binding and clearance. Use with caution in clients with a history of GI tract disorders, in fluid retention, hypertension, and heart failure.

K

Additional Side Effects: *GI:* Peptic ulcer, GI bleeding, dyspepsia, nausea, diarrhea, constipation, abdominal pain, flatulence, anorexia, vomiting, stomatitis. *CNS:* Headache. *CV:* Peripheral edema, fluid retention.

Additional Drug Interactions

Acetylsalicylic acid / ↑ Plasma ketoprofen levels due to ↓ plasma protein binding

Hydrochlorothiazide / ↓ Chloride and potassium excretion

Methotrexate / Concomitant use → toxic plasma levels of methotrexate

Probenecid / ↓ Plasma clearance of ketoprofen and ↓ plasma protein binding

Warfarin / Additive effect to cause bleeding

Dosage: Capsules. *Rheumatoid arthritis, osteoarthritis:* **Initial:** 75 mg t.i.d. or 50 mg q.i.d. Dose may be increased to 300 mg daily in divided doses, if necessary; doses above 300 mg daily are not recommended. Dosage should be decreased by one-half to one-third in clients with impaired renal function or in geriatric clients. *Analgesia, dysmenorrhea:* 25–50 mg q 6–8 hr as required, not to exceed 300 mg daily. Dosage should be reduced in geriatric clients and in those with liver or renal dysfunction.

NURSING CONSIDERATIONS

See also *Nursing Considerations for Nonsteroidal Anti-Inflammatory Drugs,* p. 189.

Administration/Storage

1. GI side effects may be minimized by taking ketoprofen with antacids, milk, or food.

2. The onset of action takes 15–30 min and lasts from 4–6 hr.

Assessment

1. Note any client history of GI disorders, cardiac failure, hypertension or fluid retention.
2. Determine if the client is pregnant.
3. Document age; the drug is not recommended for children under 12 years of age.
4. Obtain baseline bleeding profiles, liver and renal function studies.

Interventions

1. Anticipate a reduced dosage of drug in elderly clients and those with impaired renal function.
2. Monitor bleeding time and prothrombin time. The drug may prolong bleeding times by decreasing platelet aggregation.
3. Inspect the client periodically for petechiae, unexplained bruising, bleeding from the gums or nose bleeds. Document and report these to the physician.
4. Monitor urine and stools for occult blood.
5. Inspect clients for evidence of liver dysfunction such as jaundice, upper right quadrant pain, clay colored stools, or yellowing of the skin and sclera. Document findings, request a liver profile, and report.

Client/Family Teaching

1. Advise client to avoid ingesting alcoholic beverages.
2. Instruct client not to take aspirin during therapy unless physician prescribed.

3. Report any new symptoms such as rash, headaches, black stools, or disturbances in vision.
4. Provide a printed list of drug side effects, which should be reported to the physician should they occur.
5. Stress the importance of reporting for scheduled lab studies and eye exams throughout therapy.

Evaluation: Evaluate client for:
- Evidence of improvement in joint pain and mobility
- Reports of effective control of pain

Ketorolac tromethamine

(kee-toh-**ROH**-lack)

Toradol (Rx)

See also *Nonsteroidal Anti-Inflammatory Drugs,* p. 186.

Classification: Nonsteroidal anti-inflammatory drug.

Action/Kinetics: Ketorolac tromethamine is a nonsteroidal anti-inflammatory drug that possesses anti-inflammatory, analgesic, and antipyretic effects. It is completely absorbed following an IM dose. **Onset:** Within 10 min. **Peak plasma levels:** 2.2–3.0 mcg/ml 50 min after a dose of 30 mg. **t½, terminal:** 3.8–6.3 hr in young adults and 4.7–8.6 hr in geriatric clients. Over 99% is bound to plasma proteins. The drug is metabolized in the liver with over 90% excreted in the urine and the remainder excreted in the feces.

Uses: IM for short-term management of pain.

Contraindications: Hypersensitivity to the drug, incomplete or partial syndrome of nasal polyps, angioedema, and bronchospasm due to aspirin or other NSAIDs. Use as an obstetrical preoperative medication or for obstetrical analgesia. Routine use with other NSAIDs.

Special Concerns: Pregnancy category: B. Use with caution in impaired hepatic or renal function, during lactation, in geriatric clients, and in clients on high-dose salicylate regimens. Safety and effectiveness have not been determined in children.

Additional Side Effects: *CV:* Vasodilation, pallor. *GI:* Flatulence, GI fullness, stomatitis, excessive thirst. *CNS:* Nervousness, abnormal thinking, depression, euphoria. *Miscellaneous:* Purpura, asthma, abnormal vision, abnormal liver function.

Drug Interactions: Ketorolac may ↑ plasma levels of salicylates due to ↓ plasma protein binding.

Dosage: IM, initial loading dose: 30 or 60 mg; **then,** 15 or 30 mg q 6 hr as needed to control pain. **Maximum daily dose:** 150 mg for the first day and 120 mg thereafter.

NURSING CONSIDERATIONS

See also *Nursing Considerations for Nonsteroidal Anti-Inflammatory Drugs,* p. 189.

Administration/Storage

1. Ketorolac should be used as part of a regular analgesic schedule rather than on an as needed basis.
2. To minimize a time delay in reaching adequate analgesic effects, an initial loading dose is recommended equal to twice the maintenance dose.
3. If the drug is given on an as

needed basis, the size of a repeat dose should be based on the duration of pain relief from the previous dose. If the pain returns within 3–5 hr, the next dose could be increased by up to 50% (as long as the total daily dose is not exceeded). If the pain does not return for 8–12 hr, the next dose could be decreased by as much as 50% or the dosing interval could be increased to q 8–12 hr.

4. Lower doses should be considered for clients under 50 kg, over 65 years of age, and with reduced renal function.

Assessment

1. Note any previous experience with NSAIDs and the results.
2. Determine any evidence of liver or renal dysfunction.

Evaluation: Evaluate client for reports of effective pain control.

L

Labetalol hydrochloride
(lah-**BET**-ah-lohl)
Normodyne, Trandate (Rx)

Classification: Alpha- and beta-adrenergic blocking agent.

Action/Kinetics: Labetalol decreases blood pressure by blocking both alpha- and beta-adrenergic receptors. Significant reflex tachycardia and bradycardia do not occur although AV conduction may be prolonged. **Onset: PO,** 2–4 hr; **IV,** 5 min. **Peak plasma levels, PO:** 1–2 hr. **Duration: PO,** 8–12 hr. **t½: PO,** 6–8 hr; **IV,** 5.5 hr. Significant first-pass effect; metabolized in liver. Food increases bioavailability of the drug.

Uses: PO: Alone or in combination with other drugs for hypertension. **IV:** Hypertensive emergencies. *Investigational:* Pheochromocytoma, clonidine withdrawal hypertension.

Contraindications: Cardiogenic shock, cardiac failure, bronchial asthma, bradycardia, greater than first-degree heart block.

Special Concerns: Use with caution during pregnancy (category: C) and lactation, in impaired renal and hepatic function, and diabetes (may prevent premonitory signs of acute hypoglycemia). Safety and efficacy in children have not been established.

Side Effects: *CV:* Postural hypotension, edema, flushing, ventricular arrhythmias, intensification of AV block. *GI:* Nausea, vomiting, diarrhea, altered taste, dyspepsia. *CNS:* Headache, drowsiness, fatigue, sleepiness, dizziness, vertigo, paresthesias, numbness. *GU:* Impotence, urinary bladder retention, difficulty in urination, failure to ejaculate, priapism, Peyronie's disease. *Dermatologic:* Rashes, facial erythema, alopecia, urticaria, pruritus, psoriasis-like syndrome, bullous lichen planus. *Respiratory:* Bronchospasm, dyspnea, wheezing. *Musculoskele-*

tal: Muscle cramps, asthenia, toxic myopathy. *Other:* Systemic lupus erythematosus, jaundice, cholestasis, difficulties with vision, dry eyes, nasal stuffiness, tingling of skin or scalp, sweating, fever.

Possible changes in laboratory values include increased serum transaminase, positive antinuclear factor, antimitochondrial antibodies, and increases in blood urea and creatinine.

Symptoms of Overdose: Excessive hypotension and bradycardia.

Drug Interactions

Beta-adrenergic bronchodilators / Labetalol ↓ bronchodilator effect of these drugs
Cimetidine / ↑ Bioavailability of oral labetalol
Glutethimide / ↓ Effects of labetalol due to ↑ breakdown by liver
Halothane / ↑ Risk of severe myocardial depression → hypotension
Nitroglycerin / Additive hypotension
Tricyclic antidepressants / ↑ Risk of tremors

Laboratory Test Interference: False + increase in urinary catecholamines.

Dosage: Tablets. Initial: 100 mg b.i.d. alone or with a diuretic; **maintenance:** 200–400 mg b.i.d. up to 1,200–2,400 mg daily for severe cases. **IV. Individualize. Initial:** 20 mg slowly over 2 min; **then,** 40–80 mg q 10 min until desired effect occurs or a total of 300 mg has been given. **IV infusion. Initial:** 2 mg/min; **then,** adjust rate according to response. **Usual dose range:** 50–300 mg. *Transfer from IV to PO therapy:* **initial,** 200 mg; **then,** 200–400 mg

6–12 hr later, depending on response. Thereafter, dosage based on response.

NURSING CONSIDERATIONS

See also *Nursing Considerations* for *Beta-Adrenergic Blocking Agents,* p. 116.

Administration/Storage

1. When transferring to PO labetalol from other antihypertensive therapy, slowly reduce dosage of current therapy.
2. To transfer from IV to PO therapy in hospitalized clients, begin when supine blood pressure begins to increase.
3. Labetalol is not compatible with 5% sodium bicarbonate injection.
4. The full antihypertensive effect of labetalol is usually seen within the first 1–3 hr after the initial dose or dose increment.
5. When given by IV infusion, labetalol should be administered using an infusion pump, a micro-drip regulator, or similar type device that allows precise control of flow rate.
6. *Treatment of Overdose:* Induce vomiting or perform gastric lavage. Clients should be placed in a supine position with legs elevated. If required, the following treatment can be used:
   • Epinephrine or a beta-2 agonist (aerosol) to treat bronchospasm.
   • Atropine or epinephrine to treat bradycardia.
   • Digitalis glycoside and a diuretic for cardiac failure; dopamine or dobutamine may also be used.
   • Diazepam to treat seizures.
   • Norepinephrine (or another

vasopressor) to treat hypotension.

- Administration of glucagon (5–10 mg rapidly over 30 seconds), followed by continuous infusion of 5 mg/hr, may be effective in treating severe hypotension and bradycardia.

Interventions

1. The effect of labetalol on standing blood pressure should be assessed before the client is discharged from the hospital. Perform measurements with the client standing at several different times during the day to determine full effects of the drug.
2. To reduce the chance of orthostatic hypotension, clients should remain supine for 3 hr after receiving parenteral labetalol.

Evaluation: Evaluate client for a ↓ in blood pressure and control of hypertension with a minimum of adverse effects.

Lactulose
(**LAK**-tyou-lohs)
Acilac✿, Cephulac, Cholac, Chronulac, Comalose-R✿, Constilac, Constulose, Duphalac, Enulose, Gel-ose✿, Lactulax✿ Laxilose✿, PMS Lactulose✿, Rhodialax✿, Rhodialose✿ (Rx)

Classification: Ammonia detoxicant, laxative.

Action/Kinetics: Lactulose, a disaccharide containing both lactose and galactose, causes a decrease in the blood concentration of ammonia in clients suffering from portal-systemic encephalopathy. The mechanism involved is attributed to the bacteria-induced degradation of lactulose in the colon, resulting in an acid medium. Ammonia will then migrate from the blood to the colon to form ammonium ion, which is trapped and cannot be absorbed. A laxative action due to increased osmotic pressure from lactic, formic, and acetic acids then expels the trapped ammonium. The decrease in blood ammonia concentration improves the mental state, EEG tracing, and diet protein tolerance of clients. The increased osmotic pressure also results in a laxative effect, which may take up to 24 hr. The drug is partly absorbed from the GI tract. **Onset:** 24–48 hr.

Uses: Prevention and treatment of portal-systemic encephalopathy, including hepatic and prehepatic coma (Cephylac, Cholac, Enulose are used). Chronic constipation (Chronulac, Constilac, Duphalac are used).

Contraindications: Clients on galactose-restricted diets.

Special Concerns: Safe use during pregnancy (category: B) and lactation and in children has not been established. Infants who have been given lactulose have developed hyponatremia and dehydration. Use with caution in presence of diabetes mellitus.

Side Effects: *GI:* Nausea, vomiting, diarrhea, cramps, flatulence, gaseous distention, belching.

Drug Interactions

Antacids / May inhibit the drop in pH of the colon required for lactulose activity
Neomycin / May cause ↓ degradation of lactulose due to

neomycin-induced ↑ in elimination of certain bacteria in the colon

Dosage: Syrup. *Encephalopathy:* **Adults, initial,** 30–45 ml (20–30 g) t.i.d.–q.i.d.; adjust q 2–3 days to obtain 2 or 3 soft stools daily. Long-term therapy may be required in portal–systemic encephalopathy; **infants:** 2.5–10 ml/day (1.6–6.6 g/day) in divided doses; **older children and adolescents:** 40–90 ml/day (26.6–60 g/day) in divided doses. *During acute episodes:* 30–45 ml (20–30 g) q 1–2 hr to induce rapid initial laxation. *Retention enema:* 300 ml (200 g), diluted to 1,000 ml with water or saline and retained for 30–60 min; may be repeated q 4–6 hr. *Chronic constipation:* **Adults and children,** 15–30 ml/day (10–20 g/day) as a single dose after breakfast (up to 60 ml/day may be required).

NURSING CONSIDERATIONS

Administration/Storage

1. To minimize sweet taste, dilute with water or fruit juice or add to desserts.
2. When given by gastric tube, dilute well to prevent vomiting and the possibility of aspiration pneumonia.
3. When administered by enema use a rectal balloon catheter to assist with retention.
4. Store below 30°C (86°F). Avoid freezing.
5. Other laxatives should not be taken with lactulose.

Interventions

1. Report any client complaint of GI distress to the physician. The problem may subside as the therapy continues, or the dose of medication may need to be reduced.

2. Monitor the serum potassium levels of clients who have portal-systemic encephalopathy. This is to determine whether the drug is causing further potassium loss that will intensify symptoms of the disease.
3. The medication contains carbohydrate. Therefore, observe clients who have diabetes for flushed, dry skin, complaints of dry mouth and intense thirst, a fruity odor to the breath, abdominal pain and low blood pressure. These are symptoms of hyperglycemia that are more likely to occur in clients with diabetes.
4. Keep the client clean and dry. Assess the client's skin condition frequently because skin breakdown may occur rapidly.

Evaluation: Evaluate client for:
- Improvement in level of consciousness and mental status
- Laboratory evidence of a decrease in the serum ammonia level
- Reports of relief of constipation with 2–3 soft bowel movements/day

Leucovorin calcium (citrovorum factor, folinic acid)
(loo-koh-**VOR**-in)
Lederle Leucovorin ✤, Wellcovorin (Rx)

Classification: Folic acid derivative.

Action/Kinetics: Leucovorin is a formyl derivative (reduced form) of folic acid. It does not require reduction by dihydrofolate reductase to be active in intracellular metabolism; thus, it is not affected by dihydrofolate inhibitors. Leucovor in is rapidly absorbed following oral administration. **Peak serum levels, PO:** Approximately 1.7 hr; **after IM:** approximately 0.7 hr. **Onset, PO:** 20–30 min; **IM:** 10–20 min; **IV:** Less than 5 min. **t½:** 3.5 hr (PO) and 3.7 hr (IM). **Duration:** 3–6 hr. The drug is excreted by the kidney.

Uses: Megaloblastic anemias due to nutritional deficiency, sprue, pregnancy, and infancy. When oral folic acid is not appropriate. Prophylaxis and treatment of toxicity due to methotrexate, pyrimethamine, and trimethoprim. Leucovorin rescue following high doses of methotrexate. *Investigational:* Adjunct with 5-fluorouracil to treat metastatic colorectal carcinoma.

Contraindications: Pernicious anemia or megaloblastic anemia due to vitamin B_{12} deficiency.

Special Concerns: Pregnancy category: C, although it is recommended for megaloblastic anemia caused by pregnancy. Use with caution during lactation. May increase the frequency of seizures in susceptible children.

Side Effects: *Allergic:* Erythema, skin rash, itching, malaise, respiratory difficulties, bronchospasms. High doses may cause: *GI:* Anorexia, nausea, distention, flatulence, bad taste in mouth. *CNS:* Excitement, altered sleep patterns, difficulty in concentration, irritability, overactivity, mental depression, confusion, and impaired judgment.

Drug Interactions

Aminosalicylic acid / ↓ Serum folate levels → folic acid deficiency

Phenytoin / ↓ Effect of phenytoin due to ↑ rate of breakdown by liver; also, phenytoin may ↓ plasma folate levels
Primidone / ↓ Serum folate levels → folic acid deficiency
Sulfasalazine / ↓ Serum folate levels → folic acid deficiency

Dosage: For Oral Solution, Tablets, IM, IV. *Overdose of folic acid antagonists—leucovorin rescue following methotrexate:* **Adults and children:** 10 mg/m² q 6 hr until methotrexate blood level falls to less than 5 x 10⁻⁸ M; if after 24 hr serum creatinine level is 50% greater than premethotrexate serum creatinine levels, increase the dose of leucovorin to 100 mg/m² q 3 hr IV until serum methotrexate is less than 5 x 10⁻⁸ M. *Leucovorin rescue following trimethoprim or pyrimethamine:* **Adults and children,** 5–15 mg daily. *Treatment following pyrimethamine or trimethoprim:* **Adults and children,** 400 mcg–5,000 mcg (5 mg) with each dose of the folic acid antagonist. *Megaloblastic anemia:* **Adults and children,** 1 mg daily.

NURSING CONSIDERATIONS

Administration/Storage

1. If leucovorin is used for methotrexate rescue purposes, the client should be well hydrated and the urine should be alkalinized in order to reduce nephrotoxicity.
2. Leucovorin calcium injection should be diluted with 5 ml bacteriostatic water for injection and used within one week. If sterile water for injection is added, the solution should be used immediately.
3. The oral solution is stable for

14 days if refrigerated or for 7 days if stored at room temperature.

4. Doses higher than 25 mg should be given parenterally because oral absorption is saturated.

5. Leucovorin calcium injection containing benzyl alcohol should not be used for doses greater than 10 mg/m².

Assessment: Note if the client has a history of vitamin B_{12} deficiency that has resulted in pernicious anemia or megaloblastic anemia.

Interventions

1. Anticipate that leucovorin rescue is used in conjunction with methotrexate therapy.

2. Note any client complaints of skin rash, itching, malaise, or difficulty breathing. Document and report to the physician immediately.

3. If the client is receiving the drug for rescue therapy, it should be administered promptly following a high dose of folic acid antagonists. The prescribed dosage must be followed exactly to be effective.

4. Parenteral therapy generally is used following chemotherapy because nausea and vomiting may prevent oral absorption.

5. Leucovorin may obscure the diagnosis of pernicious anemia if previously undiagnosed.

6. Monitor appropriate renal, folic acid, and hematologic values. Creatinine increases of 50% over pretreatment levels indicate renal toxicity.

7. Urine pH should be greater than 7.0. Urine alkalinization with $NaHCO_3$ or acetazolamide may be necessary to prevent nephrotoxic effects.

8. When high-dose therapy is used be alert for the client exhibiting mental confusion and impaired judgment. Provide appropriate safety measures to ensure client protection.

Evaluation: Evaluate client for:

• Improved symptomatology and laboratory evidence of an ↑ production of normoblasts (with megaloblastic anemias)

• Prevention and reversal of GI, renal, and bone marrow toxicity in methotrexate therapy or during overdosage of folic acid antagonists

Leuprolide acetate
(loo-**PROH**-lyd)
Lupron, Lupron Depot (Rx)

See also *Antineoplastic Agents*, p. 85.

Classification: Antineoplastic agent, hormonal.

Action/Kinetics: Leuprolide is related to the naturally occurring gonadotropin-releasing hormone (GnRH). By desensitizing GnRH receptors, gonadotropin secretion is inhibited. Initially, however, LH and FSH levels increase, leading to increases of sex hormones. However, decreases in these hormones will be observed within 2–4 weeks. $t^{1/2}$: 3 hr. **Peak plasma level following depot injection:** 20 ng/ml after 4 hr and 0.36 ng/ml after 4 weeks.

Uses: Palliative treatment in advanced prostatic cancer when orchiectomy or estrogen treatment are not appropriate. Endometriosis (use depot form). *Investigational:* Breast, ovarian, and endometrial cancer; leiomyoma uteri; precocious puberty; prostatic hypertrophy; infertility.

Contraindications: Pregnancy category: X. Depot form is contraindicated during pregnancy in women who may become pregnant while receiving the drug, and during lactation. Clients sensitive to benzyl alcohol (found in leuprolide injection). Undiagnosed abnormal vaginal bleeding.

Special Concerns: Safety and efficacy have not been determined in children. May cause increased bone pain and difficulty in urination during the first few weeks of therapy.

Side Effects: Injection and Depot. *GI:* Nausea, vomiting, anorexia, diarrhea. *CNS:* Paresthesia, insomnia, pain. *CV:* Peripheral edema, angina, cardiac arrhythmias. *GU:* Hematuria, urinary frequency or urgency, dysuria, testicular pain. *Respiratory:* Dyspnea, hemoptysis. *Endocrine:* Gynecomastia, breast tenderness, impotency, hot flashes, sweating, decreased testicular size, decreased libido. *Other:* Myalgia, bone pain, dermatitis, asthenia, diabetes, fever, chills, increased calcium.
    Injection. *CV:* ECG changes, hypertension, ischemia, heart murmur, congestive heart failure, thrombosis, phlebitis, myocardial infarction, hypotension, pulmonary emboli. *GI:* Constipation, GI bleeding, dysphagia, taste disorders, peptic ulcer, hepatic dysfunction, rectal polyps. *CNS:* Headache, dizziness, lightheadedness, lethargy, memory disorders, mood swings, anxiety, nervousness, syncope, blackouts, depression, fatigue. *Respiratory:* Sinus congestion, pneumonia, cough, pleural rub, pulmonary fibrosis or infiltrate. *Dermatologic:* Hair loss, skin pigmentation, skin lesions, carcinoma of ear or skin, dry skin, ecchymosis. *GU:* Urinary tract infection, bladder spasms, incontinence, penile swelling, prostate pain, increased libido, urinary obstruction. *Neuromuscular:* Joint pain, ankylosing spondylitis, pelvic fibrosis, peripheral neuropathy, numbness, spinal fracture, spinal paralysis. *Miscellaneous:* Blurred vision, hypoglycemia, ophthalmologic disorders, temporal bone swelling, enlarged thyroid, inflammation, infection, hypoproteinemia, decreased white blood cells.
    Depot. *Miscellaneous:* Hair growth, weight gain, hard nodule in throat.

Laboratory Test Interferences: Injection: ↑ BUN, creatinine. **Depot:** ↑ LDH, alkaline phosphatase, AST, uric acid. Misleading results from tests of pituitary gonadotropic and gonadal function up to 4–8 weeks after discontinuing depot therapy.

Dosage: SC: *Advanced prostatic cancer:* 1 mg daily, using the syringes provided. **Depot:** *Advanced prostatic cancer:* 7.5 mg IM q 28–33 days. *Endometriosis:* 3.75 mg once a month for at least 6 months. Retreatment is not recommended.

NURSING CONSIDERATIONS

See also *Nursing Considerations for Antineoplastic Agents,* p. 88.

Administration/Storage

1. If unrefrigerated, injection should be stored below 30°C (86°F).
2. The injection should be administered using only the syringes provided.
3. Depot may be stored at room temperature. The injection should be refrigerated until used.
4. The depot should be reconstituted only with the diluent provided; after reconstitution, the preparation is stable for 24 hr. However, since there is no preservative, it should be used immediately.
5. When injecting the depot form, needles smaller than 22 gauge should not be used.

Client/Family Teaching

1. Review the appropriate method and frequency of administration. Have clients return/demonstrate.
2. Stress that hot flashes are a common side effect of drug therapy.
3. Provide a printed list of drug side effects. Stress those that require immediate reporting such as weakness, numbness, respiratory difficulty, and impaired urination.
4. Advise that increased bone pain may be evident at the start of therapy. Analgesics may be prescribed for pain control.

Evaluation: Evaluate client for:
- Clinical evidence of control of tumor size and spread
- Reports of improvement in symptoms of endometriosis

Levamisole hydrochloride
(lee-**VAM**-ih-sohl)
Ergamisol (Rx)

Classification: Antineoplastic, adjunct.

Action/Kinetics: Levamisole is used in combination with fluorouracil and is considered to be an immunomodulator. The drug is thought to restore depressed immune function. As such, it stimulates formation of antibodies, stimulates T-cell activation and proliferation, potentiates monocyte and macrophage function (including phagocytosis and chemotaxis), and increases mobility adherence and chemotaxis of neutrophils. Levamisole is rapidly absorbed from the GI tract. **Peak plasma levels:** 0.13 mcg/ml after 1.5–2 hr. **t½:** 3–4 hr. Metabolized by the liver and excreted mainly in the urine.

Uses: In combination with fluorouracil to treat clients with Dukes' stage C colon cancer following surgical resection.

Contraindications: Lactation.

Special Concerns: Pregnancy category: C. Safety and effectiveness have not been demonstrated in children. Agranulocytosis, caused by levamisole, may be accompanied by a flu-like syndrome, or it may be asymptomatic. Thus, hematologic monitoring is required.

Side Effects: *GI:* Commonly nausea and diarrhea; vomiting, stomatitis, anorexia, abdominal pain, constipation, flatulence, dyspepsia. *Hematologic:* Leukopenia, thrombocytopenia, anemia, granulocyto-penia. *Dermatologic:* Commonly, dermatitis and pruritus; alopecia, skin discoloration. *CNS:* Dizziness, headache, inability to concentrate, weakness, memory loss, paresthe-sia, ataxia, somnolence, depression, insomnia, confusion, nervousness, anxiety, forgetfulness. *Musculoskel-etal:* Arthralgia, myalgia. *Ophthal-mologic:* Abnormal tearing, con-junctivitis, blurred vision. *Miscella-neous:* Fatigue, fever, rigors, chest pain, edema, taste perversion, al-tered sense of smell, infection, hyperbilirubinemia, epistaxis.

Drug Interactions

Ethanol / Disulfiram-like reaction when used with levamisole
Phenytoin / ↑ Phenytoin plasma levels

Dosage: Tablets. Adults, initial: levamisole, 50 mg q 8 hr for 3 days (starting 7–30 days after surgery) given together with fluorouracil, 450 mg/m²/day by IV push for 5 days (starting 21–34 days after sur-gery). **Maintenance:** levamisole, 50 mg q 8 hr for 3 days q 2 weeks for 1 year; fluorouracil, 450 mg/m²/day by IV push once a week begin-ning 28 days after the beginning of the 5-day course and continuing for 1 year.

NURSING CONSIDERATIONS

Administration/Storage

1. Levamisole therapy should be started no earlier than 7 and no later than 30 days after surgery; fluorouracil therapy should be initiated no earlier than 21 days and no later than 35 days after surgery. Before fluorouracil therapy is started, the client should be out of the hospital, ambulatory, eating normally,

have well-healed wounds, and have recovered from any post-operative complications.
2. If levamisole therapy has been started 7–20 days after surgery, fluorouracil therapy should be started at the same time as the second course of levamisole (i.e., 21–34 days after surgery).

Assessment

1. Record pretreatment weight.
2. Obtain baseline CBC with dif-ferential, platelets, electrolytes, and liver function studies; monitor throughout therapy.
3. Determine if client is taking phenytoin because therapy may increase plasma levels of phenytoin and require close monitoring.

Interventions

1. Observe if client manifests sto-matitis or diarrhea after fluoro-uracil administration because the drug should be discon-tinued before the full 5 doses are given.
2. Monitor and carefully evaluate hematologic studies.
   - If the white blood count (WBC) is between 2,500 and 3,500/mm³, the dose of fluo-rouracil should be deferred until the WBC is greater than 3,500/mm³.
   - If the WBC is less than 2,500/mm³, the dose of fluoroura-cil should be deferred until the WBC is greater than 3,500/mm³ and then reinsti-tuted at a dose reduced by 20%.
   - If the WBC is less than 2,500/mm³ for more than 10 days even though fluorouracil has not been given, the adminis-

tration of levamisole should be discontinued.

- Administration of both levamisole and fluorouracil should be deferred until the platelet count is at least 100,000/mm³.

Client/Family Teaching

1. Provide a printed list of drug side effects that should be reported.
2. Instruct client to report immediately any malaise, confusion, or flu-like symptoms.
3. Avoid alcohol because drug may cause a disulfiram-like effect.
4. Stress the importance of weekly lab studies for CBC and platelets prior to therapy with fluorouracil and every 3-month electrolyte and liver function determinations for one year.
5. Advise female clients of child-bearing age to practice safe contraception.

Evaluation: Evaluate client for:

- Clinical evidence of control of tumor size and spread
- Laboratory confirmation that WBC count within desired range

---

Levarterenol bitartrate (Norepinephrine)

(lee-var-**TER**-ih-nohl)

Levophed (Rx)

See also *Sympathomimetic Drugs*, p. 218.

Classification: Direct-acting adrenergic agent, vasopressor

Action/Kinetics: Levarterenol produces vasoconstriction (in-crease in BP) by stimulating alpha-adrenergic receptors. Also causes a moderate increase in contraction of heart by stimulating beta-1 receptors. Minimal hyperglycemic effect. **Onset:** immediate; **duration:** 1–2 min. Metabolized in liver and other tissues by the enzymes MAO and catechol-O-methyltransferase; however, the pharmacologic activity is terminated by uptake and metabolism in sympathetic nerve endings. Metabolites excreted in urine.

Uses: Hypotensive states caused by trauma, septicemia, blood transfusions, drug reactions, spinal anesthesia, poliomyelitis, central vasomotor depression, and myocardial infarctions. Adjunct to treatment of cardiac arrest and profound hypotension.

Additional Contraindications: Hypotension due to blood volume deficiency (except in emergencies), mesenteric or peripheral vascular thrombosis, in halothane or cyclopropane anesthesia (due to possibilities of fatal arrhythmias). Pregnancy (may cause fetal anoxia or hypoxia).

Special Concerns: Use with caution in clients taking MAO inhibitors or tricyclic antidepressants.

Additional Side Effects: Drug may cause bradycardia that can be abolished by atropine.

Dosage: IV infusion only (effect on BP determines dosage): initial, 8–12 mcg/min or 2–3 ml of a 4 mcg/ml solution/min; **maintenance,** 2–4 mcg/min with the dose determined by client response.

NURSING CONSIDERATIONS

See also *Nursing Considerations for Sympathomimetic Drugs*, p. 220.

L

Administration/Storage

1. Discard solutions that are brown or that have a precipitate.
2. Do not administer through the same tube as blood products.
3. The infusion should be continued until blood pressure is maintained without therapy. Abrupt withdrawal of levarterenol should be avoided.
4. Levarterenol should be diluted in either 5% dextrose in distilled water or 5% dextrose in saline.
5. For IV administration, a large vein should be used, preferably the antecubital or subclavian. Veins with poor circulation should be avoided.
6. Administer IV solutions with an electronic infusion device. Monitor the rate of flow constantly.
7. Have phentolamine available for use at the site of extravasation to dilate local blood vessels and to minimize local necrosis.

Assessment: Obtain a baseline CBC, blood pressure, and pulse recording prior to initiating therapy.

Interventions

1. During the administration of levarterenol, the client should be in a closely monitored environment.
2. Monitor the blood pressure frequently during therapy. An arterial line or Dinemapp for continuous BP determinations may be of some value.
3. Monitor the pulse frequently, noting any signs of bradycardia. Have atropine available for treatment of bradycardia.

4. Monitor I&O. Urine output should be reported if less than 30 ml/hr.
5. Observe the IV infusion site frequently for evidence of extravasation because ischemia and sloughing may occur.
6. Check the area for blanching along the course of the vein. This could indicate permeability of the vein wall which could allow leakage to occur. As a result, the IV site would need to be changed and phentolamine administered to the site of the extravasation.
7. The drug should be gradually withdrawn. Avoid an abrupt withdrawal. Clients may experience an initial rebound drop in blood pressure.
8. Extra fluids parenterally may diminish rebound hypotension and help stabilize BP during withdrawal of the drug.

Evaluation: Evaluate client for:
- ↑ in blood pressure
- Evidence of improved tissue perfusion
- Adequate urinary output (30 ml/hr)

——— *COMBINATION DRUG* ———
Levlen 21 and Levlen 28
(**LEV**-len)
(Rx)

See also *Oral Contraceptives,* p. 192.

Classification: Monophasic combination oral contraceptive.

Components: Each tablet of Levlen 21 and the first 21 tablets of Levlen 28 contain ethinyl estradiol, 30 mcg and levonorgestrel, 0.15 mg; the 28s also contain 7 inert pink tablets.

Special Concerns: Pregnancy category: X.

NURSING CONSIDERATIONS

See *Nursing Considerations* for *Oral Contraceptives,* p. 195.

Levobunolol hydrochloride

(lee-voh-**BYOU**-no-lohl)

Betagan✿, Betagan C Cap Q.D., Betagan C Cap B.I.D. (Rx)

See also *Beta-Adrenergic Blocking Agents,* p. 113.

Classification: Beta-adrenergic blocking agent for glaucoma.

Action/Kinetics: Levobunolol acts on both beta-1- and beta-2-adrenergic receptors. The drug may act by decreasing the formation of aqueous humor. **Onset:** Less than 60 min. **Peak effect:** 2–6 hr. **Duration:** 24 hr.

Uses: To decrease intraocular pressure in chronic open-angle glaucoma or ocular hypertension.

Special Concerns: Use with caution during pregnancy (category: C). Safety and effectiveness have not been determined in children. Significant absorption in geriatric clients may result in myocardial depression. Also, use with caution in angle-closure glaucoma (use with a miotic), in clients with muscle weaknesses, and in those with decreased pulmonary function.

Additional Side Effects: *Ophthalmic:* Stinging and burning (transient), decreased corneal sensitivity, blepharoconjunctivitis. *Dermatologic:* Urticaria, pruritus.

Dosage: Ophthalmic Solution. Adults: usual, 1 gtt of 0.5% solution in affected eye(s) 1–2 times/day (depending on variations in diurnal intraocular pressure).

NURSING CONSIDERATIONS

See also *Nursing Considerations* for *Beta-Adrenergic Blocking Agents,* p. 116.

Administration/Storage

1. Instruct the client not to close the eyes tightly or blink more frequently than usual after instillation of the drug.
2. If other eye drops are to be administered, wait at least 5 min before instillation of other eye drops.
3. Apply gentle pressure to the inside corner of the eye for approximately 60 sec following instillation.
4. If intraocular pressure is not decreased sufficiently, pilocarpine, epinephrine, or systemic carbonic anhydrase inhibitors may be used.

Client/Family Teaching

1. Review the method and frequency for instilling eye drops.
2. Explain the reasons for the medication and the side effects that should be reported should they occur.
3. Stress the importance of return visits to evaluate intraocular pressure and the effectiveness of the medication.

Evaluation: Evaluate client for evidence of a decrease in intraocular pressure.

Levodopa

(lee-voh-**DOH**-pah)

Dopar, Larodopa, L-Dopa (Rx)

Classification: Antiparkinson agent.

Action/Kinetics: Depletion of dopamine in the striatum of the brain is thought to cause the symptoms of Parkinson's disease. Levodopa, a dopamine precursor, is able to cross the blood-brain barrier to enter the CNS. It is decarboxylated to dopamine in the basal ganglia, thus replenishing depleted dopamine stores. **Peak plasma levels:** 0.5–2 hr (may be delayed if ingested with food). **$t^{1/2}$, plasma:** 1–3 hr. Onset occurs in 2–3 weeks although some clients may require up to 6 months. Levodopa is extensively metabolized both in the GI tract and the liver and metabolites are excreted in the urine.

Uses: Idiopathic, arteriosclerotic, or postencephalitic parkinsonism. Parkinsonism due to carbon monoxide or manganese intoxication. Levodopa only provides symptomatic relief and does not alter the course of the disease. When effective it relieves rigidity, bradykinesia, tremors, dysphagia, seborrhea, sialorrhea, and postural instability. Used in combination with carbidopa. *Investigational:* Pain from herpes zoster; restless legs syndrome.

Contraindications: Concomitant use with MAO inhibitors. History of melanoma or in clients with undiagnosed skin lesions. Lactation. Hypersensitivity to drug, narrow-angle glaucoma, blood dyscrasias, hypertension, coronary sclerosis.

Special Concerns: Use with extreme caution in clients with history of myocardial infarctions, convulsions, arrhythmias, bronchial asthma, emphysema, active peptic ulcer, psychosis or neurosis, wide-angle glaucoma and in renal, hepatic, or endocrine diseases. Use during pregnancy only if benefits clearly outweigh risks. Safety has not been established in children less than 12 years of age. Geriatric clients may require a lower dose as they have a reduced tolerance for the drug and its side effects (including cardiac effects). Clients may experience an "on-off" phenomenon in which they experience an improved clinical status followed by loss of therapeutic effect.

Side Effects: The side effects of levodopa are numerous and usually dose related. Some may abate with usage. *CNS:* Choreiform and/or dystonic movements, paranoid ideation, psychotic episodes, depression (with possibility of suicidal tendencies), dementia, seizures (rare), dizziness, headache, faintness, confusion, insomnia, nightmares, hallucinations, delusions, agitation, anxiety, malaise, fatigue, euphoria. *GI:* Nausea, vomiting, anorexia, abdominal pain, dry mouth, sialorrhea, dysphagia, dysgeusia, hiccups, diarrhea, constipation, burning sensation of tongue, bitter taste, flatulence, weight gain or loss, GI bleeding (rare), duodenal ulcer (rare). *CV:* Cardiac irregularities, palpitations, orthostatic hypotension, hypertension, phlebitis, hot flashes. *Ophthalmologic:* Diplopia, dilated pupils, blurred vision, development of Horner's syndrome, oculogyric crisis. *Hematologic:* Hemolytic anemia, agranulocytosis, leukopenia. *Musculoskeletal:* Muscle twitching (early sign of overdose), tonic contraction of the muscles of mastication, increased hand tremor, ataxia. *Miscellaneous:* Blepharospasm (early sign of overdose), urinary retention, urinary incontinence, increased sweating, unusual breathing patterns, weakness, numbness, bruxism, alopecia, priapism, hoarseness, edema, dark sweat and/or urine, flushing, skin rash, sense of stimulation.

Levodopa interacts with many other drugs (see below) and must be administered cautiously.

Symptoms of Overdose: Muscle twitching, blepharospasm. Also see *Side Effects,* above.

Drug Interactions

Amphetamines / Levodopa potentiates the effect of indirectly acting sympathomimetics

Antacids / ↑ Effect of levodopa due to ↑ absorption from GI tract

Anticholinergic drugs / Possible ↓ effect of levodopa due to ↑ breakdown of levodopa in stomach (due to delayed gastric emptying time)

Antidepressants, tricyclic / ↓ Effect of levodopa due to ↓ absorption from GI tract; also, ↑ risk of hypertension

Benzodiazepines / ↓ Effect of levodopa

Clonidine / ↓ Effect of levodopa

Digoxin / ↓ Effect of digoxin

Ephedrine / Levodopa potentiates the effect of indirectly acting sympathomimetics

Furazolidone / ↑ Effect of levodopa due to ↓ breakdown by liver

Guanethidine / ↑ Hypotensive effect of guanethidine

Hypoglycemic drugs / Levodopa upsets diabetic control with hypoglycemic agents

MAO inhibitors / Concomitant administration may result in hypertension, lightheadedness, and flushing due to ↓ breakdown of dopamine and

norepinephrine formed from levodopa

Methionine / ↓ Effect of levodopa

Methyldopa / Additive effects including hypotension

Metoclopramide / ↑ Bioavailability of levodopa; ↓ effect of metoclopramide

Papaverine / ↓ Effect of levodopa

Phenothiazines / ↓ Effect of levodopa due to ↓ uptake of dopamine into neurons

Phenytoin / Phenytoin antagonizes the effect of levodopa

Propranolol / Propranolol may antagonize the hypotensive and positive inotropic effect of levodopa

Pyridoxine / Pyridoxine reverses levodopa-induced improvement in Parkinson's disease

Reserpine / Reserpine inhibits response to levodopa by ↓ dopamine in the brain

Thioxanthines / ↓ Effect of levodopa in Parkinson clients

Tricyclic antidepressants / ↓ Absorption of levodopa → ↓ effect

Laboratory Test Interferences: ↑ BUN, AST, LDH, ALT, bilirubin, alkaline phosphatase, protein-bound iodine. ↓ Hemoglobin, hematocrit, white blood cells. False + Coombs' test. Interference with tests for urinary glucose and ketones.

Dosage: Capsules, Tablets. Adults, initial: 250 mg b.i.d.–q.i.d. taken with food; **then,** increase total daily dose by 100–750 mg q 3–7 days until optimum dosage reached (should not exceed 8 g/day). Up to 6 months may be required to achieve a significant therapeutic effect.

NURSING CONSIDERATIONS

See also *Nursing Considerations* for *Cholinergic Blocking Agents*, p. 138.

Administration/Storage

1. Administer to clients unable to swallow tablets or capsules by crushing tablets or emptying the capsule into a small amount of fruit juice at the time of administration.
2. Levodopa is often administered together with an anticholinergic agent.
3. *Treatment of Overdose:* Immediate gastric lavage for acute overdose. Maintain airway and give IV fluids carefully. General supportive measures.

Assessment

1. Obtain baseline ECG, complete blood count, liver and renal function studies, and protein bound iodine tests prior to beginning therapy.
2. Review the client's medical history for contraindications to the drug therapy.

Interventions

1. Monitor vital signs, CBC, liver and renal function studies throughout drug therapy, especially when long-term.
2. If the client is to have surgery, check with the physician to determine if the drug is to be stopped 24 hr before surgery. Also, determine when the drug is to be restarted following surgery.
3. Observe and document any evidence of the client becoming depressed, psychotic, or exhibiting any other unusual behavioral changes.
4. Offer emotional support and encouragement throughout the therapy.
5. Document parkinsonism symptoms displayed and note response to drug therapy as well as any sudden change in symptoms.

Client/Family Teaching

1. Take levodopa with food.
2. Report the occurrence of headaches because these may indicate drug-induced glaucoma.
3. Stress that dosage of drug is not to exceed 8 g daily.
4. Advise clients to avoid taking multivitamin preparations containing 10–25 mg of vitamin B_6. This vitamin rapidly reverses the antiparkinson effect of levodopa.
5. Significant results may take up to 6 months to be realized. Therefore, instruct client to continue taking the drug even though immediate results are not evident.
6. Instruct the client and family how to take blood pressure and pulse readings and to monitor these during drug therapy. Provide parameters for which the physician should be notified.
7. Drug may cause dizziness or drowsiness. Do not perform tasks that require mental alertness until drug effects realized.
8. Warn clients that their sweat and urine may appear dark. This is not harmful.
9. Male clients need to be warned that priapism may occur. This should be reported to the physician.
10. Stress the importance of reporting for all scheduled lab

and medical visits so that the effectiveness of drug therapy can be evaluated and adjusted as needed.

Evaluation: Evaluate client for:
- Evidence of improvement in motor function, reflexes, gait, strength of grip, and amount of tremor
- Any adverse side effects that may require a reduction in drug dose or "drug holiday"

Levonorgestrel Implants
(**lee**-voh-nor-**JES**-trel)
Norplant System (Rx)

See also *Progesterone and Progestins,* p. 209.

Classification: Progestin, contraceptive system.

Action/Kinetics: Levonorgestrel implants are marketed in a set of six flexible Silastic capsules each containing 36 mg of levonorgestrel; an insertion kit is provided to the physician to assist with implantation. Small amounts of the drug slowly diffuse through the wall of each capsule resulting in blood levels of levonorgestrel that are lower than those seen when levonorgestrel or norgestrel are taken as oral contraceptives. The dose released is initially 85 mcg/day, followed by a decrease to approximately 50 mcg/day after 9 months, to 35 mcg/day after 18 months, and then leveling off to 30 mcg/day thereafter. Blood levels of levonorgestrel vary over a wide range and cannot be used as the sole measure of the risk of pregnancy. If used properly, the risk of pregnancy is less than one for every one hundred users. Levonorgestrel does not have any estrogenic effects. The implant system lasts up to 5 years and the contraceptive effect is rapidly reversed if the system is removed from the body.

Uses: Prevention of pregnancy.

Contraindications: Active thrombophlebitis, thromboembolic disorders, undiagnosed abnormal genital bleeding, acute liver disease, benign or malignant liver tumors, known or suspected breast carcinoma, confirmed or suspected pregnancy.

Special Concerns: Menstrual bleeding irregularities are commonly observed. Women who have a family history of breast cancer or who have breast nodules should be monitored carefully. Use with caution in individuals in whom fluid retention might be dangerous and in those with a history of depression. Women being treated for hyperlipidemias should be monitored closely because an increase in LDL levels may occur. Capsules should not be inserted until 6 weeks after parturition in women who are breast-feeding.

Side Effects: *Menstrual irregularities:* Prolonged menses, spotting, irregular onset of menses, frequent menses, amenorrhea, scanty bleeding, cervicitis, vaginitis. *At implant site:* Pain or itching, infection, bruising following insertion or removal, hyperpigmentation (reversible upon removal). *GI:* Abdominal discomfort, nausea, change of appetite, weight gain. *CNS:* Headache, nervousness, dizziness. *Dermatologic:* Dermatitis, acne, hirsutism, scalp hair loss, excess hair growth. *Miscellaneous:* Breast discharge, breast pain,

L

leukorrhea, musculoskeletal pain, fluid retention, possibility of ectopic pregnancy in long-term users.

Drug Interactions

Carbamazepine / ↓ Effectiveness → ↑ risk of pregnancy
Phenytoin / ↓ Effectiveness → ↑ risk of pregnancy

Dosage: Six levonorgestrel-containing (36 mg each) Silastic capsules implanted subdermally in the mid-portion of the upper arm (8–10 cm above the elbow crease). Capsules are distributed in a fan-like pattern 15° apart (total of 75°).

NURSING CONSIDERATIONS

See also *Nursing Considerations* for *Progesterone and Progestins,* p. 210.

Administration/Storage

1. To ensure effectiveness, the capsules should be implanted during the first 7 days of the cycle or immediately after an abortion.
2. Capsules should be inserted only by individuals instructed on the proper procedure for insertion. If capsules are placed too deeply, they may be more difficult to remove.
3. If all capsules cannot be removed at the first attempt, the site should be healed before another attempt is made.
4. Expulsion is not common but may occur if the capsules are placed too shallow, too close to the incision, or if infection occurs.
5. If infection occurs, it should be treated and cured before replacing capsules.
6. After 5 years, capsules should be removed; if the woman desires additional contraception, a new set of capsules can be inserted.

Assessment

1. A complete medical history and physical examination should be performed prior to implantation or reimplantation and annually during use.
2. Ensure that the woman is not pregnant at the time the capsules are implanted.
3. Determine if client is breast-feeding because capsules should not be inserted until 6 weeks after delivery.
4. Note any history of thromboembolic disorders or depression.
5. Assess liver function and note any evidence of hyperlipidemia and associated treatment.
6. Note any family history of breast cancer. Document the presence of breast nodules because these require careful monitoring.
7. Obtain baseline weight. Be aware that the effectiveness of levonorgestrel may be slightly decreased with weights exceeding 70.5 kg.

Client/Family Teaching

1. Review appropriate procedure for wound care post-insertion and identify symptoms of infection and rejection that should be reported to the physician. Advise that a tiny scar may be evident at the insertion site.
2. Provide a printed list of side effects associated with drug therapy and instruct clients in what requires immediate reporting.
3. Advise client to expect some

irregularity with the menstrual cycle such as longer periods, missed periods, and spotting in between during the first year of implantation.

4. Stress the importance of reporting for regularly scheduled follow-up visits so that therapy can be carefully evaluated.

5. Advise that the capsules may be removed at any time for any reason and that pregnancy can occur after the next menstrual cycle.

Evaluation: Evaluate client for:
- Effectiveness of drug as a contraceptive agent
- Freedom from complications and side effects of drug therapy

---

Levothyroxine (T$_4$) sodium

(lee-voh-thigh-**ROX**-een)

Eltroxin✲, Levothroid, Levoxine, Synthroid, L-Thyroxine Sodium (Rx)

See also *Thyroid Drugs*, p. 235.

Classification: Thyroid preparation.

Action/Kinetics: Levothyroxine is the synthetic sodium salt of the levoisomer of thyroxine (tetraiodothyronine). From 0.05–0.06 mg levothryoxine is approximately equivalent to 60 mg thyroid. Levothyroxine absorption from the GI tract is incomplete and variable, especially when taken with food. This hormone has a slower onset but a longer duration than sodium liothyronine. It is more active on a weight basis than thyroid. Is usually the drug of choice. Effect is predictable because thyroid content is standard. **Time to peak therapeutic effect:** 3–4 weeks. **t½:** 6–7 days in a euthyroid person, 9–10 days in a hypothyroid client, and 3–4 days in a hyperthyroid client. Is 99% protein bound. **Duration:** 1–3 weeks after withdrawal of chronic therapy.

Note: All levothyroxine products are not bioequivalent; thus, changing brands is not recommended.

Dosage: Tablets. *Mild hypothyroidism:* **Adults, initial,** 50 mcg as a single daily dose; **then,** increase by 25–50 mcg q 2–3 weeks until desired clinical response is attained; **maintenance, usual:** 75–125 mcg daily (although doses up to 200 mcg daily may be required in some clients). *Severe hypothyroidism:* **Adults, initial,** 12.5–25 mcg as a single daily dose; **then,** increase dose, as necessary, in increments of 25 mg at 2–3 week intervals. *Hypothyroidism:* **Pediatric, 12 years and older:** 2–3 mcg/kg daily as a single dose until the adult daily dose (usually 150 mcg) is reached. **6–12 years of age:** 4–5 mcg/kg daily or 100–150 mcg daily as a single dose. **1–5 years of age:** 5–6 mcg/kg daily or 75–100 mcg daily as a single dose. **6–12 months of age:** 6–8 mcg/kg daily or 50–75 mcg daily as a single dose. **Less than 6 months of age:** 8-10 mcg/kg daily or 25–50 mcg daily as a single dose.

IV. *Myxedematous coma without heart disease.* **Adults, initial,** 200–500 mcg even in geriatric clients. If there is no response in 24 hr, 100–300 mcg may be given on the second day. Smaller daily doses should be given until client can tolerate oral medication. *Hypothyroidism:* **Adults,** 50–100 mcg as a single daily dose; **pediatric, IV,**

IM: A dose of 75% of the usual oral pediatric dose should be given.

Transfer from liothyronine to levothyroxine: Administer replacement drug for several days before discontinuing liothyronine. *Transfer from levothyroxine to liothyronine:* Discontinue levothyroxine before starting client on low daily dose of liothyronine.

NURSING CONSIDERATIONS

See also *Nursing Considerations* for *Thyroid Drugs,* p. 237.

Administration/Storage

1. Prepare the solution for injection immediately before administration.
2. Reconstitute the injectable by adding 0.9% sodium chloride injection or bacteriostatic sodium chloride injection. Shake the solution until it is clear.
3. Discard any unused portion of the IV medication.
4. Do not mix with other IV infusion solutions.

Assessment

1. Note the age of the client. Elderly clients are likely to have undetected cardiac problems. Therefore, a baseline ECG should be taken prior to initiating drug therapy.
2. Note if the client is pregnant. The woman must continue taking thyroid preparations throughout the pregnancy.
3. Note height, weight, and psychomotor development in children.

Client/Family Teaching

1. Advise not to switch brands because bioavailability may change.

2. Do not take with food since this may interfere with absorption.
3. Stress that the drug is not a cure for hypothyroidism and will have to be taken for client's lifetime.

Evaluation: Evaluate client for:
- Reports of symptomatic improvement
- Laboratory evidence of improved levels of T_3 and T_4

———— *COMBINATION DRUG* ————
Librax
(**LIB**-rax)
(**Rx**)

Classification/Content: *Antianxiety agent:* Chlordiazepoxide, 5 mg. *Anticholinergic agent:* Clidinium bromide, 2.5 mg.

See also information on individual components.

Uses: Possibly effective as an adjunct in the treatment of irritable colon, spastic colon, mucous colitis, and acute enterocolitis.

Contraindications: Pregnancy, glaucoma, prostatic hypertrophy.

Dosage: Capsules. Individualized. Adults, usual: 1–2 capsules t.i.d.–q.i.d. before meals and at bedtime.

NURSING CONSIDERATIONS

See *Nursing Considerations* for *Benzodiazepines,* p. 111, and *Cholinergic Blocking Agents,* p. 138.

Lidocaine hydrochloride
(**LYE**-doh-kayn)
IM: Lidopen Auto-Injector, Xylocaine HCl IM for Cardiac Arrhythmias (Rx). Direct IV or IV

Admixtures: Lidocaine HCl without Preservatives, Xylocaine HCl IV for Cardiac Arrhythmias, Xylocard✿ (Rx). IV Infusion: Lidocaine HCl in 5% Dextrose (Rx)

See also *Antiarrhythmic Drugs,* p. 51.

Classification: Antiarrhythmic, type IB.

Action/Kinetics: Lidocaine shortens the refractory period and suppresses the automaticity of ectopic foci without affecting conduction of impulses through cardiac tissue. It does not affect blood pressure, cardiac output, or myocardial contractility. **IV: Onset,** 45–90 sec; **duration:** 10–20 min. **IM, Onset,** 5–15 min; **duration,** 60–90 min. **t½:** 1–2 hr. **Therapeutic serum levels:** 1.5–6 mcg/ml. **Time to steady-state plasma levels:** 3–4 hr (8–10 hr in clients with acute myocardial infarction). **Protein-binding:** 40%–80%. Since lidocaine has little effect on conduction at normal antiarrhythmic doses, it should be used in acute situations (instead of procainamide) in instances in which heart block might occur.

Uses: IV: Treatment of acute ventricular arrhythmias such as those following myocardial infarctions or occurring during surgery. The drug is ineffective against atrial arrhythmias. **IM:** Certain emergency situations (e.g., ECG equipment not available; mobile coronary care unit, under advice of a physician).

Contraindications: Hypersensitivity to amide-type local anesthetics, Adams-Stokes syndrome, or total or partial heart block. Use with caution in the presence of liver or severe kidney disease, CHF, marked hypoxia, severe respiratory depression, or shock.

Special Concerns: Use with caution during pregnancy (category: B), labor, and delivery and in children. In geriatric clients, the rate and dose for IV infusion should be decreased by one-half and slowly adjusted.

Side Effects: *CV:* Precipitation or aggravation of arrhythmias (following IV use), hypotension, bradycardia (with possible cardiac arrest), cardiovascular collapse. *CNS:* Dizziness, restlessness, apprehension, euphoria, stupor, convulsions, unconsciousness. *Respiratory:* Difficulties in breathing or swallowing, respiratory depression. *Allergic:* Rash, urticaria, edema, anaphylaxis. *Other:* Tinnitus, blurred vision, vomiting, numbness, sensation of heat or cold, twitching, tremors.

During anesthesia, cardiovascular depression may be the first sign of lidocaine toxicity. During other usage, convulsions are the first sign of lidocaine toxicity.

Symptoms of Overdose: Symptoms are dependent on plasma levels. If plasma levels range from 4–6 mcg/ml, mild CNS effects are observed. Levels from 6–8 mcg/ml may result in significant CNS and cardiovascular depression while levels greater than 8 mcg/ml cause hypotension, decreased cardiac output, respiratory depression, obtundation, seizures, and coma.

Drug Interactions

Aminoglycosides /
↑ Neuromuscular blockade
Cimetidine / ↑ Effects of
lidocaine
Metoprolol / ↓ Lidocaine
clearance

Phenytoin / IV phenytoin → excessive cardiac depression
Procainamide / Additive neurologic side effects
Propranolol / ↓ Lidocaine clearance
Succinylcholine / ↑ Action of succinylcholine by ↓ plasma protein binding
Tubocurarine / ↑ Neuromuscular blockade

Dosage: IV bolus: 50–100 mg at rate of 25–50 mg/min. Repeat if necessary after 5-min interval. Onset of action is 10 sec. **Maximum dose/hr:** 200–300 mg. **Infusion:** 20–50 mcg/kg at a rate of 1–4 mg/min. No more than 300 mg/hr should be given. **IM:** 4.5 mg/kg (approximately 300 mg for a 70-kg adult). Switch to IV lidocaine or PO antiarrhythmics as soon as possible.

Pediatric: initial IV bolus dose, *antiarrhythmic:* 1 mg/kg at a rate of 25–50 mg/min; the dose can be repeated after 5 min if needed but the total dose should not exceed 3 mg/kg. **Then,** infuse 30 mcg/kg/min (range: 20–50 mcg/min).

NURSING CONSIDERATIONS

See also *Nursing Considerations* for *Antiarrhythmic Drugs,* p. 52.

Administration/Storage

1. *Do not add lidocaine to blood transfusion assembly.*
2. Lidocaine solutions that contain epinephrine should not be used to treat arrhythmias. Make certain that vial states, "For Cardiac Arrhythmias." Check prefilled syringes closely to ensure the appropriate dose has been obtained. (Lidocaine prefilled syringes come in both milligrams and grams).

3. Use 5% dextrose in water to prepare solution; this is stable for 24 hr.
4. IV infusions should be administered with an electronic infusion device.
5. IV bolus dosage should be reduced in clients over 70 years of age, in those with CHF or liver disease, and in clients taking cimetidine or propranolol (i.e., where metabolism of lidocaine is reduced).
6. *Treatment of Overdose:* Discontinue the drug and begin emergency resuscitative procedures. Seizures can be treated with diazepam, thiopental, or thiamylal. Succinylcholine, IV, may be used if the client is anesthetized. IV fluids, vasopressors, and CPR are used to correct circulatory depression.

Assessment

1. Note the age of the client. Elderly clients who have hepatic or renal disease or who weigh less than 45.5 kg will need to be watched especially closely for adverse side effects.
2. Note any client history of hypersensitivity to amide-type local anesthetics. These clients can be expected to have adverse reactions to lidocaine.
3. Obtain blood pressure, pulse, and respirations to use as baseline data against which to measure response to the drug therapy.

Interventions

1. All clients who receive lidocaine by the IV route should be in a monitored environment.
2. Observe clients for myocardial depression, variations of

rhythm or aggravation of the arrhythmia. Document and report these changes since drug administration may need to be altered.

3. Assess BP frequently during IV therapy. Clients on antiarrhythmic drug therapy are particularly susceptible to hypotension and cardiac collapse.

4. Monitor cardiac rate. Bradycardia may be a sign of impending cardiac collapse.

5. Note evidence of CNS effects such as twitching and tremors. These symptoms may precede convulsions.

6. Assess for respiratory depression, characterized by slow, shallow respirations.

7. Note any sudden changes in the client's mental status. Notify physician immediately because the dose of drug may need to be decreased.

8. The administration of the drug should be titrated to the client's response and within the written guidelines established by the physician.

Evaluation: Evaluate client for:
- ECG evidence of termination of ventricular arrhythmias
- Laboratory confirmation that serum drug levels are within therapeutic range (1.5–6 mcg/ml)

Lincomycin hydrochloride
(link-oh-**MY**-sin)
Lincocin (Rx)

See also *Anti-Infectives,* p. 80.

Classification: Anti-infective.

Action/Kinetics: Lincomycin is isolated from *Streptomyces lincolnensis.* Its spectrum resembles that of the erythromycins and includes a variety of gram-positive organisms, in particular staphylococci, streptococci, and pneumococci, and some gram-negative organisms. Lincomycin suppresses protein synthesis by microorganisms by binding to ribosomes (50S subunit), which is essential for transmittal of genetic information. It is both bacteriostatic and bactericidal. Lincomycin is absorbed rapidly from the GI tract and is widely distributed. **Peak plasma levels: PO,** 2–4 hr; **IM,** 30 min ($t^{1/2}$: 5.4 hr). This drug should not be used for trivial infections.

Uses: Not a first-choice drug but useful for clients allergic to penicillin. Used for serious respiratory tract, skin, and soft tissue infections due to staphylococci, streptococci, or pneumococci. Septicemia. In conjunction with diphtheria antitoxin in the treatment of diphtheria.

Contraindications: Hypersensitivity to drugs. Use in infants up to 1 month of age.

Special Concerns: Safe use during pregnancy has not been established. Use with caution in clients with GI disease, liver or renal disease, or with a history of allergy or asthma. Not for use in treating viral and minor bacteria infections.

Side Effects: *GI:* Nausea, vomiting, diarrhea, abdominal pain, tenesmus, flatulence, bloating, anorexia, weight loss, esophagitis. Nonspecific colitis, pseudomembranous colitis (may be severe). *Allergic:* Morbilliform rash (most common). Also, maculopapular rash, urticaria, pruritus, fever, hypotension. Rarely, polyarteritis, anaphylaxis, erythema multiforme. *Hematologic:* Leukopenia, neutropenia, eosinophilia, thrombocytopenia, agranulocytosis. *Miscellaneous:* Superinfection.

Following IV use: Thrombophlebitis, erythema, pain, swelling. IV lincomycin may cause hypotension, syncope, and cardiac arrest (rare). *Following IM use:* Pain, induration, sterile abscesses. *Following topical use:* Erythema, irritation, dryness, peeling, itching, burning, oiliness. Also, sore throat, fatigue, urinary frequency, headache.

Note: The injection contains benzyl alcohol, which has been associated with a fatal gasping syndrome in infants.

Drug Interactions

Antiperistaltic antidiarrheals (opiates, Lomotil) / ↑ Diarrhea due to ↓ removal of toxins from colon

Erythromycin / Cross-interference → ↓ effect of both drugs

Kaolin (e.g., Kaopectate) / ↓ Effect due to ↓ absorption from GI tract

Neuromuscular blocking agents / ↑ Effect of blocking agents

Laboratory Test Interferences: ↓ Levels of AST, ALT, NPN, alkaline phosphatase, bilirubin, BSP retention, and ↓ platelet count.

Dosage: Capsules, adults: 500 mg t.i.d.–q.i.d.; **children over 1 month of age:** 30–60 mg/kg/day in 3–4 divided doses, depending on severity of infection. **IM, adults:** 600 mg q 12–24 hr; **children over 1 month of age:** 10 mg/kg/day q 12–24 hr, depending on severity of infection. **IV, adults:** 0.6–1.0 g q 8–12 hr up to 8 g daily, depending on severity of infection; **children over 1 month of age:** 10–20 mg/kg/day, depending on severity of infection. **Subconjunctival injection:** 0.75 mg/0.25 ml.

In impaired renal function, reduce dosage by 70%–75%. Total blood counts and liver function tests should be done periodically during long-term therapy.

NURSING CONSIDERATIONS

See also *General Nursing Considerations For All Anti-Infectives,* p. 83.

Administration/Storage

1. Prepare drug for administration as directed on package insert.
2. Administer slowly IM to minimize pain.
3. For IV use, carefully follow concentration and rate of administration recommendation to prevent severe cardiopulmonary reactions.

Interventions

1. Be prepared to manage colitis, which can occur 2–9 days to several weeks after initiation of therapy, by providing fluids, electrolytes, protein supplements, systemic corticosteroids, and vancomycin.
2. Do not administer, and caution client against using, antiperistaltic agents if diarrhea occurs, because these agents can prolong or aggravate condition.
3. Do not use any acne or topical mercury preparations containing a peeling agent in an area affected by medication because severe irritation can occur.
4. Do not administer kaolin concomitantly with lincomycin because kaolin will reduce absorption of the antibiotic. If kaolin is required, administer 3 hr before antibiotic.
5. Observe for adverse drug interactions caused by concur-

rent administration of neuro-muscular blocking agents. Be alert to hypotension, broncho-spasms, cardiac disturbances, hyperthermia, and respiratory depression.

6. Assess for transient flushing and sensations of warmth, and cardiac disturbances, which may accompany IV infusions. Monitor pulse rate before, during, and after infusion until rate is stable at levels normal for client.

Client/Family Teaching

1. Instruct client to take lincomy-cin on an empty stomach be-tween meals and not with a sugar substitute.
2. Administer on an empty stom-ach to ensure optimum absorp-tion. GI disturbances, including abdominal pain, diarrhea, an-orexia, nausea, vomiting, bloody or tarry stools, and excessive flatulence should be reported as discontinuation of drug may be indicated.

Evaluation: Evaluate client for:

- Evidence of negative labora-tory culture reports
- Freedom from complica-tions of drug therapy

Liothyronine sodium (T₃)

(lye-oh-**THIGH**-roh-neen)
Cytomel, Sodium-L-Triiodothyronine (Rx)

See also *Thyroid Drugs,* p. 235.

Classification: Thyroid prepara-tion.

Action/Kinetics: Synthetic sodi-um salt of levoisomer of triiodothy-ronine. Liothyronine has more pre-dictable effects due to standard hormone content. From 15–37.5 mcg is equivalent to about 60 mg of desiccated thyroid. It may be pre-ferred when a rapid effect or rapid-ly reversible effect is required. Drug has a rapid onset, which may result in difficulty in controlling the dosage as well as the possibility of cardiac side effects and changes in metabolic demands. However, its short duration allows quick adjust-ment of dosage and helps control overdosage. **t½:** 24 hr for euthyroid clients, approximately 34 hr in hypothyroid clients, and ap-proximately 14 hr in hyperthyroid clients. **Duration:** Up to 72 hr. Is 99% protein bound.

Additional Contraindications: Use of liothyronine is not recom-mended in children with cretinism because there is some question about whether the hormone cross-es the blood-brain barrier.

Dosage: Tablets. *Mild hypo-thyroidism: individualized:* **Adults,** 25 mcg daily. Increase by 12.5–25 mcg q 1–2 weeks until satisfactory response has been obtained. **Usual maintenance:** 25–75 mcg daily. Use lower initial dosage (5 mcg/day) for the elderly, children, and clients with cardiovascular disease. Increase gradually as adult dosage. *Myxedema:* **Adults, initial,** 5 mcg/day increased by 5–10 mcg daily q 1–2 weeks until 25 mcg/day is reached; **then,** increase q 1–2 weeks by 12.5–50 mcg. **Usual maintenance:** 50–100 mcg/day. *Nontoxic goiter:* **Initial,** 5 mcg/ day; **then,** increase q 1–2 weeks by 5–10 mcg until 25 mcg daily is reached; **then,** dose can be in-creased by 12.5–25 mcg weekly until the maintenance dose of 50–100 mcg daily is reached.

T_3 suppression test: 75–100 mcg/day for 7 days followed by a repeat of the I^{131} thyroid uptake test (a 50% or greater suppression of uptake indicates a normal thryoid-pituitary axis).

Congenital hypothyroidism: **initial,** 5 mcg/day; **then,** increase by 5 mcg/day q 3–4 days until the desired effect is achieved. Approximately 20 mcg/day may be sufficient for infants while children 1 year of age may require 50 mcg/day. Children above 3 years may require the full adult dose.

Transfer from other thyroid preparations to liothyronine: Discontinue old preparation before starting on low daily dose of liothyronine. *Transfer from liothyronine to another thyroid preparation:* Start therapy with replacement drug several days prior to complete withdrawal of sodium liothyronine.

NURSING CONSIDERATIONS

See also *Nursing Considerations* for *Thyroid Drugs,* p. 237.

Administration/Storage

1. If symptoms of hyperthyroidism are noted, the drug can be withdrawn for 2–3 days after which therapy can be reinstituted, but at a lower dose.
2. A *Cytomel* injection kit is available for the emergency treatment of myxedema coma.

Liotrix
(LYE-oh-trix)
Euthroid, Thyrolar (Rx)

See also *Thyroid Drugs,* p. 235.

Classification: Thyroid preparation.

General Statement: Mixture of synthetic levothyroxine sodium (T_4) and liothyronine (T_3). The mixture contains the products in a 4:1 ratio by weight and in a 1:1 ratio by biologic activity. The two commercial preparations contain slightly different amounts of each component. Because of this discrepancy, a switch from one preparation to the other must be made cautiously. Liotrix has standard hormone content; thus, the effect is predictable.

Dosage: Tablets. *Hypothyroidism:* **Adults and children, initial,** 50 mcg levothyroxine and 12.5 mcg liothyronine (Thyrolar) or 60 mcg levothyroxine and 15 mcg liothyronine (Euthroid) daily; **then,** at monthly intervals, increments of like amounts can be made until the desired effect is achieved. **Usual maintenance:** 50–100 mcg of levothyroxine and 12.5–25 mcg liothyronine daily.

Congenital hypothyroidism: **Children, 0–6 months:** 8–10 mcg T_4/kg/day (25–50 mcg daily); **6–12 months:** 6–8 mcg T_4/kg/day (50–75 mcg daily); **1–5 years:** 5–6 mcg T_4/kg/day (75–100 mcg daily); **6–12 years:** 4–5 mcg T_4/kg/day (100–150 mcg daily); **over 12 years:** 2–3 mcg T_4/kg/day (over 150 mcg daily).

NURSING CONSIDERATIONS

See also *Nursing Considerations* for *Thyroid Drugs,* p. 237.

Administration/Storage

1. The initial dose for geriatric clients should be 1/4–1/2 the usual adult dose; this dose can be doubled q 6–8 weeks until the desired effect is attained.
2. In children, dosing increments should be made q 2 weeks

until the desired response has been attained.

3. Thyroid function tests should always be done before initiating dosage changes.

4. Administer as a single dose before breakfast.

5. Protect tablets from light, heat, and moisture.

6. Due to differences in the amounts of hormones between Euthroid and Thyrolar, once started on a particular brand, the client should not be switched.

Lisinopril

(lyes-**IN**-oh-prill)

Prinivil, Zestril (Rx)

Classification: Antihypertensive, angiotensin-converting enzyme inhibitor.

Action/Kinetics: By inhibiting angiotensin-converting enzyme, lisinopril prevents the conversion of angiotensin I to angiotensin II. Inhibiting angiotensin I conversion results in decreased vasopressor activity, leading to decreased blood pressure and decreased secretion of aldosterone. Both supine and standing blood pressure are reduced, although the drug is less effective in blacks than in Caucasians. Although food does not alter the bioavailability of lisinopril, only 25% of an oral dose is absorbed. **Onset:** 1 hr. **Peak serum levels:** 7 hr. **Duration:** 24 hr. **t½:** 12 hr. 100% of the drug is excreted unchanged in the urine.

Uses: Alone or in combination with a diuretic to treat hypertension (Step I therapy). *Investigational:* In combination with digitalis and a diuretic for treating congestive heart failure not responding to other therapy.

Special Concerns: Pregnancy category: C. Use with caution during lactation. Safety and efficacy have not been established in children.

Side Effects: *CNS:* Dizziness, headache, fatigue, vertigo, insomnia, depression, sleepiness, paresthesias, vertigo, nervousness, malaise. *GI:* Diarrhea, nausea, vomiting, dyspepsia, anorexia, constipation, dysgeusia, dry mouth, abdominal pain, flatulence. *Respiratory:* Cough, dyspnea, bronchitis, upper respiratory symptoms, nasal congestion, sinusitis, pharyngeal pain. *CV:* Hypotension, orthostatic hypotension, angina, tachycardia, palpitations, rhythm disturbances, stroke, myocardial infarction. *Musculoskeletal:* Asthenia, muscle cramps, joint pain, shoulder and back pain, myalgia, arthralgia, arthritis. *Hepatic:* Hepatitis, cholestatic jaundice, pancreatitis. *Miscellaneous:* Angioedema (may be fatal if laryngeal edema occurs), hyperkalemia, neutropenia, anemia, agranulocytosis, increased sweating, rash, decreased libido, chest pain, fever, flushing, peripheral edema, oliguria, azotemia, acute renal failure, blurred vision, urticaria, pruritus, syncope, urinary tract infection, vasculitis of the legs.

Drug Interactions

Diuretics / Excess ↓ blood pressure

Indomethacin / Possible ↓ effect of lisinopril

Potassium-sparing diuretics / Significant ↑ serum potassium

Laboratory Test Interferences: ↑ Serum potassium, BUN, serum creatinine. ↓ Hemoglobin, hematocrit.

Dosage: Tablets. *Essential hypertension, used alone:* 10 mg once daily. Adjust dosage depending on response (range: 20–40 mg daily). Doses greater than 80 mg daily do not give a greater effect. *Essential hypertension in combination with a diuretic:* **Initial,** 5 mg. The blood pressure-lowering effects of the combination are additive. Dosage should be reduced in clients with renal impairment. *Congestive heart failure:* **Initial,** 2.5–5 mg daily; **maintenance:** 10–40 mg daily.

NURSING CONSIDERATIONS

See also *Nursing Considerations* for *Antihypertensive Agents,* p. 78.

Administration/Storage

1. When considering use of lisinopril in a client taking diuretics, discontinue the diuretic, if possible, 2–3 days before beginning lisinopril therapy. If the diuretic cannot be discontinued, the initial dose of lisinopril should be 5 mg and the client should be closely observed for at least 2 hr.
2. In some clients, maximum antihypertensive effects may not be observed for 2–4 weeks.
3. Clients whose blood pressure is controlled with lisinopril, 20 mg plus hydrochlorothiazide, 25 mg given separately should be given a trial of Prinzide 12.5 mg or Zestoretic 20–12.5 mg before Prinzide 25 mg or Zestoretic 20–25 mg is used.
4. The maximum recommended daily dose of lisinopril is 80 mg in a single daily dose. However, clients usually do not require hydrochlorothiazide in doses exceeding 50 mg daily, especially if combined with other antihypertensives.
5. Use of potassium supplements, potassium-sparing diuretics, or potassium salt substitutes with Prinzide or Zestoretic may lead to increases in serum potassium.
6. Prinzide or Zestoretic is recommended for those clients with a creatinine clearance greater than 30 ml/min.
7. Anticipate reduced dosage if the client has renal insufficiency.

Client/Family Teaching

1. Take medication at bedtime to minimize potential adverse side effects.
2. Explain how to avoid symptoms of orthostatic hypotension, (i.e., rise slowly from sitting or lying position and wait until symptoms subside).
3. Avoid all potassium supplements as well as foods high in potassium.
4. Stress the importance of reporting for scheduled laboratory studies.

Evaluation: Evaluate client for a ↓ in blood pressure and control of hypertension with a minimum of adverse effects.

Lithium carbonate
(**LITH**-ee-um)
Carbolith✶, Cibalith-S, Duralith✶, Eskalith, Eskalith CR, Lithane, Lithizine✶, Lithobid, Lithonate, Lithotabs (Rx)

Lithium citrate
(**LITH**-ee-um)
Cibalith-S (Rx)

Classification: Antipsychotic agent, miscellaneous.

Action/Kinetics: Although the precise mechanism for the antimanic effect of lithium is not known, various hypotheses have been put forth. These include: (a) a decrease in catecholamine neurotransmitter levels caused by lithium's effect on Na + –K + ATPase to improve transneuronal membrane transport of sodium ion; (b) a decrease in cyclic AMP levels caused by lithium which decreases sensitivity of hormonal-sensitive adenyl cyclase receptors; or (c) interference by lithium with lipid inositol metabolism ultimately leading to insensitivity of cells in the CNS to stimulation by inositol.

Lithium also affects the distribution of calcium, magnesium, and sodium ions and affects glucose metabolism. **Peak serum levels** (regular release): 1–4 hr; (slow-release): 4–6 hr. **Onset:** 5–14 days. **Therapeutic serum levels:** 0.4–1.0 mEq/L (must be carefully monitored because toxic effects may occur at these levels and significant toxic reactions occur at serum lithium levels of 2 mEq/L). **t½** (plasma): 24 hr (longer in presence of renal impairment and in the elderly). Lithium and sodium are excreted by the same mechanism in the proximal tubule. Thus, to reduce the danger of lithium intoxication, sodium intake must remain at normal levels.

Uses: Control of manic and hypomanic episodes in manic-depressive clients. Prophylaxis of bipolar depression. *Investigational:* To reverse neutropenia induced by cancer chemotherapy and in children with chronic neutropenia. Prophylaxis of cluster headaches and cyclic migraine headaches. Treatment of certain types of mental depression (e.g., schizoaffective disorder, augment the antidepressant effect of tricyclic or MAO drugs in treating unipolar depression). Also for premenstrual tension, alcoholism accompanied by depression, tardive dyskinesia, bulimia, hyperthyroidism, excess ADH secretion. Lithium succinate, in a topical form, has been used for the treatment of genital herpes and seborrheic dermatitis.

Contraindications: Cardiovascular or renal disease. Brain damage. Dehydration, sodium depletion, clients receiving diuretics. Pregnancy (category: D), lactation.

Special Concerns: Safety and efficacy have not been established for children less than 12 years of age. Use with caution in geriatric clients because lithium is more toxic to the CNS in these clients; also, geriatric clients are more likely to develop lithium-induced goiter and clinical hypothyroidism and are more likely to manifest excessive thirst and larger volumes of urine.

Side Effects: These are related to the blood lithium level. *CNS:* Fainting, drowsiness, slurred speech, confusion, dizziness, tiredness, lethargy, ataxia, dysarthria, aphasia, vertigo, stupor, restlessness, coma, seizures. Pseudotumor cerebri leading to papilledema and increased intracranial pressure. *GI:* Anorexia, nausea, vomiting, diarrhea, thirst, dry mouth, bloated stomach. *Muscular:* Tremors (especially of hand), muscle weakness, fasciculations and/or twitching, clonic movements of limbs, increased deep tendon reflexes, choreoathetoid movements, cogwheel rigidity. *Renal:* Nephrogenic diabetes insipidus (polyuria, polydypsia),

L

oliguria, albuminuria. *Endocrine:* Hypothyroidism, goiter, hyperparathyroidism. *CV:* Changes in ECG, edema, hypotension, cardiovascular collapse, irregular pulse, tachycardia. *Ophthalmologic:* Blurred vision, downbeat nystagmus. *Dermatologic:* Acneform eruptions, pruritic-maculopapular rashes, drying and thinning of hair, alopecia, paresthesia, cutaneous ulcers, lupus-like symptoms. *Miscellaneous:* Hoarseness, swelling of feet, lower legs, or neck; cold sensitivity, leukemia, leukocytosis, dyspnea on exertion.

Symptoms of Overdose: Symptoms dependent on serum lithium levels. Levels less than 2 mEq/L: nausea, vomiting, diarrhea, muscle weakness, drowsiness, loss of coordination.

Levels from 2–3 mEq/L: agitation, ataxia, blackouts, blurred vision, choreoathetoid movements, confusion, dysarthria, fasciculations, giddiness, hyperreflexia, hypertonia, manic-like behavior, myoclonic twitching or movement of entire limbs, slurred speech, tinnitus, urinary or fecal incontinence, vertigo.

Levels over 3 mEq/L: arrhythmias, coma, hypotension, peripheral vascular collapse, seizures (focal and generalized), spasticity, stupor, twitching of muscle groups.

Drug Interactions

Acetazolamide / ↓ Lithium effect by ↑ renal excretion
Aminophylline / ↓ Lithium effect by ↑ renal excretion
Bumetanide / ↑ Lithium toxicity due to ↓ renal clearance
Carbamazepine / ↑ Risk of lithium toxicity
Diazepam / ↑ Risk of hypothermia
Ethacrynic acid / ↑ Lithium toxicity due to ↓ renal clearance
Fluoxetine / ↑ Serum levels of lithium
Furosemide / ↑ Lithium toxicity due to ↓ renal clearance
Haloperidol / ↑ Risk of neurologic toxicity
Ibuprofen / ↑ Chance of lithium toxicity due to ↓ renal clearance
Indomethacin / ↑ Chance of lithium toxicity due to ↓ renal clearance
Iodide salts / Additive effect to cause hypothyroidism
Mannitol / ↓ Lithium effect by ↑ renal excretion
Mazindol / ↑ Chance of lithium toxicity due to ↑ serum levels
Methyldopa / ↑ Chance of lithium toxicity due to ↑ serum levels
Naproxen / ↑ Chance of lithium toxicity due to ↑ serum levels
Neuromuscular blocking agents / Lithium ↑ effect of these agents → respiratory depression and apnea
Phenothiazines / ↓ Levels of phenothiazines and ↑ neurotoxicity
Phenylbutazone / ↑ Chance of lithium toxicity due to ↓ renal clearance
Phenytoin / ↑ Chance of lithium toxicity
Piroxicam / ↑ Chance of lithium toxicity due to ↓ renal clearance
Probenecid / ↑ Chance of lithium toxicity due to ↑ serum levels
Sodium bicarbonate / ↓ Lithium effect by ↑ renal excretion
Sodium chloride / Excretion of lithium is proportional to amount of sodium chloride ingested; if patient is on salt-free diet, may develop lithium toxicity since less lithium excreted
Spironolactone / ↑ Chance of

lithium toxicity due to ↑ serum levels

Succinylcholine / ↑ Muscle relaxation

Sympathomimetics / ↓ Pressor effect of sympathomimetics

Tetracyclines / ↑ Chance of lithium toxicity due to ↑ serum levels

Theophyllines / ↓ Effect of lithium due to ↑ renal excretion

Thiazide diuretics, triamterene / ↑ Chance of lithium toxicity due to ↓ renal clearance

Tricyclic antidepressants / ↑ Effect of tricyclic antidepressants

Urea / ↓ Lithium effect by ↑ renal excretion

Laboratory Test Interferences: False + urinary glucose test (Benedict's). ↑ serum glucose, creatinine kinase. False (−) or ↓ serum protein bound iodine (PBI), uric acid; ↑ thyroid-stimulating hormone; ↓ thyroxine.

Dosage: Capsules, Slow-release Capsules, Tablets, Extended-release Tablets, Syrup. *Acute mania:* Individualized and according to lithium serum level (not to exceed 1.4 mEq/L) and clinical response. **Usual initial:** 300–600 mg t.i.d. or 600–900 mg b.i.d. of slow-release form; **elderly and debilitated clients:** 0.6–1.2 g daily in 3 doses. **Maintenance:** 300 mg t.i.d.–q.i.d.

Administration of drug is discontinued when lithium serum level exceeds 1.2 mEq/L and resumed 24 hr after it has fallen below that level. *To reverse neutropenia:* 300–1,000 mg/day (to achieve serum levels of 0.5–1.0 mEq/L) for 7–10 days. *Prophylaxis of cluster headaches:* 600–900 mg/day.

NURSING CONSIDERATIONS

Administration/Storage

1. To prevent toxic serum levels from occurring, blood levels should be determined 1–2 times/week during initiation of therapy, and monthly thereafter, on blood samples taken 8–12 hr after dosage.
2. Full beneficial effects of lithium therapy may not be noted for 6–10 days after initiation.
3. *Treatment of Overdose:* Early symptoms are treated by decreasing the dose or stopping treatment for 24–48 hr.
   - Use gastric lavage.
   - Restore fluid and electrolyte balance (can use saline) and maintain kidney function.
   - Increase lithium excretion by giving aminophylline, mannitol, or urea.
   - Prevent infection. Maintain adequate respiration.
   - Monitor thyroid function.
   - Institute hemodialysis.

Assessment

1. Conduct a drug history and determine if the client is taking other medications that are likely to interact with lithium.
2. If clients have arthritic conditions, determine if they are taking any anti-inflammatory agents and document.
3. Obtain pretreatment thyroid function studies and monitor throughout therapy.

Intervention: Monitor cardiovascular function periodically during drug therapy as well as serum drug levels.

Client/Family Teaching

1. Review the goals of therapy and the possible side effects asso-

ciated with this drug. Advise client not to change brands of medication.

2. Provide printed instructions regarding medication administration and side effects that require immediate reporting.

3. Caution the client and family to report any side effects that may occur. If diarrhea, vomiting, drowsiness, muscular weakness, and lack of coordination occur, lithium therapy must be discontinued immediately, and client must report for medical supervision.

4. Take drug with food or immediately after meals. Report any episodes of persistent diarrhea because these symptoms may indicate a need for supplemental fluids or salt.

5. Avoid any caffeinated beverages/foods because these may aggravate mania.

6. Explain the relationship between lithium activity and dietary sodium. Instruct clients to maintain a constant level of sodium intake to avoid fluctuations in lithium action.

7. Advise client to drink 10–12 glasses of water each day and to avoid dehydration (e.g., sunbathing, sauna).

8. Do not engage in physical activities that require alertness or physical coordination until drug effects are realized. Lithium therapy causes drowsiness and may impair these abilities.

9. Reassure the client and family that it will take several weeks to realize a benefit from lithium therapy.

10. Provide the name and telephone number of persons to contact if the client has problems or if family members note behavioral changes or physical changes contrary to expectations.

11. Establish a schedule of follow-up lab and medical appointments and stress the importance of adhering to this schedule.

12. Instruct clients to wear a Medic Alert tag or bracelet indicating the diagnosis and prescribed medication regimen.

Evaluation: Evaluate client for:
- Knowledge and understanding of illness and response to teaching; evaluate compliance with the prescribed drug regimen
- Evidence of stabilization of mood swings and affect
- Reports of reduction in symptoms of mania such as hyperactivity, sleeplessness, and/or poor judgment
- Laboratory evidence that serum drug levels are within therapeutic maintenance range (0.4–1.0 mEq/L)

——— COMBINATION DRUG ———
Loestrin 21 1/20 and Loestrin Fe 1/20
(lo-**ES**-trin)
(Rx)

Loestrin 21 1.5/30 and Loestrin Fe 1.5/30
(lo-**ES**-trin)
(Rx)

See also *Oral Contraceptives,* p. 192.

Classification: Monophasic combination oral contraceptive.

Components: Loestrin 21 1/20: Each tablet contains ethinyl estradiol, 20 mcg and norethindrone acetate, 1 mg (white tablets). Loestrin Fe 1/20: 21 tablets each containing ethinyl estradiol, 20 mcg and norethindrone acetate, 1 mg (white tablets) and 7 tablets each containing ferrous fumarate, 75 mg (brown tablets).

Loestrin 21 1.5/30: Each tablet contains ethinyl estradiol, 30 mcg and norethindrone acetate, 1.5 mg (green tablets).

Loestrin Fe 1.5/30: 21 tablets each containing ethinyl estradiol, 30 mcg and norethindrone acetate, 1.5 mg (green tablets) and 7 tablets each containing ferrous fumarate, 75 mg (brown tablets).

Special Concerns: Pregnancy category: X.

NURSING CONSIDERATIONS

See *Nursing Considerations* for *Oral Contraceptives,* p. 195.

Lomustine
(loh-**MUS**-teen)
CeeNu (Abbreviation: CCNU) (Rx)

See also *Antineoplastic Agents,* p. 85, and *Alkylating Agents,* p. 20.

Classification: Antineoplastic, alkylating agent.

Action/Kinetics: Lomustine is an alkylating agent with cross-reactivity to carmustine. The drug interferes with the function of DNA and RNA and is cell-cycle nonspecific. Lomustine also inhibits protein synthesis by inhibiting necessary enzyme reactions. Rapidly absorbed from the GI tract; crosses the blood-brain barrier resulting in concentrations higher than in plasma. **Peak plasma level:** 1–6 hr; $t\frac{1}{2}$: biphasic; **initial,** 6 hr; **post-distribution:** 1–2 days. From 15% to 20% of drug remains in body after 5 days. Fifty percent of drug excreted within 12 hr through the kidney, 75% within 4 days. Small amounts are excreted through the lungs and feces. Metabolites present in milk.

Uses: Used alone or in combination with other drugs. Primary and metastatic brain tumors. Secondary therapy in disseminated Hodgkin's disease (in combination with other antineoplastics). *Investigational:* Cancer of the lung, breast, kidney; multiple myeloma; malignant melanoma.

Contraindications: Use during lactation.

Special Concerns: Pregnancy category: D.

Additional Side Effects: High incidence of nausea and vomiting 3–6 hr after administration and lasting for 24 hr. Renal and pulmonary toxicity. Dysarthria. **Note:** Delayed bone marrow suppression may occur due to cumulative bone marrow toxicity. Thrombocytopenia and leukopenia may lead to bleeding and overwhelming infections.

Laboratory Test Interference: Elevated liver function tests (reversible).

Dosage: Capsules. Adults and children: initial, 100–130 mg/m^2 as a single dose q 6 weeks. If bone marrow function reduced, decrease dose to 100 mg/m^2 q 6 weeks. Subsequent dosage based on blood counts of clients (platelet count above 100,000/mm^3 and leukocyte count above 4,000/mm^3). Blood tests should be undertaken weekly, and repeat therapy should not be undertaken before 6 weeks.

NURSING CONSIDERATIONS

See also *Nursing Considerations* for *Antineoplastic Agents,* p. 88.

Administration/Storage

1. Store below 40°C.
2. Lomustine may be given alone or in combination with other drugs, surgery, or radiotherapy.

Client/Family Teaching

1. Client may have nausea and vomiting up to 36 hr after treatment; this period may be followed by 2–3 days of anorexia. Administer antiemetics as prescribed.
2. GI distress may be reduced by the administration of antiemetics before drug or by taking the drug after fasting.
3. The client is often depressed by prolonged nausea and vomiting; try various antiemetics and ensure that psychological support is available as needed.
4. Explain to client that intervals of 6 weeks are necessary between doses for optimum effect with minimal toxicity.
5. Inform client that medication comes in capsules of three strengths and a combination of capsules will make up the correct dose; this combination should be taken at one time.

Evaluation: Evaluate client for evidence of a ↓ in tumor size and spread.

——— COMBINATION DRUG ———
Lo/Ovral 21 and Lo/Ovral 28
(low-**OHV**-ral)
(Rx)

See also *Oral Contraceptives,* p. 192.

Classification: Monophasic combination oral contraceptive.

Components: Each tablet of Lo/Ovral 21 and the first 21 tablets of Lo/Ovral 28 contain ethinyl estradiol, 30 mcg and norgestrel, 0.3 mg (white tablets); the 28s also contain 7 inert pink tablets.

Special Concerns: Pregnancy category: X.

NURSING CONSIDERATIONS

See *Nursing Considerations* for *Oral Contraceptives,* p. 195.

Loperamide hydrochloride
(loh-**PER**-ah-myd)
Imodium, Imodium A-D (Immodium is Rx, Immodium A-D is OTC)

Classification: Antidiarrheal agent, systemic.

Action/Kinetics: Loperamide is a piperidine derivative that slows intestinal motility by acting on the nerve endings and/or intramural ganglia embedded in the intestinal wall. The prolonged retention of the feces in the intestine results in reducing the volume of the stools, increasing viscosity, and decreasing fluid and electrolyte loss. The drug is reported to be more effective than diphenoxylate. **Time to peak effect, capsules:** 5 hr; **oral solution:** 2.5 hr. **t½:** 9.1–14.4 hr.

Uses: Symptomatic relief of acute, nonspecific diarrhea, chronic diarrhea associated with inflammatory bowel disease, reduction of volume discharged from ileostomies.

Contraindications: Discontinue drug promptly if abdominal distention develops in clients with acute ulcerative colitis. In clients in whom constipation should be avoided. OTC if body temperature is over 101°F and in presence of bloody diarrhea.

Special Concerns: Safe use during pregnancy (category: B), in children under 2 years of age, and during lactation not established. Children less than 3 years of age are more sensitive to the narcotic effects of loperamide.

Side Effects: *GI:* Abdominal pain, distention, or discomfort. Constipation, dry mouth, nausea, vomiting, epigastric distress. Toxic megacolon in clients with acute colitis. *CNS:* Drowsiness, dizziness, fatigue. *Other:* Allergic skin rashes. *Symptoms of Overdose:* Constipation, CNS depression, GI irritation.

Dosage: Capsules, Liquid. *Acute diarrhea:* **Adults, initial:** 4 mg, followed by 2 mg after each unformed stool, up to maximum of 16 mg daily. *Day 1 doses,* **pediatric: 8–12 years:** 2 mg t.i.d.; **6–8 years:** 2 mg b.i.d.; **2–5 years:** 1 mg t.i.d. After day 1, 1 mg/10 kg after a loose stool (total daily dosage should not exceed day 1 recommended doses). *Chronic diarrhea:* **Adults,** 4–8 mg/day as a single or divided dose. Dosage not established for chronic diarrhea in children.
Oral Solution, Tablets (OTC). *Acute diarrhea:* **Adults,** 4 mg after the first loose bowel movement followed by 2 mg after each subsequent bowel movement to a maximum of 8 mg daily for no more than 2 days. **Pediatric, 9–11 years:** 2 mg after the first bowel movement followed by 1 mg after each subsequent loose bowel movement, not to exceed 6 mg daily for no more than 2 days. **Pediatric, 6–8 years:** 1 mg after

the first bowel movement followed by 1 mg after each subsequent loose bowel movement, not to exceed 4 mg daily for no more than 2 days.

NURSING CONSIDERATIONS

Administration/Storage

1. OTC products are not intended for use in children less than 6 years of age unless the physician prescribes.
2. If improvement is not seen within 10 days after using up to 16 mg/day for chronic diarrhea, symptoms are not likely to improve with further use. Seek medical intervention.
3. In acute diarrhea, discontinue drug after 48 hr if ineffective.
4. *Treatment of Overdose:* Give activated charcoal (it will reduce absorption up to ninefold). If vomiting has not occurred, perform gastric lavage followed by activated charcoal, 100 g, through a gastric tube. Give naloxone for respiratory depression.

Assessment: Note any history of allergy to piperidine derivatives prior to administering drug.

Client/Family Teaching

1. Since loperamide may cause a dry mouth, provide instructions suggesting methods to alleviate.
2. Use caution while driving or in undertaking other tasks requiring alertness because the drug may cause dizziness and drowsiness.
3. Record t e number and consistency of stools per day and the amount of medication consumed.

4. Contact physician if diarrhea lasts up to 10 days without relief.
5. Report to the physician if fever, nausea, abdominal pain, or abdominal distention occurs as dosage may require adjustment or drug may need to be discontinued.
6. Remind parents that dietary treatment of diarrhea is preferred, if possible, in children.

Evaluation: Note a decrease in the amount and frequency of diarrheal stools.

Lorazepam

(lor-**AYZ**-eh-pam)

Apo-Lorazepam✦, Ativan, Lorazepam Intensol, Novo-Lorazem✦, Nu-Loraz✦ (C-IV, Rx)

See also *Benzodiazepines*, p. 108.

Classification: Antianxiety agent, benzodiazepine.

Action/Kinetics: Absorbed and eliminated faster than other benzodiazepines. **Peak plasma levels: PO,** 1–6 hr; **IM,** 1–1.5 hr. **t½:** 10–20 hr. Is metabolized to inactive compounds which are excreted through the kidneys.

Uses: PO: Anxiety, tension, anxiety with depression, insomnia, acute alcohol withdrawal symptoms. **Parenteral:** Amnesic agent, anticonvulsant, antitremor drug, adjunct to skeletal muscle relaxants, preanesthetic medication, adjunct prior to endoscopic procedures, treatment of status epilepticus, relief of acute alcohol withdrawal symptoms.

Additional Contraindications: Narrow-angle glaucoma. Use cautiously in presence of renal and hepatic disease. Parenterally in children less than 18 years.

Special Concerns: Pregnancy category: D. Oral dosage has not been established in children less than 12 years of age and IV dosage has not been established in children less than 18 years of age.

Additional Drug Interactions: With parenteral lorazepam, scopolamine → sedation, hallucinations, and behavioral abnormalities.

Dosage: Tablets. Adults: *Anxiety:* 1–3 mg b.i.d.–t.i.d. *Hypnotic:* 2–4 mg at bedtime. **Geriatric/debilitated clients: initial,** 0.5–2 mg/day in divided doses. Dose can be adjusted as required.

IM. Adults: 0.05 mg/kg up to maximum of 4 mg 2 hr before surgery for maximum amnesic effect. **IV. Adults, initial:** 0.044 mg/kg or a total dose of 2 mg, whichever is less. *Amnesic effect:* 0.05 mg/kg up to a maximum of 4 mg administered 15–20 min prior to surgery.

NURSING CONSIDERATIONS

See also *Nursing Considerations* for *Benzodiazepines,* p. 111.

Administration/Storage

1. For IV use, dilute just before use with either sterile water for injection, sodium chloride injection, or 5% dextrose injection.
2. The IV rate of administration should not exceed 2 mg/min.
3. The solution should not be used if it is discolored or contains a precipitate.
4. If higher doses are required, the evening dose should be increased before the daytime doses.

Evaluation: Evaluate client for:
- Reports of symptomatic improvement in levels of anxiety, tension, and depression
- Prevention of alcohol withdrawal symptoms
- Successful attainment of muscle relaxation and amnesia

Lovastatin (Melvinolin)
(**LOW**-vah-**STAT**-in, mel-**VIN**-oh-lin)
Mevacor (Rx)

Classification: Antihyperlipidemic.

Action/Kinetics: Lovastatin is a drug isolated from a strain of *Aspergillus terreus*. It specifically inhibits HMG-coenzyme A reductase, an enzyme that is necessary to convert HMG-coenzyme A to mevalonate (an early step in the biosynthesis of cholesterol). The levels of VLDL, LDL, cholesterol, and plasma triglycerides are reduced, while the plasma concentration of HDL cholesterol is increased. Since the enzyme is not completely inhibited, mevalonate is available in amounts necessary to maintain homeostasis. Absorption is decreased by about one-third if the drug is given on an empty stomach rather than with food. **Onset:** within 2 weeks using multiple doses. **Time to peak plasma levels:** 2–4 hr. **Time to peak effect:** 4–6 weeks using multiple doses. **Duration:** 4–6 weeks after termination of therapy. The drug is metabolized in the liver (its main site of action) to active metabolites. Over 80% of an oral dose is excreted in the feces, via the bile, and approximately 10% is excreted through the urine.

Uses: As an adjunct to diet in primary hypercholesterolemia (types IIa and IIb) in clients with a significant risk of coronary artery disease and who have not responded to diet or other measures. May also be useful in clients with combined hypercholesterolemia and hypertriglyceridemia.

Contraindications: During pregnancy and lactation, active liver disease, persistent elevations of serum transaminases.

Special Concerns: Pregnancy category: X. Use in children is not recommended. Use with caution in clients who have a history of liver disease or who are known heavy consumers of alcohol.

Side Effects: *GI:* Flatus (most common), abdominal pain, cramps, diarrhea, constipation, dyspepsia, nausea, heartburn. *CNS:* Headache, dizziness. *Musculoskeletal:* Myalgia, muscle cramps. *Miscellaneous:* Blurred vision, rash, pruritus, dysgeusia, lenticular opacities.

Drug Interactions

Cholestyramine / Additive effects with lovastatin
Colestipol / Additive effects with lovastatin
Warfarin / ↑ Prothrombin time

Laboratory Test Interference: Lovastatin ↑ transaminase and creatine phosphokinase levels.

Dosage: Tablets. Adults/adolescents: initial, 20 mg once daily with the evening meal. If serum cholesterol levels are greater than 300 mg/dl, initial dose should be 40 mg daily. **Maintenance:** 20–80 mg daily, individualized and adjusted at intervals of every 4 weeks, if necessary.

NURSING CONSIDERATIONS

Administration/Storage

1. Dosage modification is not necessary in clients with renal insufficiency.
2. The maximum dose for clients on immunosuppressive therapy is 20 mg/day.

Assessment

1. Note any evidence of hepatic disease and any heavy consumption of alcohol.
2. Determine if the client has had recent eye examinations and request a report to serve as a baseline against which to measure possible eye changes in the future. Slight changes have been noted in the lens of some clients.
3. If female and of childbearing age, determine if pregnant.
4. Assess liver function tests every 4–6 weeks for the first 15 months of therapy. A threefold increase in serum transaminase or an indication of abnormal liver function is a sign the therapy should be discontinued.

Client/Family Teaching

1. Take the medication with meals.
2. If of childbearing age, advise client to practice some form of birth control.
3. Report the development of malaise, muscle spasms, or fever. These may be mistaken for the flu, but the symptoms could be serious side effects of drug therapy and should not be ignored.
4. Any right upper quadrant abdominal pain or change in color and consistency of the stool should be reported.

5. Stress the importance of periodic eye exams during therapy with lovastatin and to report any early visual disturbances.

Evaluation: Evaluate client for laboratory evidence of ↓ serum cholesterol and triglyceride levels.

Loxapine hydrochloride
(**LOX**-ah-peen)
Loxapac✳, Loxitane C, Loxitane IM (Rx)

Loxapine succinate
(**LOX**-ah-peen)
Loxapac✳, Loxitane (Rx)

See also *Phenothiazines*, p. 201.

Classification: Antipsychotic, miscellaneous.

Action/Kinetics: Loxapine belongs to a new subclass of tricyclic antipsychotic agents. The drug is thought to act by blocking dopamine at postsynaptic brain receptors. It causes significant extrapyramidal symptoms, moderate sedative effects, and a low incidence of anticholinergic effects, as well as orthostatic hypotension. **Onset:** 20–30 min. **Peak effects:** 1.5–3 hr. **Duration:** about 12 hr. $t\frac{1}{2}$: 3–4 hr. Partially metabolized in the liver; excreted in urine, and unchanged in feces.

Uses: Psychoses. *Investigational:* Anxiety neurosis with depression.

Additional Contraindications: History of convulsive disorders.

Special Concerns: Pregnancy category: C. Use with caution in clients with cardiovascular disease. Use during lactation only if benefits outweigh risks. Dosage has not been established in children less than 16 years of age. Geriatric clients may be more prone to developing orthostatic hypotension, anticholinergic, sedative, and extrapyramidal side effects.

Additional Side Effects: Tachycardia, hypertension, hypotension, lightheadedness, and syncope.

Dosage: Capsules, Oral Solution. Adults, initial, 10 mg (of the base) b.i.d. *Severe:* up to 50 mg daily. Increase dosage rapidly over 7–10 days until symptoms are controlled. **Range:** 60–100 mg up to 250 mg daily. **Maintenance:** If possible reduce dosage to 15–25 mg b.i.d.–q.i.d.

IM: 12.5–50 mg (of the base) q 4–6 hr; once adequate control has been established, switch to PO medication after control achieved (usually within 5 days).

NURSING CONSIDERATIONS

See also *Nursing Considerations* for *Phenothiazines,* p. 205.

Administration/Storage

1. Measure the dosage of the concentrate *only* with the enclosed calibrated dropper.
2. Mix oral concentrate with orange or grapefruit juice immediately before administration to disguise unpleasant taste.

Evaluation: Evaluate client for evidence of a reduction in exhibition of psychotic manifestations.

M

—— *COMBINATION DRUG* ——

Maalox Plus Extra Strength Oral Suspension
(**MAY**-lox)
(OTC)

Maalox Plus Tablets
(**MAY**-lox)
(OTC)

See also *Antacids,* p. 37.

Classification/Content: Tablets. *Antacid:* Magnesium hydroxide, 200 mg. *Antacid:* Aluminum hydroxide, 200 mg. *Antiflatulent:* Simethicone, 25 mg. **Extra Strength Oral Suspension.** *Antacid:* Magnesium hydroxide, 450 mg/5 ml. *Antacid:* Aluminum hydroxide, 500 mg/5 ml. *Antiflatulent:* Simethicone, 40 mg/5 ml. The acid neutralizing capacity is 11.4 mEq/tablet and 58.1 mEq/10 ml of the extra strength oral suspension.

See also information on individual components.

Uses: Relief of hyperacidity due to peptic ulcer, peptic esophagitis, gastric hyperacidity, gastritis, hiatal hernia, or heartburn. Also, to relieve symptoms of gas, including postoperative gas pain.

Dosage: Tablets: 1–4 tablets q.i.d. 20–60 min after meals and at bedtime. **Extra Strength Oral Suspension:** 10–20 ml q.i.d. 20–60 min after meals and at bedtime.

NURSING CONSIDERATIONS

See also *Nursing Considerations* for *Maalox Tablets, Oral Suspension, Extra Strength Tablets,* p. 819, and *Antacids,* p. 38.

Administration/Storage

1. No more than 16 tablets should be taken within a 24-hr period. The maximum dosage should not be taken for more than 14 days.
2. No more than 60 ml of the oral suspension should be taken within a 24-hr period. The maximum dosage should not be taken for more than 14 days.
3. The suspension is available in three flavors—lemon swiss creme, cherry creme, and mint creme.

—— *COMBINATION DRUG* ——
Maalox TC Suspension and Tablets
(MAY-lox)
(OTC)

Classification/Content: Maalox TC (therapeutic concentrate) is a high-potency antacid preparation. *Antacid:* Magnesium hydroxide, 300 mg (tablet or 5-ml suspension). *Antacid:* Aluminum hydroxide, 600 mg (tablet or 5-ml suspension). See also information on individual components. The acid neutralizing capacity is 27.2 mEq/5 ml of the suspension and 28 mEq/tablet.

Uses: Relief of hyperacidity due to peptic ulcer, gastritis, gastric hyperacidity, peptic esophagitis, hiatal hernia, heartburn, and other conditions where a high degree of neutralization of acid is desirable.

Dosage: Suspension: 5–10 ml q.i.d. 20–60 min after meals and at bedtime. **Tablets:** 1–2 tablets between meals and at bedtime.

NURSING CONSIDERATIONS

See *Nursing Considerations* for *Maalox Tablets, Oral Suspension, Extra Strength Tablets,* p. 819, and *Antacids,* p. 38.

Administration/Storage: No more than 40 ml of the suspension or 8 tablets should be taken within a 24-hr period. The maximum dosage should not be used for more than 14 days.

—— *COMBINATION DRUG* ——
Maalox Tablets, Oral Suspension, Extra Strength Tablets
(MAY-lox)
(OTC)

See also *Antacids,* p. 37.

Classification/Content: Maalox Tablets. *Antacids:* Aluminum hydroxide, 200 mg and magnesium hydroxide, 200 mg. **Note:** The Extra Strength Tablets contain twice the amount of each antacid per tablet. **Maalox Suspension.** *Antacids:* Aluminum hydroxide, 225 mg/5 ml and magnesium hydroxide, 200 mg/5 ml. The neutralizing capacity is 26.6 mEq/10 ml for the Suspension, 19.4 mEq/2 tablets, and 23.4 mEq/1 Extra Strength tablet.

Uses: Relief of hyperacidity due to peptic ulcer, gastritis, gastric hyperacidity, peptic esophagitis, hiatal hernia, or heartburn.

Dosage: Tablets: 2–4 tablets 20–60 min after meals and at bedtime. **Double Strength Tablets:** 1–2 tablets q.i.d. 20–60 min after meals and at bedtime. **Suspension:** 10–20 ml q.i.d. 20–60 min after meals and at bedtime.

NURSING CONSIDERATIONS

See also *Nursing Considerations* for *Antacids*, p. 38.

Administration/Storage: Tablets may be followed by milk or water.

Client/Family Teaching

1. Advise client to chew tablets well before swallowing.
2. If a suspension is to be used, shake the container thoroughly before pouring the medication.
3. Advise the client not to take more than 80 ml of the Oral Suspension in a 24-hr period.
4. If the client is taking Tablets, advise the client to take no more than 16 tablets/day. If there is no relief, notify the physician.
5. If the client is to take Double Strength Tablets, advise client to take no more than 8 tablets in a 24-hr period.
6. If the client is taking tetracycline advise the physician so that antacid therapy can be avoided.

Evaluation: Evaluate client for evidence of a ↓ in gastric acidity.

Mafenide acetate

(**MAH**-fen-eyed)
Sulfamylon (Rx)

See also *Sulfonamides*, p. 213.

Classification: Sulfonamide, topical.

Uses: Topical application in the treatment of second- and third-degree burns (prevention of infections).

Contraindication: Not to be used for already established infections.

Special Concerns: Pregnancy category: C. Use with caution during lactation. Use not recommended in infants less than 1 month of age.

Dosage: Cream: $1/16$-inch-thick film applied over entire surface of burn with gloves once or twice daily until healing is progressing satisfactorily or until site is ready for grafting.

NURSING CONSIDERATIONS

See also *Sulfonamides*, p. 213, and *General Nursing Considerations For All Anti-Infectives*, p. 83.

Administration: Mafenide, unlike other sulfonamides, is not inhibited by pus or body fluids.

Client/Family Teaching

1. Demonstrate the appropriate method for administration of medication.
2. Burns treated with mafenide are to be covered only with a thin dressing.
3. The drug causes pain upon application.

Evaluation: Evaluate burn site for response to therapy, any evidence of infection, and readiness for grafting.

Magaldrate (Hydroxymagnesium aluminate)

(**MAG**-al-drayt)
Antiflux✻, Lowsium, Riopan, Riopan Extra Strength✻ (OTC)

See also *Antacids*, p. 37.

Classification: Antacid.

Action/Kinetics: Chemical combination of aluminum hydroxide

M

and magnesium hydroxide. This compound is an effective nonsystemic antacid. It buffers (pH 3.0–5.5) without causing alkalosis. Acid-neutralizing capacity: 13.5 mEq/tablet or 15 mEq/5 ml suspension.

Use: Antacid.

Contraindication: Sensitivity to aluminum. Use with caution in clients with impaired renal function.

Side Effects: Mild constipation and hypermagnesemia. Rebound hyperacidity, milk-alkali syndrome.

Dosage: Oral Suspension, Tablets, Chewable Tablets. Adults: 480–1,080 mg q.i.d. between meals and at bedtime. Frequency of administration may have to be increased initially to every hour to control severe symptoms. The suspension contains 540 mg/5 ml.

NURSING CONSIDERATIONS

See also *Nursing Considerations* for *Antacids,* p. 38.

Assessment: Baseline renal function studies prior to administering drug therapy to determine any dysfunction.

Evaluation: Evaluate client for reports of symptomatic improvement in gastric irritation and associated pain.

Magnesium hydroxide (magnesia)

(mag-**NEE**-see-um hy-**DROX**-eyed)
Phillip's Magnesia Tablets❋, Phillips' Milk of Magnesia, M.O.M. (OTC)

See also *Antacids,* p. 37, and *Laxatives,* p. 171.

Classification: Antacid, laxative.

Action/Kinetics: Depending on dosage, drug acts as an antacid or as a laxative. Neutralizes hydrochloric acid. Does not produce alkalosis and has a demulcent effect. A dose of 1 ml neutralizes 2.7 mEq of acid. As an antacid, often alternated with aluminum hydroxide to counteract laxative effect.

As a laxative, magnesium hydroxide increases the bulk of the stools by attracting and holding large amounts of fluids. The increased bulk results in the mechanical stimulation of peristalsis. **Onset:** 2–6 hr.

Uses: Antacid. As a laxative to empty the bowel prior to diagnostic or surgical procedures, to eliminate parasites following anthelmintic therapy, to remove toxic materials following poisoning, and to collect a stool specimen for parasite examination.

Contraindications: Poor renal function.

Side Effects: Diarrhea, abdominal pain, nausea, vomiting. Hypermagnesemia and CNS depression (especially in clients with renal failure). Magnesium intoxication is manifested by drowsiness, dizziness, other signs of CNS depression, and thirst.

Additional Drug Interactions

Procainamide / Procainamide ↑ muscle relaxation produced by Mg salts
Skeletal muscle relaxants (surgical), succinylcholine, tubocurarine / ↑ Muscle relaxation

Dosage: Oral Suspension, Tablets, Chewable Tablets. Adults and children over 12 years:

Antacid, 5–15 ml liquid or 650–1,300 mg tablets q.i.d. *Laxative:* 15–40 ml liquid once daily with water. **Children, 6–12 years:** *Antacid,* 2.5–5 ml liquid with water; *laxative,* 15–30 ml (depending on age) once daily with water. **Children, 2–6 years:** *laxative,* 5–15 ml liquid once daily with water.

NURSING CONSIDERATIONS

See also *Nursing Considerations* for *Antacids,* p. 38, and *Laxatives,* p. 172.

Administration/Storage

1. Suspensions should be administered with water.
2. Administer combined magnesia magma and aluminum hydroxide gel with one-half glass of water.
3. Provide a slice of orange or glass of orange juice after administration as a laxative, to minimize the unpleasant aftertaste.
4. Administer laxative dose at bedtime because medication takes about 8 hr to be effective and, therefore, will not interfere with client's rest.

Evaluation: Evaluate client for:
- Evidence of a reduction in gastric acidity
- Successful bowel evacuation

Magnesium oxide
(mag-**NEE**-see-um **OX**-eyed)
Mag-Ox 400, Maox, Par-Mag, Uro-Mag (OTC)

See also *Antacids,* p. 37, and *Laxatives,* p. 171.

Classification: Antacid, laxative.

Action/Kinetics: Magnesium oxide is a nonsystemic antacid with a laxative effect. The compound has a rather high neutralizing capacity (1.0 g neutralizes 50 mEq acid). Magnesium oxide is slower acting than sodium bicarbonate but has a more prolonged activity.

Uses: Antacid.

Contraindication: Poor renal function.

Side Effects: Abdominal pain, nausea, diarrhea. Hypermagnesemia and CNS depression in clients with poor renal function. Symptoms of magnesium intoxication include drowsiness, dizziness, other signs of CNS depression, and thirst. Rebound hyperacidity, milk-alkali syndrome.

Drug Interactions: See *Magnesium Hydroxide,* p. 820.

Dosage: Capsules, Tablets. *Antacid:* **Capsules,** 140 mg with water or milk t.i.d.–q.i.d. **Tablets:** 400–840 mg daily.

NURSING CONSIDERATIONS

See *Nursing Considerations* for *Antacids,* p. 38, and *Laxatives,* p. 172.

Magnesium sulfate
(mag-**NEE**-see-um **SUL**-fayt)
Epsom Salts (OTC and Rx)

See also *Anticonvulsants,* p. 61, and *Laxatives,* p. 171.

Classification: Anticonvulsant, electrolyte, saline laxative.

Action/Kinetics: Magnesium is an important cation present in the extracellular fluid at a concentration of 1.5–2.5 mEq/L. Magnesium is an essential element for muscle contraction, certain enzyme systems, and nerve transmission.

Magnesium depresses the CNS and controls convulsions by blocking release of acetylcholine at the myoneural junction. Also, the drug decreases the sensitivity of the motor end plate to acetylcholine and decreases the excitability of the motor membrane. **Therapeutic serum levels:** 4–6 mEq/L (normal Mg levels: 1.5–3.0 mEq/L). **Onset: IM,** 1 hr; **IV,** immediate. **Duration: IM,** 3–4 hr; **IV,** 30 min. Magnesium is excreted by the kidneys.

Uses: Seizures associated with toxemia of pregnancy, epilepsy, or when abnormally low levels of magnesium may be a contributing factor in convulsions, such as in hypothyroidism or glomerulonephritis. Acute nephritis in children. Uterine tetany. Replacement therapy in magnesium deficiency. Adjunct in total parenteral nutrition (TPN). Laxative.

Contraindications: In the presence of heart block or myocardial damage.

Special Concerns: Pregnancy category: A. Use with caution in clients with renal disease because magnesium is removed from the body solely by the kidneys.

Side Effects: Magnesium intoxication. *CNS:* Depression. *CV:* Flushing, hypotension, circulatory collapse, depression of the myocardium. *Other:* Sweating, hypothermia, muscle paralysis, respiratory paralysis. Suppression of knee jerk reflex can be used to determine toxicity. Respiratory failure may occur if given after knee jerk reflex disappears.

Symptoms of Overdose: Serum levels can predict symptoms of toxicity. Symptoms include sharp decrease in blood pressure and respiratory paralysis, changes in ECG (increased PR interval, increased QRS complex, prolonged QT interval), asystole, heart block. At serum levels of 7–10 mEq/L there is hypotension, narcosis, and loss of deep tendon reflexes. Levels of 12–15 mEq/L result in respiratory paralysis; greater than 15 mEq/L cause cardiac conduction problems. Levels greater than 25 mEq/L cause cardiac arrest.

Drug Interactions

CNS depressants (general anesthetics, sedative-hypnotics, narcotics) / Additive CNS depression

Digitalis / Heart block when Mg intoxication is treated with calcium in digitalized clients

Neuromuscular blocking agents / Possible additive neuromuscular blockade

Dosage: IM. *Anticonvulsant:* 1–5 g of a 25%–50% solution up to 6 times daily. **Pediatric:** 20–40 mg/kg using the 20% solution (may be repeated if necessary). **IV:** 1–4 g using 10%–20% solution, not to exceed 1.5 ml/min of the 10% solution. **IV infusion:** 4 g in 250 ml 5% dextrose at a rate not to exceed 3 ml/min.

Hypomagnesemia, mild, **IM:** 1 g as a 50% solution q 6 hr for 4 times (or total of 32.5 mEq/24 hr). *Severe,* **IM:** up to 2 mEq/kg over 4 hr or **IV:** 5 g (40 mEq) in 1,000 ml dextrose 5% or sodium chloride solution by **slow** infusion over period of 3 hr. *Hyperalimentation,* **adults:** 8–24 mEq/day; **infants:** 2–10 mEq/day.

Laxative. **PO. Adults:** 10–15 g; **pediatric:** 5–10 g.

NURSING CONSIDERATIONS

See also *Nursing Considerations* for *Anticonvulsants,* p. 63, and *Laxatives,* p. 172.

Administration/Storage

1. For IV injections, administer only 1.5 ml of 10% solution per minute. Discontinue administration when convulsions cease.
2. For IV infusion, administration should not exceed 3 ml/min.
3. Dilutions for IM: deep injection of 50% concentrate is appropriate for adults. A 20% solution should be used for children. IV: dilute as specified by manufacturer.
4. When used as a laxative, dissolve in a glassful of ice water or other chilled fluid to lessen the disagreeable taste.
5. *Treatment of Overdose:*
   * Use artificial ventilation immediately.
   * Have 5–10 mEq of calcium (e.g., 10–20 ml of 10% calcium gluconate) readily available for IV injection to reverse heart block and respiratory depression.
   * Hemodialysis and peritoneal dialysis are effective.

Assessment

1. Obtain baseline serum magnesium levels and renal function.
2. Determine if the client has a history of kidney disease.
3. Assess ECG for evidence of any abnormality prior to administering drug IV.

Interventions

1. Check with the physician before administering magnesium if any of the following conditions exist:
   * Absent patellar reflexes or knee jerk reflex
   * Respirations below 16/min
   * Urinary output less than 100 ml during the past 4 hr

   * Early signs of hypermagnesemia: flushing, sweating, hypotension, or hypothermia
   * Past history of heart block or myocardial damage; prolonged PQ and widened QRS intervals
2. Anticipate that the dose of CNS depressants administered to the client receiving magnesium sulfate will be adjusted.
3. If the client is receiving digitalis preparations and magnesium sulfate, monitor the client closely. Toxicity treated with calcium is extremely dangerous and may result in heart block.
4. Do not administer magnesium sulfate for 2 hr preceding the delivery of a baby.
5. If a mother has received continuous IV therapy of magnesium sulfate during 24 hr prior to delivery, assess the newborn for neurologic and respiratory depression.

Evaluation: Evaluate client for:
   * Effective control of seizures
   * Serum magnesium levels within desired range (1.8–3 mg/dl)
   * Reports of evacuation of stool (when used as a laxative)

M

Maprotiline hydrochloride

(mah-**PROH**-tih-leen)
Ludiomil (Rx)

See also *Tricyclic Antidepressants*, p. 239.

Classification: Antidepressant, tetracyclic.

Action/Kinetics: Maprotiline is actually a tetracyclic compound but has many similarities to the tricyclic drugs. It causes moderate anticholinergic, sedative, and orthostatic hypotensive effects. **Effective plasma levels:** 200–300 ng/ml. **t½:** Approximately 21–25 hr. **Peak effect:** 12 hr. Beneficial effects may not be observed for 2–3 weeks.

Uses: Treat symptoms of depression. Depressive neuroses, depression in clients with manic-depressive illness, depression with anxiety.

Additional Contraindications: Known or suspected seizure disorders.

Special Concerns: Pregnancy category: B. Not recommended for clients under 18 years of age.

Additional Side Effects: Overdosage may cause increased incidence of seizures.

Dosage: Tablets. Adults, *mild to moderate depression,* **outpatients, initial:** 75 mg/day; can be increased to 150–225 mg/day if necessary. **Adult,** *severe depression,* **hospitalized, initial:** 100–150 mg/day; can be increased to 225 mg if necessary. Dosage should not exceed 225 mg/day. **Maintenance:** For all uses, 75–150 mg/day, adjusted depending on therapeutic response. **Geriatric clients:** 50–75 mg/day.

NURSING CONSIDERATIONS

See also *Nursing Considerations* for *Tricyclic Antidepressants,* p. 242.

Administration/Storage

1. May be given in single or divided doses.
2. Should be discontinued as long as possible before elective surgery.

Evaluation: Evaluate client for:
- Reports of symptomatic improvement of depressive episodes with lowered anxiety levels
- Laboratory evidence of serum drug levels within therapeutic range (200–300 ng/ml)

Mazindol

(MAYZ-in-dohl)

Mazanor, Sanorex (C-IV) (Rx)

See also *Amphetamines and Derivatives,* p. 29.

Classification: Anorexiant.

Action/Kinetics: Onset: 30–60 min; **duration:** 8–15 hr. **t½:** Less than 24 hr. **Therapeutic blood levels:** 0.003–0.012 mcg/ml. Excreted in urine partially unchanged.

Use: Short-term (8–12 weeks) treatment of exogenous obesity in conjunction with a weight reduction program including exercise, reduced caloric intake, and behavior modification.

Special Concerns: Pregnancy category: C.

Additional Side Effects: Testicular pain.

Dosage: Tablets. Adults, initial: 1 mg once daily 1 hr before the first meal of the day; **then,** dose can be increased to 1 mg t.i.d. or 2 mg once daily 1 hr before lunch.

NURSING CONSIDERATIONS

See also *Nursing Considerations* for *Amphetamines and Derivatives,* p. 31.

Administration/Storage: Clients may take the medication with meals if they experience GI distress.

Evaluation: Evaluate client for evidence of a reduction in body weight.

Mebendazole
(meh-**BEN**-dah-zohl)
Vermox (Rx)

See also *Anthelmintics*. p. 40.

Classification: Anthelmintic.

Action/Kinetics: Mebendazole exerts its anthelmintic effect by blocking the glucose uptake of the organisms, thereby reducing their energy until death results. It also inhibits the formation of micro-tubules in the helminth. **Peak plasma levels:** 2–4 hr. Poorly absorbed from the GI tract. Excreted in feces.

Uses: Whipworm, pinworm, roundworm, common and American hookworm infections; in single or mixed infections.

Contraindications: Hypersensitivity to mebendazole.

Special Concerns: Pregnancy category: C. Use with caution in children under 2 years of age and during lactation.

Side Effects: Transient abdominal pain and diarrhea.

Drug Interactions: Carbamazepine and hydantoin may ↓ effect due to ↓ plasma levels of mebendazole.

Dosage: Tablets, Chewable. *Whipworm, roundworm, and hookworm:* **PO, adults and children:** 1 tablet morning and evening on 3 consecutive days. *Pinworms:* 1 tablet, one time. All treatments can be repeated after 3 weeks.

NURSING CONSIDERATIONS

See also *Nursing Considerations* for *Anthelmintics,* p. 42, and *General Nursing Considerations For All Anti-Infectives,* p. 83.

Client/Family Teaching

1. Tablet may be chewed, crushed, and/or mixed with food.
2. No prior fasting, purging, or other procedures are required.

Evaluation: Evaluate client for evidence of negative stool specimens and negative perianal swabs.

Mecamylamine hydrochloride
(mek-ah-**MILL**-ah-meen)
Inversine (Rx)

M

Classification: Ganglionic blocking agent, antihypertensive.

Action/Kinetics: The drug is less apt than other ganglionic blocking agents to induce tolerance. Withdraw or substitute mecamylamine slowly because sudden withdrawal or switching to other antihypertensive agents may result in severe hypertensive rebound. Since mecamylamine reduces peristalsis, it is a useful addition to a thiazide-guanethidine regimen in clients who experience persistent diarrhea with guanethidine.

Onset (gradual): ½–2 hr. **Duration:** 6–12 hr. May take 2–3 days to achieve full therapeutic potential. Mecamylamine is excreted unchanged by the kidneys. The rate of excretion is influenced by urinary pH in that alkalinization of the urine decreases, and acidification increases, renal excretion.

Uses: Moderate to severe hypertension including uncomplicated malignant hypertension.

Contraindications: Mild, moderate, labile hypertension; coronary insufficiency, clients with recent myocardial infarction, uremia, clients being treated with antibiotics and sulfonamides, glaucoma, pyloric stenosis, uncooperative clients.

Special Concerns: Pregnancy category: C. Safe use during lactation has not been established. Dosage has not been established in children. Geriatric clients may be more sensitive to the hypotensive effects of mecamylamine; also, a decrease in dose may be required in these clients due to age-related decreases in renal function. Use with caution in marked cerebral and coronary arteriosclerosis, after recent cerebral vascular accident, prostatic hypertrophy, urethral stricture, bladder neck obstruction. Abdominal distention, decreased bowel signs, and other symptoms of adynamic ileus are reasons for discontinuing the drug.

Side Effects: *GI:* Nausea, vomiting, constipation (may be preceded by small, frequent, liquid stools), dry mouth, glossitis, anorexia, ileus. *CNS:* Sedation, weakness, fatigue. Rarely, choreiform movements, mental aberrations, tremors, seizures. *Respiratory:* Fibrosis, interstitial pulmonary edema. *CV:* Postural hypotension, orthostatic dizziness, syncope. *GU:* Urinary retention, decreased libido, impotence. *Miscellaneous:* Paresthesia, blurred vision, dilated pupils.

Symptoms of Overdose: Hypotension, peripheral vascular collapse, nausea, vomiting, diarrhea, constipation, paralytic ileus, dizziness, anxiety, dry mouth, mydriasis, blurred vision, palpitations, increased intraocular pressure, urinary retention.

Dosage: Tablets. Adults: initial, 2.5 mg b.i.d. Increase by increments of 2.5 mg every 2 or more days; **maintenance:** 25 mg daily in 3 divided doses.

NURSING CONSIDERATIONS

See also *Nursing Considerations* for *Antihypertensive Agents,* p. 78.

Administration/Storage

1. For better control of hypertension, administer after meals.
2. The morning dose may be small or omitted; larger doses are given at noon and in the evening.
3. *Treatment of Overdose:* Vasopressors to treat hypotension.

Interventions

1. Take BP and pulse at the specific times ordered.
2. Make sure that the client is in positions ordered for all readings, whether sitting or standing. If this is not possible, alterations in time and position should be indicated on the client's record.
3. Weigh the client daily and check for edema to determine if any weight gain is the result of retained fluid or due to increased appetite.
4. Measure I&O to detect evidence of oliguria, a result of excessive hypotension.
5. Note client complaint of constipation. Check with the physician regarding orders for laxatives, which can be administered if the client fails to have

regular bowel movements. If constipation persists, the drug must be discontinued; bulk-producing cathartics are ineffective.

6. Note evidence of additive hypotensive effects if any other hypotensive agents or diuretics are concomitantly administered. Adjustment in the dosage of drug may be required.

Client/Family Teaching

1. Instruct client how to take BP and pulse and assist to develop a method to maintain a written record for review by health care provider.

2. Orthostatic hypotension may occur. This is manifested by weakness, dizziness, and fainting. Since these symptoms occur when arising rapidly from a supine position, advise clients to rise slowly—first to a sitting position, dangling the legs for a few minutes, then when feeling stable, stand up. If this is a persistent problem have a family member present to assist.

3. Allow more time to prepare for the day's activities than usual to permit the body time to adjust to changes of position.

4. If weak, dizzy, or faint after standing or exercising for a long time, lie down if possible or otherwise sit down and lower head between knees.

5. Eat a diet high in fiber and provide a list of food and fluids that will help to avoid constipation.

Evaluation: Evaluate client for ↓ in blood pressure with a minimum of adverse effects.

Mechlorethamine hydrochloride (Nitrogen Mustard)

(meh-klor-**ETH**-ah-meen)
Mustargen (Rx)

See also *Antineoplastic Agents,* p. 85, and *Alkylating Agents,* p. 20.

Classification: Antineoplastic, alkylating agent.

Action/Kinetics: Mechlorethamine is cell-cycle nonspecific. It acts by forming an unstable ethylenimmonium ion, which then alkylates or binds with various compounds, including nucleic acids. The cytotoxic activity is due to cross-linking of DNA and RNA strands and protein synthesis. When used for intracavitary tumors, the drug exerts both an inflammatory reaction and sclerosis on serous membranes, which causes adherence of the drug to serosal surfaces. It reacts rapidly with tissues and within minutes after administration the active drug is no longer present. Metabolites are excreted through the urine.

Uses: IV: Bronchogenic carcinoma; chronic lymphocytic and chronic myelocytic leukemia; palliative treatment of stages III and IV of Hodgkin's disease, polycythemia vera, mycosis fungoides. **Intracavitary:** Intrapericardially, intraperitoneally, or intrapleurally for treatment of metastatic carcinoma resulting in effusion. *Investigational:* **Topical:** Cutaneous mycosis fungoides.

Contraindications: Use during lactation. During infectious disease.

Special Concerns: Pregnancy category: D. Extravasation into subcutaneous areas causes painful inflammation and induration. Use in children has been limited although the drug has been used in MOPP therapy.

Additional Side Effects: High incidence of nausea and vomiting. Amyloidosis, hyperuricemia, petechiae, subcutaneous hemorrhages, tinnitus, deafness, herpes zoster, or temporary amenorrhea. Extravasation into subcutaneous tissue causes painful inflammation.

Drug Interaction: Amphotericin B: combination increases possibility of blood dyscrasias.

Dosage: IV, Adults, children, *total dose:* 0.4 mg/kg per course of therapy given as a single dose or in 2–4 divided doses over 2–4 days. Depending on blood cell count, a second course may be given after 3 weeks. **Intracavitary:** 0.4 mg/kg. **Intrapericardial:** 0.2 mg/kg. **Topical Ointment, Solution:** Apply to entire skin surface once daily until 6–12 months after a complete response is obtained; **then,** use once to several times a week for up to 3 years.

NURSING CONSIDERATIONS

See also *Nursing Considerations* for *Antineoplastic Agents,* p. 88.

Administration/Storage

1. Because drug is highly irritating, any contact with skin should be avoided; plastic or rubber gloves should be worn during preparation.
2. Drug is best administered through tubing of a rapidly flowing IV saline infusion.
3. Prepare solution immediately before administration because it decomposes on standing.
4. Medication is available in a rubber-stoppered vial to which 10 ml of either sterile water for injection or sodium chloride injection should be added to give a concentration of 1 mg/ml.
5. Insert the needle and keep it inserted until the medication is dissolved and the required dose withdrawn. Carefully discard the vial with the remaining solution so that no one will come in contact with it.
6. For intracavitary administration, turn client every 60 sec for 5 min to the following positions: prone, supine, right side, left side, and knee-chest. Lack of effect often results from failure to move the client often enough.
7. An aqueous solution of equal parts of 5% sodium thiosulfate and 5% sodium bicarbonate should be used to clean glassware, tubings, and other articles after drug administration. Soak for 45 min.
8. Monitor IV closely because extravasation causes swelling, erythema, induration, and sloughing.
9. In case of extravasation, remove IV, assist in infusion of area with isotonic sodium thiosulfate (4.14% solution of USP salt), and apply cold compresses. If sodium thiosulfate is not available, use isotonic sodium chloride solution or 1% lidocaine. Apply ice for 6–12 hr.

Interventions

1. Administer phenothiazine and/or a sedative as ordered, prior to medication and as needed, to control severe nausea and

vomiting that usually occur 1–3 hr after administration of nitrogen mustard.

2. Administer in late afternoon, and follow with a sedative (sleeping pill) at an appropriate time to control any adverse symptoms and induce sleep.

3. Irrigate eye with copious amounts of saline solution and consult with an ophthalmologist if mechlorethamine comes in contact with eye.

4. Irrigate skin with water for 15 min and then with 2% solution of sodium thiosulfate in the event of accidental contact.

Evaluation: Evaluate client for:
- Evidence of a ↓ in tumor size and spread
- Laboratory evidence of improved hematologic parameters

Meclizine hydrochloride
(**MEK**-lih-zeen)
Antivert, Antivert/25 and /50, Antivert/25 Chewable, Antrizine, Bonamine✺, Bonine, Dizmiss, Meni-D, Ru-Vert-M (OTC and Rx)

See also *Antihistamines,* p. 71, and *Antiemetics,* p. 70.

Classification: Antihistamine (piperidine-type), antiemetic, antimotion sickness.

Action/Kinetics: The mechanism for the antiemetic effect is not known but may be due to a central anticholinergic effect to decrease vestibular stimulation and depress labyrinthine activity. The drug may also act on the chemoreceptor trigger zone to decrease vomiting. **Onset:** 30–60 min; **Duration:** 8–24 hr. **t½:** 6 hr.

Uses: Nausea, vomiting, dizziness of motion sickness, vertigo associated with diseases of the vestibular system.

Special Concerns: Pregnancy category: B. Safety for use during lactation and in children less than 12 years of age has not been determined. Pediatric and geriatric clients may be more sensitive to the anticholinergic effects of meclizine.

Side Effects: *CNS:* Drowsiness, excitation, nervousness, restlessness, insomnia, euphoria, vertigo, hallucinations (auditory or visual). *GI:* Nausea, vomiting, diarrhea, constipation, anorexia. *GU:* Urinary frequency or retention; difficulty in urination. *CV:* Hypotension, tachycardia, palpitations. *Miscellaneous:* Dry nose and throat, blurred or double vision, tinnitus, rash, urticaria.

Dosage: Capsules, Tablets, Chewable Tablets. *Motion sickness:* **Adults,** 25–50 mg 1 hr before travel; may be repeated q 24 hr during travel. *Vertigo:* **Adults:** 25–100 mg daily in divided doses.

NURSING CONSIDERATIONS

See also *Nursing Considerations* for *Antihistamines,* p. 74, and *Antiemetics,* p. 71.

Interventions

1. Assess the client for other adverse symptoms in addition to nausea. An antiemetic drug may mask signs of drug overdose as well as signs of pathology such as increased intracranial pressure or intestinal obstruction.

2. Antiemetics tend to cause drowsiness and dizziness. Therefore, caution clients

against driving or performing other hazardous tasks until individual response to the drug has been evaluated.

Evaluation: Evaluate client for:
- Prevention of motion sickness
- Control of vertigo

Meclofenamate sodium

(me-kloh-fen-**AM**-ayt)
Meclomen (Rx)

See also *Nonsteroidal Anti-Inflammatory Drugs,* p. 186.

Classification: Anti-inflammatory, nonsteroidal, analgesic.

Action/Kinetics: Peak plasma levels: 30–60 min. **t½:** 2–3.3 hr. Peak anti-inflammatory activity may not be observed for 2–3 weeks. Excreted through urine and feces.

Uses: Acute and chronic rheumatoid arthritis and osteoarthritis. Not indicated as the initial drug for rheumatoid arthritis due to GI side effects. Has been used in combination with gold salts or corticosteroids. Mild to moderate pain. Primary dysmenorrhea, excessive menstrual blood loss. *Investigational:* Sunburn, prophylaxis of migraine, migraine due to menses.

Additional Contraindications: Not recommended for use during pregnancy or lactation. Use in children less than 14 years of age.

Special Concerns: Safe use during lactation not established. Safety and efficacy not established in functional class IV rheumatoid arthritis.

Additional Side Effects: Severe diarrhea, nausea, headache, rash,

dermatitis, abdominal pain, pyrosis, flatulence, malaise, fatigue, paresthesia, insomnia, depression, taste disturbances, nocturia, blood loss (through feces: 2 ml/day).

Drug Interactions

Aspirin / ↓ Plasma levels of meclofenamate
Warfarin / ↑ Effect of warfarin

Laboratory Test Interferences: ↑ Serum transaminase, alkaline phosphatase; rarely, ↑ serum creatinine or BUN.

Dosage: Capsules. *Rheumatoid arthritis, osteoarthritis:* **usual,** 200–400 mg/day in 3–4 equal doses. Initiate at lower dose and increase to maximum of 400 mg daily if necessary. After initial satisfactory response, lower dosage to decrease severity of side effects. *Mild to moderate pain:* 50 mg q 4–6 hr (100 mg may be required in some clients), not to exceed 400 mg daily. *Excessive menstrual blood loss and primary dysmenorrhea:* 100 mg t.i.d. for up to 6 days, starting at the onset of menses.

NURSING CONSIDERATIONS

See also *Nursing Considerations* for *Nonsteroidal Anti-Inflammatory Drugs,* p. 189.

Administration/Storage

1. Lower doses may be effective for chronic use.
2. The drug can be given with food or milk to diminish GI effects.
3. Reduce dose or discontinue temporarily if diarrhea occurs.

Client/Family Teaching

1. Continue to take the drug as ordered and do not become discouraged because beneficial

effects are not readily evident and it may take 2–3 weeks to see improvement in arthritic conditions.

2. Provide a printed list of adverse side effects; emphasize those that require immediate reporting.

Evaluation: Evaluate client for:

- Reports of symptomatic improvement in joint pain and mobility
- Effective control of pain
- Control of heavy menstrual bleeding

Medroxyprogesterone acetate

(meh-**drox**-see-proh-**JESS**-ter-ohn)
Amen, Curretab, Cycrin, Depo-Provera, Provera (Rx)

See also *Progesterone/Progestins,* p. 209, and *Antineoplastic Agents,* p. 85.

Classification: Progestational hormone, synthetic.

Action/Kinetics: Medroxyprogesterone acetate, a synthetic progestin, is devoid of estrogenic and androgenic activity. The drug prevents stimulation of endometrium by pituitary gonadotropins. Also available in depot form. Priming with estrogen is necessary before response is noted.

Additional Uses: Secondary amenorrhea, abnormal uterine bleeding due to hormonal imbalance (no organic pathology). Adjunct in palliative treatment of inoperable, recurrent, or metastatic endometrial or renal carcinoma. *Investigational:* Premenopausal and menopausal symptoms (injec-

tion). To stimulate respiration in obesity–hypoventilation syndrome (oral). The depot form has been used as a long-acting contraceptive and to treat advanced breast cancer.

Contraindications: Clients with or a history of thrombophlebitis, thromboembolic disease, cerebral apoplexy. Liver dysfunction. Known or suspected malignancy of the breasts or genital organs. Missed abortion; as a diagnostic for pregnancy. Undiagnosed vaginal bleeding. Use during the first 4 months of pregnancy.

Side Effects: *GU:* Amenorrhea or infertility for up to 18 months. *CV:* Thrombophlebitis, pulmonary embolism. *GI:* Nausea (rare), jaundice. *CNS:* Nervousness, drowsiness, insomnia, fatigue, dizziness, headache (rare). *Dermatologic:* Pruritus, urticaria, rash, acne, hirsutism, alopecia, angioneurotic edema. *Miscellaneous:* Hyperpyrexia, anaphylaxis.

Dosage: Tablets. *Secondary amenorrhea:* 5–10 mg/day for 5–10 days, with therapy beginning at any time. If endometrium has been estrogen primed: 10 mg medroxyprogesterone/day for 10–13 days (beginning on day 16–13, respectively). *Abnormal uterine bleeding with no pathology:* 5–10 mg/day for 5–10 days, with therapy beginning on day 16 or 21 of the menstrual cycle. If endometrium has been estrogen primed: 10 mg/day for 10 days, beginning on day 16 of the menstrual cycle. Bleeding usually begins within 3–7 days. **IM.** *Endometrial or renal carcinoma:* **initial,** 400–1,000 mg weekly; **then, if improvement noted,** 400 mg monthly. Medroxyprogesterone is not intended to be the primary therapy. *Long-acting contraceptive:* 150 mg of depot form q 3 months or 450 mg of depot form q 6 months.

NURSING CONSIDERATIONS

See also *Nursing Considerations* for *Antineoplastic Agents,* p. 88, and *Progesterone and Progestins,* p. 210.

Assessment

1. Note any history of thromboembolic disease.
2. Obtain baseline calcium levels and liver function studies.

Interventions

1. The combined effect of the drug and osteolytic metastases may result in hypercalcemia. Therefore, note especially client complaints of insomnia, lethargy, anorexia, nausea, and vomiting. Withhold the drug, obtain serum calcium levels and report to the physician if elevated.
2. In the event the client develops severe hypercalcemia, have IV fluids, diuretics, corticosteroids, and phosphate supplements available.
3. Monitor I&O. Encourage a high fluid intake to minimize hypercalcemia.
4. Closely monitor the client who has resumed therapy after drug-induced hypercalcemia has been corrected.

Evaluation: Evaluate client for:

- Evidence of control of tumor size and spread
- Re-establishment of regular menses with laboratory evidence of normal hormone levels

Mefloquine hydrochloride
(meh-**FLOH**-kwin)
Lariam (Rx)

Classification: Antimalarial.

Action/Kinetics: Although the precise mechanism of action is not known, mefloquine is related chemically to quinine and acts as a blood schizonticide. It may increase intravesicular pH in acid vesicles of parasite. Mefloquine is a mixture of enantiomeric molecules that results in differences in the rates of release, absorption, distribution, metabolism, elimination, and activity of the drug. **t½:** 13–24 days (average 3 weeks). The drug is 98% bound to plasma proteins and is concentrated in blood erythrocytes (i.e., the target cells in treatment of malaria).

Uses: Mild to moderate acute malaria caused by mefloquine-susceptible strains of *Plasmodium falciparum* (both chloroquine susceptible and resistant strains) or *P. vivax.* Data are not available regarding effectiveness in treating *P. ovale* or *P. malariae.* Also, prophylaxis of *P. falciparum* and *P. vivax* infections, including prophylaxis of chloroquine-resistant strains of *P. falciparum.* **Note:** Clients with acute *P. vivax* malaria are at a high risk for relapse as mefloquine does not eliminate the exoerythrocytic (hepatic) parasites. Thus, these clients should also be treated with primaquine.

Contraindications: Hypersensitivity to mefloquine or related compounds.

Special Concerns: Use during pregnancy (category: C) only if potential benefits outweigh potential risks. Use with caution during lactation. Safety and effectiveness have not been determined in children.

Side Effects: Note: At the doses used, it is difficult to distinguish side effects due to the drug from symptoms attributable to the disease itself. **When used for treatment of acute malaria.** *GI:* Nausea, vomiting, diarrhea, abdominal pain, loss of appetite. *CNS:* Dizziness, fever, headache, fatigue, emotional problems, seizures. *Miscellaneous:* Myalgia, chills, skin rash, tinnitus, bradycardia, hair loss. **When used for prophylaxis of malaria.** *CNS:* Dizziness, syncope, encephalopathy of unknown etiology. *Miscellaneous:* Vomiting, extrasystoles. **Postmarketing surveillance:** *CNS:* Vertigo, psychoses, confusion, anxiety, depression, hallucinations. *Miscellaneous:* Visual disturbances. *Symptoms of Overdose:* Cardiotoxic effects, vomiting, diarrhea.

Drug Interactions

Beta-adrenergic blocking agents / ECG abnormalities or cardiac arrest
Chloroquine / ↑ Risk of seizures
Quinidine / ↑ Risk of ECG abnormalities or cardiac arrest
Quinine / ↑ Risk of seizures, ECG abnormalities, or cardiac arrest
Valproic acid / Loss of seizure control and ↓ blood levels of valproic acid

Laboratory Test Interferences: When used for prophylaxis: Transient ↑ transaminases, leukocytosis, thrombocytopenia. **When used for treatment of acute malaria:** ↓ Hematocrit, transient ↑ transaminases, leukocytosis, thrombocytopenia.

Dosage: Tablets. *Mild to moderate malaria* caused by susceptible strains of *P. falciparum* or *P. vivax:* 1,250 mg (5 tablets) as a single dose with at least 8 oz of water. *Prophylaxis of malaria:* 250 mg (1 tablet) once a week for 4 weeks; **then,** 1 tablet every other week. **Pediatric, 15–19 kg:** 1/4 tablet (62.5 mg) weekly; **20–30 kg:** 1/2 tablet (125 mg) weekly; **31–45 kg:** 3/4 tablet (187.5 mg) weekly; **over 45 kg:** 1 tablet (250 mg) weekly.

NURSING CONSIDERATIONS

See also *General Nursing Considerations For All Anti-Infectives,* p. 83

Administration

1. For prophylaxis, therapy with mefloquine should be initiated 1 week prior to travel to an endemic area and should be continued for 4 additional weeks after return from an endemic area.
2. *Treatment of Overdose:* Induce vomiting and administer fluid therapy to treat vomiting and diarrhea.

Assessment

1. Note laboratory confirmation of causative organism.
2. Determine liver function and monitor closely during long-term drug therapy.

Interventions

1. If the client has a life-threatening *P. falciparum* infection, treatment should be initiated with an IV antimalarial drug. This can be followed by mefloquine, orally, to complete therapy.
2. To reduce the potential of cardiotoxic effects, vomiting

M

should be induced in cases of overdose.

3. Periodic ophthalmic examinations are recommended.
4. Liver function tests should be performed if the drug is to be taken chronically.

Client/Family Teaching

1. Do not take the drug on an empty stomach.
2. Take the medication with at least 8 oz of water.
3. Provide a printed list of side effects and stress those that require immediate reporting.
4. Advise client to report any early evidence of visual disturbance. Stress the importance of periodic ophthalmic examinations during drug therapy.

Evaluation: Evaluate for control and prevention of acute attacks of malaria in clients with drug-sensitive malarial parasites.

Megestrol acetate
(meh-**JESS**-trohl)
Megace (Rx)

See also *Progesterone/Progestins,* p. 209, and *Antineoplastic Agents,* p. 85.

Classification: Synthetic progestin.

Action/Kinetics: The antineoplastic activity is due to suppression of gonadotropins (antiluteinizing effect). Drug contains tartrazine, which can cause allergic-type reactions, including asthma, often occurring in clients sensitive to aspirin.

Uses: Palliative treatment of endometrial or breast cancer. Should not be used instead of chemotherapy,

radiation, or surgery. *Investigational:* Appetite stimulant in HIV-related cachexia.

Additional Contraindications: Not to be used for diagnosis of pregnancy. Use during the first 4 months of pregnancy.

Special Concerns: Use with caution in clients with a history of thrombophlebitis.

Side Effects: *Few:* Abdominal pain, headache, nausea, vomiting, breast tenderness, carpal tunnel syndrome (soreness, weakness, and tenderness of muscles of thumbs), deep vein thrombosis, thrombophlebitis, pulmonary embolism, alopecia.

Dosage: Tablets. *Breast cancer:* 40 mg q.i.d. *Endometrial cancer:* 40–320 mg/day in divided doses. To determine efficacy, treatment should be continued for at least 2 months.

NURSING CONSIDERATIONS

See also *Nursing Considerations* for *Antineoplastic Agents,* p. 88, *Progesterone and Progestins,* p. 210, and *Medroxyprogesterone Acetate,* p. 832.

Assessment

1. Note any history of thromboembolic disease.
2. If female and of childbearing age, determine if pregnant.
3. Document any client history of sensitivity to tartrazines.

Melphalan (L-PAM, L-Phenylalanine mustard, L-Sarcolysin)
(**MEL**-fah-lan)
Alkeran (Abbreviation: MPL) (Rx)

See also *Antineoplastic Agents,* p. 85, and *Alkylating Agents,* p. 20.

Classification: Antineoplastic, alkylating agent.

Action/Kinetics: Melphalan is cell-cycle nonspecific. The drug forms an unstable ethylenimmonium ion which binds to or alkylates various intracellular substances including nucleic acids. It produces a cytotoxic effect by cross-linking of DNA and RNA strands as well as inhibition of protein synthesis. Absorption from GI tract is variable and incomplete. $t^{1/2}$: 90 min. The drug is inactivated in tissues and body fluids although it will remain active in the blood for approximately 6 hr. Within 24 hr, 10% is excreted unchanged in the urine.

Uses: Multiple myeloma. Epithelial carcinoma of ovary (nonresectable). *Investigational:* Cancer of the breast and testes.

Contraindications: Use during lactation. Known resistance to drug.

Special Concerns: Pregnancy category: D. Safety and efficacy have not been determined in children less than 12 years of age. Use with extreme caution in those with compromised bone marrow function due to prior chemotherapy or radiation.

Additional Side Effects: Severe bone marrow depression, chromosomal aberrations, leukemia (acute, nonlymphatic) in clients with multiple myeloma. Also, pulmonary fibrosis, interstitial pneumonia, vasculitis, hemolytic anemia. *Symptoms of Overdose:* Vomiting, diarrhea, ulceration of mouth, hemorrhage of GI tract, bone marrow toxicity.

Laboratory Test Interferences: ↑ Uric acid and urinary 5-hydroxyindole acetic acid levels.

Dosage: Tablets. *Multiple myeloma:* (1) 0.15 mg/kg daily for 7 days followed by a rest period of at least 3 weeks. During the rest period, the leukocyte count will decrease; when white blood cell and platelet counts are increasing, a maintenance dose of 0.05 mg/kg daily may be given; or, (2) 0.1–0.15 mg/kg daily for 2–3 weeks (or 0.25 mg/kg daily for 4 days) followed by a rest period of 2–4 weeks. When leukocyte counts rise to 3,000–4,000/mm³ and platelet counts increase above 100,000/mm³ a maintenance dose of 2–4 mg daily may be given; or, (3) 7 mg/m² (or 0.25 mg/kg) daily for 5 days q 5–6 weeks (dose is adjusted to produce slight leukopenia and thrombocytopenia). *Ovarian cancer:* 0.2 mg/kg daily for 5 days repeated q 4–5 weeks (as long as blood counts return to normal).

NURSING CONSIDERATIONS

See also *Nursing Considerations* for *Antineoplastic Agents,* p. 88.

Administration/Storage

1. Drug should be protected from light and dispensed in glass.
2. *Treatment of Overdose:* General supportive treatment, blood transfusions, antibiotics. Monitor hematology for up to 6 weeks.

Assessment

1. Document any previous radiation or chemotherapy.
2. Assess baseline CBC with differential prior to initiating drug therapy. Monitor hemoglobin and platelet levels and differential leukocyte count. Severe risk of infection exists if the absolute neutrophil count is

less than 1,000/mm³, hemorrhage is possible if platelet count drops below 50,000/mm³, and symptoms of anemia will develop if hemoglobin level falls below 9–10 g/day.

3. The client should be advised to use contraceptive measures during therapy.

Evaluation: Evaluate client for:

- Evidence of control of tumor size and spread
- Laboratory evidence of improved hematologic parameters

Menadiol sodium diphosphate (Vitamin K₄)

(men-ah-**DYE**-ohl)

Synkavite ✽, Synkayvite (Rx)

See also *Vitamin K,* p. 246.

Classification: Vitamin K.

Action/Kinetics: Precursors of blood-clotting factors. Menadiol sodium diphosphate is water soluble and is converted to menadione in the body. Both may be absorbed directly into the bloodstream even in the absence of bile. **Onset, IM, SC:** 8–24 hr. **Duration:** (normal prothrombin time), 8–24 hr. **IV,** onset faster than IM, SC; **duration:** shorter.

Uses: Not as safe as phytonadione in treating hemorrhagic disease of the newborn. Ineffective in treating oral anticoagulant-induced hypoprothrombinemia.

Contraindications: Last weeks of pregnancy or during labor as a prophylaxis against hypoprothrombinemia or hemorrhagic disease of the newborn. Use in infants.

Special Concerns: Pregnancy category: C. Use with caution in children due to an increased risk of hepatotoxicity and hemolytic anemia.

Additional Side Effects: Hemolysis of red blood cells in clients with glucose 6-phosphate dehydrogenase deficiency.

Laboratory Test Interference: Falsely elevated urinary 17-hydroxycorticosteroid levels (Reddy, Thorn, and Jenkins procedure).

Dosage: Tablets. *Hypoprothrombinemia due to obstructive jaundice and biliary fistulas:* **Adults,** 5 mg/day.   *Hypoprothrombinemia due to antibacterial/salicylate use:* **Adults,** 5–10 mg/day. **Pediatric, all uses:** 5–10 mg daily. **IM, SC.** *Hypoprothrombinemia,* **Adults:** 5–15 mg, 1–2 times/day; **children:** 5–10 mg, 1–2 times/day.

NURSING CONSIDERATIONS

See also *Nursing Considerations* for *Vitamin K,* p. 247.

Administration/Storage: Although the response following IV use is faster, IM or SC use leads to a more sustained effect.

Interventions

1. Monitor liver function studies and hematologic values.
2. If clients are sensitive to sulfites, caution them to avoid taking menadiol sodium diphosphate and menadione.
3. Anticipate that large doses of menadione may decrease client response to oral anticoagulants.
4. If the client has decreased bile secretion, administer bile salts to ensure the absorption of vitamin K₄ taken orally.

Evaluation: Evaluate for control or prevention of bleeding in clients with hypoprothrombinemia or impaired vitamin K absorption.

Menotropins
(men-oh-**TROH**-pinz)
Pergonal (Rx)

Classification: Ovarian stimulant.

Action/Kinetics: Menotropins is a mixture of follicle-stimulating hormone (FSH) and luteinizing hormone (LH), which cause growth and maturation of ovarian follicles. For ovulation to occur, HCG is administered the day following menotropins. **Time to peak effect, females:** 18 hr. In men, menotropins with HCG given for a minimum of 3 months induce spermatogenesis. Eliminated through the kidneys.

Uses: *Females:* In combination with HCG to induce ovulation in clients with anovulatory cycles not due to primary ovarian failure. *Males:* In combination with HCG to induce spermatogenesis in males with primary or secondary hypogonadotropic hypogonadism.

Contraindications: *Women:* Pregnancy. Primary ovarian failure as indicated by high levels of urinary gonadotropins, ovarian cysts, intracranial lesions, including pituitary tumors. *Men:* Normal gonadotropin levels, primary testicular failure, disorders of fertility other than hypogonadotropic hypogonadism. Thyroid or adrenal dysfunction. Absence of neoplastic disease should be established before treatment is initiated.

Special Concerns: Pregnancy category: X.

Side Effects: *Women:* Ovarian overstimulation, hyperstimulation syndrome (maximal 7–10 days after discontinuation of drug), ovarian enlargement (20% of clients), ruptured ovarian cysts, hemoperitoneum, thromboembolism, multiple births (20%). Fever, hypersensitivity. *Men:* Gynecomastia.

Dosage: Women, IM. *Individualized:* **initial,** 75 IU of FSH and 75 IU of LH for 9–12 days, followed by 5,000–10,000 USP units of HCG one day after last dose of menotropins. *Subsequent courses:* Same dosage schedule for two more courses, if ovulation has occurred. **Then,** dose may be increased to 150 IU of FSH and 150 IU of LH for 9 to 12 days, followed by HCG as above for 2 or more courses. **Men, IM:** To increase serum testosterone levels, it may be necessary to give HCG alone, 5,000 IU 3 times weekly, for 4–6 months prior to menotropins; **then,** 75 IU FSH and 75 IU LH **IM** 3 times weekly and HCG 2,000 IU 2 times weekly for at least 4 months. If no response after 4 months, double each dose of menotropins with the HCG dose unchanged.

NURSING CONSIDERATIONS

Administration/Storage

1. Menotropins are destroyed in the GI tract, therefore, they must be administered parenterally.
2. Reconstituted solutions must be used immediately.
3. ⸱Discard any unused portions of the reconstituted drug.
4. Have emergency drugs and equipment available to treat allergic reactions should they occur.

Assessment

1. Determine if the client has been tested for high levels of

urinary gonadotropins or evaluated for the presence of ovarian cysts. The drug is contraindicated in these instances.

2. Obtain baseline peripheral pulse assessments as data against which to compare future findings.

Interventions

1. Take the client's urinary estrogen excretion levels daily. If they are greater than 100 mcg, or if the daily estriol excretion is greater than 50 mcg, *withhold HCG* and notify the physician. These levels are signs of an impending hyperstimulation syndrome.

2. An occasional client will develop erythrocytosis. Therefore, monitor the CBC on a routine basis.

3. Observe the client for complaints of unexplained fever or abdominal pain. Withhold the medication and report these findings to the physician.

4. If the client requires hospitalization for hyperstimulation, the following interventions should be performed:
   - Place the client on bed rest.
   - Monitor I&O and weigh daily.
   - Monitor the specific gravity of the urine as well as serum and urinary electrolytes.
   - Assess for hemoconcentration. If the hematocrit rises to critical levels, have sodium heparin on hand for administration.
   - Increase fluid intake and anticipate electrolyte replacement therapy.
   - Provide analgesics as needed for comfort.

Client/Family Teaching

1. Report any pain in the extremities, if an extremity is cool to the touch, or if an extremity becomes pale blue. This is a sign of arterial thromboembolism and must be reported to the physician immediately.

2. Explain that fever or the development of lower abdominal pain may be the result of overstimulation of the ovaries that has caused cysts to form, a loss of fluid into the peritoneum, or bleeding and must be reported to the physician immediately. Discuss the need for examination for this phenomenon at least every other day during drug therapy and for 2 weeks thereafter. If overstimulation occurs, hospitalization is necessary for close monitoring.

3. Explain the need to collect a 24-hr urine daily, to be analyzed for estrogen and provide a suitable container for collection. Provide the client with printed instructions concerning the delivery of a 24-hr urine sample to the appropriate laboratory facility.

4. Instruct the client in taking her basal body temperature and charting it on a graph.

5. Describe the signs that indicate ovulation, such as an increase in the basal body temperature, and an increase in the appearance and volume of cervical mucus. Also, discuss the significance of the urinary excretion of estriol.

6. Client should engage in daily intercourse from the day before chorionic gonadotropin is administered and until ovulation occurs.

7. If symptoms indicate over-stimulation of the ovaries, a significant ovarian enlargement may have occurred. Instruct client to abstain from intercourse because of the increased possibility of rupturing the ovarian cysts.

8. Discuss with the client and family that with this therapy there is an increased possibility of multiple births.

9. Explain that pregnancy usually occurs 4–6 weeks after the completion of therapy.

Evaluation: Evaluate client for:
- Ovulation in females as evidenced by increased estrogen levels
- Spermatogenesis in males as evidenced by increased testosterone levels
- Freedom from complications of drug therapy

Meperidine hydrochloride (Pethidine hydrochloride)

(meh-**PER**-ih-deen)

Demerol Hydrochloride (C-II, Rx)

See also *Narcotic Analgesics,* p. 174.

Classification: Narcotic analgesic, synthetic.

Action/Kinetics: The pharmacologic activity of meperidine is similar to that of the opiates; however, meperidine is only one-tenth as potent an analgesic as morphine. Its analgesic effect is only one-half when given orally rather than parenterally. Meperidine has no antitussive effects and does not pro-duce miosis. The drug does produce moderate spasmogenic effects on smooth muscle. The duration of action of meperidine is less than that of most opiates, and this must be kept in mind when a dosing schedule is being established. Meperidine will produce both psychologic and physical dependence; overdosage is manifested by severe respiratory depression (see *Morphine Overdosage,* p. 174). **Onset:** 10–45 min. **Peak effect:** 30–60 min. **Duration:** 2–4 hr. **t½:** 3–4 hr.

Uses: Any situation that requires a narcotic analgesic: severe pain, hepatic and renal colic, obstetrics, preanesthetic medication, adjunct to anesthesia. These drugs are particularly useful for minor surgery, as in orthopedics, ophthalmology, rhinology, laryngology, and dentistry, and for diagnostic procedures such as cystoscopy, retrograde pyelography, and gastroscopy. Spasms of GI tract, uterus, urinary bladder. Anginal syndrome and distress of CHF.

Additional Contraindications: Hypersensitivity to drug, convulsive states as in epilepsy, tetanus and strychnine poisoning, children under 6 months, diabetic acidosis, head injuries, shock, liver disease, respiratory depression, increased cranial pressure, and before labor during pregnancy.

Special Concerns: To be used with caution in pregnancy (category: C), lactating mothers, and in older or debilitated clients. Use with extreme caution in clients with asthma. Meperidine has atropine-like effects that may aggravate glaucoma, especially when given with other drugs, which should be used with caution in glaucoma.

M

Additional Side Effects: Transient hallucinations, transient hypotension (high doses), visual disturbances. Meperidine may accumulate in clients with renal dysfunction, leading to an increased risk of CNS toxicity.

Additional Drug Interactions

Antidepressants, tricyclic / Additive anticholinergic side effects

Hydantoins / ↓ Effect of meperidine due to ↑ breakdown by liver

MAO inhibitors / ↑ Risk of severe symptoms including hyperpyrexia, restlessness, hyper- or hypotension, convulsions, or coma

Dosage: Tablets, Syrup, IM, SC: *Analgesic.* **Adults:** 50–100 mg q 3–4 hr as needed; **pediatric:** 1.1–1.8 mg/kg, up to adult dosage, q 3–4 hr as needed. *Preoperatively:* **Adults: IM, SC,** 50–100 mg 30–90 min before anesthesia; **pediatric: IM, SC,** 1–2 mg/kg 30–90 min before anesthesia. *Support of anesthesia:* **IV infusion** (1 mg/ml) or **slow IV injection** (10 mg/ml) until client needs met. *Obstetrics:* **IM, SC:** 50–100 mg q 1–3 hr.

NURSING CONSIDERATIONS

See also *Nursing Considerations for Narcotic Analgesics,* p. 177.

Administration/Storage

1. For repeated doses, IM administration is preferred over SC use.
2. Meperidine is more effective when given parenterally than when given orally.
3. The syrup should be taken with ½ glass of water to minimize

anesthetic effect on mucous membranes.
4. If used concomitantly with phenothiazines or antianxiety agents, the dose of meperidine should be reduced by 25%–50%.
5. Meperidine for IV use is incompatible with the following drugs: aminophylline, barbiturates, heparin, iodide, methicillin, morphine sulfate, phenytoin, sodium bicarbonate, sulfadiazine, and sulfisoxazole.
6. *Treatment of Overdose:* Naloxone 0.4 mg IV is effective in the treatment of acute overdosage. In oral overdose, gastric lavage and induced emesis are indicated. Treatment, however, is aimed at combating the progressive respiratory depression usually through artificial ventilation.

Assessment

1. Note any evidence of head injury or history of epileptic seizures.
2. Record any client history of asthma or other conditions that tend to compromise respirations.
3. Obtain baseline renal function studies and note any history of glaucoma.

Evaluation: Evaluate client for reports of effective analgesia.

Mephentermine sulfate
(meh-**FEN**-ter-meen)
Wyamine (Rx)

See also *Sympathomimetic Drugs,* p. 218

Classification: Indirect-acting adrenergic agent, vasopressor.

Action/Kinetics: Mephentermine acts by releasing norepinephrine from its storage sites. It has slight effects on alpha and beta-1 receptors and moderate effects on beta-2 receptors mediating vasodilation. The drug causes increased cardiac output; also elicits slight CNS effects. **IV: Onset,** immediate; **duration:** 15–30 min. **IM: Onset,** 5–15 min; **duration:** 1–4 hr. Metabolized in liver. Excreted in urine within 24 hr (rate increased in acidic urine).

Uses: Hypotension due to anesthesia, ganglionic blockade, or hemorrhage (only as emergency treatment until blood or blood substitutes can be given).

Additional Contraindications: Hypotension due to phenothiazines; in combination with MAO inhibitors.

Special Concerns: Safe use during pregnancy has not been established.

Additional Drug Interactions: Mephentermine will potentiate hypotensive effects of phenothiazines.

Dosage: Injection. *Hypotension during spinal anesthesia:* **IV,** 30–45 mg; 30-mg doses may be repeated as required; or, **IV infusion:** 0.1% mephentermine in dextrose 5% in water with the rate of infusion and duration dependent on client response. *Prophylaxis of hypotension in spinal anesthesia:* **IM,** 30–45 mg 10–20 min before anesthesia. *Shock following hemorrhage:* Not recommended, but IV infusion of 0.1% in dextrose 5% in water may maintain

BP until blood volume is replaced. **Pediatric, IM, IV:** 0.4 mg/kg (12 mg/m²) as a single dose; may be repeated if needed. **Pediatric, IV infusion:** 0.1% solution in 5% dextrose in water with the rate of infusion and duration dependent on client response.

NURSING CONSIDERATIONS

See also *Nursing Considerations for Sympathomimetics,* p. 220.

Interventions: Take an initial reading of client's BP and pulse before initiating therapy. Then, take a reading every 5 min until stable. Once BP has stabilized, take a reading every 15–30 min beyond the duration of the drug's action (IM 1-4 hr; IV 5-15 min).

Evaluation

1. Identify cause of client's hypotensive episode.
2. Evaluate client for satisfactory stabilization of BP.

Meprobamate
(meh-proh-**BAM**-ayt)
Apo-Meprobamate✿, Equanil, Equanil Wyseals, Meditran✿, Meprospan 200 and 400; Miltown 200, 400, and 600; Neuramate, Novo-Mepro✿, (C-IV) (Rx)

Classification : Antianxiety agent.

Action/Kinetics: Meprobamate is a carbamate derivative that also possesses muscle relaxant and anticonvulsant effects. It acts on the limbic system and the thalamus, as well as to inhibit polysynaptic spinal reflexes. **Onset:** 1 hr. **Blood levels, chronic therapy:** 5–20 mcg/ml. **t½:** 6–24 hr. Extensively metabolized in liver and inactive metabolites and some unchanged drug (8%–19%) are excreted in the urine. Mebrobamate is also found in *Equagesic*.

Uses: Short-term treatment (no more than 4 months) of anxiety.

Contraindications: Hypersensitivity to meprobamate or carisoprodol. Porphyria. Children less than 6 years of age.

Special Concerns: Use with caution in pregnancy, lactation, epilepsy, liver and kidney disease. Geriatric clients may be more sensitive to the depressant effects of meprobamate; also, due to age-related impaired renal function, the dose of meprobamate may have to be reduced.

Side Effects: *CNS:* Ataxia, drowsiness, dizziness, weakness headache, paradoxical excitement, euphoria, slurred speech, vertigo. *GI:* Nausea, vomiting, diarrhea. *Miscellaneous:* Visual disturbances, allergic reactions including hematologic and dermatologic symptoms, paresthesias. *Symptoms of Overdose:* Drowsiness, stupor, lethargy, ataxia, shock, coma, respiratory collapse, death. Also, arrhythmias, tachycardia or bradycardia, reduced venous return, profound hypotension, cardiovascular collapse. Excessive oronasal secretions, relaxation of pharyngeal wall leading to obstruction of airway.

Drug Interactions: Additive depressant effects when used with CNS depressants, MAO inhibitors, and tricyclic antidepressants.

Laboratory Test Interferences: *With test methods:* ↑ 17-Hydroxy-corticosteroids, 17-ketogenic steroids, and 17-ketosteroids. *Pharmacologic effects:* ↑ Alkaline phosphatase, bilirubin, serum transaminase, urinary estriol (colorimetric tests), porphobilinogen. ↓ Prothrombin time in clients on coumarin.

Dosage: Tablets. Adults, initial, 400 mg t.i.d.–q.i.d. (or 600 mg b.i.d.). May be increased, if necessary, up to maximum of 2.4 g daily. **Pediatric, 6–12 years of age:** 100–200 mg t.i.d.–t.i.d. (the 600-mg tablet is not recommended for use in children). **Extended-release Capsules:** 400–800 mg in the morning and at bedtime. **Pediatric 6–12 years:** 200 mg in the morning and at bedtime.

NURSING CONSIDERATIONS

See also *Nursing Considerations* for *Benzodiazepines,* p. 111.

Administration/Storage

1. Tablets and sustained-release capsules should not be crushed or chewed.
2. *Treatment of Overdose:* Induction of vomiting or gastric lavage if detected shortly after ingestion. It is imperative that gastric lavage be continued or gastroscopy be performed as incomplete gastric emptying can cause relapse and death.
   - Give fluids to treat hypotension. Avoid fluid overload.
   - Institute artificial respiration.
   - Use care in treating seizures due to combined CNS depressant effects.
   - Use forced diuresis and vasopressors followed by hemodialysis or hemoperfusion if condition deteriorates.

Mercaptopurine (6-Mercaptopurine)

(mer-kap-toe-**PYOUR**-een)

Purinethol (Abbreviation: 6-MP) (Rx)

See also *Antineoplastic Agents,* p. 85.

Classification: Antimetabolite, purine analog.

Action/Kinetics: Mercaptopurine is cell-cycle specific for the S phase of cell division. The drug is converted to thioinosinic acid by the enzyme hypoxanthine-guanine phosphoribosyltransferase. Thioinosinic acid then inhibits reactions involving inosinic acid. Also, both thioinosinic acid and 6-methylthioinosinate (also formed from mercaptopurine) inhibit RNA synthesis. About 50% absorbed from GI tract. **Plasma t½:** 47 min in adults and 21 min in children. Metabolites are excreted in urine with up to 39% excreted unchanged. Cross-resistance with thioguanine has been observed.

Uses: Acute lymphocytic or myelocytic leukemia. Lymphoblastic leukemia, especially in children. Acute myelogenous and myelomonocytic leukemia. Effectiveness varies depending on use. The drug is not effective for leukemia of the CNS, solid tumors, lymphomas, or chronic lymphatic leukemia. *Investigational:* Inflammatory bowel disease, chronic myelocytic leukemia, polycythemia vera, non-Hodgkin's lymphoma, psoriatic arthritis.

Contraindications: Use in resistance to mercaptopurine or thioguanine. To treat CNS leukemia, chronic lymphatic leukemia, lymphomas (including Hodgkin's disease), solid tumors. Lactation.

Special Concerns: Pregnancy category: D. Use with caution in clients with impaired renal function. Use during lactation only if benefits clearly outweigh risks. Severe bone marrow depression (anemia, leukopenia, thrombocytopenia) may occur. There is an increased risk of pancreatitis when used for inflammatory bowel disease.

Additional Side Effects: Hepatotoxicity, oral lesions, drug fever, hyperuricemia. Produces less GI toxicity than folic acid antagonists, and side effects are less frequent in children than in adults. Pancreatitis (when used for inflammatory bowel disease). *Symptoms of Overdose:* Immediate symptoms include nausea, vomiting, diarrhea, anorexia while delayed symptoms include myelosuppression, gastroenteritis, and liver dysfunction.

Drug Interaction

Allopurinol / ↑ Effect of methotrexate due to ↓ breakdown by liver (reduce dose of methotrexate by 25%–33%)

Trimethoprim–Sulfamethoxazole / ↑ Risk of bone marrow suppression

Dosage: Tablets. *Highly individualized:* 2.5 mg/kg/day. *Usual,* **adults:** 100–200 mg; **pediatric:** 50 mg. Dosage may be increased to 5 mg/kg daily after 4 weeks if beneficial effects are not noted. Dosage is increased until symptoms of toxicity appear. **Maintenance after remission:** 1.5–2.5 mg/kg daily.

NURSING CONSIDERATIONS

See also *Nursing Considerations* for *Antineoplastic Agents,* p. 88.

Administration/Storage

1. Since the maximum effect of mercaptopurine on the blood count may be delayed and the blood count may drop for several days after drug has been discontinued, therapy should be discontinued at first sign of abnormally large drop in leukocyte count.
2. Administer drug in one dose daily at any convenient time.
3. Discourage intake of alcoholic beverages.
4. *Treatment of Overdose:* Induction of emesis if detected soon after ingestion. Supportive measures.

Evaluation: Evaluate client for:
- Laboratory evidence of improved hematologic parameters
- Symptoms of disease remission

Mesalamine (5-aminosalicylic acid)

(mes-AL-ah-meen)
Rowasa, Salofalk✚ (Rx)

Classification: Anti-inflammatory agent.

Action/Kinetics: Chemically, mesalamine is related to acetylsalicylic acid. Mesalamine is believed to act locally in the colon to inhibit prostaglandin synthesis, thereby reducing inflammation of colitis. Mesalamine is administered rectally; thus, it is excreted mainly in the feces. However, between 10%–30% is absorbed and is excreted through the urine as the N-acetyl-5-aminosalicylic acid metabolite. $t\frac{1}{2}$, **mesalamine:** 0.5–1.5 hr; $t\frac{1}{2}$, **n-acetyl mesalamine:** 5–10 hr.

Uses: Mild to moderate distal ulcerative colitis, proctitis, or proctosigmoiditis.

Contraindications: Lactation.

Special Concerns: Use during pregnancy (category: B) only if benefits outweigh risks. Use with caution in clients with sulfasalazine sensitivity. Safety and efficacy have not been established in children.

Side Effects: *Sulfite sensitivity:* Hives, wheezing, itching, anaphylaxis. *Intolerance syndrome:* Acute abdominal pain, cramping, bloody diarrhea, rash, fever, headache. *GI:* Abdominal pain or discomfort, flatulence, cramps, nausea, diarrhea, hemorrhoids, rectal pain or burning, constipation. *CNS:* Headache, dizziness, insomnia, fatigue, malaise. *Miscellaneous:* Asthenia, flu-like symptoms, fever, rash, sore throat, leg or joint pain, back pain, itching, hair loss, peripheral edema, urinary burning.

Dosage: Rectal, suspension enema: 4 g in 60 ml once daily for 3–6 weeks, usually given at bedtime. For maintenance, the drug can be given on every other day or every third day at doses of 1–2 g.

NURSING CONSIDERATIONS

Administration/Storage

1. Shake the bottle well to ensure that the suspension is homogeneous.
2. Have the client lie on the left side with the lower leg extended and the upper right leg flexed forward. The knee-chest position may also be used.
3. Insert the applicator tip and squeeze the bottle steadily to allow the bottle to empty.
4. The client should retain the enema for approximately 8 hr.

Assessment

1. Prior to initiating therapy, determine if the client has a history of sulfite sensitivity.
2. Obtain baseline renal function studies.

Client/Family Teaching

1. Demonstrate the proper technique for administering the suspension enema. Have the client/family do a return demonstration to ensure that they understand the procedure.
   - Explain that prior to use, the bottle should be shaken until all contents are thoroughly mixed.
   - Review the appropriate positions that facilitate administering enemas.
   - Describe how to protect the bed linens.
2. To ensure the proper absorption of the drug it must be retained for 8 hr. This may best be accomplished by administering the enema at bedtime and retaining throughout the sleep cycle.
3. The therapy may last 3–6 weeks. Therefore, it is important to continue taking the medication therapy as prescribed.
4. If any severe abdominal pain, cramping, bloody diarrhea, rash, fever or headache occurs, discontinue the drug and report to the physician.

Evaluation: Evaluate client for:
- Reports of symptomatic improvement in pain and diarrhea of colitis
- Return to normal bowel patterns

Mesna
(**MEZ**-nah)
Mesnex, Uromitexan ✹ (Rx)

Classification: Antidote for use with ifosfamide.

Action/Kinetics: Ifosfamide is metabolized to products that cause hemorrhagic cystitis. In the kidney, mesna reacts chemically with the ifosfamide metabolites to cause their detoxification. Following IV use, mesna is rapidly oxidized to mesna disulfide (dimensa) which is eliminated by the kidneys. **$t^{1/2}$ in blood, mesna:** 0.36 hr; **dimensa:** 1.17 hr.

Uses: Prophylactically to reduce the incidence of hemorrhagic cystitis caused by ifosfamide. *Investigational:* Reduce incidence of hemorrhagic cystitis caused by cyclophosphamide.

Contraindications: Hypersensitivity to thiol compounds.

Special Concerns: Pregnancy category: B. Use with caution during lactation.

Side Effects: Since mesna is used with ifosfamide and other antineoplastic agents, it is difficult to identify those side effects due to mesna. The following symptoms are believed possible. *GI:* Nausea, vomiting, diarrhea, bad taste in mouth.

Laboratory Test Interferences: False + test for urinary ketones.

Dosage: IV bolus: *Prophylaxis of ifosfamide-induced hemorrhagic cystitis,* dosage of mesna equal to 20% of the ifosfamide dose given at the time of ifosfamide and at 4 and 8 hr after each dose of ifosfamide. Thus, the total daily dose of mesna is 60% of the ifosfamide dose (e.g., an ifosfamide dose of 1.2 g/m^2 would mean doses of mesna would be 240 mg/m^2 at the time the ifosfamide dose was given, 240 mg/m^2 after 4 hr, and 240 mg/m^2 after 8 hr). This dosage should be given on each day that ifosfamide is administered.

NURSING CONSIDERATIONS

Administration/Storage

1. If the dosage of ifosfamide is increased or decreased, the dosage of mesna should be adjusted accordingly.
2. The drug can be reconstituted to a final concentration of 20 mg mesna/ml fluid by adding either 5% dextrose injection, 5% dextrose and sodium chloride injection, 0.9% sodium chloride injection, or lactated Ringer's injection.
3. Diluted solutions are stable for 24 hr at 25°C (77°F). However, when mesna is exposed to oxygen, dimesna is formed; thus, a new ampule should be used for each administration.
4. Mesna is not compatible with cisplatin.

Interventions

1. Drug must be administered with each dose of ifosfamide to be effective against drug-induced hemorrhagic cystitis.
2. Obtain a morning urine specimen for analysis each day before ifosfamide therapy.

Client/Family Teaching

1. Client may have bad taste in the mouth during drug therapy; use hard candy to mask taste.
2. Nausea, vomiting, and diarrhea are frequent side effects of drug therapy; report if persistent or bothersome.

Evaluation: Evaluate client for the prevention of ifosfamide-induced hemorrhagic cystitis.

Mesoridazine besylate
(mez-oh-**RID**-ah-zeen)
Serentil (Rx)

See also *Phenothiazines,* p. 201.

Classification: Antipsychotic, piperidine-type phenothiazine.

Action/Kinetics: Mesoridazine has pronounced sedative and hypotensive effects, moderate anticholinergic effects, and a low incidence of extrapyramidal symptoms and antiemetic effects.

Uses: Schizophrenia, acute and chronic alcoholism, behavior problems in clients with mental deficiency and chronic brain syndrome, psychoneurosis.

Special Concerns: Use during pregnancy only if benefits clearly outweigh risks. Dosage has not been established in children less than 12 years of age. Geriatric, debilitated, and emaciated clients require a lower initial dose.

Dosage: Oral Solution, Tablets. *Psychotic disorders:* **Adults and adolescents,** 30–150 mg daily in 2–3 divided doses. *Alcoholism:* **initial,** 25 mg b.i.d.; **optimum total dose:** 50–200 mg/day. **IM.** *Psychotic disorders:* **Adults and adolescents:** 25 mg (base); **then,** repeat the dose in 30–60 min as needed.

NURSING CONSIDERATIONS

See also *Nursing Considerations for Phenothiazines,* p. 205.

Administration/Storage

1. Maintain client supine for minimum of 30 min after parenteral

administration to minimize orthostatic effect.

2. Acidified tap or distilled water, orange juice, or grape juice may be used to dilute the concentrate prior to use.
3. Bulk dilutions should not be prepared or stored.
4. For IM administration, give 25 mg initially, repeated at 30–60-min intervals as needed.

Evaluation: Evaluate client for evidence of improved patterns of behavior with changes that reflect a positive response to the medication.

Metaproterenol sulfate (Orciprenaline sulfate)

(met-ah-proh-**TER**-ih-nohl)

Alupent, Arm-A-Med Metaproterenol, Dey-Dose Metaproterenol, Dey-Lute Metaproterenol, Metaprel (Rx)

See also *Sympathomimetic Drugs,* p. 218.

Classification: Direct-acting adrenergic agent, bronchodilator.

Action/Kinetics: Metaproterenol markedly stimulates beta-2 receptors, resulting in relaxation of smooth muscles of the bronchial tree, as well as peripheral vasodilation. It is similar to isoproterenol, but it has a longer duration of action and fewer side effects. Has minimal beta-1 activity. **Onset: Inhalation aerosol,** within 1 min; **peak effect:** 1 hr; **duration:** 1–5 hr. **Onset, hand bulb nebulizer or IPPB:** 5–30 min; **duration:** 4–6 hr after repeated doses. **PO: Onset,** 15–30 min; **Peak effect:** 1 hr. **Duration:** 4 hr. Oral administration produces a marked first-pass

effect. Metabolized in the liver and excreted through the kidney.

Uses: Bronchodilator in asthma, bronchitis, emphysema, and other conditions associated with reversible bronchospasms. Treatment of acute asthmatic attacks in children over 6 years of age.

Special Concerns: Safe use during pregnancy not established (pregnancy category: C). Dosage of syrup or tablets in children less than 6 years of age. Inhalation not recommended for children under 12 years of age.

Drug Interactions: Possible potentiation of adrenergic effects if used before or after other sympathomimetic bronchodilators.

Dosage: Syrup, Tablets. Adults and children over 27.2 kg: 20 mg t.i.d.–q.i.d.; **children under 27.2 kg or 6–9 years of age:** 10 mg t.i.d.–q.i.d. **Inhalation. Hand nebulizer:** single dose, 10 inhalations of undiluted 5% solution. **Intermittent positive pressure breathing (IPPB):** 0.3 ml of 5% solution diluted to 2.5 ml saline or other diluent. **Metered-dose inhaler:** 2–3 inhalations (1.30–2.25 mg) q 3–4 hr. Total daily dose should not exceed 12 inhalations (9 mg). For acute bronchospasms, administer metaproterenol every 4 hr. For chronic bronchospasms (pulmonary disease), administer 3–4 times/day.

NURSING CONSIDERATIONS

See also *Special Nursing Considerations for Adrenergic Bronchodilators* under *Sympathomimetics,* p. 221.

Administration/Storage

1. Instruct client to shake the container.

M

2. Unit dose vials should be refrigerated at 2°C–8°C (35°F–46°F).
3. The inhalant solution can be stored at room temperature, but excessive heat and light should be avoided.
4. The solution should not be used if it is brown or shows a precipitate.

Evaluation: Evaluate client for reports of symptomatic improvement and for evidence of improved airway exchange on auscultation.

Metaraminol bitartrate

(met-ah-**RAM**-ih-nohl)

Aramine (Rx)

See also *Sympathomimetic Drugs,* p. 218.

Classification: Direct-acting adrenergic agent, vasopressor.

Action/Kinetics: Metaraminol indirectly releases norepinephrine from storage sites and directly stimulates primarily alpha receptors and, to a slight extent, beta-1 receptors. The drug causes marked increases in BP due primarily to vasoconstriction and to a slight increase in cardiac output. Reflex bradycardia is also manifested. CNS stimulation usually does not occur. **Onset: IV:** 1–2 min; **IM:** 10 min; **SC:** 5–20 min. **Duration, IV:** 20 min; **IM, SC:** About 60 min. Metabolized in the liver and excreted through the urine and feces. Urinary excretion of unchanged drug can be enhanced by acidifying the urine.

Uses: Hypotension associated with surgery, spinal anesthesia, hemorrhage, trauma, infections, and ad-

verse drug reactions. Adjunct to the treatment of either septicemia or cardiogenic shock. *Investigational:* Injected intracavernosally to treat priapism due to phentolamine, papaverine, or other causes.

Additional Contraindications: As a substitute for blood or fluid replacement.

Special Concerns: Pregnancy category: C. Use with caution in cirrhosis and malaria. Hypertension and ischemic electrocardiographic changes may occur when used to treat priapism.

Dosage: Injection: IM, SC, IV. *Prophylaxis of hypotension:* **IM, SC,** 2–10 mg; **pediatric:** 0.01 mg/kg (3 mg/m^2). *Treatment of hypotension:* **IV infusion,** 15–100 mg in 500 ml of 0.9% sodium chloride injection or 5% dextrose injection given at a rate to maintain desired blood pressure (up to 500 mg/500 ml has been used). **Pediatric: IV infusion,** 0.4 mg/kg (12 mg/m^2) in a solution containing 1 mg/25 ml 0.9% sodium chloride injection or 5% dextrose injection. *Severe shock:* **Direct IV,** 0.5–5.0 mg followed by **IV infusion** of 15–100 mg in 500 ml fluid. **Pediatric, direct IV:** 0.01 mg/kg (0.3 mg/m^2).

NURSING CONSIDERATIONS

See also *Nursing Considerations* for *Sympathomimetic Drugs,* p. 220.

Administration/Storage: Do not inject IM in areas that seem to have poor circulation because sloughing has occurred with extravasation.

Interventions

1. Take BP at frequent intervals throughout the therapy. Obtain written parameters for maintaining the systolic pressure.

2. Frequently assess the site of administration because extravasation of drug may result in sloughing.
3. Use an electronic infusion device when administering IV drug therapy for more adequate control and titration of drug.

Evaluation: Evaluate client for the prevention and management of hypotension.

Metaxalone
(meh-**TAX**-ah-lohn)
Skelaxin (Rx)

See also *Centrally Acting Skeletal Muscle Relaxants*, p. 130.

Classification: Centrally acting muscle relaxant.

Action/Kinetics: The beneficial effects of metaxalone may be due to its sedative effects. The drug resembles meprobamate. **Onset:** 1 hr. **$t^{1/2}$:** 2–3 hr. **Time to peak levels:** 2 hr (after 800 mg). **Peak serum levels:** 205 mcg/ml. **Duration:** 4–6 hr. Metabolites are excreted in the urine.

Uses: As an adjunct for acute skeletal muscle spasm associated with sprains, strains, dislocation, and other trauma.

Contraindications: Liver disease, epilepsy, impaired renal function, history of drug-induced hemolytic or other anemias, pregnancy, children under 12 years.

Special Concerns: Safe use during lactation has not been determined.

Side Effects: *CNS:* Drowsiness, dizziness, headache, nervousness, irritability. *GI:* Nausea, vomiting, gastric upset. *Miscellaneous:* Allergic reactions, jaundice, leukopenia, hemolytic anemia.

Dosage: Tablets. Adults and children over 12 years: 800 mg t.i.d.–q.i.d.

NURSING CONSIDERATIONS
Assessment

1. Obtain baseline CBC, and liver and renal function studies.
2. Note any history of drug induced hemolytic or other type anemias.
3. Determine if client has a history of epilepsy.

Client/Family Teaching

1. Complaints of high fever, nausea, or diarrhea should be reported. These are early symptoms of hepatotoxicity and require the withdrawal of metaxalone.
2. Complaints of sore throat, fever, and lassitude or of having a "cold" should be further explored because these may be symptoms of blood dyscrasias.
3. Clients with a history of grand mal epilepsy should be advised that metaxalone may precipitate seizures.
4. Avoid symptoms of a dry mouth by rinsing the mouth frequently and increasing the fluid intake. Sugarless gum and hard candy may also be of some benefit.
5. Drug causes drowsiness, so clients should not operate dangerous machinery or drive a car.
6. Report any jaundice, irritability, or allergic responses. These are adverse drug effects that may require a readjustment of the dosage or withdrawal of the drug.

M

Evaluation: Evaluate client for reports of symptomatic improvement in pain and mobility and relief of muscle spasm.

Methadone hydrochloride

(**METH**-ah-dohn)
Dolophine, Methadose (C-II, Rx)

See also *Narcotic Analgesics,* p. 174.

Classification: Narcotic analgesic, morphine type.

Action/Kinetics: Methadone produces only mild euphoria, which is the reason it is used as a heroin withdrawal substitute and for maintenance programs. Methadone produces physical dependence, but the abstinence syndrome develops more slowly upon termination of therapy; also, withdrawal symptoms are less intense but more prolonged than those associated with morphine. Methadone does not produce sedation or narcosis. Methadone is not effective for preoperative or obstetric anesthesia. When administered orally, it is only one-half as potent as when given parenterally. **Onset:** 30–60 min. **Peak effects:** 30–60 min. **Duration:** 4–6 hr. $t^{1/2}$: 15–30 hr. Both the duration and half-life increase with repeated use due to cumulative effects.

Uses: Severe pain. Drug withdrawal and maintenance of narcotic dependence.

Additional Contraindications: IV use, liver disease; give rarely, if at all, during pregnancy. Use in children. Use in obstetrics (due to long duration of action and chance of respiratory depression in the neonate).

Special Concerns: Pregnancy category: C. Use with caution during lactation.

Additional Side Effects: Marked constipation, excessive sweating, pulmonary edema, choreic movements.

Drug Interactions: Rifampin and phenytoin ↓ plasma methadone levels by ↑ breakdown by liver; thus, possible symptoms of narcotic withdrawal may develop.

Laboratory Test Interference: ↑ Immunoglobulin G.

Dosage: Tablets, Oral Solution, Oral Concentrate, IM, SC. *Analgesia:* **Adults, individualized,** 2.5–10 mg q 3–4 hr, although higher doses may be necessary for severe pain or due to development of tolerance. *Narcotic withdrawal:* **initial,** 15–20 mg/day orally (some may require 40 mg/day); **then,** depending on need of the client, slowly decrease dosage. *Maintenance (individualized):* **PO, initial,** 20–40 mg 4–8 hr after heroin is stopped; **then,** adjust dosage as required up to 120 mg daily.

NURSING CONSIDERATIONS

See also *Nursing Considerations* for *Narcotic Analgesics,* p. 177.

Administration/Storage

1. Oral concentrations of solution should be diluted in at least 90 ml of water prior to administration.
2. If the client is taking dispersible tablets, the tablets should be diluted in 120 ml of water, orange juice, citrus flavored drink, or other acidic fruit drink. Allow at least 1 min for complete dispersion of the drug.

3. For repeated analgesic doses, IM administration is preferred over SC administration.
4. Clients receiving methadone for detoxification purposes should be on the drug no longer than 21 days. The treatment should not be repeated until 4 weeks have elapsed.

Interventions

1. Inspect the injection sites for signs of irritation.
2. If the client has nausea and vomiting as a result of the medication therapy, a lower dose of drug may relieve these symptoms.

Client/Family Teaching

1. Review side effects with the client and family. Note that if the client is ambulatory and not suffering acute pain, side effects may be more pronounced.
2. If the client is on narcotic withdrawal therapy, advise that the drug should be stored out of the reach of children.

Evaluation: Evaluate client for:
- Reports of effective control of severe pain
- Successful drug withdrawal and maintenance of narcotic dependence

---

Methamphetamine hydrochloride

(meth-am-**FET**-ah-meen)
Desoxyn, (C-II) (Rx)

See also *Amphetamines and Derivatives,* p. 29.

Classification: CNS stimulant, amphetamine-type.

Action/Kinetics: t½: 4–5 hr, depending on urinary pH.

Uses: Attention deficit disorders in children over 6 years of age.

Contraindications: Use for obesity. Attention deficit disorders in children less than 6 years of age.

Special Concerns: Use during pregnancy only when benefits clearly outweigh risks (pregnancy category: C).

Dosage: Tablets. *Attention deficit disorders in children, 6 years and older:* **initial,** 5 mg 1–2 times daily; increase in increments of 5 mg daily at weekly intervals until optimum dose is reached (usually 20–25 mg daily). **Extended-release Tablets.** *Attention deficit disorders in children, 6 years and older:* 20–25 mg once daily.

NURSING CONSIDERATIONS

See also *Nursing Considerations* for *Amphetamines and Derivatives,* p. 31.

Administration/Storage

1. When used to facilitate verbalization during psychotherapeutic interview, give second dose only if the first dose has proven effective.
2. When used for attention deficit disorders, the total daily dose can be given in two divided doses or once a day using the long-acting product. The long-acting product should not be used to initiate therapy. Evaluate client progress periodically to determine the need for continued treatment.

Evaluation: Evaluate client for successful control of the symptoms of attention deficit disorder.

Methantheline bromide

(meth-**AN**-thah-eh-leen)
Banthine (Rx)

See also *Cholinergic Blocking Agents,* p. 136.

Classification: Synthetic anticholinergic, antispasmodic (quaternary ammonium compound).

Action/Kinetics: PO: Onset, 30 min; **duration:** 6 hr. **IM: Duration,** 2–4 hr. Drug has some ganglionic blocking activity.

Uses: Adjunct in peptic ulcer therapy. Urinary incontinence.

Special Concerns: Pregnancy category: C.

Additional Side Effects: Postural hypotension, impotence. Respiratory paralysis and tachycardia (overdosage).

Dosage: Tablets. Adults: 50–100 mg q.i.d. **Pediatric, over 1 year:** 12.5–50 mg q.i.d. **Infants, 1–12 months:** 12.5 up to 25 mg q.i.d. **Newborns:** 12.5 mg b.i.d.; **then,** 12.5 mg t.i.d.

NURSING CONSIDERATIONS

See also *Nursing Considerations* for *Cholinergic Blocking Agents,* p. 138.

Interventions

1. Initiate therapy for clients with duodenal ulcer while the client is on a liquid diet.
2. If the client is taking potassium chloride, anticholinergic agents may delay absorption of the potassium. Special attention should be given to client complaints that could indicate lesions in the GI mucosa. These should be reported to the physician.
3. Auscultate for bowel sounds and assess the client for abdominal distention, epigastric distress, and vomiting. The drug reduces gastric motility.

Client/Family Teaching

1. Rise slowly from a supine position to prevent hypotension from developing.
2. Remind male clients that drug-induced impotence may occur and should be reported.

Evaluation: Evaluate client for:
- Reports of ↓ GI pain and irritation
- Evidence of control of urinary incontinence

Methenamine

(meh-**THEEN**-ah-meen)
(OTC)

Methenamine hippurate

(meh-**THEEN**-ah-meen)
Hip-Rex✿, Hiprex, Urex (Rx)

Methenamine mandelate

(meh-**THEEN**-ah-meen)
Deltamine, Mandelamine, Methendelate (Rx)

Classification: Urinary tract anti-infective.

Action/Kinetics: This drug is converted in an acid medium into ammonia and formaldehyde (the active principle), which denatures protein. Thus, it is most effective when the urine has a pH value of 5.5 or less, which is maintained by using the hippurate or mandelate salt. Readily absorbed from GI tract but up to 60% may be hydrolyzed by gastric acid if tablets are not enteric-coated. To be effective, urinary formaldehyde concentration must be greater than 25 mcg/ml. **Peak levels of formaldehyde:** 2 hr if using hippurate and 3–8 hr if using mandelate (if urinary pH is 5.5 or less) **t½:** 3–6 hr. Seventy to 90% of drug and metabolites excreted in urine within 24 hr.

Uses: Acute, chronic, and recurrent urinary tract infections by susceptible organisms, especially gram-negative organisms including *Escherichia coli.* As a prophylactic before urinary tract instrumentation. Never used as sole agent in the treatment of acute infections.

Contraindications: Renal insufficiency, severe liver damage, or severe dehydration.

Special Concerns: Pregnancy category: C. Use with caution in gout (methenamine may cause urate crystals to precipitate in the urine).

Side Effects: *GI:* Nausea, vomiting, diarrhea, anorexia, cramps, stomatitis. *GU:* Hematuria, albuminuria, crystalluria, dysuria, urinary frequency or urgency, bladder irritation. *Dermatologic:* Skin rashes, urticaria, pruritus. *Other:* Tinnitus, muscle cramps, headache, dyspnea, edema, lipoid pneumonitis.

Drug Interactions

Acetazolamide / ↓ Effect of methenamine due to ↑ alkalinity of urine by acetazolamide
Sodium bicarbonate / ↓ Effect of methenamine due to ↑ alkalinity of urine by sodium bicarbonate
Sulfonamides / ↑ Chance of sulfonamide crystalluria due to acid urine produced by methenamine

Thiazide diuretics / ↓ Effect of methenamine due to ↑ alkalinity of urine produced by thiazides

Laboratory Test Interference: False + urinary glucose with Benedict's solution. Drug interferes with determination of urinary catecholamines and estriol levels by acid hydrolysis technique (enzymatic techniques not affected). False + catecholamines, hydroxycorticosteroids, vanillylmandelic acid; false (−) 5-hydroxyindoleacetic acid.

Dosage: **Tablets.** *Hippurate:* **Adults and children over 12 years:** 1 g b.i.d. in the morning and evening; **children, 6–12 years:** 0.5 g b.i.d. **Oral Solution, Oral Suspension, Tablets.** *Mandelate:* **Adults:** 1 g q.i.d. after meals and at bedtime; **children 6–12 years:** 0.5 g q.i.d.; **children under 6 years:** 0.25 g/13.6 kg q.i.d.

M

NURSING CONSIDERATIONS

See also *Nursing Considerations For All Anti-Infectives,* p. 83.

Interventions

1. An acidic urine should be maintained, especially when treating *Proteus* or *Pseudomonas* infections.
2. Oral methenamine mandelate suspensions have a vegetable oil base; particular care should thus be taken in the elderly or debilitated to prevent lipid pneumonia.
3. Clearly indicate on chart that client is receiving drug because drug will interfere with tests to determine urinary estriol, catecholamines, and hydroxyindoleacetic acid.
4. Urine may become turbid and full of sediment when methenamine mandelate is adminis-

tered concomitantly with sulfamethizole.

5. Monitor urine sample for any evidence of hematuria and/or albuminuria.

Client/Family Teaching

1. If GI upset occurs, the drug can be taken with food.
2. In order to maintain an acidic urine, alkalizing foods (e.g., milk products) or medication (e.g., acetazolamide, bicarbonate) should not be taken in excess.
3. Protein-rich foods (such as prunes, plums, and cranberry juice) may help maintain acid urine. Drugs such as ascorbic acid, methionine, ammonium chloride, or sodium diphosphate may additionally be required.
4. Instruct client in the use of Labstix or Nitrazine paper to test that pH of urine is 5.5 or lower.
5. Report any evidence of skin rash because this is an indication for drug withdrawal.
6. Clients on high dosage of drug should report any evidence of bladder irritation or painful and frequent micturition.
7. Report adverse drug effects such as nausea, vomiting, dermatologic reaction, tinnitus, and muscle cramps as these may require termination of drug therapy.
8. Advise client to maintain an adequate fluid intake of 1,500–2,500 ml daily. Instruct client on how to maintain a record of I&O.

Evaluation: Evaluate for laboratory C&S confirmation of resolution of UTI.

Methicillin sodium
(meth-ih-**SILL**-in)
Staphcillin (Rx)

See also *Anti-Infectives,* p. 80, and *Penicillins,* p. 197.

Classification: Antibiotic, penicillin.

Action/Kinetics: This drug is a semisynthetic, penicillinase-resistant salt suitable for soft tissue, penicillin G-resistant, and resistant staphylococcal infections. **Peak plasma levels: IM,** 10–20 mcg/ml after 30–60 min; **IV,** 15 min. **t½:** 30 min. Excreted chiefly in the urine.

Additional Uses: Infections by penicillinase-producing staphylococci, osteomyelitis, septicemia, enterocolitis, bacterial endocarditis.

Special Concerns: Use with caution in clients with renal failure. Safe use in neonates has not been established. Periodic renal function tests are indicated for long-term therapy.

Dosage: IM, continuous IV infusion. Adults: 4–12 g daily, depending on the infection, in divided doses q 4–6 hr. (**Note:** If creatinine clearance is less than 10 ml/min, the dose should not exceed 2 g q 12 hr.) **Pediatric:** 100–300 mg/kg daily in divided doses q 4–6 hr. **Infants over 7 days of age and weighing more than 2 kg:** 100 mg/kg daily in divided doses q 6 hr (*for meningitis:* 150–200 mg/kg daily). **Infants more than 7 days of age and weighing less than 2 kg or less than 7 days of age and weighing more than 2 kg:** 75 mg/kg daily in divided doses q 8 hr (*for meningitis:* 150 mg/kg daily). **Infants under 7 days of age and weighing less than 2 kg:** 50 mg/

kg daily in divided doses q 12 hr (*for meningitis:* 100 mg/kg daily).

NURSING CONSIDERATIONS

See also *Nursing Considerations* for *Penicillins,* p. 200.

Administration/Storage

1. Do not use dextrose solutions for diluting methicillin because their low acidity may destroy the antibiotic.
2. Inject medication slowly. Methicillin injections are particularly painful.
3. Inject deeply into gluteal muscle. Use caution to avoid sciatic nerve injury.
4. To prevent sterile abscesses at injection site, include 0.2–0.3 ml of air in syringe before starting injection so that when the needle is withdrawn the irritating solution will not leak into tissue.
5. If used IV, care should be taken as thrombophlebitis can occur, especially in geriatric clients.
6. Check for redness or edema at site of injection and for pain along the course of the vein into which the drug is administered. Methicillin is a vesicant.
7. Methicillin is sensitive to heat when dissolved. Therefore, solutions for IM administration must be used within 24 hr if standing at room temperature or within 4 days if refrigerated. Solutions for IV use must be used within 8 hr.
8. For IV administration, dilute 1 ml with 20–25 ml of sterile water for injection or sodium chloride injection USP.
9. Do not mix methicillin with any other drug in the same syringe or IV solution.

Interventions

1. Monitor renal function studies. Note any evidence of hematuria or casts in urine.
2. Observe for any evidence of pallor, ecchymosis, or bleeding tendencies; monitor CBC.
3. Monitor liver function studies. Observe for fever, nausea, and other signs of hepatotoxicity, especially with prolonged therapy.
4. Be sure blood cultures and WBC counts with differential are taken prior to start of, and weekly during, therapy. Many strains of methicillin-resistant staphylococci have been identified. It has been recommended that these clients be isolated until appropriate antibiotic therapy can be instituted to prevent major institutional outbreaks.

M

Methimazole

(meth-**IM**-ah-zohl)
Tapazole (Rx)

See also *Antithyroid Drugs,* p. 99.

Classification: Antithyroid preparation.

Action/Kinetics: Onset is more rapid but effect is less consistent than that of propylthiouracil. Bioavailability may be affected by food. $t\frac{1}{2}$: 4–14 hr. **Onset:** 10–20 days. **Time to peak effect:** 2–10 weeks. $t\frac{1}{2}$: 6–13 hr. Crosses the placenta; high levels appear in breast milk. Metabolized in the liver and excreted through the kidneys (7% unchanged).

Special Concerns: Incidence of hepatic toxicity may be greater than for propylthiouracil.

Dosage: Tablets. Adults, initial:
Mild hyperthyroidism: 15 mg/day; *moderately severe hyperthyroidism:* 30–40 mg/day; *severe hyperthyroidism:* 60 mg/day. For hyperthyroidism, the daily dose is usually given in 3 equal doses 8 hr apart. **Maintenance:** 5–15 mg daily as a single dose or divided into 2 doses. **Pediatric:** 0.4 mg/kg given once daily or divided into 2 doses; **maintenance:** 0.2 mg/kg. Alternatively, **initial,** 0.5–0.7 mg/kg/day (15–20 mg/m²/day in 3 divided doses; **maintenance:** ⅓–⅔ initial dose when client is euthyroid up to a maximum of 30 mg/day. *Thyrotoxic crisis: **Adults,** 15–20 mg q 4 hr during the first day as an adjunct to other treatments.

NURSING CONSIDERATIONS

See also *Nursing Considerations* for *Antithyroid Drugs,* p. 100.

Interventions

1. Assess the client for changes in sensation of the extremities. For example, check if the client has any strange, tingling sensations of the fingers and toes. Some clients develop paresthesias. Document and report to the physician.
2. If the client is over 40 years of age, monitor for agranulocytosis. Question the client about sore throats, fever, chills, and unexplained bleeding.
3. Observe for any evidence of hair loss and if evident, report to the physician.

Client/Family Teaching

1. Take the medication at evenly spaced times and with evenly spaced doses during the day.

2. Advise the client to take the medication with a snack to reduce gastric irritation and to report if GI upset persists.
3. Report any unexpected symptoms immediately. The effects of the medication may not be evident for weeks after the therapy begins, and the physician may need to adjust the dosage of drug.

Evaluation: Evaluate client for:
- Evidence of control of symptoms of hyperthyroidism
- Laboratory evidence that serum thyroid levels within desired range

Methocarbamol
(meth-oh-**KAR**-bah-mohl)
Delaxin, Marbaxin 750, Robamol, Robaxin, Robaxin-750, Robomol-500 and -750 (Rx)

See also *Centrally Acting Skeletal Muscle Relaxants,* p. 130.

Classification: Centrally acting muscle relaxant.

Action/Kinetics: The beneficial action of methocarbamol may be related to the sedative properties of the drug. Of limited usefulness. The drug may be given IM or IV in polyethylene glycol 300 (50% solution). PO therapy should be initiated as soon as possible. **Onset:** 30 min. **Peak plasma levels:** 2 hr. **t½:** 1–2 hr. Inactive metabolites are excreted in the urine.

Uses: Muscle spasms associated with sprains and/or trauma, acute back pain due to nerve irritation or discogenic disease, postoperative orthopedic procedures, bursitis, and torticollis. Acute phase muscle spasms. Adjunct in tetanus.

Contraindications: Hypersensitivity, when muscle spasticity is required to maintain upright position, pregnancy, lactation, children under 12 years. Renal disease (parenteral dosage form only).

Special Concerns: Use with caution in epilepsy.

Side Effects: *Following PO use. CNS:* Dizziness, drowsiness, lightheadedness, vertigo, lassitude, headache. *GI:* Nausea. *Miscellaneous:* Allergic symptoms including rash, urticaria, pruritus, conjunctivitis, nasal congestion, blurred vision, fever. *Following IV use (in addition to above). CV:* Fainting, hypotension, bradycardia. *Miscellaneous:* Metallic taste, GI upset, flushing, nystagmus, double vision, thrombophlebitis, pain at injection site, anaphylaxis.

Drug Interaction: CNS depressants (including alcohol) may increase the effect of methocarbamol.

Laboratory Test Interferences: Color interference in 5-hydroxyindoleacetic acid (5-HIAA) and vanillylmandelic acid (VMA).

Dosage: Tablets. Adults, initial: 1.5 g q.i.d. for the first 2–3 days (for severe conditions, 8 g daily may be given); **maintenance:** 1 g q.i.d., 0.75 g q 4 hr, or 1.5 g t.i.d. **IM, IV: usual initial,** 1 g; in severe cases, up to 2–3 g may be necessary. **IV administration should not exceed 3 days.** *Tetanus:* **IV, Adults** 1–3 g given into tube of previously inserted indwelling needle. May be given q 6 hr (up to 24 g daily may be needed) until **PO** administration is feasible. **Pediatric, initial:** 15 mg/kg given into tube of previously inserted indwelling needle. Dose may be repeated q 6 hr.

NURSING CONSIDERATIONS
Administration/Storage
1. If the drug is to be administered IV, the rate should not exceed 3 ml/min.
2. For IV drip, one ampule may be added to no more than 250 ml of sodium chloride or 5% dextrose injection.
3. If the client is to receive the drug by IV, check frequently for infiltration. Extravasation of fluid may cause sloughing or thrombophlebitis.
4. Before removing IV, clamp off the tubing to prevent extravasation of the hypertonic solution, which may cause thrombophlebitis.
5. If the drug is to be administered IM, inject no more than 5 ml into each gluteal region.
6. When administering IM to an adult, select a large muscle mass. When administering the drug IM to a child, use the vastus lateralis. Document and rotate sites.

Interventions
1. Position the client in a recumbent position during IV administration. Have client maintain this position for 10–15 min after injection to minimize the side effects of postural hypotension.
2. Have side rails in place unless the client is attended during IV administration. Observe seizure precautions.
3. Monitor BP and pulse. If the heart rate drops below 60 beats/min, notify the physician.
4. Supervise the ambulation of elderly clients or those who have been immobilized prior to drug therapy.

Client/Family Teaching

1. Advise that urine may turn black, brown, or green. This side effect will disappear once the drug is discontinued.
2. Rise slowly from a recumbent position and dangle legs before standing up to minimize hypotensive effects.
3. Drug causes drowsiness; do not operate dangerous machinery and equipment or drive a car.
4. Avoid the use of alcohol.
5. Nausea, anorexia, and a metallic taste may occur with drug therapy. If these symptoms become severe or interfere with nutrition notify the physician.
6. Diplopia, blurred vision, and nystagmus may occur. These side effects usually disappear with continued use of the medication. Clients should, however, report these symptoms to the physician.
7. Report any urticaria, skin eruptions, rash, or pruritus. These are allergic responses and may necessitate the withdrawal of the drug.

Evaluation: Evaluate client for reports of symptomatic improvement in muscle spasticity, pain, and mobility.

Methotrexate, Methotrexate sodium
(meth-oh-**TREKS**-ayt)
Amethopterin, Folex, Folex PFS, Rheumatrex Dose Pack (Abbreviation: MTX) (Rx)

See also *Antineoplastic Agents,* p. 85.

Classification: Antimetabolite, folic acid analog.

Action/Kinetics: Methotrexate is cell-cycle specific for the S phase of cell division. The drug acts by inhibiting dihydrofolate reductase, which prevents reduction of dihydrofolate to tetrahydrofolate; this results in decreased synthesis of purines and consequently DNA. The most sensitive cells are bone marrow, fetal cells, dermal epithelium, urinary bladder, buccal mucosa, intestinal mucosa, and malignant cells. The mechanism of action for use in rheumatoid arthritis is not known although the drug may affect immune function. Variable absorption from GI tract. **Peak serum levels, IM:** 30–60 min; **PO:** 1–2 hr. **t½:** initial, 1 hr; intermediate, 2–3 hr; final, 8–12 hr. Drug may accumulate in the body. Excreted by kidney (55%–92% in 24 hr). Renal function tests are recommended before initiation of therapy; daily leukocyte counts should be taken during therapy.

Uses: Uterine choriocarcinoma (curative), chorioadenoma destruens, hydatidiform mole, acute lymphocytic and lymphoblastic leukemia, lymphosarcoma, and other disseminated neoplasms in children; meningeal leukemia, some beneficial effect in regional chemotherapy of head and neck tumors, breast tumors, and lung cancer. In combination for advanced stage non-Hodgkin's lymphoma. Advanced mycosis fungoides. High doses followed by leucovorin rescue in combination with other drugs for prolonging relapse-free survival in nonmetastatic osteosarcoma in individuals who have had surgical resection or amputation for the primary tumor. Severe, recalcitrant, disabling psoriasis. Rheumatoid arthritis (severe, active, classical or definite) in clients who have had inadequate response to NSAIDs and at least one or more antirheumatic drugs (disease modifying). *Investigational:* Severe corticosteroid-dependent asthma to reduce corticosteroid dosage; adjunct to treat osteosarcoma.

Contraindications: Psoriasis clients with kidney or liver disease; blood dyscrasias as hypoplasia, thrombocytopenia, anemia, or leukopenia. Alcoholism, alcoholic liver disease or other chronic liver disease. Immunodeficiency syndromes. Pregnancy and lactation.

Special Concerns: Pregnancy category: D (category X for pregnant psoriatic or rheumatoid arthritis clients). Use with caution in impaired renal function and elderly clients. Use with extreme caution in the presence of active infection and in debilitated clients. Safety and efficacy have not been established for juvenile rheumatoid arthritis.

Additional Side Effects: Severe bone marrow depression. Hepatotoxicity. Hemorrhagic enteritis, intestinal ulceration or perforation, acne, ecchymosis, hematemesis, melena, increased pigmentation, diabetes, leukoencephalopathy, chronic interstitial obstructive pulmonary disease, acute renal failure. Intrathecal use may result in chemical arachnoiditis, transient paresis, or seizures. Concomitant exposure to sunlight may aggravate psoriasis.

Drug Interactions

Alcohol, ethyl / Additive hepatotoxicity; combination can result in coma

Aminoglycosides, oral / ↓ Absorption of oral methotrexate

Anticoagulants, oral / Additive hypoprothrombinemia

Chloramphenicol / ↑ Effect of methotrexate by ↓ plasma protein binding

Etretinate / Possible hepatotoxicity if used together for psoriasis

Folic acid-containing vitamin preparations / ↓ Response to methotrexate

Ibuprofen / ↑ Effect of methotrexate by ↓ renal secretion

NSAIDs / Possible fatal interaction

PABA / ↑ Effect of methotrexate by ↓ plasma protein binding

Phenylbutazone / ↑ Effect of methotrexate by ↓ renal secretion

Phenytoin / ↑ Effect of methotrexate by ↓ plasma protein binding

Probenecid / ↑ Effect of methotrexate by ↓ renal clearance

Procarbazine / Possible ↑ nephrotoxicity

Pyrimethamine / ↑ Methotrexate toxicity

Salicylates (aspirin) / ↑ Effect of methotrexate by ↓ plasma protein binding; also, salicylates ↓ renal excretion of methotrexate

Smallpox vaccination / Methotrexate impairs immunologic response to smallpox vaccine

Sulfonamides / ↑ Effect of methotrexate by ↓ plasma protein binding

Tetracyclines / ↑ Effect of methotrexate by ↓ plasma protein binding

Thiopurines / ↑ Plasma levels of thiopurines

Dosage: *Cancer chemotherapy. Methotrexate is administered* **PO**

(**Tablets**); *methotrexate sodium is administered* **IM, IV, intra-arterially** or **intrathecally.** *Dose individualized. Choriocarcinoma, and similar trophoblastic diseases:* **PO, IM:** 15–30 mg/day for 5 days. May be repeated 3–5 times with 1-week rest period between courses. *Acute lymphatic (lymphoblastic) leukemia,* **initial:** 3.3 mg/m² (with 60 mg/m² prednisone daily); **maintenance: PO, IM,** 30 mg/m² 2 times weekly or **IV,** 2.5 mg/kg q 14 days. *Meningeal leukemia,* **intrathecal:** 12 mg/m² q 2–5 days until cell count returns to normal. *Lymphomas,* **PO:** 10–25 mg/day for 4–8 days for several courses of treatment with 7- to 10-day rest periods between courses. *Mycosis fungoides,* **PO,** 2.5–10 mg/day for several weeks or months; **alternatively, IM:** 50 mg once weekly or 25 mg twice weekly. *Lymphosarcoma:* 0.625–2.5 mg/kg/day in combination with other drugs. *Osteosarcoma:* Used in combination with other drugs, including doxorubicin, cisplatin, bleomycin, cyclophosphamide, and dactinomycin. **Usual IV starting dose for methotrexate:** 12 g/m²; dose may be increased to 15 g/m² to achieve a peak serum level of 10⁻³ mol/L at the end of the methotrexate infusion. *Psoriasis.* **Individualized: usual (average adult): PO, IM, IV,** 10–25 mg weekly, continued until beneficial response observed. Weekly dose should not exceed 50 mg. **Alternate regimens: PO,** 2.5 mg q 12 hr for 3 doses or q 8 hr for 4 doses each week (not to exceed 30 mg weekly); **or** 2.5 mg **PO** daily for 5 days followed by 2 days of rest (dose should not exceed 6.25 mg daily). Once beneficial effects are noted, reduce dose to lowest possible level with longest rest periods between doses. *Rheumatoid arthri-*

tis: **initial,** single oral doses of 7.5 mg/week or divided PO doses of 2.5 mg at 12 hr intervals for 3 doses given once a week; **then,** adjust dosage to achieve optimum response, not to exceed a total weekly dose of 20 mg. Once response has been reached, the dose should be reduced to the lowest possible effective dose.

NURSING CONSIDERATIONS

See also *Nursing Considerations* for *Antineoplastic Agents,* p. 88.

Administration/Storage

1. Use only sterile, preservative-free sodium chloride injection to reconstitute powder for intrathecal administration.
2. Prevent inhalation of particles of medication and skin exposure.
3. When used for rheumatoid arthritis, improvement is thought to be maintained for up to 2 years with continuous therapy. When the drug is discontinued, the arthritis usually worsens within 3–6 weeks.
4. Methotrexate products containing preservatives should not be used intrathecally.
5. Six hours prior to initiation of a methotrexate infusion, the client should by hydrated with 1 L/m² of IV fluid. Hydration should be continued at 125 ml/m²/hr during the methotrexate infusion and for 2 days after the infusion has been completed.
6. The urine should be alkalinized (see sodium bicarbonate) to a pH above 7 during methotrexate infusion.
7. Follow guidelines provided for leucovorin rescue schedule following high doses of methotrexate.

8. *Treatment of Overdose:* Leucovorin, given as soon as possible, may decrease toxic effects. The dose used is 10 mg/m² PO or parenterally followed by 10 mg/m² PO q 6 hr for 72 hr. Charcoal hemoperfusion will reduce serum levels. In massive overdosage, hydration and urinary alkalinization are needed to prevent precipitation of methotrexate and metabolites in the renal tubules.

Assessment

1. Determine if client is receiving other organic acids, such as aspirin, phenylbutazone, probenecid, and/or sulfa drugs, because these agents affect renal clearance of methotrexate and increase thrombocytopenia and GI side effects.
2. List drugs client currently prescribed to determine if any interact unfavorably with methotrexate.
3. Assess for oral ulcerations, one of the first signs of toxicity.
4. Note any evidence of acute infections.
5. Obtain baseline CBC and renal function studies. Document adequate renal function.

Interventions

1. Monitor I&O, and encourage fluid intake to facilitate excretion of drug.
2. Report oliguria, since this symptom may indicate need to discontinue drug.
3. Have calcium leucovorin—a potent antidote for folic acid antagonists—readily available in case of overdosage. Antidotes are ineffective if not administered within 4 hr of overdosage. Corticosteroids are sometimes given concomitantly with initial dose of methotrexate.

4. Advise client to avoid ingestion of alcohol when receiving methotrexate because coma may result.
5. Do not vaccinate for smallpox when the client is receiving methotrexate because the impaired immunologic response may result in vaccinia.
6. Anticipate reduction in anticoagulant dosage if administered concomitantly.
7. Advise client to avoid salicylates and prolonged exposure to sunlight or sunlamps.
8. Test the urine pH and maintain a pH above 7 during drug therapy.

Evaluation: Evaluate client for:
- Evidence of a positive chorionic response
- Evidence of a ↓ in size and spread of tumor
- Laboratory evidence of improved hematologic parameters
- Visual improvement in psoriatic lesions
- Reports of improvement in resistant arthritic joint pain and mobility

Methsuximide
(meth-**SUCKS**-ih-myd)
Celontin (Rx)

See also *Anticonvulsants,* p. 61, and *Succinimides,* p. 212.

Classification: Anticonvulsant, succinimide type.

Action/Kinetics: Peak levels: 1–4 hr. **t½:** 1–3 hr for methsuximide and 36–45 hr for the active metabolite. **Therapeutic serum levels:** 10–40 mcg/ml.

Uses: Methsuximide is used for absence seizures refractory to other drugs. May be given with other anticonvulsants when absence seizures coexist with other types of epilepsy.

Additional Side Effects: Most common are ataxia, dizziness, and drowsiness.

Additional Drug Interaction: Methsuximide may ↑ the effect of primidone.

Dosage: Capsules. Adults and children: initial, 300 mg daily for first week; **then,** if necessary, increase dosage by 300 mg/day at weekly intervals until control established. **Maximum daily dose:** 1.2 g in divided doses.

NURSING CONSIDERATIONS

See also *Nursing Considerations* for *Anticonvulsants,* p. 63, and *Succinimides,* p. 213.

Administration/Storage: The 150-mg dosage form can be used for children.

Evaluation: Evaluate client for evidence of control of seizures.

Methylcellulose
(meth-ill-**SELL**-you-lohs)
Citrucel, Cologel (OTC)

Classification: Bulk-forming laxative.

Action/Kinetics: Methylcellulose is composed of indigestible fibers that form a colloidal, bulky gelatinous mass on contact with water. The fibers pass through the stomach and increase the bulk of the feces, stimulating peristalsis. The drug is usually effective within 12–24 hr.

Uses: Prophylaxis of constipation in clients who should not strain during defecation. Short-term treatment of constipation; useful in geriatric clients with diminished colonic motor response and during pregnancy and postpartum to reestablish normal bowel function. To soften feces during fecal impaction.

Contraindications: Intestinal obstruction, ulceration, and severe abdominal pain.

Dosage: Capsules, Tablets. Adults: 2–3 capsules or tablets t.i.d.; **pediatric, over 6 years:** 1–2 capsules or tablets b.i.d. **Powder. Adults:** 1–1.5 g t.i.d. **pediatric:** 1–1.5 g daily. **Citrucel Granules: Adults and pediatric over 12 years:** 1 19 g packet in 8 oz water 1–3 times daily; **pediatric, 6–12 years:** 1 level teaspoon in 4 oz water t.i.d.–q.i.d. **Cologel Oral Solution: Adults,** 5–20 ml t.i.d. with a glass of water; **pediatric, over 6 years:** 5 ml b.i.d.

NURSING CONSIDERATIONS

See also *Nursing Considerations* for *Laxatives,* p. 172.

Administration/Storage: Follow each dose of medication with a full glass of water or milk to prevent impaction.

Evaluation: Evaluate client for evidence of the prevention and/or the relief of constipation.

Methyldopa
(meth-ill-**DOH**-pah)
Aldomet, Apo-Methyldopa✤, Dopamet✤, Novo–Medopa✤, Nu-Medopa✤, PMS Dopazide✤, Supres✤ (Rx)

Methyldopate hydrochloride

(meth-ill-**DOH**-payt)

Aldomet Ester✾, Aldomet Hydrochloride (Rx)

Classification: Antihypertensive, centrally acting antiadrenergic.

Action/Kinetics: Primary mechanism thought to be that the active metabolite, alpha-methyl-norepinephrine, lowers BP by stimulating central inhibitory alpha-adrenergic receptors, false neurotransmission, and/or reduction of plasma renin. It causes little change in cardiac output. **PO: Onset:** 7–12 hr. **Duration:** 12–24 hr. All effects terminated within 48 hr. Absorption is variable. **IV: Onset:** 4–6 hr. **Duration:** 10–16 hr. Seventy percent of drug excreted in urine. **Full therapeutic effect:** 1–4 days. **t½:** 1.7 hr. **Note:** Methyldopa is a component of Aldoril.

Uses: Moderate to severe hypertension. Particularly useful for clients with impaired renal function, renal hypertension, resistant cases of hypertension complicated by stroke, coronary artery disease, or nitrogen retention, and for hypertensive crisis (parenterally).

Contraindications: Sensitivity to drug, labile and mild hypertension, pregnancy, active hepatic disease, or pheochromocytoma.

Special Concerns: Use with caution in clients with a history of liver or kidney disease. Use during pregnancy only if benefits clearly outweigh risks (pregnancy category: B). Geriatric clients may be more sensitive to the hypotensive and sedative effects of guanabenz; also, it may be necessary to decrease the dose in these clients due to age-related decreases in renal function.

Side Effects: *CNS:* Sedation (disappears with use), weakness, headache, asthenia, dizziness, paresthesias, Parkinson-like symptoms, psychic disturbances, choreoathetotic movements, Bell's palsy, decreased mental acuity, verbal memory impairment. *CV:* Bradycardia, orthostatic hypotension, hypersensitivity of carotid sinus, worsening of angina, hypertensive response (paradoxical), myocarditis. *GI:* Nausea, vomiting, abdominal distention, diarrhea or constipation, flatus, colitis, dry mouth, "black tongue," pancreatitis, sialoadenitis. *Hematologic:* Hemolytic anemia, leukopenia, granulocytopenia, thrombocytopenia, bone marrow depression. *Endocrine:* Gynecomastia, amenorrhea, galactorrhea, lactation, hyperprolactinemia. *Miscellaneous:* Edema, jaundice, hepatitis, liver disorders, abnormal liver function tests, rash (eczema, lichenoid eruption), toxic epidermal necrolysis, fever, lupus-like symptoms, impotence, failure to ejaculate, decreased libido, nasal stuffiness, joint pain, myalgia, septic shock-like syndrome. *Symptoms of Overdose:* CNS, GI, and CV effects including sedation, weakness, lightheadedness, dizziness, coma, bradycardia, acute hypotension, impairment of atrioventricular conduction, constipation, diarrhea, distention, flatus, nausea, vomiting.

Drug Interactions

Anesthetics, general / Additive hypotension

Antidepressants, tricyclic / Tricyclic antidepressants may block hypotensive effect of methyldopa

M

Ephedrine / Action of ephedrine ↓ in methyldopa-treated clients

Fenfluramine / ↑ Effect of methyldopa

Haloperidol / Methyldopa ↑ toxic effects of haloperidol

Levodopa / ↑ Effect of both drugs

Lithium / ↑ Possibility of lithium toxicity

MAO inhibitors / May reverse hypotensive effect of methyldopa and cause headache and hallucinations

Methotrimeprazine / Additive hypotensive effect

Norepinephrine / ↑ Pressor response to norepinephrine

Phenoxybenzamine / Urinary incontinence

Phenylpropanolamine / ↑ Pressor response to phenylpropanolamine

Propranolol / Paradoxical hypertension

Sympathomimetics / Potentiation of hypertensive effect of sympathomimetics

Thiazide diuretics / Additive hypotensive effect

Thioxanthines / Additive hypotensive effect

Tolbutamide / ↑ Hypoglycemia due to ↓ breakdown by liver

Tricyclic antidepressants / ↓ Effect of methyldopa

Vasodilator drugs / Additive hypotensive effect

Verapamil / ↑ Effect of methyldopa

Laboratory Test Interferences: False + or ↑ : Alkaline phosphatase, bilirubin, BUN, BSP, cephalin flocculation, creatinine, AST, ALT, uric acid, Coombs' test, prothrombin time. Positive lupus erythematosus (LE) cell preparation and antinuclear antibodies.

Dosage: *Methyldopa:* **Oral Suspension, Tablets. Initial:** 250 mg b.i.d.–t.i.d. for 2 days. Adjust dose every 2 days. If increased, start with evening dose. **Usual maintenance:** 0.5–3.0 g daily in 2–4 divided doses; **maximum:** 3 g daily. Transfer to and from other antihypertensive agents should occur gradually, with initial dose of methyldopa not exceeding 500 mg. **Note:** Do not use combination medication to initiate therapy. **Pediatric: initial,** 10 mg/kg daily in 2–4 divided doses, adjusting maintenance to a maximum of 65 mg/kg/day (or 3 g daily, whichever is less). *Methyldopate HCl:* **IV infusion, adults:** 250–500 mg q 6 hr; **maximum:** 1 g q 6 hr for *hypertensive crisis.* Switch to oral methyldopa, at same dosage level, when blood pressure is brought under control. **Pediatric:** 20–40 mg/kg daily in divided doses q 6 hr; **maximum:** 65 mg/kg/day (or 3 g daily, whichever is less).

NURSING CONSIDERATIONS

See also *Nursing Considerations* for *Antihypertensive Agents,* p. 78.

Administration/Storage

1. If the drug is to be administered by IV, methyldopate HCl should be mixed with 100 ml of 5% dextrose or administered in 5% dextrose in water at a concentration of 10 mg/ml.
2. The IV should be administered over a 30- to 60-min period.
3. Tolerance may occur following 2–3 months of therapy.
4. Increasing the dose or adding a diuretic often restores effect on blood pressure.
5. *Treatment of Overdose:* Induction of vomiting or gastric lavage if detected early. General supportive treatment with

special attention to heart rate, cardiac output, blood volume, urinary function, electrolyte imbalance, paralytic ileus, and CNS activity. In severe cases, hemodialysis is effective.

Assessment

1. Ascertain that hematologic studies, liver function tests, and a Coombs' test are done before and during drug therapy.
2. If the client requires a blood transfusion, ascertain that both direct and indirect Coombs' tests are done. If the indirect and direct Coombs' tests are positive, anticipate consultation with a hematologist.
3. Assess for signs of drug tolerance. These may occur during the second or third month of drug therapy.
4. Note any evidence of jaundice. The drug is contraindicated when the client has hepatic disease.

Client/Family Teaching

1. To prevent dizziness and fainting, rise from bed slowly to a sitting position and dangle legs over the edge of the bed.
2. Sedation may occur when therapy is first started, but it disappears once the maintenance dose is established.
3. In rare cases, methyldopa may darken urine or turn it blue, but this reaction is not harmful.
4. Withhold drug and report to the physician any of the following symptoms: tiredness, fever, or yellowing of skin and whites of eyes.
5. Always carry a card detailing current medication regimen.

Evaluation: Evaluate client for evidence of control of hypertension.

—— COMBINATION DRUG ——

Methyldopa and Hydrochlorothiazide

(meth-ill-**DOH**-pah, hy-droh-klor-oh-**THIGH**-ah-zyd)
Aldoril 15, Aldoril 25, Aldoril D30, Aldoril D50, Novodoparil✶, PMS Dopazide✶ (Rx)

See also *Methyldopa,* p. 862, and *Hydrochlorothiazide,* p. 718.

Content/Classification: *Antihypertensive:* Methyldopa, 250–500 mg. *Diuretic/antihypertensive:* Hydrochlorothiazide, 15–50 mg.

Uses: Hypertension (not for initial treatment).

Contraindications: Active hepatic disease.

Special Concerns: Use in pregnancy only if benefits outweigh risks.

Dosage: Tablets. Adults: one tablet b.i.d.–t.i.d. for first 48 hr; **then,** increase or decrease dose, depending on response, in intervals of not less than 2 days. Maximum daily dosage: methyldopa, 3.0 g; hydrochlorothiazide, 100–200 mg.

NURSING CONSIDERATIONS

See also *Nursing Considerations* for *Methyldopa,* p. 864, and *Thiazide and Related Diuretics,* p. 233.

Administration/Storage

1. If Aldoril is given together with antihypertensives other than thiazides, the initial dose of methyldopa should not be more than 500 mg daily in divided doses.

2. Additional methyldopa may be given separately if Aldoril alone does not control blood pressure adequately.
3. If tolerance is observed after 2–3 months of therapy, the dose of either methyldopa and/or hydrochlorothiazide may be increased to restore control.

Methylene Blue
(METH-ih-leen)
Urolene Blue (Rx)

Classification: Urinary germicide, antidote, oxidizing agent.

Action/Kinetics: Methylene blue is a dye possessing bacteriostatic activity. High doses oxidize Fe^2 (ferrous ion) of reduced hemoglobin to Fe^3 (ferric ion), resulting in methemoglobinemia (basis for use in cyanide poisoning). Lower doses increase the conversion of methemoglobin to hemoglobin.

Uses: Mild GU tract antiseptic, drug-induced methemoglobinemia, antidote for cyanide poisoning, treatment of urinary tract calculi (oxalate). *Investigational:* Diagnosis of ruptured amniotic membranes; by its dye effect can determine body structures and fistulas.

Contraindications: Hypersensitivity to drug. Renal insufficiency.

Special Concerns: Use with caution in clients with glucose-6-phosphate dehydrogenase deficiency because hemolysis may result.

Side Effects: *GI:* Nausea, vomiting, diarrhea. *GU:* Dysuria, bladder irritation, may cause urine or feces to turn blue-green. *Other:* Anemia, fever, cyanosis, CV abnormalities.

Dosage: Tablets. *GU antiseptic:* 55–130 mg t.i.d. after meals with a full glass of water. **IV.** *Antidote:* 1–2 mg/kg slowly over several minutes.

NURSING CONSIDERATIONS

Client/Family Teaching: Stress that medication may turn urine and stools a blue-green color and will stain body tissues.

Evaluation: Review appropriate lab data and assess for symptoms of GI or GU dysfunction and resolution of underlying problem.

Methylergonovine maleate
(meth-ill-er-GON-oh-veen)
Methergine (Rx)

Classification: Oxytocic agent.

Action/Kinetics: Methylergonovine is a closely related synthetic drug of ergonovine, a natural alkaloid obtained from ergot. Methylergonovine stimulates the rate, tone, and amplitude of uterine contractions. The uterus becomes more sensitive to the drug toward the end of pregnancy. **Onset** (uterine contractions): **PO,** 5–10 min; **IM,** 2–5 min; **IV,** immediate. **t½, IV:** 2–3 min (initial) and 20–30 min (final). **Duration, PO, IM:** 3 hr; **IV:** 45 min.

Uses: Management and prevention of postpartum and postabortal hemorrhage by producing firm uterine contractions and decreasing uterine bleeding. Incomplete abortion. *Investigational:* Ergonovine has been used to diagnose Prinzmetal's angina (variant angina).

Contraindications: Pregnancy, toxemia, hypertension. Ergot hypersensitivity. Should be given with caution in sepsis, obliterative vascular disease, impaired renal or hepatic function. To induce labor or threatened spontaneous abortions. Administration prior to delivery of the placenta.

Side Effects: *GI:* Nausea, vomiting. *CNS:* Dizziness, headache, tinnitus. *Miscellaneous:* Sweating, chest pain, dyspnea, palpitations, transient hypertension.

Note: Use of methylergonovine during labor may result in uterine tetany with rupture, cervical and perineal lacerations, embolism of amniotic fluid as well as hypoxia and intracranial hemorrhage in the infant.

Symptoms of Overdose: Initially, nausea, vomiting, abdominal pain, increase in blood pressure, tingling of extremities, numbness. Symptoms of severe overdose include hypotension, hypothermia, respiratory depression, seizures, coma.

Dosage: IM, IV (emergencies only): 0.2 mg q 2–4 hr following delivery of placenta, of the anterior shoulder, or during the puerperium. **Tablets.** 0.2–0.4 mg b.i.d.–q.i.d. until danger of hemorrhage and uterine atony is over (usually within 2 days, although treatment for up to 7 days may be necessary).

NURSING CONSIDERATIONS

Administration/Storage

1. IV methylergonovine should be administered slowly over 1 min. After IV administration, check the client's vital signs for evidence of shock or hypertension. Have emergency drugs available.
2. Ampules of discolored methylergonovine should be discarded.
3. *Treatment of Overdose:* Induce vomiting or perform gastric lavage. Administer a cathartic; institute diuresis. Maintain respiration, especially if seizures or coma occur. Treat seizures with anticonvulsant drugs. Warm extremities to control peripheral vasospasm.

Assessment

1. Determine the location of the fundus, its height, and consistency.
2. Observe and record the amount and characteristics of lochia.

Interventions

1. Note the character and amount of lochia; document and report to the physician if the amount remains abnormal.
2. Continue to assess the uterus, palpate the fundus, and note findings.
3. Monitor BP, pulse, and respirations. If there is any abnormal elevation or decrease in BP, or if the pulse and respirations assume a pattern unusual for the client, document and report to the physician.
4. If the client complains of severe cramping, report because this adverse effect suggests the need for a reduction in dosage of the drug.
5. Question the client about the presence of dizziness, headache, or ringing in the ears. Note if the client has nausea, complains of drowsiness, if she appears to be confused, or has diarrhea. These are early signs of accidental ergotism (the drug is a derivative of lysergic acid). GI and CNS effects may occur before disturbances to

M

the circulation of the hands and feet. Document and report to the physician immediately.

Evaluation: Evaluate client for evidence of a decrease in the amount and frequency of uterine bleeding.

Methylphenidate hydrochloride

(meth-ill-**FEN**-ih-dayt)

PMS-Methylphenidate ✤, Ritalin, Ritalin-SR (C-II) (Rx)

Classification: CNS stimulant.

Action/Kinetics: The mechanism of action of methylphenidate is not known with certainty although it may act by blocking the reuptake mechanism of dopaminergic neurons. In children with attention deficit disorders, methylphenidate causes decreases in motor restlessness with an increased attention span. In narcolepsy the drug acts on the cerebral cortex and subcortical structures (e.g., thalamus) to increase motor activity and mental alertness and decrease fatigue. **Peak blood levels, children:** 1.9 hr for tablets and 4.7 hr for extended-release tablets. **Duration:** 4–6 hr. **t½:** 1–3 hr. The drug is metabolized by the liver and excreted by the kidney.

Uses: Attention deficit disorders in children as part of overall treatment regimen. Narcolepsy.

Contraindications: Marked anxiety, tension and agitation, glaucoma. Severe depression, use for preventing normal fatigue. Tourette's syndrome, motor tics. Should not be used in children who manifest symptoms of primary psychiatric disorders (psychoses) or acute stress.

Special Concerns: Use during pregnancy only if benefits clearly outweigh risks. Use with caution during lactation. Safety and efficacy in children less than 6 years of age have not been established. Use with great caution in clients with history of hypertension or convulsive disease.

Side Effects: *CNS:* Nervousness, insomnia, headaches, dizziness, drowsiness, chorea. Toxic psychoses, dyskinesia, Tourette's syndrome. Psychologic dependence. *CV:* Palpitations, tachycardia, angina, arrhythmias, hyper- or hypotension. *GI:* Nausea, anorexia, abdominal pain, weight loss (chronic use). *Allergic:* Skin rashes, fever, urticaria, arthralgia, dermatoses, erythema. *Hematologic:* Thrombocytopenic purpura, leukopenia, anemia. *Miscellaneous:* Hair loss.

In children, the following side effects are more common: anorexia, abdominal pain, weight loss (chronic use), tachycardia, insomnia.

Symptoms of Overdose: Characterized by cardiovascular symptoms (hypertension, cardiac arrhythmias, tachycardia), mental disturbances, agitation, headaches, vomiting, hyperreflexia, hyperpyrexia, convulsions, and coma.

Drug Interactions

Anticoagulants, oral / ↑ Effect of anticoagulants due to ↓ breakdown by liver

Anticonvulsants (phenobarbital, phenytoin, primidone) / ↑ Effect of anticonvulsants due to ↓ breakdown by liver

Guanethidine / ↓ Effect of guanethidine by displacement from its site of action

MAO inhibitors / Possibility of hypertensive crisis, hyperthermia, convulsions, coma

Phenylbutazone / ↑ Effect of phenylbutazone due to ↓ breakdown by liver

Tricyclic antidepressants / ↑ Effect of antidepressants due to ↓ breakdown by liver

Laboratory Test Interference: ↑ Urinary excretion of epinephrine.

Dosage: Tablets. Adults: 5–20 mg b.i.d.–t.i.d. preferably 30–45 min before meals. *Attention deficit disorders,* **pediatric, 6 years and older: initial,** 5 mg b.i.d. before breakfast and lunch; **then,** increase by 5–10 mg/week to a maximum of 60 mg daily.

Extended-release   Tablets. Adults: 20 mg 1–3 times daily q 8 hr, preferably on an empty stomach. *Attention deficit disorders,* **pediatric, 6 years and older:** 20 mg 1–3 times daily.

NURSING CONSIDERATIONS

Administration/Storage

1. Administer the drug before breakfast and lunch to avoid interference with sleep.
2. If the client is receiving the medication for attention deficit disorders and no improvement is noticed in 1 month, or if stimulation occurs, discontinue the medication.
3. The drug should be discontinued periodically to assess the condition of the client because drug therapy is not considered to be indefinite.

Drug therapy should be terminated at the time of puberty.

4. Sustained-release tablets are effective for 8 hr and may be substituted for regular release tablets if the 8-hr dosage of the sustained-release tablets is the same as the titrated 8-hr dosage of regular tablets.
5. *Treatment of Overdose:* Symptomatic. Excess CNS stimulation may be treated by keeping the client in quiet, dim surroundings to reduce external stimuli. Protect the client from self-injury. A short-acting barbiturate may be used. Emesis or gastric lavage should be undertaken if the client is conscious. Adequate circulatory and respiratory function must be maintained. Hyperpyrexia may be treated by cooling the client (e.g., cool bath, hypothermia blanket).

Assessment

1. Obtain baseline CNS evaluation and ECG prior to starting therapy.
2. Note other drugs the client is prescribed that may interact unfavorably with methylphenidate.

Interventions

1. Monitor BP and pulse b.i.d. to detect any changes that may occur.
2. Monitor the client for skin rashes, exfoliative dermatitis, fever, or pain in the joints. Report any such symptoms to the physician because they may signal the development of Stevens-Johnson syndrome.

M

Client/Family Teaching

1. Advise that caution must be used when driving or when operating hazardous machinery during methylphenidate therapy. Drug may mask fatigue and/or cause physical incoordination, dizziness, or drowsiness.
2. Record weight two times per week and report any significant loss. Clients tend to lose weight while they are taking the medication.
3. Note any changes in client mood and report to the physician.
4. Advise that children who do respond to the therapy may have the therapy interrupted every few months ("drug holiday") to determine if the drug therapy is still necessary.

Evaluation: Evaluate client for:

- Evidence of control of symptoms of attention deficit disorder
- Reports of prevention of narcolepsy

Methylprednisolone

(meth-ill-pred-**NISS**-oh-lohn)

Tablets: Medrol, Meprolone (Rx)

Methylprednisolone acetate

(meth-ill-pred-**NISS**-oh-lohn)

Cream: Medrol Veriderm Cream ✤. Enema: Medrol Enpak (Rx). Parenteral: depMedalone-40 and -80, Depoject 40 and 80, Depo-Medrol, D-Med 80, Duralone-40 and -80, Medralone-40 and -80, M-Prednisol-40 and -80, Rep-Pred 40 and 80 (Rx). Topical Ointment: Medrol (Rx)

Methylprednisolone sodium succinate

(meth-ill-pred-**NISS**-oh-lohn)

Parenteral: A-methaPred, Solu-Medrol (Rx)

See also *Adrenocorticosteroids and Analogs,* p. 8.

Classification: Adrenocorticosteroid, synthetic, glucocorticoid-type.

Action/Kinetics: Low incidence of increased appetite, peptic ulcer, and psychic stimulation. Also, low degree of sodium and water retention. May mask negative nitrogen balance. **Onset:** Slow, 12–24 hr. **t½, plasma:** 78–188 min. **Duration:** Long, up to 1 week. The sodium succinate product has a rapid onset by both the IM and IV routes. Methylprednisolone acetate has a long duration of action.

Additional Uses: Severe hepatitis due to alcoholism. Within 8 hr of severe spinal cord injury (to improve neurologic function). Septic shock (controversial).

Special Concerns: Use during pregnancy only if benefits outweigh risks.

Additional Drug Interactions

Erythromycin / ↑ Effect of methylprednisolone due to ↓ breakdown by liver
Troleandomycin / ↑ Effect of methylprednisolone due to ↓ breakdown by liver

Laboratory Test Interference: ↓ Immunoglobulins A, G, M.

Dosage: *Highly individualized. Methylprednisolone,* **Tablets:** *Rheumatoid arthritis,* 6–16 mg daily. Decrease gradually when condition is under control. **Pediatric:** 6–10 mg daily. *Systemic lupus* *erythematosus:* **acute:** 20–96 mg daily; **maintenance:** 8–20 mg daily. *Acute rheumatic fever:* 1 mg/kg body weight daily. Drug is always given in 4 equally divided doses after meals and at bedtime.

Methylprednisolone acetate, **not for IV use. IM:** *Adrenogenital syndrome:* 40 mg q 2 weeks. *Rheumatoid arthritis:* 40–120 mg/week. *Dermatologic lesions, dermatitis:* 40–120 mg/week for 1–4 weeks; for severe cases, a single dose of 80–120 mg should provide relief. *Seborrheic dermatitis:* 80 mg/week. *Asthma, rhinitis:* 80–120 mg. **Intra-articular, soft tissue and intralesional injection:** 4–80 mg, depending on site. **Retention enema:** 40 mg 3 to 7 times/week for 2 or more weeks. **Topical, ointment:** 0.25%–1% applied sparingly b.i.d.–q.i.d.

Methylprednisolone sodium succinate. **IV: initial,** 10–40 mg, depending on the disease; **then,** adjust dose depending on response, with subsequent doses given either **IM, IV.** *Severe conditions:* 30 mg/kg infused IV over 10–20 min; may be repeated q 4–6 hr for 2–3 days only. **Pediatric:** not less than 0.5 mg/kg/day.

NURSING CONSIDERATIONS

See also *Nursing Considerations* for *Adrenocorticosteroids,* p. 15.

Administration/Storage

1. Solutions of methylprednisolone sodium succinate should be used within 48 hr after preparation.
2. For alternate day therapy using methylprednisolone, twice the usual oral dose is given every other morning (the client receives the beneficial effect while minimizing side effects).

Methysergide maleate
(meth-ih-**SIR**-jyd)
Sansert (Rx)

Classification: Prophylactic for vascular headaches.

Action/Kinetics: Methysergide is an ergot alkaloid derivative structurally related to LSD. It is thought to act by directly stimulating smooth muscle leading to vasoconstriction. The drug blocks the effects of serotonin, a powerful vasodilator believed to play a role in vascular headaches; it also inhibits the release of histamine from mast cells and prevents the release of serotonin from platelets. It has weak emetic and oxytocic activity. **Onset:** 1–2 days. **Peak plasma levels:** 60 ng/ml. **Duration:** 1–2 days. Excreted through the urine as unchanged drugs and metabolites.

M

Uses: Prophylaxis of vascular headache (in clients having one or more per week or in cases where headaches are so severe preventive therapy is indicated). Clients should remain under supervision.

Contraindications: Severe renal or hepatic disease, severe hypertension, coronary artery disease, peripheral vascular disease, or tendency toward thromboembolic disease, cachexia (profound ill health or malnutrition), severe arteriosclerosis, phlebitis or cellulitis of lower limbs, collagen diseases, valvular heart disease, infectious disease, or peptic ulcer. Pregnancy, lactation, use in children.

Special Concerns: Geriatric clients may be more affected by peripheral vasoconstriction leading to the possibility of hypothermia.

Side Effects: The drug is associated with a high incidence of side effects. *Fibrosis:* Retroperitoneal fibrosis, cardiac fibrosis, pleuropulmonary fibrosis, Peyronies-like disease. The fibrotic condition may result in vascular insufficiency in the lower legs. *CV:* Vasoconstriction of arteries leading to paresthesia, chest pain, abdominal pain, or extremities that are cold, numb, or painful. Tachycardia, postural hypotension. *CNS:* Dizziness, ataxia, drowsiness, vertigo, insomnia, euphoria, lightheadedness, and psychic reactions such as depersonalization, depression, and hallucinations. *GI:* Nausea, vomiting, diarrhea, heartburn, abdominal pain, increased gastric acid, constipation. *Hematologic:* Eosinophilia, neutropenia. *Other:* Peripheral edema, flushing of face, skin rashes, transient alopecia, myalgia, arthralgia, weakness, weight gain, telangiectasia.

Drug Interactions: Narcotic analgesics are inhibited by methysergide.

Dosage: Tablets. Administer 4–8 mg daily in divided doses. Continuous administration should not exceed 6 months. Drug may be readministered after a 3- to 4-week rest period.

NURSING CONSIDERATIONS

Administration/Storage

1. Administer the drug with meals or milk to minimize irritation due to increased hydrochloric acid production.
2. The drug must be discontinued gradually to avoid migraine headache rebound.
3. If the drug is not effective after 3 weeks, it is not likely to be beneficial.

Assessment

1. Note any history of renal or hepatic disease. Obtain baseline liver and renal function studies prior to initiating therapy.
2. Obtain baseline eosinophil and neutrophil count prior to beginning therapy.
3. Note the frequency and severity of the client's headaches and efforts made in the past to control them.
4. Assess the client's behavior prior to initiating therapy.

Interventions

1. Compare behavior after the client has been taking methysergide maleate to ascertain changes, such as hallucinations, that would indicate an adverse response to the drug.
2. Closely observe the client for the presence of vascular headaches, lightheadedness, nervousness, or insomnia and report these symptoms to the physician.
3. A client who develops general malaise, fatigue, weight loss, low grade fever, or urinary tract problems may be developing fibrosis (cardiac or pleuropulmonary fibrosis), and the drug should be discontinued.
4. If the client has no effect from the drug within 3 weeks, there is likely to be no response and the drug should be discontinued.

Client/Family Teaching

1. Report symptoms of nervousness, weakness, rashes, alopecia, and peripheral edema to the physician.

2. Weigh daily, record, and report any unusual weight gain.
3. If the weight gain becomes excessive, instruct the client on how to adjust the caloric intake.
4. Check the extremities for edema and report if evident.
5. Administration of methysergide should not be continued on a regular basis for longer than 6 months.
6. Maintain a low-salt diet, if prescribed, and refer to a dietitian as needed.
7. Remind the client to remain under medical supervision. Stress that blood tests must be done at periodic intervals to detect complications of drug therapy.
8. Report to the physician immediately any chest or flank pain and dyspnea because the drug should be discontinued.
9. Do not drive a car or engage in other hazardous tasks until drug effects are realized because drug may cause drowsiness.
10. Discuss with the family psychologic changes that may occur and advise them to report these to the physician.
11. Be alert to signs of circulatory disturbances that should be reported to the physician.
12. If dizziness or lightheadedness occurs upon arising, rise slowly from a supine position and dangle the legs for a few minutes before standing erect.
13. If feeling faint, lie down with the legs elevated.
14. Avoid alcohol as this may precipitate vascular headaches.
15. Do not discontinue medication abruptly. Rebound migraine headaches may occur. Medication must be discontinued gradually.

Evaluation: Evaluate client for reports of decreased frequency and incidence of severe vascular headaches.

Metipranolol hydrochloride
(met-ih-**PRAN**-oh-lohl)
OptiPranolol (Rx)

See also *Beta-Adrenergic Blocking Agents,* p. 113.

Classification: Beta-adrenergic blocking agent.

Action/Kinetics: Metipranolol blocks both beta-1- and beta-2-adrenergic receptors. The mechanism for causing a reduction in intraocular pressure is not known but may be related to a decrease in production of aqueous humor and a slight increase in the outflow of aqueous humor. A decrease of from 20% to 26% in intraocular pressure may be seen if the intraocular pressure is greater than 24 mm Hg at baseline. The drug may be absorbed and exert systemic effects. When used topically, metipranolol does not have any local anesthetic effect and exerts no action on pupil size or accommodation. **Onset:** 30 min. **Maximum effect:** 1–2 hr. **Duration:** 12–24 hr.

Uses: To reduce intraocular pressure in clients with ocular hypertension and chronic open-angle glaucoma.

Special Concerns: Pregnancy category: C. Use with caution during lactation. Safety and effectiveness have not been determined in children.

Side Effects: *Ophthalmologic:* Local discomfort, dermatitis of the eyelid, blepharitis, conjunctivitis, browache, tearing, blurred vision, abnormal vision, photophobia, edema.

Due to absorption, the following systemic side effects have been reported. *CV:* Hypertension, myocardial infarction, atrial fibrillation, angina, bradycardia, palpitation. *CNS:* Headache, dizziness, anxiety, depression, somnolence, nervousness. *Respiratory:* Dyspnea, rhinitis, bronchitis, coughing. *Miscellaneous:* Allergic reaction, asthenia, nausea, epistaxis, arthritis, myalgia, rash.

Dosage: Ophthalmic Solution. Adults: 1 gtt in the affected eye(s) b.i.d. Increasing the dose or more frequent administration does not increase the beneficial effect.

NURSING CONSIDERATIONS

See also *Nursing Considerations* for *Beta-Adrenergic Blocking Agents,* p. 116.

Administration/Storage

1. Other drugs to lower intraocular pressure may be used concomitantly with metipranolol.
2. Due to diurnal variation in response, intraocular pressure should be measured at different times during the day.

Assessment

1. Note ocular condition that requires drug therapy.
2. Obtain baseline ECG and vital signs.
3. Record pretreatment intraocular pressure.

Client/Family Teaching

1. Demonstrate and review appropriate method for administration.

2. Transient burning or stinging is common during administration but should be reported if severe.
3. Take only as directed and report any persistent bothersome side effects.
4. Stress the importance of reporting for follow-up visits to assess for systemic effects and to measure intraocular pressures in order to determine drug effectiveness.

Evaluation: Evaluate client for evidence of a significant lowering of intraocular pressures.

Metoclopramide

(meh-toe-kloh-**PRAH**-myd)

Apo-Metoclop❋, Clopra, Emex❋, Maxeran❋, Maxolon, Octamide, Reclomide, Reglan (Rx)

Classification: Gastrointestinal stimulant.

Action/Kinetics: Metoclopramide, by increasing sensitivity to acetylcholine, increases motility of the upper GI tract and relaxes the pyloric sphincter and duodenal bulb. This results in shortened gastric emptying and GI transit time. Metoclopramide is considered a dopamine antagonist. The drug facilitates intubation of the small bowel and speeds transit of a barium meal. **Onset, IV:** 1–3 min; **IM,** 10–15 min; **PO,** 30–60 min. **Duration:** 1–2 hr. $t\frac{1}{2}$: 4–6 hr. Significant first-pass effect following PO use; unchanged drug and metabolites excreted in urine.

Uses: PO: Acute and recurrent diabetic gastroparesis, gastroesophageal reflux. **Parenteral:** Facilitate small bowel intubation, stimulate gastric emptying, and increase intestinal transit of barium to aid in radiologic examination of stomach and small intestine, prophylaxis of nausea and vomiting in cancer chemotherapy. *Investigational:* Postoperative drug-related nausea and vomiting, treatment of slow gastric emptying time, gastric stasis in premature infants, prophylaxis of aspiration pneumonitis, vascular headaches, increase milk secretion.

Contraindications: Gastrointestinal hemorrhage, obstruction, or perforation; epilepsy, clients taking drugs likely to cause extrapyramidal symptoms, such as phenothiazines. Pheochromocytoma.

Special Concerns: Safe use during pregnancy (category: B) and lactation not established. Extrapyramidal effects are more likely to occur in children and geriatric clients.

Side Effects: *CNS:* Restlessness, drowsiness, fatigue, lassitude, insomnia. Headaches, dizziness, extrapyramidal symptoms, Parkinson-like symptoms, dystonia, myoclonus, depression, dyskinesia. *GI:* Nausea, bowel disturbances. *CV:* Hypertension (transient).

Symptoms of Overdose: Agitation, irritability, hypertonia of muscles, drowsiness, disorientation, extrapyramidal symptoms.

Drug Interactions

Acetaminophen / ↑ GI absorption of acetaminophen
Anticholinergics / ↓ Effect of metoclopramide
Cimetidine / ↓ Effect of cimetidine due to ↓ absorption from GI tract

CNS depressants / Additive sedative effects
Digoxin / ↓ Effect of digoxin due to ↓ absorption from GI tract
Ethanol / ↑ GI absorption of ethanol
Levodopa / ↑ GI absorption of levodopa
Narcotic analgesics / ↓ Effect of metoclopramide
Tetracyclines / ↑ GI absorption of tetracyclines

Dosage: Tablets, Syrup. *Diabetic gastroparesis:* **Adults,** 10 mg 30 min before meals and at bedtime for 2–8 weeks (therapy should be reinstituted if symptoms recur). *Gastroesophageal reflux:* 10–15 mg q.i.d. 30 min before meals and at bedtime.

Delayed GI emptying, peristaltic stimulant: **Pediatric, 5–14 years:** 2.5–5 mg t.i.d. 30 min before meals.

IV. *Prophylaxis of vomiting due to chemotherapy:* **initial,** 1–2 mg/kg for 2 doses, with the first dose 30 min before chemotherapy; **then,** 10 mg or more q 3 hr for 3 doses. Inject slowly IV over 15 min. *Facilitate small bowel intubation:* **Adults,** 10 mg given over 1–2 min; **pediatric, 6–14 years:** 2.5–5 mg; **pediatric, less than 6 years:** 0.1 mg/kg. *Radiologic examinations to increase intestinal transit time:* 10 mg as a single dose given over 1–2 min. *Delayed GI emptying, peristaltic stimulant:* **Pediatric, up to 6 years:** 0.1 mg/kg; **pediatric, 6–14 years:** 2.5–5 mg as a single dose. Pediatric dosage should not exceed 0.5 mg/kg.

NURSING CONSIDERATIONS

Administration/Storage

1. Inject slowly over 1–2 min to prevent transient feelings of anxiety and restlessness.

2. After oral use, absorption of certain drugs from the GI tract may be affected (see *Drug Interactions*).

3. Metoclopramide is physically and/or chemically incompatible with a number of drugs; check package insert if drug is to be admixed.

4. For IV use, doses greater than 10 mg should be diluted in 50 ml of either dextrose 5% in water, dextrose 5% in 0.45% sodium chloride, lactated Ringer's injection, Ringer's injection, or sodium chloride injection.

5. *Treatment of Overdose:* Treat extrapyramidal effects by giving anticholinergic, antiparkinson, or antihistamines with anticholinergic effects. General supportive treatment.

Client/Family Teaching

1. Metoclopramide will have an added sedative effect if client is taking any other CNS depressants such as tranquilizers or sleeping pills.

2. Avoid alcohol.

3. Operating a car or hazardous machinery should not be attempted because medication has a sedative effect.

4. Discuss the side effects related to this drug. Instruct the client to keep a record of events to share with the physician so the adverse side effects can be properly evaluated and counteracted.

Evaluation: Evaluate client for:

• Reports of effective control of nausea and vomiting in cancer chemotherapy
• Evidence of return of normal GI function

Metoprolol
(me-toe-**PROH**-lohl)
Apo-Metoprolol✦, Apo-Metaprolol (Type L)✦, Betaloc✦, Lopressor, Novo–Metoprolol✦, Nu-Metop✦ (Rx)

See also *Beta-Adrenergic Blocking Agents,* p. 113.

Action/Kinetics: Exerts mainly beta-1-adrenergic blocking activity although beta-2 receptors are blocked at high doses. Has no membrane stabilizing or intrinsic sympathomimetic effects. Moderate lipid solubility. **Onset:** 15 min. **Peak plasma levels:** 90 min. **t½:** 3–7 hr. Effect of drug is cumulative. Food increases bioavailability. Exhibits significant first-pass effect. Metabolized in liver and excreted in urine.

Uses: Hypertension (either alone or with other antihypertensive agents, such as thiazide diuretics). Acute myocardial infarction in hemodynamically stable clients. Angina pectoris. *Investigational:* IV to suppress atrial ectopy in chronic obstructive pulmonary disease, aggressive behavior, prophylaxis of migraine, ventricular arrhythmias, enhancement of cognitive performance in geriatric clients, essential tremors.

Additional Contraindications: Myocardial infarction in clients with a heart rate of less than 45 beats/min, in second- or third-degree heart block, or if systolic blood pressure is less than 100 mm Hg. Cardiac failure.

Special Concerns: Pregnancy category: B. Dosage has not been established in children.

Additional Drug Interactions

Cimetidine / May ↑ plasma levels of metoprolol

Contraceptives, oral / May ↑ effects of metoprolol

Methimazole / May ↓ the effects of metoprolol

Phenobarbital / ↓ Effect of metoprolol due to ↑ breakdown by liver

Propylthiouracil / May ↓ the effects of metoprolol

Quinidine / May ↑ effects of metoprolol

Rifampin / ↓ Effect of metoprolol due to ↑ breakdown by liver

Laboratory Test Interferences: ↑ Serum transaminase, LDH, alkaline phosphatase.

Dosage: Tablets. *Hypertension:* **initial,** 100 mg daily in single or divided doses; **then,** dose may be increased weekly to maintenance level of 100–450 mg daily. A diuretic may also be used. *Prophylaxis of myocardial infarction:* **early treatment,** 50 mg q 6 hr beginning 15 min after the last IV dose (or as soon as client's condition allows). This dose is continued for 48 hr followed by **late treatment: PO,** 100 mg b.i.d. as soon as feasible; continue for 1–3 months (although data suggest treatment should be continued for 1–3 years). *Aggressive behavior:* 200–300 mg daily. *Essential tremors:* 50–300 mg daily. *Prophylaxis of migraine:* 50–100 mg b.i.d. *Ventricular arrhythmias:* 200 mg daily. **IV.** *Myocardial infarction,* **early treatment:** 5 mg as an IV bolus q 2 min for a total of 3 doses (15 mg); **then,** if this dose is tolerated, give 50 mg PO q 6 hr for 48 hr, beginning 15 min after the last IV dose (see above). If client cannot tolerate full IV dose, begin PO dose at 25 or 50 mg q 6 hr.

NURSING CONSIDERATIONS

See also *Nursing Considerations* for *Beta-Adrenergic Blocking Agents,* p. 116, and *Antihypertensive Agents,* p. 78.

Assessment

1. Document any history of cardiac disease.
2. Obtain baseline ECG and BP prior to initiating therapy.

Client/Family Teaching: Doses of metoprolol should be taken at the same time each day.

Evaluation: Evaluate client for:
- Evidence of a ↓ in blood pressure
- Reports of a ↓ in frequency of anginal attacks

M

Metronidazole

(meh-troh-**NYE**-dah-zohl)

Apo-Metronidazole ✶, Femazole, Flagyl, Flagyl I.V., Flagyl I.V. RTU, Metizol, Metric 21, MetroGel, Metro I.V., Metryl, Metryl-500, Metryl I.V., Neo-Metric ✶, Novo-Nidazol ✶, PMS Metronidazole ✶, Protostat, Satric, Satric 500, Trikacide ✶ (Rx)

See also *Anti-Infectives,* p. 80.

Classification: Systemic trichomonacide, amebicide.

Action/Kinetics: Effective against anaerobic bacteria and protozoa. Specifically inhibits growth of trichomonae and amebae by binding to DNA, resulting in loss of helical structure, strand breakage, inhibition of nucleic acid synthesis, and cell death. Well absorbed from GI tract and widely distributed in body tissues. **Peak serum concentration: PO,** 6–40 mcg/ml, depending on the dose, after 1–2 hr. **t½: PO,** 6–12 hr average: 8 hr. Eliminated primarily in urine (20% unchanged), which may be red-brown in color following either PO or IV use.

Uses: Systemic. Amebiasis. Symptomatic and asymptomatic trichomoniasis; to treat asymptomatic partner. Amebic dysentery and amebic liver abscess. To reduce postoperative anaerobic infection following colorectal surgery, elective hysterectomy, and emergency appendectomy. Anaerobic bacterial infections of the abdomen, female genital system, skin or skin structures, bones and joints, lower respiratory tract, and CNS. Also, septicemia, endocarditis, hepatic encephalopathy. Orally for Crohn's disease and pseudomembranous colitis. *Investigational:* giardiasis, *Gardnerella vaginalis.* **Topical.** Inflammatory papules, pustules, and erythema of rosacea.

Contraindications: Blood dyscrasias; active organic disease of the CNS. Not recommended for trichomoniasis during the first trimester of pregnancy. During lactation. For topical use: hypersensitivity to parabens or other ingredients of the formulation.

Special Concerns: Pregnancy category: B. Safety and efficacy have not been established in children.

Side Effects: *GI:* Following PO use, nausea, dry mouth, metallic taste, vomiting, diarrhea, abdominal discomfort, constipation. *CNS:* Headache, dizziness, vertigo, incoordination, ataxia, confusion, irritability, depression, weakness, insomnia, syncope, seizures, peripheral neuropathy including paresthesias. *Hematologic:* Leukopenia, bone marrow aplasia. *GU:* Burning, dysuria, cystitis, polyuria, incontinence, dryness of vagina or vulva, dyspareunia, decreased libido. *Allergic:* Urticaria, pruritus, erythematous rash, flushing, nasal congestion, fever, joint pain. *Miscellaneous:* Furry tongue, glossitis, stomatitis (due to overgrowth of *Candida.*) ECG abnormalities, thrombophlebitis.

Topical Use: Watery eyes if gel applied too closely to this area; transient redness; mild burning, dryness, and skin irritation.

Symptoms of Overdose: Ataxia, nausea, vomiting, peripheral neuropathy, seizures up to 5–7 days.

Drug Interactions

Alcohol, ethyl / Disulfiram-like reaction possible
Anticoagulants, oral /
↑ Anticoagulant effect due to ↓ breakdown by liver
Disulfiram / Additive effects

Dosage: Capsules, Tablets. *Amebiasis: Acute amebic dysentery or amebic liver abscess:* **Adult:** 500–750 mg t.i.d. for 5–10 days; **pediatric:** 35–50 mg/kg daily in 3 divided doses for 10 days. *Trichomoniasis, female:* 250 mg t.i.d. for 7 days or 2 g given on 1 day in single or divided doses. **Pediatric:** 5 mg/kg t.i.d. for 7 days. An interval of 4–6 weeks should elapse between courses of therapy. **Note:** Pregnant women should not be treated during the first trimester. *Male:* Individualize dosage; usual, 250 mg t.i.d. for 7 days. *Giardiasis:* 250 mg t.i.d. for 7 days. *Gardnerella vaginalis:* 500 mg b.i.d. for 7 days. **IV.** *Anaerobic bacterial infections:* **Initially:** 15 mg/kg infused over 1 hr;

then, after 6 hr, 7.5 mg/kg q 6 hr for 7–10 days (daily dose should not exceed 4 g). Treatment may be necessary for 2–3 weeks, although PO therapy should be initiated as soon as possible. *Prophylaxis of anaerobic infection during surgery:* **IV,** 15 mg/kg given over a 30- to 60-min period, with completion 1 hr prior to surgery and 7.5 mg/kg infused over 30–60 min 6 and 12 hr after the initial dose.

Topical. *Rosacea:* After washing, apply a thin film and rub in well in the morning and evening for 9 weeks.

NURSING CONSIDERATIONS

See also *General Nursing Considerations For All Anti-Infectives,* p. 83.

Administration/Storage

1. If used IV, drug should not be given by IV bolus.
2. Syringes with aluminum needles or hubs should not be used.
3. If a primary IV fluid setup is used, discontinue the primary solution during infusion of metronidazole.
4. The order of mixing to prepare the Powder for Injection is important:
   - Reconstitute.
   - Dilute in IV solutions (in glass or plastic containers).
   - Neutralize pH with sodium bicarbonate solution. Neutralized solutions should not be refrigerated.
5. For topical use, therapeutic results should be seen within 3 weeks with continuing improvement through 9 weeks of therapy.
6. Cosmetics may be used after application of topical metronidazole.

7. IV metronidazole has a high sodium content.
8. *Treatment of Overdose:* Supportive treatment.

Client/Family Teaching

1. Take with food or milk to reduce GI upset.
2. Report any symptoms of CNS toxicity immediately, such as ataxia or tremor, that may necessitate withdrawal of drug.
3. Do not perform tasks that require mental alertness until drug effects are realized as dizziness may occur.
4. During treatment for trichomoniasis, explain the necessity for the male partner to have therapy also, since organisms also may be located in the male urogenital tract.
5. Sexual partners should use a condom throughout therapy to prevent reinfection.
6. The drug may turn urine brown; do not be alarmed.
7. Do not drink alcohol when on metronidazole therapy because a disulfiram-like reaction may occur. Symptoms include abdominal cramps, vomiting, flushing, and headache.

Evaluation: Evaluate client for:
- Reports of symptomatic improvement
- Evidence of negative laboratory culture reports

Mexiletine hydrochloride

(mex-**ILL**-eh-teen)
Mexitil (Rx)

See also *Antiarrhythmic Drugs,* p. 51.

Classification: Antiarrhythmic, type IB.

Action/Kinetics: Mexiletine is similar to lidocaine but is effective orally. The drug inhibits the flow of sodium into the cell, thereby reducing the rate of rise of the action potential. Blood pressure and pulse rate are not affected following use, but there may be a small decrease in cardiac output and an increase in peripheral vascular resistance. The drug also has both local anesthetic and anticonvulsant effects. **Onset:** 30–120 min. **Peak blood levels:** 2–3 hr. **Therapeutic plasma levels:** 0.5–2 mcg/ml. **Plasma t½:** 10–12 hr. Approximately 10% excreted unchanged in the urine; acidification of the urine enhances excretion, whereas alkalinization decreases excretion.

Uses: Frequent premature ventricular contractions, unifocal or multifocal couplets, and ventricular tachycardia.

Contraindications: Cardiogenic shock, preexisting second- or third-degree AV block (if no pacemaker is present). Lactation.

Special Concerns: Pregnancy category: C. Use with caution in hypotension and severe congestive heart failure. Dosage has not been established in children.

Side Effects: *CV:* Worsening of arrhythmias, palpitations, chest pain. *GI:* Nausea, vomiting, heartburn, diarrhea or constipation, changes in appetite. *CNS:* Lightheadedness, dizziness, tremor, coordination difficulties, changes in sleep habits, fatigue, weakness, tinnitus, paresthesias, depression, confusion, difficulty with speech, headache. *Miscellaneous:* Blurred vision, dyspnea, rash, edema, arthralgia, dry mouth, elevated liver AST. *Symptoms of Overdose:* Ataxia, seizures, other CNS effects.

Drug Interactions

Cimetidine / ↑ Plasma levels of mexiletine
Phenobarbital / ↓ Plasma levels of mexiletine
Phenytoin / ↓ Plasma levels of mexiletine
Rifampin / ↓ Plasma levels of mexiletine

Dosage: Capsules. Adults, individualized, initial: 200 mg q 8 hr if rapid control of arrhythmia not required; **then,** 300–400 mg q 8 hr, depending on response and tolerance of client. If adequate response is achieved with 300 mg or less q 8 hr, the same total daily dose may be given in divided doses q 12 hr (i.e., 450 mg q 12 hr). *Rapid control of arrhythmias,* **initial loading dose:** 400 mg followed by a 200-mg dose in 8 hr.

If transferring to mexiletine from other class I antiarrhythmics, mexiletine may be initiated at a dose of 200 mg and then titrated according to the response at the following times: 6–12 hr after the last dose of quinidine sulfate, 3–6 hr after the last dose of procainamide, 6–12 hr after the last dose of disopyramide, or 8–12 hr after the last dose of tocainide.

NURSING CONSIDERATIONS

See also *Nursing Considerations* for *Antiarrhythmic Drugs,* p. 52.

Administration/Storage

1. Two to three days should elapse between dosage adjustments; the dose may be adjusted in 50- to 100-mg increments up or down.

2. When transferring to mex-iletine, the client should be hospitalized if there is a chance that withdrawal of the previous antiarrhythmic may produce life-threatening arrhythmias.
3. *Treatment of Overdose:* General supportive treatment. Give atropine to treat hypotension or bradycardia. Acidification of the urine may increase rate of excretion.

Assessment

1. Determine baseline CBC, liver and renal function studies and monitor throughout therapy.
2. Note any evidence of CHF and assess ECG for evidence of AV block.

Interventions

1. Review ECG for increased arrhythmias and report.
2. Observe for adverse CNS effects such as dizziness, tremor, impaired coordination, nausea, and vomiting.
3. Obtain urinary pH to determine alkalinity or acidity. Alkalinity decreases renal excretion and acidity increases renal excretion of the drug.

Client/Family Teaching

1. Take medication with food or an antacid.
2. Report any bruising, bleeding, fevers, or sore throat.
3. Note any increase in heart palpitations, irregularity, or rate less than 50 bpm and report immediately.
4. Do not perform tasks that require mental alertness until drug effects are realized.
5. Wear a Medic Alert bracelet and carry identification that lists drugs currently prescribed.

Evaluation: Evaluate client for ECG evidence of succesful control of ventricular arrhythmias.

Mezlocillin sodium

(mez-low-**SILL**-in)
Mezlin (Rx)

See also *Anti-Infectives,* p. 80, and *Penicillins,* p. 197.

Classification: Antibiotic, penicillin.

Action/Kinetics: Mezlocillin is a broad-spectrum (gram-negative and gram-positive organisms, including aerobic and anaerobic strains) antibiotic used parenterally. **Therapeutic serum levels:** 35–45 mcg/ml. **t½: IV,** 55 min. Excreted mostly unchanged by the kidneys. Penetration to CSF is poor unless meninges are inflamed.

Uses: Septicemia and infections of the lower respiratory tract, urinary tract, abdomen, skin, and female genital tract caused by *Klebsiella, Proteus, Pseudomonas, Escherichia coli, Bacteroides, Peptococcus, Streptococcus faecalis* (enterococcus), *Peptostreptococcus,* and *Enterobacter.* Also, *Neisseria gonorrhoeae* infections of the urinary tract and female genital system. Infections caused by *Streptococcus pneumoniae* and group A beta-hemolytic streptococcus.

Additional Side Effects: Bleeding abnormalities. Decreased hemoglobin or hematocrit values.

Laboratory Test Interferences: ↑ AST, ALT, serum alkaline phosphatase, serum bilirubin, serum creatinine, and/or BUN. ↓ Serum potassium.

Dosage: IV, IM. Adults: *Serious infections:* 200–300 mg/kg/day in

4–6 divided doses; **usual:** 3 g q 4 hr or 4 g q 6 hr. *Life-threatening infections:* up to 350 mg/kg/day, not to exceed 24 g daily. *Gonococcal urethritis:* single dose of 1–2 g with probenecid, 1 g. *Prophylaxis of postoperative infection:* 4 g 30–90 min prior to start of surgery; **then,** 4 g, IV, 6 and 12 hr later. *Prophylaxis of infection in clients undergoing cesarean section:* **first dose,** 4 g IV when cord is clamped; **second and third doses:** 4 g IV 4 and 8 hr after the first dose. **IV, IM. Infants and children:** *Serious infections:* **1 month–12 years,** 50 mg/kg q 4 hr given **IM** or **IV** over 30 min; **infants more than 2 kg and less than 1 week of age or less than 2 kg and less than 1 week of age:** 75 mg/kg q 12 hr; **infants less than 2 kg and more than 1 week of age:** 75 mg/kg q 8 hr; **infants more than 2 kg and more than 1 week of age:** 75 mg/kg q 6 hr.

NURSING CONSIDERATIONS

See also *Nursing Considerations for Penicillins,* p. 200.

Administration/Storage

1. When given by IV infusion (including piggyback), administration of other drugs should be discontinued during administration of mezlocillin.
2. For pediatric IV administration, infuse over 30 min.
3. Vials and infusion bottles should be stored at temperatures below 30°C (86°F).
4. The powder and reconstituted solution may darken slightly, but potency is not affected.
5. IM doses should not exceed 2 g/injection. Mezlocillin should be continued for at least 2 days after symptoms of infection have disappeared.

6. For group A beta-hemolytic streptococcus, therapy should continue for at least 10 days.
7. Dosage should be reduced in clients with impaired renal function (based on creatinine clearance).

Interventions: Monitor CBC, PT, PTT, electrolytes, and renal function studies.

Client/Family Teaching

1. Immediately report any increased bruising and/or bleeding from any orifice to the physician.
2. Advise that symptoms of drug-induced anemia may be manifested by fatigue, pallor, weakness, vertigo, headache, dyspnea, and palpitations and to report if evident.

Evaluation: Evaluate client for:
- Laboratory evidence of negative culture reports
- Reports of symptomatic improvement
- Evidence that serum drug levels are within therapeutic range (35–45 mcg/ml)

Miconazole

(my-**KON**-ah-zohl)

Systemic: Monistat I.V. Topical: Micatin, Monistat-Derm. Vaginal: Monistat❀, Monistat 3, Monistat 5❀, Monistat 7 (Rx and OTC)

See also *Anti-Infectives,* p. 80.

Classification: Antifungal agent.

Action/Kinetics: Miconazole may be fungistatic or fungicidal, depending on the concentration. It is a broad-spectrum fungicide that alters the permeability of the fungal membrane by inhibiting synthesis of sterols; thus, essential intracellular materials are lost. The drug also inhibits biosynthesis of triglycerides and phospholipids and also inhibits oxidative and peroxidative enzyme activity. **Peak blood levels:** 1 mcg/ml. The drug is eliminated in three phases; **t½ of each phase:** 0.4, 2.1, and 24 hr. More than 90% of miconazole is bound to serum proteins. Excretion of the drug is unaltered in clients with renal insufficiency, including those on hemodialysis.

Uses: Systemic fungal infections caused by coccidioidomycosis, candidiasis, cryptococcosis, paracoccidioidomycosis, chronic mucocutaneous candidiasis, pseudoallescheriosis. When used for the treatment of either fungal meningitis or urinary bladder infection, IV infusion must be supplemented with intrathecal administration or bladder irrigation of the drug. *Topical:* Tinea pedis, tinea cruris, tinea corporis caused by *Trichophyton rubrum, T. mentagrophytes,* and *Epidermophyton floccosum* (both OTC and Rx). Moniliasis and tinea versicolor (Rx only).

Contraindications: Hypersensitivity. Use of topical products in or around the eyes.

Special Concerns: Pregnancy category: C. Safe use in children less than 1 year of age has not been established.

Side Effects: Following topical use: Vulvovaginal symptoms, pelvic cramps, hives, skin rash, headache, burning, irritation, maceration. **Following systemic use.** *GI:* Nausea, vomiting, diarrhea, anorexia. *Hematologic:* Thrombocytopenia, aggregation of erythrocytes, rouleaux formation on blood smears. Transient decrease in hematocrit. *Dermatologic:* Pruritus, rash, flushing, phlebitis at injection site. *CV:* Transient tachycardia or arrhythmias following rapid injection of undiluted drug. *Miscellaneous:* Fever, chills, drowsiness, transient decrease in serum sodium values. Hyperlipemia due to the vehicle (PEG 40 and castor oil).

Drug Interactions

Amphotericin B / ↓ Activity of miconazole of each drug
Coumarin anticoagulants / Miconazole ↑ anticoagulant effect

Dosage: IV infusion, adults: *Candidiasis:* 600–1,800 mg daily for 1–more than 20 weeks. *Coccidioidomycosis:* 1,800–3,600 mg for 3–more than 20 weeks. *Cryptococcosis:* 1,200–2,400 mg daily for 3 to more than 12 weeks. *Paracoccidioidomycosis:* 200–1,200 mg daily for 2 to more than 16 weeks. *Pseudoallescheriosis:* 600–3,000 mg daily for 5 to more than 20 weeks. **Pediatric, less than 1 year of age:** 15–30 mg/kg daily; **1–12 years of age:** 20–40 mg/kg daily, not to exceed 15 mg/kg per dose. **Intrathecal:** 20 mg/dose of the undiluted solution as an adjunct to **IV** therapy. **Bladder instillation:** 200 mg of diluted solution as adjunct in treatment of fungal infections of urinary bladder. **Topical, Aerosol Powder, Aerosol Solution, Cream, Lotion, Powder:** Apply to cover affected areas in morning and evening (once daily for tinea versicolor). **Vaginal, Monistat 3:** One suppository daily at bedtime for 3 days. **Vaginal, Monistat 7:** One applicatorful of cream or one suppository at bed-

M

time daily for 7 days. Course may be repeated after presence of other pathogens has been ruled out.

NURSING CONSIDERATIONS

See also *General Nursing Considerations For All Anti-Infectives*, p. 83.

Administration/Storage

1. For IV infusion, the drug should be diluted in at least 200 ml of either 0.9% sodium chloride or 5% dextrose solution and administered over a period of 30–60 min.
2. The IV dose may be divided over 3 infusions daily.
3. The lotion is preferred for intertriginous areas.
4. To reduce recurrence of symptoms, tinea cruris, tinea corporis, and candida should be treated for 2 weeks; tinea pedis should be treated for 1 month.
5. For intrathecal use, the drug is given as the undiluted solution (20 mg/dose) as an adjunct to IV treatment for fungal meningitis. Doses are alternated between lumbar, cervical, and cisternal punctures every 3–7 days; document sites.

Assessment

1. Obtain baseline CBC, electrolytes and liver function studies and monitor throughout therapy.
2. Determine any previous client experience with this drug and document response obtained and any evidence of sensitivity.
3. Obtain appropriate pretreatment lab studies as IV therapy may be required for periods ranging from 1 to more than 20 weeks, depending on the organism.

Client/Family Teaching

1. Demonstrate appropriate technique for medication administration and instruct client to take/use medication only as directed.
2. Use sanitary pads to protect clothing and linens when using cream or suppositories.
3. When used for vaginal infections, the client should refrain from intercourse to prevent reinfection.
4. When used vaginally, miconazole treatment should be continued during menses.
5. Persistent nausea, vomiting, diarrhea, dizziness, and pruritus should be reported.

Evaluation: Evaluate client for:
- Laboratory evidence of negative culture results
- Reports of symptomatic improvement
- Evidence of compliance with prescribed medication regimen and the need for continued treatment

Microfibrillar Collagen Hemostat

(my-kroh-**FIB**-rih-lar **KOLL**-ah-jen **HEE**-moh-stat)

Avitene (Rx)

Classification: Hemostatic, topical.

Action/Kinetics: This product is purified bovine corium collagen prepared as the partial hydrochloric acid salt. Attracts platelets, which then release clotting factors that initiate formation of a fibrinous mass. Absorbable, water insoluble.

Uses: During surgery to control

capillary bleeding and as an adjunct to hemostasis when conventional procedures are ineffectual or insufficient. It is ineffective in controlling systemic coagulation disorders.

Contraindications: Closure of skin incisions, because preparation may interfere with healing. On bone surfaces to which prosthetic materials will be attached. Intraocular use or for injection.

Special Concerns: Use during pregnancy only when benefits clearly outweigh risks.

Side Effects: Potentiation of infections, abscess formation, hematomas, wound dehiscence, mediastinitis. Formation of adhesions, foreign body or allergic reactions. *Following dental use:* Alveolalgia. *Following tonsillectomy:* Laryngospasm due to inhalation of dry material.

Dosage: *Individualized,* depending on severity of bleeding. *Usual for capillary bleeding:* 1 g for 50 cm². More for heavier flow.

NURSING CONSIDERATIONS

Administration/Storage

1. Before applying dry product, compress surface to be treated with dry sponge. Use dry smooth forceps to handle.
2. Apply collagen hemostat directly to source of bleeding.
3. Once in place, apply pressure with a dry sponge (not a gloved hand) for up to 5 min, depending on severity of bleeding.
4. When controlling oozing from porous (cancellous) bone, pack collagen hemostat tightly into affected area. Tease off excess material after 5–10 min. Apply more in case of breakthrough bleeding.
5. Avoid spillage on nonbleeding surfaces, especially in the abdomen or thorax.
6. Remove excess material after a few minutes.
7. Do not reautoclave. Discard any unused portion.
8. Avoid contacting nonbleeding surfaces with microfibrillar collagen hemostat.
9. Dry forceps should be used to handle collagen hemostat as it will adhere to wet gloves or instruments.

Intervention: Monitor BP and pulse and assess for shock because collagen hemostat may mask a deeper hemorrhage by sealing off its exit site.

Evaluation: Evaluate for the control of capillary bleeding that does not respond to normal control mechanisms during surgery.

Midazolam HCl
(my-**DAYZ**-oh-lam)
Versed (Rx, C-IV)

See also *Benzodiazepines,* p. 108.

Classification: Sedative benzodiazepine; adjunct to general anesthesia.

Action/Kinetics: Midazolam is a short-acting benzodiazepine with sedative–general anesthetic properties. The drug depresses the response of the respiratory system to carbon dioxide stimulation; this effect is more pronounced in clients with chronic obstructive pulmonary disease. There may be mild to moderate decreases in cardiac output, mean arterial BP, stroke volume, and systemic vascular resistance. The effect on heart rate may rise somewhat in clients with slow heart rates (less than 65/min) and decrease in others (especially those with heart rates more than 85/min). **Onset, IM:** 15 min; **IV:** 2–2.5 min for induction (if combined with a preanesthetic narcotic, induction is about 1.5 min). If preanesthetic medication (morphine) is given, the **Peak plasma levels, IM:** 45 min. **Maximum effect:** 30–60 min. About 97% bound to plasma protein. **t½, elimination:** 1.2–12.3 hr. The drug is rapidly metabolized in the liver and excreted through the liver.

Uses: IV: Induction of general anesthesia; before administration of other anesthetics; supplement to balanced anesthesia for surgical procedures of short duration. Midazolam should be used for conscious sedation only by personnel skilled in early detection of underventilation, maintaining a patent airway, and supporting ventilation. **IM:** Preoperative sedation; to impair memory of events surrounding surgery.

Contraindications: Hypersensitivity to benzodiazepines. Acute narrow-angle glaucoma. Use in obstetrics. Not to be given to clients in coma, shock, or in acute alcohol intoxication where vital signs are depressed. Intra-arterial injection.

Special Concerns: Pregnancy category: D. Use with caution during lactation. Safety and effectiveness have not been determined in children less than 18 years of age. Hypotension may be more common in conscious sedation clients who have received a preanesthetic narcotic. Geriatric and debilitated clients require lower doses to induce anesthesia and they are more prone to side effects. IV midazolam should be used with extreme caution in clients with severe fluid or electrolyte disturbances.

Side Effects: Fluctuations in vital signs (including decreased respiratory rate and tidal volume) are common. The following are general side effects regardless of the route of administration. *Respiratory:* IV use has resulted in respiratory depression and respiratory arrest when used for conscious sedation. *CV:* Hypotension, cardiac arrest. *CNS:* Confusion, retrograde amnesia, euphoria, nervousness, agitation, anxiety, argumentativeness, restlessness, emergence delirium, increased time for emergence, dreaming during emergence, nightmares, insomnia, tonic/clonic seizures, ataxia, muscle tremor, involuntary or athetoid movements, dizziness, dysphoria, dysphonia, slurred speech, paresthesia. *GI:* Acid taste, retching, excessive salivation. *Ophthalmologic:* Double vision, blurred vision, nystagmus, pinpoint pupils, visual disturbances, cyclic eyelid movements, difficulty in focusing. *Dermatologic:* Hives, swelling or feeling of burning, warmth or cold feeling at injection site, hive-like wheal at injection site, pruritus, rash. *Miscellaneous:* Blocked ears, loss of balance, chills, weakness, faint feeling, lethargy, yawning, toothache, hematoma.

More common following IM use: Pain at injection site, headache, induration and redness, muscle stiffness.

More common following IV use: *Respiratory:* Bronchospasm, dyspnea, laryngospasm, hyperventilation, shallow respirations, tachypnea, airway obstruction, wheezing.

CV: Premature ventricular contractions, bigeminy, tachycardia, vasovagal episode, nodal rhythm. *GI:* Hiccoughs, nausea, vomiting. *At injection site:* Tenderness, pain, redness, induration, phlebitis. *Miscellaneous:* Drowsiness, oversedation, coughing, headache.

Drug Interactions

Alcohol / ↑ Risk of apnea or underventilation
Anesthetics, inhalation / Dose should be reduced if midazolam used as an induction agent
CNS Depressants / ↑ Risk of apnea or underventilation
Droperidol / ↑ Hypnotic effect of midazolam when used as a premedication
Fentanyl / ↑ Hypnotic effect of midazolam when used as a premedication
Meperidine / See *Narcotics;* also, ↑ Risk of hypotension
Narcotics / ↑ Hypnotic effect of midazolam when used as premedications

Dosage: IM, IV. *Preoperative sedation, memory impairment for events surrounding surgery:* **IM, Adults,** 0.08 mg/kg (average: 5 mg) 1 hr before surgery. *Conscious sedation for endoscopic or cardiovascular procedures:* **IV, Healthy adults, less than 60 years of age,** Using the 1 mg/ml (can be diluted with 0.9% sodium chloride or 5% dextrose in water) product, titrate slowly to the desired effect (usually slurred speech); dose may be as low as 1 mg. No more than 2.5 mg should be given within a 2-min period, after which an additional 2 min should be waited to evaluate the sedative effect. If additional sedation is necessary, small increments should be given waiting an additional 2 min or more after each increment to evaluate the effect. Total doses greater than 5 mg are usually not required.

IV, Debilitated or chronically ill clients or clients aged 60 or over: Slowly titrate to the desired effect using as little as 1 mg. No more than 1.5 mg should be given over a 2-min period after which an additional 2 min or more should be waited to evaluate the effect. If additional sedation is needed, no more than 1 mg should be given over 2 min; wait an additional 2 min or more after each increment in dose. Total doses greater than 3.5 mg are usually not needed. If preanesthetic medications with a depressant component are given, the midazolam dosage should be reduced by 50% compared with healthy, young unmedicated clients. Maintenance doses to all clients should be given in increments of 25% of the dose first required to achieve the sedative endpoint.

Induction of general anesthesia, before use of other anesthetics: **Adults, unmedicated clients, IV, initial:** 0.3–0.35 mg/kg given over 20–30 sec waiting 2 min for effects to occur. If needed, increments of about 25% of the initial dose can be used to complete induction; or, induction can be completed using a volatile liquid anesthetic. Up to 0.6 mg/kg may be used but recovery will be prolonged. *Induction of general anesthesia, before use of other anesthetics:* **Adults, premedicated, IV, initial:** 0.15–0.35 mg/kg. If less than 55 years of age, 0.25 mg/kg may be given over 20–30 sec allowing 2 min for effect. In clients with severe systemic disease or debilitation, 0.15 mg/kg may be sufficient.

Maintenance of balanced anesthesia for short surgical procedures:

M

IV, Incremental injections about 25% of the dose used for induction when signs indicate anesthesia is lightening.

Note: Narcotic preanesthetic medication may include fentanyl, 1.5–2 mcg/kg IV 5 min before induction; morphine, up to 0.15 mg/kg IM; meperidine, up to 1 mg/kg IM; or, Innovar, 0.02 ml/kg IM. Sedative preanesthetic medication may include secobarbital sodium, 200 mg PO or hydroxyzine pamoate, 100 mg PO. Except for fentanyl, all preanesthetic medications should be given 1 hr prior to midazolam. Doses should always be individualized.

NURSING CONSIDERATIONS

See also *Nursing Considerations* for *Benzodiazepines,* p. 111.

Administration/Storage

1. When used for conscious sedation, the drug should not be given by rapid or single bolus IV administration.
2. When used for induction of general anesthesia, the initial dose of midazolam should be given over 20–30 sec.
3. When used for procedures via the mouth, a topical anesthetic should also be used.
4. A narcotic preanesthetic should be given for bronchoscopic procedures.
5. All IV doses should be carefully monitored with the immediate availability of oxygen, resuscitative equipment, and personnel who are skilled in maintaining a patent airway and for support of ventilation.
6. IM doses should be given in a large muscle mass.

Interventions: The client should be monitored constantly for early signs of respiratory distress or apnea which can lead to cardiac arrest or hypoxia. Monitoring should continue during the recovery period.

Evaluation: Evaluate client for reports of effective sedation and amnesia.

Mineral Oil
Agoral Plain, Fleet Mineral Oil, Kondremul✸, Kondremul Plain, Lansoyl✸, Milkinol, Neo-Cultrol (OTC)

Classification: Emollient laxative.

Action/Kinetics: This mixture of liquid hydrocarbons obtained from petroleum lubricates the intestine; it also decreases absorption of fecal water from the colon. **Onset: PO,** 6–8 hr; **Enema,** 2–15 min.

Uses: Constipation, to avoid straining under certain conditions, such as rectal surgery, hemorrhoidectomy, and certain cardiovascular conditions. Short-term treatment of constipation; useful in geriatric clients with diminished colonic motor response and during pregnancy and postpartum to reestablish normal bowel function. To soften feces during fecal impaction.

Contraindications: Nausea, vomiting, abdominal pain, or intestinal obstruction.

Special Concerns: Mineral oil may decrease absorption of fat-soluble vitamins (vitamins A, D, E, K).

Side Effects: Acute or chronic lipid pneumonia due to aspiration of mineral oil; young, elderly, and dysphagic clients are at greatest risk. Pruritus ani, which may interfere with healing following anorectal surgery. Use during pregnancy may decrease vitamin K absorption sufficiently to cause hypoprothrombinemia in the newborn.

Drug Interactions

Anticoagulants, oral / ↑ Hypoprothrombinemia by ↓ absorption of vitamin K from GI tract; also, mineral oil could ↓ absorption of anticoagulant from GI tract

Sulfonamides / ↓ Effect of nonabsorbable sulfonamide in GI tract

Surface-active laxatives / ↑ Absorption of mineral oil

Vitamins A, D, E, K / ↓ Absorption following prolonged use of mineral oil

Dosage: Emulsion, Gel, Oral Suspension. Adults: 15–45 ml at bedtime; **children:** 5–20 ml at bedtime.

NURSING CONSIDERATIONS

See also *Nursing Considerations* for *Laxatives,* p. 172.

Administration/Storage

1. Administer mineral oil at bedtime and cautiously as there is the possibility of lipid pneumonitis. Unless contraindicated, give the client orange juice or a piece of orange to suck on after taking the mineral oil.
2. The emulsion form is pleasant tasting and does not require anything to make it more palatable. However, when taken at bedtime, there is an increased risk of developing lipid pneumonia.
3. Store in the refrigerator to make the medication more palatable.
4. Administer mineral oil slowly to elderly, debilitated clients to prevent aspiration. Aspiration could result in lipid pneumonia.
5. Administer mineral oil carefully and slowly to children to prevent aspiration.
6. Do not administer mineral oil with food or vitamin preparations. The medication may delay digestion and prevent absorption of fat-soluble vitamins, A, D, E, and K.

Assessment: Note if the client is of childbearing age and likely to be pregnant. Mineral oil may cause hypoprothrombinemia in the newborn and therefore should be avoided.

Interventions: If the client is taking more than 30 ml of mineral oil, check the perianal area for leakage of feces. These clients require more frequent cleansing and a perianal pad to prevent soiling of clothes and bedding.

Client/Family Teaching

1. Sit upright when taking mineral oil to avoid the possibility of aspiration.
2. If the client is taking mineral oil in large amounts and over extended periods of time, caution of the potential problem of leakage of fecal matter.
3. Warn pregnant women not to take the medication to relieve constipation, but rather, to check with their physician for suitable alternatives.

M

Evaluation: Evaluate client for evidence of successful evacuation of a soft, formed stool.

Minoxidil, oral
(mih-**NOX**-ih-dil)
Loniten, Minodyl (Rx)

Classification: Antihypertensive, depresses sympathetic nervous system.

Action/Kinetics: Decreases elevated BP by decreasing peripheral resistance. Drug causes increase in renin secretion, increase in cardiac rate and output, and salt/water retention. It does not cause orthostatic hypotension. **Onset:** 30 min. **Peak plasma levels:** reached within 60 min; **plasma t½:** 4.2 hr. **Duration:** 24–48 hr. Ninety percent absorbed from GI tract; excretion: renal (90% metabolites). The time needed to reach the maximum effect is inversely related to the dose.

Minoxidil can produce severe side effects; it should be reserved for resistant cases of hypertension. Use generally requires concomitant administration of beta-adrenergic blocking agents and diuretics. Close medical supervision required, including possible hospitalization during initial administration.

Use: Hypertension not controllable by the use of a diuretic plus two other antihypertensive drugs. Usually taken with at least two other antihypertensive drugs (a diuretic and a drug to minimize tachycardia such as a beta-adrenergic blocking agent). Topically to promote hair growth in balding men (see p. 891).

Contraindications: Pheochromocytoma. Within 1 month after a myocardial infarction.

Special Concerns: Safe use during pregnancy (category: C) and lactation not established. Use with caution and at reduced dosage in impaired renal function. Geriatric clients may be more sensitive to the hypotensive and hypothermic effects of minoxidil; also, it may be necessary to decrease the dose in these clients due to age-related decreases in renal function.

Side Effects: *CV:* Edema, pericardial effusion, tamponade (acute compression of heart caused by fluid or blood in pericardium), CHF, angina pectoris, increased heart rate. *GI:* Nausea, vomiting. *CNS:* Headache, fatigue. *Other:* Hypertrichosis (enhanced hair growth, pigmentation and thickening of fine body hair 3–6 weeks after initiation of therapy), skin rashes (hypersensitivity), breast tenderness.

Symptom of Overdose: Excessive hypotension.

Drug Interactions: Concomitant use with guanethidine may result in severe hypotension.

Laboratory Test Interferences: Nonspecific changes in ECG. ↓ Hematocrit, erythrocyte count, and hemoglobin. ↑ Alkaline phosphatase, serum creatinine, and BUN.

Dosage: Tablets. Adults and children over 12 years: Initial, 5 mg once daily. For optimum control, dose can be increased to 10, 20, and then 40 mg in single or divided doses/day. Daily dosage should not exceed 100 mg. **Children under 12 years: Initial,** 0.2 mg/kg once daily. Effective dose range: 0.25–1.0 mg/kg/day. Dosage must be titrated to individual response. Daily dosage should not exceed 50 mg.

NURSING CONSIDERATIONS

See *Nursing Considerations* for *Antihypertensive Agents*, p. 78.

Administration/Storage

1. Can be taken with fluids and without regard to meals.
2. *Treatment of Overdose:* Give normal saline IV (to maintain blood pressure and urine output). Vasopressors, such as phenylephrine and dopamine, can be used but only in under-perfusion of a vital organ.

Interventions

1. Anticipate that minoxidil therapy will be initiated in the hospital. After medication administration, BP decreases within 30 min and the client reaches minimum BP within 2–3 hr.
2. Anticipate the clients receiving guanethidine concomitantly may experience severe hypotensive effects that may be precipitated by drug interaction.

Client/Family Teaching

1. Review the technique for monitoring pulse and BP. Assist the client to develop and maintain a written record and instruct client to report any abnormal reading to the physician.
2. Record weight daily and report any weight gain of over 2.3 kg within 3 days, as well as edema of extremities, face, and abdomen.
3. Report any dyspnea that occurs especially when lying down.
4. Report angina, dizziness, or fainting.
5. Explain that the medication may cause elongation, thickening, and increased pigmentation of body hair, but that there is generally a return to pre-treatment norm when the drug is discontinued.
6. Use drug only in the dose and form prescribed.

Evaluation: Evaluate client for evidence of control of hypertension.

Minoxidil topical solution

(mih-**NOX**-ih-dill)
Rogaine (Rx)

Classification: Hair growth stimulant.

Action/Kinetics: Minoxidil topical solution stimulates vertex hair growth in clients with male pattern baldness. The mechanism is unknown, but may be related to the fact that minoxidil dilates arterioles and stimulates resting hair follicles into active growth. Oral minoxidil is used to treat hypertension and, when used systemically, is associated with a significant number of potential side effects. Following topical administration, approximately 1.4% is absorbed into the systemic circulation. **Onset:** 4 months but is variable. **Duration:** New hair growth may be lost 3–4 months after withdrawal of therapy. Minoxidil and its inactive metabolites are excreted in the urine.

Uses: To treat male and female pattern baldness (alopecia androgenetica). In males this is manifested by baldness of the vertex of the scalp and in females as thinning of the frontoparietal areas or diffuse hair loss. *Investigational:* Alopecia areata.

Contraindications: Lactation.

Special Concerns: Pregnancy category: C. Use with caution in clients with hypertension, coronary heart disease, or predisposition to heart failure. Safety and efficacy in clients under 18 years of age have not been determined. Increased systemic absorption may occur if the scalp is irritated or there are abrasions.

Side Effects: *Dermatologic:* Allergic contact dermatitis, irritant dermatitis, pruritus, dry skin, flaking of scalp, alopecia, hypertrichosis, erythema, worsening of hair loss. *Allergic:* Hives, facial swelling, allergic rhinitis. *CNS:* Dizziness, lightheadedness, headache, faintness, anxiety, depression, fatigue. *Respiratory:* Sinusitis, bronchitis, respiratory infection. *Miscellaneous:* Conjunctivitis, vertigo, decreased visual acuity, vertigo. **Note:** The incidence of side effects due to placebos is often similar to the incidence of side effects due to the drug itself.

Drug Interactions

Corticosteroids, topical / Enhance absorption of topical minoxidil
Guanethidine / Possible ↑ risk of orthostatic hypotension
Petrolatum / Enhances absorption of topical minoxidil
Retinoids / Enhance absorption of topical minoxidil

Dosage: Topical Solution. Adult, 1 ml of the 2% solution is applied to the affected area of the scalp in the morning and before bedtime. The total daily dose should not exceed 2 ml.

NURSING CONSIDERATIONS

Administration/Storage

1. Only clients with normal, healthy scalps should use topical minoxidil. Dermatitis, scalp abrasions, scalp psoriasis, or severe sunburn may increase the absorption of topical minoxidil and lead to systemic side effects (See *Minoxidil, oral*).

2. Hair may be shampooed before treatment, but the hair and scalp should be dry prior to application of topical minoxidil.

3. The product comes with a metered spray attachment (for application to large areas of the scalp), extender spray attachment (for application to small scalp areas or under the hair), and a rub-on applicator tip (to spread the solution on the scalp). The directions on the package insert should be followed carefully for each of these methods of application.

4. If the fingertips are used to apply the drug, the hands should be washed thoroughly after application.

5. At least 4 months of continuous therapy is necessary before evidence of hair growth can be expected. Further hair growth continues through one year of treatment.

6. The alcohol base in topical minoxidil will cause irritation and burning of the eyes, abraded skin, or mucous membranes. If there is contact with any of these areas, wash the site with copious amounts of water.

7. The client should avoid inhaling the spray mist.

Interventions: Clients on topical minoxidil therapy should be monitored 1 month after starting therapy and every 6 months thereafter for any systemic effects. These should be documented and reported to the physician.

Client/Family Teaching

1. Review appropriate method and frequency for application.
2. Advise that more frequent than prescribed applications will not enhance hair growth but will increase systemic side effects.
3. Advise the client that the new hair growth is not permanent. Cessation of therapy will lead to hair loss within a few months. Thus, the topical minoxidil must be used for an indefinite period of time.
4. Discuss the fact that the treatment has positive benefits for only approximately one-half the population. Assist the client to set realistic goals.
5. Explain that it may take up to 4 months of continuous therapy before any response is noted.
6. Instruct client to report any evidence of irritation or rash at the site of treatment.
7. Do not apply any other topical products to the scalp without physician consent.

Evaluation: Evaluate client for evidence of hair regrowth in a previously bald scalp area.

Misoprostol

(my-soh-**PROST**-ohl)
Cytotec (Rx)

Classification: Prostaglandin.

Action/Kinetics: Misoprostol is a synthetic prostaglandin E_1 analog that inhibits gastric acid secretion, protects the gastric mucosa by increasing bicarbonate and mucous production, and decreases pepsin levels during basal conditions. The drug may also stimulate uterine contractions that may endanger pregnancy. Misoprostol is rapidly converted to the active misoprostol acid. **Time for peak levels of misoprostol acid:** 12 min. **t½, misoprostol acid:** 20–40 min. Misoprostol acid is less than 90% bound to plasma protein. **Note:** Misoprostol does not prevent development of duodenal ulcers in clients on NSAIDs.

Uses: Prevention of aspirin and other nonsteroidal anti-inflammatory-induced gastric ulcers in clients with a high risk of gastric ulcer complications (e.g., geriatric clients with debilitating disease) or in those with a history of ulcer. Prevent duodenal ulcers in clients who use nonsteroidal anti-inflammatory drugs chronically.

Contraindications: Allergy to prostaglandins, pregnancy (category: X), during lactation (may cause diarrhea in nursing infants).

Special Concerns: Use with caution in clients with renal impairment and in clients older than 64 years of age. Safety and efficacy have not been established in children less than 18 years of age.

Side Effects: *GI:* Diarrhea, abdominal pain, nausea, dyspepsia, flatulence, vomiting, constipation. *Gynecologic:* Cramps, dysmenorrhea, hypermenorrhea, menstrual disorders, postmenopausal vaginal bleeding. *Miscellaneous:* Headache. *Symptoms of Overdose:* Abdominal pain, diarrhea, dyspnea, sedation, tremor, fever, palpitations, bradycardia, hypotension, seizures.

Dosage: Tablets. Adults: 200 mcg q.i.d. with food. Dose can be reduced to 100 mcg if the larger dose cannot be tolerated. In renal impairment, the 200 mcg dose can be reduced if necessary.

NURSING CONSIDERATIONS

Administration/Storage

1. The incidence of diarrhea can be reduced by giving the drug after meals and at bedtime as well as by avoiding magnesium-containing antacids. Diarrhea is usually self-limiting, however.
2. Maximum plasma levels of misoprostol are decreased if the drug is taken with food.
3. Misoprostol should be taken for the duration of nonsteroidal anti-inflammatory therapy.
4. Drug may increase gastric bicarbonate and mucous production.
5. Available in both 100-mcg and 200-mcg tablets.
6. *Treatment of Overdose:* Use supportive therapy.

Assessment

1. Obtain a negative pregnancy test on females of childbearing age prior to initiating drug therapy.
2. Document any history of ulcer disease.

Client/Family Teaching

1. Provide both oral and written warnings of adverse drug effects. Instruct client to keep a record of events to share with the physician so that side effects and drug therapy can be evaluated.
2. Remind clients not to share medications with anyone.
3. Take misoprostol exactly as prescribed for the duration of aspirin or NSAID therapy.
4. Stress that all women of childbearing age must practice effective contraceptive measures because drug has abortifacient properties.
5. Clients may experience abdominal discomfort and/or diarrhea. Instruct them to take misoprostol after meals and at bedtime to minimize these side effects.
6. Persistent diarrhea or increased menstrual bleeding should be reported to the physician.

Evaluation: Evaluate for the prevention of drug-induced gastric ulcers during therapy with NSAIDs or ASA.

Mitomycin
(my-toe-**MY**-sin)
Mutamycin (Abbreviation: MTC) (Rx)

See also *Antineoplastic Agents,* p. 85.

Classification: Antineoplastic, antibiotic.

Action/Kinetics: Antibiotic produced by *Streptomyces caespitosus* that inhibits DNA synthesis. At high doses both RNA and protein synthesis are inhibited. Most active during late G_1 and early S stages. Not recommended as a single agent for primary treatment or in place of surgery and/or radiotherapy. $t\frac{1}{2}$, **initial:** 5–15 min; **final:** 50 min. Metabolized in liver; 10% excreted unchanged in urine, more when dose is increased.

Uses: Palliative treatment and adjunct to surgical or radiologic treatment of disseminated adenocarcinoma of the stomach and pancreas. Used in combination with other agents. *Investigational:* Superficial bladder cancer; cancer of the breast, head and neck, lung, cervix; colorectal cancer; biliary cancer; chronic myelocytic leukemia. Ophthalmic solution used as an adjunct to surgical excision to treat primary or recurrent pterygia.

Contraindications: Pregnancy and lactation. Thrombocytopenia, coagulation disorders, increase in bleeding tendency due to other causes. In clients with a serum creatinine level greater than 1.7 mg/dl.

Special Concerns: Use with extreme caution in presence of impaired renal function.

Additional Side Effects: Severe bone marrow depression, especially leukopenia and thrombocytopenia. Pulmonary toxicity including dyspnea with nonproductive cough. Microangiopathic hemolytic anemia with renal failure and hypertension (hemolytic uremic syndrome), especially when used long-term in combination with fluorouracil. Cellulitis. Extravasation causes severe necrosis of surrounding tissue. Respiratory distress syndrome in adults especially when used with other chemotherapy.

Drug Interaction: Severe bronchospasm and shortness of breath when used with vinca alkaloids.

Dosage: IV only: 10–20 mg/m^2 as a single dose via infusion q 6–8 wk. Subsequent courses of treatment are based on hematologic response and should not be repeated until leukocyte count is at least 4,000/mm^3 and platelet count is at least 100,000/mm^3.

NURSING CONSIDERATIONS

See also *Nursing Considerations for Antineoplastic Agents,* p. 88.

Administration/Storage

1. Drug is toxic, and extravasation is to be avoided.
2. Reconstitute 5-, 20-, or 40-mg vial with 10, 40, or 80 ml sterile water for injection respectively, as indicated on label. Medication will dissolve if allowed to remain at room temperature.
3. Drug at concentration of 0.5 mg/ml is stable for 14 days under refrigeration or for 7 days at room temperature.
4. Diluted to a concentration of 20–40 mcg/ml, the drug is stable for 3 hr in D$_5$W, for 12 hr in isotonic saline, and for 24 hr in sodium lactate injection.
5. Mitomycin (5–15 mg) and heparin (1,000–10,000 units) in 30 ml of isotonic saline is stable for 48 hr at room temperature.

Assessment

1. Obtain baseline CBC, PT, PTT, and platelets, and note any evidence of abnormalities.
2. Assess renal function and do not initiate drug therapy if serum creatinine level is greater than 1.7 mg/dl.

Interventions

1. Observe closely for early evidence of pulmonary complications, such as dyspnea, nonproductive cough, and abnormal lung sounds and ABGs.
2. Monitor CBC and renal function studies carefully throughout therapy.
3. Observe infusion site closely for any evidence of erythema or client complaints of discomfort.

Evaluation: Evaluate client for evidence of a ↓ in tumor size and spread.

M

Mitotane (O,P'-DDD)
(MY-toe-tayn)
Lysodren (Rx)

See also *Antineoplastic Agents,* p. 85.

Classification: Antihormone.

Action/Kinetics: Mitotane directly suppresses activity of adrenal cortex. It also changes the peripheral metabolism of corticosteroids resulting in a decrease in 17-hydroxycorticosteroids. About 40% of drug absorbed from GI tract; detectable in serum for long periods of time (6–9 weeks after administration). Drug, however, mostly stored in adipose tissue. **t½:** After therapy terminated, 18–159 days. Unchanged drug and metabolites are excreted in the bile and eventually the feces. Steroid replacement therapy may have to be instituted (i.e., increased) to correct adrenal insufficiency. Therapy is continued as long as drug seems effective. Beneficial results may not become apparent until after 3 months of therapy.

Use: Inoperable cancer of the adrenal cortex. *Investigational:* Cushing's syndrome.

Contraindications: Hypersensitivity to drug. Discontinue temporarily after shock or severe trauma.

Special Concerns: Pregnancy category: C. Use with caution in the presence of liver disease other than metastatic lesions. Long-term usage may cause brain damage and functional impairment. Use during lactation only if benefits outweigh risks.

Additional Side Effects: Adrenal insufficiency. *CNS:* Depression, sedation, vertigo, lethargy. *Ophthalmic:* Blurring, diplopia, retinopathy, opacity of lens. *Renal:* Hemorrhagic cystitis, hematuria, proteinuria. *Cardiovascular:* Flushing, orthostatic hypotension, hypertension. *Miscellaneous:* Hyperpyrexia, skin rashes, aching of body.

Drug Interactions: Mitotane may ↑ rate of metabolism of heparin requiring an increase of dosage.

Laboratory Test Interferences: ↓ PBI and urinary 17-hydroxycorticosteroids.

Dosage: Tablets: Adults, initial, 8–10 g/day in 3–4 equally divided doses (maximum tolerated dose may range from 2–16 g daily). Adjust dosage upward or downward according to severity of side effects or lack thereof. **Usual maintenance:** 8–10 g/day. **Pediatric, initial:** 1–2 g/day in divided doses; **then,** dose can be increased gradually to 5–7 g daily. *Cushing's syndrome:* **initial,** 3–6 g daily in 3–4 divided doses; **then,** 0.5 mg two times a week to 2 g daily.

NURSING CONSIDERATIONS

See also *Nursing Considerations* for *Antineoplastic Agents,* p. 88.

Administration/Storage

1. Institute treatment in hospital until stable dosage schedule is achieved.
2. Treatment should be continued for 3 months to determine beneficial effects.
3. To counteract shock or trauma, be prepared to administer steroid medications in high doses, because depressed adrenals may not produce sufficient steroids.

Assessment

1. Assess for evidence of brain damage by performing behavioral and neurologic assessments of client.
2. Note any history of sensitivity to mitotane and document any episodes of shock or severe trauma that would necessitate discontinuation of drug therapy.

Client/Family Teaching

1. Symptoms of adrenal insufficiency, such as weakness, increased fatigue, lethargy, and GI effects (including weight loss and anorexia) should be reported to the physician.
2. Stress the importance of wearing Medic Alert identification in case of trauma or shock, and carrying a list of drugs currently prescribed.
3. Avoid tasks that require mental alertness until drug effects are realized.

Evaluation: Evaluate client for evidence of a ↓ in tumor size and spread.

Mitoxantrone hydrochloride
(my-toe-**ZAN**-trohn)
Novantrone (Rx)

Classification: Antineoplastic agent, antibiotic.

Action/Kinetics: Mitoxantrone is most active in the late S phase of cell division but is not cell-cycle specific. The drug appears to bind to DNA by intercalation between base pairs and a nonintercalative electrostatic interaction; this results in inhibition of DNA and RNA synthesis. Distribution to tissues such as the brain, spinal cord, spinal fluid, and eyes is low. **t½:** Approximately 6 days. Mitoxantrone is highly bound to plasma proteins. The drug is excreted through both the feces (via the bile) and the urine (up to 65% unchanged).

Uses: In combination with other drugs, for the initial treatment of acute nonlymphocytic leukemias, including monocytic, promyelocytic, myelocytic, and acute erythroid leukemias. *Investigational:* Alone or in combination with other drugs to treat breast and liver cancer; non-Hodgkin's lymphomas.

Contraindications: Preexisting myelosuppression (unless benefits outweigh risks). During lactation. Intrathecal use.

Special Concerns: Pregnancy category: D. Safety and efficacy have not been established in children. The drug may be mutagenic.

Side Effects: *Hematologic:* Severe myelosuppression, ecchymosis, petechiae. *GI:* Nausea, vomiting, diarrhea, stomatitis, mucositis, abdominal pain, GI bleeding. *CNS:* Headache, seizures. *CV:* Congestive heart failure, decreases in left ventricular ejection fraction, arrhythmias, tachycardia, chest pain, hypotension. *Respiratory:* Cough, dyspnea. *Miscellaneous:* Conjunctivitis, urticaria, rashes, renal failure, hyperuricemia, alopecia, fever, phlebitis (at infusion site), tissue necrosis (as a result of extravasation), jaundice. In addition, there is an increased risk of pneumonia, urinary tract and fungal infections, and sepsis. *Symptoms of Overdose:* Severe leukopenia with infection.

Laboratory Test Interference: Transient ↑ AST and ALT.

Dosage: IV infusion. *Initial therapy for acute nonlymphocytic leukemia, induction:* mitoxantrone, 12 mg/m²/day on days 1–3 combined with cytosine arabinoside, 100 mg/m² as a continuous 24-hr infusion on days 1–7. If the response is incomplete, a second induction course may be given using the same daily dosage, but giving mitoxantrone for 2 days and cytosine arabinoside for 5 days. *Consolidation therapy, approximately 6 weeks after final induction therapy:* mitoxantrone, 12 mg/m²/day on days 1 and 2 combined with cytosine arabinoside, 100 mg/m² as a continuous 24-hr infusion on days 1–5. A second consolidation course of therapy may be given 4 weeks after the first.

NURSING CONSIDERATIONS

See also *Administration* and *Nursing Considerations* for *Antineoplastic Agents,* p. 88.

Administration/Storage

1. The drug should not be frozen.
2. The client must be closely monitored for chemical, laboratory, and hematologic values.
3. Mitoxantrone should not be mixed in the same infusion with other drugs.
4. Mitoxantrone must be diluted prior to use with a minimum of 50 ml of either 5% dextrose injection or 0.9% sodium chloride injection.
5. The diluted solution is given into a freely running IV infusion of either 5% dextrose injection or 0.9% sodium chloride injection over a period of at least 3 min.
6. Maintain infusion on an electronic infusion device.
7. Care should be taken to avoid extravasation at the injection site. Also, the solution should not come in contact with the eyes, mucous membranes, or skin.
8. Hospital procedures for the handling and disposal of antineoplastic drugs should be followed closely.
9. *Treatment of Overdose:* Antibiotic therapy. Monitor hematology.

Assessment

1. Obtain baseline hematologic and chemistry studies and monitor throughout therapy; drug causes severe myelosuppression.
2. Note any history of cardiac disease; perform baseline ECG.
3. Assess liver and renal function and determine uric acid level.

Interventions

1. Monitor vital signs and closely observe client during therapy for any adverse side effects.
2. Initiate appropriate precautions for clients with severe myelosuppression.
3. Anticipate nausea, vomiting, mucositis, and stomatitis as side effects, and initiate appropriate protocol.
4. Monitor uric acid levels and, if elevated, determine the need for allopurinol therapy.

Client/Family Teaching

1. Advise females of childbearing age to practice conception during drug therapy.
2. Drug may discolor urine and/or sclera a greenish blue color 24 hr after therapy. This is only temporary.
3. Provide a printed list of drug side effects stressing those that require immediate reporting such as persistent diarrhea, nausea and vomiting, abnormal bruising and bleeding, severe dyspnea, and any evidence of infection.

Evaluation: Evaluate client for:

- Laboratory evidence of improved hematologic parameters
- Evidence of a ↓ in tumor size and spread

—— COMBINATION DRUG ——
Modicon 21 Day and Modicon 28 Day
(MOD-ih-kon)
(Rx)

See also *Oral Contraceptives,* p. 192.

Classification: Monophasic combination oral contraceptive.

Components: Each tablet of Modicon 21 Day and the first 21 tablets of Modicon 28 day contains ethinyl estradiol, 35 mcg and norethindrone, 0.5 mg (white tablets); the 28s also contain 7 inert green tablets.

Special Concerns: Pregnancy category: X.

NURSING CONSIDERATIONS

See *Nursing Considerations* for *Oral Contraceptives,* p. 195.

Monoctanoin
(mahn-**OCK**-tah-noyn)
Moctanin (Rx)

Classification: Solubilizer for gallstones.

Action/Kinetics: Monoctanoin is a semisynthetic esterified glycerol that causes complete dissolution of gallstones in approximately one-third of treated clients, with an additional one-third manifesting a decrease in the size of stones. The decreased size may allow the stone to pass spontaneously.

Uses: To solubilize cholesterol gallstones located in the biliary tract, especially when other treatments have failed or cannot be undertaken. Most effective if the stones are radiolucent.

Contraindications: Biliary tract infection, recent duodenal ulcer or jejunitis, clinical jaundice, impaired hepatic function, acute pancreatitis, porto-systemic shunting.

Special Concerns: Use with caution during pregnancy (category: C) and lactation. Safety and effectiveness in children have not been established.

Side Effects: *GI:* Irritation of GI and biliary tracts, ascending cholangitis, erythema in antral and duodenal mucosa, ulceration or irritation of the mucosa of the common bile duct, duodenal erosion, abdominal pain or discomfort, nausea, vomiting, diarrhea, indigestion, anorexia, burning, bile shock. *CNS:* Fever, fatigue, lethargy, depression, headache. *Other:* Leukopenia, pruritus, chills, diaphoresis, hypokalemia, allergic symptoms.

Dosage: Infusion via catheter inserted into common bile duct. Perfuse at rate not to exceed 3–5 ml/hr at a pressure of 10 cm water (to minimize irritation) for 7–21 days.

NURSING CONSIDERATIONS

Administration/Storage

1. The drug should not be administered IM or IV.
2. The drug should be maintained at a temperature of 37°C (98.6°F) for maximum effects.
3. To reduce viscosity and enhance the bathing effect on the stones, the drug should be diluted with 120 ml sterile water for injection.
4. Perfusion pressure should never exceed 15 cm water (use overflow manometer or peristaltic pump).
5. The perfusion should be continued for approximately 9–10 days after which X-ray or endoscopy studies should be conducted. If tests do not show a reduction in size or dissolution of stones, the drug should be discontinued.
6. Irritation of the GI and biliary tracts may occur. These usually disappear within 2–7 days after the termination of therapy.
7. The drug is intended only for direct biliary duct infusion.

Assessment

1. Note if the client has a history of biliary tract infection or recent duodenal ulcer.
2. If the client has a history of hepatic dysfunction, obtain baseline liver function studies.

Interventions

1. Note any client complaint of GI irritation.
2. Monitor stools for occult blood. Document and report to the physician.
3. Observe the client for fever, lethargy, depression, pruritus, diaphoresis, and hypokalemia. Document and report these findings to the physician.

Evaluation: Evaluate client for:
- Radiographic evidence of a complete dissolution of gallstones or a marked decrease in the size of stones
- Evidence of freedom from complication of prolonged direct bile duct infusion

---

Moricizine hydrochloride

(mor-**IS**-ih-zeen)

Ethmozine (Rx)

Classification: Antiarrhythmic, type I.

Action/Kinetics: Moricizine causes a stabilizing effect on the myocardial membranes as well as local anesthetic activity. The drug shortens phase II and III repolarization leading to a decreased duration of the action potential and an effective refractory period. Also, there is a decrease in the maximum rate of phase O depolarization and a prolongation of AV conduction in clients with ventricular tachycardia. Whether the client is at rest or is exercising, moricizine has minimal effects on cardiac index, stroke index volume, systemic or pulmonary vascular resistance or ejection fraction, and pulmonary capillary wedge pressure. There is a small increase in resting blood pressure and heart rate. Neither the time, course, nor intensity of antiarrhythmic and electrophysiologic effects is related to plasma levels of the drug. **Peak plasma levels:** 30–120 min. **t½:** 2–3 hr. Significant first-pass effect. Metabolized almost completely by the liver with metabolites excreted through both the urine and feces; the drug induces its own metabolism. Food delays the rate of absorption resulting in lower peak plasma levels; however, the total amount absorbed is not changed.

Uses: Documented life-threatening ventricular arrhythmias (e.g., sustained ventricular tachycardia) where benefits of the drug are determined to outweigh the risks.

Contraindications: Preexisting second- or third-degree block, right bundle branch block when associated with bifascicular block (unless the client has a pacemaker), cardiogenic shock. Use during lactation.

Special Concerns: Pregnancy category: B. Safety and effectiveness in children less than 18 years of age have not been determined. Geriatric clients have a higher rate of side effects. Increased survival rates following use of antiarrhythmic drugs have not been proven in clients with ventricular arrhythmias. Use with caution in clients with sick sinus syndrome due to the possibility of sinus bradycardia, sinus pause, or sinus arrest. Use with caution in clients with congestive heart failure.

Side Effects: *CV:* Proarrhythmias, including new rhythm disturbances or worsening of existing arrhythmias; ECG abnormalities, including conduction defects, sinus pause, function rhythm, AV block; palpitations, sustained ventricular tachy-cardia, cardiac chest pain, congestive heart failure, cardiac death, hypotension, hypertension, atrial fibrillation, atrial flutter, syncope, bradycardia, cardiac arrest, myocardial infarction, pulmonary embolism, vasodilation, thrombophlebitis, cerebrovascular events. *CNS:* Dizziness (common), anxiety, headache, fatigue, nervousness, paresthesias, sleep disorders, tremor, hypoesthesias, depression, euphoria, somnolence, agitation, confusion, seizures, hallucinations, loss of memory, vertigo, coma. *GI:* Nausea, dry mouth, abdominal pain, vomiting, diarrhea, dyspepsia, anorexia, ileus, flatulence, dysphagia, bitter taste. *Musculoskeletal:* Asthenia, abnormal gait, akathisia, ataxia, abnormal coordination, dyskinesia, pain. *GU:* Urinary retention, dysuria, urinary incontinence, urinary frequency, impotence, kidney pain, decreased libido. *Respiratory:* Dyspnea, apnea, asthma, hyperventilation, pharyngitis, cough, sinusitis. *Opthalmologic:* Nystagmus, diplopia, blurred vision, eye pain, periorbital edema. *Dermatologic:* Rash, pruritus, dry skin, urticaria. *Miscellaneous:* Sweating, drug fever, hypothermia, temperature intolerance, swelling of the lips and tongue, jaundice. *Symptoms of Overdose:* Vomiting, hypotension, lethargy, worsening of congestive heart failure, myocardial infarction, conduction disturbances, arrhythmias, sinus arrest, respiratory failure.

Drug Interactions

Cimetidine / ↑ Plasma levels of mori023cizine due to ↓ excretion

Digoxin / Additive prolongation of the PR interval (but no significant increase in the rate of second- or third-degree AV block)

Propranolol / Additive prolongation of the PR interval

Theophylline / ↓ Plasma levels of theophylline due to ↑ rate of clearance

Laboratory Test Interferences: ↑ Bilirubin and liver transaminases.

Dosage: Tablets. Adults: 600–900 mg daily in equally divided doses q 8 hr. If needed, the dose can be increased in increments of 150 mg daily at 3-day intervals until the desired effect is obtained.

NURSING CONSIDERATIONS

See also *Nursing Considerations* for *Antiarrhythmic Drugs*, p. 52.

Administration/Storage

1. When transferring clients from other antiarrhythmics to moricizine, the previous drug should be withdrawn for 1–2 plasma half-lives before starting moricizine. For example, when transferring from quinidine or disopyramide, moricizine can be started 6–12 hr after the last dose; when transferring from procainamide, moricizine can be initiated 3–6 hr after the last dose, and when transferring from encainide, mexiletine, propafenone, or tocainide, moricizine can be started 8–12 hr after the last dose.
2. If clients are well controlled on an 8-hr regimen, they might be given the same total daily dose q 12 hr in order to increase compliance.
3. *Treatment of Overdose:* In acute overdose, induce vomiting, taking care to prevent aspiration. Client should be hospitalized and closely monitored for cardiac, respiratory, and CNS changes. Provide life support, including an intracardiac pacing catheter, if necessary.

Assessment

1. Document cardiac history and note any preexisting conditions and ECG abnormalities.
2. Obtain baseline ECG, electrolytes, liver and renal function studies.
3. List drugs client currently taking to determine any potential adverse interactions.

Interventions

1. Monitor cardiac rhythm closely to observe for drug-induced rhythm disturbances during therapy.
2. Anticipate lower initial doses in clients with impaired hepatic or renal function.
3. Clients should be hospitalized for initial dosing because they will be at high risk. Antiarrhythmic response may be determined by cardiac rhythm monitoring, ECG intervals, exercise testing, or programmed electrical stimulation testing.
4. Correct any electrolyte imbalance before initiating drug therapy.
5. Document and monitor pacing parameters in clients with pacemakers.
6. Monitor vital signs and report any persistent temperature elevations.

Client/Family Teaching

1. Take before meals because food delays the rate of absorption.
2. Provide a printed list of side effects that require immediate reporting to the physician.

3. Drug may cause dizziness. Use care when rising from a lying or sitting position.

Evaluation: Evaluate client for:
- ECG evidence of termination of life-threatening ventricular arrhythmias
- Freedom from complications of drug therapy

Morphine hydrochloride
Morphitec✤, M.O.S.✤, M.O.S.-S.R.✤ (RxO

Morphine sulfate
(MOR-feen SUL-fayt)
Astramorph PF, Duramorph, Epimorph✤, Infumorph, Morphine H P✤, MS Contin, MSIR, Oramorph SR, RMS, RMS Rectal Suppositories, Roxanol, Roxanol 100, Roxanol SR, Roxanol UD, Statex✤ (C-II, Rx)

See also *Narcotic Analgesics,* p. 174.

Classification: Narcotic analgesic, morphine type.

Action/Kinetics: Morphine is the prototype for opiate analgesics. **Onset:** approximately 15–60 min. **Peak effect:** 30–60 min. **Duration:** 3–7 hr. **t½:** 1.5–2 hr. Oral morphine is only one-third to one-sixth as effective as parenteral products.

Uses: Intrathecally, epidurally, orally, or by continuous IV infusion for acute or chronic pain. In low doses, morphine is more effective against dull, continuous pain than against intermittent, sharp pain. Large doses, however, will dull almost any kind of pain. Preoperative med-

ication. To facilitate induction of anesthesia and reduce dose of anesthetic. *Investigational:* Acute left ventricular failure (for dyspneic seizures) and pulmonary edema. Morphine should not be used with papaverine for analgesia in biliary spasms but may be used with papaverine in acute vascular occlusions.

Additional Contraindications: Epidural or intrathecal morphine if infection is present at injection site, in clients on anticoagulant therapy, bleeding diathesis, if client has received parenteral corticosteroids within the past 2 weeks.

Special Concerns: Pregnancy category: C. Morphine may increase the length of labor. Clients with known seizure disorders may be at greater risk for morphine-induced seizure activity.

Dosage: Tablets, Oral Solution, Soluble Tablets. 10–30 mg q 4 hr. **Sustained-Release Tablets:** 30 mg q 8–12 hr, depending on client needs and response. **IM, SC: Adults,** 5–20 mg/70 kg q 4 hr as needed; **pediatric:** 100–200 mcg/kg up to a maximum of 15 mg. **IV infusion: Adults,** 2.5–15 mg/70 kg in 4–5 ml of water for injection (should be administered slowly over 4–5 min). **IV infusion, continuous:** 0.1–1 mg/ml in 5% dextrose in water by a controlled-infusion pump. **Rectal:** 10–20 mg q 4 hr. **Intrathecal: Adults,** 0.2–1 mg as a single daily injection. **Epidural: initial,** 5 mg daily in the lumbar region; if analgesia is not manifested in 1 hr, increasing doses of 1–2 mg can be given, not to exceed 10 mg daily. For continuous infusion, 2–4 mg daily with additional doses of 1–2 mg if analgesia is not satisfactory. Dose may be lower in geriatric clients or those with respiratory disease.

NURSING CONSIDERATIONS

See also *Nursing Considerations* for *Narcotic Analgesics,* p. 177.

Administration/Storage

1. Controlled-release tablets should not be crushed or chewed. May be administered with food to diminish GI upset.
2. Rapid IV administration increases the risk of adverse effects; a narcotic antagonist (e.g., naloxone) should be available at all times if morphine is given IV.
3. For intrathecal use, no more than 2 ml of the 5 mg/10 ml preparation or 1 ml of the 10 mg/10 ml product should be given.
4. Intrathecal administration should be only in the lumbar region; repeated injections are not recommended.
5. To reduce the chance of side effects with intrathecal administration, a constant IV infusion of naloxone (0.6 mg/hr for 24 hr after intrathecal injection) is recommended.
6. In certain circumstances (e.g., tolerance, severe pain), the physician may prescribe doses higher than those listed under dosage.
7. Use an electronic infusion device for IV solutions.
8. Obtain written parameters for BP and respirations during IV infusions.
9. Have naloxone available in the event of overdose.

Evaluation: Evaluate client for reports of effective control of pain.

Moxalactam disodium
(mox-ah-**LACK**-tam)
Moxam, Oxalactam ✱ (Rx)

See also *Anti-Infectives,* p. 80, and *Cephalosporins,* p. 132.

Classification: Antibiotic, third-generation cephalosporin.

Action/Kinetics: Broad-spectrum semisynthetic cephalosporin that is stable in the presence of beta-lactamase, penicillinase, and cephalosporinase. Cross-sensitivity with penicillin has not been observed; in selected cases, it can be used instead of chloramphenicol or aminoglycosides. Well absorbed into pleural, interstitial, and cerebrospinal (both normal and inflamed meninges) fluids, aqueous humor. **Peak serum concentrations (dose-dependent): IM,** 15 mcg/ml 1–2 hr after 500 mg; **IV infusion,** 57 mcg/ml after 500 mg. **t½, IM:** 2.1 hr (longer in clients with impaired renal function). From 60% to 90% of the drug is excreted by the kidneys within 24 hr.

Uses: Infections of the urinary tract, CNS (including ventriculitis and meningitis), skin and skin structures, bones, joints, and lower respiratory tract (including pneumonia). Intra-abdominal infections (including endometritis, pelvic cellulitis, peritonitis), bacterial septicemia, *Pseudomonas* infections. Used concomitantly with aminoglycosides in gram-positive or gram-negative sepsis or other serious infections in which the causative organism is not known.

Contraindications: Hypersensitivity to drug.

Special Concerns: Safe use during pregnancy not established (pregnancy category: C). Use with caution in individuals with history of sensitivity to penicillins or other cephalosporins.

Additional Side Effects: Hypoprothrombinemia resulting in bleeding and/or bruising.

Drug Interactions: Moxalactam may induce an Antabuse-like reaction if used with alcohol.

Laboratory Test Interferences: False + test for proteinuria with acid and denaturization-precipitation tests.

Dosage: Deep IM, IV. Adults, usual: 2–4 g daily in divided doses q 8–12 hr for 5–10 days (or up to 14 days). *Mild to moderate infections:* 0.5–2 g q 12 hr. *Mild skin and skin structure infections, uncomplicated pneumonia:* 0.5 g q 8 hr. *Mild, uncomplicated urinary tract infections:* 0.25 g q 12 hr. *Persistent or serious urinary tract infections:* 0.5 g q 8–12 hr. *Life-threatening infections or infections due to less susceptible organisms:* up to 4 g q 8 hr may be required. **Neonates up to 1 week:** 50 mg/kg q 12 hr; **1–4 weeks:** 50 mg/kg q 8 hr. **Infants:** 50 mg/kg q 6 hr. **Children:** 50 mg/kg q 6–8 hr. Pediatric dosage may be increased up to 200 mg/kg but should not exceed the maximum adult dosage. *For pediatric gram-negative meningitis:* initial loading dose, 100 mg/kg; **then,** follow above dosage regimen. *For clients with impaired renal function:* **initially,** 1–2 g; **maintenance:** see recommendations of manufacturer.

NURSING CONSIDERATIONS

See also *Nursing Considerations* for *Cephalosporins,* p. 134.

Administration/Storage

1. *IM:* 1 g moxalactam should be diluted with 3 ml of either sterile water for injection, bacteriostatic water for injection, 0.9% sodium chloride injection, bacteriostatic sodium chloride injection, or 0.5% lidocaine injection.
2. *Intermittent IV:* 1 g moxalactam should be diluted with 10 ml sterile water for injection, 5% dextrose injection, or 0.9% sodium chloride injection. Inject slowly over 3–5 min by physician. (**Note:** IV solutions containing alcohol should be avoided.) If a Y-tube administration set is used, the other solution should be discontinued while moxalactam is being administered.
3. *Continuous IV infusion:* 1 g moxalactam should be diluted with 10 ml sterile water for injection and added to appropriate IV solution.
4. Rotate frequently and observe IV site for phlebitis during IV administration.
5. Anticipate that 10 mg/week of vitamin K should be given to clients receiving moxalactam.
6. Anticipate different dosing technique for clients with altered renal function.
7. Reconstituted moxalactam is stable for 96 hr when refrigerated (5°C, 41°F) and for 24 hr at room temperature.

Assessment

1. Assess for bleeding during therapy, caused by eradication of intestinal bacteria that produce vitamin K.
2. If drug administered with aminoglycosides, monitor renal

M

function studies for potentiation of nephrotoxic effect.

Client/Family Teaching: Alcohol should not be ingested while on therapy with moxalactam, because an Antabuse-like reaction may occur.

Evaluation

1. Review PT/PTT for evidence of impairment related to drug therapy and determine if weekly dose of vitamin K is effective.
2. Review status of pretreatment symptoms and C&S results to determine effectiveness of therapy.

Mupirocin

(myou-**PEER**-oh-sin)
Bactroban (Rx)

Classification: Anti-infective, topical.

Action/Kinetics: Mupirocin exerts its antibacterial action by binding to bacterial isoleucyl transfer-RNA synthetase, which results in inhibition of protein synthesis by the organism. The drug is not absorbed into the systemic circulation. Serum present in exudative wounds decreases the antibacterial activity. Mupirocin is metabolized to the inactive monic acid in the skin and is then removed by normal skin desquamation. There is no cross resistance with other antibiotics such as chloramphenicol, erythromycin, gentamicin, lincomycin, methicillin, neomycin, novobiocin, penicillin, streptomycin, or tetracyclines.

Uses: Topically to treat impetigo

due to *Staphylococcus aureus, Streptococcus pyogenes,* and beta-hemolytic streptococcus.

Contraindications: Ophthalmic use. Lactation.

Special Concerns: Pregnancy category: B. Superinfection may result from chronic use.

Side Effects: Superinfection, rash, burning, stinging, pain, nausea, tenderness, erythema, swelling, dry skin, contact dermatitis, and increased exudate.

Dosage: Topical Ointment. A small amount of ointment is applied to the affected area t.i.d.

NURSING CONSIDERATIONS

Administration/Storage: A gauze dressing may be used if desired.

Client/Family Teaching

1. Demonstrate the appropriate technique for applying topical medications. Review hygienic measures and stress the importance of hand washing to prevent spread.
2. Report any symptoms of chemical irritation or hypersensitivity such as increased rash, itching, or pain at the site.
3. If no improvement is noted after 3–5 days of therapy, notify physician.
4. Notify school nurse to ensure appropriate screening is performed when treating school-aged children.

Evaluation: Evaluate client for evidence of healing with a decrease in lesions and reports of symptomatic improvement.

Muromonab-CD3

(myour-oh-**MON**-ab)

Orthoclone OKT3 (Rx)

Classification: Immunosuppressive agent.

Action/Kinetics: Muromonab-CD3 is a murine monoclonal antibody; the antibody is a purified IgG_{2a} immunoglobulin. The antibody acts to prevent rejection of transplanted kidney tissue by blocking the action of T cells, which play a significant role in acute rejection. Specifically, the CD3 molecule in the membrane of T cells is blocked; this molecule is necessary for signal transduction. The drug does not cause myelosuppression. Antibodies to muromonab-CD3 have been observed after approximately 20 days. **Average serum levels after 3 days:** 0.9 mcg/ml. **Time to steady-state trough levels:** 3 days. **Duration:** 1 week for return of circulating CD3 positive T cells to pretreatment levels.

Uses: To reverse acute allograft rejection in kidney transplant clients; used in combination with azathioprine, cyclosporine, corticosteroids. *Investigational:* Treat acute rejection of liver and heart transplants.

Contraindications: Hypersensitivity to drug (or any product of murine origin), clients with edema (fluid overload). Use during lactation.

Special Concerns: Use during pregnancy only if benefits outweigh risks (pregnancy category: C). Although used in children, safety and effectiveness have not been assessed.

Side Effects: Significant and serious side effects may occur within 0.5–6 hr following the first dose. Thus, therapy must be initiated in a hospital by physicians experienced in immunosuppressive therapy and where equipment is available to perform cardiopulmonary resuscitation. *First-dose symptoms:* Fever, chills (can be minimized by giving 1 mg/kg methylprednisolone sodium succinate; can be reversed by giving acetaminophen and/or by using a cooling blanket); dyspnea (can be minimized or reversed by giving 100 mg hydrocortisone sodium succinate injection within 30 min after muromonab-CD3 administration, with an additional 100 mg as needed); pulmonary edema (can be minimized by ensuring a clear chest, using X ray within 24 hr of injection, or by ensuring that less than a 3% weight gain has occurred in the week prior to drug injection; can be reversed by prompt intubation and use of oxygen). *Within first 2 days of therapy:* Fever, chills, dyspnea, wheezing, chest pain, nausea, vomiting, diarrhea, tremor, severe pulmonary edema. *Within 45 days of therapy:* Infections (which may be life-threatening) due to cytomegalovirus, herpes simplex virus, *Staphylococcus epidermidis, Pneumocystis carinii, Legionella, Cryptococcus, Serratia,* and other gram-negative bacteria.

Dosage: IV bolus. Adults: 5 mg daily for 10–14 days; **pediatric, less than 12 years:** 0.1 mg/kg daily for 10–14 days.

NURSING CONSIDERATIONS

Administration/Storage

1. Treatment should be initiated as soon as acute renal rejection is diagnosed.

2. The bolus should be given in less than 1 min.

3. The drug is not to be given by IV infusion or with any other drug solutions.

4. If the body temperature of the client is 100°F (37.8°C), drug therapy should not be initiated.

5. The solution (which is a protein) should be drawn into a syringe through a 0.2- or 0.22-μm filter; the filter is then discarded and the needle attached.

6. The appearance of a few translucent particles of protein does not affect the potency of the preparation.

7. The dose of other immunosuppressant drugs should be decreased as follows during muromonab-CD3 use: prednisone, 0.5 mg/kg daily; azathioprine, 25 mg daily. Cyclosporine should be discontinued. Maintenance doses of these drugs can be resumed approximately 3 days prior to termination of muromonab-CD3 therapy.

8. The drug should be stored at 2°C–8°C (36°F–46°F) and should not be frozen or shaken.

Assessment

1. Determine if client has received this drug therapy in the past and assess closely for evidence of antibodies.

2. Note any history of sensitivity to murine derivatives.

Interventions

1. Monitor the client's intake and output, assess for positive fluid balance, and report.

2. Obtain CXR and report any evidence of congestion.

3. Weigh the client daily and document and report any evidence of rapid weight gain in excess of 3%/week.

4. Take the client's temperature every 4 hr. If the temperature goes above 100°F (37.7°C), withhold the drug until the temperature goes below 100°F (37.7°C). Monitor CBC with differential and circulating T cells.

5. Monitor the client's renal status for a decrease in urine volume and a decrease in creatinine clearance. These are signs of transplant rejection and should be reported to the physician immediately.

6. Administer acetaminophen for flu-like symptoms and febrile reaction. This is usually noted after the first dose.

7. Symptoms of aseptic meningitis are usually evident within 3 days. Fever, headache, nuchal rigidity, and photophobia characterize this condition.

Client/Family Teaching

1. Explain to the client that chills, fever, shortness of breath, and malaise are first-dose symptoms that will diminish on consecutive treatment days.

2. Any symptoms of dyspnea, chest pain, nausea and vomiting, or infection require immediate reporting to the physician.

Evaluation: Evaluate client for clinical and laboratory evidence of successful treatment of acute rejection of organ transplant.

—— *COMBINATION DRUG* ——
Mylanta Liquid and Tablets
(my-**LAN**-tah)
(OTC)

Mylanta-II Liquid and Tablets
(my-**LAN**-tah)
(OTC)

See also *Antacids,* p. 37.

Classification/Content: Mylanta. Each tablet or 5 ml contains: *Antacid:* Aluminum hydroxide, 200 mg; *Antacid:* Magnesium hydroxide, 200 mg; and, *Antiflatulent:* Simethicone, 20 mg. The acid neutralizing capacity is 25.4 mEq/20 ml of the liquid and 23.0 mEq/2 tablets. **Mylanta-II.** Each tablet or 5 ml contains: *Antacid:* Aluminum hydroxide, 400 mg; *Antacid:* Magnesium hydroxide, 400 mg; and, *Antiflatulent:* Simethicone, 40 mg. The acid neutralizing capacity is 50.8 mEq/10 ml of the liquid and 46 mEq/2 tablets. See also information on individual components.

Uses: Symptoms due to heartburn, gastritis, peptic ulcer, hiatal hernia, and peptic esophagitis. The product also relieves accompanying distress due to gas and swallowed air.

Dosage: Oral Suspension, Chewable Tablets. *Mylanta or* *Mylanta-II.* **Adults:** 10–20 ml of the liquid or 2–4 tablets between meals and at bedtime.

NURSING CONSIDERATIONS

See also *Nursing Considerations* for *Antacids,* p. 38.

Administration/Storage: The gastric acid output and gastric emptying time vary greatly; thus, the dosage schedule should be individualized.

Client/Family Teaching

1. Chew tablets well before swallowing.
2. If a suspension is to be used, shake the container well before pouring the medication.
3. Do not take more than 120 ml of the Oral Mylanta Suspension or 60 ml of the Oral Mylanta II suspension in a 24-hr period.
4. If the client is taking Mylanta Tablets, advise the client to take no more than 24 Mylanta tablets or 12 Mylanta II tablets per day. If there is no relief, notify the physician.
5. If the client is taking tetracycline, advise the physician so that therapy with these products can be avoided.

Evaluation: Evaluate client for reports of improvement in symptoms of GI irritability.

M

N

—— COMBINATION DRUG ——
N.E.E. 1/35 21 Day and N.E.E. 1/35 28 Day
(Rx)

See also *Oral Contraceptives*, p. 192.

Classification: Monophasic combination oral contraceptive.

Components: Each tablet of N.E.E. 1/35 21 day and the first 21 tablets of N.E.E. 1/35 28 Day contains ethinyl estradiol, 35 mcg and norethindrone, 1 mg (yellow tablets); the 28s also contain 7 inert peach tablets.

Special Concerns: Pregnancy category: X.

NURSING CONSIDERATIONS

See *Oral Contraceptives*, p. 192.

Nadolol
(NAY-doh-lohl)
Apo-Nadol✲, Corgard, Syn-Nadolol✲ (Rx)

See also *Beta-Adrenergic Blocking Agents*, p. 113.

Classification: Beta-adrenergic blocking agent.

Action/Kinetics: Manifests both beta-1 and beta-2 adrenergic blocking activity. Has no membrane stabilizing or intrinsic sympathomimetic activity. Low lipid solubility. **Peak serum concentration:** 3–4 hr. **t½:** 20–24 hr (permits once-daily dosage). **Duration:** 17–24 hr. Absorption variable, averaging 30%; steady plasma level achieved after 6–9 days of administration. Excreted unchanged by the kidney.

Uses: Hypertension, either alone or with other drugs (e.g., thiazide diuretic). Angina pectoris. *Investigational:* Prophylaxis of migraine, ventricular arrhythmias, treatment of lithium-induced tremors, aggressive behavior, essential tremor, tremors associated with lithium or parkinsonism, antipsychotic-induced akathisia, rebleeding of esophageal varices, situational anxiety, reduce intraocular pressure.

Special Concerns: Pregnancy category: C. Dosage has not been established in children.

Dosage: Tablets. *Hypertension:* **initial,** 40 mg once daily; **then,** may be increased in 40- to 80-mg intervals until optimum response obtained. **Maintenance:** 40–80 mg once daily although up to 320 mg once daily may be needed. *Angina:* **initial,** 40 mg once daily; **then,** increase dose in 40-to 80-mg increments q 3–7 days until optimum response obtained. **Maintenance:** 40–80 mg once daily, although up to 240 mg once daily may be needed. *Aggressive behavior:* 40–160 mg daily. *Antipsychotic-induced akathisia:* 40–80 mg daily. *Essential tremor:* 120–240 mg daily. *Lithium-induced tremors:* 20–40 mg daily. *Tremors associated with parkinsonism:* 80–320 mg daily. *Prophylaxis of migraine:* 40–80 mg daily. *Rebleeding from esophageal varices:* 40–160 mg daily. *Situational anxiety:* 20 mg. *Ventricular arrhythmias:* 10–640 mg daily. *Reduction of intraocular pressure:* 10–20 mg b.i.d. Dosage for all uses should be decreased in clients with renal failure.

NURSING CONSIDERATIONS

See *Nursing Considerations* for *Beta-Adrenergic Blocking Agents,* p. 116.

Client/Family Teaching

1. Report any evidence of rapid weight gain, increased shortness of breath, or swelling of extremities.
2. Do not perform tasks that require mental alertness until drug effects realized. Nadolol may cause dizziness.
3. Drug may cause an increased sensitivity to cold.

Evaluation: Evaluate client for:
- Evidence of a reduction in blood pressure
- Reports of ↓ in frequency and intensity of angina attacks

Nafarelin acetate

(**NAF**-ah-rel-in)
Synarel (Rx)

Classification: Gonadotropin-releasing hormone.

Action/Kinetics: Nafarelin is a hormone produced through biotechnology; it differs by only one amino acid from naturally occurring gonadotropin-releasing hormone. The drug stimulates the release of luteinizing hormone (LH) and follicle-stimulating hormone (FSH) from the adenohypophysis. These hormones cause estrogen and progesterone synthesis in the ovary, resulting in the maturation and subsequent release of an ovum. With repeated use of the drug, however, the pituitary becomes desensitized and no longer produces endogenous LH and FSH; thus endogenous estrogen is not produced leading to a regression of endometrial tissue, cessation of menstruation, and a menopausal-like state. The drug is broken down by the enzyme peptidase. **Peak serum levels:** 10–40 min. **t½:** 3 hr; 80% is bound to plasma proteins.

Uses: Endometriosis (including reduction of endometriotic lesions) in clients aged 18 or older; use restricted to no more than 6 months.

Contraindications: Hypersensitivity to gonadotropin-releasing hormone or analogs. Abnormal vaginal bleeding of unknown origin. Pregnancy or possibility of becoming pregnant. Lactation.

Special Concerns: Pregnancy category: X. Use of nafarelin in pregnancy is not recommended; pregnancy should be ruled out before initiating therapy. Safety and effectiveness in children have not been established.

Side Effects: *Due to hypoestrogenic effects:* Hot flashes (common), decreased libido, vaginal dryness, headaches, emotional lability, insomnia. *Due to androgenic effects:* Acne, myalgia, reduced breast size, edema, seborrhea, weight gain, increased libido, hirsutism. *Musculoskeletal:* Decrease in vertebral trabecular bone density and total vertebral bone mass. *Miscellaneous:* Nasal irritation, depression, weight loss.

Laboratory Test Interference: ↑ Cholesterol and triglyceride levels, plasma phosphorus, eosinophils. ↓ Serum calcium, white blood cell counts.

Dosage: Nasal spray: 200 mcg into one nostril in the morning and 200 mcg into the other nostril at

N

night (400 mcg b.i.d. may be required by some women).

NURSING CONSIDERATIONS

Administration/Storage

1. Treatment with nafarelin should be initiated between days 2 and 4 of the menstrual cycle.
2. Use for longer than 6 months is not recommended due to the lack of safety data.
3. The product should be stored at room temperature in an upright position protected from light.

Assessment

1. Perform a complete client history and note any evidence of chronic alcohol, tobacco, or corticosteroid use. Query about any family history of osteoporosis. Conditions such as these are major risk factors for loss of bone mineral content and would deter repeated courses of treatment with this drug.
2. Note client description of menstrual cycles. Document any incidence of abnormal vaginal bleeding of unknown origin because drug is contraindicated in this event.
3. Determine if the client is pregnant prior to administering therapy because drug is teratogenic.
4. Review the method of contraception being practiced. A nonhormonal method should be advised and practiced during drug therapy.

Client/Family Teaching

1. Treatment should begin between the second and fourth day of the menstrual cycle.

Stress the importance of accurate record keeping in relation to menstrual patterns and cycles.
2. Teach the client how to administer the nasal spray and remind her to use only as directed. The client should be encouraged to take the spray upon arising and just before bedtime. Stress the importance of alternating the nostrils to decrease mucosal irritation.
3. Explain that menses should cease while on nafarelin therapy. If regular menses continues the physician should be notified.
4. Remind the client that breakthrough bleeding may occur if successive doses are missed.
5. Stress the importance of using a nonhormonal form of contraception. Explain the potential hazards to the fetus should one become pregnant during therapy with nafarelin acetate.
6. If a topical nasal decongestant is required during treatment with nafarelin, the decongestant should be used at least 30 min after nafarelin to decrease the chances of reducing the absorption of nafarelin.
7. Provide a printed list of the hypoestrogenic and androgenic side effects that may occur with this drug therapy. Report these symptoms to the physician because a change in drug dosage or drug therapy may be indicated.

Evaluation: Evaluate client for:
- Restoration of normal function of the pituitary-gonadal system in 4–8 weeks
- Evidence of a reduction in the number and size of endometriotic lesions

Nafcillin sodium
(naf-**SILL**-in)
Nafcil, Nallpen, Unipen (Rx)

See also *Anti-Infectives,* p. 80, and *Penicillins,* p. 197.

Classification: Antibiotic, penicillin.

Action/Kinetics: Nafcillin is penicillinase-resistant and acid stable. Used for resistant staphylococcal infections. Parenteral therapy is recommended initially for severe infections. **Peak plasma levels: PO,** 7 mcg/ml after 30–60 min; **IM,** 14–20 mcg/ml after 30–60 min. **t½:** 60 min. Significantly bound to plasma proteins.

Uses: Infections by penicillinase-producing staphylococci; also certain pneumococci and streptococci. As initial therapy if staphylococcal infection is suspected (i.e., until results of culture have been obtained).

Additional Side Effects: Sterile abscesses and thrombophlebitis occur frequently, especially in the elderly.

Dosage: IV. Adults: 0.5–1 g q 4 hr. **IM. Adults:** 0.5 g q 4–6 hr. **Children and infants:** 25 mg/kg b.i.d. **Neonates:** 10 mg/kg b.i.d. Or, for neonates weighing less than 2,000 g and less than 7 days of age, a dose of 25 mg/kg b.i.d. can be given; for neonates weighing less than 2,000 g but older than 7 days, a dose of 75 mg/kg daily divided every 6 hr. **Capsules, Oral Solution, Tablets. Adults:** 250–500 mg q 4–6 hr for mild to moderate infections (up to 1 g q 4–6 hr for severe infections). **Pediatric:** *Pneumonia/scarlet fever:* 25 mg/kg/day in 4 divided doses. *Staphylococcal infections:* 50 mg/kg/day in 4 divided doses. **Neonates:** 10 mg/kg t.i.d.–q.i.d. *Streptococcal pharyngitis:* 250 mg t.i.d. IV administration is not recommended for neonates or infants.

NURSING CONSIDERATIONS

See also *Nursing Considerations* for *Penicillins,* p. 200.

Administration/Storage

1. Reconstitute for oral use by adding powder to bottle of diluent. Replace cap tightly. Then *shake* thoroughly until all powder is in solution. Check carefully for undissolved powder at the bottom of bottle. Solution must be stored in refrigerator and unused portion discarded after 1 week.
2. Reconstitute for parenteral use by adding required amount of sterile water. Shake vigorously. Date, time and initial bottle. Refrigerate after reconstitution and discard unused portion after 48 hr.
3. For direct IV administration, dissolve powder in 15–30 ml of sterile water for injection or isotonic sodium chloride solution and inject over 5- to 10-min period into the tubing of flowing IV infusion. For IV drip, dissolve the required amount in 100–150 ml of isotonic sodium chloride injection and administer by IV drip over a period of 15–90 min.
4. IV use should be reserved for therapy of 24–48 hr duration due to the possibility of thrombophlebitis, especially in geriatric clients.
5. Administer IM by deep intragluteal injection.
6. Serum levels after oral administration are low and unpredictable.

N

Interventions

1. Do not administer IV to newborn infants.
2. Reduce rate of flow and report any pain, redness, or edema at site of IV administration.
3. Assess client for GI distress after oral administration.

Evaluation: Evaluate client for:

- Laboratory evidence of a decrease in the number of colonies of the infecting organism
- Reports of symptomatic improvement

Naftifine hydrochloride

(NAF-tih-feen)
Naftin (Rx)

Classification: Antifungal agent.

Action/Kinetics: Naftifine is a synthetic antifungal agent with a broad spectrum of activity. The drug is thought to inhibit squalene 2,3-epoxidase, which is responsible for synthesis of sterols. The decreased levels of sterols (especially ergosterol) and the accumulation of squalene in cells result in fungicidal activity. Although used topically, approximately 6% of the drug is absorbed. Naftifine and its metabolites are excreted via the feces and urine. **t½:** 2–3 days.

Uses: Naftifine is effective against *Candida albicans, Epidermophyton floccosum, Microsporum canis, M. audouinii, M. gypseum, Trichophyton rubrum, T. mentagrophytes,* and *T. tonsurans.* Used to treat tinea cruris, tinea pedis, and tinea corporis caused by organisms listed above.

Contraindications: Ophthalmic use.

Special Concerns: Pregnancy category: B. Consideration should be given to discontinuing nursing while using naftifine and for several days after the last application. Safety and efficacy in children have not been determined.

Side Effects: *Topical cream:* Burning, stinging, dryness, itching, local irritation, erythema. *Topical gel:* Burning, stinging, itching, rash, tenderness, erythema.

Dosage: Topical Cream (1%), Topical Gel (1%): Massage into affected area and surrounding skin once daily if using the cream and twice daily (morning and evening) if using the gel.

NURSING CONSIDERATIONS

Client/Family Teaching

1. Demonstrate the appropriate technique for topical application.
2. Wash hands before and after applying medication.
3. Use care to avoid contact with the eyes, nose, mouth, or other mucous membranes.
4. Occlusive dressings or wrappings should not be used. Area should not be covered unless directed by the physician.
5. Beneficial effects are usually observed within 1 week; treatment should be continued as prescribed for 1–2 weeks after symptoms have decreased.
6. Medication is for external use only.
7. Report any excessive itching or burning.
8. Advise that the client should be reevaluated if beneficial effects are not evident after 4 weeks of treatment.

Evaluation: Evaluate client for:
- A positive response to drug therapy as evidenced by negative lab culture reports
- Reports of symptomatic improvement

Nalbuphine hydrochloride

(**NAL**-byou-feen)
Nubain (Rx)

See also *Narcotic Analgesics,* p. 174.

Classification: Narcotic analgesic—agonist-antagonist.

Action/Kinetics: Nalbuphine, a synthetic compound resembling oxymorphone and naloxone, is a potent analgesic with both narcotic agonist and antagonist actions. Its analgesic potency is approximately equal to that of morphine, while its antagonistic potency is approximately one-fourth that of nalorphine. **Onset:** IV, 2–3 min; **SC or IM,** less than 15 min. **Peak effect:** 30–60 min. **Duration:** 3–6 hr; t½: 5 hr.

Uses: Moderate to severe pain. Preoperative analgesia, anesthesia adjunct, obstetric analgesia.

Contraindications: Hypersensitivity to drug. Children under 18 years.

Special Concerns: Safe use during pregnancy (except for delivery) and lactation not established. Use with caution in presence of head injuries and asthma, myocardial infarction (if client is nauseous or vomiting), biliary tract surgery (may induce spasms of sphincter of Oddi), renal insufficiency. Clients dependent on narcotics may experience withdrawal symptoms following use of nalbuphine.

Additional Side Effects: Even though nalbuphine is an agonist-antagonist, it may cause dependence and may precipitate withdrawal symptoms in an individual physically dependent on narcotics. *CNS:* Sedation is common. Crying, feelings of unreality, and other psychologic reactions. *GI:* Cramps, dry mouth, bitter taste, dyspepsia. *Skin:* Itching, burning, urticaria, sweaty, clammy skin. *Other:* Blurred vision, difficulty with speech, urinary frequency.

Drug Interactions: Concomitant use with CNS depressants, other narcotics, phenothiazines, may result in additive depressant effects.

Dosage: SC, IM, IV. Adults: 10 mg for 70-kg client q 3–6 hr as needed (single dose should not exceed 20 mg q 3–6 hr; total daily dose should not exceed 160 mg).

Overdosage: See *Narcotic Analgesics,* p. 174, and *Narcotic Antagonists,* p. 181.

NURSING CONSIDERATIONS

See also *Nursing Considerations* for *Narcotic Analgesics,* p. 177.

Administration: Nalbuphine hydrochloride may be administered IV, undiluted. Administer each 10 mg or less over a 3–5-min period.

Assessment

1. Take a complete client history, noting any evidence of dependence on narcotics. Nalbuphine may precipitate withdrawal symptoms in clients with narcotic addiction.
2. Note client history of head injuries, asthma or cardiac dysfunction because the drug may be contraindicated.

Interventions: Note any client symptoms of withdrawal such as extreme restlessness, lacrimation, rhinorrhea, yawning, perspiration, and dilation of the pupils. These are indications of narcotic dependence. Document and report these symptoms to the physician.

Evaluation: Evaluate client for reports of effective control of pain.

—— COMBINATION DRUG ——
Naldecon Syrup, Tablets, Pediatric Drops, and Pediatric Syrup
(**NAL**-deh-kon)
(Rx)

Classification/Content: Each sustained-action tablet contains the following (one-half for immediate release and one-half for delayed action):
Antihistamine: Chlorpheniramine maleate, 5 mg.
Decongestant: Phenylpropanolamine HCl, 40 mg.
Decongestant: Phenylephrine HCl, 10 mg.
Antihistamine: Phenyltoloxamine citrate, 15 mg.
Note: The syrup contains one-half the amount of the above components in each 5 ml, whereas the pediatric syrup (in each 5 ml) and pediatric drops (in each 1 ml) contain chlorpheniramine maleate, 0.5 mg; phenylpropanolamine HCl, 5 mg; phenylephrine HCl, 1.25 mg; and phenyltoloxamine citrate, 2 mg. See also information on individual components.

Uses: Nasal congestion and eustachian tube congestion observed with the common cold, acute upper respiratory tract infections, or sinusitis. Also, seasonal or perennial allergic rhinitis or vasomotor rhinitis. Also used to relieve eustachian tube congestion associated with serous otitis media, acute eustachian salpingitis, or aerotitis.

Special Concerns: Pregnancy category: C. Use with caution during lactation.

Dosage: Pediatric Drops and Syrup, Syrup, Tablets. Adults and children over 12 years: 1 tablet on arising, in midafternoon, and at bedtime; or 5 ml syrup q 3–4 hr not to exceed 4 doses daily. **Pediatric, 6–12 years:** 10 ml pediatric syrup q 3–4 hr, not to exceed 4 doses daily; or, 2.5 ml syrup q 3–4 hr not to exceed 4 doses daily; or ½ tablet on arising, in midafternoon, and at bedtime. **1–6 years:** 5 ml pediatric syrup or 1 ml pediatric drops q 3–4 hr, not to exceed 4 doses daily; **6–12 months:** 2.5 ml pediatric syrup or 0.5 ml pediatric drops q 3–4 hr, not to exceed 4 doses daily; **3–6 months:** 0.25 ml pediatric drops q 3–4 hr, not to exceed 4 doses daily.

NURSING CONSIDERATIONS
See *Nursing Considerations* for *Antihistamines,* p. 74.

Evaluation: Evaluate client for reports of relief of congestion and allergic manifestations.

Nalidixic acid
(nah-lih-**DICKS**-ick **AH**-sid)
NegGram (Rx)

Classification: Urinary germicide.

Action/Kinetics: Nalidixic acid is believed to inhibit the DNA synthesis of the microorganism, probably by interfering with DNA polymerization. The drug is either bacteriostatic or bactericidal. Nalidixic acid is rapidly absorbed from the GI tract. **Peak plasma concentration:** 20–40 mcg/ml after 1–2 hr; **peak urine levels:** 150–200 mcg/ml after 3–4 hr **t½:** 1.1–2.5 hr, increased to 21 hr in anuric clients). The drug is extensively protein bound, partially metabolized in liver, and rapidly excreted in urine.

Sensitivity determinations are recommended before and periodically during prolonged administration of nalidixic acid. Renal and liver function tests are advisable if course of therapy exceeds 2 weeks.

Uses: Acute and chronic urinary tract infections caused by susceptible gram-negative organisms, including *Escherichia coli, Proteus, Enterobacter,* and *Klebsiella.*

Contraindications: To be used with caution in clients with liver disease, severely impaired kidney function, epilepsy, and severe cerebral arteriosclerosis. Lactation. Use not recommended in infants and children.

Special Concerns: Safety in pregnancy has not been established.

Side Effects: *GI:* Nausea, vomiting, diarrhea, pain. *CNS:* Drowsiness, headache, dizziness, weakness, vertigo, toxic psychoses, seizures (rare). *Allergic:* Photosensitivity, skin rashes, arthralgia, pruritus, urticaria, angioedema, eosinophilia. *Hematologic:* Leukopenia, thrombocytopenia, hemolytic anemia (especially in clients with glucose-6-phosphate dehydrogenase deficiency). *Other:* Metabolic acidosis, cholestatic jaundice, paresthesia.

Drug Interactions

Antacids, oral / ↓ Effect of nalidixic acid due to ↓ absorption from GI tract

Anticoagulants, oral / ↑ Effect of anticoagulants due to ↓ in plasma protein binding
Nitrofurantoin / ↓ Effect of nalidixic acid

Laboratory Test Interferences: False + for urinary glucose with Benedict's solution, Fehling's solution, or Clinitest Reagent tablets. Falsely elevated 17-ketosteroids.

Dosage: Oral Suspension, Tablets. Adults: initially, 1 g q.i.d. for 1–2 weeks; **maintenance,** if necessary, 2 g daily.

NURSING CONSIDERATIONS

See also *Nursing Considerations For All Anti-Infectives,* p. 83.

Assessment

1. Note any history of liver or renal dysfunction.
2. Determine that baseline CBC and urine cultures have been performed.

Interventions

1. Use Clinistix Reagent Strips or Tes-Tape for urinary glucose tests because other methods may result in a false + reaction. Finger sticks are the most reliable for glucose determinations.
2. Monitor for adverse CNS effects, e.g., seizures, psychosis, or evidence of increased ICP. Withhold drug and report if evident.

Client/Family Teaching

1. Take drug 1 hr before meals, on an empty stomach unless GI upset occurs. May be taken with food in this event.
2. Encourage to drink at least 2 quarts of water a day during drug therapy.

3. Do not perform tasks that require mental alertness until drug effects realized. Drug may cause drowsiness, confusion, blurred vision, and dizziness.
4. Avoid prolonged exposure to sunlight or ultraviolet light. Wear protective clothing and sunscreen if exposure is necessary.

Evaluation: Evaluate client for:
- Laboratory evidence of negative urine culture reports
- Reports of symptomatic improvement

Naloxone hydrochloride
(nal-**OX**-ohn)
Narcan (Rx)

See also *Narcotic Antagonists,* p. 181.

Classification: Narcotic antagonist.

Action/Kinetics: Naloxone, administered by itself, does not produce significant pharmacologic activity. Since the duration of action of naloxone is shorter than that of the narcotic analgesics, the respiratory depression may return when the narcotic antagonist has worn off. **Onset: IV,** 2 min; **SC, IM:** less than 5 min. **Time to peak effect:** 5–15 min. **Duration:** Dependent on dose and route of administration but may be as short as 45 min. **t½:** 60–100 min. Metabolized in the liver to inactive products that are eliminated through the kidneys.

Uses: Respiratory depression induced by natural and synthetic narcotics, including butorphanol, methadone, nalbuphine, pentazocine, and propoxyphene. Drug of choice when nature of depressant drug is not known. Diagnosis of acute opiate overdosage. Not effective when respiratory depression is induced by hypnotics, sedatives, or anesthetics and other nonnarcotic CNS depressants. *Investigational:* Refractory shock to improve circulation. Treatment of Alzheimer's dementia, alcoholic coma, and schizophrenia.

Contraindications: Sensitivity to drug. Narcotic addicts (drug may cause severe withdrawal symptoms). Not recommended for use in neonates.

Special Concern: Pregnancy category: B. Safe use during lactation and in children is not established.

Side Effects: Nausea, vomiting, sweating, hypertension, tremors, sweating due to reversal of narcotic depression. If used postoperatively, excessive doses may cause tachycardia, fibrillation, hypo- or hypertension, pulmonary edema.

Dosage: IV, IM, SC. *Narcotic overdosage:* **Initial,** 0.4–2 mg; if necessary, additional IV doses may be repeated at 2- to 3-min intervals. If no response after 10 mg, reevaluate diagnosis. *To reverse postoperative narcotic depression:* **IV, initial,** 0.1- to 0.2-mg increments at 2- to 3-min intervals; **then,** repeat at 1- to 2-hr intervals if necessary. Supplemental IM dosage increases the duration of reversal. **Pediatric.** *Narcotic overdosage:* **IV, IM, SC, initial,** 0.01 mg/kg; **then,** 0.1 mg/kg, if needed. *To reverse postoperative narcotic depression:* **initial,** increments of 0.005–0.01 mg **IV** q 2–3 min to desired effect. *To reverse narcotic depression:* **IV, IM, SC,** initial 0.01 mg/kg; may be repeated if necessary.

NURSING CONSIDERATIONS

See also *Nursing Considerations* for *Narcotic Antagonists,* p. 181.

Administration/Storage

1. If the drug is to be administered IV, 2 mg total may be added to 500 ml of normal saline or 5% dextrose to provide a concentration of 0.004 mg/ml. The rate of administration varies with the response of the client.
2. Do not mix naloxone with preparations containing bisulfite, metabisulfite, long-chain or high molecular weight anions, or solutions with an alkaline pH.
3. When naloxone is mixed with other solutions they should be used within 24 hr.
4. Naloxone is effective within 2 min after IV administration.

Interventions

1. The duration of the effects of the narcotic may exceed the effects of naloxone. Therefore, more than one dose of drug may be necessary to counteract the effects of the narcotic.
2. Monitor the client's BP, pulse, and respirations at 5-min intervals, then every 30 min once vital signs have stabilized.
3. Have emergency drugs and equipment available for resuscitation.
4. For acutely ill clients or those who are in a coma, have a suction machine immediately available. These clients additionally should be attached to a cardiac monitor.

Evaluation: Evaluate client for:
• Evidence of restoration of normal respiratory patterns following narcotic overdosage
• Improved level of consciousness

Naltrexone
(nal-**TREX**-ohn)
Trexan (Rx)

See also *Narcotic Antagonists,* p. 181.

Classification: Narcotic antagonist.

Action/Kinetics: Naltrexone binds to opiate receptors, thereby reversing or preventing the effects of narcotics. This is an example of competitive inhibition. **Peak plasma levels:** 1 hr. **Duration:** 24–72 hr. Metabolized in the liver; a major metabolite—6-beta-naltrexol—is active. **Peak serum levels, after 50 mg: naltrexone,** 8.6 ng/ml; **6-beta-naltrexol,** 99.3 ng/ml. **t½: naltrexone,** approximately 4 hr; **6-beta-naltrexol,** 13 hr. Naltrexone and its metabolites are excreted in the urine.

Uses: To prevent narcotic use in former narcotic addicts. *Investigational:* To treat eating disorders and postconcussional syndrome not responding to other approaches.

Contraindications: Clients taking narcotic analgesics, those dependent on narcotics, those in acute withdrawal from narcotics. Liver disease, acute hepatitis.

Special Concerns: Safety during pregnancy (category: C) and lactation and in children under 18 years of age has not been established.

Side Effects: *CNS:* Headache, anx-

N

iety, nervousness, sleep disorders, dizziness, change in energy level, depression, confusion, restlessness, disorientation, hallucinations, nightmares, paranoia, fatigue, drowsiness. *GI:* Nausea, vomiting, diarrhea, constipation, anorexia, abdominal pain or cramps, flatulence, ulcers, increased appetite, weight gain or loss, increased thirst, xerostomia. *CV:* Phlebitis, edema, increased blood pressure, changes in ECG, palpitations, epistaxis, tachycardia. *GU:* Delayed ejaculation, increased urinary frequency or urinary discomfort, changes in interest in sex. *Respiratory:* Cough, sore throat, nasal congestion, rhinorrhea, sneezing, excess secretions, hoarseness, shortness of breath, heaving breathing, sinus trouble. *Dermatologic:* Rash, oily skin, itching, pruritus, acne, cold sores, alopecia, athlete's foot. *Musculoskeletal:* Joint/muscle pain, muscle twitches, tremors, pain in legs, knees, or shoulders. *Other:* Hepatotoxicity, blurred vision, tinnitus, painful ears, aching or strained eyes, chills, swollen glands, inguinal pain, cold feet, "hot" spells, "pounding" head, fever.

A severe narcotic withdrawal syndrome may be precipitated if naltrexone is administered to a dependent individual. The syndrome may begin within 5 min and last for up to 2 days.

Dosage: Tablets. *To produce blockade of opiate actions:* **Initial:** 25 mg followed by an additional 25 mg in 1 hr if no withdrawal symptoms occur. **Maintenance:** 50 mg daily. *Alternate dosing schedule:* The weekly dose of 350 mg may be given as: (a) 50 mg daily on weekdays and 100 mg on Saturday; (b) 100 mg q 48 hr; (c) 100 mg every Monday and Wednesday and 150 mg on Friday; or, (d) 150 mg q 72 hr.

NURSING CONSIDERATIONS

See also *Nursing Considerations* for *Narcotic Antagonists,* p. 181.

Administration/Storage

1. Naltrexone therapy should **never** be initiated until it has been determined that the individual is not dependent on narcotics (i.e., a naloxone challenge test should be completed).
2. The client should be opiate free for at least 7–10 days before beginning naltrexone therapy.
3. When initiating naltrexone therapy, begin with 25 mg and observe for 1 hr for any signs of narcotic withdrawal.
4. The blockade produced by naltrexone may be overcome by taking large doses of narcotics. Such doses may be fatal.
5. Clients taking naltrexone may not respond to preparations containing narcotics for use in coughs, diarrhea, or pain.

Assessment

1. Determine if the client is addicted to opiates and when he had the last dose of this drug. Client must be opiate free for 7–10 days before initiating therapy.
2. Obtain a baseline BP, pulse, respirations, and ECG prior to initiating therapy.
3. Ensure that liver function studies have been performed prior to administering drug therapy.
4. Determine that urinalysis confirms absence of opiates and that naloxone challenge test

has been performed before initiating drug therapy.

Interventions

1. Note client complaints of headache, restlessness, and irritability. These are usually due to the effects of naltrexone.
2. Monitor BP, pulse, and respirations daily. If the respirations are severely lowered or if the client complains of difficulty breathing, notify the physician.
3. Routinely order liver function studies while the client is receiving drug therapy. Monitor monthly during the first 6 months of therapy.
4. Note client complaints of abdominal pain or difficulty with bowel function. If the discomfort becomes severe, notify the physician and anticipate a reduction in the dosage of naltrexone.

Client/Family Teaching

1. Review the goals of therapy.
2. Provide printed information outlining the adverse side effects, such as loss of appetite, unusual fatigue, yellowing of skin or sclera or itching, to be reported to the physician.
3. Inform health care providers that they are taking naltrexone.
4. May take with food or milk to diminish GI upset.
5. Encourage clients to remain drug free. Provide clients with the names of health care agencies and support groups that may assist them in remaining drug free.
6. Wear a medical identification tag or bracelet and carry identification indicating that client is taking naltrexone.

Evaluation: Evaluate for effectiveness in discouraging narcotics use in former addicts.

Naproxen
(nah-**PROX**-en)
Apo-Naproxen✤, Naprosyn, Naxen✤, Novo–Naprox✤, Nu-Naprox✤ (Rx)

Naproxen sodium
(nah-**PROX**-en)
Anaprox, Anaprox DS, Apo-Napro-Na✤, Neo-Prox✤, Novo–Naprox✤, Synflex✤ (Rx)

See also *Nonsteroidal Anti-Inflammatory Drugs,* p. 186.

Classification: Nonsteroidal, anti-inflammatory analgesic.

Action/Kinetics: Peak serum levels of naproxen: 2–4 hr; **for sodium salt:** 1–2 hr. **t½ for naproxen:** 12–15 hr; **for sodium salt:** 12–13 hr. **Onset, analgesia:** 1 hr. **Duration, analgesia:** Approx. 7 hr. The onset of anti-inflammatory effects may take up to 2 weeks and may last 2–4 weeks. Naproxen is more than 90% bound to plasma protein. Food delays the rate but not the amount of drug absorbed. Clinical improvement for inflammatory disease may not be observed for 2 weeks.

Uses: Mild to moderate pain. Musculoskeletal and soft tissue inflammation including rheumatoid arthritis, osteoarthritis, bursitis, tendinitis, ankylosing spondylitis. Primary dysmenorrhea, acute gout. Juvenile rheumatoid arthritis (naproxen only). *Investigational:* Antipyretic in cancer clients, sunburn, acute migraine (sodium salt only), prophylaxis of migraine, migraine due to menses, premenstrual syndrome (sodium salt only).

Contraindications: Use of naproxen and naproxen sodium simultaneously. Lactation.

Special Concerns: Pregnancy category: B. Safety and effectiveness of naproxen have not been determined in children less than 2 years of age; the safety and effectiveness of naproxen sodium have not been established in children. Geriatric clients may manifest increased total plasma levels of naproxen.

Drug Interactions

Methotrexate / Possibility of a fatal interaction
Probenecid / ↓ Plasma clearance of naproxen

Laboratory Test Interferences: Naproxen may increase urinary 17-ketosteroid values. Both forms may interfere with urinary assays for 5-hydroxyindoleacetic acid.

Dosage: Naproxen: Oral Suspension, Tablets. *Antirheumatic (rheumatoid arthritis, osteoarthritis, ankylosing spondylitis):* **Adults, individualized. Usual:** 250, 375, or 500 mg b.i.d. in the morning and evening. Improvement should be observed within 2 weeks; if no improvement is seen, an additional 2-week course of therapy should be considered. May increase to 1.5 g for short periods of time. *Acute gout:* **initial,** 750 mg; **then,** 250 mg naproxen q 8 hr until symptoms subside. *Pain, dysmenorrhea, bursitis, tendinitis:* **initial,** 500 mg; **then,** 250 mg q 6–8 hr. Total daily dosage should not exceed 1,250 mg. *Juvenile rheumatoid arthritis:* Naproxen only, 10 mg/kg daily in 2 divided doses. If the suspension is

used, the following dosage can be used: **13 kg:** 2.5 ml b.i.d.; **25 kg:** 5 ml b.i.d.; **38 kg:** 7.5 ml b.i.d.

Naproxen Sodium: Tablets. Adults: *Anti-rheumatic,* 275 mg b.i.d. in the morning and evening (alternate dosage: 275 mg in the morning and 550 mg at night). *Acute gout:* **initial,** 825 mg; **then,** 275 mg q 8 hr until symptoms subside. *Pain, dysmenorrhea, tendinitis, bursitis:* **initial,** 550 mg; **then,** 275 mg q 6–8 hr as needed. Total daily dose should not exceed 1,375 mg.

NURSING CONSIDERATIONS

See also *Nursing Considerations* for *Nonsteroidal Anti-Inflammatory Drugs,* p. 189.

Administration/Storage

1. The onset of action is 1–2 hr. The duration of action is 7 hr.
2. It is recommended that the medication be taken in the morning and in the evening. The doses do not have to be equal.
3. Naproxen sodium should not be administered to children.
4. Naproxen suspension can be used to treat children with rheumatoid arthritis.

Assessment

1. Note any client history of hypersensitivity to naproxen or other NSAID.
2. Review the client's medical history. The drug is contraindicated for persons with GI bleeding or ulcers.

Client/Family Teaching: Report any persistent abdominal pain or dark colored stools to the physician immediately.

Evaluation: Evaluate client for:
- Reports of improvement in joint pain and mobility
- Reports of relief of headache and control of pain

Natamycin
(nah-tah-**MY**-sin)
Natacyn (Rx)

See also *Anti-Infectives*, p. 80.

Classification: Antifungal (ophthalmic).

General Statement: Discontinue drug if toxicity is suspected. Review therapy if no improvement noted after 7–10 days.

Action/Kinetics: Natamycin is an antifungal antibiotic derived from *Streptomyces natalensis*. The drug binds to the fungal cell membrane, resulting in alteration of permeability and loss of essential intracellular materials. It is fungicidal. After topical administration, the drug reaches therapeutic levels in the corneal stroma but not in the intraocular fluid. It is not absorbed systemically.

Uses: For ophthalmic use only. Drug of choice for *Fusarium solanae* keratitis. For treatment of fungal blepharitis, conjunctivitis, and keratitis caused by susceptible organisms. It is active against a variety of yeasts and filamentous fungi including *Candida, Aspergillus, Cephalosporium, Fusarium,* and *Penicillium*. Before initiating therapy, determine the susceptibility of the infectious organism to drug in smears and cultures of corneal scrapings. Effectiveness of natamycin for use as single agent in fungal endophthalmitis not established.

Contraindications: Hypersensitivity to drug.

Special Concerns: Safe use during pregnancy not established.

Side Effects: Eye irritation, occasional allergies.

Dosage: Ophthalmic Suspension: *Fungal keratitis:* **Initially,** 1 gtt of 5% suspension in conjunctival sac q 1–2 hr; can be reduced usually, after 3–4 days to 1 gtt 6–8 times/day. Continue therapy for 14–21 days, during which dosage can be reduced gradually at 4- to 7-day intervals. *Blepharitis/conjunctivitis:* 1 gtt 4–6 times daily.

NURSING CONSIDERATIONS

See also *General Nursing Considerations For All Anti-Infectives,* p. 83.

Administration/Storage

1. Store natamycin at room temperature or in refrigerator.
2. Shake well before using.
3. Avoid contamination of dropper.

Client/Family Teaching

1. Stress the importance of close medical supervision (initially twice weekly) to regulate dosage.
2. Demonstrate proper administration technique.
3. Continue therapy for 14–21 days as ordered, even though condition may appear to be under control.

Evaluation: Evaluate client for:
- Laboratory evidence of negative lab culture reports
- Improved ophthalmic exams and reports of symptomatic improvement

—— *COMBINATION DRUG* ——
Nelova 0.5/35E 21 Day and Nelova 0.5/35E 28 Day
(neh-**LOV**-vah)
(Rx)

Nelova 1/35E 21 Day and Nelova 1/35E 28 Day
(ne-**LOV**-vah)
(Rx)

Nelova 1/50M 21 Day and Nelova 1/50M 28 Day
(neh-**LOV**-vah)
(Rx)

See also *Oral Contraceptives*, p. 192.

Classification: Monophasic combination oral contraceptive.

Components: Each tablet of Nelova 0.5/35E 21 Day and the first 21 tablets of Nelova 0.5/35E 28 Day contains ethinyl estradiol, 35 mcg and norethindrone, 0.5 mg (light yellow tablets); the 28s also contain 7 inert white tablets.

Each tablet of Nelova 1/35E 21 Day and the first 21 tablets of Nelova 1/35E 28 Day contains ethinyl estradiol, 35 mcg and norethindrone, 1 mg (dark yellow tablets); the 28s also contain 7 inert white tablets.

Each tablet of Nelova 1/50M 21 Day and the first 21 tablets of Nelova 1/50M 28 Day contains mestranol, 50 mcg and norethindrone, 1 mg (light blue tablets); the 28s also contain 7 inert white tablets.

Special Concerns: Pregnancy category: X.

NURSING CONSIDERATIONS
See *Oral Contraceptives*, p. 192.

—— *COMBINATION DRUG* ——
Nelova 10/11 21 Day and Nelova 10/11 28 Day
(neh-**LOV**-vah)
(Rx)

See also *Oral Contraceptives*, p. 192.

Classification: Biphasic combination oral contraceptive.

Components: The first 10 tablets (first phase) of Nelova 10/11 21 Day and 28 Day each contain ethinyl estradiol, 35 mcg and norethindrone 0.5 mg (light yellow tablets). The next 11 tablets (second phase) each contain ethinyl estradiol, 35 mcg and norethindrone, 1 mg (dark yellow tablets). Nelova 10/11 28 Day also contain 7 inert white tablets.

Special Concerns: Pregnancy category: X.

NURSING CONSIDERATIONS
See *Oral Contraceptives*, p. 192.

Neomycin sulfate
(nee-oh-**MY**-sin)
Mycifradin Sulfate, Myciguent, Neobiotic, Neo-IM (Rx)

See also *Anti-Infectives*, p. 80, and *Aminoglycosides*, p. 23.

Classification: Antibiotic, aminoglycoside.

Action/Kinetics: Peak plasma levels: PO, 1–4 hr; **Therapeutic serum level:** 5–10 mcg/ml. **t½:** 2–3 hr.

Uses: PO: Hepatic coma, sterilization of gut prior to surgery, inhibition of ammonia-forming bacteria in GI tract in hepatic encephalopathy. Therapy of intestinal infections due to pathogenic strains of *Escherichia coli,* primarily in children. *Investigational:* Hypercholesterolemia.

Topical: Used for itching, burning, inflamed skin conditions that are threatened by, or complicated by, a secondary bacterial infection.

Additional Contraindications: Intestinal obstruction (PO). Topical products should not be used in or around the eyes.

Special Concerns: Safe use during pregnancy has not been determined. Due to the possibility of toxicity, some experts do not recommend the parenteral use of neomycin for any purpose. Use with caution in clients with extensive burns, trophic ulceration, or other conditions where significant systemic absorption is possible.

Additional Side Effects: Ototoxicity, nephrotoxicity. Sprue-like syndrome with steatorrhea, malabsorption, and electrolyte imbalance. Skin rashes after topical or parenteral administration. Chronic use in allergic contact dermatitis and chronic dermatoses increases the risk of sensitization.

Additional Drug Interactions

Digoxin / ↓ Effect of digoxin due to ↓ absorption from GI tract
Penicillin V / ↓ Effect of penicillin due to ↓ absorption from GI tract
Procainamide / ↑ Muscle relaxation produced by neomycin

Dosage: Oral solution. *Preoperatively in colorectal surgery:* 1 g each of neomycin and erythromycin base

for a total of three doses: the first two doses 1 hr apart the afternoon before surgery and the third dose the night before surgery at bedtime. *Hepatic coma, adjunct:* **Adults,** 4–12 g/day in divided doses for 5–6 days; **children:** 50–100 mg/kg/day in divided doses for 5–6 days.

IM. Adults: 15 mg/kg/day in four equal doses, not to exceed 1 g/day. The IM preparation should not be used in infants and children. Maximum course of therapy is 10 days.

Topical Cream, Ointment. Neomycin alone or in combination with other antibiotics (bacitracin or gramicidin) and/or an anti-inflammatory agent (corticosteroid). Apply ointment (0.5%) or cream (0.5%) 1–5 times daily to affected area. If necessary, a bandage may be used to cover the area.

NURSING CONSIDERATIONS

See also *Nursing Considerations* for *Aminoglycosides,* p. 25. N

Administration/Storage

1. For IM use, sterile normal saline should be added to the vial to obtain a concentration of 250 mg/ml.
2. Reconstituted neomycin sulfate for IM use should be refrigerated at 2°C–8°C (36°F–46°F) and used within 1 week.
3. The recommended procedure should be followed to prepare the GI tract for surgery.

Interventions

1. Monitor I&O and serum electrolyte levels. Encourage fluid intake of 2–3 L/day unless contraindicated.
2. Have available neostigmine to counteract renal failure, respir-

atory depression and arrest, side effects that may occur when neomycin is administered intraperitoneally.

3. Anticipate a slight laxative effect produced by oral neomycin. Withhold the drug and consult with physician in case of suspected intestinal obstruction.

4. Anticipate a low-residue diet for preoperative disinfection and, unless contraindicated, a laxative immediately preceding PO administration of neomycin sulfate.

5. Clean the affected area before applying ointment or solution of neomycin topically.

Evaluation: Evaluate client for:

- Improved levels of consciousness in hepatic coma
- Prevention of infection to skin wounds
- Evidence of effective bowel sterilization before intestinal surgery
- Laboratory evidence of negative culture reports

Neostigmine bromide
(nee-oh-**STIG**-meen)
Prostigmin Bromide (Rx)

Neostigmine methylsulfate
(nee-oh-**STIG**-meen)
PMS-Neostigmine Methylsulfate Injection ✱, Prostigmin (Rx)

Classification: Indirectly acting cholinergic-acetylcholinesterase inhibitor.

Action/Kinetics: By inhibiting the enzyme acetylcholinesterase, these drugs cause an increase in the concentration of acetylcholine at the myoneural junction, thus facilitating transmission of impulses across the myoneural junction. In myasthenia gravis, muscle strength is increased. The drug may also act on the autonomic ganglia of the CNS. Neostigmine also prevents or relieves postoperative distention by increasing gastric motility and tone and prevents or relieves urinary retention by increasing the tone of the detrusor muscle of the bladder. Shorter acting than ambenonium chloride and pyridostigmine. Atropine is often given concomitantly to control side effects. **Onset: PO,** 45–75 min; **IM,** 20–30 min; **IV,** 4–8 min. **Time to peak effect, parenteral:** 20–30 min. **Duration:** All routes, 2–4 hr. **t½, PO:** 42–60 min; **IM:** 51–90 min; **IV:** 47–60 min. Eliminated through the urine (about 40% unchanged).

Uses: Diagnosis and treatment of myasthenia gravis. Prophylaxis and treatment of postoperative GI ileus or urinary retention. Antidote for tubocurarine and other nondepolarizing drugs.

Contraindications: Hypersensitivity, mechanical obstruction of GI or urinary tract, peritonitis, history of bromide sensitivity. Vesical neck obstruction of urinary bladder.

Special Concerns: Safe use during pregnancy (category: C) and lactation not established. Safety and effectiveness in children have not been established. Use with caution in clients with bronchial asthma, bradycardia, vagotonia, epilepsy, hyperthyroidism, peptic ulcer, cardiac arrhythmias, or recent coronary occlusion. May cause uterine irritability and premature labor if given IV to pregnant women near term. In geriatric clients, the duration of action may be increased.

Side Effects: *GI:* Nausea, vomiting, diarrhea, abdominal cramps, involuntary defecation, salivation, dysphagia, flatulence, increased gastric and intestinal secretions. *CV:* Bradycardia, tachycardia, hypotension, ECG changes, nodal rhythm, cardiac arrest, syncope, AV block, substernal pain, thrombophlebitis after IV use. *CNS:* Headache, seizures, malaise, weakness, dysarthria, dizziness, drowsiness, loss of consciousness. *Respiratory:* Increased oral, pharyngeal, and bronchial secretions; bronchospasms, skeletal muscle paralysis, laryngospasm, central respiratory paralysis, respiratory depression or arrest, dyspnea. *Ophthalmologic:* Miosis, double vision, lacrimation, accommodation difficulties, hyperemia of conjunctiva, visual changes. *Musculoskeletal:* Muscle fasciculations or weakness, muscle cramps or spasms, arthralgia. *Other:* Skin rashes, urinary frequency and incontinence, sweating, flushing, allergic reactions, anaphylaxis, urticaria. These effects can usually be reversed by parenteral administration of 0.6 mg of atropine sulfate, which should be readily available.

Cholinergic crisis, due to overdosage, must be distinguished from myasthenic crisis (worsening of the disease), since cholinergic crisis involves removal of drug therapy, while myasthenic crisis involves an increase in anticholinesterase therapy.

Symptoms of Overdose: Abdominal cramps, vomiting, diarrhea, epigastric distress, excessive salivation, cold sweating, pallor, blurred vision, urinary urgency, fasciculation and paralysis of voluntary muscles (including the tongue), miosis, increased blood pressure (may be accompanied by bradycardia), sensation of internal trembling, panic, severe anxiety.

Drug Interactions

Aminoglycosides /
  ↑ Neuromuscular blockade
Atropine / Atropine suppresses symptoms of excess GI stimulation caused by cholinergic drugs
Corticosteroids / ↓ Effect of neostigmine
Magnesium salts / Antagonize the effects of anticholinesterases
Mecamylamine / Intense hypotensive response
Organophosphate-type insecticides/ pesticides / Added systemic effects with cholinesterase inhibitors
Succinylcholine /
  ↑ Neuromuscular blocking effects

Dosage: Tablets: Neostigmine bromide. *Treat myasthenia gravis:* **Adults,** 15 mg q 3–4 hr; adjust dose and frequency as needed. **Usual maintenance,** 150 mg/day with dosing intervals determined by client response. **Pediatric,** 2 mg/ kg (60 mg/m²) daily in 6–8 divided doses. **IM, IV, SC: Neostigmine methylsulfate.** *Treat myasthenia gravis:* **Adults: IM, SC,** 0.5 mg. **Pediatric: IM, SC,** 0.01–0.04 mg/ kg q 2–3 hr. *Diagnosis of myasthenia gravis:* **Adults: IM, SC,** 1.5 mg given with 0.6 mg atropine; **pediatric, IM:** 0.04 mg/kg (1 mg/m²); or, **IV:** 0.02 mg/kg (0.5 mg/m²). *Antidote for tubocurarine,* **Adults: IV,** 0.5–2 mg slowly with 0.6–1.2 mg atropine sulfate. Can repeat if necessary up to total dose of 5 mg. **Pediatric: IV,** 0.04 mg/kg with 0.02

N

mg/kg atropine sulfate. *Prevention of postoperative GI distention or urinary retention:* **Adults: IM, SC,** 0.25 mg (1 ml of the 1:4000 solution) immediately after surgery repeated q 4–6 hr for 2–3 days. *Treatment of postoperative GI distention:* **Adults: IM, SC,** 0.5 mg (1 ml of the 1:2000 solution) as required. *Treatment of urinary retention:* **Adults: IM, SC,** 0.5 mg (1 ml of the 1:2000 solution). If urination does not occur within 1 hr after 0.5 mg, the client should be catheterized. After the bladder is emptied, 0.5 mg is given q 3 hr for at least 5 injections.

NURSING CONSIDERATIONS

Administration/Storage

1. The interval between doses must be individually determined to achieve optimum effects.
2. If greater fatigue occurs at certain times of the day, a larger part of the daily dose can be administered at these times.
3. Neostigmine should not be given if high concentrations of halothane or cyclopropane are present.
4. *Treatment of Overdose:* Discontinue medication temporarily. Give atropine, 0.5–1 mg IV (up to 5–10 or more mg may be needed to get heart rate to 80 beats/min). Supportive treatment including artificial respiration and oxygen.

Assessment

1. Note any history of hypersensitivity to drugs in this category.
2. Identify any drugs the client is taking to determine if they are interactant with neostigmine.
3. Note any history of bromide

sensitivity. The drug is contraindicated in these instances.
4. Take the client's pulse prior to administering the drug. If the client's pulse is less than 80, the drug should be withheld and the physician notified.

Interventions

1. Observe the client for generalized cholinergic stimulation. This is evidence of a toxic reaction and the physician should be notified immediately.
2. Assess the client for stability and vision. If the client has difficulty with coordination or vision caution him to avoid use of heavy machinery until the effects of the medication wear off. If the effects become severe, notify the physician.
3. Monitor the pulse and BP for the first hour after drug administration. If hypotension occurs, have the client remain recumbent until the BP stabilizes.
4. When the medication is used as an antidote for tubocurarine, assist in the ventilation of the client and maintain a patent airway.
5. If the client is taking the medication for treatment of myasthenia gravis, any onset of weakness 1 hr after administration usually indicates overdosage of drug. Notify the physician immediately. The onset of weakness 3 hr or more after administration usually indicates underdosage and/or resistance and should also be documented and reported to the physician. Also note any associated difficulty with respirations or increase in muscle weakness.

Client/Family Teaching

1. Provide a printed list of adverse drug effects, stressing those that require immediate reporting to the physician.
2. Advise clients with myasthenia to maintain a written record of periods of muscle strength or weakness so that dosage can be evaluated and adjusted accordingly. Encourage client to space activities to avoid excessive fatigue.
3. Stress that any increasing weakness should be reported immediately because drug tolerance can develop.
4. Wear a Medic Alert bracelet and carry identification indicating that clients are receiving neostigmine and for what reasons.

Evaluation: Evaluate client for:

- Evidence of increased muscle strength and reports of symptomatic improvement in myasthenia gravis
- Clinical evidence of relief of postoperative ileus or urinary retention
- Successful reversal of nondepolarizing drugs

Niacin (Nicotinic Acid)

(**NYE**-ah-sin, nih-koh-**TIN**-ick **AH**-sid)
Nia-Bid, Niac, Niacels, Nico-400, Nicobid, Nicolar, Nicotinex, Novo–Niacin✱, Slo-Niacin, Span-Niacin, Tega-Span, Tri-B3✱
(Rx and OTC)

Niacinamide

(nye-ah-**SIN**-ah-myd)
(Rx: Injection; OTC: Tablets)

Classification: Vitamin B complex.

Action/Kinetics: Niacin (nicotinic acid) and niacinamide are water-soluble, heat-resistant vitamins prepared synthetically. Niacin (after conversion to the active niacinamide) is a component of the coenzymes NAD and NADP, which are essential for oxidation-reduction reactions involved in lipid metabolism, glycogenolysis, and tissue respiration. Deficiency of niacin results in pellagra, the most common symptoms of which are dermatitis, diarrhea, and dementia. In high doses niacin also produces vasodilation and a reduction in serum lipids. **Peak serum levels:** 45 min; **$t^{1/2}$:** 45 min.

Uses: Prophylaxis and treatment of pellagra; niacin deficiency. Niacin is also used to treat hyperlipidemia in clients not responding to either diet or weight loss.

Contraindications: Hypotension, hemorrhage, liver dysfunction, peptic ulcer. Use with caution in diabetics, gall bladder disease, and clients with gout.

Special Concerns: Pregnancy category: C. The extended-release tablets and capsules are not recommended for use in children.

Side Effects: *GI:* Nausea, vomiting, diarrhea, peptic ulcer activation, abdominal pain. *Dermatologic:* Flushing, warm feeling, skin rash, pruritus, dry skin, itching and tingling feeling, keratosis nigricans. *Other:* Hypotension, headache, macular cystoid edema, amblyopia. **Note:** Megadoses are accompanied by serious toxicity including the symptoms listed above as well as liver damage, hyperglycemia, hyperuricemia, arrhythmias, tachycardia, and dermatoses.

N

Drug Interactions

Chenodiol / ↓ Effect of chenodiol
Probenecid / Niacin may ↓
   uricosuric effect of probenecid
Sulfinpyrazone / Niacin ↓
   uricosuric effect of
   sulfinpyrazone
Sympathetic blocking agents /
   Additive vasodilating effects →
   postural hypotension

Dosage: *Niacin.* **Extended-release Capsules, Oral Solution, Tablets, Extended-release Tablets.** *Vitamin:* **Adults,** Up to 500 mg daily; **pediatric,** Up to 300 mg daily. *Antihyperlipidemic:* **Adults, initial,** 1 g t.i.d.; **then,** increase dose in increments of 500 mg daily q 2–4 weeks as needed. **Maintenance:** 1–2 g t.i.d. (up to a maximum of 6 g daily). **IM, IV.** *Pellagra:* **Adults, IM,** 50–100 mg 5 or more times daily; **IV, slow,** 25–100 mg 2 or more times daily. **Pediatric, IV slow,** Up to 300 mg daily.

Niacinamide. **Capsules, Tablets.** *Vitamin:* **Adults,** Up to 500 mg daily. **Pediatric:** Up to 300 mg daily. Capsules not recommended for use in children. **IM, IV.** *Pellagra:* **Adults, IM,** 50–100 mg 5 or more times daily; **IV, slow,** 25–100 mg 2 or more times daily. **Pediatric, IV, slow:** Up to 300 mg daily.

NURSING CONSIDERATIONS

Administration/Storage

1. Nicotinic acid should be taken orally only with cold water (no hot beverages).
2. Can be taken with meals if GI upset occurs.

Assessment

1. Obtain baseline plasma lipids and monitor periodically throughout therapy.

2. Note any history of liver dysfunction, gallbladder disease, or peptic ulcers.

Client/Family Teaching

1. Client may feel a warm flushing in the face and ears within 2 hr after taking the medication. Alcohol may increase these effects. One aspirin may reduce effect.
2. Clients who feel weak and dizzy after taking niacin should be instructed to lie down until this feeling passes and to inform the physician of this occurrence.
3. Report for all scheduled lab studies.
4. Clients who have diabetes mellitus should not take niacin unless specifically ordered. Then the blood glucose levels must be closely monitored for hyperglycemia. Clients must also be monitored for ketonuria and glucosuria. Advise clients taking antidiabetic agents that they may require an increase in dosage of these agents when taken in combination with niacin.
5. Instruct clients with hepatic dysfunction to report any skin color change or yellowing of the sclera.
6. Clients who are predisposed to gout may experience flank, joint, or stomach pains. Report this to the physician immediately.
7. Advise that some clients may develop blurred vision. If this occurs they should remain out of direct sunlight.
8. Review foods high in niacin (dairy products, meats, and eggs) and determine levels of consumption.

9. Advise against unsupervised excessive vitamin ingestion.

Evaluation: Evaluate client for:
- Laboratory evidence of a decrease in serum cholesterol and triglyceride levels
- Evidence of compliance with prescribed dietary and exercise program
- Improvement or prevention of symptoms of pellagra and other vitamin B deficiency states

Nicardipine hydrochloride
(nye-**KAR**-dih-peen)
Cardene (Rx)

See also *Calcium Channel Blocking Agents,* p. 118.

Classification: Calcium channel blocking agent (antianginal, antihypertensive).

Action/Kinetics: The drug moderately increases cardiac output and significantly decreases peripheral vascular resistance. **Onset of action:** 20 min. **Maximum plasma levels:** 30–120 min. Significant first-pass metabolism by the liver. Steady-state plasma levels are reached after 2–3 days of therapy. **Therapeutic serum levels:** 0.028–0.050 mcg/ml. **t½, at steady state:** 8.6 hr. **Duration:** 8 hr. The drug is highly bound to plasma protein (>95%) and is metabolized by the liver with excretion through both the urine and feces.

Uses: Chronic stable angina (effort-associated angina) alone or in combination with beta-adrenergic blocking agents. Hypertension alone or in combination with other antihypertensive drugs. *Investigational:* Congestive heart failure.

Contraindications: Clients with advanced aortic stenosis due to the effect on reducing afterload. During lactation.

Special Concerns: Use during pregnancy only if the potential benefits outweigh potential risks (pregnancy category: C). Safety and efficacy in children less than 18 years of age have not been established. Use with caution in clients with CHF, especially in combination with a beta-blocker. Use with caution in clients with impaired liver function, reduced hepatic blood flow, or impaired renal function.

Side Effects: *CV:* Pedal edema, flushing, increased angina, palpitations, tachycardia, other edema, abnormal ECG, hypotension, postural hypotension, syncope, myocardial infarction, AV block, ventricular extrasystoles, peripheral vascular disease. *CNS:* Dizziness, headache, somnolence, malaise, nervousness, insomnia, abnormal dreams, vertigo, depression, confusion, amnesia, anxiety, weakness, psychoses, hallucinations, paranoia. *GI:* Nausea, vomiting, dyspepsia, dry mouth, constipation, sore throat. *Neuromuscular:* Asthenia, myalgia, paresthesia, hyperkinesia, arthralgia. *Miscellaneous:* Rash, dyspnea, shortness of breath, nocturia, polyuria, allergic reactions, abnormal liver chemistries, hot flashes, impotence, rhinitis, sinusitis, nasal congestion, chest congestion, tinnitus, equilibrium disturbances, abnormal or blurred vision, infection, atypical chest pain.

N

Drug Interactions

Cimetidine / ↑ Bioavailability of nicardipine
Cyclosporine / ↑ Plasma levels of cyclosporine possibly leading to renal toxicity
Digoxin / Nicardipine may ↑ blood levels of digoxin
Ranitidine / ↑ Bioavailability of nicardipine

Dosage: Capsules, individualized. *Angina or hypertension:* **initial:** 20 mg t.i.d.; **maintenance:** ranges from 20–40 mg t.i.d. In renal impairment, the initial dose should be 20 mg t.i.d. In hepatic impairment, the initial dose should be 20 mg b.i.d.

NURSING CONSIDERATIONS

See also *Nursing Considerations* for *Calcium Channel Blocking Agents,* p. 119.

Administration/Storage

1. When used for treating clients with angina, nicardipine may be administered safely along with sublingual nitroglycerin, prophylactic nitrates, or beta-blockers.
2. When used to treat clients with hypertension, nicardipine may be administered safely along with diuretics or beta-blockers.
3. When used to treat clients with both angina and hypertension, at least 3 days should elapse before increasing the dose of nicardipine so that steady-state plasma levels can be attained.
4. During initial therapy and when dosage is increased, clients may experience an increase in the frequency, duration, or severity of angina.

Assessment

1. Note any history of CHF and if the client is taking beta-blockers. This indicates the drug should be used with caution and demands particularly close monitoring.
2. Determine other drugs the client may be taking that could cause unfavorable drug interactions.
3. Assure that renal and liver studies have been conducted prior to initiating therapy.
4. Take BP reading prior to initiating therapy to obtain baseline data against which to measure results of therapy.

Interventions

1. When used for hypertension, the maximum lowering of BP occurs 1–2 hr after dosing. Thus, during initiation of therapy BP should be monitored at this interval. Also, BP should be evaluated at the trough (8 hr after dosing).
2. Obtain lab studies to determine renal or hepatic dysfunction. Use cautiously and anticipate reduced dosage with these conditions.

Client/Family Teaching

1. Remind client to take the medication at the same time each day.
2. Report any persistent and/or bothersome side effects such as dizziness, flushing, or increased incidents of angina or evidence of weight gain or edema.
3. Maintain a proper intake of fluids to avoid constipation.
4. Male clients may experience impotence. If this occurs, they

should discuss with the physician.

5. Explain that anginal attacks may persist up to 30 min following drug ingestion due to reflex tachycardia; advise to use nitrates as prescribed.

6. Report any evidence of change in the client's psychological state—depression, anxiety, or decreased mental acuity. This may be particularly important when working with elderly clients since there may be a tendency to misdiagnose the problem as senility.

7. Advise client to report any altered sleep patterns. Notify the physician there has been a change so he/she may ascertain if the change could be drug related.

Evaluation: Evaluate client for:

- Laboratory evidence that serum drug levels are within therapeutic range (0.028–0.050 mcg/ml)
- Evidence of control of hypertension
- Reports of ↓ frequency and intensity of anginal attacks

Nicotine polacrilex (nicotine resin complex)

(NIK-oh-teen)

Nicorette (Rx)

Classification: Smoking deterrent.

Action/Kinetics: Following chewing, nicotine is released from an ion exchange resin in the gum product, providing blood nicotine levels approximating those produced by smoking cigarettes. The amount of nicotine released depends on the rate and duration of chewing. Following repeated administration every 30 min, nicotine blood levels reach 25–50 ng/ml. If the gum is swallowed, only a minimum amount of nicotine is released. Nicotine is metabolized mainly by the liver, with about 10%–20% excreted unchanged in the urine.

Uses: Adjunct with behavioral modification in smokers wishing to give up the smoking habit. Is considered only as an initial aid, with the ultimate goal being abstention from all forms of nicotine. Most likely to benefit are individuals with the following characteristics:

a. smoke brands of cigarettes containing > 0.9 mg nicotine;
b. smoke > 15 cigarettes daily;
c. inhale cigarette smoke deeply and frequently;
d. smoke most frequently during the morning;
e. smoke the first cigarette of the day within 30 min of arising;
f. indicate cigarettes smoked in the morning are the most difficult to give up;
g. smoke even if the individual is ill and confined to bed;
h. find it necessary to smoke in places where smoking is not allowed.

Contraindications: Pregnancy (category: X), lactation, nonsmokers, serious arrhythmias, angina, vasospastic disease, active temporomandibular joint disease.

Special Concerns: Safety and effectiveness in children and adolescents who smoke have not been determined. Use with caution in hypertension, peptic ulcer disease, oral or pharyngeal inflammation, gastritis, stomatitis, hyperthyroidism, insulin-dependent diabetes, and pheochromocytoma.

Side Effects: *CNS:* Dizziness, irritability, headache. *GI:* Nausea, vomiting, indigestion, GI upset, salivation, eructation. *Other:* Sore mouth or throat, hiccoughs, sore jaw muscles.

Symptoms of Overdose: GI: Nausea, vomiting, diarrhea, salivation, abdominal pain. *CNS:* Headache, dizziness, confusion, weakness, fainting, seizures. *Respiratory:* Labored breathing, respiratory paralysis (cause of death). *Other:* Cold sweat, disturbed hearing and vision, hypotension, and rapid, weak pulse.

Drug Interactions

Caffeine / Possibly ↓ blood levels of caffeine due to ↑ rate of breakdown by liver

Catecholamines / ↑ Levels of catecholamines

Cortisol / ↑ Levels of cortisol

Furosemide / Possible ↓ diuretic effect of furosemide

Glutethimide / Possible ↓ absorption of glutethimide

Imipramine / Possibly ↓ blood levels of imipramine due to ↑ rate of breakdown by liver

Pentazocine / Possibly ↓ blood levels of pentazocine due to ↑ rate of breakdown by liver

Theophylline / Possibly ↓ blood levels of theophylline due to ↑ rate of breakdown by liver

Dosage: Gum. Initial: one piece of gum chewed whenever the urge to smoke occurs; **maintenance:** about 10 pieces of gum daily during the first month, not to exceed 30 pieces daily.

NURSING CONSIDERATIONS

Administration/Storage

1. The individual must want to stop smoking and should do so immediately.
2. Each piece of gum should be chewed slowly for about 30 min.
3. Clients should be evaluated monthly and if the individual has not smoked for 3 months, the gum should be slowly withdrawn. Nicotine should not be used for longer than 6 months.
4. *Treatment of Overdose:* Syrup of ipecac if vomiting has not occurred, saline laxative, gastric lavage followed by activated charcoal (if client is unconscious), maintenance of respiration, maintenance of cardiovascular function.

Client/Family Teaching

1. Use the gum only as directed. When client has the urge to smoke, chew one piece very slowly. When a slight tingling becomes evident, stop chewing until sensation subsides.
2. Advise that too vigorous chewing can increase adverse effects. Provide a printed list of drug (gum) side effects. Instruct the client to report to the physician any that are bothersome.
3. Discuss with the client the local support groups that can help the client to stop smoking and provide emotional and psychologic support throughout the endeavor.

Evaluation: Evaluate client for evidence of control of nicotine withdrawal symptoms with a decrease in the number of cigarettes smoked per day or complete smoking cessation.

Nicotine transdermal system
(NIK-oh-teen)
Habitrol, Nicoderm, Prostep (Rx)

Classification: Smoking deterrent.

Action/Kinetics: Nicotine transdermal system is a multilayered film that provides systemic delivery of 7 mg, 14 mg, or 21 mg of nicotine over a 24-hr period after applying to the skin. Nicotine's reinforcing activity is due to two CNS effects. The first is stimulation of the cortex (via the locus ceruleus), producing increased alertness and cognitive performance. Secondly, there is a "reward" effect due to an action in the limbic system. At low doses the stimulatory effects predominate, whereas at high doses the reward effects predominate. The nicotine transdermal system produces an initial (first day of use) increase in blood pressure, an increase in heart rate (3%–7%), and a decrease in stroke volume after 10 days. Nicotine is metabolized in the liver to a large number of metabolites, all of which are less active than nicotine. **$t\frac{1}{2}$, following removal of the system from the skin:** 3–4 hr.

Uses: As an aid to stopping smoking for the relief of nicotine withdrawal symptoms. Should be used in conjunction with a comprehensive behavioral smoking cessation program.

Contraindications: Hypersensitivity or allergy to nicotine or any components of the therapeutic system. Use in children and during labor and delivery. Use in the immediate postmyocardial period, in clients with serious arrhythmias, and in those with severe or worsening angina pectoris. Use with severe renal impairment.

Special Concerns: Pregnancy category: D; pregnant smokers should be encouraged to try to stop smoking using educational and behavioral interventions before using the nicotine transdermal system. The product should only be used during pregnancy if the potential benefit outweighs the potential risk of nicotine to the fetus. The use of nicotine transdermal systems for longer than 3 months has not been studied. Clients with coronary heart disease (history of myocardial infarction and/or angina pectoris), serious cardiac arrhythmias, or vasospastic diseases (e.g., Buerger's disease, Prinzmetals variant angina) should be screened carefully before using the transdermal system. Use with caution in clients with hyperthyroidism, pheochromocytoma, or insulin-dependent diabetes (nicotine causes the release of catecholamines). Use with caution in clients with active peptic ulcers, in accelerated hypertension, and during lactation.

Side Effects: *Note:* The incidence of side effects is complicated by the fact that clients manifest effects of nicotine withdrawal or by concurrent smoking.
Dermatologic: Erythema, pruritus, or burning at the site of application; cutaneous hypersensitivity, sweating. *Body as a whole:* Allergy, back pain. *GI:* Diarrhea, dyspepsia, dry mouth, abdominal pain, constipation, nausea, vomiting. *Musculoskeletal:* Arthralgia, myalgia. *CNS:* Abnormal dreams, somnolence,

N

dizziness, impaired concentration, headache, insomnia. *CV:* Tachycardia, hypertension. *Respiratory:* Increased cough, pharyngitis, sinusitis. *GU:* Dysmenorrhea.

Symptoms of Overdose: Pallor, cold sweat, nausea, vomiting, abdominal pain, salivation, diarrhea, headache, dizziness, disturbed hearing and vision, mental confusion, weakness, tremor. Large overdoses may cause prostration, hypotension, respiratory failure, seizures, and death.

Dosage: Transdermal System.
Healthy clients: **initial dose,** 21 mg/day for 4–8 weeks; **first weaning dose,** 14 mg/day for 2–4 weeks; **second weaning dose:** 7 mg/day for 2–4 weeks. *Clients weighing less than 45.5 kg, those who smoke fewer than 10 cigarettes daily, or clients with cardiovascular disease:* **initial dose,** 14 mg/day for 4–8 weeks; **first weaning dose:** 7 mg/day for 2–4 weeks.

NURSING CONSIDERATIONS

Administration/Storage

1. The transdermal system should be applied promptly after its removal from the protective pouch to prevent loss of nicotine due to evaporation. Systems should only be used when the pouch is intact.
2. The system should be applied once daily to a non-hairy, clean, and dry site on the trunk or upper, outer arm. After 24 hr, the system should be removed and a new system applied to an alternate skin site. Skin sites should not be reused for at least a week.
3. When a used system is removed, it should be folded over and placed in the protective pouch that contained the new system. The used system should be disposed of to ensure access is prevented by children or pets.
4. The goal of therapy with nicotine transdermal systems is complete abstinence. If the client has not stopped by the fourth week of therapy, treatment should be discontinued.
5. The need for adjustment of the dose should be assessed during the first 2 weeks of therapy.
6. Nicotine will continue to be absorbed from the skin for several hours after removal of the system.
7. Clients who have successfully refrained from smoking should have the dose of nicotine decreased after each 2–4 weeks of treatment until the 7 mg/day dose has been used for 2–4 weeks.
8. *Treatment of Overdose:* Remove the transdermal system immediately. The surface of the skin may be flushed with water and dried; soap should not be used as it may increase the absorption of nicotine. Diazepam or barbiturates may be used to treat seizures and atropine can be given for excessive bronchial secretions or diarrhea. Respiratory support for respiratory failure and fluid support for hypotension and cardiovascular collapse. If transdermal systems are ingested orally, activated charcoal should be given to prevent seizures. If the client is unconscious, the charcoal should be administered by a nasogastric tube. A saline cathartic or sorbital added to the first dose of activated charcoal may hasten

GI passage of the system. Doses of activated charcoal should be repeated as long as the system remains in the GI tract as nicotine will continue to be released for many hours.

Assessment

1. Determine any evidence of renal or liver dysfunction.
2. Note any history of coronary artery disease.
3. List all medications client currently prescribed. Cessation of smoking, with or without nicotine replacement, may alter the response to certain drugs. For example, a decrease in the dosage of acetaminophen, caffeine, imipramine, insulin, oxazepam, pentazocine, propranolol, theophylline, and certain adrenergic blockers (e.g., prazosin, labetalol) may be required. An increase in the dose of adrenergic agonists (e.g., isoproterenol, phenylephrine) may be required.
4. Document any skin disorders as nicotine transdermal systems may be irritating for clients with skin disorders such as atopic or eczematous dermatitis.

Interventions: Use extreme caution during application and advise all to avoid contact with active systems. If contact does occur, wash the area with water only. The eyes should not be touched.

Client/Family Teaching

1. Follow the manufacturer's guidelines for proper system application. Review the information sheet that comes with the product as it contains instructions on how to use and dispose of the transdermal systems properly.
2. Stop smoking completely when initiating the nicotine transdermal system. If smoking continues, advise clients that they may experience side effects due to higher nicotine levels in the body.
3. Encourage participation in a formal smoking cessation program. The success or failure of smoking cessation depends on the quality, intensity, and frequency of supportive care. Stress that clients are more likely to stop smoking if they are seen frequently and are active in a formal smoking cessation program.
4. Advise client that nicotine in any form can be toxic and addictive. Review the risks of therapy and stress that the use of nicotine transdermal systems may lead to dependence. To minimize this risk, clients should be encouraged to withdraw use of the transdermal system gradually after 4–8 weeks of use.
5. Any persistent skin irritations such as erythema, edema, or pruritus at the application site as well as any generalized skin reactions such as hives, urticaria, or a generalized rash should be reported to the physician and the system should be removed.
6. Review the symptoms of nicotine withdrawal, which include craving, nervousness, restlessness, irritability, mood lability, anxiety, drowsiness, sleep disturbances, impaired concentration, increased appetite, headache, myalgia, constipation, fa-

tigue, and weight gain and advise client to report if evident as dosage may require adjustment.

7. Keep all products used and unused away from children and pets. Advise that sufficient nicotine is still present in used systems to cause toxicity.

Evaluation

1. Evaluate client for successful smoking cessation with control of symptoms of nicotine withdraw.

2. If therapy is unsuccessful after 4 weeks, discontinue and identify reasons for failure so that a later attempt may be more successful.

Nicotinic acid (Niacin)

(nih-koh-**TIN**-ick **AH**-sid, **NYE**-ah-sin)
Nia-Bid, Niac, Niacels, Niacor, Nico-400, Nicobid, Nicolar, Nicotinex, Slo-Niacin (Both Rx and OTC)

Classification: Vitamin, antihyperlipidemic.

Action/Kinetics: Nicotinic acid is present in two coenzymes—nicotinamide adenine dinucleotide (NAD) and nicotinamide adenine dinucleotide phosphate (NADP)—which are essential for oxidation-reduction reactions for tissue respiration. By altering fat metabolism in adipose cells (increasing lipolysis, stimulating lipoprotein lipase), nicotinic acid decreases serum cholesterol, triglycerides, VLDL, and LDL in types II, III, IV, and V hyperlipoproteinemia, while levels of HDL increase. It stimulates the release of histamine from mast cells and increases gastric secretion. **Onset:** 30 min. **Peak plasma concentration:** 45 min. **t½:** 45 min. **Therapeutic plasma concentration:** 0.5–1.0 mcg/ml. **Onset, decreased cholesterol levels:** several days. **Onset, decreased triglyceride levels:** several hours. Excreted by the kidneys.

Uses: Primary hyperlipidemia (types IIa, IIb, III, IV, or V hyperproteinemia) in clients with a significant risk of coronary artery disease and who have not responded to weight loss and diet. Prevention and treatment of pellagra.

Contraindications: Active peptic ulcer, hemorrhage, severe hypotension, hepatic dysfunction.

Special Concerns: Pregnancy category: C. Use with caution in gallbladder disease and in clients with a history of jaundice, liver disease, arterial bleeding, glaucoma, gout, or diabetes. Safety and efficacy have not been determined in children or geriatric clients.

Side Effects: *GI:* Nausea, vomiting, diarrhea, GI distress, activation of peptic ulcer, abdominal pain, hepatotoxicity. These reactions can be severe but usually respond to dosage reduction. Concomitant administration of antacids helps. *Ophthalmologic:* Blurred vision, amblyopia, ocular edema. *CNS:* Panic reactions, nervousness. *Dermatologic:* Flushing, pruritus, urticaria, dry skin, sensation of warmth, keratosis nigricans, skin rashes, itching and tingling of skin. *Alteration of glucose metabolism:* Hyperglycemia, glycosuria, precipitation of diabetes. *Other:* Hypotension, atrial fibrillation, cardiac arrhythmias, headache (transient).

Drug Interactions

Adrenergic blocking agents / Additive vasodilating effect → hypotension

Anticoagulants / Aluminum nicotinate ↑ effect

Antidiabetic agents / Change in sugar metabolism caused by aluminum nicotinate may require change in dosage of antidiabetic drugs

Probenecid / Nicotinic acid ↓ uricosuric effect of probenecid

Sulfinpyrazone / Nicotinic acid ↓ uricosuric effect of sulfinpyrazone

Tetracyclines / Effect ↓ by aluminum nicotinate

Laboratory Test Interferences: ↓ Glucose tolerance. Hyperuricemia, abnormal liver function tests.

Dosage: Extended-release Capsules/Tablets, Oral Solution, Tablets. Adults/adolescents: *antihyperlipidemic:* 1–2 g t.i.d. The dose can be increased in increments of 500 mg daily q 2–4 weeks as needed. **Maintenance:** 1–2 g t.i.d. (maximum dose: 6 g/day). **Pediatric:** Up to 300 mg daily using the oral solution or tablets. *Niacin deficiency:* Up to 100 mg daily. *Pellagra:* Up to 500 mg daily. *Recommended dietary allowance:* **Adults, males:** 15–20 mg daily; **females:** 13–15 mg daily.

NURSING CONSIDERATIONS

Administration/Storage

1. When used for hyperlipidemia, nicotinic acid is taken with or following meals and taken with cold water.
2. If flushing is persistent or bothersome, one aspirin, given 30 min prior to each dose of nicotinic acid, may assist the client.

3. Parenteral use (IV, SC, IM) is intended only when oral therapy is not possible and for treating vitamin deficiencies. The parenteral route is not to be used for treating hyperlipidemias.

Client/Family Teaching

1. Limit alcohol intake.
2. Take drug in *divided* doses with cold water at mealtime. If GI side effects persist, report to physician, who may reduce dosage and/or order an antacid.
3. Avoid taking aluminum nicotinate on an empty stomach, because in addition to gastric side effects, the likelihood of flushing is increased.
4. Flushing, pruritus, and nausea may subside with continued therapy. Aspirin may assist to reduce discomfort from the flushing response.
5. Clients with diabetes should be alert to symptoms of hyperglycemia precipitated by nicotinic acid. Monitor finger sticks and report hyperglycemia to the physician because a change in antidiabetic agents may be indicated.
6. Clients on anticoagulant therapy need to observe for increased bruising or bleeding and to report this to the physician.
7. In clients where acanthosis nigricans develops as a side effect, instruct that growths generally disappear 2 months after discontinuing drug therapy.

Evaluation: Evaluate client for laboratory evidence a decrease in serum cholesterol and triglyceride levels.

N

Nifedipine

(nye-**FED**-ih-peen)

Adalat, Adalat FT❋, Adalat P.A. 10 and 20❋, Apo-Nifed❋, Novo-Nifedin❋, Nu-Nifed❋, Procardia, Procardia XL (Rx)

See also *Calcium Channel Blocking Agents*, p. 118.

Classification: Calcium channel blocking agent (antianginal, antihypertensive).

Action/Kinetics: Variable effects on AV node effective and functional refractory periods. Cardiac output is moderately increased while peripheral vascular resistance is significantly decreased. **Onset:** 20 min. **Peak plasma levels:** 30 min (up to 4 hr for extended-release). **t½:** 2–5 hr. **Therapeutic serum levels:** 0.025–0.1 mcg/ml. **Duration:** 4–8 hr (12 hr for extended-release). Metabolized in the liver to inactive metabolites.

Uses: Angina due to coronary artery spasm, chronic stable angina including angina due to increased effort (especially in clients who cannot take beta-blockers or nitrates or who remain symptomatic following clinical doses of these drugs). Essential hypertension (sustained-release only). *Investigational:* Orally, sublingually, or chewed in hypertensive emergencies. Also prophylaxis of migraine headaches, primary pulmonary hypertension, severe pregnancy-associated hypertension, esophageal diseases, Raynaud's phenomenon, congestive heart failure, asthma, premature labor, biliary and renal colic, and cardiomyopathy.

Contraindications: Hypersensitivity. Lactation.

Special Concerns: Use during pregnancy only if benefits outweigh risks (pregnancy category: C). Use with caution in impaired hepatic or renal function and in elderly clients.

Side Effects: *CV:* Peripheral and pulmonary edema, myocardial infarction, hypotension, palpitations, syncope, congestive heart failure, decreased platelet aggregation, arrhythmias, tachycardia. Increased frequency, length, and duration of angina when beginning nifedipine therapy. *GI:* Nausea, diarrhea, constipation, flatulence, abdominal cramps, dysgeusia, vomiting, dry mouth, eructation, gastroesophageal reflux, melena. *CNS:* Dizziness, lightheadedness, giddiness, nervousness, sleep disturbances, headache, weakness, depression, migraine, psychoses, hallucinations, disturbances in equilibrium, somnolence, insomnia, abnormal dreams, malaise, anxiety. *Dermatologic:* Rash, dermatitis, urticaria, pruritus, photosensitivity, erythema multiforme, Stevens-Johnson syndrome. *Respiratory:* Dyspnea, cough, wheezing, shortness of breath, respiratory infection, throat, nasal, or chest congestion. *Musculoskeletal:* Muscle cramps or inflammation, joint pain or stiffness, arthritis, ataxia, myoclonic dystonia, hypertonia, asthenia. *Hematologic:* Thrombocytopenia, leukopenia, purpura, anemia. *Other:* Fever, chills, sweating, blurred vision, sexual difficulties, flushing, transient blindness, hyperglycemia, hypokalemia, gingival hyperplasia, hepatitis, tinnitus, gynecomastia, polyuria, nocturia, erythromelalgia, weight gain, epistaxis, facial and periorbital edema, hypoesthesia, gout, abnormal lacrimation, breast pain, dysuria, hematuria.

Additional Drug Interactions

Anticoagulants, oral / Possibility of ↑ prothrombin time

Cimetidine / ↑ Bioavailability of nifedipine

Digoxin / ↑ Effect of digoxin by ↓ excretion by kidney

Quinidine / Possible ↓ effect of quinidine due to ↓ plasma levels; ↑ risk of hypotension, bradycardia, AV block, pulmonary edema, and ventricular tachycardia

Ranitidine / ↑ Bioavailability of nifedipine

Theophylline / Possible ↑ effect of theophylline

Laboratory Test Interferences: ↑ Alkaline phosphatase, CPK, LDH, AST, ALT. Positive Coombs' test.

Dosage: Capsules. Individualized. Initial: 10 mg t.i.d. (range: 10–20 mg t.i.d.); **maintenance:** 10–30 mg t.i.d.–q.i.d. Clients with coronary artery spasm may respond better to 20–30 mg t.i.d.–q.i.d. Doses greater than 180 mg daily are not recommended. **Sustained-release Tablets, initial:** 30 or 60 mg once daily. Dosage can be increased as required and as tolerated. *Investigational, hypertensive emergencies:* 10–20 mg given orally, sublingually (by puncturing capsule and squeezing contents under the tongue), or chewed (capsule is punctured several times and then chewed).

NURSING CONSIDERATIONS

See also *Nursing Considerations* for *Calcium Channel Blocking Agents,* p. 119.

Administration/Storage

1. A single dose (other than sustained-released) should not exceed 30 mg.

2. Before increasing the dose of drug, BP should be carefully monitored.

3. Only the sustained-release tablets should be used to treat hypertension.

4. Sublingual nitroglycerin and long-acting nitrates may be used concomitantly with nifedipine.

5. Concomitant therapy with beta-adrenergic blocking agents may be used. In these cases, note any potential drug interactions.

6. Clients withdrawn from beta-blockers may manifest symptoms of increased angina which cannot be prevented by nifedipine; in fact, nifedipine may increase the severity of angina in this situation.

7. Clients with angina may be switched to the sustained-release product at the nearest equivalent total daily dose. However, doses greater than 90 mg daily should be used with caution.

8. Protect capsules from light and moisture and store at room temperature in the original container.

9. During initial therapy and when dosage is increased, clients may experience an increase in the frequency, duration, or severity of angina.

10. Food may decrease the rate, but not the extent, of absorption. Thus, the drug can be taken without regard to meals.

Assessment

1. Note any evidence of pulmonary edema, ECG abnormalities, or client complaint of palpitations.

2. Record any history of hypersensitivity to other calcium channel blocking agents.
3. When working with women of childbearing age, determine if pregnant because drug is contraindicated.

Interventions

1. During the titration period, note evidence of hypotensive response and increased heart rate that results from peripheral vasodilation. These side effects may precipitate angina.
2. Although beta-blocking drugs may be used concomitantly in clients with chronic stable angina, the combined effects of the drugs cannot be predicted (especially in clients with compromised left ventricular function or cardiac conduction abnormalities). Thus, BP should be monitored closely since severe hypotension may occur.
3. If therapy with a beta-blocker is to be discontinued, gradually decrease dosage to prevent withdrawal syndrome.
4. Determine if client is able to swallow before administering sublingually.

Client/Family Teaching

1. Sustained-release tablets should not be chewed or divided.
2. There is no cause for concern if an empty tablet appears in the stool.
3. Instruct clients to maintain a fluid intake of 2,000–3,000 ml/day to avoid constipation, unless contraindicated.
4. Caution not to use OTC drugs unless first discussed with the physician.

5. Report any symptoms of persistent headache, flushing, nausea, palpitations, weight gain, dizziness, or lightheadedness.
6. For clients also receiving beta-adrenergic blocking agents, review symptoms and advise to report any evidence of hypotension, exacerbation of angina, or evidence of heart failure.
7. Advise that once beta-blocking agents have been discontinued they may experience increased anginal pain. This is a common withdrawal symptom and should be reported to the physician.
8. Perform daily weights and note any extremity swelling. Advise that peripheral edema may result from arterial vasodilation that is precipitated by nifedipine or that swelling may indicate increasing ventricular dysfunction and should be reported to the physician.

Evaluation: Evaluate client for:
- Laboratory evidence that serum levels are within therapeutic range (0.025–0.1 mcg/ml)
- Reports of a reduction in the frequency and intensity of anginal episodes
- Evidence of a ↓ in blood pressure

Nimodipine

(nye-**MOH**-dih-peen)
Nimotop (Rx)

See also *Calcium Channel Blocking Agents,* p. 118.

Classification: Calcium channel blocking agent.

Action/Kinetics: Nimodipine acts similarly to other calcium channel blocking agents although it has a greater effect on cerebral arteries than arteries elsewhere in the body (probably due to its highly lipophilic properties). Its mechanism, however, is not known when used to reduce neurologic deficits following subarachnoid hemorrhage. **Peak plasma levels:** 1 hr. **$t^{1/2}$:** 1–2 hr. Significantly bound (over 95%) to plasma protein. Undergoes first-pass metabolism in the liver; metabolites are excreted through the urine.

Uses: Improvement of neurologic deficits due to spasm following subarachnoid hemorrhage from ruptured congenital intracranial aneurysms; clients should have Hunt and Hess grades of I–III. *Investigational:* Migraine headaches and cluster headaches.

Contraindications: Lactation.

Special Concerns: Use during pregnancy only if the potential benefits outweigh potential risks (pregnancy category: C). Safety and efficacy have not been established in children. Use with caution in clients with impaired hepatic function. The half-life may be increased in geriatric clients.

Side Effects: *CV:* Hypotension, peripheral edema, congestive heart failure, ECG abnormalities, tachycardia, bradycardia, palpitations, rebound vasospasm, hypertension, hematoma, disseminated intravascular coagulation, deep vein thrombosis. *GI:* Nausea, dyspepsia, diarrhea, abdominal discomfort, cramps, GI hemorrhage, vomiting. *CNS:* Headache, depression, lightheadedness, dizziness. *Hepatic:* Abnormal liver function test, hepatitis, jaundice. *Hematologic:* Thrombocytopenia, anemia, purpura, ecchymosis. *Dermatologic:* Rash, dermatitis, pruritus, urticaria. *Miscellaneous:* Dyspnea, muscle pain or cramps, acne, itching, flushing, diaphoresis, wheezing, hyponatremia.

Laboratory Test Interference: ↑ Nonfasting serum glucose, LDH, alkaline phosphatase, ALT. ↓ Platelet count.

Dosage: Capsules, Adults: 60 mg q 4 hr beginning within 96 hr after subarachnoid hemorrhage and continuing for 21 consecutive days. The dosage should be reduced to 30 mg q 4 hr in clients with hepatic impairment.

NURSING CONSIDERATIONS

See also *Nursing Considerations for Calcium Channel Blocking Agents,* p. 119.

Administration/Storage

1. If the client cannot swallow the capsule (e.g., unconscious or at time of surgery), a hole should be made in both ends of the capsule (soft gelatin) with an 18-gauge needle and the contents withdrawn into a syringe. The medication can then be administered into the nasogastric tube of the client and washed down the tube with 30 ml of normal saline.
2. Adult clients should be given 60 mg q 4 hr for 21 consecutive days after subarachnoid hemorrhage. The drug dosage should be reduced to 30 mg q 4 hr if the client has hepatic failure.

Assessment

1. Determine that laboratory studies for hepatic dysfunction have been performed.

2. If the client is of childbearing age, ascertain if pregnant.

Interventions

1. Anticipate initiation of nimodipine therapy within 96 hr of subarachnoid hemorrhage.
2. Perform baseline neuro scores and thoroughly document deficits.
3. Monitor I&O, BP, and pulse throughout therapy.
4. Anticipate reduction of dosage in clients with impaired liver function.

Client/Family Teaching

1. Inform the client that it is important to give the drug on time. Therefore, sleep must be interrupted to give the medication every 4 hr around the clock (RTC) for 21 days.
2. Explain the importance of reporting any side effects of the drug therapy, such as nausea, lightheadedness, dizziness, muscle cramps, or muscle pain.
3. Advise client to report any shortness of breath, the need to take deep breaths on occasion, wheezing or any other evidence of adverse effects.

Evaluation: Evaluate client for:

- Improved neuro scores and reduction of neurologic deficits due to venospasm following subarachnoid hemorrhage
- Reports of effective termination of migraine and cluster headaches

---

Nitrofurantoin

(nye-troh-fyour-AN-toyn)
Apo-Nitrofurantoin✤, Furadantin, Furalan, Furan, Furanite, Furatoin,

Furaton, Nitrofan, Nitrofor, Nitrofuracot, Novo–Nifedin✤, Nu-Nifed✤, Ro-Antoin (Rx)

Nitrofurantoin macrocrystals

(nye-troh-fyour-AN-toyn)
Macrodantin (Rx)

See also *Anti-Infectives,* p. 80.

Classification: Urinary germicide.

Action/Kinetics: Nitrofurantoin interferes with bacterial carbohydrate metabolism by inhibiting acetyl coenzyme A; the drug also interferes with bacterial cell wall synthesis. It is bacteriostatic at low concentrations and bactericidal at high concentrations. Tablets are readily absorbed from the GI tract. $t^{1/2}$: 20 min. **Urine levels:** 50–250 mcg/ml. From 30%–50% excreted unchanged in the urine. Nitrofurantoin macrocrystals (Macrodantin) are available; this preparation maintains effectiveness while decreasing GI distress.

Uses: Severe urinary tract infections refractory to other agents. Useful in the treatment of pyelonephritis, pyelitis, or cystitis caused by susceptible organisms, including *Escherichia coli, Staphylococcus aureus,* and *Streptococcus faecalis* and certain strains of *Enterobacter, Proteus,* and *Klebsiella.*

Contraindications: Anuria, oliguria, and clients with impaired renal function (creatinine clearance below 40 ml/min); pregnant women, especially near term; infants less than 1 month of age; and nursing mothers.

Special Concerns: To be used with extreme caution in clients with anemia, diabetes, electrolyte imbalance, avitaminosis B, or a debilitating disease.

Side Effects: Nitrofurantoin is a potentially toxic drug with many side effects. *GI:* Nausea, vomiting, anorexia, diarrhea, abdominal pain, parotitis, pancreatitis. *CNS:* Headache, dizziness, vertigo, drowsiness, nystagmus. *Hematologic:* Leukopenia, thrombocytopenia, eosinophilia, megaloblastic anemia, agranulocytosis, granulocytopenia, hemolytic anemia (especially in clients with glucose-6-phosphate dehydrogenase deficiency). *Allergic:* Drug fever, skin rashes, pruritus, urticaria, angioedema, exfoliative dermatitis, erythema multiforme (rarely, Stevens-Johnson syndrome), anaphylaxis, arthralgia, asthma symptoms in susceptible clients. *Respiratory:* Dyspnea, cough, chest pain, permanent impairment of pulmonary function with chronic therapy. *Hepatic:* Hepatitis, cholestatic jaundice, cholestatic hepatitis, liver dysfunction. *Miscellaneous:* Peripheral neuropathy, alopecia, superinfections of the GU tract, hypotension, muscle pain.

Drug Interactions

Acetazolamide / ↓ Effect of nitrofurantoin due to ↑ alkalinity of urine produced by acetazolamide

Antacids, oral / ↓ Effect of nitrofurantoin due to ↓ absorption from GI tract

Anticholinergic drugs / ↑ Effect of nitrofurantoin due to ↑ absorption from stomach

Magnesium trisilicate / ↓ Absorption of nitrofurantoin from GI tract

Nalidixic acid / Nitrofurantoin ↓ effect of nalidixic acid

Probenecid / High doses ↓ secretion of nitrofurantoin → toxicity

Sodium bicarbonate / ↓ Effect of nitrofurantoin due to ↑ alkalinity of urine produced by sodium bicarbonate

Dosage: Capsules, Oral Suspension, Tablets. Adults: 50–100 mg q.i.d., not to exceed 400 mg/day; **prolonged therapy:** 50–100 mg at bedtime. **Pediatric:** 5–7 mg/kg/day in 4 equal doses; **prolonged therapy:** 1 mg/kg/day in 1–2 doses.

NURSING CONSIDERATIONS

See also *General Nursing Considerations For All Anti-Infectives,* p. 83.

Administration/Storage

1. Administer oral medication with meals or milk to reduce gastric irritation.
2. Preferably, administer capsules containing crystals, instead of tablets, because crystals cause less GI intolerance.
3. Store oral medications in amber-colored bottles.
4. The medication should be continued for a minimum of three days after obtaining a negative urine culture.

Interventions

1. Observe client for acute or delayed anaphylactic reaction and have emergency equipment readily available.
2. Clearly label chart to show that client is on drug because it may alter certain laboratory determinations.
3. Monitor for recurrent UTI symptoms and report because urinary superinfections may occur.
4. Blacks and ethnic groups of Mediterranean and Near Eastern origin should be assessed for symptoms of anemia.

N

Client/Family Teaching

1. Drug may turn urine a dark yellow or brown color.
2. Increase fluid intake, drink at least 2 quarts of water a day, unless contraindicated
3. Take as prescribed and complete the full course of therapy.
4. Take with food or milk to minimize GI upset.
5. Report any persistent or bothersome side effects.
6. Immediately report any symptoms of numbness and tingling in the extremities. These side effects are indications for drug withdrawal because the condition may worsen and become irreversible.
7. Persistent nausea, vomiting, and diarrhea may be symptoms of a GI superinfection. Notify physician of these symptoms.

Evaluation: Evaluate client for laboratory evidence of negative urine cultures and for reports of symptomatic improvement.

Nitroglycerin IV
(nye-troh-**GLIH**-sir-in)
Nitro-Bid IV, Nitroject✿, Nitrostat IV, Tridil (Rx)

See also *Antianginal Drugs,* p. 47

Classification: Coronary vasodilator.

Action/Kinetics: Onset: 1–2 min; **duration:** 3–5 min (dose-dependent).

Uses: Hypertension associated with surgery and congestive heart failure associated with acute myocardial infarction. Angina unresponsive to usual doses of organic nitrate or beta-adrenergic blocking agents. Cardiac-load reducing agent.

Special Concerns: Pregnancy category: C. Dosage has not been established in children.

Dosage: IV infusion only. Initial: 5 mcg/min delivered by precise infusion pump. May be increased by 5 mcg/min q 3–5 min until response seen. If no response seen at 20 mcg/min, dose can be increased by 10–20 mcg/min until response noted. Monitor titration continuously until client reaches desired level of response.

NURSING CONSIDERATIONS

See also *Nursing Considerations* for *Antianginal Drugs,* p. 49.

Administration/Storage

1. Dilute with 5% dextrose USP, or 0.9% sodium chloride injection. Nitroglycerin injection is not for direct IV use; it must first be diluted.
2. Use only a glass IV bottle and administration set provided by the manufacturer because nitroglycerin is readily adsorbed onto many plastics. Avoid adding unnecessary plastic to IV system.
3. Aspirate medication into a syringe and then inject immediately into a glass bottle (or polyolefin bottle) to minimize contact with plastic.
4. Administer with a volumetric infusion pump rather than a peristaltic pump to regulate flow more accurately.
5. Do not administer with any other medications in the IV system.
6. Do not interrupt IV nitroglycerin for administration of a bolus of any other medication.
7. To provide correct dosage,

remove 15 ml of solution from the IV tubing if concentration of solution is changed.

Interventions

1. Obtain written parameters for BP and pulse and monitor closely throughout drug therapy.
2. Be prepared to monitor central venous pressure and/or pulmonary artery pressures as ordered.
3. Have emergency drugs readily available.
4. Administer IV solution with an electronic infusion device and in a closely monitored environment.
5. Monitor vital signs. Note any evidence of hypotension, client complaint of nausea, sweating and/or vomiting. Document presence of tachycardia or bradycardia. These symptoms may indicate that the dosage of drug is more than the client can tolerate.
   - Elevate the legs to restore BP.
   - Be prepared to reduce the rate of flow of the solution or to administer additional IV fluids.
6. Assess for thrombophlebitis at the IV site. Remove the IV from the reddened area.
7. Anticipate that after the initial positive response to therapy the dosage increments will be smaller. Adjustments in dosage will also be made at longer intervals.
8. Sinus tachycardia may occur in a client with angina pectoris who is receiving a maintenance dose of nitroglycerin. Notify physician, because a heart rate of 80 beats/min or less reduces myocardial demand.

9. Check that topical, oral, or sublingual doses are adjusted if client is on concomitant therapy with IV nitroglycerin.
10. Anticipate that client will be weaned from IV nitroglycerin by gradually decreasing doses to avoid posttherapy or cardiovascular distress. Tapering off is usually initiated when the client is receiving the peak effect from oral or topical vasodilators. The IV flow is usually reduced, and the client is monitored for hypertension and angina, which would require increased titration.
11. Obtain p.r.n. order for a non-narcotic analgesic (usually acetaminophen) because headache is a common side effect of drug therapy.

Evaluation: Evaluate client for:
- Reports of effective control of angina
- Evidence of a ↓ in blood pressure

Nitroglycerin sublingual

(nye-troh-**GLIH**-sir-in)
Nitrostat (Rx)

See also *Antianginal Drugs,* p. 47.

Classification: Antianginal agent.

Action/Kinetics: Sublingual. Onset: 1–3 min; **duration:** 30–60 min.

Uses: Agents of choice for prophylaxis and treatment of angina pectoris.

Special Concerns: Pregnancy category: C. Dosage has not been established in children.

Dosage: Sublingual Tablets: 150–600 mcg under the tongue or in the buccal pouch at first sign of attack; may be repeated in 5 min if necessary (no more than 3 tablets should be taken within 15 min). For prophylaxis, tablets may be taken 5–10 min prior to activities that may precipitate an attack.

NURSING CONSIDERATIONS

See also *Nursing Considerations* for *Antianginal Drugs,* p. 49.

Administration/Storage

1. Sublingual tablets should be placed under the tongue and allowed to dissolve; they should not be swallowed.
2. Sublingual tablets should be stored in the original container at room temperature protected from moisture. Unused tablets should be discarded if 6 months has elapsed since the original container was opened.

Client/Family Teaching

1. Instruct to date sublingual container upon opening.
2. Advise that if pain is not controlled, the physician should be contacted immediately.

Evaluation: Evaluate client for:
- Evidence of angina prophylaxis prior to strenuous activities
- Reports of effective termination of anginal attack

Nitroglycerin sustained-release capsules

(nye-troh-**GLIH**-sir-in)
Nitro-Bid Plateau Caps, Nitrocine Timecaps, Nitroglyn (Rx)

Nitroglycerin sustained-release tablets

(nye-troh-**GLIH**-sir-in)
Nitrogard-SR✹, Nitrong, Nitrong SR✹ (Rx)

See also *Antianginal Drugs,* p. 47.

Classification: Antianginal agent.

Action/Kinetics: Sustained-release: Onset: 20–45 min; **duration:** 3–8 hr.

Uses: To prevent anginal attacks. "Possibly effective" for the prophylaxis or treatment of anginal attacks.

Special Concerns: Pregnancy category: C. Dosage has not been established in children.

Dosage: Sustained-release capsules: 2.5, 6.5, or 9 mg q 8–12 hr. **Sustained-release tablets:** 1.3, 2.6, or 6.5 mg q 8–12 hr.

NURSING CONSIDERATIONS

See also *Nursing Considerations* for *Antianginal Drugs,* p. 49.

Administration/Storage

1. Sustained-release tablets and capsules should not be chewed and are not intended for sublingual use.
2. The smallest effective dose should be given 2–4 times daily.
3. Tolerance may develop.

Nitroglycerin, topical ointment

(nye-troh-**GLIH**-sir-in)
Nitro-Bid, Nitrol, Nitrol TSAR Kit✹, Nitrong✹ (Rx)

See also *Antianginal Drugs,* p. 47.

Classification: Antianginal agent.

Action/Kinetics: Topical ointment. Onset: 30–60 min; **duration:** 2–12 hr (depending on amount used per unit of surface area).

Special Concerns: Pregnancy category: C. Dosage has not been established in children.

Uses: Prophylaxis and treatment of angina pectoris.

Dosage: Topical ointment (2%): 1–2 inches (15–30 mg) q 8 hr [up to 5 (75 mg) inches q 4 hr may be necessary]. One inch equals approximately 15 mg nitroglycerin. Determine optimum dosage by starting with ½ inch q 8 hr and increasing by ½ inch with each successive dose until headache occurs; then, decrease to largest dose that does not cause headache. When ending treatment, reduce both the dose and frequency of administration over 4–6 weeks to prevent sudden withdrawal reactions.

NURSING CONSIDERATIONS

See also *Nursing Considerations* for *Antianginal Drugs,* p. 49.

Administration/Storage

1. Squeeze ointment carefully onto dose-measuring application papers, which are packaged with the medicine. Use applicator to spread ointment or fold paper in half and rub back and forth.
2. Use the paper to spread the ointment onto a nonhairy area of skin. Many clients find application to the chest psychologically helpful, but ointment may be applied to other nonhairy areas.
3. Rotate sites to prevent irritation. Keep a record of areas used to avoid unnecessary repetitive use of sites.
4. Apply ointment in a thin, even layer covering an area of skin 5–6 inches in diameter. Remember to remove last dose.
5. Tape the application paper over the area, or cover the area with a piece of plastic wrap-type material. A clear plastic cover causes less leakage of ointment, decreases skin irritation, increases the amount absorbed, and prevents clothing stains. Date, time, and initial tape at site.
6. Once the dose is established, use the same type of covering to ensure that the same amount of drug is absorbed during each application.
7. Clean around tube opening and tightly cap tube after use.
8. To prevent systemic absorption into nurse's system, the nurse should protect her own skin from contact with the ointment. Wash hands thoroughly after application to prevent headache.
9. Remove at bedtime or as directed to prevent tolerance or loss of drug effect.

Evaluation: Evaluate client for reports of effective termination and prevention of acute anginal episodes.

Nitroglycerin transdermal system

(nye-troh-**GLIH**-sir-in)

Deponit 0.2 mg/hr and 0.4 mg/hr, Minitran 0.1 mg/hr, 0.2 mg/hr, 0.4 mg/hr, and 0.6 mg/hr; Nitrocine 0.6 mg/hr; Nitrodisc 0.2 mg/hr, 0.3 mg/hr, and 0.4 mg/hr; Nitro-Dur 0.1 mg/hr, 0.2 mg/hr, 0.3 mg/hr, 0.4 mg/hr,

and 0.6 mg/hr; Transderm-Nitro 0.1 mg/hr, 0.2 mg/hr, 0.4 mg/hr, and 0.6 mg/hr (Rx)

See also *Antianginal Drugs,* p. 47.

Classification: Antianginal agent.

Action/Kinetics: Onset: 30–60 min; **duration:** 8–24 hr. The amount released each hour is indicated in the name.

Uses: Prophylaxis of angina pectoris due to coronary artery disease.

Special Concerns: Pregnancy category: C. Dosage has not been established in children.

Dosage: Initial: 0.2–0.4 mg/hr (initially the smallest available dose in the dosage series) applied each day to skin site free of hair and free of excessive movement (e.g., chest, upper arm). **Maintenance:** Additional systems or strengths may be added depending on the clinical response.

NURSING CONSIDERATIONS

See also *Nursing Considerations* for *Antianginal Drugs,* p. 49.

Administration/Storage

1. Follow instructions for specific products on package insert.
2. To avoid skin irritation, the application site should be slightly different each day.
3. Do not apply to distal areas of extremities.
4. If the pad loosens, apply a new pad.
5. It is important to note that there is a wide variety between clients in the actual amount of nitroglycerin absorbed each day. Physical exercise and increased ambient temperatures may increase the amount absorbed.
6. When terminating therapy, the dose and frequency of application should be gradually reduced over 4–6 weeks.
7. Tolerance is a significant factor affecting efficacy if the system is used continuously for more than 12 hr each day. Thus, a dosage regimen would include a daily period where the patch is on for 12–14 hr and a period of 10–12 hr when the patch is off.

Client/Family Teaching

1. Apply only as directed. Make sure skin is completely dry before applying.
2. Remember to remove old pad.
3. Rotate sites of application.
4. Date patch as a reminder that drug has been administered.
5. Once applied, do not disturb or open patch.
6. Remove at bedtime or as directed to prevent a diminished response (tolerance) to the drug.
7. Bathing or swimming should not interfere with therapy.

Evaluation: Evaluate client for reports of effective control and prevention of anginal episodes.

Nitroglycerin, translingual spray
(nye-troh-**GLIH**-sir-in)
Nitrolingual (Rx)

See also *Antianginal Drugs,* p. 47.

Classification: Coronary vasodilator.

Action/Kinetics: Onset: 2–4 min; **duration:** 30–60 min.

Uses: Coronary artery disease to relieve an acute attack or used prophylactically 10–15 min before beginning activities that can cause an acute anginal attack.

Special Concerns: Pregnancy category: C. Dosage has not been established in children.

Dosage: Spray. *Termination of acute attack:* 1–2 metered doses (400–800 mcg) on or under the tongue q 5 min as needed; no more than 3 metered doses should be administered within a 15-min period. *Prophylaxis:* 1–2 metered doses 5–10 min before beginning activities that might precipitate an acute attack.

NURSING CONSIDERATIONS

See also *Nursing Considerations* for *Antianginal Drugs,* p. 49.

Administration/Storage

1. The spray should *not* be inhaled.
2. Immediate medical attention should be sought if chest pain persists.

Evaluation: Evaluate client for reports of effective control and prevention of acute anginal episodes.

Nitroglycerin transmucosal

(nye-troh-**GLIH**-sir-in)
Nitrogard, Nitrogard-SR✸ (Rx)

See also *Antianginal Drugs,* p. 47

Classification: Coronary vasodilator.

Action/Kinetics: Onset: 3 min; **duration:** 3–5 hr.

Uses: Treatment and prophylaxis of angina.

Special Concerns: Pregnancy category: C. Dosage has not been established in children.

Dosage: Initial: 1 mg q 3–5 hr during time client is awake. Dose may be increased if necessary.

NURSING CONSIDERATIONS

See also *Nursing Considerations* for *Antianginal Drugs,* p. 49.

Administration/Storage

1. Tablet should be placed either between the lip and gum above the upper incisors or between the gum and cheek in the buccal area.
2. Allow tablet to dissolve in the mouth. The client should be warned not to swallow the tablet.
3. From 3–5 hr is required for tablet dissolution.
4. Store properly to maintain potency.
   - Do not expose to light, heat or air.
   - Keep in a tightly closed container below 30°C (86°F).
   - *Do not* keep cotton in the container once the bottle has been opened.

Client/Family Teaching

1. Demonstrate and review the appropriate method for buccal administration and proper storage of medication to maintain potency.
2. Instruct not to chew or swallow tablet and to expect 3–5 hr for complete dissolution.
3. Advise that drinking hot liquids or touching tablet with tongue will increase the rate of dissolution.

Evaluation: Evaluate client for reports of a ↓ frequency and ↓ intensity of anginal episodes.

N

Nitroprusside sodium
(nye-troh-**PRUS**-eyed)
Nipride, Nitropress (Rx)

Classification: Antihypertensive, direct action on vascular smooth muscle.

Action/Kinetics: Direct action on vascular smooth muscle, leading to peripheral vasodilation. The drug acts on excitation-contraction coupling of vascular smooth muscle by interfering with both influx and intracellular activation of calcium. Nitroprusside has no effect on smooth muscle of the duodenum or uterus and is more active on veins than on arteries. The drug may also improve congestive heart failure by decreasing systemic resistance, preload and afterload reduction, and improved cardiac output. **Onset** (drug must be given by IV infusion): 0.5–1 min; **peak effect:** 1–2 min; **t½:** 2 min; **duration:** Up to 10 min after infusion stopped. Nitroprusside reacts with hemoglobin to produce cyanmethemoglobin and cyanide ion. Caution must be exercised as nitroprusside injection can result in toxic levels of cyanide. However, when used briefly or at low infusion rates, the cyanide produced reacts with thiosulfate to produce thiocyanate, which is excreted in the urine.

Uses: Hypertensive crisis to reduce BP immediately. To produce controlled hypotension during anesthesia to reduce bleeding. *Investigational:* Severe refractory congestive heart failure (may be combined with dopamine); in combination with dopamine for acute myocardial infarction.

Contraindications: Compensatory hypertension. Use to produce controlled hypotension during surgery in clients with known inadequate cerebral circulation. Clients with congenital optic atrophy or tobacco amblyopia (both of which are rare).

Special Concerns: Use with caution in hypothyroidism, liver or kidney impairment, during pregnancy (category: C) and lactation, and in the presence of increased intracranial pressure. Geriatric clients may be more sensitive to the hypotensive effects of nitroprusside; also, a decrease in dose may be necessary in these clients due to age-related decreases in renal function.

Side Effects: Excessive hypotension. Large doses may lead to cyanide toxicity. *Following rapid injection:* Dizziness, nausea, restlessness, headache, sweating, muscle twitching, palpitations, abdominal pain, apprehension, retching, retrosternal discomfort. *Other symptoms:* Bradycardia, tachycardia, increased intracranial pressure, ECG changes, venous streaking, rash, methemoglobinemia, decreased platelet aggregation, flushing, hypothyroidism, ileus. *Symptoms of thiocyanate toxicity:* Blurred vision, tinnitus, confusion, hyperreflexia, seizures. *CNS symptoms (transitory):* Restlessness, agitation, and muscle twitching. Vomiting or skin rash.

Symptoms of Overdose: Excessive hypotension, cyanide toxicity, thiocyanate toxicity.

Drug Interaction: Concomitant use of other antihypertensives, volatile liquid anesthetics, or certain depressants ↑ response to nitroprusside.

Dosage: IV infusion only.
Adults: average, 3 mcg/kg/min. **Range:** 0.5–10 mcg/kg/min. Smaller dose is required for clients receiving other antihypertensives. **Pediatric:** 1.4 mcg/kg/min adjusted slowly depending on the response.

Monitor BP and use as guide to regulate rate of administration to maintain desired antihypertensive effect. Rate of administration should not exceed 10 mcg/kg/min.

NURSING CONSIDERATIONS

Administration/Storage

1. Protect drug from heat, light, and moisture.
2. Protect dilute solutions during administration by wrapping flask with opaque material, such as aluminum foil.
3. The contents of the vial (50 mg) should be dissolved in 2–3 ml of 5% dextrose in water. This stock solution must be diluted further in 250–1,000 ml 5% dextrose in water.
4. If properly protected from light, the reconstituted solution is stable for 24 hr.
5. Discard solutions that are any color but light brown.
6. Do not add any other drug or preservative to solution.
7. Cover IV bag and tubing with aluminum foil or foil-lined bags and change setup every 24 hr, unless otherwise indicated. Explain to client that covering the IV bag protects the medication from light and maintains drug stability. Administer IV solution with an electronic infusion device in a monitored environment.
8. Cyanide toxicity is possible if

more than 500 mcg/kg nitroprusside is given faster than 2 mcg/kg/min. To reduce this possibility, sodium thiosulfate can be co-infused with nitroprusside at rates of 5–10 times that of nitroprusside.
9. *Treatment of Overdose:*
    • Measure cyanide levels and blood gases to determine venous hyperoxemia or acidosis.
    • To treat cyanide toxicity, discontinue nitroprusside and give sodium nitrite, 4–6 mg/kg (about 0.2 ml/kg) over 2–4 min (to convert hemoglobin into methemoglobin); follow by sodium thiosulfate, 150–200 mg/kg (about 50 ml of the 25% solution). This regimen can be given again, at half the original doses, after 2 hr.

Assessment

1. Obtain baseline liver and renal function studies to assess function.
2. Note any history of hypothyroidism or vitamin B_{12} deficiency.

Interventions

1. Obtain written parameters for BP and monitor closely throughout drug therapy. Titrate infusion accordingly.
2. Observe for symptoms of thiocyanate toxicity listed under side effects. Evaluate laboratory values for thiocyanate levels every 24 hr or as directed during therapy.
3. Metabolic acidosis may be an early indicator of cyanide toxi-

N

city. Monitor closely and interrupt infusion and report to physician when toxicity evident.

Evaluation: Evaluate client for:
- Successful treatment of hypertensive crisis with a return of client BP to desired level
- Freedom from complications of drug therapy such as drug toxicity and overdosage

---

Nizatidine
(nye-**ZAY**-tih-deen)
Axid (Rx)

Classification: Histamine H_2-receptor antagonist.

Action/Kinetics: Nizatidine decreases gastric acid secretion by blocking the effect of histamine on histamine H_2-receptors. Does not affect the P-450 and P-448 drug metabolizing enzymes. **Peak plasma levels:** 0.5–3 hr after an oral dose. **Time to peak effect:** 0.5–3 hr. **Duration, nocturnal:** Up to 12 hr; **basal:** Up to 8 hr. **t½:** 1–2 hr. Approximately 60% of an oral dose is excreted unchanged in the urine. Clients with moderate to severe renal impairment manifest a significant prolongation of t½ with decreased clearance.

Uses: Acute duodenal ulcer. Prophylaxis of duodenal ulcer following healing of an active ulcer. *Investigational:* Benign gastric ulcer, gastroesophageal reflux disease.

Contraindications: Hypersensitivity to H_2-receptor antagonists. Cirrhosis of the liver, impaired renal or hepatic function. Lactation.

Special Concerns: Pregnancy category: C. Safety and efficacy have not been determined in children.

Side Effects: *CNS:* Headache, fatigue, somnolence, insomnia, confusion (rare). *GI:* Nausea, vomiting, diarrhea, pancreatitis, constipation, abdominal discomfort. *Dermatologic:* Exfoliative dermatitis, erythroderma, pruritus, urticaria, erythema multiforme. *CV:* Asymptomatic ventricular tachycardia; rarely, cardiac arrhythmias or arrest following rapid IV use. *Miscellaneous:* Impotence, loss of libido, thrombocytopenia, sweating, gynecomastia, hyperuricemia, eosinophilia, gout, and cholestatic or hepatocellular effects (resulting in ↑ AST, ALT, or alkaline phosphatase).

Drug Interactions: Following high doses of aspirin, nizatidine → ↑ salicylate serum levels.

Laboratory Test Interference: False + test for urobilinogen.

Dosage: Capsules. *Active duodenal ulcer:* Either 300 mg once daily at bedtime or 150 mg b.i.d. *Prophylaxis following healing of duodenal ulcer:* 150 mg once daily at bedtime. Dosage must be decreased for clients with moderate to severe renal insufficiency. *Treatment of gastric ulcer:* 150 mg b.i.d. or 300 mg h.s. *Gastroesophageal reflux disease:* 150 mg b.i.d.

NURSING CONSIDERATIONS

Administration/Storage

1. Treatment for active duodenal ulcer should be maintained for up to 8 weeks.
2. Gastric malignancy may be present even though a clinical response to nizatidine has occurred.

3. Doses of 150 and 300 mg can be mixed with commercial juices (apple juice, *Gatorade,* and others); such preparations are stable for 48 hr when refrigerated.

Assessment

1. Take a drug history to determine if the client has any allergies to H_2-receptor antagonists.
2. Obtain baseline laboratory studies including hepatic and renal function studies prior to initiating therapy.

Interventions

1. Assess the client for evidence of renal insufficiency. Document and report to the physician. Anticipate reduced dosage in clients with renal insufficiency.
2. Drug may cause a false + test for urobilinogen. If this test has been ordered, notify the lab that the client is taking nizatidine.

Client/Family Teaching

1. Notify the physician of any side effects, such as rashes, flaking of skin, or extreme sleepiness.
2. Take the medication at bedtime due to potential sedative effects.
3. Use caution when performing tasks that require mental alertness until drug effects realized.
4. Continue to take the medication as ordered even if symptoms subside.
5. Avoid alcohol, spicy foods, and aspirin products.
6. Do not smoke as this interferes with drug effects.

Evaluation: Evaluate client for reports of symptomatic improvement in gastric pain and irritation.

―――― *COMBINATION DRUG* ――――
Norcept-E 1/35 21 Day and Norcept-E 1/35 28 Day
(**NOR**-sept)
(Rx)

See also *Oral Contraceptives,* p. 192.

Components: Each tablet of Norcept-E 1/35 21 Day and the first 21 tablets of Norcept-E 1/35 28 Day contains ethinyl estradiol, 35 mcg and norethindrone, 1 mg (white tablets); the 28s also contain 7 inert green tablets.

Special Concerns: Pregnancy category: X.

NURSING CONSIDERATIONS
See *Oral Contraceptives,* p. 192.

N

―――― *COMBINATION DRUG* ――――
Nordette 21 Day and Nordette 28 Day
(**NOR**-dett)
(Rx)

See also *Oral Contraceptives,* p. 192.

Classification: Monophasic combination oral contraceptive.

Components: Each tablet of Nordette 21 and the first 21 tablets of Nordette 28 contains ethinyl estradiol, 30 mcg and levonorgestrel, 0.15 mg (light orange tablets); the 28s also contain 7 inert pink tablets.

Special Concerns: Pregnancy category: X.

NURSING CONSIDERATIONS
See *Oral Contraceptives,* p. 192.

—— *COMBINATION DRUG* ——
Norethin 1/35E 21 Day and Norethin 1/35E 28 Day
(NOR-eh-thin)
(Rx)

Norethin 1/50M 21 Day and Norethin 1/50M 28 Day
(NOR-eh-thin)
(Rx)

See also *Oral Contraceptives*, p. 192.

Classification: Monophasic combination oral contraceptive.

Components: Each tablet of Norethin 1/35E 21 Day and the first 21 tablets of Norethin 1/35E 28 Day contains ethinyl estradiol, 35 mcg and norethindrone, 1 mg (white tablets); the 28s also contain 7 inert blue tablets.

Each tablet of Norethin 1/50M 21 Day and the first 21 tablets of Norethin 1/50M 28 Day contains mestranol, 50 mcg and norethindrone, 1 mg (white tablets); the 28s also contain 7 inert blue tablets.

Special Concerns: Pregnancy category: X.

NURSING CONSIDERATIONS
See *Oral Contraceptives*, p. 192.

Norfloxacin
(nor-**FLOX**-ah-sin)
Chibroxin, Noroxin (Rx)

See also *Anti-Infectives*, p. 80 and *Fluoroquinolones*, p. 152.

Classification: Urinary anti-infective.

Action/Kinetics: Norfloxacin manifests activity against gram-positive and gram-negative organisms by inhibiting bacterial DNA synthesis. It is not effective against obligate anaerobes. **Peak plasma levels:** 1.4–1.6 mcg/ml after 1–2 hr following a dose of 400 mg and 2.5 mcg/ml 1–2 hr after a dose of 800 mg. **$t^{1/2}$:** 3–4 hr. Approximately 30% excreted unchanged in the urine and 30% through the feces.

Uses: *Systemic:* Complicated and uncomplicated urinary tract infections caused by *Escherichia coli, Klebsiella pneumoniae, Enterobacter cloacae, Proteus mirabilis, P. vulgaris, Providencia rettgeri, Pseudomonas aeruginosa, Citrobacter freundii, Morganella morganii, Staphylococcus aureus, S. epidermidis,* and group D streptococci. *Investigational:* Urethral gonorrhea and endocervical gonococcal infections due to penicillinase or nonpenicillinase-producing *Neisseria gonorrhoeae.*

Ophthalmic: Superficial ocular infections due to staphylococcal, klebsiella, streptococcal, proteus, enterobacter, and vibrio species; *S. aureus, E. coli, H. aegyptius, H. influenzae, K. pneumoniae, N. gonorrhoeae, Acinetobacter calcoaceticus, Enterobacter aerogenes, Pseudomonas aeruginosa, Aeromonas hydrophilia.*

Contraindications: Hypersensitivity to nalidixic acid, cinoxacin, or norfloxacin. Lactation, infants, and children.

Special Concerns: Pregnancy category: C. Use with caution in clients with a history of seizures and in impaired renal function.

Side Effects: *GI:* Nausea, abdominal pain, dyspepsia, heartburn, constipation, flatulence, diarrhea, vomiting, dry mouth, stomatitis, pseudomembranous colitis. *CNS:* Dizziness, headache, fatigue, depression, insomnia, somnolence, malaise, confusion, psychoses, paresthesia, seizures (rare). *Hematologic:* Decreased hematocrit, eosinophilia, decreased WBC count or neutrophil count, either increased or decreased platelets. *Dermatologic:* Rash, pruritus, exfoliative dermatitis, toxic epidermal necrolysis, erythema, erythema multiforme, Stevens-Johnson syndrome. *Other:* Hypersensitivity, fever, visual disturbances, hearing loss, crystalluria, cylindruria, candiduria, myoclonus (rare), hepatitis, pancreatitis, arthralgia.

Following ophthalmic use: Conjunctival hyperemia, photophobia, chemosis, bitter taste in mouth.

Additional Drug Interactions

Nitrofurantoin ↓ antibacterial effect of norfloxacin.

Laboratory Test Interferences: ↑ AST, ALT, alkaline phosphatase, BUN, serum creatinine, and LDH.

Dosage: Tablets. *Uncomplicated urinary tract infections:* 400 mg b.i.d. for 7–10 days. *Complicated urinary tract infections:* 400 mg b.i.d. for 10–21 days. Maximum dose for urinary tract infections should not exceed 800 mg daily. *Impaired renal function, with creatinine clearance equal to or less than 30 ml/min/1.73 m²:* 400 mg once daily for 7–10 days.

Ophthalmic solution. *Acute infections:* **initially,** 1–2 gtt q 15–30 min; **then,** reduce frequency as infection is controlled. *Moderate infections:* 1–2 gtt 4–6 times daily.

NURSING CONSIDERATIONS

See also *General Nursing Considerations For All Anti-Infectives,* p. 83.

Assessment

1. Note any history of seizure disorder or impaired renal function and anticipate reduced dosage with impaired renal function.
2. Obtain baseline CBC and urine cultures prior to initiating therapy.
3. Determine if client is pregnant. The drug is not for use in pregnant women or in children.

Client/Family Teaching

1. The medication should be taken 1 hr before or 2 hr after meals, with a glass of water.
2. To prevent crystalluria, clients should be well hydrated. Encourage intake of 2–3 L/day unless contraindicated.
3. Antacids should not be taken with or for 2 hr after a dose of norfloxacin.
4. Use caution while operating equipment or in driving a motor vehicle because the drug may cause dizziness.
5. Advise females of childbearing age to practice contraception during drug therapy.
6. Avoid prolonged sun exposure and wear sunglasses when exposed to prevent photophobia reactions.

Evaluation: Evaluate client for:
- Laboratory evidence of negative urine culture reports
- Reports of symptomatic improvement

─── *COMBINATION DRUG* ───
Norinyl 1 + 35 21-Day and Norinyl 1 + 35 28-Day
(**NOR**-ih-nill)
(Rx)

Norinyl 1 + 50 21-Day and Norinyl 1 + 50 28-Day

(**NOR**-ih-nill)

(Rx)

See also *Oral Contraceptives*, p. 192.

Classification: Monophasic combination oral contraceptive.

Components: Each tablet of Norinyl 1 + 35 21 and the first 21 tablets of Norinyl 1 + 35 28 Day contains ethinyl estradiol, 35 mcg and norethindrone, 1 mg (green tablets); the 28s also contain 7 inert orange tablets.

Each tablet of Norinyl 1 + 50 21 and the first 21 tables of Norinyl 1 + 50 28 Day contains mestranol, 50 mcg and norethindrone, 1 mg (white tablets); the 28s also contain 7 inert orange tablets.

Special Concerns: Pregnancy category: X.

NURSING CONSIDERATIONS

See *Oral Contraceptives*, p. 192.

――――― COMBINATION DRUG ―――――
Norlestrin 21 1/50 and Norlestrin 28 1/50

(nor-**LESS**-trin)

(Rx)

Norlestrin 21 2.5/50

(nor-**LESS**-trin)

(Rx)

Norlestrin Fe 1/50 and Norlestrin Fe 2.5/50

(nor-**LESS**-trin)

(Rx)

See also *Oral Contraceptives*, p. 192.

Classification: Monophasic combination oral contraceptive.

Components: Norlestrin 21 1/50 and Norlestrin 28 1/50: Each tablet of Norlestrin 21 1/50 and the first 21 tablets of Norlestrin 28 1/50 contains ethinyl estradiol, 50 mcg and norethindrone acetate, 1 mg (yellow tablets); the 28s also contain 7 inert white tablets.

Norlestrin Fe 1/50: The first 21 tablets each contain ethinyl estradiol, 50 mcg and norethindrone acetate, 1 mg (yellow tablets); the last 7 tablets each contain ferrous fumarate, 75 mg (brown tablets).

Norlestrin Fe 2.5/50: The first 21 tablets each contain ethinyl estradiol, 50 mcg and norethindrone acetate, 2.5 mg (pink tablets); the last 7 tablets each contain ferrous fumarate, 75 mg (brown tablets).

Norlestrin 21 2.5/50: Each tablet contains ethinyl estradiol, 50 mcg and norethindrone acetate, 2.5 mg (pink tablets).

Special Concerns: Pregnancy category: X.

NURSING CONSIDERATIONS

See *Oral Contraceptives*, p. 192.

Nortriptyline hydrochloride

(nor-**TRIP**-tih-leen)

Aventyl, Pamelor (Rx)

See also *Tricyclic Antidepressants*, p. 239.

Classification: Antidepressant, tricyclic.

Action/Kinetics: Nortriptyline manifests moderate anticholinergic and sedative effects but slight orthostatic hypotensive effects. **Effective plasma levels:** 50–150 ng/ml. **t½:** 18–44 hr.

Uses: Treatment of symptoms of depression. Chronic, severe neurogenic pain. Dermatologic disorders including chronic urticaria, angioedema, and nocturnal pruritus in atopic eczema.

Special Concerns: Use with caution during pregnancy. Safety and efficacy have not been determined in children.

Laboratory Test Interference: ↓ Urinary 5-hydroxyindole acetic acid (5-HIAA).

Dosage: Capsules, Oral Solution. Adults: *Depression:* 25 mg t.i.d.–q.i.d. Dose individualized. **Doses above 150 mg daily are not recommended. Elderly clients:** 30–50 mg/day in divided doses. **Not recommended for children.** *Dermatologic disorders:* 75 mg daily.

NURSING CONSIDERATIONS

See also *Nursing Considerations* for *Tricyclic Antidepressants,* p. 242.

Administration/Storage: Give after meals and at bedtime.

Evaluation: Evaluate client for:
- Reports of improvement in the levels of depression experienced
- Reports of effective control of neurogenic pain

—— COMBINATION DRUG ——
Novahistine Elixir
(no-vah-**HISS**-teen)
(OTC)

Classification/Content: *Antihistamine:* Chlorpheniramine maleate, 2 mg/5 ml. *Decongestant:* Phenylephrine HCl, 5 mg/5 ml.

See also information on individual components.

Uses: To treat congestion of the nose and eustachian tubes manifested by hay fever, the common cold, and sinusitis. Also useful for relief of other symptoms (e.g., runny nose, sneezing, itchy nose and throat, water eyes) due to hay fever or the common cold.

Dosage: Elixir. Adults: 10 ml q 4 hr; **pediatric, 6–12 years:** 5 ml q 4 hr; **pediatric, 2–6 years:** 2.5 ml q 4 hr. Use only on advice of physician if child is less than 2 years of age.

NURSING CONSIDERATIONS

See *Nursing Considerations* for *Antihistamines,* p. 74, and *Sympathomimetics,* p. 220.

Evaluation: Evaluate client for reports of symptomatic improvement in congestion and allergic manifestations.

N

Nylidrin
(**NYE**-lih-drin)
Arlidin, Arlidin Forte✲, PMS Nylidrin✲ (Rx)

Classification: Peripheral vasodilator.

Action/Kinetics: Vasodilation, primarily of skeletal muscle, by beta-adrenergic receptor stimulation and by direct relaxation of vascular smooth muscle. The drug also increases cardiac output. **Onset:** 10 min; **time to peak effect:** 30 min. **Duration:** 2 hr. Excreted in urine.

Uses: "Possibly effective" in peripheral vascular disease, including Raynaud's disease, thromboangiitis obliterans, arteriosclerosis obliterans, diabetic vascular disease, frostbite, night leg cramps, ischemic ulcer, acrocyanosis, acroparesthesia, thrombophlebitis. Circulatory disturbances of inner ear. Not a drug of choice. *Investigational:* To treat cognitive, emotional, and physical impairment in elderly clients.

Contraindications: Acute myocardial infarctions, angina pectoris, paroxysmal tachycardia, thyrotoxicosis.

Special Concerns: Use with caution in all clients with cardiac disease. Safety for use during pregnancy has not been determined. Risk of drug-induced hypothermia may be increased in geriatric clients. Clients intolerant to lactose, milk, or milk products may also be intolerant to nylidrin tablets because they contain lactose.

Side Effects: *CV:* Palpitations, orthostatic hypotension. *CNS:* Tremors, weakness, dizziness, nervousness. *GI:* Nausea, vomiting.

Dosage: Tablets: *Peripheral vascular disease, circulatory disturbances of the inner ear:* 3–12 mg t.i.d.–q.i.d. *Elderly clients to treat cognitive, emotional, and physical impairment:* 6–24 mg daily.

NURSING CONSIDERATIONS

Assessment

1. Note any history of heart disease. This drug must be used cautiously with clients who have cardiac dysfunction.
2. Assess BP and determine any evidence of pulse-pressure deficit.
3. Determine extent of client discomfort with alteration of vascularity.
4. Note any evidence of edema, numbness, and assess skin color prior to initiating drug therapy.

Client/Family Teaching

1. Review mutually set goals of therapy.
2. Avoid wearing restrictive garments.
3. Heart palpitations may occur but they should subside as therapy continues. Complaints of palpitations or persistent weakness or tremors should be reported as this may necessitate discontinuation of drug therapy.
4. Improvement may not be apparent for several weeks, but continue to take medication as prescribed.
5. Report any persistent bothersome symptoms to the physician.
6. Warn that possible circulatory disorders could cause client to have ringing in the ears or feelings of dizziness.
7. Sit up slowly and dangle legs a few minutes on the side of the bed before standing up to avoid hypotensive effects.
8. Take nylidrin with meals or with an antacid to avoid gastric distress.

Evaluation: Evaluate client for:
- Improved coloring with evidence of increased warmth in extremities
- Reports of symptomatic improvement with evidence of improved quality of pedal pulses

Nystatin
(nye-STAT-in)
Tablets: Mycostatin, Nilstat. Oral Suspension: Mycostatin, Nadostine ✤, Nilstat, Nystex, PMS Nystatin. Troches: Mycostatin

**Pastilles. Vaginal Tablets:
Mycostatin, Nadostine ✿, Nilstat,
O-V Statin. Topical: Mycostatin,
Nadostine ✿, Nilstat,
Nyaderm ✿, Nystex (Rx)**

See also *Anti-Infectives,* p. 80.

Classification: Antibiotic, antifungal.

Action/Kinetics: This natural antifungal antibiotic is derived from *Streptomyces noursei* and is both fungistatic and fungicidal against all species of *Candida.* Nystatin binds to fungal cell membranes (sterols), resulting in altered cellular permeability and leakage of potassium and other essential intracellular components. Nystatin is poorly absorbed from the GI tract; unabsorbed nystatin is excreted in the feces.

Uses: *Candida* infections of the skin, mucous membranes, GI tract, vagina, and mouth (thrush). The drug is too toxic for systemic infections although it can be given PO for intestinal moniliasis infections as it is not absorbed from the GI tract.

Contraindications: Use of topical products in or around the eyes.

Special Concerns: Pregnancy category: A (for vaginal use). Occlusive dressings should not be used when treating candidiasis. Lozenges should not be used in children less than 5 years of age.

Side Effects: Nystatin has few toxic effects. *GI:* Epigastric distress, nausea, vomiting, diarrhea. *Other:* Rarely, irritation.

Dosage: Lozenge, Oral Suspension, Tablets. *Intestinal candidiasis:* **Tablets,** 500,000–1,000,000 units t.i.d.; continue treatment for 48 hr after cure to prevent relapse. *Oral candidiasis:* **Oral Suspension, adults and children:** 400,000–600,000 units q.i.d. (½ dose in each side of mouth, held as long as possible before swallowing); **infants:** 200,000 units q.i.d. (same procedure as with adults); **premature or low birth weight infants:** 100,000 units q.i.d. **Lozenge, adults and children:** 200,000–400,000 units 4–5 times daily, up to 14 days. **Note:** Lozenges should not be chewed or swallowed. **Vaginal Cream, tablets:** 100,000 units (one tablet) inserted in vagina once or twice each day for 2 weeks. **Topical (ointment, cream, powder**—contains 100,000 units/g): Apply to affected areas b.i.d.–t.i.d., or as indicated, until healing is complete.

NURSING CONSIDERATIONS

See also *General Nursing Considerations For All Anti-Infectives,* p. 83.

N

Administration/Storage

1. A powder for extemporaneous compounding of the oral suspension is available. To reconstitute, add ⅛ tsp of the powder (about 500,000 units) to approximately ½–1 cup water and stir well. This product is administered immediately after mixing.
2. Protect drug from heat, light, moisture, and air.
3. The suspension can be stored for 7 days at room temperature or for 10 days in the refrigerator without loss of potency.
4. For *Candida* infections of the feet, the powder can be freely dusted on the feet as well as in socks and shoes.
5. The cream is generally used in *Candida* infections involving

intertriginous areas; however, very moist lesions should be treated with powder.

Interventions

1. Anticipate that vaginal tablets may be continued in the gravid client for 3–6 weeks before term to reduce incidence of thrush in the newborn.
2. Do not mix oral suspension in foods because the medication will be inactivated.
3. Apply cream or ointment to mycotic lesions with a swab or wear gloves to avoid direct contact with hands as contact dermatitis may ensue.
4. Drop 1 ml of oral suspension in each side of mouth or apply with a swab to treat oral moniliasis. Instruct client to swish around and keep medication in the mouth as long as possible before swallowing.
5. Vaginal tablets may be administered orally for candidiasis. These should be sucked on as a lozenge and not chewed or swallowed.
6. For pediatric use, 250,000 units of cherry flavor nystatin has been given frozen in the form of popsicles.
7. Insert vaginal tablets high in vagina with an applicator.
8. For fungal infections of the feet, the powder should be used freely on the feet, as well as in the shoes and socks.
9. For intertriginous areas, the cream should be used; however, for moist lesions, the powder is best.

Client/Family Teaching

1. Provide written guidelines and review the appropriate method and technique for administration and associated instructions according to area being treated as delineated under *Interventions*.
2. Continue using vaginal tablets even when menstruating because the treatment should be continued for 2 weeks. Avoid tampons.
3. To prevent reinfection, avoid intercourse during therapy or use condoms to prevent reinfection.
4. Provide a printed list of drug side effects. Advise to report any bothersome or persistent symptoms to physician.
5. Discontinue drug and notify physician if vaginal tablets cause irritation, redness, or swelling.
6. Drug may stain; sanitary pads may help protect clothing and linens.

Evaluation: Evaluate client for:
- Laboratory evidence of negative culture results
- Reports of improvement in skin and mucous membrane irritation with less associated discomfort

O

Octreotide acetate
(ock-**TREE**-oh-tyd)
Sandostatin (Rx)

Classification: Antineoplastic.

Action/Kinetics: Octreotide exerts effects similar to the natural hormone somatostatin. It suppresses secretion of serotonin and GI peptides including gastrin, insulin, glucagon, secretin, motilin, vasoactive intestinal peptide, and pancreatic polypeptide. The drug stimulates fluid and electrolyte absorption from the GI tract. It also inhibits growth hormone. The drug is rapidly absorbed from injection sites. **Peak levels:** Approximately 25 min. **t½:** 1.5 hr. **Duration:** Up to 12 hr. About one-third of a dose is excreted unchanged in the urine.

Uses: Metastatic carcinoid tumors; vasoactive intestinal tumors (VIPomas). The drug inhibits severe diarrhea in both situations and causes improvement in hypokalemia in VIPomas. *Investigational:* Life-threatening hypotension, acromegaly.

Special Concerns: Use during pregnancy only if clearly needed (pregnancy category: B). Use with caution during lactation. Use with caution in diabetics, in clients with gallbladder disease, and in clients with severe renal failure requiring dialysis.

Side Effects: *GI:* Nausea, diarrhea or loose stools, abdominal pain, malabsorption of fat, vomiting; less commonly, constipation, anorexia, dry mouth, flatulence, rectal spasm, GI bleeding, swollen stomach, heartburn, cholelithiasis. *CNS:* Headache, dizziness, lightheadedness, fatigue; less commonly, anxiety, seizures, depression, vertigo, hyperesthesia, drowsiness, pounding in head, irritability, decrease in libido, drowsiness, malaise, forgetfulness, nervousness, syncope, tremor, shakiness, Bell's palsy. *CV:* Flushing, edema; less commonly, hypertension, thrombophlebitis, shortness of breath, congestive heart failure, ischemia, palpitations, orthostatic hypotension, chest pain. *Metabolic:* Hyperglycemia or hypoglycemia, hyperosmolarity of urine, increase in CPK. *Musculoskeletal:* Asthenia, weakness; less commonly, muscle pain or cramping, back pain; joint, shoulder, arm, and leg pain; leg cramps. *Dermatologic:* Less commonly, thinning or flaking of skin, bruising, bleeding from superficial wounds, hair loss, rash, pruritus. *GU:* Prostatitis, oliguria, pollakiuria. *Other:* Pain, wheal, or erythema at injection site; less commonly, rhinorrhea, galactorrhea, hypothyroidism, numbness, hyperhidrosis, hyperdipsia, warm feeling or burning sensation, visual disturbance, chills, fever, throat discomfort, eyes burning.

Symptoms of Overdose: Hyperglycemia and hypoglycemia manifested by dizziness, drowsiness, loss of sensory or motor function, incoordination, disturbed consciousness, and visual blurring.

Drug Interactions: Octreotide may interfere with drugs such as diazoxide, insulin, beta-adrenergic blocking agents, or sulfonylureas. Close monitoring is necessary.

Dosage: SC (recommended), IV

bolus (emergencies). Initial, SC: 50 mcg 1–2 times daily. **Then,** *for carcinoid tumors:* 100–600 mcg daily in 2–4 divided doses for the first two weeks; **maintenance, usual:** 450 mcg daily (range: 50–1,500 mcg daily). *VIPomas:* 200–300 mcg daily in 2–4 divided doses for the first two weeks; **maintenance:** 150–750 mcg daily. **Pediatric, SC:** 1–10 mcg/kg daily.

NURSING CONSIDERATIONS

Administration/Storage

1. Experience is lacking for doses greater than 750 mcg daily.
2. Ampules should be inspected for particulate matter and discoloration; if present, the ampule must not be used.
3. Multiple injections at the same site should be avoided within a short period of time. Preferred sites for injection are the abdomen, hip, and thigh.
4. Reactions at the site of injection can be minimized by letting the solution warm to room temperature before administering the injection and by giving the injection slowly.
5. GI side effects can be minimized by giving the drug between meals and at bedtime.
6. Ampules should be stored for long periods at 2°C–8°C (36°F–46°F) although they may be stored at room temperature the day they will be used.
7. *Treatment of Overdose:* Withdraw drug temporarily and treat symptomatically.

Interventions

1. Monitor serum electrolyte and blood glucose levels. The drug alters serum glucose levels and may require an adjustment of antidiabetic drug dosage in clients with diabetes.
2. Obtain baseline thyroid function studies and monitor throughout therapy. The drug may cause biochemical hypothyroidism, necessitating replacement therapy.
3. Because the drug may alter fat absorption and gallbladder function, monitor the appropriate laboratory values, e.g., quantitative 72-hr fecal fat and serum carotene (fat malabsorption), and ultrasonography studies during long-term therapy.
4. Monitor the client's intake and output. Perform abdominal assessments routinely during therapy. Document and report any abnormal findings to the physician.

Client/Family Teaching

1. Provide a printed list of side effects and advise of the more frequent side effects, such as nausea, vomiting, dizziness, headache, diarrhea, abdominal pain, and weakness. If any of these symptoms persist, advise the client to report them to the physician.
2. Explain that the drug is usually administered SC. There may be pain at the site of injection. Discuss the need to rotate administration sites and provide written guidelines for the administration, dose, and site rotation.
3. Demonstrate the appropriate technique for SC injection and have the client do a return demonstration.
4. Explain that the dosage of drug is highly individualized. Therefore, it is important to take only as prescribed.

5. Keep the medication refrigerated.
6. Clients with diabetes should monitor blood sugars frequently and report variations.

Evaluation: Evaluate client for:
- Evidence of a ↓ in tumor size and spread
- Reports of a reduction in number of diarrheal stools and laboratory evidence of control of secondary electrolyte imbalance

Ofloxacin
(oh-**FLOX**-ah-zeen)
Floxin (Rx)

See also *Anti-Infectives,* p. 80.

Classification: Antibacterial, fluoroquinolone.

Action/Kinetics: Ofloxacin has activity against a wide range of gram-positive and gram-negative aerobic and anaerobic bacteria. Its bactericidal effect is thought to be due to inhibition of DNA gyrase, an essential bacterial enzyme necessary in the duplication, transcription, and repair of bacterial DNA. The production of penicillinase should have no effect on the activity of ofloxacin. The drug is widely distributed to body fluids. **Maximum serum levels:** 1–2 hr. **t½, first phase:** 4–5 hr; **second phase:** 20–25 hr. **Peak serum levels at steady state:** 1.5 mcg/ml after 200 mg doses, 2.4 mcg/ml after 300 mg doses, and 2.9 mcg/ml after 400 mg doses. Between 70%–80% is excreted unchanged in the urine.

Uses: Pneumonia or acute bacterial exacerbations of chronic bronchitis due to *Haemophilus influenzae* or *Streptococcus pneumoniae.* Not a drug of first choice in the treatment of presumed or confirmed pneumococcal pneumonia. Acute, uncomplicated urethral and cervical gonorrhea due to *Neisseria gonorrhoeae;* nongonococcal urethritis, and cervicitis due to *Chlamydia trachomatis.* Mixed infections of the urethra and cervix due to *Neisseria gonorrhoeae* and *Chlamydia trachomatis.* Mild to moderate skin and skin structure infections due to *Staphylococcus aureus, Streptococcus pyogenes,* or *Proteus mirabilis.* Uncomplicated cystitis due to *Citrobacter diversus, Enterobacter aerogenes, Escherichia coli, Klebsiella pneumoniae, Proteus mirabilis,* or *Pseudomonas aeruginosa.* Complicated urinary tract infections due to *Escherichia coli, Klebsiella pneumoniae, Proteus mirabilis, Citrobacter diversus,* or *Pseudomonas aeruginosa.* Prostatitis due to *Escherichia coli.*

Contraindications: Hypersensitivity to quinolone antibacterial agents. Use during lactation.

Special Concerns: Pregnancy category: C. Safety and effectiveness have not been established in children, adolescents under the age of 18 years, pregnant women, and lactating women. Use with caution in clients with known or suspected CNS disorders such as severe cerebral atherosclerosis, epilepsy, or factors that predispose to seizures.

Side Effects: *Hypersensitivity reactions:* Urticaria, dyspnea, pharyngeal or facial edema, itching, tingling, cardiovascular collapse, loss of consciousness, anaphylaxis. *GI:* Nausea (common), diarrhea, vomiting, GI distress, flatulence, dry mouth, dysgeusia, decreased appetite, constipation, dyspepsia, dysgeusia. *CNS:* Insomnia, headache, seizures, dizziness, fatigue, somnolence, sleep disorders, nervousness, anxiety, depression, cognitive change, dream abnormality, euphoria, hallucinations, paresthesia, syncope, vertigo. *CV:* Chest pain, edema, hypertension, palpitations, vasodilation. *GU:* External genital pruritus in women, vaginitis, vaginal discharge; burning, irritation, pain, and rash of the female genitalia; glucosuria, proteinuria, hematuria, pyuria, crystalluria, cylindruria, dysmenorrhea, menorrhagia, metrorrhagia, urinary frequency or pain. *Respiratory:* Cough, rhinorrhea. *Dermatologic:* Pruritus, rash, diaphoresis, vasculitis. *Hematologic:* Leukocytosis, pancytopenia, eosinophilia. *Musculoskeletal:* Asthenia, extremity pain, arthralgia, myalgia, possibility of osteochondrosis. *Miscellaneous:* Chills, malaise, hyperglycemia or hypoglycemia, whole body pain, thirst, weight loss, decreased hearing acuity, visual disturbances, photophobia, trunk pain.

Laboratory Test Interferences: ↑ ALT, AST.

Dosage: Tablets. *Pneumonia, exacerbation of chronic bronchitis:* 400 mg q 12 hr for 10 days. *Acute uncomplicated gonorrhea:* One 400 mg dose. *Cervicitis/urethritis* due to *C. trachomatis* or *C. trachomatis* and *N. gonorrhoeae:* 300 mg q 12 hr for 7 days. *Mild to moderate skin and skin structure infections:* 400 mg q 12 hr for 10 days. *Cystitis due to E. coli or K. pneumoniae:* 200 mg q 12 hr for 3 days. *Cystitis due to other organisms:* 200 mg q 12 hr for 7 days. *Complicated urinary tract infections:* 200 mg q 12 hr for 10 days. *Prostatitis:* 300 mg q 12 hr for 6 weeks.

The dose should be adjusted in clients with a creatinine clearance of 50 ml/min or less. If the creatinine clearance is 10–50 ml/min the dosage interval should be q 24 hr and if creatinine clearance is less than 10 ml/min the dose should be ½ the recommended dose given q 24 hr.

NURSING CONSIDERATIONS

See also *General Nursing Considerations For All Anti-Infectives,* p. 83.

Administration/Storage: The drug should be stored in tightly closed containers at a temperature below 30°C (86°F).

Assessment

1. Note any client history of hypersensitivity to quinolone derivatives.
2. Determine that baseline CBC, liver and renal function studies as well as necessary cultures have been performed prior to administering drug.
3. Assess client and history carefully and document any evidence of CNS disorders.

Interventions

1. Anticipate reduced dosage with altered renal function.
2. Perform culture and sensitivity studies throughout therapy to assess for any evidence of bacterial resistance.
3. Observe client with CNS disorders closely. Document and report any evidence of CNS effects such as tremors, restlessness, confusion, and hallucinations as drug therapy may need to be discontinued.

Client/Family Teaching

1. Do not take with food. Take medication 1 hr before or 3 hr after meals.
2. Drink 2–3 quarts of fluids per day to assist in drug elimination.
3. Do not take any vitamins, iron or mineral combinations, or aluminum- or magnesium-based antacids for 2 hr before or 2 hr after ingestion of ofloxacin.
4. Provide a printed list of drug side effects, and stress the ones that require immediate reporting to the physician.
5. Avoid direct sunlight as a photosensitivity reaction may occur. If exposure is necessary wear protective clothing and sunscreens.
6. Clients with diabetes should be advised to monitor their blood sugars consistently during drug therapy as extreme variations may develop.
7. Do not perform activities that require mental alertness until drug effects are realized as drug may cause drowsiness and lightheadedness.

Evaluation: Evaluate client for:
- Laboratory evidence of negative culture reports
- Reports of symptomatic improvement

Olsalazine Sodium
(ohl-**SAL**-ah-zeen)
Dipentum (Rx)

Classification: Anti-inflammatory drug.

Action/Kinetics: Olsalazine is a salicylate that is converted by bacteria in the colon to 5-aminosalicylic acid, which exerts an anti-inflammatory effect for the treatment of ulcerative colitis. The 5-aminosalicylic acid is slowly absorbed resulting in a high concentration of drug in the colon. The anti-inflammatory activity is likely due to inhibition of synthesis of prostaglandins in the colon. After oral use the drug is only slightly absorbed (2.4%) into systemic circulation where it has a short half-life (less than 1 hr) and is more than 99% bound to plasma proteins.

Uses: To maintain remission of ulcerative colitis in clients who cannot take sulfasalazine.

Contraindications: Hypersensitivity to salicylates.

Special Concerns: Pregnancy category: C. Use with caution during lactation. Safety and efficacy have not been established in children. May cause worsening of symptoms of colitis.

Side Effects: *GI:* Diarrhea (common), pain or cramps, nausea, dyspepsia, bloating, anorexia, vomiting, stomatitis. *CNS:* Headache, drowsiness, lethargy, fatigue, dizziness, vertigo. *Miscellaneous:* Arthralgia, rash, itching, upper respiratory tract infection. **Note:** The following symptoms have been reported upon withdrawal of therapy: diarrhea, nausea, abdominal pain, rash, itching, headache, heartburn, insomnia, anorexia, dizziness, lightheadedness, rectal bleeding, depression.

Symptoms of Overdose: Diarrhea, decreased motor activity.

Dosage: Capsules. Adults: Total of 1 g daily in 2 divided doses.

NURSING CONSIDERATIONS

Assessment

1. Note any history of sensitivity to salicylates and/or an intolerance to sulfasalazine.
2. In clients with renal disease, obtain pretreatment urinalysis, BUN, and creatinine and monitor throughout drug therapy.

Client/Family Teaching

1. Drug should be taken with food and in evenly divided doses.
2. Provide a printed list of drug side effects and stress those, such as persistent diarrhea, that should be immediately reported to the physician.

Evaluation: Evaluate client for:

- Evidence of the maintenance of remission of symptoms in ulcerative colitis
- Freedom from complications of side effects of drug therapy

Omeprazole

(oh-**MEH**-prah-zohl)
Prilosec (Rx)

Classification: Agent to suppress gastric acid secretion.

Action/Kinetics: Omeprazole does not possess either anticholinergic or histamine H_2-receptor antagonist effects. Rather, the drug is thought to be a gastric pump inhibitor in that it blocks the final step of acid production by inhibiting the $H^+ - K^+$ ATPase system at the secretory surface of the gastric parietal cell. Both basal and stimulated acid secretions are inhibited.

Serum gastrin levels are increased during the first one or two weeks of therapy and are maintained at such levels during the course of therapy. Because omeprazole is acid-labile, the product contains an enteric-coated granule formulation; however, absorption is rapid. **Peak plasma levels:** 0.5–3.5 hr. **Onset:** Within 1 hr. **t½:** 0.5–1 hr. **Duration:** Up to 72 hr (due to prolonged binding of the drug to the parietal $H^+ - K^+$ ATPase enzyme). The drug is significantly bound (95%) to plasma protein. Omeprazole is metabolized in the liver and inactive metabolites are excreted through the urine. Although plasma levels of omeprazole are increased in clients with chronic hepatic disease and in the elderly, dosage adjustment is not necessary.

Uses: Short-term (4–8 wk) treatment of duodenal ulcer, severe erosive esophagitis, and poorly responsive gastroesophageal reflux disease. Long-term treatment of pathologic hypersecretory conditions such as Zollinger-Ellison syndrome, multiple endocrine adenomas, and systemic mastocytosis. *Investigational:* Gastric ulcers, including healing gastric ulcers in clients receiving nonsteroidal anti-inflammatory drugs.

Contraindications: Long-term treatment of gastroesophageal reflux disease and esophagitis. Lactation.

Special Concerns: Use during pregnancy (category: C) only if potential benefits outweigh potential risks. Safety and effectiveness have not been determined in children.

Side Effects: *CNS:* Headache, dizziness. Possibly, anxiety disorders, abnormal dreams, vertigo, insomnia, nervousness, apathy, paresthesia, somnolence, hemifacial dysesthesia. *GI:* Diarrhea, nausea, abdominal pain, vomiting, constipation, flatulence, acid regurgitation, abdominal swelling. Possibly, anorexia, fecal discoloration, esophageal candidiasis, mucosal atrophy of the tongue, dry mouth, irritable colon. *CV:* Angina, chest pain, tachycardia, bradycardia, palpitation, peripheral edema. *Respiratory:* Upper respiratory infection, pharyngeal pain, epistaxis. *Skin:* Inflammation, alopecia, urticaria, pruritus, dry skin, hyperhidrosis. *GU:* Urinary tract infection, urinary frequency, hematuria, proteinuria, glycosuria, testicular pain, microscopic pyuria. *Hematologic:* Pancytopenia, thrombocytopenia, anemia, leukocytosis, neutropenia. *Musculoskeletal:* Asthenia, back pain, myalgia, joint pain, muscle cramps, leg pain. *Miscellaneous:* Rash, cough, fever, pain, fatigue, malaise, hypoglycemia, weight gain, tinnitus, abdominal swelling, alteration in taste.

Note: Data are lacking on the effect of long-term hypochlorhydria and hypergastrinemia on the risk of developing tumors.

Drug Interactions

Ampicillin (esters) / Possible ↓ absorption of ampicillin esters due to ↑ pH of stomach
Diazepam / ↑ Plasma levels of diazepam due to ↓ rate of metabolism by the liver
Iron salts / Possible ↓ absorption of iron salts due to ↑ pH of stomach
Ketoconazole / Possible ↓

absorption of ketoconazole due to ↑ pH of stomach
Phenytoin / ↑ Plasma levels of phenytoin due to ↓ rate of metabolism of the liver
Warfarin / Prolonged rate of elimination of warfarin due to ↓ rate of metabolism by the liver

Dosage: Capsules, sustained-release. *Active duodenal ulcer, severe erosive esophagitis, poorly responsive gastroesophageal reflux disease:* **Adults,** 20 mg daily for 4–8 wk. *Pathologic hypersecretory conditions:* **Adults, initial,** 60 mg once daily; **then,** dose individualized although doses up to 120 mg t.i.d. have been used. Daily doses greater than 80 mg should be divided. *Gastric ulcers:* 20–40 mg daily.

NURSING CONSIDERATIONS

Administration/Storage

1. Antacids can be administered with omeprazole.
2. The capsule should be taken before eating and is to be swallowed whole; it should not be opened, chewed, or crushed.

Assessment

1. Assess if female of childbearing age, to determine if pregnant.
2. Obtain baseline CBC, prior to initiating therapy.
3. Note any history of hepatic dysfunction.

Client/Family Teaching

1. Review the list of side effects associated with drug therapy. Instruct client to report any adverse effects to the physician.
2. Take drug as prescribed and

before meals. Do not crush or chew drug.

3. Report any changes in urinary elimination or pain and discomfort associated with voiding.

Evaluation: Evaluate client for:
- Evidence of a reduction in gastric acidity due to ↓ HCl production
- Reports of symptomatic improvement

Ondansetron hydrochloride
(on-**DAN**-sih-tron)
Zofran (Rx)

Classification: Antiemetic.

Action/Kinetics: Ondansetron is a 5-HT$_3$ (serotonin) antagonist. Serotonin receptors of the 5-HT$_3$ type are found centrally in the chemoreceptor trigger zone and peripherally on vagal nerve terminals. It is believed that cytotoxic chemotherapy results in the release of serotonin from enterochromoffin cells of the small intestine. The released serotonin may stimulate the vagal afferent nerves through the 5-HT$_3$ receptors thus stimulating the vomiting reflex. It is not known, however, whether the drug acts centrally and/or peripherally to antagonize the effect of serotonin. **t½:** 3.5–4.7 hr. A decrease in clearance and increase in half-life are observed in clients over 75 years of age, although no dosage adjustment is recommended. Clients less than 15 years of age show a shortened plasma half-life (2.4 hr). The drug is significantly metabolized with 5% of a dose excreted unchanged in the urine.

Uses: Prevent nausea and vomiting resulting from initial and repeated courses of cancer chemotherapy, including high-dose cisplatin.

Special Concerns: Pregnancy category: B. Use with caution during lactation. Data on safety and effectiveness in children 3 years of age and younger are not available.

Side Effects: *GI:* Diarrhea (most common), constipation. *CNS:* Headache, clonic-tonic seizures. *CV:* Tachycardia, chest pain, ECG alterations. *Miscellaneous:* Rash, bronchospasm, hypokalemia.

Dosage: IV. Adults and children, 4–18 years: Three doses of 0.15 mg/kg each. The first dose is infused over 15 min starting 30 min before the start of chemotherapy; the second and third doses are given 4 hr and 8 hr, respectively, after the first dose.

NURSING CONSIDERATIONS

See also *Nursing Considerations* for *Antiemetics,* p. 71.

Administration/Storage

1. The injection (containing 2 mg/ml) should be diluted in 50 ml of 5% dextrose injection or 0.9% sodium chloride injection before administration.
2. The diluted drug is stable at room temperature, with normal lighting, for 48 hr after dilution with 0.9% sodium chloride injection, 5% dextrose injection, 5% dextrose and 0.9% sodium chloride injection, 5% dextrose and 0.45% sodium chloride injection, and 3% sodium chloride injection.

Assessment: Determine that the initial dose of drug has been administered 30 min before the start of cancer chemotherapy; anticipate continuation of oral antiemetics for several days following a course of ondansetron therapy.

Evaluation: Evaluate client for:
- Evidence of the prevention of chemotherapy-induced emesis
- Reports of the effective control of refractory nausea and vomiting R/T chemotherapy

———— COMBINATION DRUG ————
Ornade
(OR-nayd)
(Rx)

Classification/Content: Each capsule contains: *Antihistamine:* Chlorpheniramine maleate, 12 mg. *Decongestant:* Phenylpropanolamine HCl, 75 mg.
See also information on individual components.

Uses: Symptoms of seasonal or perennial allergic rhinitis or the common cold including runny nose, nasal congestion, sneezing, itching throat or nose, itchy and watery eyes.

Contraindications: Lactation.

Special Concerns: Pregnancy category: B. Safety and effectiveness in children less than 12 years of age have not been determined.

Dosage: Capsules. Adults and children over 12 years: One capsule q 12 hr. Not to be used in children under 12 years of age.

NURSING CONSIDERATIONS

See *Nursing Considerations* for *Antihistamines,* p. 74, and *Sympathomimetics,* p. 220.

Evaluation: Evaluate client for reports of symptomatic improvement in allergic manifestations and symptoms of congestion.

Orphenadrine citrate
(or-**FEN**-ah-dreen)
Banflex, Blanex, Flexagin, Flexain, Flexoject, Flexon, K-Flex, Marflex, Myolin, Myotrol, Neocyten, Noradex, Norflex, O-Flex, Orflagen, Orfro, Orphenate, Tega-Flex (Rx)

See also *Centrally Acting Skeletal Muscle Relaxants,* p. 130.

Classification: Centrally acting muscle relaxant.

Action/Kinetics: Action may be related, in part, to its centrally mediated analgesic effects. It also possesses anticholinergic activity. **Onset, PO:** Within 1 hr; **IM:** 5 min; **IV:** immediate. **Peak effect:** 2 hr. **Peak serum levels:** 60–120 ng/ml (after 100 mg). **Duration:** 4–6 hr. **t½:** 14 hr. Excretion of a small amount of unchanged drug and metabolites is via both urine and feces.

Uses: Adjunct to the treatment of acute musculoskeletal disorders.

Contraindications: Angle-closure glaucoma, stenosing peptic ulcers, prostatic hypertrophy, pyloric or duodenal obstruction, cardiospasm, and myasthenia gravis. Use in children.

Special Concerns: Use with caution during pregnancy and lactation. Use with caution in cardiac disease.

Side Effects: Most side effects are anticholinergic in nature. *GI:* Dry mouth (first to appear), nausea, vomiting, constipation, gastric irritation. *CV:* Tachycardia, transient syncope, palpitation. *CNS:* Headache, dizziness, drowsiness, lightheadedness, agitation, tremor, hallucinations, weakness, confusion (in geriatric clients). *GU:* Urinary retention or hesitancy. *Ophthalmologic:* Dilated pupils, blurred vision, increased intraocular tension (especially in closed-angle glaucoma). *Miscellaneous:* Hypersensitivity reactions. Rarely, aplastic anemia, urticaria, anaphylaxis.

Symptoms of Overdose: Cardiac rhythm disturbances, seizures, shock, coma, respiratory arrest. Death can occur within 3–5 hr.

Drug Interactions

Anticholinergics / Additive anticholinergic effects
Contraceptives, oral / Orphenadrine ↑ breakdown by liver
Griseofulvin / Orphenadrine ↑ breakdown by liver
Propoxyphene / Concomitant use may result in anxiety, tremors, and confusion

Dosage: Extended-release Tablets. Adults: 100 mg b.i.d. in the morning and evening. **IV or IM:** 60 mg. May be repeated q 12 hr.

NURSING CONSIDERATIONS

See also *Nursing Considerations for Centrally Acting Skeletal Muscle Relaxants,* p. 130.

Administration/Storage

1. If the drug is to be administered IV, it should be given over a period of 5 min. The client should be in a supine position and should remain supine for 5–10 min following IV administration.

2. Sustained-release tablets should not be chewed or crushed.
3. *Treatment of Overdose:* Gastric lavage. Treat symptoms.

Assessment

1. Note any client history of angle-closure glaucoma. The drug is contraindicated when this condition exists.
2. Note any evidence of the disorders listed under contraindications; document and report.

Interventions: Observe the client for the presence of dry mouth. This is an indication that the dosage of drug should be reduced.

Client/Family Teaching

1. Encourage frequent rinsing of mouth and more fluids in the diet to relieve dry mouth.
2. Caution not to operate dangerous machinery or to drive a car because drug causes drowsiness.
3. Report any adverse side effects to the physician immediately.

Evaluation: Evaluate client for reports of effective control of musculoskeletal pain and discomfort.

—— *COMBINATION DRUG* ——
Ortho Cyclen-21 and Ortho Cyclen-28
(**OR**-thoh)
(**SIGH**-klen)
(**Rx**)

See also *Oral Contraceptives,* p. 192.

Components: Each tablet of Ortho Cyclen-21 and the first 21 tablets of Ortho Cyclen-28 contains ethinyl estradiol, 35 mcg and norgestimate, 0.25 mg. Ortho Cyclen-28s also contain 7 inert tablets.

Special Concerns: Pregnancy category: X.

NURSING CONSIDERATIONS

See *Oral Contraceptives*, p. 192.

See *Oral Contraceptives*, p. 192.

—— *COMBINATION DRUG* ——
Ortho-Novum 1/35 21 Day and Ortho-Novum 1/35 28 Day
(OR-thoh NO-vum)
(Rx)

Ortho-Novum 1/50 21 Day and Ortho-Novum 1/50 28 Day
(OR-thoh NO-vum)
(Rx)

See also *Oral Contraceptives*, p. 192.

Classification: Monophasic combination oral contraceptives.

Components: Ortho-Novum 1/35 21 and 1/35 28: Each tablet of Ortho-Novum 1/35 21 and the first 21 tablets of Ortho-Novum 1/35 28 contains ethinyl estradiol, 35 mcg and norethindrone, 1 mg (peach tablets); the 28s also contain 7 inert green tablets.

Ortho-Novum 1/50 21 and 1/50 28: Each tablet of Ortho-Novum 1/50 21 and the first 21 tablets of Ortho-Novum 1/50 28 contains mestranol, 50 mcg and norethindrone, l mg (yellow tablets); the 28s also contain 7 inert green tablets.

Special Concerns: Pregnancy category: X.

NURSING CONSIDERATIONS

See *Oral Contraceptives*, p. 192.

—— *COMBINATION DRUG* ——
Ortho-Novum 10/11 21 Day and Ortho-Novum 10/11 28 Day
(OR-thoh NO-vum)
(Rx)

See also *Oral Contraceptives*, p. 192.

Classification: Biphasic combination oral contraceptives.

Components: The first 10 tablets (first phase) of both Ortho-Novum 10/11 21 Day and 10/11 28 Day each contain ethinyl estradiol, 35 mcg and norethindrone, 0.5 mg (white tablets); the next 11 tablets (second phase) each contain ethinyl estradiol, 35 mcg and norethindrone, 1 mg (peach tablets). Ortho-Novum 10/11–28 Day also contains 7 inert green tablets.

Special Concerns: Pregnancy category: X.

NURSING CONSIDERATIONS

See *Oral Contraceptives*, p. 192.

—— *COMBINATION DRUG* ——
Ortho-Novum 7/7/7
(OR-thoh NO-vum)
(Rx)

See also *Oral Contraceptives*, p. 192.

Classification: Triphasic combination oral contraceptive.

Components: Phase 1 (first seven tablets): Each tablet contains ethinyl estradiol, 35 mcg and norethindrone, 0.5 mg (white tablets). Phase 2 (next 7 tablets): Each tablet contains ethinyl estradiol, 35 mcg and norethindrone, 0.75 mg (light peach tablets). Phase 3 (seven tablets): Each tablet contains ethinyl estradiol, 35 mcg and norethindrone, 1 mg (peach tablets). This product is packaged in both 21- and 28-tablet (with 7 inert green tablets) packs.

Special Concerns: Pregnancy category: X.

NURSING CONSIDERATIONS

See *Oral Contraceptives,* p. 192.

──── COMBINATION DRUG ────
Ovcon-35 21 Day and Ovcon-35 28 Day
(OV-kon)
(Rx)

Ovcon-50 21 Day and Ovcon-50 28 Day
(OV-kon)
(Rx)

See also *Oral Contraceptives,* p. 192.

Classification: Monophasic combination oral contraceptive.

Components: Ovcon-35: Each tablet of Ovcon-35 21 Day and the first 21 tablets of Ovcon-35 28 Day contains ethinyl estradiol, 35 mcg and norethindrone, 0.4 mg (peach tablets); the 28s also contain 7 inert green tablets.

Ovcon-50: Each tablet of Ovcon-50 21 Day and the first 21 tablets of Ovcon-50 28 Day contains ethinyl estradiol, 50 mcg and norethindrone, 1 mg (yellow tablets); the 28s also contain 7 inert green tablets.

Special Concerns: Pregnancy category: X.

NURSING CONSIDERATIONS

See *Oral Contraceptives,* p. 192.

──── COMBINATION DRUG ────
Ovral 21 Day and Ovral 28 Day
(OV-ral)
(Rx)

See also *Oral Contraceptives,* p. 192.

Classification: Monophasic combination oral contraceptives.

Components: Each tablet of Ovral 21 Day and the first 21 tablets of Ovral 28 Day contains ethinyl estradiol, 50 mcg and norgestrel, 0.5 mg (white tablets); the 28s also contain 7 inert pink tablets.

Special Concerns: Pregnancy category: X.

NURSING CONSIDERATIONS

See *Oral Contraceptives,* p. 192.

Oxacillin sodium
(ox-ah-**SILL**-in)
Bactocill, Prostaphlin (Rx)

See also *Anti-Infectives,* p. 80, and *Penicillins,* p. 197.

Classification: Antibiotic, penicillin.

Action/Kinetics: This is a penicillinase-resistant, acid-stable drug used for resistant staphylococcal infections. **Peak plasma levels: PO,** 1.6–10 mcg after 30–60 min; **IM,** 5–11 mcg/ml after 30 min. **t½:** 30 min.

Uses: Infections caused by penicillinase-producing staphylococci; also certain pneumococci and streptococci.

Dosage: Capsules, Oral Solution. Adults and children (over 20 kg): *Mild to moderate infections of the upper respiratory tract,* *skin, soft tissue:* 500 mg q 4–6 hr for at least 5 days. **Children less than 20 kg:** 50 mg/kg daily in equally divided doses q 6 hr for at least 5 days. *Septicemia, deep-seated infections:* Parenteral therapy (see below) followed by oral therapy. **Adults:** 1 g q 4–6 hr; **children:** 100 mg/kg daily in equally divided doses q 4–6 hr.

IM, IV. Adults and children (over 40 kg): 250–500 mg q 4–6 hr (up to 1 g q 4–6 hr in severe infections of the lower respiratory tract or disseminated infections); **children (less than 40 kg):** 50 mg/kg/day in equally divided doses q 6 hr (up to 100 mg/kg/day in severe infections). **Neonates and premature infants, less than 2,000 g:** 50 mg/kg daily divided q 12 hr if less than 7 days of age and 100 mg/kg daily divided q 8 hr if more than 7 days of age. **Neonates and premature infants, more than 2,000 g:** 75 mg/kg daily divided q 8 hr if less than 7 days of age and 150 mg/kg daily divided q 6 hr if more than 7 days of age. Maximum daily dose: **Adults,** 12 g; **children,** 100–300 mg/kg.

NURSING CONSIDERATIONS

See also *Nursing Considerations* for *Penicillins,* p. 200.

Administration/Storage

1. Administer IM by deep intragluteal injection, rotate injection sites, and observe for pain and swelling at IM injection site.
2. Reconstitution: Add sterile water for injection or sodium chloride injection in amount indicated on vial. Shake until solution is clear. For parenteral use, reconstituted solution may be kept for 3 days at room temperature or 1 week in refrigerator. Discard outdated solutions.
3. IV administration (two methods):
   - For rapid, direct administration, add an equal amount of sterile water or isotonic saline to reconstituted dosage and administer over a period of 10 min.
   - For IV infusion, add reconstituted solution to either dextrose, saline, or invert sugar solution and administer over a 6-hr period, during which time drug remains potent.
   - Observe for pain, redness, and edema at the site of IV injection and along the course of the vein.
4. Treatment of osteomyelitis may require several months of intensive oral therapy.

Evaluation: Evaluate client for:
- Clinical evidence of improvement in signs and symptoms of infection and for reports of improvement
- Laboratory evidence of negative culture reports
- Any reports of GI distress after oral administration, which may require alterations in therapy

Oxamniquine
(ox-**AM**-nih-kwin)
Vansil (Rx)

Classification: Anthelmintic, antischistosomal.

Action/Kinetics: *Schistosoma mansoni* is a trematode parasite found in Egypt, elsewhere in Africa, South America, and the West Indies, including Puerto Rico. The agent is found in water and is transmitted by snails. The drug causes the worms to shift from the mesenteric veins to the liver, where they are destroyed. Oxamniquine is more effective against male than against female schistosomes, but females cease laying eggs following treatment; thus, the infection eventually subsides due to decreased reproduction. **Peak plasma concentration:** 1–1.5 hr. **t½:** 1–2.5 hr. The drug is well absorbed after PO administration. Inactive metabolites are excreted in urine.

Uses: All stages of *S. mansoni* infections (acute and chronic), including involvement of the liver and spleen. *Investigational:* With praziquantel to treat neurocysticercosis (single dose only).

Special Concerns: Pregnancy category: C. Use during pregnancy and lactation only when potential benefits outweigh risks.

Side Effects: Well tolerated. *CNS:* Transient drowsiness and dizziness, headaches. Convulsions have been observed, but mostly in epileptics; therefore, closely monitor clients with history of convulsive disorders. *GI:* Nausea, vomiting, abdominal pain, anorexia. *Dermatologic:* Urticaria.

Dosage: Capsules. Adults: 12–15 mg/kg as single oral dose. **30–40 kg:** 500 mg; **41–60 kg:** 750 mg; **61–80 kg:** 1,000 mg; **81–100 kg:** 1,250 mg. **Children (under 30 kg):** 10 mg/kg followed in 2–8 hr with a second 10 mg/kg dose.

NURSING CONSIDERATIONS

See also *Nursing Considerations For All Anti-Infectives,* p. 83, and *Anthelmintics,* p. 42.

Client/Family Teaching

1. Do not drive a car or operate hazardous machinery because drug may cause dizziness and/or drowsiness.
2. Administer after food to minimize GI distress.

Evaluation: Evaluate for laboratory evidence of eradication of *Schistosoma mansoni* parasite.

Oxazepam
(ox-**AY**-zeh-pam)
Apo-Oxazepam ❋, Novoxapam ❋, Serax, Zapex ❋ (C-IV, Rx)

See also *Benzodiazepines,* p. 108.

Classification: Antianxiety agent, benzodiazepine.

Action/Kinetics: Absorbed more slowly than most benzodiazepines. **Peak plasma levels:** 2–4 hr. **t½:** 5–20 hr. Broken down in the liver to inactive metabolites, which are excreted through both the urine and feces. Drug is reputed to cause less drowsiness than chlordiazepoxide.

Uses: Anxiety, tension, anxiety with depression. Adjunct in acute alcohol withdrawal.

Special Concerns: Pregnancy category: D. Dosage has not been established in children less than 12 years of age; use is not recommended in children less than 6 years of age.

Additional Side Effects: Paradoxical reactions characterized by sleep disorders and hyperexcitability during first weeks of therapy. Hypotension has occurred with parenteral administration.

Dosage: Capsules, Tablets. Adults: *Anxiety, mild to moderate:* 10–30 mg t.i.d.–q.i.d. **Geriatric**

and debilitated clients, *anxiety, tension, irritability, agitation:* 10 mg t.i.d.; can be increased to 15 mg t.i.d.–q.i.d. *Alcohol withdrawal:* 15–30 mg t.i.d.–q.i.d.

NURSING CONSIDERATIONS

See *Nursing Considerations* for *Benzodiazepines,* p. 111.

Evaluation: Evaluate client for:

- Reports of ↓ levels of anxiety and tension
- Evidence of effective control of alcohol withdrawal symptoms

---

Ox Bile Extract (Bile Salts)
(OX BYEL)
Bilron (OTC)

Classification: Digestant (choleretic).

Action/Kinetics: Natural dried extract of ox bile, which allegedly increases the flow of bile as well as exerting a laxative effect. Effectiveness has not been shown, however.

Uses: Bile deficiency states. Laxative.

Contraindications: Severe jaundice, complete mechanical biliary obstruction. If symptoms of appendicitis are present (e.g., nausea, vomiting, abdominal pain).

Special Concerns: Use with caution in clients with obstructive jaundice.

Side Effects: Nausea, vomiting, diarrhea, and cramping.

Dosage: Bilron Capsules: 150–600 mg 1–3 times daily with or after meals. **Ox Bile Extract Enseal Tablets:** 324–648 mg (2 tablets)

daily with meals, up to a total of 6 tablets daily.

NURSING CONSIDERATIONS
Assessment

1. Determine if complete biliary obstruction is present and assess for any symptoms of obstruction because drug is contraindicated in this event.
2. Obtain baseline liver function studies and monitor throughout therapy.

Client/Family Teaching

1. Instruct client not to chew tablets because they taste bitter.
2. Take the medication with water either with or after meals.
3. Report any symptoms of nausea, vomiting, cramping, and diarrhea as dose may require adjustment.

Evaluation: Evaluate client for reports of improved digestion with desired laxative effect.

O

Oxiconazole nitrate
(ox-ee-**KON**-ah-zohl)
Oxistat (Rx)

Classification: Antifungal agent, topical.

Action/Kinetics: Oxiconazole acts by inhibiting ergosterol synthesis, which is required for cytoplasmic membrane integrity of fungi. It is active against a broad range of organisms including many strains of *Trichophyton rubrum* and *T. mentagrophytes.* Systemic absorption of the drug is low.

Uses: Topical treatment of tinea pedis, tinea cruris, and tinea corporis due to *T. rubrum* and *T. mentagrophytes.*

Contraindications: Ophthalmic use.

Special Concerns: Pregnancy category: B. Use with caution during lactation.

Side Effects: *Dermatologic:* Burning, itching, irritation, erythema, fissuring, maceration.

Dosage: Cream, topical: Apply 1% cream to cover affected areas once daily in the evening. To prevent recurrence, treatment should continue for 2 weeks for tinea corporis and tinea cruris and for 1 month for tinea pedis.

NURSING CONSIDERATIONS

Client/Family Teaching

1. Demonstrate how to apply the medication and instruct client/family to use only as directed.
2. Report any itching and/or burning associated with therapy because treatment should be discontinued if symptoms suggesting sensitivity or chemical irritation appear.
3. Stress the importance of following prescribed therapy as some infections may require 2 weeks to a month of daily treatments to ensure there is no recurrence.
4. Oxiconazole is intended for external use only and should not be introduced into the eye.

Evaluation

1. Evaluate client for reports of improvement in signs and symptoms of infection.
2. The diagnosis should be reviewed if the client shows no clinical response after the designated treatment period (tinea corporis and tinea cruris require 2 weeks of therapy; tinea pedis requires 1 month of therapy to prevent recurrence).

Oxybutynin chloride
(ox-ee-**BYOU**-tih-nin)
Ditropan (Rx)

Classification: Antispasmodic.

Action/Kinetics: Oxybutynin causes increased vesicle capacity and delay of initial urgency to void by exerting a direct antispasmodic effect. Has no effect at either the neuromuscular junction or autonomic ganglia. Has four to ten times the antispasmodic effect of atropine but only one-fifth the anticholinergic activity. **Onset:** 30–60 min; **Time to peak effect:** 3–6 hr; **duration:** 6–10 hr. Eliminated through the urine.

Use: Neurogenic bladder disease characterized by urinary retention, urinary overflow, incontinence, nocturia, urinary frequency or urgency, reflex neurogenic bladder.

Contraindications: Glaucoma (angle closure), GI obstruction, paralytic ileus, intestinal atony, megacolon, severe colitis, myasthenia gravis, obstructive urinary tract disease, acute hemorrhage.

Special Concerns: *Use with caution when increased cholinergic effect is undesirable and in the elderly.* Safe use during pregnancy (category: B) and in children less than 5 years of age has not been determined. Use with caution in geriatric clients; in clients with autonomic neuropathy, renal, or hepatic disease; and in clients with hiatal hernia with reflex esophagitis. Heat stroke and fever (due to decreased sweating) may occur if given at high environmental temperatures.

Side Effects: *GI:* Nausea, vomiting, constipation, bloated feeling, decreased GI motility. *CNS:* Drowsiness, insomnia, weakness, dizziness, restlessness, hallucinations. *EENT:* Dry mouth, blurred vision, dilation of pupil, cycloplegia, increased ocular tension. *CV:* Tachycardia, palpitations, vasodilation. *Miscellaneous:* Decreased sweating, urinary hesitancy and retention, impotence, suppression of lactation, severe allergic reactions, drug idiosyncrasies, urticaria, and other dermal manifestations. **Note:** The drug may aggravate symptoms of prostatic hypertrophy, hypertension, coronary heart disease, congestive heart failure, hyperthyroidism, cardiac arrhythmias, and tachycardia.

Symptoms of Overdose: Intense CNS disturbances (restlessness, psychoses), circulatory changes (flushing, hypotension) and failure, respiratory failure, paralysis, coma.

Dosage: Syrup, Tablets. Adults: 5 mg b.i.d.–t.i.d.; maximum dosage, 20 mg daily. **Children, over 5 years:** 5 mg b.i.d.–t.i.d.; maximum dosage, 15 mg daily.

NURSING CONSIDERATIONS

See also *Nursing Considerations* for *Cholinergic Blocking Agents,* p. 138.

Administration/Storage

1. Store in tight containers at 15°C–30°C (59°F–86°F).
2. *Treatment of Overdose:* Stomach lavage, physostigmine (0.5–2 mg IV; repeat as necessary up to maximum of 5 mg). Supportive therapy, if necessary. Counteract excitement with sodium thiopental (2%) or chloral hydrate (100–200 ml of 2% solution) rectally. Artifi-

cial respiration may be necessary if respiratory muscles become paralyzed.

Client/Family Teaching

1. Review prescription and instruct client to take only as directed.
2. Provide a printed list of side effects, stressing those that require immediate reporting to the physician.
3. Use caution driving a car or in operating dangerous machinery because drug may cause drowsiness and blurred vision.
4. Consult with physician before continuing with medication if diarrhea occurs (especially in clients with an ileostomy or colostomy) because diarrhea may be an early symptom of intestinal obstruction.
5. Wear sunglasses, sunscreens, and protective clothing during sunlight exposure as drug may cause a photosensitivity reaction.
6. Avoid overexposure to heat and acknowledge the body's need for increased fluids in hot weather because sweating is inhibited by the drug and heat stroke may occur.
7. Occasionally rinse mouth with water and increase fluid intake unless contraindicated, to relieve dryness of mouth.
8. Return as scheduled for cystometry to evaluate response to therapy and to determine the need for continuation of medication.

Evaluation: Evaluate client for:
- Reports of relief of spasms and associated GU pain
- Evidence of positive cystometry findings

Oxycodone hydrochloride

(ox-ee-**KOH**-dohn)
Roxicodone, Roxicodone Intensol, Supeudol✿ (C-II, Rx)

Oxycodone terephthalate

(ox-ee-**KOH**-dohn teh-ref-**THAL**-ayt)
(C-II, Rx)

See also *Narcotic Analgesics,* p. 174.

Classification: Narcotic analgesic, morphine type.

Action/Kinetics: A semisynthetic opiate, oxycodone produces mild sedation with little or no antitussive effect. It is most effective in relieving acute pain. **Onset:** 15–30 min. **Peak effect:** 60 min. **Duration:** 4–6 hr. Dependence liability is moderate. Oxycodone terephthalate is only available in combination with aspirin (e.g., Percodan) or acetaminophen.

Uses: Moderate to severe pain.

Additional Contraindications: Use in children.

Special Concerns: Pregnancy category: C.

Additional Drug Interactions: Clients with gastric distress, such as colitis or gastric or duodenal ulcer, and clients who have glaucoma should not receive Percodan, which also contains aspirin.

Dosage: Oral Solution, Concentrated Solution, Tablets. Adults: 5 mg q 6 hr. Use for children not recommended.

NURSING CONSIDERATIONS

See also *Nursing Considerations* for *Narcotic Analgesics,* p. 177.

Client/Family Teaching: Advise client to take medication with food to minimize GI upset.

Evaluation: Evaluate client for reports of effective control of pain.

Oxymetazoline hydrochloride

(ox-ee-meh-**TAZ**-oh-leen)
Nasal: 4-Way Long-Acting Nasal, Afrin Children's Strength 12 Hour Nose Drops and Regular Drops, Afrin 12 Hour Nasal Spray, Afrin Menthol Nasal Spray, Afrin Nasal Spray, Afrin Nose Drops, Coricidin Nasal Mist, Dristan Long Lasting Nasal Spray, Duramist Plus, Duration 12 Hour Nasal Spray, Nafrine Decongestant Nasal Drops and Spray, Neo-Synephrine 12 Hour Spray and Drops, Nostrilla 12 Hour Nasal Decongestant, Nostril Nasal Decongestant Mild and Regular, NTZ Long Acting Decongestant Nose Drops and Spray, Sinarest 12 Hour Nasal Spray, Vicks Sinex 12-Hour Spray. Ophthalmic: Ocu-Clear (OTC)

See also *Nasal Decongestants,* p. 182.

Classification: Nasal decongestant, topical.

Uses: Nasal decongestant, relieve eye redness due to minor irritations.

Special Concerns: Pregnancy category: C.

Dosage: Intranasal. Adults and children over 6 years: 2–3 sprays or 2–4 drops of 0.05% solution (regular or menthol) in each nostril in the morning and at night. **Pediatric, 2–6 years:** 2–3 gtt of the 0.025% solution in each nostril in the morning and at night. Available as a 0.025% solution for pediatric use and a 0.05% spray (regular or menthol) and drops for adult use.

Ophthalmic. 1–2 gtt into affected eye(s) q 6 hr.

NURSING CONSIDERATIONS

See *Nursing Considerations* for *Nasal Decongestants,* p. 182.

Evaluation: Evaluate client for:
- Reports of relief of nasal congestion
- Evidence of resolution of conjunctivitis

Oxytetracycline
(ox-ee-**teh**-trah-**SYE**-kleen)
Terramycin IM (Rx)

Oxytetracycline hydrochloride
(ox-ee-**teh**-trah-**SYE**-kleen)
E.P. Mycin, Terramycin, Uri-Tet (Rx)

See also *Anti-Infectives,* p. 80, and *Tetracyclines,* p. 222.

Classification: Antibiotic, tetracycline.

Action/Kinetics: $t^{1/2}$: 6–12 hr. 70% excreted unchanged in urine. From 20%–40% bound to serum proteins.

Dosage: Capsules, Tablets. See oral dosage for tetracycline hydrochloride. **IM. Adults, usual,** 250 mg once daily or 300 mg daily in divided doses q 8–12 hr. Up to 800 mg daily may be used. **Pediatric over 8 years:** 15–25 mg/kg up to maximum of 250 mg in single daily injection or divided and given q 8–12 hr. **IV infusion. Adults:** 250–500 mg (as the base) q 12 hr up to 2 g daily. **Pediatric 8 years of age and older:** 5–10 mg (as the base)/kg q 12 hr.

NURSING CONSIDERATIONS

See also *General Nursing Considerations For All Anti-Infectives,* p. 83, and *Tetracyclines,* p. 224.

Administration/Storage
1. Do not give with food or antacids.
2. Pediatric dosage should not be administered with milk or calcium-containing foods.
3. Check dilutions for IV administration.

Oxytocin, parenteral
(ox-eh-**TOE**-sin)
Pitocin (Rx)

Oxytocin, synthetic, nasal
(ox-eh-**TOE**-sin)
Syntocinon (Rx)

Classification: Oxytocic agent.

Action/Kinetics: These products are synthetic compounds identical to the natural hormone isolated from the posterior pituitary. Oxytocin has uterine stimulant, vasopressive, and antidiuretic properties. It acts by an indirect effect to mimic contractions of normal labor. Uterine sensitivity to oxytocin, as well as amplitude and duration of uterine contractions, increases gradually during gestation and just before parturition increases rapidly. The hormone facilitates ejection of milk from the breasts by stimulating smooth muscle. **Onset, IV:** immediate; **IM,** 3–5 min; **Nasal,** several minutes. **Peak effects:** 40 min. $t^{1/2}$: 1–6 min (decreased in late pregnancy and lactation). **Duration, IV:** 20 min after infusion is stopped; **IM:** 30–60 min; **nasal:** 20 min. Eliminated through the urine, liver, and functional mammary gland.

O

Uses: *Antepartum:* Induction or stimulation of labor at term. Used to overcome true primary or secondary uterine inertia. Induction of labor with oxytocin is indicated only under certain *specific* conditions and is not usual because serious toxic effects can occur.

Oxytocin is indicated

1. for uterine inertia.
2. for induction of labor in cases of erythroblastosis fetalis, maternal diabetes mellitus, preeclampsia, and eclampsia.
3. for induction of labor after premature rupture of membranes in last month of pregnancy when labor fails to develop spontaneously within 12 hr.
4. for routine control of postpartum hemorrhage and uterine atony.
5. to hasten uterine involution.
6. to complete inevitable abortions after the 20th week of pregnancy.
7. intranasally for initial letdown of milk.

Investigational: Breast engorgement, oxytocin challenge test for determining antepartum fetal heart rate.

Contraindications: Hypersensitivity to drug, cephalopelvic disproportion, malpresentation of the fetus, undilated cervix, overdistention of the uterus, hypotonic uterine contractions, and history of cesarean section or other uterine surgery. Also, predisposition to thromboplastin and amniotic fluid embolism (dead fetus, abruptio placentae), history of previous traumatic deliveries, or women with four or more deliveries. Oxytocin should never be given IV undiluted or in high concentrations. Oxytocin citrate is contraindicated in severe toxemia, cardiovascular or renal disease. Intranasal oxytocin is contraindicated during pregnancy (category: X).

Side Effects: *Mother:* Tetanic uterine contractions, rupture of the uterus, hypertension, tachycardia, and ECG changes after IV administration of concentrated solutions. Also, rarely, anxiety, dyspnea, precordial pain, edema, cyanosis or reddening of the skin, and cardiovascular spasm. Water intoxication from prolonged IV infusion, maternal deaths due to hypertensive episodes, subarachnoid hemorrhage, or uterine rupture.

Fetus: Death, premature ventricular contractions, bradycardia, tachycardia, hypoxia, intracranial hemorrhage due to overstimulation of the uterus during labor leads to uterine tetany with marked impairment of uteroplacental blood flow.

Note: Hypersensitivity reactions occur rarely. When they do, they occur most often with natural oxytocin administered IM or in concentrated IV doses and least frequently after IV infusion or diluted doses. Accidental swallowing of buccal tablets is not harmful.

Symptoms of Overdose: Hyperstimulation of the uterus resulting in hypertonic or tetanic contractions. Or, a resting tone of 15–20 cm water between contractions can result in uterine rupture, cervical and vaginal lacerations, tumultuous labor, uteroplacental hypoperfusion, postpartum hemorrhage, and a variable deceleration of fetal heart, fetal hypoxia, hypercapnia, or death. Water intoxication with seizures can occur if large doses (40–50 ml/min) of the drug are infused for long periods of time.

Drug Interactions: Severe hypertension and possible stroke when used with sympathomimetic pressor amines.

Dosage: IV infusion, IM. *Induction or stimulation of labor:* **IV infusion,** dilute 10 units (1 ml) to 1,000 ml isotonic saline or 5% dextrose. **Initial:** 0.001–0.002 unit/min (0.1–0.2 ml/min); dose can be gradually increased at 15–30 min intervals by 0.001 unit/min (0.1 ml/min) to maximum of 0.02 unit/min (2 ml/min). *Reduction of postpartum bleeding:* **IV infusion,** dilute 10–40 units (1–4 ml) to 1,000 ml with isotonic saline or 5% dextrose. Administer at a rate to control uterine atony, usually at a rate of 0.02–0.1 unit/min. *Incomplete or therapeutic abortion:* **IV infusion,** 10 units at a rate of 0.02–0.04 unit/min. **IM:** 10 units after placental delivery.

Synthetic, nasal (*for milk letdown*): one spray into one or both nostrils 2–3 min before nursing or pumping breasts.

NURSING CONSIDERATIONS

Administration/Storage

1. For *IV* use: Use Y-tubing system, with one bottle containing IV solution and oxytocin, and the other containing only the IV solution. This allows for the discontinuation of the drug while maintaining the patency of the vein when it is decided to change to the drug-free infusion bottle. Parenteral oxytocin infusions should be administered only with an electric infusion device.
2. As a *nasal spray:* Have the client sit upright and hold the bottle upright. Apply gentle pressure while spraying medication into the nostril. The nasal spray may be administered in drop form by applying gentle pressure to the bottle.
3. Oxytocin is rapidly broken down by sodium bisulfite. Have magnesium sulfate immediately available.
4. The physician should be immediately available during the administration of the drug.
5. *Treatment of Overdose:* Discontinue the drug and restrict fluid intake. Diuresis should be initiated and a hypertonic saline solution administered IV. Electrolyte imbalance should be corrected and seizures controlled with a barbiturate. If the client is comatose, special nursing care should be provided.

Assessment

1. Note if the client has any history of hypersensitivity to the drug.
2. Determine fetal maturity, pelvic adequacy, and fetal presentation prior to drug administration.
3. Check for dilation of the uterus and time the duration and frequency of the uterine contractions. Note fetal heart rate.
4. Carefully review the client's history for any contraindications prior to administering oxytocin.

(For induction and stimulation of labor and/or oxytocin challenge test):

Interventions

1. Before initiating therapy, inform the client of the rationale for using oxytocic agents and reassure the client that the procedure is not unusual.

2. Remain with the client during the induction period and throughout the stimulation of labor. The client must be attended by a qualified registered nurse.

3. Take the vital signs and check the I&O every 15 min.

4. Check the resting uterine tone and assess the uterine contractions for frequency, duration, and strength of the contraction.

5. Monitor the fetal heart rate and rhythm at least every 10 min. Document and immediately report any alterations from the normal pattern.

6. Prevent uterine rupture and fetal damage by clamping off IV oxytocin, starting medication-free IV fluids, turning client on her side, providing oxygen, and notifying the physician when the following events occur:
   - If the contractions occur more frequently than every 2 min and last longer than 60–90 sec with no period of uterine relaxation between contractions.
   - If the contractions are excessively strong and/or exceed 50 mm Hg, as measured either on an external monitor or by an internal uterine catheter with an electronic monitor.
   - If the fetal heart rate indicates bradycardia, tachycardia, or irregularities of rhythm, as measured by the fetoscope, Dopptone, or other type of electronic monitor.

7. Assess for water intoxication following prolonged administration of oxytocin. Monitor the client's I&O and serum electrolytes closely.

8. Observe the client for lethargy, confusion, and stupor. Note if the client has developed neuromuscular hyperexcitability with increased reflexes and muscular twitching. These symptoms should be reported immediately since convulsions and coma may occur if left untreated. Magnesium sulfate should be readily available for IV administration.

(During the fourth stage of labor when oxytocin is administered for prevention or control of hemorrhage):

Interventions

1. Describe the location, size, and firmness of the uterus. Report to the physician if the uterus is displaced or boggy and follow designated hospital protocol.

2. Note the amount and color of the lochia. Report any bright red lochia, excessive bleeding, or the passage of clots.

3. Monitor the client's vital signs until they remain stable.

4. Closely monitor I&O.

5. Observe the client for signs of water intoxication, document, and report to the physician immediately.

Evaluation: Evaluate client for:
- A positive clinical response based on indications for drug therapy such as induction of labor with effective contractions or increase in uterine tone
- Freedom from complications of drug therapy

P

Pamidronate disodium
(pah-**MIH**-droh-nayt)
Aredia (Rx)

Classification: Bone growth regulator, antihypercalcemic.

Action/Kinetics: Pamidronate inhibits both normal and abnormal bone resorption without inhibiting bone formation and mineralization. The precise mechanism is not known, but the drug may inhibit dissolution of hydroxyapatite crystal or have an effect on bone resorbing cells. The drug causes decreased serum phosphate levels probably due to a decreased release of phosphate from bone and increased renal excretion as parathyroid levels return to normal. Urinary calcium/creatinine and urinary hydroxyproline/creatinine ratios decrease and usually return to normal or below normal after treatment. **t½:** Biphasic, 1.6 hr (alpha) and 27.3 hr (beta). Approximately 50% of an IV infused dose is excreted unchanged in the urine within 72 hr.

Uses: In conjunction with hydration to treat moderate to severe hypercalcemia associated with malignancy (with or without bone metastases). *Investigational:* Paget's disease of the bone; postmenopausal osteoporosis; bone metastases from breast cancer to prevent further development of tumor-related hypercalcemia and to reduce the incidence of pathological fractures and severe bone pain; hyperparathyroidism; prophylaxis of glucocorticoid-induced osteoporosis; reduce bone pain in clients with

prostatic carcinoma and multiple myeloma osteolytic lesions; treat immobilization-induced hypercalcemia.

Contraindications: Hypersensitivity to biophosphonates.

Special Concerns: Pregnancy category: C. Use with caution during lactation. Safety and effectiveness have not been determined in children. Pamidronate has not been tested in clients who have creatinine levels greater than 5 mg/dl.

Side Effects: *Metabolic/Electrolytes:* Hypocalcemia, hypokalemia, hypomagnesemia, hypophosphatemia. *Body as a whole:* Slight increase in body temperature, fluid overload, generalized pain, fatigue, moniliasis. *GI:* Nausea, vomiting, constipation, abdominal pain, anorexia, GI hemorrhage, ulcerative stomatitis. *CNS:* Somnolence, insomnia, abnormal vision, slight possibility of seizures. *CV:* Hypertension, atrial fibrillation, syncope, tachycardia. *Respiratory:* Rales, rhinitis, upper respiratory tract infection. *GU:* Urinary tract infection. *Musculoskeletal:* Bone pain. *At site of administration:* Redness, swelling or induration, pain on palpation. *Miscellaneous:* Anemia, hypothyroidism.

Dosage: IV infusion. Initial therapy. *Moderate hypercalcemia (corrected serum calcium of about 12–13.5 mg/dl):* 60–90 mg. *Severe hypercalcemia (corrected serum calcium greater than 13.5 mg/dl):* 90 mg. If retreatment is necessary, use the same dose as for initial therapy.

NURSING CONSIDERATIONS

Administration/Storage

1. Initially, give as a single dose IV infusion over 24 hr.
2. If hypercalcemia recurs, re-treatment can be instituted provided a minimum of 7 days has elapsed to allow full response to the initial dose.
3. The drug is reconstituted by adding 10 ml sterile water for injection, which results in a concentration of 30 mg/10 ml with a pH of 6–7.4.
4. The drug is given over a 24-hr period by diluting in 1,000 ml of sterile 0.45% or 0.9% sodium chloride or 5% dextrose injection.
5. The solution for infusion is stable for up to 24 hr at room temperature. If reconstituted with sterile water for injection, the drug may be stored in the refrigerator for up to 24 hr at 2°–8°C (36°–46°F).
6. The drug should not be mixed with calcium-containing infusion solutions such as Ringer's solution.

Assessment

1. Document any history of bi-phosphonate hypersensitivity.
2. Note any evidence of cardiac disease.
3. Obtain baseline serum calcium, magnesium, potassium, and phosphorus levels.
4. Determine that CBC with differential and renal function studies have been performed.
5. Note indications for therapy, i.e., hypercalcemia of malignancy, symptomatic Paget's disease, postmenopausal osteoporosis, bone pain.

Interventions

1. Monitor I&O. Ensure adequate administration of fluids to correct hypovolemia and correct any volume deficits before administering diuretics.
2. At the time of drug administration, vigorous saline hydration should be undertaken for moderate to severe hypercalcemia to restore the urine output to about 2 L/day. For less severe hypercalcemia, more conservative approaches can be taken including saline hydration with or without loop diuretics. Overhydration should be avoided, however, especially in clients with heart failure.
3. Weigh client and observe for any evidence of edema.
4. Observe for any evidence of seizure activity and incorporate seizure precautions.
5. Monitor laboratory data. The following parameters should be monitored carefully: serum calcium, phosphate, magnesium, electrolytes, and creatinine as well as CBC and differential. Clients with pre-existing anemia, leukopenia, or thrombocytopenia should be carefully monitored during the first 2 weeks following treatment.

Client/Family Teaching

1. Review dietary sources of calcium (dark green vegetables, yogurt, cheese, milk, etc.) and vitamin D (herring, sardines, salmon, tuna) and encourage adequate intake. Determine need for supplements.
2. Advise clients they may experience transient mild temperature elevations for up to 48 hr following therapy.

3. Stress the importance of maintaining adequate hydration. A daily log of intake and output may assist to ensure compliance.

Evaluation: Evaluate client for laboratory evidence that serum calcium levels are within desired range (8.8–10.4 mg/dl).

Pancrelipase

(pan-kree-**LY**-payz)

Cotazym, Cotazym-S, Creon, Entolase, Entolase-HP, Festal II, Ilozyme, Ku-Zyme HP, Pancoate, Pancrease, Pancrease MT 4, Pancrease MT 10, Pancrease MT 16, Protilase, Viokase, Zymase (OTC and Rx)

Classification: Digestant.

Action/Kinetics: Enzyme concentrate from hog pancreas, which contains lipase, amylase, and protease, enzymes that replace or supplement naturally occurring enzymes. The product is more active at neutral or slightly alkaline pH. Pancrelipase has 12 times the lipolytic activity and 4 times both the proteolytic and amylolytic activity of pancreatin.

Uses: Replacement therapy for clients with pancreatic insufficiency, chronic pancreatitis, cystic fibrosis, ductal obstructions due to pancreatic cancer, postpancreatectomy, steatorrhea or malabsorption syndrome, postgastrectomy. Also, for presumptive test for pancreatic function.

Contraindications: Hog protein sensitivity.

Special Concerns: Use with cau-tion during pregnancy (category: C). Safety for use during lactation and in children less than 6 months of age not established.

Side Effects: *GI:* Nausea, diarrhea, abdominal cramps. Inhalation of the powder is irritating to the skin and mucous membranes and may result in an asthma attack. High doses cause hyperuricemia and hyperuricosuria.

Symptoms of Overdose: Diarrhea, intestinal upset.

Drug Interactions: Antacids containing calcium carbonate or magnesium hydroxide may reverse the beneficial effect of pancrelipase.

Dosage: Capsules, Delayed-release Capsules, Powder, Tablets. Adults and children: Dosage should be calculated according to fat content of the diet. Products contain varying amounts of the enzymes. **Usual dose:** 1–3 capsules or tablets before or with meals and snacks (severe deficiencies may require up to 8 capsules or tablets if no GI side effects occur). The dose of the powder is 1 packet (containing 0.7 g) before or with meals and snacks. For treatment of steatorrhea, the dose may be increased up to 3 capsules with meals.

NURSING CONSIDERATIONS

Administration/Storage

1. When administering to young children, the contents of the capsule can be sprinkled on food.
2. After several weeks of use, the dosage should be adjusted according to the therapeutic response.
3. Unopened preparations should

be stored in tight containers at a temperature not to exceed 25°C (77°F).

4. Enteric-coated products should not be crushed or chewed. Also, enteric-coated products that come in contact with foods with a pH greater than 5.5 will dissolve.

5. Generally, 300 mg of pancrelipase is required to digest every 17 g of dietary fat.

Assessment

1. Obtain a thorough nursing history.

2. Determine if the client has any sensitivity or allergy to hog protein. Hog protein is the main constituent of pancrelipase.

Client/Family Teaching

1. Review the appropriate dietary recommendations (usually low fat, high calorie, high protein) and refer to a dietitian for appropriate dietary counseling and assistance in meal planning.

2. The medication should be taken just before or with meals and snacks and with plenty of liquids to prevent oral irritation.

3. Report any nausea, cramping, or diarrhea. The dosage of medication may need to be adjusted to control steatorrhea.

4. Discuss the importance of reporting for follow-up laboratory studies as scheduled.

Evaluation: Evaluate for:

• Improved nutritional status following replacement in deficiency states

• Control of diarrhea in clients with steatorrhea

Pancuronium bromide
(pan-kyou-**ROH**-nee-um)
Pavulon (Rx)

See also *Neuromuscular Blocking Agents,* p. 183.

Classification: Nondepolarizing neuromuscular blocking agent.

Action/Kinetics: Effects similar to *d*-tubocurarine although pancuronium is 5 times as potent. Drug effects can be reversed by anticholinesterase agents. Pancuronium possesses vagolytic activity although it is not likely to cause histamine release. **Onset:** Within 45 sec. **Time to peak effect:** 3–4.5 min (depending on the dose). **Duration:** 35–45 min (increased with multiple doses). **t½, elimination:** 114–116 min. Ninety percent of the total dose is excreted through the urine either unchanged or as metabolites; 10% is excreted through the bile. In clients with renal failure, the t½ is doubled. Significantly bound to plasma protein.

Uses: Muscle relaxation during anesthesia, endotracheal intubation, management of clients undergoing mechanical ventilation.

Special Concerns: Pregnancy category: C. Children up to 1 month of age may be more sensitive to the effects of atracurium.

Additional Side Effects: *Respiratory:* Apnea, respiratory insufficiency. *CV:* Increased heart rate and increased mean arterial pressure. *Miscellaneous:* Salivation, skin rashes, hypersensitivity reactions (e.g., bronchospasm, flushing, hypotension, redness, tachycardia).

Additional Drug Interactions

Azathioprine / Reverses effects of pancuronium

Bacitracin / Additive muscle relaxation

Enflurane / ↑ Muscle relaxation

Isoflurane / ↑ Muscle relaxation

Quinine / ↑ Effect of pancuronium

Succinylcholine / ↑ Intensity and duration of action of pancuronium

Tetracyclines / Additive muscle relaxation

Theophyllines / ↓ Effects of pancuronium; also, possible cardiac arrhythmias

Dosage: IV only. Adults and children over 1 month of age, initial: 0.04–0.1 mg/kg. Additional doses of 0.01 mg/kg may be administered as required (usually q 20–60 min). **Neonates:** A test dose of 0.02 mg/kg should be administered first to determine responsiveness. *Endotracheal intubation:* 0.06–0.1 mg/kg as a bolus dose. *When used with enflurane or isoflurane anesthesia and/or after succinylcholine-assisted endotracheal intubation:* 0.05 mg/kg initially; **then,** adjust to client response.

NURSING CONSIDERATIONS

See also *Nursing Considerations* for *Neuromuscular Blocking Agents,* p. 184.

Administration/Storage

1. Additional doses of pancuronium significantly increase the duration of skeletal muscle relaxation.
2. The drug may be mixed with 5% dextrose, 5% dextrose and sodium chloride, lactated Ringer's injection, and 0.9% sodium chloride injection. When mixed with any of these solutions, the drug is stable for 2 days.
3. Anticipate the medication will act within 3 min upon administration and last 35–45 min.
4. Administer IV drug in a continuously monitored environment.

Interventions

1. Provide ventilatory support.
2. Monitor and record vital signs, I&O.
3. A peripheral nerve stimulator should be used to evaluate neuromuscular response intraoperatively.
4. Consciousness is not affected by pancuronium. Explain all procedures and provide emotional support.
5. Reassure clients that they will be able to talk and move once the drug effects are reversed.
6. Position the client for comfort and so that the body is in proper alignment. Turn and perform mouth care and eye care frequently.
7. Assess the client's airway at frequent intervals. Have a suction machine at the bedside.
8. Check to be certain that the ventilator alarms are set and on at all times.
9. Determine client need for medication for anxiety and/or for sedation.

Evaluation: Evaluate client for evidence of effective muscle relaxation with desired level of paralysis.

Pantothenic Acid (Vitamin B₅)

(pan-toe-**THEHN**-ick **AH**-sid)

Calcium Pantothenate (OTC)

Classification: Vitamin B complex.

Action/Kinetics: Pantothenic acid is a precursor of coenzyme A, which is a cofactor required for oxidative metabolism of carbohydrates, synthesis and breakdown of fatty acids, sterol synthesis, gluconeogenesis, and steroid synthesis. Pantothenic acid is found in many foods; thus, deficiency in human beings has not been observed.

Uses: There is no therapeutic indication for pantothenic acid alone because deficiency has not been observed. However, it is included in vitamin preparations for the prophylaxis and treatment of vitamin deficiency.

Contraindication: Hemophilia. Should not be used to treat diabetic neuropathy, increasing GI peristalsis, Addison's disease, allergies, respiratory disorders, improvement of mental processes, prevention of birth defects, or treatment of toxicity due to salicylate or streptomycin.

Side Effects: Allergic symptoms have occurred occasionally.

Dosage: Tablets. Adults and children: Up to 100 mg daily has been used.

NURSING CONSIDERATIONS

Assessment: Review client history to determine any evidence of conditions for which drug is contraindicated.

Client/Family Teaching: Report any allergic symptoms such as rash, erythema, or itching to the physician, as this is an indication to discontinue drug therapy.

Papaverine

(pah-**PAV**-er-een)

Cerespan, Genabid, Pavabid HP Capsulet, Pavabid Plateau Caps, Pavacap, Pavacen, Pavagen, Pavarine Spancaps, Pavased, Pavatine, Pavatym, Paverolan Lanacaps (Rx)

Classification: Peripheral vasodilator.

Action/Kinetics: Direct spasmolytic effect on smooth muscle, possibly by inhibiting cyclic nucleotide phosphodiesterase, thus increasing levels of cyclic AMP. This effect is seen in the vascular system, bronchial muscle, and in the GI, biliary, and urinary tracts. Large doses produce CNS sedation and sleepiness as well as depressing AV nodal and intraventricular conduction. The drug may also directly relax cerebral vessels as it increases cerebral blood flow and decreases cerebral vascular resistance. Absorbed fairly rapidly. Localized in fat tissues and liver. Steady plasma concentration maintained when drug is given q 6 hr. **Peak plasma levels:** 1–2 hr. **t½:** 30–120 min. Sustained-release products may be poorly and erratically absorbed. Metabolized in the liver and inactive metabolites excreted in the urine.

Uses: PO. Cerebral and peripheral ischemia due to arterial spasm and myocardial ischemia complicated by arrhythmias. Smooth muscle relaxant. **Parenteral.** Various conditions in which muscle spasm is observed including acute myocardial infarction, angina pectoris, peripheral vascular disease (with a vasospastic element), peripheral and pulmonary embolism, certain cerebral angiospastic states; ureteral, biliary, and GI colic. *Investigational:* Alone or with phentolamine as an intracavernous injection for impotence.

Contraindications: Complete AV block; administer with extreme caution in presence of coronary insufficiency and glaucoma.

Special Concerns: Safe use during pregnancy (category: C) and lactation or for children not established.

Side Effects: *CV:* Flushing of face, hypertension, increase in heart rate. *GI:* Nausea, anorexia, abdominal distress, constipation or diarrhea, dry mouth and throat. *CNS:* Headache, drowsiness, sedation, vertigo. *Miscellaneous:* Sweating, malaise, pruritus, skin rashes, increase in depth of respiration, hepatitis, jaundice, eosinophilia, altered liver function tests.

Note: Both acute and chronic poisoning may result from use of papaverine. Symptoms are extensions of side effects.

Symptoms of Acute Poisoning: Nystagmus, diplopia, drowsiness, weakness, lassitude, incoordination, coma, cyanosis, respiratory depression.

Symptoms of Chronic Poisoning: Ataxia, blurred vision, drowsiness, anxiety, headache, GI upset, depression, urticaria, erythematous macular eruptions, blood dyscrasias, hypotension.

Drug Interactions

Diazoxide IV / Additive hypotensive effect
Levodopa / Papaverine ↓ effect of levodopa by blocking dopamine receptors

Laboratory Test Interferences: ↑ AST, ALT, and bilirubin.

Dosage: Tablets: 100–300 mg 3–5 times/day; **Capsules, extended-release:** 150 mg q 12 hr up to 150 mg q 8 hr or 300 mg q 12 hr for severe cases. **IM, IV:** 30–120 mg given slowly (over 1–2 min, if IV) q 3 hr. *Cardiac extrasystoles:* Two doses 10 min apart either IM or IV (given slowly over 2 min). **Pediatric:** 6 mg/kg. **Intra-arterial:** 40 mg given slowly over 1–2 min. **Intracavernosal:** *impotence therapy:* 30 mg (of the injectable) mixed with 0.5–1 mg phentolamine mesylate for injection.

NURSING CONSIDERATIONS

Administration/Storage

1. IV injections must be given by the physician or under physician's immediate supervision.
2. Do not mix with Ringer's lactate solution because a precipitate will form.
3. Have emergency drugs and equipment readily available.
4. *Treatment of Acute Poisoning:* Delay absorption by giving tap water, milk, or activated charcoal followed by gastric lavage or induction of vomiting and then a cathartic. Blood pressure should be maintained and measures taken to treat respiratory depression and coma. Hemodialysis is effective.
5. *Treatment of Chronic Poisoning:* Discontinue medication. Monitor and treat blood dyscrasias. Provide symptomatic treatment. Treat hypotension by IV fluids, elevation of legs, and a vasopressor with inotropic effects.

Assessment

1. Note in the drug history if client is taking any drugs that would interact with papaverine therapy.
2. Determine any evidence of cardiac dysfunction and obtain baseline ECG.

Interventions

1. Closely monitor pulse, respirations, and BP for at least 30 min after IV injection of papaverine.
2. Report any symptoms of autonomic nervous system distress such as nystagmus, diplopia, or blurred vision to the physician.
3. Assess for GI reactions such as nausea or anorexia that should be reported to the physician. These may be symptoms of acute poisoning and require the immediate withdrawal of the drug and institution of emergency measures.

Client/Family Teaching

1. Advise not to perform activities that require mental alertness until drug effects are realized as drug may cause dizziness or drowsiness.
2. Avoid tobacco products as nicotine may cause vasospasm.

Evaluation: Evaluate client for:

- Evidence of control of vasospasm as demonstrated by absence of symptoms of peripheral, cerebral, or myocardial ischemia
- Reports of suppression of ureteral, biliary, and GI colic as demonstrated by a reduction in associated pain symptoms

---

Paraldehyde
(par-**AL**-deh-hyd)
Paral (C-IV) (Rx)

Classification: Nonbarbiturate sedative-hypnotic.

Action/Kinetics: Paraldehyde is bitter tasting (liquid) and has a strong, unpleasant odor. In usual doses, it has little effect on either respiration or BP. In the presence of pain, paraldehyde may induce excitement or delirium; it is not analgesic. **Onset:** 10–15 min. **Duration:** 8–12 hr. **Peak serum levels:** After PO, 30–60 min; after rectal administration, 2.5 hr. Approximately 70%–90% is detoxified in the liver, with the remainder excreted unchanged by the lungs. **t½:** 3.4–9.8 hr.

Uses: Sedative and hypnotic, although such use has generally been replaced by other sedative-hypnotics. Delirium tremens and other excited states. Prior to EEG to induce artificial sleep. Emergency treatment of seizures, eclampsia, tetanus, status epilepticus, and overdose of stimulant or convulsant drugs.

Contraindications: Gastroenteritis, bronchopulmonary disease, hepatic insufficiency. Use with caution during labor and during lactation.

Special Concerns: Pregnancy category: C. Use during labor may lead to respiratory depression in the neonate.

Side Effects: *Dermatologic:* Skin rash, redness, swelling or pain at injection site; nerve damage (may be severe and permanent), especially of the sciatic nerve if drug injected too close to nerve. *Respiratory:* Rarely, difficulty in breathing, shortness of breath. *Miscellaneous:* Bradycardia, strong odor to breath up to 24 hr following use. *Following IV use:* Coughing; right heart edema, dilation and failure; massive pulmonary hemorrhage. *Following prolonged use:* Dependence, similar to alcoholism leading to withdrawal syndrome including hallucinations and delirium tremens. Also, prolonged use may result in hepatitis.

Symptoms of Overdose: See *Barbiturates,* p. 101.

Drug Interactions

Disulfiram / Combination may produce an Antabuse-like-reaction
Sulfonamides / ↑ Chance of sulfonamide crystalluria

Laboratory Test Interference: 17-hydroxycorticosteroids, 17-ketogenic steroids.

Dosage: Liquid, Oral or Rectal. *Hypnotic:* **Adults, PO,** 10–30 ml; **rectal,** 10–20 ml with 1–2 parts olive oil or isotonic sodium chloride. **Pediatric, PO, rectal:** 0.3 ml/kg. *Sedation:* **Adults, PO, rectal,** 5–10 ml. **Pediatric, PO, rectal,** 0.15 ml/kg. *Delirium tremens:* **Adults, PO,** 10–35 ml. *Anticonvulsant:* **Adults, PO,** Up to 12 ml via gastric tube q 4 hr, if needed; **rectal,** 10–20 ml. **Pediatric, PO, rectal,** 0.3 ml/kg.

IM, IV. *Anticonvulsant:* **Adults, IM,** 5–10 ml; **IV infusion,** 5 ml diluted with at least 100 ml 0.9% sodium chloride given at a rate not to exceed 1 ml/min. **Pediatric, IM, IV,** 0.1–0.15 ml/kg.

NURSING CONSIDERATIONS

See also *Nursing Considerations* for *Chloral Hydrate,* p. 424.

Administration/Storage

1. *PO:* Drug should be cold to minimize odor and taste as well as gastric irritation. Mask the taste and odor by mixing drug with syrup, milk, or fruit juice.
2. *Rectal:* Mix with olive oil, cottonseed oil, or isotonic sodium chloride solution to minimize irritation—1 part medication to 2 parts diluent.
3. *IM:* A pure sterile preparation should be used. Inject deeply into gluteus maximus and avoid extravasation into subcutaneous tissue because drug is irritating and may cause sterile abscesses and nerve injury and paralysis.
4. *IV:* Only in an emergency, dilute with 20 volumes of 0.9% sodium chloride injection and inject at a rate not to exceed 1 ml/min because circulatory collapse or pulmonary edema may occur. Use glass syringe and metal needles because the drug may react with the plastic used in disposable syringes and needles.
5. Store in a tight, light-resistant container, at temperatures not to exceed 25°C (77°F).
6. Should not be used if paraldehyde has a strong vinegar odor or is brownish in color.
7. Paraldehyde should not be used if the container has been opened for more than 24 hr.
8. *Treatment of Overdose:* See *Barbiturates,* p. 101.

Assessment

1. Document baseline neuro and mental status.
2. Obtain baseline liver and renal function studies. Monitor periodically to measure future organ function as the therapy progresses.

Interventions

1. Ensure that the room is well ventilated so as to remove exhaled paraldehyde.
2. Offer reassurance if the client is disturbed by the odor of the drug.

3. Assess the client for evidence of dependency and toxicity. Do not withdraw the drug abruptly.
4. Report any evidence of coughing during IV administration. This symptom can indicate deleterious effects on pulmonary capillaries.
5. Note evidence of pulmonary edema or respiratory depression, document and report to the physician immediately.
6. Assess the client for symptoms of overdosage as evidenced by labored breathing, a fast, feeble pulse, low blood pressure, and a characteristic odor of paraldehyde on the breath.

Evaluation: Evaluate client for:
- Reports of effective sedation
- Evidence of control of delirium tremens
- Evidence of termination of seizures

Paregoric (Camphorated Opium Tincture)
(pair-eh-**GOR**-ick)
(C-III, Rx)

See also *Narcotic Analgesics,* p. 174.

Classification: Antidiarrheal agent, systemic.

Action/Kinetics: The active principle of the mixture is opium (0.04% morphine). The preparation also contains benzoic acid, camphor, and anise oil. Morphine increases the muscular tone of the intestinal tract, decreases digestive secretions, and inhibits normal peristalsis. The slowed passage of the feces through the intestines promotes desiccation, which is a function of the time the feces spend in the intestine. **t½:** 2–3 hr. **Duration:** 4–5 hr.

Uses: Acute diarrhea.

Contraindications: See *Morphine Sulfate,* p. 903. Do not use in clients with diarrhea caused by poisoning until toxic substance has been eliminated. Treatment of pseudomembranous colitis due to lincomycin, penicillins, and cephalosporins. Rubbing paregoric on the gums of a teething child is no longer recommended.

Special Concerns: Pregnancy category: C. Many physicians do not recommend use of paregoric in treating neonatal opioid dependence.

Side Effects: See *Morphine Sulfate,* p. 903.

Drug Interactions: See *Narcotic Analgesics,* p. 174.

Dosage: Liquid. Adult: 5–10 ml 1–4 times daily (5 ml contains 2 mg of morphine). **Pediatric:** 0.25–0.5 ml/kg 1–4 times daily.

NURSING CONSIDERATIONS

See also *Nursing Considerations* for *Narcotics,* p. 177.

Administration/Storage

1. Administer paregoric with water to ensure that it will reach the stomach. The mixture will have a milky appearance.
2. Store the medication in a light-resistant container.
3. Carefully distinguish between paregoric and tincture of opium. Tincture of opium contains 25 times more morphine than paregoric.
4. Paregoric preparations are sub-

ject to the Controlled Substances Act and must be charted accordingly.

5. Have naloxone available to treat any overdosage.

Assessment

1. Note the length of time the client has been taking paregoric, the reasons for taking, and its level of effectiveness.
2. Note any history of hepatic dysfunction or drug dependence.

Client/Family Teaching

1. Advise the client to adhere to the prescribed regimen.
2. If the diarrhea persists, consult with the physician.
3. Stop medication once diarrhea has abated. Continued use of paregoric may result in constipation.

Evaluation: Evaluate client for reports of a decrease in the frequency and number of diarrheal stools.

Paromomycin sulfate
(pair-oh-moh-**MY**-sin)
Humatin (Rx)

See also *Aminoglycosides*, p. 23.

Classification: Antibiotic, aminoglycoside.

Action/Kinetics: Paromomycin is obtained from *Streptomyces rimosus forma paromomycina*. Its spectrum of activity resembles that of neomycin and kanamycin. The drug is poorly absorbed from the GI tract and is ineffective against systemic infections when given orally.

Additional Uses: Inhibition of ammonia-forming bacteria in GI tract in hepatic encephalopathy, intestinal amebiasis, preoperative suppression of intestinal flora. *Investigational:* Anthelmintic, to treat *Dientamoeba fragilis, Diphyllobothrium latum, Taenia saginata, T. solium, Dipylidium caninum,* and *Hymenolepis nana.*

Contraindications: Intestinal obstruction.

Special Concerns: Use during pregnancy only if benefits outweigh risks. To be used with caution in the presence of GI ulceration because of possible systemic absorption.

Additional Side Effects: Diarrhea or loose stools. Heartburn, emesis, and pruritus ani. Superinfections, especially by monilia.

Drug Interaction: Penicillin is inhibited by paromomycin.

Dosage: Capsules. *Hepatic coma:* **Adults:** 4 g daily in divided doses for 5–6 days. *Intestinal amebiasis:* **Adults and children:** 25–35 mg/kg/day administered in three doses with meals for 5–10 days. *D. fragilis:* 25–30 mg/kg daily in three divided doses for 1 week. *H. nana:* 45 mg/kg daily for 5–7 days. *D. latum, T. saginata, T. solium, D. caninum:* **Adults:** 1 g q 15 min for a total of four doses; **pediatric:** 11 mg/kg q 15 min for four doses.

NURSING CONSIDERATIONS

See also *Nursing Considerations* for *Aminoglycosides*, p. 25.

Administration/Storage: Do not administer parenterally and do not administer concurrently with penicillin.

Client/Family Teaching

1. Take before or after meals.
2. Report any diarrhea, dehydra-

tion, and general weakness because drug therapy may need to be interrupted if symptoms are excessive.

—— *COMBINATION DRUG* ——
Pediazole
(PEE-dee-ah-zohl)
(Rx)

Classification/Content: This product is available as granules that, when reconstituted, provide an oral suspension.

Antibacterial, antibiotic: Erythromycin ethylsuccinate, 200 mg/5 ml erythromycin activity. *Antibacterial, sulfonamide:* Sulfisoxazole, 600 mg/5 ml.

See also information on individual components.

Use: Acute otitis media in children caused by *Haemophilus influenzae.*

Contraindications: Pregnancy at term and in children less than 2 months of age. Use with caution during other times of pregnancy.

Dosage: Oral Suspension. Usual: Equivalent of 50 mg/kg daily of erythromycin and 150 mg/kg daily of sulfisoxazole, up to a maximum of 6 g daily. **Over 45 kg:** 10 ml q 6 hr; **24 kg:** 7.5 ml q 6 hr; **16 kg:** 5 ml q 6 hr; **8 kg:** 2.5 ml q 6 hr; **less than 8 kg:** Calculate dose according to body weight.

NURSING CONSIDERATIONS

See *General Nursing Considerations For All Anti-Infectives,* p. 83, and *Sulfonamides,* p. 216.

Administration/Storage

1. The reconstituted suspension should be refrigerated and used within 14 days.
2. Therapy should be continued for 10 days.
3. May be taken without regard to meals.

Evaluation: Evaluate client for clinical evidence of improvement in signs and symptoms of infection.

Pegademase Bovine
(peg-AD-eh-mace BOH-veen)
Adagen (Rx)

Classification: Enzyme.

Action/Kinetics: Pegademase is derived from bovine intestine and is the conjugate of numerous strands of monomethoxypolyethylene glycol, which is attached covalently to the enzyme adenosine deaminase. In deficiency clients, adenosine, 2'-deoxyadenosine, and their metabolites are toxic to lymphocytes. Replacement with pegademase bovine improves immune function and decreases the frequency of opportunistic infections. The time required to correct the metabolic abnormalities may range from a few weeks to 6 months. Adequate dosage may be evaluated by measuring adenosine deaminase levels and by monitoring the level of deoxyadenosine triphosphate in erythrocytes. **Peak plasma levels, after IM:** 2–3 days. **t½:** 3 to more than 6 days. After initiation of therapy, the trough level should be between 15–35 micromol/hr/ml before a maintenance injection is given.

Uses: Enzyme replacement for the treatment of severe combined immunodeficiency disease (SCID) in which there is a deficiency of adenosine deaminase. Pegademase bovine may be used in infants from birth and in children of any age at the time of diagnosis of deficiency. The drug is ineffective in clients with immunodeficiency due to other causes.

Contraindications: Severe thrombocytopenia. IV use.

Special Concerns: Pregnancy category: C. Use with caution during lactation. There is no evidence to support the safety and effectiveness of pegademase bovine either prior to or as support therapy for bone marrow transplantation. Use with caution in mild to moderate thrombocytopenia.

Side Effects: Data are limited but pain at the injection site and headache have been reported.

Drug Interactions: Since vidarabine is a substrate for adenosine deaminase, use of vidarabine with pegademase bovine may alter the activities of both drugs.

Dosage: IM: Individualized. Dose is given q 7 days. *First dose:* 10 U/kg. *Second dose:* 15 U/kg. *Third dose:* 20 U/kg. *Maintenance doses:* 20 U/kg/week. If necessary, the weekly dose may be increased by 5 U/kg but the maximum single dose should not exceed 30 U/kg.

NURSING CONSIDERATIONS

Administration/Storage

1. Pegademase bovine should not be mixed with any other drug prior to administration.
2. Pegademase should be stored in the refrigerator between 2°C and 8°C (36°F–46°F). It should not be stored frozen or at room temperature.
3. Pegademase should not be used if there is any chance the vial has been frozen.

Assessment

1. Document onset of SCID with adenosine deaminase (ADA) deficiency. Record baseline level of ADA activity in plasma and erythrocyte dATP.
2. Note if client has a failed bone marrow transplant or if client is not suitable for transplant because this is the usual cure for ADA deficiency.
3. Obtain baseline CBC to determine if thrombocytopenia is present.

Interventions

1. Antibodies to pegademase bovine may develop and should be suspected if the preinjection level of adenosine deaminase is less than 10 micromol/hr/ml and if other causes for the decrease have been ruled out (e.g., improper storage of vials, improper handling of plasma samples).
2. Protect client from opportunistic infections until immune response/function has returned.
3. Monitor plasma ADA activity and red blood cell dATP levels to determine drug response and adequate dosing levels of pegademase bovine.

Client/Family Teaching

1. Review early signs and symptoms of infection. Instruct client to report any such symptoms immediately.
2. Explain that after initial therapy, adenosine deaminase activity should be measured every 1–2 weeks during the first 8–12 weeks of therapy. Between 3 and 9 months, activity should be measured twice a month and then monthly until after 18–24 months of therapy. Adenosine deaminase activity

can then be monitored every 2–4 months.

3. Advise that laboratory studies of deoxyadenosine triphosphate, once it has decreased to acceptable levels, should be measured 2–4 times during the remainder of the first year of therapy and 2–3 times yearly thereafter provided that therapy has not been interrupted.

Evaluation: Evaluate client for:

- Laboratory evidence of effective enzyme replacement as evidenced by plasma adenosine deaminase activity in the range of 15–35 micromol/hr/ml
- Laboratory confirmation of a decrease in erythrocyte dATP to less than or equal to 0.005–0.015 micromol/ml packed erythrocytes or less than or equal to 1% of the total erythrocyte adenine nucleotide (ATP + dATP) content, with a normal ATP level (as measured in a preinjection sample)
- Freedom from complications of drug therapy

Pemoline

(PEM-oh-leen)
Cylert, Cylert Chewable (C-IV) (Rx)

Classification: CNS stimulant.

Action/Kinetics: Although pemoline resembles amphetamine and methylphenidate pharmacologically, its mechanism of action is not fully known. Pemoline is believed to act by dopaminergic mechanisms. The drug will result in a decrease in hyperactivity and a prolonged attention span in children. **Peak serum levels:** 2–4 hr. **t½:** 12 hr. Steady state reached in 2–3 days, and beneficial effects may not be noted for 3–4 weeks. Approximately 50% is bound to plasma protein. Pemoline is metabolized by the liver, and approximately 50% is excreted unchanged by the kidneys.

Uses: Attention deficit disorders. *Investigational:* Narcolepsy.

Contraindications: Hypersensitivity to drug. Tourette's syndrome. Children under 6 years of age.

Special Concerns: Pregnancy category: B. Safe use during lactation has not been established. Use with caution in impaired renal or kidney function. Chronic use in children may cause growth suppression.

Side Effects: *CNS:* Insomnia (most common). Dyskinesia of the face, tongue, lips, and extremities; precipitation of Tourette's syndrome. Mild depression, headache, nystagmus, dizziness, hallucinations, irritability, seizures. Exacerbation of behavior disturbances and thought disorders in psychotic children. *GI:* Transient weight loss, gastric upset, nausea. *Miscellaneous:* Skin rash.

Symptoms of Overdose: Symptoms of CNS stimulation and sympathomimetic effects including agitation, confusion, delirium, euphoria, headache, muscle twitching, mydriasis, vomiting, hallucinations, flushing, sweating, tachycardia, hyperreflexia, tremors, hyperpyrexia, hypertension, seizures (may be followed by coma).

Laboratory Test Interference: ↑ AST, ALT, serum LDH.

Dosage: Tablets, Chewable Tablets. Children, 6 years and

older, initial: 37.5 mg/day as a single dose in the morning; increase at 1-week intervals by 18.75 mg until desired response is attained up to maximum of 112.5 mg/day. **Usual maintenance:** 56.25–75 mg daily. *Narcolepsy:* 50–200 mg/day in 2 divided doses.

NURSING CONSIDERATIONS

Administration/Storage

1. Administer as a single dose in the morning.
2. Interrupt treatment once or twice annually to determine whether behavioral symptoms still necessitate drug therapy.
3. Anticipate the drug will reach peak activity in 2–4 hr and last up to 8 hr.
4. *Treatment of Overdose:* Reduce external stimuli. If symptoms are not severe, induce vomiting or undertake gastric lavage. Chlorpromazine can be used to decrease the CNS stimulation and sympathomimetic effects.

Client/Family Teaching

1. Measure the height of the child every month, and weigh child twice a week. Record all measurements on a chart, and bring this chart to each follow-up medical visit so the physician can evaluate the child's growth pattern.
2. Report any noted weight loss or failure to grow to the physician as soon as evident.
3. Advise child's school health department of medication regimen.
4. Administer the drug early in the morning to minimize insomnia associated with drug therapy.
5. Advise family to continue with therapy, because behavioral changes take 3–4 weeks to occur.
6. Instruct the family when to interrupt drug administration, as recommended by the physician. Then, observe and record behavior without the medication, to help the physician decide whether therapy should be resumed.
7. Stress the importance of bringing the child in periodically for liver function tests to detect adverse effects that would necessitate withdrawal of pemoline.
8. Provide a printed list of drug side effects. Instruct family to note signs of overdosage, such as agitation, restlessness, hallucinations, and tachycardia. If these symptoms occur, instruct parents to withhold the drug, to protect child and give supportive care, and to report immediately to the physician.
9. Advise not to perform activities that require mental alertness until drug effects are realized.
10. Avoid excessive consumption of caffeine-containing products.

Evaluation

1. Evaluate client for:
   - Attainment of desired behavioral changes in order to determine drug effectiveness and dosage levels
   - Evidence of a prolonged attention span (in attention deficit disorder)
   - Reports of a calming effect and ↓ in hyperactivity
2. Weight and height will progress normally in the medicated child. Evaluate recordings.

P

Penbutolol sulfate

(pen-**BYOU**-toe-lohl)
Levatol (Rx)

See also *Beta-Adrenergic Blocking Agents,* p. 113.

Action/Kinetics: Penbutolol has both beta-1 and beta-2 receptor blocking activity. It has no membrane-stabilizing activity but does possess minimal intrinsic sympathomimetic activity. High lipid solubility. **t½:** 5 hr. 80%–98% protein bound. Penbutolol is metabolized in the liver and excreted through the urine.

Uses: Mild to moderate arterial hypertension.

Special Concerns: Pregnancy category: C. Dosage has not been established in children. Geriatric clients may manifest increased or decreased sensitivity to the usual adult dose.

Dosage: Tablets. *Hypertension:* **initial,** 20 mg once daily either alone or with other antihypertensive agents. **Maintenance:** Same as initial dose. Doses greater than 40 mg daily do not result in a greater antihypertensive effect.

NURSING CONSIDERATIONS

See also *Nursing Considerations* for *Beta-Adrenergic Blocking Agents,* p. 116, and *Antihypertensive Agents,* p. 78.

Administration/Storage

1. The full effect of a 20–40 mg dose may not be observed for 2 weeks.
2. Doses of 10 mg daily are effective but full effects are not evident for 4–6 weeks.

Client/Family Teaching

1. Review the signs and symptoms associated with postural hypotension and instruct client to rise slowly from a sitting or lying position.
2. Take medication only as prescribed because full effects may not be realized for a month or more.
3. Drug may cause an increased sensitivity to cold.

Evaluation: Evaluate client for evidence of control of hypertension.

Penicillamine

(pen-ih-**SILL**-ah-meen)
Cuprimine, Depen (Rx)

Classification: Antirheumatic, heavy metal antagonist, to treat cystinuria.

Action/Kinetics: Penicillamine, a degradation product of penicillin, is a chelating agent for mercury, lead, iron, and copper thus decreasing toxic levels of the metal (e.g., copper in Wilson's disease). The anti-inflammatory activity of penicillamine may be due to its ability to inhibit T-lymphocyte function and therefore decrease cell-mediated immune response. It may also protect lymphocytes from hydrogen peroxide generated at the site of inflammation by inhibiting release of lysosomal enzymes and oxygen radicals. In cystinuria, penicillamine is able to reduce excess cystine excretion, probably by disulfide interchange between penicillamine and cystine. This results in penicillamine-cysteine disulfide, which is a complex that is more soluble than cystine and is thus readily excreted. Penicillamine is well absorbed from the GI tract and is excreted in urine. **Peak plasma levels:** 1–3 hr. About 80% is bound to plasma albumin. **t½:** Approximately 2 hr. Metabolites are excreted through the urine. **It may take 2–3 months for positive responses to become apparent when treating rheumatoid arthritis.**

Uses: Wilson's disease, cystinuria, and rheumatoid arthritis—severe active disease unresponsive to conventional therapy. Heavy metal antagonist. *Investigational:* Primary biliary cirrhosis. Rheumatoid vasculitis. Felty's syndrome.

Contraindications: Pregnancy, lactation, penicillinase-related aplastic anemia or agranulocytosis, hypersensitivity to drug. Clients allergic to penicillin may cross-react with penicillamine. Renal insufficiency or history thereof.

Special Concerns: The use of penicillamine for juvenile rheumatoid arthritis has not been established. Clients older than 65 years may be at greater risk of developing hematologic side effects.

Side Effects: This drug manifests a large number of potentially serious side effects. Clients should be carefully monitored. *GI:* Altered taste perception (common), nausea, vomiting, diarrhea, anorexia, GI pain, stomatitis, oral ulcerations, reactivation of peptic ulcer, glossitis, cheilosis, colitis. *Hematologic:* Thrombocytopenia, leukopenia, agranulocytosis, aplastic anemia, eosinophilia, monocytosis, red cell aplasia, thrombocytopenia, hemolytic anemia, leukocytosis, throm-

bocytosis. *Renal:* Proteinuria, hematuria, nephrotic syndrome, Goodpasture's syndrome (a severe and ultimately fatal glomerulonephritis). *Allergic:* Rashes (common), lupus-like syndrome, pruritus, pemphigoid-type symptoms (e.g., bullous lesions), drug fever, arthralgia, lymphadenopathy, dermatoses, urticaria, obliterative bronchiolitis, thyroiditis, hypoglycemia, migratory polyarthralgia, polymyositis, allergic alveolitis. *Other:* Tinnitus, optic neuritis, neuropathy, thrombophlebitis, alopecia, precipitation of myasthenia gravis, increased body temperature, pulmonary fibrosis, pneumonitis, bronchial asthma, renal vasculitis (may be fatal), hot flashes, increased skin friability, pancreatitis, hepatic dysfunction, intrahepatic cholestasis.

Drug Interactions

Antacids / ↓ Effect of penicillamine due to ↓ absorption from GI tract
Digoxin / Penicillamine ↓ effect of digoxin
Iron salts / ↓ Effect of penicillamine due to ↓ absorption from GI tract
Antimalarials, cytotoxic drugs, gold therapy, oxyphenbutazone, phenylbutazone / ↑ Risk of blood dyscrasias and adverse renal effects

Laboratory Test Interferences: ↑ Serum alkaline phosphatase, LDH. + Thymol turbidity test and cephalin flocculation test.

Dosage: Capsules, Tablets. *Wilson's disease:* Dosage is usually calculated on the basis of the urinary excretion of copper. One gram of penicillamine promotes excretion of 2 mg of copper. **PO, adults and adolescents:** *usual, initial,* 250 mg q.i.d. Dosage may have to be increased to 2 g daily. A further increase does not produce additional excretion. **Pediatric, 6 months—young children:** 250 mg as a single dose given in fruit juice.

Antidote for heavy metals: **Adults,** 0.5–1.5 g daily for 1–2 months; **pediatric:** 30–40 mg/kg daily (600–750 mg/m² daily) for 1–6 months.

Cystinuria: individualized and based on excretion rate of cystine (100–200 mg/day in clients with no history of stones, below 100 mg with clients with history of stones or pain). Initiate at low dosage (250 mg/day) and increase gradually to minimum effective dosage. **Adult:** *Usual,* 2 g/day (range: 1–4 g/day); **pediatric:** 7.5 mg/kg q.i.d. If divided in fewer than 4 doses, give larger dose at night.

Rheumatoid arthritis: **PO,** *individualized:* **initial,** 125–250 mg/day. Dosage may be increased at 1- to 3-month intervals by 125- to 250-mg increments until adequate response is attained. **Maximum:** 500–750 mg/day. Up to 500 mg/day can be given as a single dose; higher dosages should be divided. **Maintenance:** Individualized. **Range:** 500–750 mg daily.

Primary biliary cirrhosis: 600–900 mg daily.

NURSING CONSIDERATIONS

Administration/Storage

1. Give penicillamine on an empty stomach 1 hr before or 2 hr after meals. Also wait 1 hr after ingestion of any other food, milk, or drug.
2. If client cannot tolerate dosage for cystinuria, the bedtime dosage should be larger and should be continued.
3. Administer the contents of the capsule in 15–30 ml of chilled juice or pureed fruit if client is unable to swallow capsules or tablets.
4. The drug should be discontinued if doses of penicillamine up to 1.5 g/day for 2–3 months do not produce improvement when treating rheumatoid arthritis.

Assessment

1. Determine if the client has any allergies to penicillin. Document and report.
2. Obtain baseline CBC, platelet count, and urinalysis prior to beginning therapy.
3. Ensure that liver function tests are conducted prior to the start of therapy.
4. Determine if the client is taking any medication with which penicillamine will interact unfavorably.
5. Assess the client's hearing to detect any evidence of hearing loss and to serve as a baseline for further auditory testing throughout drug therapy.
6. Women of childbearing age, who are sexually active should be tested for pregnancy. Penicillamine is contraindicated during pregnancy because it can cause fetal damage.

Interventions

1. Note client complaints of nausea, vomiting, or diarrhea. Check for any alterations in taste. Monitor weight, I&O and report persistent side effects to the physician.
2. Inspect the client's mucosal

surfaces at regular intervals throughout the therapy. If ulcers appear and are severe or persistent, it may be necessary for the physician to reduce the dose of the drug.

3. Routinely monitor the client's WBC and platelet counts. If the WBC falls below 3,500/mm³ or the platelet count falls below 100,000/mm³, withhold the penicillamine and report these findings to the physician. If the counts are low for 3 successive laboratory tests, a temporary interruption of therapy is indicated.

4. Monitor liver function studies, especially if the client develops jaundice or demonstrates other signs of hepatic dysfunction.

5. White papules appearing at the site of venipuncture or at surgical sites may indicate sensitivity to penicillamine or the presence of infection. Check for signs of infection.

6. If the client is to undergo surgery, anticipate that the dosage of medication will be reduced to 250 mg/day until wound healing is complete. Anticipate that the physician may order vitamin B$_6$ prophylactically prior to and following surgery.

7. Penicillamine increases the body's need for pyridoxine. Therefore, pyridoxine (25 mg/day) should be ordered as a supplement.

8. Clients may develop symptoms that suggest an antinuclear antibody test be conducted. A positive test indicates that the client may develop a lupus-like syndrome in the future. The drug need not be discontinued. Rather, the practitioner needs

to be aware of the potential and report any symptoms to the physician should they occur.

9. If the client develops cystinuria, encourage a high fluid intake throughout the day and at bedtime.

10. For clients being treated for Wilson's disease, avoid multivitamin preparations containing copper.

Client/Family Teaching

1. Review the goals of the therapy and the anticipated benefits, and provide clients with a printed list of possible side effects.

2. Instruct clients to take their temperature nightly during the first few months of therapy. A fever may indicate a hypersensitivity reaction. Stress that the physician should be notified.

3. Any incidents of fever, sore throat, chills, bruising, or bleeding need to be reported to the physician immediately. These are early symptoms of granulocytopenia.

4. If stomatitis occurs, it needs to be reported immediately and the drug discontinued. Instruct the client on oral hygiene such as brushing the teeth with a soft tooth brush, flossing daily, and using mouth rinses free of alcohol.

5. Taste perception may become altered. This may last for 2 months or more. Encourage the client to maintain adequate nutrition throughout, noting that nutrition is important and that the condition is usually self-limiting.

6. If the client is to receive an oral iron preparation, at least 2 hr

should elapse between ingestion of penicillamine and the dose of therapeutic iron. Iron decreases the cupruretic effects of penicillamine.

7. The skin of clients taking penicillamine tends to become friable and susceptible to injury. Caution clients to avoid activities that could injure the skin. When working with elderly clients teach them how to avoid excessive pressure on the shoulders, elbows, knees, toes, and buttocks. Report all skin changes to the physician for evaluation.

8. Report cloudy urine or urine that is smoky brown in color. These are signs of proteinuria and hematuria and may require withdrawal of the drug.

9. Women of childbearing age should be instructed to practice a safe form of birth control. If the client misses a menstrual period or has other symptoms of pregnancy, they should report this to the physician.

10. If the drug is used to treat clients with Wilson's disease, they should be advised as follows:
   - Eat a diet low in copper. Exclude foods such as chocolate, nuts, shellfish, mushrooms, liver, molasses, broccoli, and copper-enriched cereals.
   - Use distilled or demineralized water if the drinking water contains more than 0.1 mg/L copper.
   - Unless the client is taking iron supplements, take sulfurated potash or Carbo-Resin with meals to minimize the absorption of copper.

- It may take 1–3 months for neurologic improvements to occur. Therefore, continue the therapy even if no improvements seem evident.
- Check any vitamin preparations being used to ensure that they do not contain copper.

11. If a client develops cystinuria advise the following:
   - Drink large amounts of fluid to prevent the formation of renal calculi. Drink 500 ml of fluid at bedtime, and another pint during the night, when the urine tends to be the most concentrated and most acidic.
   - Teach client how to measure specific gravity and determine pH. The urine specific gravity should be maintained at less than 1.010 and the pH maintained at 7.5–8.0.
   - Advise clients to have a yearly X ray of the kidneys to detect the presence of renal calculi.
   - Eat a diet low in methionine, a major precursor of cystine. Exclude from the diet foods high in cystine such as rich meat soups and broths, milk, eggs, cheeses, and peas.
   - If the client is pregnant or is a child, a diet low in methionine is also low in calcium. Therefore, such a diet is contraindicated in these instances.

12. If clients have rheumatoid arthritis, advise them to continue using other approaches to achieve relief from their symptoms because penicillamine may take up to 6 months to have a therapeutic effect.

Evaluation

1. Review the goals of therapy and prescribed therapeutic regimen and assess client compliance. Stress the need to adhere to all aspects of the program to obtain a positive clinical response.
2. Assess client for evidence of control of symptoms of copper toxicity in Wilson's disease.
3. Evaluate client for laboratory evidence of a reduction of cystine excretion and prevention of renal calculi in cystinuria.
4. Evaluate client for reports of improvement in symptoms of severe rheumatoid arthritis.

Penicillin G benzathine, parenteral

(pen-ih-**SILL**-in, **BEN**-zah-theen)

Bicillin ✿, Bicillin L-A, Megacillin Suspension ✿, Permapen (Rx)

See also *Anti-Infectives*, p. 80, and *Penicillins*, p. 197.

Classification: Antibiotic, penicillin.

Action/Kinetics: Penicillin G is neither penicillinase resistant nor acid stable. The product is a long-acting (repository) form of penicillin in an aqueous vehicle; it is administered as a sterile suspension. **Peak plasma levels: IM** 0.03–0.05 unit/ml.

Uses: Most gram-positive (streptococci, staphylococci, pneumococci) and some gram-negative (gonococci, meningococci) organisms. Syphilis. Prophylaxis of glomerulonephritis and rheumatic fever. Surgical infections, secondary infections following tooth extraction, tonsillectomy.

Dosage: Parenteral Suspension (IM only). Adults: *Upper respiratory tract infections, erysipeloid, yaws:* 1,200,000 units as a single dose; **older children:** 900,000 units as a single dose; **children under 27 kg:** 300,000–600,000 units as a single dose; **Neonates:** 50,000 units/kg as a single dose. *Early syphilis:* 2,400,000 units as a single dose. *Late syphilis:* 2,400,000 units q 7 days for 3 weeks. *Neurosyphilis:* Penicillin G, 12,000,000–24,000,000 units IV/day for 10–14 days followed by penicillin G benzathine, 2,400,000 units IM q week for 3 weeks. *Congenital syphilis, older children:* 50,000 units/kg IM (up to adult dose of 2,400,000 units). *Prophylaxis of rheumatic fever:* **Adults and children over 27.3 kg:** 1,200,000 units q 4 weeks; **children and infants less than 27.3 kg:** 50,000 units/kg as a single dose.

NURSING CONSIDERATIONS

See also *Nursing Considerations* for *Penicillins*, p. 200.

P

Administration/Storage

1. Shake multiple-dose vial vigorously before withdrawing the desired dose because medication tends to clump on standing. Check that all medication is dissolved and that there is no residue at bottom of bottle.
2. Use a 20-gauge needle and do not allow medication to remain in the syringe and needle for long periods of time before administration because the needle may become plugged and the syringe "frozen."

3. Inject slowly and steadily into the muscle and *do not massage* injection site.
4. For adults, use the upper outer quadrant of the buttock; for infants and small children, the midlateral aspect of the thigh should be used. Benzathine penicillin should not be administered in the gluteal region in children less than 2 years of age.
5. Before injection of medication, aspirate needle to ascertain that needle is not in a vein.
6. Rotate and chart site of injections.
7. *Do not administer IV.*
8. Divide between two injection sites if dose is large or available muscle mass is small.

Client/Family Teaching

1. Explain why it is necessary to return for repository penicillin injections.
2. Evaluate the need for sexual counseling or referral in clients being treated for venereal disease. Stress the importance of the sexual partner undergoing treatment.

──── *COMBINATION DRUG* ────
Penicillin G, benzathine and procaine combined
(pen-ih-**SILL**-in, **BEN**-zah-theen, **PROH**-kain)
Bicillin C-R, Bicillin C-R 900/300 (Rx)

See also *Anti-Infectives,* p. 80, and *Penicillins,* p. 197.

Classification: Antibiotic, penicillin.

Uses: Streptococcal infections (A, C, G, H, L, and M) without bacteremia, of the upper respiratory tract, skin, and soft tissues. Scarlet fever, erysipelas, pneumococcal infections, and otitis media.

Contraindications: Use to treat syphilis, gonorrhea, yaws, bejel, and pinta.

Special Concerns: Pregnancy category: B.

Dosage: IM only. *Streptococcal infections:* **Adults and children over 27 kg:** 2,400,000 units, given at a single session using multiple injection sites or, alternatively, in divided doses on days 1 and 3; **children 13.5–27 kg:** 900,000–1,200,000 units; **infants and children under 13.5 kg:** 600,000 units. *Pneumococcal infections, except meningitis:* **Adults,** 1,200,000 units; **pediatric:** 600,000 units. Give q 2–3 days until temperature is normal for 48 hr.

NURSING CONSIDERATIONS

See *Nursing Considerations* for *Penicillin G Benzathine Parenteral,* p. 1005, and *Penicillins,* p. 200.

Administration/Storage

1. For adults, administer by deep IM injection in the upper outer quadrant of the buttock. For infants and children, use the midlateral aspect of the thigh.
2. Injection sites should be rotated for repeated doses.

Penicillin G Potassium for Injection
(pen-ih-**SILL**-in)
Pfizerpen (Rx)

Penicillin G Potassium, Oral

(pen-ih-**SILL**-in)

Megacillin✻, Novo–Pen G✻, Pentids '400' for Syrup, Pentids '400' Tablets, and '800' Tablets (Rx)

Penicillin G (Aqueous) Sodium for Injection

(pen-ih-**SILL**-in)

Crystapen✻ (Rx)

See also *Anti-Infectives*, p. 80, and *Penicillins*, p. 197.

Classification: Antibiotic, penicillin.

Action/Kinetics: The low cost of penicillin G still makes it the first choice for treatment of many infections. Rapid onset makes it especially suitable for fulminating infections. Penicillin G is neither penicillinase resistant nor acid stable. **Peak plasma levels: IM or SC,** 6–20 units/ml after 15–30 min **t½:** 30 min.

Uses: Streptococci of groups A, C, G, H, L, and M are sensitive to penicillin G. High serum levels are effective against streptococci of the D group.

Additional Side Effects: Rapid IV administration may cause hyperkalemia and cardiac arrhythmias. Renal damage occurs rarely.

Dosage: Penicillin G Potassium and Sodium Parenteral (IM, continuous IV infusion). Adults: 300,000–30 million units daily, depending on the use. **Pediatric:** 100,000–250,000 units/kg daily (given in divided doses q 4 hr). **Infants over 7 days of age weighing more than 2 kg:** 100,000 units/kg daily (given in divided doses q 6 hr). *For meningitis:* 200,000 units/kg. **Infants over 7 days of age weighing less than 2 kg:** 75,000 units daily (given in divided doses q 8 hr). *For meningitis:* 150,000 units/kg. **Infants less than 7 days of age weighing more than 2 kg:** 50,000 units/kg daily (given in divided doses q 8 hr). *For meningitis:* 150,000 units/kg. **Infants less than 7 days of age weighing less than 2 kg:** 50,000 units/kg daily (given in divided doses q 12 hr). *For meningitis:* 100,000 units/kg daily for 14 days.

Parenteral, for specific diseases. *Gram-negative bacillary bacteremia:* 20 million or more units daily. *Anthrax:* A minimum of 5 million units daily (up to 12–20 million units have been used). *Clostridial infections:* 20 million units daily used with an antitoxin. *Actinomycosis, cervicofacial:* 1–6 million units daily; *thoracic and abdominal disease:* **initial,** 12–20 million units daily IV for 6 weeks followed by penicillin V, PO, 500 mg q.i.d. for 2–3 months. *Rat-bite fever, Haverhill fever:* 12–20 million units daily for 3–4 weeks. *Endocarditis due to Listeria:* 15–20 million units daily for 4 weeks (in adults). *Endocarditis due to Erysipelothrix rhusiopathiae:* 12–20 million units daily for 4–6 weeks. *Meningitis due to Listeria:* 15–20 million units daily for 2 weeks (in adults). *Pasturella infections causing bacteremia and meningitis:* 4–6 million units daily for 2 weeks. *Severe fusospirochetal infections of the oropharynx, lower respiratory tract, and genital area:* 5–10 million units daily. *Pneumococcal infections causing empyema:* 5–24 million units daily in

P

divided doses q 4–6 hr; *pneumococcal infections causing meningitis:* 20–24 million units daily for 14 days; *pneumococcal infections causing endocarditis, pericarditis, peritonitis, suppurative arthritis, osteomyelitis, mastoiditis:* 12–20 million units daily for 2–4 weeks. *Adjunct with antitoxic to prevent diphtheria:* 2–3 million units daily in divided doses for 10–12 days. *Meningococcal meningitis:* 20–30 million units daily by continuous IV drip for 14 days (or until there is no fever for 7 days) or 200,000–300,000 units/kg daily q 2–4 hr in divided doses for a total of 24 doses. *Neurosyphilis:* 12–24 million units daily for 10–14 days (can be followed by benzathine penicillin G, 2.4 million units IM weekly for 3 weeks). *Congenital syphilis in newborns:* 50,000 units/kg daily (IV) in divided doses q 8–12 hr for 10–14 days; *in infants after newborn period:* 50,000 units/kg q 4–6 hr for 10–14 days. *Gonococcal infections in infants:* 100,000 units/kg daily in 2 equal doses.

Oral Solution, Tablets. Adults: Depending on the use, 200,000–500,000 units q 6–8 hr; **pediatric under 12 years of age:** 25,000–90,000 units/kg/day in 3–6 divided doses. **Note:** 250 mg Penicillin G potassium, oral, is equivalent to 400,000 units. *Upper respiratory tract infections due to streptococci:* 200,000–250,000 units q 6–8 hr for 10 days (for severe infections, use 400,000–500,000 units q 8 hr for 10 days or 800,000 units q 12 hr). *Infections of the respiratory tract due to pneumococci:* 400,000–500,000 units q 6 hr until client has no fever for 48 hr. *Infections of the skin and skin structures due to staphylococci:*

200,000–500,000 units q 6–8 hr until cured. *Infections of the oropharynx due to fusospirochetes:* 400,000–500,000 units q 6–8 hr. *Prophylaxis of rheumatic fever and/or chorea:* 200,000–250,000 units b.i.d. chronically.

NURSING CONSIDERATIONS

See also *Nursing Considerations* for *Penicillins,* p. 200.

Administration/Storage

1. IM administration is preferred; discomfort is minimized by using solutions of up to 100,000 units/ml.
2. Use sterile water, isotonic saline USP, or 5% D_5W and mix with volume recommended on label for desired strength.
3. Loosen powder by shaking bottle before adding diluent.
4. Hold vial horizontally and rotate slowly while directing the stream of the diluent against the wall of the vial.
5. Shake vigorously after addition of diluent.
6. Solutions may be stored at room temperature for 24 hr or in refrigerator for 1 week. Discard remaining solution.
7. Use 1%–2% lidocaine solution as diluent for IM (if ordered by physician) to lessen pain at injection site. Do not use procaine as diluent for aqueous penicillin.
8. The oral products should be taken at least 1 hr before or 2 hr after meals.
9. Note the drugs that should *not* be mixed with penicillin during IV administration: Aminophylline, Amphotericin B, Ascorbic acid, Chlorpheniramine, Chlorpromazine, Genta-

micin, Heparin, Hydroxyzine, Lincomycin, Metaraminol, Novobiocin, Oxytetracycline, Phenylephrine, Phenytoin, Polymyxin B, Prochlorperazine, Promazine, Promethazine, Sodium bicarbonate, Sodium salts of barbiturates, Sulfadiazine, Tetracycline, Tromethamine, Vancomycin, Vitamin B complex

Interventions

1. Order drug by specifying sodium or potassium salt.
2. Monitor I&O. Dehydration decreases the excretion of the drug by the kidneys and may raise the blood level of penicillin G to dangerously high levels that can cause kidney damage.
3. Assess client for GI disturbances, which may lead to dehydration.

Evaluation: Evaluate client for:
- Clinical evidence and reports of improvement in symptoms
- Laboratory evidence of negative culture reports

Penicillin G Procaine Aqueous, Sterile

(pen-ih-**SILL**-in, **PROH**-kain)
Ayercillin❋, Crysticillin 300 A.S. and 600 A.S., Pfizerpen-AS, Wycillin, Wycillin 5 Million❋ (Rx)

See also *Anti-Infectives,* p. 80, and *Penicillins,* p. 197.

Classification: Antibiotic, penicillin.

Action/Kinetics: Long-acting (repository) form in an aqueous ve-

hicle. Is neither penicillinase resistant nor acid stable. Because of slow onset, a soluble penicillin is often administered concomitantly for fulminating infections.

Uses: Penicillin-sensitive staphylococci, pneumococci, streptococci, and bacterial endocarditis. Gonorrhea, all stages of syphilis. *Prophylaxis:* Rheumatic fever, pre- and postsurgery. Diphtheria, anthrax, fusospirochetosis (Vincent's infection), erysipeloid, rat-bite fever.

Dosage: IM only. Adults, usual: *Pneumococcccal, staphylococcal, streptococcal infections; erysipeloid, rat-bite fever, anthrax, fusospirochetosis:* 600,000–1,200,000 units daily for 10–14 days. **Newborns, usual:** 50,000 units/kg in a single daily dose. *Bacterial endocarditis:* **Adults:** 1,200,000 units penicillin G procaine q.i.d. for 2–4 weeks with streptomycin, 500 mg b.i.d. for the first 14 days. *Diphtheria carrier state:* 300,000 units/day for 10 days. *Gonococcal infections:* 4.8 million units divided into at least 2 doses (at one visit) given with 1 g PO probenecid (given 30 min before penicillin injections). *Neurosyphilis:* 2.4 million units daily for 10 days (given at two sites) with 1 g PO probenecid; **then,** benzathine penicillin G, 2.4 million units/week for 3 weeks. *Congenital syphilis in infants:* 50,000 units/kg daily for at least 10 days. *Acute pelvic inflammatory disease:* Single dose of 4.8 million units (given at two sites) with 1 g PO probenecid; **then,** doxycycline, PO, 100 mg b.i.d. for 10–14 days. *Sexually transmitted epididymo-orchitis, urethritis:* 4.8 million units (given at two sites) with 1 g PO probenecid; **then,** tetracycline, PO, 500 mg q.i.d. for 10 days.

P

NURSING CONSIDERATIONS

See also *Nursing Considerations* for *Penicillins,* p. 200.

Administration/Storage

1. Note on package whether medication is to be refrigerated, since some brands require this to maintain stability.
2. Shake multiple-dose vial thoroughly to ensure uniform suspension before injection. If the medication is clumped at the bottom of the vial, it must be shaken until clump dissolves.
3. Use a 20-gauge needle and aspirate immediately after withdrawing medication from the vial; otherwise needle may become clogged and syringe may "freeze."
4. Administer into two sites if dose is large or available muscle mass is small.
5. Aspirate to check that the needle is not in a vein.
6. Inject deep into muscle at a slow rate.
7. Do not massage after injection.
8. Rotate and chart injection sites.
9. Drug is for IM use only.

Client/Family Teaching

1. Observe for wheal or other skin reactions at site of injection that may indicate a reaction to procaine as well as to penicillin and report.
2. Determine need for sexual counseling/referral in clients being treated for venereal disease. Stress importance of the sexual partner undergoing treatment.

Evaluation: Evaluate client for:
- Laboratory confirmation of

control and treatment of underlying infection
- Prophylaxis pre- and post-surgery (with hx of rheumatic fever)

Penicillin V Potassium (Phenoxymethylpenicillin potassium)
(pen-ih-SILL-in)
Apo-Pen-VK✽, Beepen-VK, Betapen-VK, Ledercillin VK, Nadopen-V✽, Novo-Pen-VK✽, Nu-Pen-VK✽, Penicillin VK, Pen-V, Pen-Vee K, PVF K✽, Robicillin VK, V-Cillin K, VC-K 500✽, Veetids 125, 250, and 500 (Rx)

See also *Anti-Infectives,* p. 80, and *Penicillins,* p. 197.

Classification: Antibiotic, penicillin.

Action/Kinetics: These preparations are related closely to penicillin G. They are not penicillinase resistant but are acid stable and resist inactivation by gastric secretions. They are well absorbed from the GI tract and are not affected by foods. **Peak plasma levels:** Penicillin V, **PO:** 2.7 mcg/ml after 30–60 min; penicillin V potassium, **PO:** 1–9 mcg/ml after 30–60 min. **t½:** 30 min.

Periodic blood counts and renal function tests are indicated during long-term usage.

Uses: Penicillin-sensitive staphylococci, pneumococci, streptococci, gonococci. Vincent's infection of the oropharynx. Lyme disease. *Prophylaxis:* Rheumatic fever, chorea, bacterial endocarditis, pre- and postsurgery. Should *not* be used as prophylaxis for GU instrumentation or surgery, sigmoidoscopy, or childbirth or during the acute stage of severe pneumonia, bacteremia, arthritis, empyema, pericarditis, and meningitis. Penicillin G, IV, should be used for treating neurologic complications due to Lyme disease.

Special Concerns: More and more strains of staphylococci are resistant to penicillin V, necessitating culture and sensitivity studies.

Additional Drug Interactions

Contraceptives, oral /
 ↓ Effectiveness of oral contraceptives
Neomycin, oral / ↓ Absorption of penicillin V

Dosage: Oral Solution, Tablets. Adults and children over 12 years: *Streptococcal infections:* 125–250 mg q 6–8 hr for 10 days. *Pneumococcal or staphylococcal infections, fusospirochetosis of oropharynx:* 250–500 mg q 6–8 hr. *Prophylaxis of rheumatic fever / chorea:* 125–250 mg b.i.d. *Prophylaxis of bacterial endocarditis.* **Adults and children over 27 kg:** 2 g 30–60 min prior to procedure; **then,** 1 g q 6 hr. **Pediatric:** 1 g 30–60 min prior to procedure; **then,** 500 mg q 6 hr. *Anaerobic infections:* 250 mg q.i.d. See also *Penicillin G, Procaine, Aqueous, Sterile,* p. 1009.

    Pediatric, usual: 25–50 mg/kg daily in divided doses q 6–8 hr. *Prophylaxis of septicemia caused by Staphylococcus pneumoniae in children with sickle cell anemia:* 125 mg b.i.d. *Streptococcal pharyngitis in children:* 250 mg b.i.d. for 10 days. *Steptococcal otitis media and sinusitis:* 250–500 mg q 6 hr for 14 days. *Lyme disease:* 250–500 mg q.i.d. for 10–20 days (for children less than 2 years of age, 50 mg/kg daily in 4 divided doses for 10–20 days).

    Note: 250 mg penicillin V is equivalent to 400,000 units.

NURSING CONSIDERATIONS

See also *Nursing Considerations* for *Penicillins,* p. 200.

Administration / Storage

1. Administer without regard to meals.
2. Do not administer at the same time as neomycin because malabsorption of penicillin V may occur.

Client / Family Teaching

1. Clients with a history of rheumatic fever or congenital heart disease need to understand the importance of using antibiotic prophylaxis prior to any invasive medical or dental procedure.
2. Use an additional nonhormonal form of birth control if taking oral contraceptives because their effectiveness may be diminished.
3. Report for all scheduled laboratory studies and explain their importance during long-term therapy.

Evaluation: Evaluate client for:
- Reports of symptomatic improvement
- Laboratory evidence of drug effectiveness

Pentaerythritol tetranitrate Sustained-release Capsules

(pen-tah-er-**ITH**-rih-toll)
Duotrate, Duotrate 45 (Rx)

Pentaerythritol tetranitrate Sustained-release Tablets

(pen-tah-er-**ITH**-rih-toll)

Peritrate SA (Rx)

Pentaerythritol tetranitrate Tablets

(pen-tah-er-**ITH**-rih-toll)

Pentylan, Peritrate, Peritrate Forte ✺ (Rx)

See also *Antianginal Drugs,* p. 47.

Classification: Coronary vasodilator.

Action/Kinetics: Onset, Tablets: 20–60 min; **Sustained-release Capsules/Tablets:** 30 min. **Duration, Tablets:** 4–6 hr; **Extended-release Capsules/Tablets:** 12 hr. Excreted in urine and feces.

Use: Prophylaxis of anginal attacks, but is not to be used to terminate acute attacks.

Special Concerns: Pregnancy category: C. Dosage has not been established in children.

Additional Side Effects: Severe rash, exfoliative dermatitis.

Additional Drug Interactions

Acetylcholine / Pentaerythritol antagonizes the effect of acetylcholine
Norepinephrine / Pentaerythritol antagonizes the effect of norepinephrine

Dosage: PO, Tablets. Initial, 10–20 mg t.i.d.–q.i.d.; **then,** up to 40 mg q.i.d. **Sustained-release:** One capsule of tablets (30, 45, or 80 mg) mg q 12 hr.

NURSING CONSIDERATIONS

See also *Nursing Considerations* for *Antianginal Drugs,* p. 49.

Client/Family Teaching

1. Drug is to be taken 30 min before or 1 hr after meals, as well as at bedtime.
2. Sustained-release tablets are to be taken on an empty stomach and are not to be chewed or crushed.
3. Advise client to take only as directed and to report any rash or bothersome side effects.
4. Remind client that this product is not for acute anginal attacks and advise to use other nitrates specifically prescribed in this event.

Evaluation: Evaluate client for reports of a ↓ in the frequency and severity of anginal attacks.

Pentamidine isethionate

(pen-**TAM**-ih-deen)

NebuPent, Pentacarinate ✺, Pentam, Pneumopent ✺ (Rx)

Classification: Antibiotic, miscellaneous (antiprotozoal).

Action/Kinetics: The drug inhibits synthesis of DNA, RNA, phospholipids, and proteins, thereby interfering with cell metabolism. It may interfere also with folate transformation. About one-third of the dose may be excreted unchanged in the urine. Plasma levels following inhalation are significantly lower than after a comparable IV dose.

Uses: Parenteral. Pneumonia caused by *Pneumocystis carinii.*

Inhalation. Prophylaxis of *P. carinii* in high-risk HIV-infected clients defined by one or both of the following: (a) a history of one or more cases of pneumonia caused by *P. carinii* and/or (b) a peripheral CD4 + lymphocyte count less than 200/mm³. *Investigational:* Trypanosomiasis, visceral leishmaniasis.

Contraindications: Clients manifesting anaphylaxis to inhaled or parenteral pentamidine.

Special Concerns: Pregnancy category: C. Use with caution in clients with hepatic or kidney disease, hypertension or hypotension, hyperglycemia or hypoglycemia, hypocalcemia, leukopenia, thrombocytopenia, anemia, ventricular tachycardia, pancreatitis, Stevens-Johnson syndrome.

Side Effects: Parenteral. *CV:* Hypotension, ventricular tachycardia, phlebitis. *GI:* Nausea, anorexia, bad taste in mouth. *Hematologic:* Leukopenia, thrombocytopenia, anemia. *Electrolytes/glucose:* Hypoglycemia, hypocalcemia, hyperkalemia. *CNS:* Dizziness without hypotension, confusion, hallucinations. *Miscellaneous:* Acute renal failure, Stevens-Johnson syndrome, elevated serum creatinine, elevated liver function tests, pain or induration at IM injection site, sterile abscess at injection site, rash, neuralgia.

Inhalation. Most frequent include the following. *GI:* Decreased appetite, nausea, vomiting, metallic taste, diarrhea, abdominal pain. *CNS:* Fatigue, dizziness, headache. *Respiratory:* Shortness of breath, cough, pharyngitis, chest pain, chest congestion, bronchospasm, pneu-

mothorax. *Miscellaneous:* Rash, night sweats, chills, myalgia, headache, anemia, edema.

Dosage: IV, Deep IM. Adults and children: 4 mg/kg once daily for 14 days. Dosage should be reduced in renal disease.

 Aerosol. *Prevention of P. carinii pneumonia:* 300 mg q 4 weeks given via the Respirgard II nebulizer.

NURSING CONSIDERATIONS

See also *General Nursing Considerations For All Anti-Infectives,* p. 83.

Administration/Storage

1. To prepare IM solution, dissolve one vial in 3 ml of sterile water for injection.
2. To prepare IV solution, dissolve one vial in 3–5 ml of sterile water for injection or 5% dextrose injection. The drug is then further diluted in 50–250 ml of 5% dextrose solution. This solution then can be infused slowly over 60 min.
3. IV solutions in concentrations of 1 and 2.5 mg/ml in 5% dextrose injection are stable for 48 hr at room temperature.
4. The dose using the nebulizer should be delivered until the chamber is empty (30–45 min). The suggested flow rate is 5–7 l/min from a 40–50 pounds per sq inch (psi) air or oxygen source.
5. Reconstitution for use in the nebulizer is accomplished by dissolving the contents of the vial in 6 ml sterile water for injection. Saline solution cannot be used because it causes the drug to precipitate.
6. When used for nebulization,

P

pentamidine should not be mixed with any other drug.

7. The solution for nebulization is stable at room temperature for 48 hr if protected from light.

Assessment

1. Assess extent of infection and document.
2. Determine history of kidney disease, hypertension, and past blood disorders.
3. Note results of tuberculosis screening tests.

Interventions

1. Obtain baseline blood sugar, calcium, electrolytes, CBC, renal and liver function studies, and monitor throughout therapy.
2. Observe for symptoms of hypoglycemia, hypocalcemia, and/or hyperkalemia.
3. Monitor and record vital signs and I&O.
4. Obtain apical pulse and auscultate for any evidence of arrhythmia if client not monitored.
5. During administration of aerosolized pentamidine, appropriate precautions should be followed to protect the health care worker. Wear:
   - Eye protection with side shields
   - Disposable gowns
   - Respiratory protective equipment such as an organic mist respirator unless client under hood-stalls or in a ventilated booth
   - Gloves
6. Follow appropriate institutional guidelines and OSHA standards for administration of drug.

7. Incorporate Universal Precautions to protect immunocompromised clients.
8. The manufacturer has a 24-hr emergency assistance hot line available: (312) 345–9746.

Client/Family Teaching

1. Advise client to report any adverse effects such as bruising, hematuria, blood in stools, or other evidence of bleeding.
2. Avoid aspirin-containing compounds, alcohol, IM injections, or rectal thermometers.
3. Advise to use a soft toothbrush, electric razor, and night light to prevent injury and falls.
4. Be alert for signs and symptoms of hypoglycemia (which may be severe) and report immediately after consuming juice with sugar.
5. Report early signs of Stevens-Johnson syndrome (characterized by high fever, severe headaches, stomatitis, conjunctivitis, rhinitis, urethritis, and balanitis), all of which may necessitate the discontinuation of drug therapy.
6. Intake of fluids should be increased to 2 qt/day during drug therapy.
7. Rise from a prone position slowly and dangle legs before rising as drug may cause dizziness.
8. During inhalation, advise that a metallic taste may be experienced.
9. Stress the importance of completing the prescribed course of therapy.

Evaluation: Evaluate client for:
   - (Parenterally) clinical evidence and reports of improvement in symptoms of *P. carinii* pneumonia
   - (Inhalation) evidence of pro-

phylaxis of *P. carinii* pneumonia in HIV-infected at risk individuals

―――― *COMBINATION DRUG* ――――
Pentazocine hydrochloride with Naloxone
(pen-**TAZ**-oh-seen, nah-**LOX**-ohn)
Talwin NX (C-IV,Rx)

Pentazocine lactate
(pen-**TAZ**-oh-seen)
Talwin (C-IV, Rx)

See also *Narcotic Analgesics,* p. 174.

Classification: Narcotic analgesic–agonist-antagonist.

General Statement: When administered preoperatively for pain, pentazocine is approximately one-third as potent as morphine. It is a weak antagonist of the analgesic effects of meperidine, morphine, and other narcotic analgesics. It also manifests sedative effects.

Pentazocine has been abused by combining it with the antihistamine tripelennamine (a combination known as *T's and Blues*). This combination has been injected IV as a substitute for heroin. To reduce this possibility, the oral dosage form of pentazocine has been combined with naloxone (Talwin NX), which will prevent the effects of IV administered pentazocine but will not affect the efficacy of pentazocine when taken orally.

Action/Kinetics: Pentazocine manifests both narcotic agonist and antagonist properties. **Onset: IM,** 15–20 min; **PO,** 15–30 min; **IV,** 2–3 min. **Peak effect: IM,** 15–60 min; **PO,** 60–180 min. **Duration, all routes:** 3 hr. However, onset, dura-

tion, and degree of relief depend on both dose and severity of pain. **t½:** 2–3 hr.

Uses: PO: Moderate to severe pain. **Parenteral:** Preoperative or preanesthetic medication, obstetrics, supplement to surgical anesthesia.

Additional Contraindications: Increased intracranial pressure or head injury. Not recommended for use in children under 12 years of age. Avoid using methadone or other narcotics for pentazocine withdrawal.

Special Concerns: Pregnancy category: C. Use with caution in impaired renal or hepatic function, as well as after myocardial infarction, when nausea and vomiting are present. Use with caution in women delivering premature infants.

Additional Side Effects: Edema of the face, syncope, dysphoria, nightmares, and hallucinations. Also, decreased white blood cells, paresthesia, chills. Both psychologic and physical dependence are possible, although the addiction liability is thought to be no greater than for codeine.

Dosage: Tablets. *Pentazocine hydrochloride with naloxone.* **Adults,** 50 mg q 3–4 hr, up to 100 mg. Daily dose should not exceed 600 mg. **IM, IV, SC.** *Pentazocine lactate.* 30 mg q 3–4 hr; doses exceeding 30 mg IV or 60 mg IM not recommended. Total daily dosage should not exceed 360 mg. *Obstetric analgesia:* **IM,** 30 mg; **IV,** 20 mg. Dosage may be repeated 2–3 times at 2- to 3-hr intervals.

NURSING CONSIDERATIONS

See also *Nursing Considerations* for *Narcotic Analgesics,* p. 177.

Administration/Storage

1. Do not mix soluble barbiturates in the same syringe with pentazocine. It will form a precipitate.
2. IV pentazocine may be administered undiluted. However, if the drug is to be diluted, place 5 mg of drug into 5 ml of sterile water for injection. Administer each 5 mg of drug or less over a 1-min period.
3. Review the list of drugs with which the medication interacts.

Assessment

1. Note any evidence of head injury or increased ICP.
2. Determine any history of hepatic, renal, or cardiac dysfunction.

Evaluation: Evaluate client for reports of effective control of pain.

Pentobarbital
(pen-toe-**BAR**-bih-tal)
Nembutal (C-II, Rx)

Pentobarbital sodium
(pen-toe-**BAR**-bih-tal)
Carbrital✿, Nembutal Sodium, Nova-Rectal✿, Novo–Pentobarb✿ (C-II, Rx)

See also *Barbiturates,* p. 101.

Classification: Sedative-hypnotic, barbiturate type.

Action/Kinetics: Short-acting. t½: 19–34 hr. Is 60%–70% protein bound.

Uses: Short-term treatment of insomnia. Sedative. Anticonvulsant (parenteral use only). *Investigational:* Parenterally to induce coma to protect the brain from ischemia and increased intracranial pressure following stroke and head trauma.

Special Concerns: Pregnancy category: D.

Dosage: Elixir, Capsules. *Sedation:* **Adults,** 20 mg t.i.d.–q.i.d. **Pediatric:** 2–6 mg/kg daily (use elixir). *Preoperative sedation:* **Adults,** 100 mg. *Hypnotic:* **Adults,** 100 mg at bedtime. **Suppositories, rectal.** *Hypnotic:* **Adults,** 120–200 mg; **infants, 2–12 months:** 30 mg; **1–4 years:** 30–60 mg; **5–12 years:** 60 mg; **12–14 years:** 60–120 mg. **IV (slow). Adults (70 kg),** 100 mg. **IM. Adults,** *hypnotic/preoperative sedation:* 150–200 mg; **pediatric:** 2–6 mg/kg (not to exceed 100 mg).

IV. Adults, *sedative/hypnotic:* 100 mg followed in 1 min by additional small doses, if required, up to a total of 500 mg. *Anticonvulsant:* **Adults, initial,** 100 mg; **then,** after 1 min, additional small doses may be given, if needed, up to a total of 500 mg.

IM, IV. Pediatric, *Anticonvulsant:* **initially,** 50 mg; **then,** after 1 min, additional small doses may be given, if needed, until the desired effect is achieved.

NURSING CONSIDERATIONS

See also *Nursing Considerations* for *Barbiturates,* p. 104.

Administration/Storage

1. The IV dose is given in fractions because pentobarbital is a potent CNS depressant that may cause adverse respiratory and circulatory responses. Adults generally receive 100 mg initially; children and debilitated clients, 50 mg. Subsequent fractions are administered after 1-min observation periods. Over-

dose or too rapid administration may cause spasms of the larynx or pharynx, or both.

2. Pentobarbital solutions are highly alkaline.

3. The parenteral product is not for SC use.

4. Parental pentobarbital is incompatible with most other drugs; therefore, do not mix other drugs in the same syringe.

5. Administer no more than 5 ml at one site **IM** because of possible tissue irritation (pain, necrosis, gangrene).

6. Suppositories are not to be divided.

Interventions

1. Observe for signs of respiratory depression. This is usually the first sign of drug overdose.

2. If the medication is administered IV, assess site for patency.

3. Note client complaint of pain at the site of injection or in the limb. Interrupt the injection, document and report to the physician.

4. Note any pallor, cyanosis, patchy discoloration of the skin, or delay in the onset of hypnosis. These are all signs of intra-arterial injection and can cause gangrene. The IV injection should be halted immediately, the observations recorded on the client's chart and the incident reported to the physician.

5. During treatment of cerebral edema (barbiturate coma), monitor and document intracranial pressure readings and client level of consciousness.

6. Initiate appropriate safety measures once the medication has been administered. This is particularly important when working with confused or elderly clients.

Evaluation: Evaluate client for:
- Reports of improved sleeping patterns with less frequent awakenings
- Evidence of desired level of sedation
- Evidence of control of seizures

Pentostatin (2'-deoxycoformycin; DCF)

(**PEN**-toh-stah-tin)
Nipent (Rx)

Classification: Antineoplastic, antibiotic.

Action/Kinetics: Pentostatin is isolated from *Streptomyces antibioticus;* the drug inhibits the enzyme adenosine deaminase (ADA). Inhibition of ADA, especially in the presence of adenosine or deoxyadenosine, results in cellular toxicity (T cells, B cells) due to elevated intracellular levels of dATP; this blocks the synthesis of DNA through inhibition of ribonucleotide reductase. Pentostatin also inhibits RNA synthesis and causes increased DNA damage. **t½, distribution,** 11 min; **terminal,** 5.7 hr. Approximately 90% is excreted in the urine as unchanged pentostatin or metabolites.

Uses: Hairy cell leukemia in adults who are refractory to alpha-interferon; such individuals have progressive disease after a minimum of 3 months of alpha-interferon therapy or no response after a minimum

P

of 6 months of alpha-interferon therapy. During lactation.

Contraindications: In combination with fludarabine phosphate.

Special Concerns: Pregnancy category: D. Treat clients with infection only if the potential benefit outweighs the risk; infection should be treated before pentostatin therapy is initiated or resumed. Safety and effectiveness have not been determined in children.

Side Effects: *Hematologic:* Leukopenia, anemia, thrombocytopenia, ecchymosis, lymphadenopathy, petechia, abnormal erythrocytes, leukocytosis, pancytopenia, purpura, splenomegaly, eosinophilia, hematologic disorder, hemolysis, lymphoma-like reaction. *GI:* Nausea, vomiting, anorexia, abdominal pain, diarrhea, constipation, flatulence, stomatitis, colitis, dysphagia, dyspepsia, eructation, gastritis, GI hemorrhage, gum hemorrhage, intestinal obstruction, leukoplakia, melena, periodontal abscess, proctitis, abnormal stools, esophagitis, gingivitis, mouth disorder. *Hepatic:* Hepatitis, hepatomegaly, hepatic failure. *CNS:* Headache, anxiety, abnormal thinking, confusion, depression, dizziness, insomnia, nervousness, paresthesia, somnolence, agitation, amnesia, ataxia, abnormal dreams, depersonalization, emotional lability, hyperesthesia, hypoesthesia, hypertonia, incoordination, decreased libido, neuropathy, stupor, tremor, vertigo, coma, seizures. *CV:* Arrhythmia, abnormal ECG, hemorrhage, thrombophlebitis, aortic stenosis, arterial anomaly, cardiomegaly, congestive heart failure, cardiac arrest, flushing, hypertension, myocardial infarct, palpitation, varicose vein, shock. *Dermatologic:* Rash, skin disorder, eczema, dry skin, herpes simplex, herpes zoster, maculopapular rash, pruritus, seborrhea, skin discoloration, sweating, vesiculobullous rash, acne, alopecia, exfoliative dermatitis, contact dermatitis, fungal dermatitis, benign skin neoplasm, psoriasis, subcutaneous nodule, skin hypertrophy, urticaria. *GU:* Genitourinary disorder, dysuria, hematuria, fibrocystic breast(s), gynecomastia, hydronephrosis, oliguria, polyuria, pyuria, hydronephrosis, toxic nephropathy, urinary frequency, urinary retention, urinary urgency, urinary tract infection, impaired urination, urolithiasis, vaginitis. *Musculoskeletal:* Myalgia, arthralgia, asthenia, facial paralysis, abnormal gait, arthritis, bone pain, osteomyelitis, neck rigidity, pathological fracture. *Respiratory:* Cough, upper respiratory infection, lung disorder, bronchitis, dyspnea, epistaxis, lung edema, pneumonia, pharyngitis, rhinitis, sinusitis, asthma, atelectasis, hemoptysis, hyperventilation, hypoventilation, increased sputum, laryngitis, larynx edema, lung fibrosis, pleural effusion, pneumothorax, pulmonary embolus. *Body as a whole:* Fever, infection, fatigue, weight loss or gain, peripheral edema, pain, allergic reaction, chills, sepsis, chest pain, back pain, flu syndrome, malaise, neoplasm, abscess, enlarged abdomen, ascites, acidosis, dehydration, diabetes mellitus, gout, abnormal healing, cellulitis, facial edema, cyst, fibrosis, granuloma, hernia, hemorrhage or inflammation of the injection site, moniliasis, pelvic pain, photosensitivity, anaphylaxis, mucous membrane disorder, immune system disorder, neck pain. *Ophthalmic:* Abnormal vision, conjunctivitis, eye pain, blepharitis, cataract, diplopia, exophthalmos, lacrimation disorder, optic neuritis, retinal detachment. *Miscellaneous:* Ear pain, deafness, otitis media, parosmia, taste perversion, tinnitus.

Symptoms of Overdose: Severe renal, hepatic, pulmonary, and CNS toxicity; death can result.

Drug Interactions

Fludarabine / Use with pentostatin may cause ↑ risk of fatal pulmonary toxicity

Vidarabine / ↑ Effect of vidarabine, including side effects

Laboratory Test Interferences:
↑ Liver function test, BUN, creatinine, LDH, creatine phosphokinase, gamma globulins. Albuminuria, glycosuria, hyponatremia, hypocholesterolemia.

Dosage: IV bolus, IV infusion.
Alpha-interferon-refractory hairy cell leukemia: 4 mg/m^2 every other week.

NURSING CONSIDERATIONS

See also *Nursing Considerations* for *Antineoplastic Agents,* p. 88.

Administration/Storage

1. To reconstitute, 5 ml of sterile water for injection is added to the vial; the vial is mixed thoroughly to obtain complete dissolution for a concentration of 2 mg/ml.
2. Pentostatin may be given by IV bolus or diluted in 25–50 ml of 5% dextrose injection or 0.9% sodium chloride injection. Dilution of the entire contents of the reconstituted vial with 25 or 50 ml provides a concentration of diluted pentostatin of 0.33 or 0.18 mg/ml, respectively. Such a dilution does not interact with PVC infusion containers or administration sets.
3. Pentostatin vials can be stored in the refrigerator at temperatures of 2°–8°C (36°–46°F). Reconstituted vials or reconstituted vials further diluted may be stored at room temperature and ambient light for up to 8 hr.
4. The optimum duration of treatment has not been determined; if major toxicity has not occurred, treatment should continue until a complete response has been achieved. This should be followed by two additional doses and then treatment should be stopped. If, after 12 months, there is only a partial response, treatment should be discontinued.
5. A dose should be withheld if there is severe rash, CNS toxicity, infection, or elevated serum creatinine.
6. Pentostatin should be temporarily withheld if the absolute neutrophil count falls below 200 cells/mm^3 during treatment in a client who had an initial neutrophil count greater than 500 cells/mm^3. Treatment may be continued when the count returns to pretreatment levels.
7. *Treatment of Overdose:* General supportive measures.

Assessment

1. Note any previous experience with alpha-interferon and describe the response.
2. Obtain baseline hematologic parameters and renal function studies.
3. Question client and note any symptoms of infection prior to initiating therapy.

Client/Family Teaching

1. Advise client to report the development of rashes as these may progress and require discontinuation of drug therapy.
2. Practice effective birth control during drug therapy.
3. Stress the importance of reporting for scheduled laboratory studies to evaluate hematologic parameters. Advise that periodic bone marrow aspirates and biopsies may be necessary.

Evaluation: Evaluate for laboratory evidence of improved hematologic parameters (↑ Hb, granulocyte and platelet counts) in the management of clients with hairy cell leukemia.

Pentoxifylline
(pen-tox-**EYE**-fih-leen)
Trental (Rx)

Classification: Agent affecting blood viscosity.

Action/Kinetics: Pentoxifylline and its active metabolites decrease the viscosity of blood. This results in increased blood flow to the microcirculation and an increase in tissue oxygen levels. Although not known with certainty, the mechanism may include (1) decreased synthesis of thromboxane A$_2$ thus decreasing platelet aggregation, (2) increased blood fibrinolytic activity (decreasing fibrinogen levels), and (3) decreased red blood cell aggregation and local hyperviscosity by increasing cellular ATP. **Peak plasma levels:** 1 hr. Significant first-pass effect. **t½:** pentoxifylline, 0.4–0.8 hr; metabolites, 1–1.6 hr. **Time to peak levels;** 2–4 hr. Excretion is via the urine.

Uses: Peripheral vascular disease including intermittent claudication. The drug is not intended to replace surgery. *Investigational:* To improve circulation in clients with cerebrovascular insufficiency, transient ischemic attacks, sickle cell thalassemia, diabetic angiopathies and neuropathies, high-altitude sickness, strokes, hearing disorders, circulation disorders of the eye, and Raynaud's phenomenon.

Contraindications: Intolerance to pentoxifylline, caffeine, theophylline, or theobromine.

Special Concerns: Pregnancy (category: C). Use with caution in impaired renal function and during lactation. Safety and efficacy in children less than 18 years of age not established. Geriatric clients may be at greater risk for manifesting side effects.

Side Effects: *CV:* Angina, chest pain, hypotension, edema. *GI:* Abdominal pain, flatus/bloating, dyspepsia, salivation, bad taste in mouth, nausea/vomiting, anorexia, constipation, dry mouth and thirst. *CNS:* Dizziness, headache, tremor, malaise, anxiety, confusion. *Ophthalmologic:* Blurred vision, conjunctivitis, scotomata. *Dermatologic:* Pruritus, rash, urticaria, brittle fingernails. *Respiratory:* Dyspnea, laryngitis, nasal congestion, epistaxis. *Miscellaneous:* Flu-like symptoms, leukopenia, sore throat, swollen neck glands, change in weight.

Symptoms of Overdose: Agitation, fever, flushing, hypotension, nervousness, seizures, somnolence, tremors, loss of consciousness.

Drug Interaction: Prothrombin times should be monitored carefully if the client is on warfarin therapy.

Dosage: Extended-release Tablets. Adults: 400 mg t.i.d. with meals. Treatment should be continued for at least 8 weeks. If side effects occur, dosage can be reduced to 400 mg b.i.d.

NURSING CONSIDERATIONS

Administration/Storage: *Treatment of Overdose:* Gastric lavage followed by activated charcoal. Monitor blood pressure and ECG. Support respiration, control seizures, and treat arrhythmias.

Assessment

1. Note any client history of sensitivity to caffeine, theophylline, or theobromine.
2. If client is female, sexually active, and of childbearing age, determine if pregnant.
3. Obtain baseline CBC and renal function studies and monitor during therapy.

Client/Family Teaching

1. Provide written instructions concerning adverse side effects, such as angina and palpitations, that should be reported to the physician.
2. Discuss the need to continue the treatment for at least 8 weeks, even though effectiveness is not yet apparent.
3. Take the medication with meals to minimize GI upset.
4. Do not perform activities that require mental alertness until drug effects are realized as dizziness and blurred vision may occur.
5. Avoid nicotine-containing products as nicotine constricts blood vessels.
6. Explain the importance of follow-up visits and reporting for laboratory studies to evaluate the effectiveness of the drug.

Evaluation: Evaluate client for reports of ↓ pain and cramping in lower extremities during activity.

—— *COMBINATION DRUG* ——
Percocet
(**PER**-koh-set)
(C-II, Rx)

See also *Acetaminophen,* p. 250, and *Narcotic Analgesics,* p. 174.

Classification/Content: Each tablet contains: *Nonnarcotic analgesic:* Acetaminophen, 325 mg. *Narcotic analgesic:* Oxycodone HCl, 5 mg. Also see information on individual components.

Uses: Moderate to moderately severe pain.

Special Concerns: Pregnancy category: C. Use with caution during lactation. Safety and effectiveness have not been determined in children. Dependence to oxycodone can occur.

Dosage: Tablets. Adults, usual: One tablet q 6 hr as required for pain.

NURSING CONSIDERATIONS

See *Nursing Considerations* for *Narcotic Analgesics,* p. 177, and *Acetaminophen,* p. 252.

Administration/Storage

1. It may be necessary to increase the dose if tolerance occurs or if the pain is severe.
2. Dosage should be adjusted depending on the response of the client and the severity of the pain.

Evaluation: Evaluate client for reports of effective control of pain.

—— *COMBINATION DRUG* ——
Percodan and Percodan-Demi
(PER-koh-dan, PER-koh-dan DEH-mee)
(C-II, Rx)

See also *Aspirin,* p. 260, and *Narcotic Analgesics,* p. 174.

Classification/Content: Each tablet contains: Percodan: *Nonnarcotic Analgesic:* Aspirin, 325 mg. *Narcotic Analgesics:* Oxycodone HCl, 4.5 mg; Oxycodone Terephthalate, 0.38 mg. Percodan-Demi contains the same amount of aspirin as Percodan but one-half the amount of oxycodone HCl and oxycodone terephthalate.

Uses: Treatment of moderate to moderately severe pain.

Contraindications: Percodan should not be used in children although Percodan-Demi may be considered for use in children from 6–12 years of age.

Special Concerns: Use during pregnancy only if benefits outweigh risks. Dependence to oxycodone can occur.

Dosage: *Percodan.* **Tablets. Adults, usual:** One tablet q 6 hr as required for pain. *Percodan-Demi.* **Tablets, Adults, usual:** 1–2 tablets q 6 hr; **pediatric, over 12 years:** ½ tablet q 6 hr; **pediatric, 6–12 years:** ¼ tablet q 6 hr.

NURSING CONSIDERATIONS

See also *Nursing Considerations for Narcotic Analgesics,* p. 177, and *Aspirin,* p. 264.

Administration/Storage

1. It may be necessary to increase the dose if tolerance occurs or if the pain is severe.

2. Dosage should be adjusted depending on the response of the client and the severity of the pain.

Evaluation: Evaluate client for reports of effective control of pain.

Pergolide mesylate
(PER-go-lyd)
Permax (Rx)

Classification: Antiparkinson agent.

Action/Kinetics: Pergolide is a potent dopamine receptor (both D_1 and D_2) agonist. The drug is believed to act by directly stimulating postsynaptic dopamine receptors in the nigrostriatal system, thus relieving symptoms of parkinsonism. The drug also inhibits prolactin secretion, causes a transient rise in serum levels of growth hormone, and a decrease in serum levels of luteinizing hormone. About 90% of the drug is bound to plasma proteins. The drug is metabolized in the liver and excreted through the urine.

Uses: Adjunctive treatment to levodopa/carbidopa in Parkinson's disease.

Special Concerns: Use during pregnancy only if clearly needed (pregnancy category: B). Benefit versus risk should be assessed when considered for use during lactation. Use with caution in clients prone to cardiac dysrhythmias, in preexisting dyskinesia, and preexisting states of confusion or hallucinations. Safety and efficacy have not been determined in children.

Side Effects: The most common side effects are listed. *CV:* Postural hypotension, palpitation, vasodilation, syncope, hypotension, hypertension, arrhythmias, myocardial infarction. *GI:* Nausea (common), vomiting, diarrhea, constipation, dyspepsia, anorexia, dry mouth. *CNS:* Dyskinesia (common), dizziness, dystonia, hallucinations, confusion, insomnia, somnolence, anxiety, tremor, depression, abnormal dreams, psychosis, personality disorder, extrapyramidal syndrome, akathisia, paresthesia, incoordination, akinesia, neuralgia, hypertonia, speech disorders. *Musculoskeletal:* Arthralgia, bursitis, twitching, myalgia. *Respiratory:* Rhinitis, dyspnea, hiccup, epistaxis. *Dermatologic:* Sweating, rash. *Ophthalmologic:* Abnormal vision, double vision, eye disorders. *GU:* Urinary tract infection, urinary frequency, hematuria. *Whole body:* Pain in chest, abdomen, neck, or back; headache, asthenia, flu syndrome, chills, facial edema, infection. *Miscellaneous:* Taste alteration, peripheral edema, anemia, weight gain. *Symptoms of Overdose:* Might include agitation, hypotension, vomiting, hallucinations, involuntary movements, palpitations, tingling of arms and legs.

Drug Interactions

Butyrophenones / ↓ Effect of pergolide due to dopamine antagonist effect
Metoclopramide / ↓ Effect of pergolide due to dopamine antagonist effect
Phenothiazines / ↓ Effect of pergolide due to dopamine antagonist effect
Thioxanthines / ↓ Effect of pergolide due to dopamine antagonist effect

Dosage: Tablets. Adults, initial: 0.05 mg daily for the first two days;

then, increase dose gradually by 0.1 or 0.15 mg/day every third day over the next 12 days. The dosage may then be increased by 0.25 mg/day every third day until the therapeutic dosage level is reached. The mean therapeutic daily dosage is 3 mg daily used concurrently with levodopa/carbidopa (expressed as levodopa) at a dose of 650 mg daily. The effectiveness of doses of pergolide greater than 5 mg daily has not been evaluated.

NURSING CONSIDERATIONS

See also *Nursing Considerations* for *Antiparkinson Agents,* p. 99.

Administration/Storage

1. Pergolide is usually given in divided doses 3 times daily.
2. When determining the therapeutic dose for pergolide, the dosage of concurrent levodopa/carbidopa may be decreased cautiously.
3. *Treatment of Overdose:* Activated charcoal (usually recommended instead of or in addition to gastric lavage or induction of vomiting). Maintain blood pressure. An antiarrhythmic drug may be helpful. A phenothiazine or butyrophenone may help any CNS stimulation. Support ventilation.

Assessment

1. Note any sensitivity to ergot.
2. Document any evidence of cardiac arrhythmias.

Client/Family Teaching

1. Pergolide is to be taken concurrently with a prescribed dose of levodopa/carbidopa.
2. Do not exceed prescribed daily dose.

3. Review the list of side effects associated with pergolide therapy and instruct the client and family to report any persistent and/or bothersome symptoms.
4. Rise slowly from a sitting or lying position to minimize hypotensive effects of pergolide.
5. Stress the importance of reporting for all scheduled lab and medical appointments so that drug therapy may be evaluated and adjusted as needed.
6. Do not perform tasks that require mental alertness until drug effects realized. Drug may cause drowsiness or dizziness.

Evaluation: Evaluate client for improved response to levidopa/carbidopa as evidenced by ↓ muscle weakness, ↓ rigidity, ↓ salivation, and improved mobility.

Perphenazine
(per-FEN-ah-zeen)
**Apo-Perphenazine✹,
Phenazine✹, PMS
Perphenazine✹, Trilafon (Rx)**

See also *Phenothiazines,* p. 201.

Classification: Antipsychotic, antiemetic, piperazine-type phenothiazine.

Action/Kinetics: Resembles chlorpromazine. Use accompanied by a high incidence of extrapyramidal effects; strong antiemetic effects; moderate anticholinergic effects; and a low incidence of orthostatic hypotension and sedation. Perphenazine is also found in Triavil. **Onset, IM:** 10 min. **Maximum effect, IM:** 1–2 hr. **Duration, IM:** 6 hr (up to 24 hr).

Uses: Psychotic disorders. To treat severe nausea and vomiting.

Special Concerns: Use during pregnancy only if benefits clearly outweigh risks. Dosage has not been established in children less than 12 years of age. Geriatric, emaciated, or debilitated clients usually require a lower initial dose.

Dosage: Oral Solution, Syrup, Tablets. *Psychoses:* **Nonhospitalized clients:** 4–8 mg t.i.d. or 8–16 mg repeat-action tablets b.i.d. **Hospitalized clients:** 8–16 mg b.i.d.–q.i.d. or 8–32 mg repeat-action tablets b.i.d. Total daily dosage should not exceed 64 mg. *Severe nausea and vomiting:* 8–16 mg/day in divided doses (24 mg daily may be required in some clients). **IM. Adults and adolescents:** *Psychotic disorders,* **Nonhospitalized clients:** 5 mg q 6 hr, not to exceed 15 mg daily. **Hospitalized clients: initial,** 5–10 mg; total daily dose should not exceed 30 mg. *Severe nausea and vomiting:* 5 mg (initially, 10 mg in severe cases) q 6 hr, not to exceed 15 mg in ambulatory clients or 30 mg in hospitalized clients. **IV.** *Severe nausea and vomiting:* Up to 5 mg diluted to 0.5 mg/ml with 0.9% sodium chloride injection. Should be given in divided doses of not more than 1 mg q 1–3 hr. Can also be given as an infusion at a rate not to exceed 1 mg/min. Use should be restricted to hospitalized recumbent adults. Maximum single dose should not exceed 5 mg.

NURSING CONSIDERATIONS

See also *Nursing Considerations* for *Phenothiazines,* p. 205.

Administration/Storage

1. Each 5.0 ml of oral concentrate should be diluted with 60 ml of diluent, such as water, milk, carbonated beverage, or orange juice.

2. Do not mix with tea, coffee, cola, grape juice, or apple juice.
3. When rapid action is required, administer IM using 5 mg. Inject deep into the muscle, and repeat at 6-hr intervals as needed. The client should be in a recumbent position and remain in that position for at least 1 hr after IM administration.
4. Protect from light.
5. Store solutions in an amber-colored container.

Interventions

1. Monitor the client's BP since the drug may cause hypotension.
2. Assess pulse rate for evidence of tachycardia and/or bradycardia.

Evaluation: Evaluate client for:
- Evidence of a reduction in paranoia, excitability, or withdrawn behaviors
- Reports of effective control of severe nausea and vomiting

——— COMBINATION DRUG ———
Phenaphen with Codeine No. 2, No. 3, and No. 4
(FEN-ah-fen, KOH-deen)
(C-III, Rx)

Phenaphen-650 with Codeine Tablets
(FEN-ah-fen, KOH-deen)
(C-III, Rx)

See also *Acetaminophen,* p. 250, and *Narcotic Analgesics,* p. 174.

Classification/Content: *Nonnarcotic analgesic:* Acetaminophen,

325 mg (in each strength). *Narcotic analgesic:* Codeine phosphate, 15 mg (No. 2), 30 mg (No. 3), and 60 mg (No. 4). Each Phenaphen-650 with Codeine tablet contains: Acetaminophen, 650 mg and codeine phosphate, 30 mg. Also see information on individual components.

Uses: Mild to moderately severe pain.

Special Concerns: Pregnancy category: C. Use with caution during lactation.

Dosage: Phenapen with Codeine Capsules. Individualized. Adults, usual: 1–2 capsules of Phenaphen with Codeine No. 2 or No. 3 q 4 hr as required for pain. Or, 1 capsule of Phenaphen No. 4 q 4 hr as required for pain. Maximum 24-hr adult dose is 360 mg codeine and 4000 mg acetaminophen. **Pediatric:** Dose of codeine equivalent to 0.5 mg/kg q 4 hr as required for pain. **Phenaphen-650 with Codeine Tablets. Individualized. Adults, usual:** 1–2 tablets q 4 hr as needed for pain up to a maximum of 360 mg codeine and 4000 mg acetaminophen in a 24-hr period.

NURSING CONSIDERATIONS

See also *Nursing Considerations* for *Narcotic Analgesics,* p. 177, and *Acetaminophen,* p. 252.

Administration/Storage

1. Dosage should be based on the response of the client and the severity of the pain.
2. Doses of codeine greater than 60 mg do not increase the analgesic effect but may increase the incidence of unpleasant side effects.

Evaluation: Evaluate client for reports of effective control of pain.

Phenazopyridine hydrochloride (Phenylazo Diamino Pyridine HCl)

(fen-AY-zoh-PEER-ih-deen)

Azo-Standard, Baridium, Eridium, Geridium, Phenazo✻, Phenazodine, Pyridiate, Pyridium, Pyronium✻, Urodine, Urogesic (Rx)

Classification: Urinary analgesic.

Action/Kinetics: Phenazopyridine HCl is an azo dye with local anesthetic effects on the urinary tract. 65% excreted unchanged or as metabolites within 24 hr.

Uses: Relief of pain, urgency or frequency, and burning in chronic urinary tract infections or irritation, including cystitis, urethritis and pyelitis, trauma, surgery, or urinary tract instrumentation. May also be used as an adjunct to antibacterial therapy.

Contraindications: Renal insufficiency. Use in children less than 12 years of age. Chronic use to treat undiagnosed pain of the urinary tract.

Special Concerns: Pregnancy category: B.

Side Effects: *GI:* Nausea. *Hematologic:* Methemoglobinemia, hemolytic anemia (especially in clients with glucose-6-phosphate dehydrogenase deficiency). *Dermatologic:* Yellowish tinge of the skin or sclerae may indicate accumulation of drug due to renal insufficiency. *Miscellaneous:* Renal and hepatic toxicity, headache, pruritus, rash. *Symptoms of Overdose:* Methemoglobinemia following massive overdoses. Hemolysis due to glucose-6-phosphate dehydrogenase deficiency.

Laboratory Test Interferences: Clinistix or Tes-Tape, colorimetric laboratory test procedures.

Dosage: Tablets. Adults: 200 mg t.i.d. with or after meals. **Pediatric, 6–12 years:** 4 mg/kg t.i.d. with food.

NURSING CONSIDERATIONS

Administration/Storage: *Treatment of Overdose:* Methylene blue, 1–2 mg/kg IV or 100–200 mg PO of ascorbic acid to treat methemoglobinemia.

Assessment: Note any history of liver and/or renal dysfunction.

Client/Family Teaching

1. Take medication with or after meals to prevent GI upset.
2. Should be used for only 2 days when taken together with an antibacterial agent for urinary tract infections.
3. Monitor I&O, and record.
4. In clients with diabetes, finger sticks should be performed to evaluate blood sugar levels.
5. Drug turns urine orange-red; may stain fabrics. Wear a sanitary napkin to avoid staining garments. A 0.25% sodium dithionate or sodium hydrosulfite solution, available from a pharmacy, will remove these stains.
6. Provide a printed list of side effects that indicate toxicity. Report to physician if evident.

Evaluation: Evaluate client for reports of relief of pain upon urination with UTI.

Phendimetrazine tartrate

(fen-dye-**ME**-trah-zeen)

Adphen, Anorex, Bacarate, Bontrol PDM and Slow-Release, Dital, Dyrexan-OD, Marlibar A, Melfiat-105 Unicelles, Metra, Neocurab, Obalan, Obe-Del, Obeval, Obezine, Panrexin M, Panrexin MTP, Parzine, Phendiet, Phendiet-105, Phendimet, Phentra, Phenzine, Plegine, Prelu-2, PT 105, Rexigen, Rexigen Forte, Slyn-LL, Statobex, Tega-Nil, Trimcaps, Trimstat, Trimtabs, Uni Trim, Wehless Timecelles, Weightrol, Wescoid, X-Trozine, X-Trozine LA (C-III) (Rx)

See also *Amphetamines and Derivatives,* p. 29.

Classification: Anorexiant.

Action/Kinetics: Duration, tablets: 4 hr. **t½:** 5.5 hr (average).

Use: Short-term (8–12 weeks) treatment of exogenous obesity in conjunction with a weight reduction program including exercise, reduced caloric intake, and behavior modification.

Special Concerns: Pregnancy category: C.

Dosage: Capsules, Tablets. Adults: 17.5–35 mg 2–3 times daily 1 hr before meals. **Maximum daily dose:** 70 mg t.i.d. **Extended-release Capsules, Extended-release Tablets. Adults:** 105 mg once daily 30–60 min before the morning meal.

NURSING CONSIDERATIONS

See *Nursing Considerations* for *Amphetamines and Derivatives,* p. 31.

Evaluation: Evaluate client for evidence of weight loss.

———— *COMBINATION DRUG* ————
Phenergan with Codeine Syrup

(**FEN**-er-gan, **KOH**-deen)
(Rx) (C-V)

Classification/Content: *Antihistamine:* Promethazine HCl, 6.25 mg/5 ml. *Antitussive, narcotic:* Codeine phosphate, 10 mg/5 ml. See also information on individual components.

Uses: Relief of coughs and other upper respiratory tract problems associated with the common cold or with allergy.

Contraindications: Clients with lower respiratory tract symptoms, including asthma. Use in children less than 2 years of age.

Special Concerns: Pregnancy category: C. Use with caution during lactation.

Dosage: Syrup. Adults: 5 ml q 4–6 hr, not to exceed 30 ml daily; **pediatric, 6–12 years:** 2.5–5 ml q 4–6 hr, not to exceed 30 ml daily; **pediatric, 2–6 years:** 1.25–2.5 ml q 4–6 hr.

NURSING CONSIDERATIONS

See also *Nursing Considerations* for *Antihistamines,* p. 74.

Administration/Storage

The maximum daily dose of medication for children between 2 and 6 years of age depends on body weight. The amount of drug administered should not exceed:

• 9 ml for 18 kg of body weight, or

- 8 ml for 16 kg of body weight, or
- 7 ml for 14 kg of body weight, or
- 6 ml for 12 kg of body weight.

Assessment: Take a thorough nursing history to determine how long the client has had the symptoms and assess whether or not the problem may be related to an allergy.

Client/Family Teaching

1. Notify the physician if the symptoms persist or intensify.
2. Advise that constipation may be a side effect of the medication. To avoid, instruct the client to drink approximately 2,500 ml of fluid per day and to include additional roughage in the diet.
3. Explain that the drug may be habit-forming and is not for long-term indiscriminate use.

Evaluation: Evaluate client for:
- Reports of ↓ allergic manifestations
- Reports of effective control of cough with fewer nighttime awakenings

—— COMBINATION DRUG ——
Phenergan with Dextromethorphan Syrup
(FEN-er-gan, dex-troh-meth-OR-fan)
(Rx)

Classification/Content: *Antihistamine:* Promethazine HCl, 6.25 mg/5 ml. *Nonnarcotic antitussive:* Dextromethorphan HCl, 15 mg/5 ml. See also information on individual components.

Uses: To treat symptoms of cough and upper respiratory problems observed with the common cold and allergies.

Contraindications: Use in children less than 2 years of age.

Special Concerns: Pregnancy category: C. Use with caution during lactation.

Dosage: Syrup. Adults: 5 ml q 4–6 hr, not to exceed 30 ml daily. **Pediatric, 6–12 years:** 2.5–5 ml q 4–6 hr, not to exceed 20 ml daily; **2–6 years:** 1.25–2.5 ml q 4–6 hr, not to exceed 10 ml daily.

NURSING CONSIDERATIONS

See *Nursing Considerations* for *Antihistamines,* p. 74, and *Dextromethorphan,* p. 525.

—— COMBINATION DRUG ——
Phenergan-D
(FEN-er-gan-D)
(Rx)

Classification/Content: Each tablet contains: *Antihistamine:* Promethazine HCl, 6.25 mg and *Decongestant:* Pseudoephedrine HCl, 60 mg. Also see information on individual components.

Uses: Relief of upper respiratory tract symptoms, such as nasal congestion, associated with the common cold or allergies.

Contraindications: Use to treat lower respiratory tract symptoms, including asthma. Use in children less than 12 years of age.

Special Concerns: Pregnancy category: C. Use with caution during lactation.

Dosage: Tablets. Adults: 1 tablet q 4–6 hr, not to exceed 4 tablets daily.

NURSING CONSIDERATIONS

See *Nursing Considerations* for *Antihistamines,* p. 74, and *Pseudoephedrine Hydrochloride,* p. 1107.

———— COMBINATION DRUG ————
Phenergan VC with Codeine Syrup
(FEN-er-gan, KOH-deen)
(C-V) (Rx)

Phenergan VC Syrup
(FEN-er-gan)

Classification/Content: Phenergan VC contains the following: *Antihistamine:* Promethazine HCl, 6.25 mg/5 ml. *Decongestant:* Phenylephrine HCl, 5 mg/5 ml. Phenergan VC with Codeine contains the above plus: *Narcotic antitussive:* Codeine phosphate, 10 mg/5 ml.

Uses: Phenergan VC: Nasal congestion accompanying allergy or the common cold. Phenergan VC with Codeine: Cough and nasal congestion accompanying allergy or the common cold.

Contraindications: Use for lower respiratory tract symptoms, including asthma. Use in children less than 2 years of age.

Special Concerns: Pregnancy category: C. Use with caution during lactation.

Dosage: *Phenergan VC Syrup, Phenergan VC with Codeine Syrup.* **PO. Adults:** 5 ml q 4–6 hr, not to exceed 30 ml daily. **Pediatric, 6–12 years:** 2.5–5 ml q 4–6 hr not to exceed 30 ml daily; **2–6 years:** 1.25–2.5 ml q 4–6 hr (the maximum daily dose of Phenergan VC with Codeine ranges from 6 to 9 ml depending on the body weight).

NURSING CONSIDERATIONS

See *Nursing Considerations* for *Antihistamines,* p. 74, *Phenylephrine,* p. 1038, and *Codeine,* p. 477.

Adminsitration/Storage: The maximum daily dose of medication for children between 2 and 6 years of age depends on body weight. The amount of drug administered should not exceed:

- 9 ml for 18 kg of body weight, or
- 8 ml for 16 kg of body weight, or
- 7 ml for 14 kg of body weight, or
- 6 ml for 12 kg of body weight

Phenobarbital
(fee-no-**BAR**-bih-tal)
Ancalixir✤, Barbita, Gardenal✤, Solfoton (C-IV, Rx)

Phenobarbital sodium
(fee-no-**BAR**-bih-tal)
Luminal Sodium (C-IV, Rx)

See also *Barbiturates,* p. 101.

Classification: Sedative, anticonvulsant, barbiturate type.

Action/Kinetics: Long-acting. **t½:** 24–140 hr. **Anticonvulsant therapeutic serum levels:** 10–40 mcg/ml. **Time for peak effect, after IV:** up to 15 min. Distributed more slowly than other barbiturates due to lower lipid solubility. Is 50%–60% protein bound.

Uses: Sedative, preanesthetic, postoperative sedation, hypnotic, anticonvulsant (tonic-clonic or cortical focal seizures); emergency control of acute seizure disorders such as status epilepticus, meningitis, tetanus, eclampsia, toxicity of local anesthetics. Phenobarbital is considered a drug of choice for tonic-clonic seizures. *Investigational:* Prophylaxis and treatment of hyperbilirubinemia.

Special Concerns: Pregnancy category: D.

Additional Side Effects: Chronic use may result in headache, fever, and megaloblastic anemia.

Dosage: *Phenobarbital, Phenobarbitol Sodium.* **Capsules, Elixir, Tablets.** *Sedation:* **Adults,** 30–120 mg daily in 2–3 divided doses. **Pediatric,** 2 mg/kg (60 mg/m²) t.i.d. *Hypnotic:* **Adults,** 100–320 mg at bedtime. **Pediatric,** Dose should be determined by physician. *Preoperative sedation:* **Pediatric,** 1–3 mg/kg. *Anticonvulsant:* **Adults,** 60–250 mg daily in single or divided doses. **Pediatric,** 1–6 mg/kg daily in single or divided doses. *Antihyperbilirubinemia:* **Adults,** 30–60 mg t.i.d. **Pediatric, up to 12 years of age:** 1–4 mg/kg t.i.d. **Neonates,** 5–10 mg/kg for the first few days after birth. **IM, IV.** *Sedation:* **Adults,** 30–120 mg daily in 2–3 divided doses. *Preoperative sedation:* **Pediatric,** 1–3 mg/kg 60–90 min prior to surgery. *Hypnotic:* **Adults,** 100–325 mg. **Pediatric:** dose to be determined by physician. **IV.** *Anticonvulsant:* **Adults,** 100–320 mg, repeated, if necessary to a total daily dose of 600 mg. **Pediatric, initial loading dose,** 10–20 mg/kg; **then,** 1–6 mg/kg daily. *Status epilepticus:* **Adults,** 10–20 mg/kg (given slowly); may be repeated if needed. **Pediatric,** 15–20 mg/kg given over a 10–15 min period. **IM only.** *Preoperative sedation:* **Adults,** 130–200 mg 60–90 min before surgery. *Antihyperbilirubinemic:* **Pediatric,** 5–10 mg/kg daily for the first few days after birth.

NURSING CONSIDERATIONS

See also *Nursing Considerations* for *Barbiturates,* p. 104.

Administration/Storage

1. When used for seizures, give the major fraction of the dose according to when seizures are likely to occur, (i.e., on arising for daytime seizures and at bedtime when seizures occur at night).
2. In most cases, when used for epilepsy, drug must be taken regularly to avoid seizures, even when no seizures are imminent.
3. The aqueous solution for injection must be freshly prepared.
4. Some ready-dissolved solutions for injection are available; the vehicle is propylene glycol, water, and alcohol.
5. For IV administration, inject slowly at a rate of 50 mg/min.

Client/Family Teaching

1. Provide a printed list of side effects. Report any that are bothersome or persistent.
2. Phenobarbital may require an increase in vitamin D consumption. Review and encourage intake of foods that are high in vitamin D.
3. Drug decreases the effect of oral contraceptives. Other forms of birth control should be practiced during drug therapy.
4. Take only as directed and do not stop abruptly without physician knowledge.

Evaluation: Evaluate client for:
- Attainment of desired level of sedation
- Evidence of control of seizures

Phenolphthalein

(fee-nohl-**THAY**-leen)

Alophen Pills No. 973, Espotabs, Evac-U-Gen, Evac-U-Lax, Ex-Lax, Feen-A-Mint Chocolated, Feen-A-Mint Gum, Feen-A-Mint Tablets, Fructines-Vichy✿, Lax Pills, Laxative Pills, Medilax, Modane, Phenolax, Prulet (OTC)

See also *Laxatives,* p. 171.

Classification: Laxative, stimulant.

Action/Kinetics: Phenolphthalein acts directly on the intestinal mucosa. It also stimulates the myenteric plexus and alters water and electrolyte absorption. It produces a semifluid stool with little or no accompanying colic. Available products contain either white or yellow phenolphthalein with yellow phenolphthalein being 2–3 times more potent than the white. **Onset:** 6–10 hr. **Duration:** May be 3–4 days due to residual effect.

Use: Short-term use for constipation.

Additional Side Effects: Hypersensitivity reactions: Dermatitis, pruritus, rarely, nonthrombocytopenic purpura or anaphylaxis. Phenolphthalein may color alkaline urine pink-red and acidic urine yellow-brown.

Dosage: Gum, Tablets, Chewable Tablets, Wafers. Adults: 60–194 mg/day; **pediatric, over 6 years:** 30–60 mg/day; **2–5 years:** 15–20 mg/day. Usually taken at bedtime.

NURSING CONSIDERATIONS

See also *Nursing Considerations* for *Laxatives,* p. 172.

Administration/Storage: Oral doses take 6–10 hr to be effective.

Client/Family Teaching

1. Phenolphthalein colors alkaline stools and urine a reddish color.
2. Store medication out of the reach of children. This is particularly important when the laxative looks like chocolate and may be accidentally ingested as candy.
3. Remind clients that Ex-Lax is a medication and to use only as directed.

Evaluation: Evaluate client for reports of relief of constipation with successful evacuation of a soft, formed stool.

Phenoxybenzamine hydrochloride

(fen-ox-ee-**BEN**-zah-meen)

Dibenzyline (Rx)

Classification: Alpha-adrenergic blocking agent.

Action/Kinetics: Phenoxybenzamine is an irreversible alpha-adrenergic blocking agent. The drug increases blood flow to the skin, mucosa, and abdominal viscera as well as lowers BP. Beneficial effects may not be noted for 2–4 weeks. **Onset:** gradual. **Peak effect:** 4–6 hr. **Duration:** 3–4 days after one dose. **$t^{1/2}$:** 24 hr. Metabolized slowly and excreted in urine and feces.

Uses: To control hypertension and sweating in pheochromocytoma prior to surgery, when surgery is contraindicated, or in malignant pheochromocytoma.

Contraindications: Conditions in which a decrease in BP is not desired. Essential hypertension.

Special Concerns: Geriatric clients may be more sensitive to the hypotensive hypothermic effects. Use with caution in coronary or cerebral arteriosclerosis, respiratory infections, and renal disease.

Side Effects: Due to adrenergic blockade and include miosis, postural hypotension, tachycardia, nasal congestion, and inhibition of ejaculation. Also, drowsiness, fatigue, GI upset. *Symptoms of Overdose:* Dizziness or fainting due to postural hypotension. Also, tachycardia, GI irritation, drowsiness, fatigue, vomiting, lethargy, and shock.

Dosage: Capsules. Adults: initial, 10 mg b.i.d.; may be increased every other day until desired effect is obtained. **Maintenance:** 20–40 mg b.i.d.–t.id. **Pediatric, initial:** 0.2 mg/kg (6 mg/m²) up to a maximum of 10 mg once daily; dose may be increased q 4 days until desired effect is reached. **Maintenance:** 0.4 mg (1.2 mg/m²) daily in 3–4 divided doses.

P **NURSING CONSIDERATIONS**

Administration/Storage

1. Observe the client closely before increasing the dosage of drug.
2. Since phenoxybenzamine is irreversible, the drug is usually started in low doses and gradually increased.
3. It may take 2 weeks to titrate the medication to the optimum dosage.
4. *Treatment of Overdose:* Discontinue the drug and consider one or more of the following:
   - Have client lie down with legs elevated to restore cerebral circulation.
   - In severe overdose, institute measures to treat shock.
   - Leg bandages and an abdominal binder may shorten the time the client needs to lie down.
   - Severe hypotension may be helped by IV norepinephrine.

Assessment

1. Obtain baseline renal function studies prior to beginning therapy.
2. Note and report any evidence of hypotension.
3. Obtain BP and pulse measurements to serve as baseline data against which to measure drug effects.

Interventions

1. Take BP every 4 hr with the client in both supine and erect positions to check for excessive hypotension.
2. Note the quality of peripheral pulses, and assess the extremities for increased warmth for 4 days after a change in drug dosage. The results may help determine whether the client needs an adjustment in dosage.
3. If the client has a preexisting respiratory infection, it may be aggravated by the drug. Increased supportive care may be required.
4. Keep the client in a supine position for 24 hr after overdosage. Wrap the legs in Ace bandages, and apply an abdominal binder, unless contraindicated.

Client/Family Teaching

1. Rise slowly from a supine position to a sitting position and dangle feet for a few minutes before standing erect.

2. If the client feels faint, lie down immediately and elevate the legs.
3. Avoid alcohol because this may enhance hypotensive effects.
4. Take a radial pulse and report tachycardia to the physician. This is a sign of autonomic blockade and requires medical intervention. Concurrent use of a beta-adrenergic blocking agent may be necessary.
5. It may take up to a month before the desired effects are obtained. Therefore, it is important to take medications as prescribed. If there are no changes after that time, report to the physician.
6. The drug affects mental alertness. Therefore, tasks that require mental alertness should be avoided until the drug effects are evident.
7. Do not take any OTC drugs without physician consent.

Evaluation: Evaluate for evidence of control of hypertension and ↓ sweating in clients with pheochromocytoma.

Phensuximide
(fen-**SUCKS**-ih-myd)
Milontin (Rx)

See also *Anticonvulsants,* p. 61, and *Succinimides,* p. 212.

Classification: Anticonvulsant, succinimide type.

Action/Kinetics: Phensuximide is said to be less effective as well as less toxic than other succinimides. May color the urine pink, red, or red-brown. **t½:** 5–12 hr. **Peak effect:** 1–4 hr.

Special Concerns: Use with caution in clients with intermittent porphyria.

Additional Side Effects: Kidney damage, hematuria, urinary frequency.

Dosage: Capsules. Adults and children, initial: 0.5 g b.i.d.; **then,** dose can be increased by 0.5 g daily at 1-week intervals until seizures are controlled or the daily dosage reaches 3 g. May be used with other anticonvulsants in the presence of multiple types of epilepsy.

NURSING CONSIDERATIONS

See *Nursing Considerations* for *Anticonvulsants,* p. 63, and *Succinimides,* p. 213.

Client/Family Teaching
1. Drug may discolor urine a pink-brown color.
2. Report any changes in urinary elimination such as pain, frequency, or blood.

Evaluation: Evaluate client for evidence of control of seizures.

Phentermine
(FEN-ter-meen)
Adipex-P, Anoxine-AM, Dapex-37.5, Fastin, Obe-Mar, Obe-Nix 30, Obephen, Obermine, Obestin-30, Oby-Trim, Panshape, Parmine, Phentercot, Phenterxene, Phentride, Phentrol, Phentrol 2, 4, and 5, Span-RD, T-Diet, Teramin, Wilpowr, Zatryl (C-IV) (Rx)

Phentermine resin
(FEN-ter-meen)
Ionamin (C-IV) (Rx)

See also *Amphetamines and Derivatives,* p. 29.

Classification: Anorexiant.

Action/Kinetics: Duration, 8-mg tablets: 4 hr; **duration, 30-mg capsules, 37.5-mg tablets, resin:** 12–14 hr.

Use: Short-term (8–12 weeks) treatment of exogenous obesity in conjunction with a weight reduction program including exercise, reduced caloric intake, and behavior modification.

Special Concerns: Pregnancy category: C.

Dosage: Capsules, Tablets. Adults: 15–37.5 mg once daily either before breakfast, 1–2 hr after breakfast, or in divided doses 30 min before meals.

Resin Capsules. Adults: 15–30 mg once daily before breakfast.

NURSING CONSIDERATIONS

See *Nursing Considerations* for *Amphetamines and Derivatives*, p. 31.

Evaluation: Evaluate client for reports of a ↓ appetite and evidence of weight loss.

Phentolamine mesylate

(fen-**TOLL**-ah-meen)
Regitine, Rogitine ✤ (Rx)

Classification: Alpha-adrenergic blocking agent.

Action/Kinetics: Phentolamine competitively blocks both presynaptic (alpha-2) and postsynaptic (alpha-1) adrenergic receptors producing vasodilation and a decrease in peripheral resistance. The drug has little effect on BP. In congestive heart failure, phentolamine reduces afterload and pulmonary arterial pressure as well as increases cardiac output. **Onset** (parenteral): Immediate. **Duration:** Short. Poorly absorbed from the GI tract. About 10% excreted unchanged in the urine after parenteral use.

Uses: Treatment of hypertension caused by pheochromocytoma prior to or during surgery. Dermal necrosis and sloughing following IV use or extravasation of norepinephrine. To test for pheochromocytoma (not the method of choice). *Investigational:* Treatment of congestive heart failure. In combination with papaverine as an intracavernous injection for impotence.

Contraindications: Coronary artery disease including angina, myocardial infarction, or coronary insufficiency.

Special Concerns: Use during pregnancy and lactation only if benefits clearly outweigh risks. Geriatric clients may have a greater risk of developing hypothermia. Use with great caution in the presence of gastritis, ulcers, and in clients with a history thereof.

Side Effects: *CV:* Acute and prolonged hypotension, tachycardia, and arrhythmias, especially after parenteral administration. Orthostatic hypotension, flushing. *GI:* Nausea, vomiting, diarrhea. *Other:* Dizziness, weakness, nasal stuffiness.

Symptoms of Overdose: Hypotension, shock.

Drug Interactions

Ephedrine / Phentolamine antagonizes vasoconstrictor and hypertensive effect
Epinephrine / Phentolamine antagonizes vasoconstrictor and hypertensive effect

Norepinephrine / Suitable antagonist to treat overdosage induced by phentolamine

Propranolol / Concomitant use during surgery for pheochromocytoma is indicated

Dosage: *Prevent hypertension in pheochromocytoma, preoperative:* **Adults, IV:** 5 mg 1–2 hr before surgery; dose may be repeated if needed. **Pediatric, IV, IM:** 1 mg (or 0.1 mg/kg) 1–2 hr before surgery; dose may be repeated if needed. *Prevent or control hypertension during surgery:* **Adults, IV:** 5 mg. **IV infusion:** 0.5–1 mg/min. **Pediatric, IV:** 0.1 mg/kg (3 mg/m²). May be repeated, if necessary. During surgery 5 mg for adults and 1 mg for children may be given to prevent or control symptoms of epinephrine intoxication (e.g., paroxysms of hypertension, respiratory depression, seizures, tachycardia). *Dermal necrosis/sloughing following IV or extravasation of norepinephrine: Prevention,* 10 mg/1,000 ml norepinephrine solution; *treatment:* 5–10 mg/10 ml saline injected into area of extravasation within 12 hr. **Pediatric:** 0.1–0.2 mg/kg to a maximum of 10 mg. *Congestive heart failure:* **Adults, IV infusion:** 0.17–0.4 mg/min. *Impotence:* **Adults, intracavernosal:** papaverine, 30 mg and 0.5–1 mg phentolamine; adjust dose according to response. *Diagnosis of pheochromocytoma:* **Adults, rapid IV, initial,** 2.5 mg (if response is negative, a 5-mg test should be undertaken before concluding the test is negative); **children:** 1 mg. **Adults, IM:** 5 mg; **children:** 3 mg.

NURSING CONSIDERATIONS

Administration/Storage: *Treatment of Overdose:* Maintain blood pressure by giving IV norepinephrine.

Assessment

1. Note any history of coronary artery disease.
2. Determine any evidence of gastritis or peptic ulcer disease.

Interventions

1. Monitor the BP and pulse before and after parenteral administration, until stabilized.
2. To avoid postural hypotension, keep clients supine for at least 30 min after injection. Then have clients dangle their legs over the side of the bed and rise slowly to avoid orthostatic hypotension.
3. If clients show signs of drug overdose, place them in the Trendelenburg position. Assist with the administration of parenteral fluids. Have levarterenol available to minimize hypotension. *Do not use epinephrine.*
4. If the IV administration of norepinephrine or dopamine results in infiltration, administer subcutaneous solutions of phentolamine at the site and within 12 hr for beneficial effects.

(For the diagnosis of pheochromocytoma)

1. The test for pheochromocytoma should not be undertaken on normotensive clients.
2. Sedatives, analgesics, and other nonessential medication should be withheld for 24 hr (and preferably 72 hr) prior to the test.
3. When testing for pheochromocytoma, the client should be kept in a supine position, preferably in a dark, quiet room.
4. If the IV test is used, the blood pressure should be measured

P

immediately after the injection, at 30-sec intervals for the first 3 min, and at 60-sec intervals for the next 7 min. If the IM test is used, blood pressure should be measured every 5 min for 30–45 min.

5. The pheochromocytoma test is most reliable in clients with sustained hypertension and least reliable in clients with paroxysmal hypertension.

Evaluation

1. A positive response for pheochromocytoma is a drop in BP of more than 35 mm Hg systolic and 25 mm Hg diastolic pressure. Maximal decreases in BP usually occur within 2 min after injection of phentolamine and return to preinjection pressure within 15–30 min. A negative response is indicated when the BP is unchanged, elevated, or reduced less than 35 mm Hg systolic and 25 mm Hg diastolic pressure.

2. Evaluate client for:
   - Evidence of control of hypertension R/T pheochromocytoma before or during surgery
   - The prevention of skin sloughing following extravasation with norepinephrine or dopamine infusions

Phenylephrine hydrochloride
(fen-ill-**EF**-rin)

Nasal: Alconefrin 12, 25, and 50, Doktors, Duration, Neo-Synephrine Jelly and Solution, Nostril, Rhinall, Rhinall-10, Children's Flavored Nose Drops, St. Joseph, Vicks Sinex.

Ophthalmic: AK-Dilate, AK-Nefrin, Dilatari, I-Phrine, Isopto Frin, Mydfrin, Neo-Synephrine, Ocugestrin, Ocu-Phrin, Phenylephrine Minims ✿, Prefrin Liquifilm, Relief, Spersaphrine ✿, Vital Eyes ✿. **Systemic:** Neo-Synephrine. (**Rx: Injection and Ophthalmic Solutions 2.5% or greater; OTC: Nasal products and ophthalmic solutions 0.12% or less**)

See also *Sympathomimetic Drugs*, p. 218, and *Nasal Decongestants*, p. 182.

Classification: Alpha-adrenergic agent.

Action/Kinetics: Phenylephrine stimulates alpha-adrenergic receptors, producing pronounced vasoconstriction and hence an increase in both systolic and diastolic BP; reflex bradycardia results from increased vagal activity. The drug also acts on alpha receptors producing vasoconstriction in the skin, mucous membranes, and the mucosa as well as mydriasis by contracting the dilator muscle of the pupil. It resembles epinephrine, but it has more prolonged action and few cardiac effects. **IV: Onset,** immediate; **duration:** 15–20 min. **IM. SC: Onset,** 10–15 min; **duration:** 1/2–2 hr for IM and 50–60 min for SC. *Nasal decongestion (topical):* **Onset:** 15–20 min; **duration:** 30 min–4 hr. *Ophthalmic:* **Time to peak effect for mydriasis,** 15–60 min for 2.5% solution and 10–90 min for 10% solution. **Duration:** 3 hr for 2.5%; 3–7 hr with 10%. Excreted in urine.

Phenylephrine is also found in Chlor-Trimetron Expectorant, Naldecon, Dimetane, and Dimetapp.

Uses: Systemic: Acute hypotensive states caused by peripheral circulatory collapse. To maintain BP during spinal anesthesia; to prolong spinal anesthesia. Paroxysmal supraventricular tachycardia. **Nasal:** Nasal congestion due to allergies, sinusitis, common cold, or hay fever. **Ophthalmologic: 0.08%–0.12%:** Temporary relief of redness of the eye associated with colds, hay fever, wind, dust, sun, smog, smoke, contact lens. **2.5%:** Produce mydriasis for refraction, retinoscopy, blanching test, and ophthalmoscopy. **2.5% and 10%:** Treatment of uveitis with posterior synechiae, prophylaxis of posterior synechiae, preoperative mydriasis.

Special Concerns: Use with caution in geriatric clients, severe arteriosclerosis, and during pregnancy (category: C) and lactation. Nasal and ophthalmic use of phenylephrine may be systemically absorbed. Use of the 2.5% or 10% ophthalmic solutions in children may cause hypertension and irregular heart beat. In geriatric clients, chronic use of the 2.5% or 10% ophthalmic solutions may cause rebound miosis and a decreased mydriatic effect.

Side Effects: Reflex bradycardia. Overdosage may cause ventricular extrasystoles and short paroxysm or ventricular tachycardia, tingling of the extremities and a sensation of heavy head. *Ophthalmologic:* Rebound miosis and decreased mydriatic response in geriatric clients, blurred vision.

Dosage: Injection: IM, IV, SC. *Vasopressor, mild–moderate hypotension:* **Adults, IM, SC,** 2–5 mg repeated no more often than q 10–15 min. **IV,** 0.2 mg repeated no more often than q 10–15 min. **Pediatric, IM, SC:** 0.1 mg/kg (3 mg/m²) repeated in 1–2 hr if needed. *Vasopressor, severe hypotension and shock:* **Adults, IV infusion,** 10 mg in 500 ml 5% dextrose injection or 0.9% sodium chloride injection given at a rate of 0.1–0.18 mg/min initial; **then,** give at a rate of 0.04–0.06 mg/min. *Prophylaxis of hypotension during spinal anesthesia:* **Adults, IM, SC,** 2–3 mg 3–4 min before anesthetic given; **pediatric, IM, SC:** 0.044–0.088 mg/kg. *Hypotensive emergencies during spinal anesthesia:* **Adults, IV, initial,** 0.2 mg; dose can be increased by no more than 0.2 mg for each subsequent dose not to exceed 0.5 mg/dose.

Nasal Jelly. Adults: small amount of 0.5% jelly inserted into the nostril and sniffed well back into the nasal passages q 3–4 hr as necessary. Use not recommended in children. **Nasal Solution. Adults, Drops:** 2–3 drops of the 0.25%–0.5% solution into each nostril q 3–4 hr as needed. **Spray:** 1–2 sprays of the 0.25%–0.5% solution into each nostril; blow nose after 3–5 min and repeat dose; then, repeat dose q 3–4 hr. **Pediatric, infants and children up to 2 years:** 2–3 drops of the 0.125% solution q 3–4 hr as needed. **2–6 years:** 2–3 drops of the 0.125% or 0.167% solution into each nostril q 4 hr as needed. **6–12 years:** 2–3 drops or 1–2 sprays of the 0.25% solution into each nostril q 3–4 hr as needed.

Ophthalmic Solution. *Mydriasis, vasoconstriction, uveitis, preoperative mydriasis:* **Adults,** 1 drop of the 2.5% or 10% solution (for children use 1 drop of the 2.5% solution). *Mydriasis in diagnostic procedures:* **Adults and children,**

1 drop of the 2.5% solution. *Refraction:* **Adults,** 1 drop of a cycloplegic followed in 5 min by one drop of the 2.5% solution of phenylephrine and in 10 min another drop of cycloplegic (eyes are ready for refraction in 50–60 min). **Pediatric:** 1 drop of a 1% solution of atropine followed in 10–15 min by 1 drop of 2.5% phenylephrine and in 5–10 min by another drop of 1% atropine solution (eyes are ready for refraction in 1–2 hr).

NURSING CONSIDERATIONS

See also *Nursing Considerations* for *Sympathomimetic Drugs,* p. 220, and *Nasal Decongestants,* p. 182.

Administration/Storage

1. Store drug in a brown bottle and away from light.
2. Anticipate that before administering Neo-Synephrine Ophthalmic Solution, instillation of a drop of local anesthetic will be necessary.
3. When the drug is used as a nasal decongestant, instruct the clients to blow their nose before administration.
4. When drug is used parenterally, monitor infusion site closely to avoid extravasation.

Interventions

1. During IV administration monitor blood pressure continuously until stabilized.
2. Perform baseline ECG and monitor cardiac rhythm continuously during IV administration noting any evidence of bradycardia or arrhythmias.

Client/Family Teaching

1. Demonstrate and review the appropriate method for drug administration.

2. Advise that ophthalmic instillations and nasal decongestants may produce systemic sympathomimetic effects. Stress that chronic excessive use may cause rebound congestion. Provide with printed material explaining how to identify these effects and instruct the client to notify the physician should they occur.
3. Wear sunglasses in bright light. Symptoms of photosensitivity and blurred vision should be reported if they persist after 12 hr.
4. When using ophthalmic solution, if there is no relief of symptoms within 2 days, notify the physician.
5. When using the drug for nasal decongestion, if there is no relief of symptoms within 3 days, notify the physician. Rebound nasal congestion may occur with longer therapy.

Evaluation: Evaluate for:
- (Parenteral) evidence of a ↑ blood pressure
- Termination of supraventricular tachyarrhythmias on ECG
- (Nasal) reports of improvement in symptoms of nasal congestion
- (Ophthalmic) evidence of a reduction in conjunctivitis and allergic manifestations
- Mydriasis during diagnostic procedures

Phenylpropanolamine hydrochloride

(fen-ill-**proh**-pah-**NOHL**-ah-meen)
Acutrim 16 Hour, Acutrim Late Day, Acutrim II Maximum

Strength, Control, Dex-A-Diet Maximum Strength and Maximum Strength Caplets, Dexatrim, Dexatrim Maximum Strength and Maximum Strength Caplets, Dexatrim Maximum Strength Pre-Meal Caplets, Efed II Yellow, Maigret-50, Phenyldrine, Prolamine, Propagest, Rhindecon, Unitrol (OTC except Maigret-50 and Rhindecon)

See also *Amphetamines and Derivatives,* p. 29, and *Sympathomimetic Drugs,* p. 218.

Classification: Decongestant, appetite suppressant.

Action/Kinetics: Phenylpropanolamine is thought to stimulate both alpha and beta receptors, as well as to act indirectly through release of norepinephrine from storage sites. Increases in BP are due mainly to increased cardiac output rather than to vasoconstriction; has minimal CNS effects. The drug acts on alpha-adrenergic receptors to produce a decongestant effect in the nasal mucosa. **Onset, decongestant:** 15–30 min; **peak plasma levels:** 1–2 hr; **duration, capsules and tablets:** 3 hr; **extended-release tablets:** 12–16 hr. **Peak plasma levels:** 100 ng. $t^{1/2}$: 3–4 hr. 80%–90% excreted in the urine unchanged.

Uses: Nasal congestion due to colds, hay fever, allergies. Short-term (8–12 weeks) treatment of exogenous obesity in conjunction with a weight reduction program including reduced caloric intake, exercise, and behavior modification. *Investigational:* Mild to moderate stress incontinence in women.

Contraindications: Arteriosclerosis, depression, glaucoma, hypertension, diabetes, kidney disease, hyperthyroidism, during or within 14 days of use of MAO inhibitors, hypersensitivity to sympathomimetics. Not recommended as an anorexiant for children less than 12 years of age.

Special Concerns: Safety and efficacy during pregnancy and lactation and for children not established. Children less than 6 years of age may be at greater risk for developing psychiatric disorders when using phenylpropanolamine. The anorexiant dose must be individualized for children 12–18 years of age.

Side Effects: *CNS:* Dizziness, headache, insomnia, restlessness, bizarre behavior. Serious effects due to abuse include: agitation, tremor, increased motor activity, hallucinations, seizures, stroke, and death. *CV:* Palpitations, hypertension (may be severe and lead to crisis), tachycardia. *Miscellaneous:* Dry mouth, dysuria, renal failure, nausea, nasal dryness.

Drug Interactions

Furazolidone / Possibility of hypertensive crisis and intracranial hemorrhage
Guanethidine / Phenylpropanolamine ↓ hypotensive effect
Indomethacin / Possibility of severe hypertensive episode
MAO inhibitors / Possibility of hypertensive crisis and intracranial hemorrhage

Dosage: Capsules, Tablets. *Decongestant:* **Adults,** 25 mg q 4 hr or 50 mg q 6–8 hr (not to exceed 150 mg/day); **Children, 2–6 years:**

6.25 mg q 4 hr, not to exceed 37.5 mg in 24 hr; **6–12 years:** 12.5 mg q 4 hr, not to exceed 75 mg in 24 hr. *Anorexiant:* **Adults,** 25 mg t.i.d. 30 min before meals, not to exceed 75 mg in 24 hr.

Extended-release Capsules, Extended-release Tablets. *Decongestant:* **Adults,** 75 mg q 12 hr. *Anorexiant:* **Adults,** 75 mg once daily in the morning.

NURSING CONSIDERATIONS

See also *Nursing Considerations* for *Amphetamines and Derivatives,* p. 31, and *Sympathomimetic Drugs,* p. 220.

Client/Family Teaching: Caution older men to report difficulties in voiding because they are more susceptible to drug-induced urinary retention. Ensure that these clients understand the importance of taking the medication only as directed.

Evaluation: Evaluate client for:
- Reports of ↓ in symptoms of nasal congestion
- Reports of a ↓ in appetite and evidence of weight loss

Phenytoin (Diphenylhydantoin)

(FEN-ih-toyn, dye-**fen**-ill-hy-**DAN**-toyn)

Dilantin Infatab, Dilantin-30 Pediatric, Dilantin-125 (Rx)

Phenytoin sodium, extended

(FEN-ih-toyn)

Dilantin Kapseals (Rx)

Phenytoin sodium, parenteral

(FEN-ih-toyn)

Dilantin Sodium (Rx)

Phenytoin sodium prompt

(FEN-ih-toyn)

Diphenylan Sodium (Rx)

See also *Anticonvulsants,* p. 61, and *Antiarrhythmic Drugs,* p. 51.

Classification: Anticonvulsant, hydantoin type; antiarrhythmic (type I).

Action/Kinetics: Phenytoin acts in the motor cortex of the brain to reduce the spread of electrical discharges from the rapidly firing epileptic foci in this area. This is accomplished by stabilizing hyperexcitable cells possibly by affecting sodium efflux. Also, phenytoin decreases activity of centers in the brain stem responsible for the tonic phase of grand mal seizures. This drug has few sedative effects.

Serum levels must be monitored because the serum concentrations of phenytoin increase disproportionately as the dosage is increased. Phenytoin extended is designed for once-a-day dosage. It has a slow dissolution rate—no more than 35% in 30 min, 30%–70% in 60 min, and less than 85% in 120 min. Absorption is variable following oral dosage. **Peak serum levels: PO,** 4–8 hr. Since the rate and extent of absorption depend on the particular preparation, the same product should be used for a particular client. **Peak serum levels (following IM):** 24 hr (wide variation). **Therapeutic serum levels:** 10–20 mcg/ml. **$t^{1/2}$:** 8–60 hr (average: 20–30 hr). Steady state attained 7–10 days after initiation. Phenytoin is biotransformed in the liver. Both inactive metabolites and unchanged drug are excreted in the urine.

As an antiarrhythmic, phenytoin increases the electrical stimulation threshold of heart muscle although it is less effective than quinidine, procainamide, or lidocaine. **Onset:** 30–60 min. **Duration:** 24 hr or more. **t½:** 22–36 hr. **Therapeutic serum level:** 10–20 mcg/ml.

Uses: Chronic epilepsy, especially of the tonic-clonic, psychomotor type. Not effective against absence seizures and may even increase the frequency of seizures in this disorder. Parenteral phenytoin is sometimes used to treat status epilepticus and to control seizures during neurosurgery.

Orally for certain premature ventricular contractions and IV for premature ventricular contractions and tachycardia. The drug is particularly useful for arrhythmias produced by digitalis overdosage.

Investigational: Paroxysmal choreoathetosis; to treat blistering and erosions in clients with recessive dystrophic epidermolysis bullosa; episodic dyscontrol; trigeminal neuralgia; as a muscle relaxant in neuromyotonia, myotonia congenita, or myotonic muscular dystrophy; to treat cardiac symptoms in overdosage of tricyclic antidepressants. Severe preeclampsia.

Contraindications: Hypersensitivity to hydantoins, exfoliative dermatitis, sinus bradycardia, second and third degree AV block, clients with Adams-Stokes syndrome, sinoatrial block. Lactation.

Special Concerns: Use with caution in acute, intermittent porphyria. Administer with extreme caution to clients with a history of asthma or other allergies, impaired renal or hepatic function, and heart disease (hypotension, severe myocardial insufficiency). Abrupt withdrawal may cause status epilepticus. Combined drug therapy is required if petit mal seizures are also present.

Side Effects: *CNS:* Most commonly, drowsiness, ataxia, dysarthria, confusion, insomnia, nervousness, irritability, depression, tremor, numbness, headache, psychoses, increased seizures. Choreoathetosis following IV use. *GI:* Gingival hyperplasia, nausea, vomiting, either diarrhea or constipation. *Dermatologic:* Various dermatoses including a measles-like rash (common), scarlatiniform, maculopapular, and urticarial rashes. Rarely, drug-induced lupus erythematosus, Stevens-Johnson syndrome, exfoliative or purpuric dermatitis, and toxic epidermal necrolysis. Alopecia, hirsutism. Skin reactions may necessitate withdrawal of therapy. *Hematopoietic:* Leukopenia, granulocytopenia, thrombocytopenia, pancytopenia, agranulocytosis, macrocytosis, megaloblastic anemia, leukocytosis, monocytosis, eosinophilia, simple anemia, aplastic anemia, hemolytic anemia. *Hepatic:* Liver damage, toxic hepatitis, hypersensitivity reactions involving the liver including hepatocellular degeneration and fatal hepatocellular necrosis. *Ophthalmic:* Diplopia, nystagmus, conjunctivitis. *Miscellaneous:* Hyperglycemia, chest pain, edema, fever, photophobia, weight gain, pulmonary fibrosis, lymph node hyperplasia, gynecomastia, periarteritis nodosa, depression of IgA, soft tissue injury at injection site, coarsening of facial features, Peyronie's disease, enlarged lips.

Rapid parenteral administration may cause serious cardiovascular effects, including hypotension, arrhythmias, cardiovascular collapse, and heart block, as well as CNS depression.

P

Many clients have a partial deficiency in the ability of the liver to degrade phenytoin, and as a result, toxicity may develop after a small oral dose. Liver and kidney function tests and hematopoietic studies are indicated prior to and periodically during drug therapy.

Symptoms of Overdose: Initially, ataxia, dysarthria, and nystagmus followed by unresponsive pupils, hypotension, and coma. Plasma levels greater than 40 mcg/ml result in significant decreases in mental capacity.

Drug Interactions

Acetaminophen / ↓ Effect of acetaminophen due to ↑ breakdown by liver; however, hepatotoxicity may be ↑

Alcohol, ethyl / In alcoholics, ↓ effect of phenytoin due to ↑ breakdown by liver

Allopurinol / ↑ Effect of phenytoin due to ↓ breakdown in liver

Amiodarone / ↑ Effect of phenytoin or amiodarone due to ↓ breakdown by liver

Antacids / ↓ Effect of phenytoin due to ↓ GI absorption

Anticoagulants, oral / ↑ Effect of phenytoin due to ↓ breakdown by liver. Also, possible ↑ in anticoagulant effect due to ↓ plasma protein binding

Antidepressants, tricyclic / May ↑ incidence of epileptic seizures or ↑ effect of phenytoin by ↓ plasma protein binding

Barbiturates / Effect of phenytoin may be ↑, ↓, or not changed; possible ↑ effect of barbiturates

Benzodiazepines / ↑ Effect of phenytoin due to ↓ breakdown by liver

Carbamazepine / ↓ Effect of phenytoin or carbamazepine due to ↑ breakdown by liver

Charcoal / ↓ Effect of phenytoin due to ↓ absorption from GI tract

Chloramphenicol / ↑ Effect of phenytoin due to ↓ breakdown by liver

Chlorpheniramine / ↑ Effect of phenytoin

Cimetidine / ↑ Effect of phenytoin due to ↓ breakdown by liver

Clonazepam / ↓ Plasma levels of clonazepam or phenytoin; or, ↑ risk of phenytoin toxicity

Contraceptives, oral / Estrogen-induced fluid retention may precipitate seizures; also, ↓ effect of contraceptives due to ↑ breakdown by liver

Corticosteroids / Effect of corticosteroids ↓ due to ↑ breakdown by liver; also, corticosteroids may mask hypersensitivity reactions due to phenytoin

Cyclosporine / ↓ Effect of cyclosporine due to ↑ breakdown by liver

Diazoxide / ↓ Effect of phenytoin due to ↑ breakdown by liver

Dicumarol / Phenytoin ↓ effect of dicumarol due to ↑ breakdown by liver

Digitalis glycosides / ↓ Effect of digitalis glycosides due to ↑ breakdown by liver

Disopyrimide / ↓ Effect of disopyramide due to ↑ breakdown by liver

Disulfiram / ↑ Effect of phenytoin due to ↓ breakdown by liver

Dopamine / IV phenytoin results in hypotension and bradycardia; also, effect of dopamine ↓

Doxycycline / ↓ Effect of doxycycline due to ↑ breakdown by liver

Estrogens / See *Contraceptives, Oral*

Fluconazole / ↑ Effect of phenytoin due to ↓ breakdown by liver

Folic acid / ↓ Effect of phenytoin

Furosemide / ↓ Effect of furosemide due to ↓ absorption

Haloperidol / ↓ Effect of haloperidol due to ↑ breakdown by liver

Ibuprofen / ↑ Effect of phenytoin

Isoniazid / ↑ Effect of phenytoin due to ↓ breakdown by liver

Levodopa / Phenytoin ↓ effect of levodopa

Levonorgestrel / ↓ Effect of norgestrel

Lithium / ↑ Risk of lithium toxicity

Loxapine / ↓ Effect of phenytoin

Mebendazole / ↓ Effect of mebendazole

Meperidine / ↓ Effect of meperidine due to ↑ breakdown by liver; toxic effects of meperidine may ↑ due to accumulation of active metabolite (normeperidine)

Methadone / ↓ Effect of methadone due to ↑ breakdown by liver

Metronidazole / ↑ Effect of phenytoin due to ↓ breakdown by liver

Metyrapone / ↓ Effect of metyrapone due to ↑ breakdown by liver

Mexiletine / ↓ Effect of mexiletine due to ↑ breakdown by liver

Miconazole / ↑ Effect of phenytoin due to ↓ breakdown by liver

Nitrofurantoin / ↓ Effect of phenytoin

Omeprazole / ↑ Effect of phenytoin due to ↓ breakdown by liver

Phenacemide / ↑ Effect of phenytoin due to ↓ breakdown by liver

Phenothiazines / ↑ Effect of phenytoin due to ↓ breakdown by liver

Phenylbutazone / ↑ Effect of phenytoin due to ↓ breakdown by liver and ↓ plasma protein binding

Primidone / Possible ↑ effect of primidone

Pyridoxine / ↓ Effect of phenytoin

Quinidine / ↓ Effect of quinidine due to ↑ breakdown by liver

Rifampin / ↓ Effect of phenytoin due to ↑ breakdown by liver

Salicylates / ↑ Effect of phenytoin by ↓ plasma protein binding

Sucralfate / ↓ Effect of phenytoin due to ↓ absorption from GI tract

Sulfonamides / ↑ Effect of phenytoin due to ↓ breakdown in liver

Sulfonylureas / ↓ Effect of sulfonylureas

Theophylline / ↓ Effect of both drugs due to ↑ breakdown by liver

Trimethoprim / ↑ Effect of phenytoin due to ↓ breakdown by liver

Valproic acid / ↑ Effect of phenytoin due to ↓ breakdown by liver and ↓ plasma protein binding; phenytoin may also ↓ effect of valproic acid due to ↑ breakdown by liver

Laboratory Test Interferences: Alters liver function tests, ↑ blood glucose values, and ↓ PBI values. ↑ Gamma globulins. Phenytoin ↓ immunoglobulins A and G. False + Coombs' test.

Dosage: Oral   Suspension, Chewable   Tablets. *Seizures.* **Adults:** 125 mg t.i.d. initially; adjust dosage at 7–10 day intervals until seizures   are   controlled; **usual,**

maintenance: 300–400 mg/day, although 600 mg/day may be required in some. **Pediatric: initial,** 5 mg/kg/day in 2–3 divided doses; **maintenance,** 4–8 mg/kg (up to maximum of 300 mg/day). Children over 6 years may require up to 300 mg/day. **Geriatric:** 3 mg/kg initially in divided doses; **then,** adjust dosage according to serum levels and response. Once dosage level has been established, the extended capsules may be used for once-a-day dosage.

Capsules, Extended-release Capsules. *Seizures:* **Adults, initial** 100 mg t.i.d.; adjust dose at 7–10 day intervals until control is achieved. An initial loading dose of 12–15 mg/kg divided into 2–3 doses over 6 hr followed by 100 mg t.i.d. on subsequent days may be preferred if seizures are frequent. **Pediatric:** See dose for oral suspension and chewable tablets.

IV. *Status epilepticus:* **Adults, loading dose,** 10–15 mg/kg at a rate not to exceed 50 mg/min; **then,** 100 mg q 6–8 hr at a rate not exceeding 50 mg/min. Oral administration at a dose of 5 mg/kg daily divided into 2–4 doses should begin 12–24 hr after a loading dose is given. **Pediatric, loading dose:** 15–20 mg/kg given at a rate of 1 mg/kg, not to exceed 50 mg/min. **IM** dose should be 50% greater than the PO dose. *Neurosurgery:* 100–200 mg IM q 4 hr during and after surgery (during first 24 hr, no more than 1,000 mg should be administered; after first day, give maintenance dosage).

Arrhythmias: **PO:** 200–400 mg daily. **IV:** 100 mg q 5 min up to maximum of 1 g.

Full effectiveness of orally administered hydantoins is delayed and may take 6–9 days to be fully established. A similar period of time will elapse before effects disappear completely.

When hydantoins are substituted for or added to another anticonvulsant medication, their dosage is gradually increased, while dosage of the other drug is decreased proportionally.

NURSING CONSIDERATIONS

See also *Nursing Considerations* for *Anticonvulsants,* p. 63, and *Antiarrhythmic Drugs,* p. 52.

Administration/Storage

1. For parenteral preparations:
   - Only a clear solution of the drug may be used.
   - Dilute with special diluent supplied by manufacturer.
   - Shake the vials until the solution is clear. It may take about 10 min for the drug to dissolve.
   - To hasten the process, warm the vial in warm water after adding the diluent.
   - The drug is incompatible with acid solutions.
2. IV phenytoin may form a precipitate. Therefore, flush tubing thoroughly with sodium chloride before and after IV administration. *Do not* use dextrose solutions. Use an in-line filter to collect microscopic particulate matter.
3. Following the IV administration of the drug, administer sodium chloride injection through the same needle or IV catheter to avoid local irritation of the vein. This is caused by alkalinity of the solution.
4. For treatment of status epilepticus, inject the IV slowly at a rate not to exceed 50 mg/min. If necessary, the dose may be

repeated 30 min after the initial administration.

5. Avoid subcutaneous or perivascular injections. Pain, inflammation, and necrosis may be caused by the highly alkaline solutions.

6. *Do not* add phenytoin to an already running IV solution.

7. If the client is receiving tube feedings of Isocal or Osmolite, there may be interference with the absorption of oral phenytoin. Therefore, do not administer them together.

8. *Treatment of Overdose:* Treat symptoms. Hemodialysis may be effective. In children, total exchange transfusion has been used.

Assessment

1. Note the history and nature of the client's epileptic seizures, addressing location, duration, and characteristics.

2. Determine if the client is hypersensitive to hydantoins or has exfoliative dermatitis.

3. If the client is female and pregnant, note that she should not breast-feed the baby following delivery.

4. Obtain CBC, liver and renal function studies as baseline data against which to measure alterations once therapy is initiated.

5. Perform baseline ECG, noting any evidence of AV block.

Interventions

1. Monitor serum drug levels on a routine basis.

2. Seven to 10 days may be required to achieve recommended serum levels. The drug is metabolized much more lowly by elderly clients.

3. If the client is receiving drugs that interact with hydantoins or has impaired liver function, the serum phenytoin level should be done more frequently. The clinically effective range is 10–20 mcg/ml.

4. Monitor the CBC and WBC differential throughout drug therapy.

5. During the IV administration, monitor BP closely for hypotension.

6. If client complains of weakness, ease of fatigue, headaches, or feeling faint, assess for signs of folic acid deficiency or megaloblastic anemia. Document and report to the physician. Invite a dietitian to review food intake and diet with the client.

7. Note if the client is developing an overgrowth of hair, coarse hair, or acne. Document and report these symptoms to the physician. Provide emotional support and discourage the client from discontinuing therapy because of these side effects. Consult a dermatologist as needed.

8. The drug may alter thyroid function results. If thyroid studies are conducted, for ensured accuracy, they should be repeated 10 days after therapy has been discontinued.

Client/Family Teaching

1. Review symptoms of overdose and instruct client to notify the physician should any of these occur.

2. Do not substitute phenytoin products or exchange brands because bioavailability of phenytoin may vary. Seizure con-

trol may be lost, or toxic blood levels may develop if a substitution is made.

3. Prompt-release forms of the medication cannot be substituted for another unless the dosage is also adjusted.
    - If the client is taking phenytoin extended, do not substitute chewable tablets for capsules. The strengths of the medications are not equal.
    - Clients taking phenytoin extended should check the labels of the bottle carefully. Chewable tablets are never in the extended form.
    - Clients taking phenytoin extended should take only a single dose of medication a day. It should be taken as directed by the physician. Also, take only the brand prescribed by the physician.

4. If the client misses a dose of medication, take the dose as soon as it is remembered. Then resume the usual schedule. Do not, however, double up to make up for the missed dose of drug. If the doses of drug are scheduled throughout the day, and one of the doses is missed, take the drug as soon as it is realized that the dose has been missed unless it is within 4 hr of the next dose of drug. In that case, omit the missed dose unless otherwise instructed.

5. Take with food to minimize GI upset. Do not take within 2–3 hr of antacid ingestion.

6. Avoid ingestion of alcohol.

7. Do not take any other medication without medical supervision. Hydantoins interact with many other medications, and the addition of other drugs may require adjustment of the anticonvulsant dose.

8. If the client has diabetes mellitus, blood glucose levels should be monitored frequently when initiating therapy or if the client is having the dosage of phenytoin adjusted. It may be necessary to adjust insulin dosage and/or the client's diet.

9. Clients with diabetes should report any changes in glucose determinations with urine tests and/or finger sticks to the physician.

10. Warn that hydantoin may cause the urine to appear pink, red, or brown and not to be alarmed.

11. To minimize bleeding from the gums, practice good oral hygiene. Client should be encouraged to brush teeth with a soft toothbrush, massage the gums, and floss every day. Advise dentist of prescribed drug.

12. Hydantoin has an androgenic effect on the hair follicle. Clients may develop acne. They should be encouraged to practice good skin care.

13. Report any excessive growth of hair on the face and trunk and any discolorations or skin rash to the physician.

14. Stress the importance of reporting for laboratory studies as ordered including a CBC, drug levels, and renal and liver function studies on a regular basis.

15. Do not abruptly stop medications without physician consent.

16. Report all bothersome side effects because these effects may be dose-related.

17. Provide sexually active women of childbearing age with birth

control information while receiving phenytoin therapy.

18. Use care when performing tasks that require mental alertness. Drug may cause drowsiness, dizziness, and blurred vision.

Evaluation: Evaluate client for:
- Evidence of control of seizures
- ECG evidence of termination of ventricular arrhythmias
- Freedom from complications of drug therapy
- Serum drug level within therapeutic range (10–20 mcg/ml)

Phosphorated carbohydrate solution

(**FOS**-for-ay-ted kar-boh-**HIGH**-drayt)

Calm-X, Emetrol, Naus-A-Way, Nausetrol (OTC)

Classification: Antiemetic.

Action/Kinetics: Phosphorated carbohydrate solution contains fructose, dextrose, and orthophosphoric acid with controlled hydrogen ion concentration. It relieves nausea and vomiting due to a direct action on the wall of the GI tract that decreases smooth muscle contraction and delays gastric emptying time; the effect is directly related to the amount used. There is some question as to the effectiveness of this product.

Uses: Relief of nausea and vomiting.

Contraindications: Diabetic clients due to the presence of carbohydrates. Individuals with hereditary fructose intolerance.

Special Concerns: Since nausea may be a symptom of a serious condition, a physician should be consulted if symptoms are not relieved or recur often.

Side Effects: *GI:* Abdominal pain and diarrhea due to large doses of fructose.

Dosage: Oral Solution. *Nausea and vomiting due to psychogenic factors, functional vomiting:* **Adults,** 15–30 ml at 15 min intervals until vomiting ceases; if the first dose is rejected, the same dosage should be given in 5 min. Should not be taken for more than 5 doses (1 hr). **Infants and children:** 5–10 ml at 15 min intervals in the same manner as adults. *Regurgitation in infants:* 5 or 10 ml, 10–15 min before each feeding; in refractory cases, 10 or 15 ml, 30 min before feeding. *Morning sickness:* 15–30 ml on arising; repeat q 3 hr or when nausea threatens. *Nausea and vomiting due to drug therapy or inhalation anesthesia, motion sickness:* **Adults and older children:** 15 ml; **young children:** 5 ml.

NURSING CONSIDERATIONS

See also *Nursing Considerations* for *Antiemetics,* p. 71.

Assessment: Note any history of diabetes or hereditary fructose intolerance as drug is contraindicated in this setting.

Client/Family Teaching

1. Provide printed guidelines for the frequency of administration.
2. Advise client to notify physician if symptoms persist, recur often, or become worse.
3. Stress the importance of increasing the intake of fluids to

prevent the development of dehydration.

Evaluation: Evaluate client for reports of effective control of nausea and vomiting.

Physostigmine salicylate

(fye-zoh-**STIG**-meen)
Antilirium, Eserine Salicylate, Isopto Eserine (Rx)

Physostigmine sulfate

(fye-zoh-**STIG**-meen)
Eserine Sulfate (Rx)

See also *Neostigmine,* p. 926, and *Ophthalmic Cholinergic Agents,* p. 190.

Classification: Indirectly acting cholinergic-acetylcholinesterase inhibitor.

Action/Kinetics: Physostigmine is a reversible acetylcholinesterase inhibitor, resulting in an increased concentration of acetylcholine at nerve endings, which can antagonize anticholinergic drugs. It produces miosis, increased accommodation, and a decrease in intraocular pressure with decreased resistance to outflow of aqueous humor. When used for chronic open-angle glaucoma, ciliary muscle contraction may open the intertrabecular spaces, facilitating aqueous humor outflow. **Onset, IV:** 3–5 min. **Duration, IV:** 1–2 hr. **t½:** 1–2 hr. No dosage alteration is necessary in clients with renal impairment. **Onset, miosis:** 10–30 min; **duration, miosis:** 12–48 hr.

Uses: Overdosage due to cholinergic blocking drugs (e.g., atropine) and tricyclic antidepressant overdosage. Reduce intraocular pressure in open-angle glaucoma.

Freidreich's and other inherited ataxias (FDA has granted orphan status for this use). *Investigational:* Angle-closure glaucoma during or after iridectomy, secondary glaucoma if no inflammation present.

Special Concerns: Use during pregnancy (category: C) only when benefits clearly outweigh risks.

Additional Side Effects: If IV administration is too rapid, bradycardia, hypersalivation, breathing difficulties, and seizures may occur. Conjunctivitis when used for glaucoma.
Symptoms of Overdose: Cholinergic crisis.

Dosage: IM, IV. *Anticholinergic drug overdosage:* **Adults, IM, IV,** 0.5–2 mg at a rate of 1 mg/min; may be repeated if necessary. **Pediatric, IV:** 0.5 mg given over a period of at least 1 min. Dose may be repeated at 5–10 min if needed to a maximum of 2 mg if no toxic effects are manifested.
    Ophthalmic Solution. Adults and children: 1 gtt of the 0.25% or 0.5% salicylate solution in the eye b.i.d.–t.i.d. **Ophthalmic Ointment. Adults and children:** 1 cm of the 0.25% sulfate ointment in the conjunctiva 1–3 times daily.

NURSING CONSIDERATIONS

See also *Nursing Considerations* for *Neostigmine,* p. 928, *Cholinergic Blocking Agents,* p. 138, and *Ophthalmic Cholinergic Agents,* p. 191.

Administration/Storage

1. Following use of the ophthalmic solution, the lacrimal sac should be pressed for 1–2 min to avoid excessive systemic absorption.
2. The ophthalmic ointment may

be used at night for prolonged effect of the medication.

3. Due to the possibility of allergic reactions, atropine should always be available as an antidote.

4. *Treatment of Overdose:* Administer atropine.

Interventions

1. During IV administration, monitor and record the heart rate and report any evidence of bradycardia, hypersalivation, respiratory difficulty, or seizure activity.

2. Determine cause of overdosage (drug or plant ingestion), amount, and time ingested.

3. Have the client void prior to administering the medication. If the client develops incontinence, it may be caused by too high a dose. Document and notify the physician.

4. During ophthalmic instillation, wipe away any excess solution from around the eyes.

5. Wash hands after administration to prevent systemic absorption.

Client/Family Teaching

1. Nausea and vomiting may occur. If the symptoms are severe, the physician should be notified.

2. Some stinging and burning of the eyes may occur. Reassure the client that these symptoms should disappear as the use of the drug continues. If the client experiences painful spasms, apply cold compresses. If itching, pain or tearing persists, do not continue using the medication until the physician has been consulted.

3. Do not use the ophthalmic solution if it is discolored.

4. Advise that night vision may be impaired.

Evaluation: Evaluate client for:

- Clinical evidence of successful reversal of CNS symptoms of overdosage with cholinergic blocking agents or tricyclic antidepressants
- Evidence of ↓ intraocular pressures

Phytonadione (Vitamin K₁)

(fye-toe-nah-**DYE**-ohn)

Aqua-Mephyton, Konakion, Mephyton (Rx)

Classification: Fat-soluble vitamin.

Action/Kinetics: Phytonadione is similar to natural vitamin K. It has a more rapid and more prolonged effect than menadiol sodium diphosphate and is generally more effective. GI absorption requires the presence of bile salts. Heparin may be used to reverse overdosage of phytonadione. Frequent determinations of prothrombin time are indicated during therapy. **IM: Onset,** 1–2 hr. *Control of bleeding:* Parenteral, 3–6 hr. *Normal prothrombin time:* 12–14 hr. **PO: Onset,** 6–12 hr.

Additional Uses: Prophylaxis of hemorrhagic disease of the newborn.

Special Concerns: Pregnancy category: C.

Additional Side Effects: IV administration may cause severe reactions leading to death. May be transient flushing of the face, sweating, a sense of constriction of the chest, and weakness. Cramp-like pain, weak and rapid pulse, convulsive movements, chills and fever, hypotension, cyanosis, or hemoglobinuria have been reported occasionally. Shock, cardiac, and respiratory failure may be observed.

Dosage: Tablets. *Hypoprothrombinemia, drug-induced:* **Adults:** 2.5–10 mg (up to 25 mg); dose may be repeated after 12–48 hr if needed. *Vitamin supplement, prothrombogenic, drug-induced hypoprothrombinemia:* **Pediatric:** 5–10 mg.

IM, SC. *Vitamin supplement, prothrombogenic, drug-induced hypoprothrombinemia:* **Adults:** 2.5–10 mg (up to 25 mg) which may be repeated after 6–8 hr if needed. **Infants:** 1–2 mg; **children:** 5–10 mg. *Prophylaxis of hypoprothrombinemia during prolonged TPN:* **Adults, IM:** 5–10 mg once weekly; **pediatric:** 2–5 mg once weekly. *Infants receiving milk substitutes or who are breast-fed:* 1 mg monthly if vitamin K in diet is less than 0.1 mg/L. *Prevention of hemorrhagic disease in the newborn:* 0.5–1 mg immediately after delivery; dose may be repeated in 6–8 hr if needed. Higher doses may be required for infants whose mothers took anticonvulsants or anticoagulants during pregnancy.

NURSING CONSIDERATIONS

See also *Nursing Considerations* for *Vitamin K,* p. 247.

Administration/Storage

1. Store injectable emulsion or colloidal solutions in cool, 5°C–15°C (41°F–59°F), dark place.
2. Do not freeze.
3. Protect vitamin K from light.
4. Mix emulsion only with water or D₅W.

5. Mix colloidal solution with D₅W, isotonic sodium chloride injection, or dextrose and sodium chloride injection.

Interventions

1. Monitor liver function studies and prothrombin time while the client is receiving drug therapy.
2. Observe the client during parenteral administration for evidence of sweating, transient facial flushing, client complaints of weakness, and constriction of the chest. Notify the physician, especially if the client develops tachycardia, and hypotension because this may progress to shock, cardiac arrest, and respiratory failure.
3. If the client has decreased bile secretion, administer bile salts to ensure the absorption of oral phytonadione.

Evaluation: Evaluate client for:

- Successful control of bleeding in hypoprothrombinemia
- Effective prophylaxis of hypoprothrombinemia during prolonged TPN
- Evidence of prevention of hemorrhagic disease in the newborn

——— COMBINATION DRUG ———

Pilocarpine and Epinephrine

(pie-low-**CAR**-peen, ep-ih-**NEF**-rin)

E-Pilo-1, E-Pilo-2, E-Pilo-3, E-Pilo-4, E-Pilo-6, P1E1, P2E1, P3E1, P4E1, P6E1 (Rx)

See also *Ophthalmic Cholinergic Agents,* p. 190, and *Pilocarpine Hydrochloride,* p. 1051.

Classification: Miotic (pilocarpine) and mydriatic (epinephrine).

Action/Kinetics: Pilocarpine and epinephrine exert an additive effect to reduce intraocular pressure; the combination exerts opposite effects on the pupil which prevents significant mydriasis or miosis. The solutions all contain epinephrine, 1%, with varying concentrations of pilocarpine, indicated by the number in the name (e.g., E-Pilo-1 contains 1% pilocarpine and P2E1 contains 2% pilocarpine).

Uses: Glaucoma.

Dosage: Solution: 1–2 gtt into the eye(s) 1–4 times daily.

NURSING CONSIDERATIONS

See *Ophthalmic Cholinergic Agents*, p. 191, and *Pilocarpine*, p. 1052.

Client/Family Teaching: Advise that blurred vision will occur for a short time after drug administration and not to drive or attempt to operate machinery until vision clears.

Evaluation: Evaluate client for evidence of reduction of intraocular pressures.

Pilocarpine hydrochloride
(pie-low-**CAR**-peen)
Adsorbocarpine, Akarpine, Almocarpine, K-Pilopine, Isopto Carpine, Miocarpine✶, Ocu-Carpine, Pilocar, Pilocarpine Minims✶, Pilokair, Pilopine✶, Piloptic-1, -2, and -4, Spersacarpine✶ (Rx)

Pilocarpine nitrate
(pie-low-**CAR**-peen)
Minims Pilocarpine✶, P.V. Carpine Liquifilm, Spectro-Pilo (Rx)

Pilocarpine ocular therapeutic system
(pie-low-**CAR**-peen)
Ocusert Pilo-20 and -40 (Rx)

See also *Ophthalmic Cholinergic Agents*, p. 190.

Classification: Direct-acting cholinergic agent (miotic).

Action/Kinetics: *Hydrochloride, Nitrate:* **Onset:** 10–30 min; **peak effect:** 2–4 hr; **duration:** 4–8 hr. The ocular therapeutic system is a unit designed to be placed in the cul-de-sac of the eye for release of pilocarpine. The drug is released from the ocular therapeutic system three times faster during the first few hours and then decreases (within 6 hr) to a rate of 20 or 40 mcg/hr for 1 week.

Uses: *HCl:* Chronic simple glaucoma (especially open-angle). Chronic angle-closure glaucoma, including after iridectomy. Acute closed-angle glaucoma (alone or with other miotics, epinephrine, beta-adrenergic blocking agents, carbonic anhydrase inhibitors, or hyperosmotic agents). To reverse mydriasis (i.e., after cycloplegic and mydriatic drugs). *Nitrate:* Similar to the hydrochloride salt. Also, used for emergency miosis. *Ocular Therapeutic System:* Glaucoma alone or with other ophthalmic medications. *Investigational:* Hydrochloride used to test xerostomia in clients with malfunctioning salivary glands.

Special Concerns: Pregnancy category: C.

Dosage: *Pilocarpine hydrochloride:* **Gel. Adults and children:** ½-inch strip of 4% gel once daily at bedtime. **Solution. Adults and children,** *chronic glaucoma:* 1 gtt of a 0.5%–4% solution q.i.d. *Acute* *angle-closure glaucoma:* 1 gtt of a 1% or 2% solution q 5–10 min for 3–6 doses; **then,** 1 gtt q 1–3 hr until pressure is decreased. *Miotic, to counteract sympathomimetics:* 1 gtt of a 1% solution. *Miosis, prior to surgery:* 1 gtt of a 2% solution q 4–6 hr for 1 or 2 doses before surgery. *Miosis before iridectomy:* 1 gtt of a 2% solution for 4 doses before surgery.

Pilocarpine nitrate: **Solution. Adults and children,** *chronic glaucoma:* 1 gtt of a 1%–4% solution q.i.d. *Acute angle-closure glaucoma:* 1 gtt of a 1% or 2% solution q 5–10 min for 3–6 doses; **then,** 1 gtt q 1–3 hr until pressure is decreased. *Miosis, to counteract sympathomimetics:* 1 gtt of a 1% solution. *Miosis, before surgery for glaucoma:* 1 gtt of a 2% solution q 4–6 hr before surgery. *Miosis, before surgery for iridectomy:* 1 gtt of a 2% solution for 4 doses.

Ocular Therapeutic System: Insert and remove as directed by physician or package insert. Ocusert Pilo-20 is approximately equal to the 0.5% or 1% drops, while Ocusert Pilo-40 is approximately equal to the 2% or 3% solution.

NURSING CONSIDERATIONS

See also *Nursing Considerations for Ophthalmic Cholinergic Agents,* p. 191.

Administration/Storage

1. The hydrochloride is available as 0.25%, 0.5%, 1%, 2%, 3%, 4%, 5%, 6%, 8%, and 10% solutions and as a 4% gel.
2. Concentrations greater than 4% of pilocarpine HCl may be more effective in clients with dark pigmented eyes; however, the incidence of side effects increases.
3. The nitrate is available as 1%, 2%, and 4% solutions.
4. Myopia may be observed during the first several hours of therapy with the ocular therapeutic system.
5. Client should check for presence of the ocular therapeutic system before bed and upon arising.
6. For acute, narrow-angle glaucoma, pilocarpine should also be administered in the unaffected eye to prevent angle-closure glaucoma.

Client/Family Teaching

1. Review how to insert drug and to check the conjunctival sac for presence of the ocular system.
2. Advise client to follow these general guidelines for insertion:
   - Wash hands.
   - Do not permit drug to touch any surface.
   - Rinse with cool water.
   - Pull down lower eyelid.
   - Place according to manufacturer's directions.
   - System may be moved under closed eyelids to upper eyelid for sleep.
3. Instruct to insert drug at bedtime to diminish side effects. Advise to check for the presence of ocular system at bedtime and also upon awakening each day.
4. Explain the importance of periodic tonometric readings to evaluate effectiveness of the drug.

Evaluation: Evaluate client for:
- Tonometric evidence of a ↓ in intraocular pressures
- Evidence of successful reversal of sympathomimetic drug effects

—— *COMBINATION DRUG* ——
Pilocarpine and Physostigmine

(pie-low-**CAR**-peen, fye-zoh-**STIG**-meen)

Isopto P-ES (Rx)

Action/Kinetics: This product contains pilocarpine hydrochloride, 2%, and physostigmine salicylate, 0.25%. No evidence suggests that this combination exerts greater effect to lower intraocular pressure than either drug alone.

Uses: Treatment of glaucoma.

Dosage: Solution: 2 gtt into the eye(s) up to q.i.d.

NURSING CONSIDERATIONS

See *Ophthalmic Cholinergic Agents,* p. 191, *Pilocarpine,* p. 1052, and *Physostigmime,* p. 1048.

Evaluation: Evaluate client for tonometric evidence of a ↓ in intraocular pressure.

Pindolol

(**PIN**-doh-lohl)

Apo-Pindol✱, Novo–Pindol✱, Nu-Pindol✱, Syn-Pindolol✱, Visken (Rx)

See also *Beta-Adrenergic Blocking Agents,* p. 113.

Action/Kinetics: Manifests both beta-1 and beta-2 adrenergic blocking activity. Pindolol also has significant intrinsic sympathomimetic effects and minimal membrane-stabilizing activity. Moderate lipid solubility. $t^{1/2}$: 3–4 hr; however, geriatric clients have a variable half-life ranging from 7–15 hr, even with normal renal function. The drug is metabolized by the liver, and the metabolites and unchanged (35%–40%) drug are excreted through the kidneys.

Uses: Hypertension (alone or in combination with other antihypertensive agents as thiazide diuretics). *Investigational:* Ventricular arrhythmias and tachycardias, antipsychotic-induced akathisia, situational anxiety.

Special Concerns: Pregnancy category: B. Dosage has not been established in children.

Laboratory Test Interferences: ↑ AST and ALT. Rarely, ↑ LDH, uric acid, alkaline phosphatase.

Dosage: Tablets. *Hypertension:* **Initial,** 5 mg b.i.d. (alone or with other antihypertensive drugs). If no response in 3–4 weeks, increase by 10 mg/day q 3–4 weeks to a maximum of 60 mg daily. *Antipsychotic-induced akathisia:* 5 mg daily.

NURSING CONSIDERATIONS

See also *Nursing Considerations* for *Beta-Adrenergic Blocking Agents,* p. 116, and *Antihypertensive Agents,* p. 78.

Intervention: Anticipate reduced dosage in clients with liver dysfunction.

Evaluation: Evaluate client for:
- Evidence of a ↓ blood pressure
- Reports of a reduction in anxiety
- ECG evidence of control of ventricular arrhythmias

P.

Pipecuronium bromide

(pih-peh-kyour-**OHN**-ee-um)
Arduan (Rx)

Classification: Neuromuscular blocking agent, nondepolarizing.

Action/Kinetics: Pipecuronium is similar to tubocurarine in that it competes for cholinergic receptors at the motor end-plate and is antagonized by acetylcholinesterase inhibitors. **Maximum time for blockade:** 5 min following single doses of 70–85 mcg/kg. **Time to recovery to 25% of control:** 30–175 min under balanced anesthesia following single doses of 70 mcg/kg. **t½, distribution:** 6.22 min; **t½, elimination:** 1.7 hr. Increased plasma levels are seen in clients with impaired renal function. The drug is metabolized in the liver and metabolites as well as unchanged drug are eliminated in the urine.

Uses: Adjunct to general anesthesia to provide relaxation of skeletal muscle during surgery. Skeletal muscle relaxation for endotracheal intubation.

Contraindications: Use for procedures anticipated to last 90 min or longer. Due to the long duration of action, the drug should not be used in myasthenia gravis or Eaton-Lambert syndrome. Clients undergoing cesarean section. Use of pipecuronium before succinylcholine.

Special Concerns: Pregnancy category: C. Although the drug is used in infants and children, no information is available on maintenance dosing. Also, children from 1–14 years of age under balanced or halothane anesthesia may be less sensitive to the drug than adults.

Use with caution in clients with impaired renal function. The drug should be administered only if there are adequate facilities for intubation, artificial respiration, oxygen therapy, and administration of an antagonist. Obesity may prolong the duration of action. Conditions resulting in an increased volume of distribution (e.g., old age, edematous states, slower circulation time in cardiovascular disease) may cause a delay in the time of onset.

Side Effects: *Neuromuscular:* Prolongation of blockade including skeletal muscle paralysis resulting in respiratory insufficiency or apnea. Muscle atrophy, difficult intubation. *CV:* Hypotension, bradycardia, hypertension, cerebrovascular accident, thrombosis, myocardial ischemia, atrial fibrillation, ventricular extrasystole. *CNS:* Hypesthesia, CNS depression. *Respiratory:* Dyspnea, respiratory depression, laryngismus, atelectasis. *Metabolic:* Hypoglycemia, hyperkalemia, increased creatinine. *Miscellaneous:* Rash, urticaria, anuria.

Symptoms of Overdose: Skeletal muscle paralysis including depressed respiration.

Drug Interactions

Aminoglycosides / ↑ Intensity and duration of neuromuscular blockade

Bacitracin / ↑ Intensity and duration of neuromuscular blockade

Colistin/Sodium colistimethate / ↑ Intensity and duration of neuromuscular blockade

Enflurane / ↑ Duration of action of pipecuronium

Halothane / ↑ Duration of action of pipecuronium

Isoflurane / ↑ Duration of action of pipecuronium

Magnesium salts / ↑ Intensity of neuromuscular blockade when used for toxemia of pregnancy

Polymyxin B / ↑ Intensity and duration of neuromuscular blockade

Quinidine / ↑ Risk of recurrent paralysis

Tetracyclines / ↑ Intensity and duration of neuromuscular blockade

Dosage: IV only; dosage individualized. Adults: Initial dose may be based on the creatinine clearance and the ideal body weight (see information provided by manufacturer). The dose range is 50–100 mcg/kg. *Endotracheal intubation using balanced anesthesia:* 70–85 mcg/kg with halothane, isoflurane, or enflurane in clients with normal renal function who are not obese; duration of muscle relaxation is 1–2 hr using this dosage range. *Use following recovery from succinylcholine:* 50 mcg/kg in clients with normal renal function who are not obese; duration of muscle relaxation using this dose is 45 min. *Maintenance:* 10–15 mcg/kg given at 25% recovery of control T_1 will provide muscle relaxation for an average of 50 min using balanced anesthesia; lower doses should be used in clients receiving inhalation anesthetics. **Pediatric:** The duration of action in infants following a dose of 40 mcg/kg ranged from 10–44 min while the duration in children following a dose of 57 mcg/kg ranged from 18–52 min.

NURSING CONSIDERATIONS

Administration/Storage

1. Pipecuronium should be administered only under the supervision of individuals experienced with the use of neuromuscular blocking agents.

2. Pipecuronium can be reconstituted using 0.9% sodium chloride, 5% dextrose in saline, 5% dextrose in water, lactated Ringer's, sterile water for injection, and bacteriostatic water for injection.

3. If used in newborns, the drug should not be reconstituted with bacteriostatic water for injection because it contains benzyl alcohol.

4. When reconstituted with bacteriostatic water for injection, the solution may be stored at room temperature or in the refrigerator; it should be used within 5 days.

5. When reconstituted with sterile water for injection or other IV solutions, the vial should be refrigerated and used within 24 hr.

6. Pipecuronium should not be diluted with or administered from large volumes of IV solutions.

7. The drug should be stored at 2°C–30°C (35°F–86°F) and protected from light.

8. *Treatment of Overdose:* Artificial respiration until effects of drug have worn off. Antagonize neuromuscular blockade by administration of neostigmine, 0.04 mg/kg. Use of edrophonium is not recommended.

Assessment

1. Review client history for evidence of myasthenia gravis or Eaton-Lambert syndrome because drug is not recommended with these conditions.

2. List drugs client currently prescribed because many interact unfavorably with pipecuronium.

3. Obtain baseline electrolytes and renal function studies.

4. Document height, weight and note any evidence of obesity because drug dose should be correlated for *ideal* body weight.

5. Determine if diarrhea is present and the duration because this may alter neuromuscular blockade.

Interventions

1. Anticipate that individuals administering pipecuronium should use a peripheral nerve stimulator. This device will assist to monitor drug response, to assess the need for additional doses of the drug, and to evaluate the adequacy of spontaneous recovery or antagonism.

2. The twitch response should be used to evaluate recovery from pipecuronium and minimize overdosage potential.

3. Allow more time for pipecuronium to achieve maximum effect in older clients with slowed circulation, cardiovascular diseases, and/or edematous states. *Do not* increase drug dose because this will produce a longer duration of action.

4. Monitor BP and pulse closely and observe postrecovery for adequate clinical evidence of antagonism:
   - 5-sec head lift
   - Adequate pronation
   - Effective airway and ventilatory patterns

Evaluation: Evaluate client for:
- Evidence of desired level of skeletal muscle relaxation
- Effective suppression of twitch response when tested with a peripheral nerve stimulator

---

Piperacillin sodium
(pie-PER-ah-sill-in)
Pipracil (Rx)

See also *Penicillins,* p. 197.

Classification: Antibiotic, penicillin.

Action/Kinetics: Piperacillin is a semisynthetic, broad-spectrum penicillin for parenteral use. It is not penicillinase resistant. The drug penetrates CSF in the presence of inflamed meninges. **Peak serum level:** 244 mcg/ml. **t½:** 36–72 min. Excreted unchanged in urine and bile.

Uses: Intra-abdominal infections, gynecologic infections, septicemia, skin and skin structure infections, bone and joint infections, urinary tract infections, lower respiratory tract infections, gonococcal infections, streptococcal infections. Mixed infections prior to the identification of the causative organisms. Prophylaxis in surgery including GI, biliary, hysterectomy, cesarean section.

Aminoglycosides have been used with piperacillin sodium, especially in clients with impaired host defenses.

Additional Side Effects: Rarely, prolonged muscle relaxation.

Laboratory Test Interference: Positive Comb's test; ↑ (especially in infants) AST, ALT, LDH, bilirubin.

Dosage: IM, IV. *Serious infections,* **IV:** 3–4 g q 4–6 hr (12–18 g/day) as a 20–30 min infusion. *Complicated urinary tract infections,* **IV:** 8–16 g/day (125–200 mg/kg/day) in divided doses q 6–8 hr. *Uncomplicated urinary tract infections and most community-acquired pneumonias,* **IM, IV:** 6–8 g/day (100–125 mg/kg/day) in divided doses q 6–12 hr. *Uncomplicated gonorrhea infections:* 2 g **IM** with 1 g probenecid **PO** 30 min before injection (both given as single dose). *Prophylaxis in surgery,* **First dose: IV,** 2 g prior to surgery; **second dose:** 2 g either during surgery (abdominal) or 4–6 hr after surgery (hysterectomy, cesarean); **third dose:** 2 g at an interval depending on use. Dosage should be decreased in renal impairment. Dosages have not been established in infants and children under 12 years of age although the following doses have been suggested: **Neonates,** 100 mg/kg q 12 hr; **children,** 200–300 mg/kg/day (up to a maximum of 24 g daily) divided q 4–6 hr. *For cystic fibrosis,* 350–500 mg/kg/day divided q 4–6 hr.

NURSING CONSIDERATIONS

See also *Nursing Considerations* for *Penicillins,* p. 200.

Administration/Storage

1. No more than 2 g should be administered IM at any one site.
2. For IM administration, use upper, outer quadrant of gluteus or well-developed deltoid muscle. Do not use lower or mid-third of upper arm.
3. For IV administration reconstitute each gram with at least 5 ml diluent, such as sterile or bacteriostatic water for injec-

tion, sodium chloride for injection, or bacteriostatic sodium chloride for injection. Shake until dissolved.
4. Inject IV slowly over a period of 3–5 min to avoid vein irritation.
5. Administer by intermittent IV infusion in at least 50 ml over a period of 20–30 min via "piggyback" or soluset.
6. After reconstitution, solution may be stored at room temperature for 24 hr, refrigerated for 1 week, or frozen for 1 month.

Interventions

1. Monitor CBC, liver and renal function studies throughout therapy.
2. Report any diarrhea or other evidence of superinfection.

Evaluation: Evaluate client for:
- Clinical evidence and reports of symptomatic improvement
- Laboratory evidence of negative culture reports

P

Piperazine citrate
(pie-**PER**-ah-zeen)
(Rx)

See also *Anthelmintics,* p. 40.

Classification: Anthelmintic.

Action/Kinetics: The drug is believed to paralyze the muscles of parasites; this dislodges the parasites and promotes their elimination by peristalsis. The drug has little effect on larvae in tissues. The drug is readily absorbed from the GI tract, is partially metabolized by the liver, and the remainder is excreted in urine. Rate of elimination differs among clients although it is excreted nearly unchanged in the urine within 24 hr.

Uses: Pinworm (oxyuriasis) and roundworm (ascariasis) infestations. Particularly recommended for pediatric use.

Contraindications: Impaired liver or kidney function, seizure disorders, hypersensitivity. Lactation.

Special Concerns: Safe use during pregnancy has not been established. Due to neurotoxicity, prolonged, repeated, or excessive use in children should be avoided.

Side Effects: Piperazine has low toxicity. *GI:* Nausea, vomiting, diarrhea, cramps. *CNS:* Tremors, headache, vertigo, decreased reflexes, paresthesias, seizures, ataxia, chorea, memory decrement. *Ophthalmologic:* Nystagmus, blurred vision, cataracts, strabismus. *Allergic:* Urticaria, fever, skin reactions, purpura, lacrimation, rhinorrhea, arthralgia, bronchospasm, cough. *Miscellaneous:* Muscle weakness.

Drug Interactions: Concomitant administration of piperazine and phenothiazines may result in an increase in extrapyramidal effects (including violent convulsions) caused by phenothiazines.

Laboratory Test Interference: False (−) or ↓ uric acid values.

Dosage: Syrup, Tablets. *Pinworms:* **Adults and children,** 65 mg/kg as a single daily dose for 7 days up to a maximum daily dose of 2.5 g. *Roundworms:* **Adults,** one dose of 3.5 g/day for 2 consecutive days; **pediatric,** one dose of 75 mg/kg/day for 2 consecutive days, not to exceed 3.5 g daily. For severe infections, repeat therapy after 1 week.

NURSING CONSIDERATIONS

See also *Nursing Considerations for Anthelmintics,* p. 42.

Assessment

1. Note any evidence of impaired hepatic or renal function.
2. Document history of seizure disorder as drug is contraindicated.
3. Determine previous treatments and length of therapy as excessive drug therapy should be avoided in children due to neurotoxic effects.

Client/Family Teaching

1. Keep pleasant-tasting medication out of reach of children.
2. Take medication after breakfast or in two divided doses.
3. Report any adverse drug effects to physician immediately.
4. The drug should be taken on an empty stomach
5. Strict hygiene is required to prevent reinfection.

Evaluation

1. Evaluate client for evidence of negative stool examinations and perianal swabs.
2. Determine cause for repeated infestation and/or reinfection and assess need for further treatment.

Pipobroman

(pip-oh-**BROH**-man)
Vercyte (Rx)

See also *Antineoplastic Agents,* p. 85, and *Alkylating Agents,* p. 20.

Classification: Antineoplastic, alkylating agent.

Action/Kinetics: The mechanism, metabolism, and excretion are not known. Well absorbed from the GI tract.

Uses: Polycythemia vera; chronic granulocytic leukemia in clients refractory to busulfan.

Additional Contraindication: Children under 15 years of age. Lactation. Bone marrow depression due to chemotherapy or X rays.

Special Concerns: Pregnancy category: D. Bone marrow depression may not occur for 4 or more weeks after therapy is started.

Side Effects: *Hematologic:* Leukopenia, anemia, thrombocytopenia. *GI:* Nausea, vomiting, diarrhea, abdominal cramps. *Dermatologic:* Skin rashes.

Symptoms of Overdose: Hematologic toxicity.

Dosage: Tablets. *Polycythemia vera:* 1 mg/kg daily (up to 1.5–3 mg/kg daily may be required in clients refractory to other treatment). When hematocrit has been reduced to 50%–55%, **maintenance dosage** of 100–200 mcg/kg is instituted. *Chronic granulocytic leukemia:* **initial,** 1.5–2.5 mg/kg daily; **maintenance,** 7–175 mg daily, to be instituted when leukocyte count approaches 10,000/mm³.

NURSING CONSIDERATIONS

See also *Nursing Considerations* for *Antineoplastic Agents,* p. 88.

Administration/Storage: *Treatment of Overdose:* Monitor hematologic status; if necessary, begin vigorous supportive treatment.

Interventions

1. Administer drug in divided doses.
2. Be alert to persistent side effects that may necessitate withdrawal of the drug.
3. Monitor CBC for dosing parameters. Be aware that bone marrow depression may occur latently in therapy (after 4 weeks) so assess client carefully.

Evaluation

1. In polycythemia vera, evaluate client for laboratory evidence of a ↓ in hematocrit to 50%-55%.
2. Evaluate for laboratory evidence of hematologic recovery in clients with leukemia.

Pirbuterol acetate
(peer-**BYOU**-ter-ohl)
Maxair (Rx)

See also *Sympathomimetic Drugs,* p. 218.

Classification: Sympathomimetic, bronchodilator.

Action/Kinetics: Pirbuterol causes bronchodilation by stimulating beta-2 adrenergic receptors. The drug also inhibits histamine release from mast cells, causes vasodilation, and increases ciliary motility. It has minimal beta-1 activity. **Onset, inhalation:** Approximately 5 min. **Time to peak effect:** 30–60 min. **Duration:** 5 hr.

Uses: Alone or with theophylline or steroids, for prophylaxis and treatment of bronchospasm in asthma and other conditions with reversible bronchospasms, including bronchitis, emphysema, bronchiectasis, obstructive pulmonary disease.

Contraindications: Cardiac arrhythmias due to tachycardia; tachycardia caused by digitalis toxicity.

Special Concerns: Pregnancy category: C.

Dosage: Inhalation Aerosol. Adults and children over 12 years: 0.2–0.4 mg (1–2 inhalations) q 4–6 hr, not to exceed 12 inhalations (2.4 mg) daily.

NURSING CONSIDERATIONS

See also *Nursing Considerations* for *Sympathomimetic Drugs,* p. 220, and *Special Nursing Considerations for Adrenergic Bronchodilators* under *Sympathomimetic Drugs,* p. 221.

Client/Family Teaching: Contact the physician immediately if the client does not obtain relief with doses of medication that have previously been effective.

Evaluation: Evaluate client for clinical evidence of a reduction in bronchoconstriction and bronchospasm with reports of improved airway exchange.

Piroxicam
(peer-**OX**-ih-kam)
Apo-Piroxicam✤, Feldene, Novo–Pirocam✤, Nu-Pirox✤ (Rx)

See also *Nonsteroidal Anti-Inflammatory Drugs,* p. 186.

Classification: Nonsteroidal anti-inflammatory, analgesic, antipyretic.

Action/Kinetics: Piroxicam may inhibit prostaglandin synthesis. **Peak plasma levels:** 1.5–2 mcg/ml after 3–5 hr (single dose). **Steady-state plasma levels** (after 7–12 days): 3–8 mcg/ml. **t½:** 50 hr. **Analgesia, onset:** 1 hr; **duration:** 2–3 days. **Anti-inflammatory activity, onset:** 7–12 days; **duration:** 2–3 weeks. Metabolites and unchanged drug excreted in urine and feces.

The effect of piroxicam is comparable to that of aspirin, but with fewer GI side effects and less tinnitus. May be used with gold, corticosteroids, and antacids.

Uses: Acute and chronic treatment of rheumatoid arthritis and osteoarthritis. *Investigational:* Juvenile rheumatoid arthritis, primary dysmenorrhea, sunburn.

Contraindications: Safe use during pregnancy has not been determined. Lactation.

Special Concerns: Safety and efficacy have not been established in children. Increased plasma levels and elimination half-life may be observed in geriatric clients (especially women).

Laboratory Test Interference: Reversible ↑ BUN.

Dosage: Capsules. Adults: *Anti-inflammatory, antirheumatic,* 20 mg daily in 1 or more divided doses. Effect of therapy should not be assessed for 2 weeks.

NURSING CONSIDERATIONS

See also *Nursing Considerations* for *Nonsteroidal Anti-Inflammatory Drugs,* p. 189.

Administration/Storage

1. Steady-state plasma levels may not be reached for 2 weeks.
2. Clients over 70 years of age usually require one-half the usual adult dose of medication.
3. The drug is not recommended for children under 14 years of age.
4. Review the list of drugs with which piroxicam interacts, p. 189.

Client/Family Teaching

1. Remind client that the therapeutic effects of the medication

cannot be evaluated fully for at least 2 weeks after beginning treatment with piroxicam.

2. Aspirin decreases the effectiveness of piroxicam and may increase the occurrence of side effects. Therefore, avoid taking aspirin while receiving piroxicam.

3. Report any increased abdominal pain or changes in the color of the stool to the physician immediately.

Evaluation: Evaluate client for reports of control of joint pain and improved joint mobility.

Plicamycin (Mithramycin)

(plye-kah-**MY**-sin, mith-rah-**MY**-sin)
Mithracin (Abbreviation: MTH) (Rx)

See also *Antineoplastic Agents,* p. 85.

Classification: Antineoplastic, antibiotic.

Action/Kinetics: Antibiotic produced by *Streptomyces plicatus, S. argillaceus,* and *S. tanashiensis.* Plicamycin complexes with DNA in the presence of magnesium (or other divalent cations), resulting in inhibition of cellular and enzymatic RNA synthesis. The drug decreases blood calcium by blocking the hypercalcemic effect of vitamin D, acting on osteoclasts, and preventing the action of parathyroid hormone. Plicamycin is cleared rapidly from the blood and is concentrated in the Kupffer cells of the liver, renal tubular cells, and along formed bone surfaces. The drug crosses the blood-brain barrier. It is excreted through the urine.

Uses: Malignant testicular tumors

usually associated with metastases and when radiation or surgery is not an alternative. Hypercalcemia and hypercalciuria associated with advanced malignancy and not responsive to other therapy.

Additional Contraindications: Thrombocytopenia, thrombocytopathy, coagulation disorders, and increased tendency to hemorrhage. Impaired bone marrow function. Pregnancy (category: X). Lactation. Do not use for children under 15 years of age.

Special Concerns: Pregnancy category: X. Use with caution in impaired liver or kidney function.

Additional Side Effects: Severe thrombocytopenia, hemorrhagic tendencies. Facial flushing. Hepatic and renal toxicity. Extravasation may cause irritation or cellulitis. Electrolyte imbalance including hypocalcemia, hypokalemia, and hypophosphatemia.
Symptoms of Overdose: Hematologic toxicity.

Laboratory Test Interferences: ↓ Serum calcium, potassium, and phosphorus. ↑ Serum BUN, creatinine, AST, ALT, alkaline phosphatase, bilirubin, isocitric dehydrogenase, ornithine carbamyltransferase, lactic dehydrogenase. ↑ BSP retention.

Dosage: IV only. *Individualized. Testicular tumor:* 25–30 (maximum) mcg/kg (given over a period of 4–6 hr) daily for 8–10 (maximum) days. A second approach is to use 25–50 mcg/kg on alternate days for an average of 8 doses. *Hypercalcemia, hypercalciuria:* 15–25 mcg/kg (given over a period of 4–6 hr) daily for 3–4 days. Additional courses of therapy may be warranted at weekly intervals if initial course is unsuccessful.

NURSING CONSIDERATIONS

See also *Nursing Considerations* for *Antineoplastic Agents*, p. 88.

Administration/Storage

1. *Store vials of medication in refrigerator at temperatures below 10°C (36°F–46°F). Discard unused portion of drug.*
2. Reconstitute fresh for each day of therapy.
3. Drug is unstable in acid solution (pH 5 and below) and in reconstituted solutions (pH 7) and thus deteriorates rapidly.
4. Add sterile water to the vial as recommended on the package insert and shake the vial to dissolve the drug.
5. Add the calculated dosage of the drug to the IV solution ordered (recommended 1 L of D_5W) and adjust the rate of flow as ordered (recommended time is 4–6 hr for 1 L).
6. Should be used only for hospitalized clients.
7. *Treatment of Overdose:* Monitor hematologic status, especially clotting factors. Also, closely monitor serum electrolytes and hepatic and renal functions.

Assessment

1. Assess clients for evidence of hemorrhage, such as epistaxis, hemoptysis, hematemesis, purpura, or ecchymoses.
2. Obtain baseline CBC, platelets, PT, calcium, potassium, hepatic and renal function studies.

Interventions

1. Therapy should be interrupted if WBC count goes below 3,000/mm³ or if prothrombin time is more than 4 sec higher than that of the control. Daily platelet count should be performed on clients who have had x-ray films taken of abdomen and mediastinum.
2. If antiemetic drugs are ordered, administer before or during therapy with mithramycin.
3. Closely check peripheral IV for extravasation. Stop IV if extravasation occurs; apply moderate heat to disperse drug and to reduce pain and tissue damage. Restart IV at another site.
4. Monitor I&O. Prevent excessively rapid IV flow, because it precipitates more severe GI side effects.
5. During therapy monitor electrolytes, liver and renal function for any evidence of imbalance or toxicity.

Evaluation: Evaluate client for:

- Evidence of a ↓ in tumor size and spread
- Laboratory confirmation of a reduction in serum and urinary calcium levels

---

Podofilox
(poh-**DAHF**-ih-lox)
Condylox (Rx)

Classification: Keratolytic.

Action/Kinetics: Podofilox is derived either from species of *Juniperus* or *Podophyllum* or chemically synthesized. It is an antimitotic agent that causes necrosis of visible wart tissue when applied topically. Small amounts are absorbed into the system 1–2 hr after application. **t½:** 1–4.5 hr. The drug does not accumulate following multiple treatments.

Uses: Topical treatment of *Condyloma acuminatum* (external genital warts). *Investigational:* Systemically for treatment of cancer.

Contraindications: Use for perianal or mucous membrane warts. Lactation.

Special Concerns: Pregnancy category: C. It is essential that genital warts be distinguished from squamous cell carcinoma prior to initiation of treatment. Safety and effectiveness have not been demonstrated in children.

Side Effects: Topical Use. *Dermatologic:* Commonly, burning, pain, inflammation, erosion, and itching. Also, tenderness, chafing, scarring vesicle formation, dryness and peeling, tingling, bleeding, ulceration, malodor, crusting edema, foreskin irretraction. *Miscellaneous:* Pain with intercourse, insomnia, dizziness, hematuria, vomiting.

Systemic Use. *GI:* Nausea, vomiting, diarrhea, oral ulcers. *Hematologic:* Bone marrow depression, leukocytosis, pancytosis. *CNS:* Altered mental status, lethargy, coma, seizures. *Miscellaneous:* Peripheral neuropathy, tachypnea, respiratory failure, hematuria, renal failure.

Symptoms of Overdose: Nausea, vomiting, diarrhea, fever, altered mental status, hematologic toxicity, peripheral neuropathy, lethargy, tachypnea, respiratory failure, hematuria, leukocytosis, pancytosis, renal failure, seizures, coma.

Dosage: Topical Solution. Adults, initial: Apply b.i.d. in the morning and evening (i.e., q 12 hr) for three consecutive days; **then,** withhold use for four consecutive days. The one week cycle of treatment may be repeated up to four times until there is no visible sign of wart tissue. Alternative treatment should be considered if the response is incomplete after four treatments.

NURSING CONSIDERATIONS

Administration/Storage

1. Apply podofilox to the warts with the cotton-tipped applicator supplied with the drug.
2. Apply only the minimum amount of solution required to cover the lesion. Treatment should be limited to less than 10 cm² of wart tissue and to 0.5 ml or less of the solution/day. Higher amounts do not increase efficacy but may increase the incidence of side effects.
3. The solution should be allowed to dry before allowing the return of opposing skin surfaces to their normal positions.
4. After each treatment, the used applicator should be disposed of properly and the individual instructed to wash hands thoroughly.
5. The solution should not be frozen or exposed to excessive heat.
6. *Treatment of Overdose:* General supportive therapy to treat symptoms.

Assessment

1. Determine if differentiation of lesion from squamous cell carcinoma has been performed by histologic confirmation.
2. Document the number and size of condyloma, location, and condition of pretreatment area.

Client/Family Teaching

1. Demonstrate the appropriate method for topical administra-

tion and have client return demonstrate procedure.

2. Stress the importance of adhering to the exact dosing instructions (on for three days, off for four days) because the incidence of side effects may otherwise increase.

3. Avoid contact of the solution with the eyes. If contact does occur, instruct the individual to immediately flush the eye with large amounts of water and to report to the physician.

4. Review the appropriate procedure for handling the medication and for the disposal of applicators.

5. Provide a printed list of side effects that should be reported to the physician should they occur.

Evaluation: Evaluate client for evidence of a decrease (or absence) in the number and size of condylomas (determine further treatment needs based on these findings).

Polyestradiol phosphate
(pol-ee-es-trah-**DYE**-ohl)
Estradurin (Rx)

See also *Estrogens,* p. 147.

Classification: Estrogen, steroidal, synthetic.

Action/Kinetics: Estradiol is slowly split off from the parent compound, thus providing continuous levels for long periods of time. Increasing the dose will increase the duration of action rather than increasing the blood levels. The estradiol combines with androgen receptors; 90% of the dose leaves the plasma in 24 hr and is stored in

the reticuloendothelial system and slowly released.

Use: Palliation of cancer of the prostate. If there is a positive response, the hormone should be given until the disease progresses again. The drug should then be discontinued; at this time the client may show another period of improvement (called "rebound regression").

Contraindications: Pregnancy (category: X).

Additional Side Effects: Burning at injection site (transient).

Dosage: Deep IM: 40–80 mg q 2–4 weeks. Response should be noted in approximately 3 months and drug continued until the disease begins progressing again.

NURSING CONSIDERATIONS

See also *Nursing Considerations* for *Estrogens,* p. 150.

Administration/Storage

1. Add sterile diluent to the vial with a 20-gauge needle and 5-ml syringe. Swirl *gently* to dissolve.

2. Inject deeply. IM administration is painful, and may require concomitant administration of local anesthetic.

3. Stable at room temperature for 10 days. Shield from light.

4. Do not use solutions that have a deposit or are cloudy.

Assessment

1. Assess for symptoms of hypercalcemia: insomnia, lethargy, anorexia, nausea, vomiting, coma, and vascular collapse.

2. Steroids and osteolytic metastases may cause hypercalcemia. Thus, ascertain that serum calcium concentrations are

routinely done; assess results (normal: 4.5–5.5 mEq/L).

3. Monitor serum acid phosphatase levels and the client's symptomatic improvement to determine dosage requirements.

Interventions

1. For severe hypercalcemia, be prepared to assist with administration of IV fluids, diuretics, adrenocorticosteroids, and phosphate supplements.
2. Encourage bedridden clients to participate in passive and modified active exercises to prevent calcium loss from the bone.

Client/Family Teaching

1. Review S&S of hypercalcemia, and advise to report if evident.
2. Avoid eating foods high in calcium, such as dairy products, cheese, and enriched products.
3. Increase fluid intake to dilute calcium and to prevent urinary calculi.
4. Advise to remain active and ambulatory as long as possible.

Evaluation: Evaluate client for evidence of control of prostatic cancer progression.

Polymyxin B sulfate, parenteral
(pol-ee-**MIX**-in)
Aerosporin (Rx)

Polymyxin B sulfate, sterile ophthalmic
(pol-ee-**MIX**-in)
(Rx)

See also *Anti-Infectives,* p. 80.

Classification: Antibiotic, polymyxin.

Action/Kinetics: Polymyxin B sulfate is derived from the spore-forming soil bacterium *Bacillus polymyxa*. It is bactericidal against most gram-negative organisms and rapidly inactivated by alkali, strong acid, and certain metal ions. Polymyxin increases the permeability of the plasma cell membrane of the bacterium (i.e., similar to detergents), causing leakage of essential metabolites and ultimately inactivation. **Peak serum levels: IM,** 2 hr. **t½:** 4.3–6 hr. Longer in presence of renal impairment. Sixty percent of drug excreted in urine. It is virtually unabsorbed from the GI tract except in newborn infants. After parenteral administration, polymyxin B seems to remain in the plasma.

Uses: Acute infections of the urinary tract and meninges, septicemia caused by *Pseudomonas aeruginosa*. Meningeal infections caused by *Hemophilus influenzae,* urinary tract infections caused by *Escherichia coli,* bacteremia caused by *Enterobacter aerogenes* or *Klebsiella pneumoniae*. Combined with neomycin for irrigation of the urinary bladder to prevent bacteriuria and bacteremia from indwelling catheters.

Ophthalmic: Conjunctival and corneal infections. Blepharitis and keratitis due to bacterial infections. Used with systemic agents for anterior intraocular infections and corneal ulcers caused by *Pseudomonas aeruginosa*. Is also effective against *Escherichia coli, Hemophilus influenzae,* and *Enterobacter aerogenes*. Used alone or in combination for ear infections.

Contraindications: Hypersensitivity. Polymyxin B sulfate is a potentially toxic drug to be reserved for the treatment of severe, resistant infections in hospitalized clients. The drug is not indicated for clients with severely impaired renal function or nitrogen retention.

Special Concerns: Safe use during pregnancy has not been established.

Side Effects: *Nephrotoxic:* Albuminuria, cylindruria, azotemia, hematuria, proteinuria, leukocyturia, electrolyte loss. *Neurologic:* Dizziness, flushing of face, mental confusion, irritability, nystagmus, muscle weakness, drowsiness, paresthesias, blurred vision, slurred speech, ataxia, coma, seizures. Neuromuscular blockade may lead to respiratory paralysis. *GI:* Nausea, vomiting, diarrhea, abdominal cramps. *Miscellaneous:* Fever, urticaria, skin exanthemata, eosinophilia, anaphylaxis.

Following intrathecal use: Meningeal irritation with fever, stiff neck, headache, increase in leukocytes and protein in the CSF. Nerve-root irritation may result in neuritic pain and urine retention. *Following IM use:* Irritation, severe pain. *Following IV use:* Thrombophlebitis. *Following ophthalmic use:* Burning, stinging, irritation, angioneurotic edema, itching, urticaria, vesicular and maculopapular dermatitis.

Drug Interactions

Aminoglycoside antibiotics /
    Additive nephrotoxic effects
Cephalosporins / ↑ Risk of renal
    toxicity
Phenothiazines / ↑ Risk of
    respiratory depression
*Skeletal muscle relaxants
    (surgical)* / Additive muscle
    relaxation

Laboratory Test Interferences: False + or ↑ levels of urea nitrogen and creatinine. Casts and RBCs in urine.

Dosage: IV: Adults and children, 15,000–25,000 units/kg/day (maximum) in divided doses q 12 hr. **Infants,** up to 40,000 units/kg/day. **IM** (not usually recommended due to pain at injection site): **Adults and children,** 25,000–30,000 units/kg/day in divided doses q 4–6 hr. **Infants,** up to 40,000 units/kg/day. Both IV and IM doses should be reduced in renal impairment. **Intrathecal** (*meningitis*): **Adults and children over 2 years,** 50,000 units once daily for 3–4 days; **then,** 50,000 units every other day until 2 weeks after cultures are negative; **children under 2 years,** 20,000 units once daily for 3–4 days or 25,000 units once every other day; dosage of 25,000 units should be continued every other day for 2 weeks after cultures are negative. **Ophthalmic solution:** 1–2 gtt 2–6 times daily, depending on the infection. Treatment may be necessary for 1–2 months or longer.

NURSING CONSIDERATIONS

See also *General Nursing Considerations For All Anti-Infectives,* p. 83.

Administration/Storage

1. Store and dilute as directed on package insert.
2. Pain on IM injection can be lessened by reducing drug concentration as much as possible. It is preferable to give drug more frequently in more dilute doses. If ordered, procaine hydrochloride (2 ml of a 0.5%–1.0% solution per 5 units of dry powder) may be used for mixing the drug for IM injection.

3. *Never use preparations containing procaine hydrochloride for IV or intrathecal use.*

Assessment

1. Determine kidney function and urinary output. Rule out edema or any other evidence of urinary tract problems.
2. Assess respiratory function and note any history of problems.
3. Utilize assessment information as a baseline against which to measure possible outcomes of the use of the medication.

Interventions

1. Note any muscle weakness, an early sign of muscle paralysis related to neuromuscular blockade. Assess closely for evidence of respiratory paralysis and withhold drug. Neuromuscular blockade may respond to calcium chloride. Have emergency equipment readily available.
2. Monitor intake and output.
3. Anticipate reduced dose in clients with impaired renal function; observe for nephrotoxicity, characterized by albuminuria, urinary casts, nitrogen retention, and hematuria.
4. Use safety precautions for ambulatory or bedridden clients with neurologic disturbances.
5. Anticipate a prolonged regimen of topical application of polymyxin B solution because drug is not toxic when used in wet dressings, and the physician may wish to prevent emergence of resistant strains.

Client/Family Teaching

1. Avoid hazardous tasks because the drug may cause dizziness, vertigo, and ataxia.

2. Report any neurologic disturbances, demonstrated by dizziness, blurred vision, irritability, circumoral and peripheral numbness and tingling, weakness, and ataxia. These symptoms usually disappear within 24–48 hr after the drug is discontinued.

Evaluation: Evaluate client for laboratory evidence of negative culture reports and clinical evidence of symptom improvement.

Potassium acetate, parenteral (Rx)

Potassium acetate, Potassium bicarbonate, and Potassium citrate (Trikates)
Oral Solution: Tri-K (Rx)

Potassium bicarbonate and citric acid
Effervescent Tablets: K + Care ET, Klor-Con/EF (Rx)

Potassium bicarbonate and Potassium chloride
Effervescent Granules: Klorvess Effervescent Granules, Neo-K✹ (Rx). Effervescent Tablets: Klorvess, K-Lyte/Cl, K-Lyte/Cl 50, Potassium-Sandoz✹ (Rx)

Potassium bicarbonate and Potassium citrate
Effervescent Tablets: K-Lyte, K-Lyte DS (Rx)

Potassium chloride

Extended-release Capsules: K-Norm, Micro-K, Micro-K 10 (Rx). **Oral Solution:** Cena-K, K-10✿, Kaochlor-10 and -20✿, Kaochlor 10%, Kaochlor S-F 10%, Kaon-Cl 20% Liquid, Kay Ciel, KCl 5%✿, Klorvess 10% Liquid, Potachlor 10% and 20%, Potasalan, Roychlor-10% and -20%, Rum-K (Rx). **Powder for Oral Solution:** Kato, Kay Ciel, K + Care, K-Lor, Klor-Con Powder, Klor-Con/25 Powder, K-Lyte/Cl Powder, Potage (Rx). **Extended-release Tablets:** Apo-K✿, K + 10, Kalium Durules✿, Kaon-Cl, Kaon-Cl-10, K-Dur, K-Long✿, Klor-Con 8 and 10, Klotrix, K-Tab, Novolente-K✿, Slow-K, Slo-Pot 600✿, Slow-K✿, Ten-K (Rx)

Potassium chloride, Potassium bicarbonate, and Potassium citrate

Effervescent Tablets: Kaochlor-Eff (Rx)

Potassium gluconate

Elixir: Kaon, Kaylixir, K-G Elixir, Potassium-Rougier✿, Royonate✿ (Rx). **Tablets:** Kaon✿ (Rx)

Potassium gluconate and Potassium chloride

Oral Solution and Powder for Oral Solution: Kolyum (Rx)

Potassium gluconate and Potassium citrate

Oral Solution: Twin-K (Rx)

Classification: Electrolyte.

General Statement: Potassium is the major cation of the body's intracellular fluid. It is essential for the maintenance of important physiologic processes, including cardiac, smooth, and skeletal muscle function, acid-base balance, gastric secretions, renal function, protein and carbohydrate metabolism. Symptoms of hypokalemia include weakness, cardiac arrhythmias, fatigue, ileus, hyporeflexia or areflexia, tetany, polydipsia, and, in severe cases, flaccid paralysis and inability to concentrate urine. Loss of potassium is usually accompanied by a loss of chloride resulting in hypochloremic metabolic alkalosis.

The usual adult daily requirement of potassium is 40–80 mg. In adults, the normal plasma concentration of potassium ranges from 3.5 to 5 mEq/L. Concentrations of up to 5.6 mEq/L are normal in children.

Both hypokalemia and hyperkalemia, if uncorrected, can be fatal; thus, potassium must always be administered cautiously.

Potassium is readily and rapidly absorbed from the GI tract. Though a number of salts can be used to supply the potassium cation, potassium chloride is the agent of choice since hypochloremia frequently accompanies potassium deficiency. Dietary measures (bananas, orange juice) can often prevent and even correct potassium deficiencies.

Potassium is excreted by the kidney and is partially reabsorbed from the glomerular filtrate.

Uses: Correction of potassium deficiency caused by vomiting, diarrhea, excess loss of GI fluids, hyperadrenalism, malnutrition, debilitation, prolonged negative nitrogen balance, dialysis, metabolic alkalosis, diabetic acidosis, certain renal conditions, cardiac arrhythmias, cardiotonic glycoside toxicity, and myasthenia gravis (experimentally).

Long-term electrolyte replacement regimen or total parenteral nutrition with potassium-free solutions. Correction of potassium deficiency possibly caused by certain drugs, including many diuretics, adrenal corticosteroids, testosterone, or corticotropin.

Prophylaxis after major surgery when urine flow has been reestablished.

Contraindications: Severe renal function impairment, postoperatively before urine flow has been reestablished. Crush syndrome, Addison's disease, hyperkalemia from any cause, oliguria or azotemia, anuria, heat cramps, acute dehydration, severe hemolytic reactions, adynamia episodica hereditaria.

Special Concerns: Safety during pregnancy (category: C) and lactation and in children has not been established. Geriatric clients are at greater risk of developing hyperkalemia due to age-related changes in renal function. Administer with caution in the presence of cardiac and renal disease and in clients receiving potassium-sparing drugs.

Side Effects: Hypokalemia. *CNS:* Dizziness, mental confusion. *CV:* Arrhythmias; weak, irregular pulse; hypotension, heart block, ECG abnormalities, cardiac arrest. *GI:* Abdominal distention, anorexia, nausea, vomiting, diarrhea. *Neuromuscular:* Weakness, paresthesia of extremities, flaccid paralysis, areflexia, muscle or respiratory paralysis, weakness and heaviness of legs. *Other:* Malaise.

Hyperkalemia. *CV:* Bradycardia, then tachycardia, cardiac arrest. *GI:* Nausea, vomiting, diarrhea, abdominal cramps, GI bleeding or obstruction. Ulceration or perforation of the small bowel from enteric-coated potassium chloride tablets. *GU:* Oliguria, anuria. *Neuromuscular:* Weakness, tingling, paralysis. *Other:* Skin rashes, hyperkalemia.

Drug Interactions

Angiotensin-converting enzyme (ACE) inhibitors / May cause potassium retention $\rightarrow$ hyperkalemia

Digitalis glycosides / Cardiac arrhythmias

Potassium-sparing diuretics / Severe hyperkalemia with possibility of cardiac arrhythmias or arrest

Dosage: Highly individualized. Oral administration is preferred because the slow absorption from the GI tract prevents sudden, large increases in plasma potassium levels. Dosage is usually expressed as mEq/L of potassium. The bicarbonate, chloride, citrate, and gluconate salts are usually administered orally. The chloride, acetate, and phosphate may be administered by **slow IV** infusion.

IV infusion. *Serum K less than 2.0 mEq/L:* 400 mEq/day at a rate not to exceed 40 mEq/hr. *Serum K more than 2.5 mEq/L:* 200 mEq/day at a rate not to exceed 20 mEq/hr.

PO. Pediatric, IV infusion: Up to 3 mEq potassium/kg (or 40 mEq/m^2) daily.

Prophylaxis of hypokalemia: 16–24 mEq/day. *Potassium depletion:* 40–100 mEq/day. **Note:** Usual dietary intake of potassium is 40–250 mEq/day.

For clients with accompanying metabolic acidosis, an alkalizing potassium salt (potassium bicarbonate, potassium citrate, or potassium acetate) should be selected.

P

NURSING CONSIDERATIONS

Administration/Storage: PO

1. Dilute or dissolve liquid potassium in fruit or vegetable juice if not already in flavored base.
2. Chill to increase palatability.
3. Give oral doses 2–4 times daily. Hypokalemia should be corrected slowly over a period of 3–7 days to minimize the development of hyperkalemia.
4. Salt substitutes should not be used concomitantly with potassium preparations.
5. Administer dilute liquid solutions of potassium rather than tablets to clients with esophageal compression.

Parenteral

1. Administer slowly as ordered by the physician for each individual client.
2. Potassium should not be administered IV undiluted. Usual method is to administer by slow IV infusion in dextrose solution at a concentration of 40–80 mEq/L.
3. Ensure uniform distribution of potassium by inverting infusion container during addition of potassium solution and then by agitating the container. Squeezing the plastic container will not prevent potassium chloride from settling to the bottom.
4. Check site of administration frequently for pain and redness because drug is extremely irritating.
5. In critical clients, potassium chloride may be given slow IV in a solution of saline (unless contraindicated) because dextrose may lower serum potassium levels by producing an intracellular shift.
6. Administer all concentrated potassium infusions and riders with an infusion control device.
7. Have available sodium bicarbonate, calcium gluconate, and regular insulin for parenteral use to treat clients who develop hyperkalemia.
8. Have sodium polystyrene sulfonate (Kayexalate) available for oral/rectal administration in the event of hyperkalemia.
9. *Treatment of Overdose:* (Plasma potassium levels greater than 6.5 mEq/L.) All measures must be monitored by ECG. Measures consist of actions taken to shift potassium ions from plasma into cells by:
   - **Sodium bicarbonate:** IV infusion of 50–100 mEq over period of 5 min. May be repeated after 10–15 min if ECG abnormalities persist.
   - **Glucose and insulin:** IV infusion of 3 g glucose to 1 unit regular insulin to shift potassium into cells.
   - **Calcium gluconate–or other calcium salt** (only for clients not on digitalis or other cardiotonic glycosides): IV infusion of 0.5–1 g (5–10 ml of a 10% solution) over period of 2 min. Dosage may be repeated after 1–2 min if ECG remains abnormal. When ECG is approximately normal, the excess potassium should be removed from the body by administration of polystyrene sulfonate, hemodialysis or peritoneal dialysis (clients with renal insufficiency), or other means.
   - **Sodium polystyrene sulfonate, hemodialysis, peritoneal dialysis:** To remove potassium from the body.

Assessment

1. Obtain baseline serum electrolyte levels and ECG.
2. Note any prior history of impaired renal function.
3. Monitor the client's intake and output for adequate urinary flow before administering potassium. Impaired renal function can lead to hyperkalemia.

Interventions

1. Once parenteral potassium administration is initiated, discontinue administering potassium-rich foods and oral potassium medication to the client.
2. If the client develops abdominal pain, distention, or GI bleeding, withhold oral potassium medication and report to the physician.
3. Note client complaints of weakness, fatigue, or the presence of cardiac arrhythmias. These may be symptoms of hypokalemia indicating a low *intracellular* potassium level although the serum potassium level may appear to be within normal limits.
4. Monitor intake and output. If the client develops oliguria, anuria, or azoturia, withhold the drug, document and report to the physician.
5. Observe the client for symptoms of adrenal insufficiency or extensive tissue breakdown. Withhold potassium, document findings, and report to the physician.
6. Note client complaints of weakness or heaviness of the legs, the presence of a gray pallor, cold skin, listlessness, mental confusion, flaccid paralysis, hypotension, or cardiac arrhythmias. These are symptoms of hyperkalemia. The medication should be stopped and the physician notified immediately because the client may go into cardiovascular collapse.
7. While the client is on parenteral potassium, monitor ECG for signs of hyperkalemia, as evidenced by peaked T waves and a widened QRS.
8. Monitor the serum potassium levels while the client is receiving parenteral potassium. The normal level is 3.5–5.0 mEq/L. Any variation should be reported to the physician.

Client/Family Teaching

1. Clients receiving potassium-sparing diuretics, such as spironolactone or triamterene, should not take potassium supplements or eat foods high in potassium unless specifically designated by the physician.
2. Provide printed information explaining the symptoms of hypo- and hyperkalemia and stress when to call the physician.
3. Review the importance of potassium in the diet and to other medications prescribed for the client.
4. Explain that once the parenteral potassium is discontinued it is important to ingest potassium-rich foods such as citrus juices, bananas, apricots, raisins, and nuts. The daily requirement is usually 3–4 g or 40 to 60 mEq/L. Have a dietitian work with the client to ensure a proper dietary regimen and to assist with meal planning.
5. Instruct the client to swallow enteric-coated tablets and not to dissolve them in the mouth.

P

Evaluation: Evaluate client for:

- Laboratory evidence of successful correction of serum potassium deficiency
- Laboratory confirmation that serum potassium levels are within desired range, 3.5–5.0 mEq/L

Pravastatin sodium

(prah-vah-**STAH**-tin)
Pravachol (Rx)

Classification: Antihyperlipidemic agent.

Action/Kinetics: Pravastatin competitively inhibits 3-hydroxy-3-methyl-glutaryl-coenzyme A (HMG-CoA) reductase, the enzyme catalyzing the conversion of HMG-CoA to mevalonate in the biosynthesis of cholesterol. This results in an increased number of low-density lipoprotein (LDL) receptors on cell surfaces and enhanced receptor-mediated catabolism and clearance of circulating LDL. The drug also inhibits LDL production by inhibiting hepatic synthesis of very low-density lipoproteins (VLDL), the precursor of LDL. Elevated levels of total cholesterol, low-density lipoprotein cholesterol, and apolipoprotein B (a membrane transport complex for LDL) promote development of atherosclerosis and are lowered by pravastatin. Pravastatin is rapidly absorbed from the GI tract. **Peak plasma levels:** 1–1.5 hr. The drug undergoes significant first-pass extraction and metabolism in the liver, which is the site of action of the drug; thus, plasma levels may not correlate well with lipid-lowering effectiveness. **t½, elimination:** 77 hr. The drug is metabolized in the liver and ap-

proximately 20% of an oral dose is excreted through the urine and 70% in the feces.

Uses: Adjunct to diet for reducing elevated total and LDL-cholesterol levels in clients with primary hypercholesterolemia (type IIa and IIb) when the response to a diet with restricted saturated fat and cholesterol has not been effective.

Contraindications: Use to treat hypercholesterolemia due to hyperalphaproteinemia. Active liver disease; unexplained, persistent elevations in liver function tests. Use during pregnancy (pregnancy category: X), lactation, and in children less than 18 years of age.

Special Concerns: Use with caution in clients with a history of liver disease, renal insufficiency, or heavy alcohol use.

Side Effects: *Musculoskeletal:* Rhabdomyolysis with renal dysfunction secondary to myoglobinuria, myalgia, myopathy, muscle cramps. *CNS:* CNS vascular lesions characterized by perivascular hemorrhage, edema, and mononuclear cell infiltration of perivascular spaces; headache, dizziness, psychic disturbances. *GI:* Nausea, vomiting, diarrhea, constipation, abdominal pain, flatulence, heartburn, anorexia. *Respiratory:* Common cold, rhinitis, cough. *Neurologic:* Dysfunction of certain cranial nerves resulting in alteration of taste, impairment of extraocular movement, and facial paresis; paresthesia, peripheral neuropathy, tremor, vertigo, memory loss peripheral nerve palsy. *Hepatic:* Hepatitis, including chronic active hepatitis; cholestatic jaundice, fatty change in liver, fulminant hepatic necrosis, cirrhosis, hepatoma. *GU:* Urinary abnormality, erectile dysfunction, loss of libido, gynecomastia. *Hypersensitivity reaction:* Vasculitis, purpura, polymyalgia rheumatica, angioedema, lupus erythematosus-like syndrome, thrombocytopenia, hemolytic anemia, leukopenia, positive ANA, arthritis, arthralgia, urticaria, asthenia, ESR increase, fever, chills, photosensitivity, malaise, dyspnea, toxic epidermal necrolysis, Stevens-Johnson syndrome. *Ophthalmic:* Lens opacities, ophthalmoplegia. *Miscellaneous:* Rash, pruritus, cardiac chest pain, fatigue, influenza.

Drug Interactions

Bile acid sequestrants /
 ↓ Bioavailability of pravastatin
Clofibrate / ↑ Risk of myopathy
Cyclosporine / ↑ Risk of
 myopathy or rhabdomyolysis
Erythromycin / ↑ Risk of
 myopathy or rhabdomyolysis
Gemfibrozil / ↑ Risk of myopathy
 or rhabdomyolysis
Niacin / ↑ Risk of myopathy or
 rhabdomyolysis
Warfarin / ↑ Anticoagulant effect
 of warfarin

Laboratory Test Interferences: ↑ Creatine phosphokinase, AST, ALT.

Dosage: Tablets. Initial: 10–20 mg once daily at bedtime (geriatric clients should take 10 mg once daily at bedtime). **Maintenance dose:** 10–40 mg once daily at bedtime (maximum dose for geriatric clients is 20 mg daily).

NURSING CONSIDERATIONS

Administration/Storage

1. Client should be placed on a standard cholesterol-lowering diet for 3–6 months before beginning pravastatin therapy.

The diet should be continued during therapy.
2. Drug may be taken without regard to meals.
3. The maximum effect is seen within 4 weeks during which time periodic lipid determinations should be undertaken.

Assessment

1. Assess for any evidence of liver disease or alcohol abuse.
2. Obtain baseline labs including a lipid profile, serum cholesterol level, CBC, liver and renal function studies.
3. Determine that secondary causes for hypercholesterolemia are ruled out. Secondary causes include hypothyroidism, poorly controlled diabetes mellitus, dysproteinemias, obstructive liver disease, nephrotic syndrome, alcoholism, and other drug therapy.
4. If female of childbearing age and sexually active, determine if pregnant.

Interventions

1. Liver function tests should be performed prior to pravastatin therapy, every 6 weeks during the first 3 months of therapy, every 8 weeks during the remainder of the first year, and at about 6- month intervals thereafter.
2. Pravastatin should be discontinued if markedly elevated creatine phosphokinase levels occur or myopathy is diagnosed or suspected.
3. Pravastatin should be discontinued temporarily in clients experiencing an acute or serious condition (e.g., sepsis, hypotension, major surgery,

P

trauma, uncontrolled epilepsy, or severe metabolic, endocrine, or electrolyte disorders) predisposing to the development of renal failure secondary to rhabdomyolysis.

Client/Family Teaching

1. Review the prescribed dietary recommendations (restricted cholesterol and saturated fats), assess client understanding of dietary guidelines, and refer to a dietitian as needed.
2. Instruct client to report any unexplained muscle pain, tenderness, or weakness, especially if accompanied by malaise or fever.
3. Advise client to practice birth control and to notify physician if pregnancy is suspected. Review potential hazards of drug therapy to a developing fetus.

Evaluation: Evaluate client for laboratory evidence of effective reduction of total cholesterol and LDL levels.

Prazepam
(PRAY-zeh-pam)
Centrax (C-IV, Rx)

See also *Benzodiazepines,* p. 108.

Classification: Antianxiety agent, benzodiazepine type.

Action/Kinetics: Significant first-pass effect results in biotransformation to the active metabolites desmethyldiazepam and oxazepam. **Peak plasma levels:** 2.5–6 hr for desmethyldiazepam. Slow onset. **t½, desmethyldiazepam:** 30–100 hr; **oxazepam,** 5–15 hr.

Uses: Antianxiety agents. Psycho-

neurosis associated with various disease states.

Special Concerns: Pregnancy category: D. Dosage has not been established in children less than 18 years of age.

Dosage: Capsules, Tablets. Adults: 10 mg t.i.d. (range 20–60 mg daily); or may be administered in a single dose at night: 20–40 mg at bedtime. **Geriatric and debilitated clients: initial,** 10–15 mg daily in divided doses.

NURSING CONSIDERATIONS

See *Nursing Considerations* for *Benzodiazepines,* p. 111.

Evaluation: Evaluate client for reports of a reduction in anxiety levels.

Praziquantel
(pray-zih-**KWON**-tell)
Biltricide (Rx)

Classification: Anthelmintic.

Action/Kinetics: Praziquantel causes increased cell permeability in the helminth, resulting in a loss of intracellular calcium with massive contractions, and paralysis of musculature with breakdown of the integrity of the organism. Thus, phagocytes can attack the parasite and death follows. **Maximum serum levels:** 1–3 hr. **t½:** 0.8–1.5 hr. Levels in the cerebrospinal fluid are approximately 14%–20% of the total amount of the drug in the plasma. Significant first-pass effect. Excreted primarily in the urine.

Uses: Schistosomal infections due to *Schistosoma japonicum, S. mansoni, S. mekongi,* and *S. hematobium.* Liver flukes (*Chonorchis* *sinensis, Opisthorchis viverrni). Investigational:* Neurocysticercosis, other tissue flukes, and intestinal cestodes.

Contraindications: Ocular cysticercosis. Lactation.

Special Concerns: Pregnancy category: B (use with caution in pregnancy). Safety in children less than 4 years of age not established.

Side Effects: *GI:* Nausea, abdominal discomfort. *CNS:* Malaise, headache, dizziness, drowsiness. *Miscellaneous:* Fever, urticaria (rare). **Note:** These side effects may also be due to the helminth infection itself. *Symptoms of Overdose:* Extention of side effects.

Dosage: Tablets. *Schistosomiasis:* Three doses of 20 mg/kg with an interval between doses not less than 4 hr or more than 6 hr. *Chonorchiasis and opisthorchiasis:* Three doses of 25 mg/kg as a one-day treatment.

NURSING CONSIDERATIONS

See *Nursing Considerations* for *Anthelmintics,* p. 42.

Administration/Storage: *Treatment of Overdose:* Administer a fast-acting laxative.

Assessment: Determine if the schistosomiasis or fluke infection is accompanied by cerebral cysticercosis. In this event, the client should be hospitalized for treatment.

Client/Family Teaching

1. Due to dizziness and drowsiness, caution should be exercised while driving or performing tasks requiring alertness.
2. The tablets should be taken as directed, during meals with

liquids. The tablets should not be chewed.

Evaluation: Evaluate client for evidence of successful treatment of parasitic infestation with laboratory evidence of negative culture reports.

Prazosin hydrochloride
(PRAY-zoh-sin)
Apo-Prazo✦, Minipress (Rx)

Classification: Antihypertensive, alpha-1 adrenergic blocking agent.

Action/Kinetics: Produces selective blockade of postsynaptic alpha-1 adrenergic receptors. Dilates arterioles and veins, thereby decreasing total peripheral resistance and decreasing diastolic blood pressure more than systolic blood pressure. Cardiac output, heart rate, and renal blood flow are not affected. Can be used to initiate antihypertensive therapy and is most effective when used with other agents (e.g., diuretics, beta-adrenergic blocking agents). **Onset:** 2 hr. **Maximum effect:** 2–3 hr; **duration:** 6–12 hr. **t½:** 2–4 hr. Full therapeutic effect: 4–6 weeks. Metabolized extensively; excreted primarily in feces.

Uses: Mild to moderate hypertension. *Investigational:* Congestive heart failure refractory to other treatment. Raynaud's disease, ergot alkaloid toxicity, pheochromocytoma.

Special Concerns: Safe use during pregnancy (category: C) and childhood has not been established. Use with caution during lactation. Geriatric clients may be more sensitive to the hypotensive and hypothermic effects of prazosin; also, it may be necessary to decrease the dose in these clients due to age-related decreases in renal function.

Side Effects: First-dose effect: Marked hypotension and syncope 30–90 min after administration of initial dose (usually 2 or more mg), increase of dosage, or addition of other **antihypertensive agent.** *CNS:* Dizziness, drowsiness, headache, fatigue, paresthesias, depression, vertigo, nervousness, hallucinations. *CV:* Palpitations, syncope, tachycardia, orthostatic hypotension, aggravation of angina. *GI:* Nausea, vomiting, diarrhea or constipation, dry mouth, abdominal pain, pancreatitis. *GU:* Urinary frequency or incontinence, impotence, priapism. *Miscellaneous:* Asthenia, sweating, symptoms of lupus erythematosus, blurred vision, tinnitus, epistaxis, nasal congestion, reddening of sclera, rash, alopecia, pruritus, dyspnea, edema, fever.

Drug Interactions

Antihypertensives (other) / ↑ Antihypertensive effect
Diuretics / ↑ Antihypertensive effect
Indomethacin / ↓ Effect of prazosin
Nifedipine / ↑ Hypotensive effect
Propranolol / Especially pronounced additive hypotensive effect
Verapamil / ↑ Hypotensive effect

Laboratory Test Interferences: ↑ Urinary metabolites of norepinephrine, VMA.

Dosage: Capsules/Tablets: *individualized,* always initiate with 0.5–1 mg b.i.d.–t.i.d.; **maintenance:** if necessary, increase gradually to 6–15 mg daily in 2–3 divided doses.

Daily dose should not exceed 20 mg. If used with diuretics or other antihypertensives, reduce dose to 1–2 mg t.i.d. **Pediatric, less than 7 years of age, initial:** 0.25 mg b.i.d.–t.i.d. adjusted according to response. **Pediatric, 7–12 years of age, initial:** 0.5 mg b.i.d.–t.i.d. adjusted according to response.

NURSING CONSIDERATIONS

See also *Nursing Considerations* for *Antihypertensive Agents,* p. 78

Administration/Storage

1. The first dose should be taken at bedtime.
2. Due to the first-dose effect, clients should not drive or operate machinery for 24 hr after the first dose.
3. In the event of overdosage, treat for shock with plasma volume expanders and vasopressor drugs as necessary.
4. *Treatment of Overdose:* Keep client supine to restore blood pressure and heart rate. If shock is manifested, use volume expanders and vasopressors; maintain renal function.

Client/Family Teaching

1. Food may delay absorption and minimize side effects of the drug.
2. Comply with prescribed drug regimen because the full effect of drug may not be evident for 4–6 weeks.
3. Report any bothersome side effects because reduction in dosage may be indicated.
4. Do not discontinue medication unless directed by medical supervision.
5. Avoid cold, cough, and allergy medications, unless physician

approves. The sympathomimetic component of such medications will interfere with the action of prazosin.

6. Do not engage in activities requiring alertness, such as operating machinery or driving a car, until drug effects are determined. The drug may cause dizziness and drowsiness.

7. Avoid rapid postural changes that may precipitate weakness, dizziness, and syncope.

8. Lie down or sit down and put head below knees to avoid fainting if a rapid heartbeat is felt.

9. Avoid dangerous situations that may lead to fainting.

Evaluation: Evaluate client for:
- Evidence of a reduction in blood pressure
- Improvement in symptoms of refractory CHF

Prednisolone
(pred-**NISS**-oh-lohn)
Syrup: Prelone. Tablets: Delta-Cortef (Rx)

Prednisolone acetate
(pred-**NISS**-oh-lohn)
Parenteral: Articulose-50, Key-Pred 25 and 50, Predaject-50, Predalone 50, Predcor-25 and -50, Predicort-50 (Rx). Ophthalmic Suspension: AK-Tate, Econopred, Econopred Plus, Ocu-Pred-A, Ophtho-Tate✿, Predair A, Pred Forte, Pred Mild, Ultra Pred (Rx)

Prednisolone acetate and Prednisolone sodium phosphate
(pred-**NISS**-oh-lohn)
(Rx)

Prednisolone sodium phosphate
(pred-**NISS**-oh-lohn)
Oral Solution: Pediapred (Rx). Ophthalmic Solution: AK-Pred, Inflamase✿, Inflamase Forte, Inflamase Mild, I-Pred, Lite Pred, Ocu-Pred, Ocu-Pred Forte, Predair, Predair Forte (Rx). Parenteral: Hydeltrasol, Key-Pred-SP (Rx)

Prednisolone tebutate
(pred-**NISS**-oh-lohn)
Hydeltra-T.B.A., Predalone T.B.A., Prednisol TPA (Rx)

See also *Adrenocorticosteroids and Analogs,* p. 8.

Classification: Adrenocorticosteroid, synthetic.

Action/Kinetics: Intermediate-acting. Prednisolone is five times more potent than hydrocortisone and cortisone. Side effects are minimal except for GI distress. Has moderate mineralocorticoid activity. **Plasma t½:** over 200 min.

Contraindications: Lactation.

Special Concerns: Use during pregnancy only if benefits outweigh risks. Use with particular caution in diabetes.

Dosage: *Prednisolone.* **PO:** 5–60 mg/day, depending on disease being treated. *Multiple sclerosis (exacerbation):* 200 mg/day for 1 week; **then,** 80 mg on alternate days for 1 month. *Pleurisy of tuberculosis:* 0.75 mg/kg daily (then taper) given concurrently with antituberculosis therapy. *Prednisolone acetate.* **IM:** 4–60 mg daily. **Not for IV use. Intralesional, intra-articular, soft tissue injection:** 4–100 mg (larger doses for large joints). *Multiple sclerosis*

P

(exacerbation): See *Prednisolone.*
Ophthalmic (0.12%–1% suspension): 1–2 drops in the conjunctival sac q hr during the day and q 2 hr during the night; **then,** after response obtained, decrease dose to 1 drop q 6–8 hr. *Prednisolone acetate and prednisolone sodium phosphate. Systemic.* **IM only:** 20–80 mg acetate and 5–20 mg sodium phosphate q several days for 3–4 weeks. **Intra-articular, intrasynovial:** 20–40 mg prednisolone acetate and 5–10 mg prednisolone sodium phosphate. *Prednisolone sodium phosphate.* **Oral Solution:** 5–60 mg daily in single or divided doses. *Adrenocortical insufficiency:* **Pediatric,** 0.14 mg/kg (4 mg/m²) daily in 3–4 divided doses. *Other uses:* **Pediatric:** 0.5–2 mg/kg (15–60 mg/m²) daily in 3–4 divided doses. **IM, IV:** 4–60 mg/day. *Multiple sclerosis (exacerbation):* See *Prednisolone.* **Intralesional, intra-articular, soft tissue injection:** 2–30 mg, depending on site and severity of disease. **Ophthalmic** (0.125%–1% solution): See *Prednisolone Acetate. Prednisolone tebutate.* **Intra-articular, intralesional, soft tissue injection:** 4–30 mg, depending on site and severity of disease. Doses higher than 40 mg are not recommended.

NURSING CONSIDERATIONS

See also *Nursing Considerations* for *Adrenocorticosteroids and Analogs,* p. 15.

Administration/Storage

1. Before administering prednisolone, check spelling and dose carefully; this drug is frequently confused with prednisone.
2. Check to see if physician wants

oral form of drug administered with an antacid.
3. Prednisolone sodium phosphate oral solution produces a 20% higher peak plasma level of prednisolone than is seen with tablets.

Evaluation: Evaluate client for:
- Reports of symptomatic improvement
- Reports of a reduction in allergic, immune, and inflammatory manifestations

---

Prednisone

(PRED-nih-sohn)

Oral Solution: Prednisone Intensol Concentrate (Rx). Syrup: Liquid Pred (Rx). Tablets: Apo-Prednisone ✳, Deltasone, Meticorten, Novo-Prednisone ✳, Orasone 1, 5, 10, 20, and 50, Panasol-S, Prednicen-M, Sterapred, Sterapred DS, Winpred ✳ (Rx)

See also *Adrenocorticosteroids and Analogs,* p. 8.

Classification: Adrenocorticosteroid, synthetic.

Action/Kinetics: Drug is three to five times as potent as cortisone or hydrocortisone. May cause moderate fluid retention. Prednisone is metabolized in the liver to prednisolone, the active form.

Special Concerns: Use during pregnancy only if benefits outweigh risks.

Dosage: *Highly individualized.* **Oral Solution, Syrup, Tablets: (acute, severe conditions): initial,** 5–60 mg daily, in 4 equally divided doses after meals and at bedtime. Decrease gradually by 5–10 mg q 4–5 days to establish minimum maintenance dosage (5–10 mg) or discontinue altogether until symptoms recur. **Pediatric:** *Replacement,* 0.1–0.15 mg/kg daily. *Chronic obstructive pulmonary disease:* 30–60 mg daily for 1–2 weeks; then taper. *Ophthalmopathy due to Graves' disease:* 60 mg daily; **then,** taper to 20 mg daily. *Duchenne's muscular dystrophy:* 0.75–1.5 mg/kg daily (used to improve strength).

NURSING CONSIDERATIONS

See *Nursing Considerations* for *Adrenocorticosteroids and Analogs,* p. 15.

Primaquine phosphate
(**PRIM**-ah-kwin)
(Rx)

Classification: 8-Aminoquinoline, antimalarial.

Action/Kinetics: Mechanism of action not known, but the drug binds to and may alter the properties of DNA leading to decreased protein synthesis. Both the gametocyte and exoerythrocyte forms are inhibited. Well absorbed from GI tract. **Peak plasma levels:** 2 hr. Poorly distributed in body tissues. **t½ elimination:** 4 hr.

Uses: It produces a radical cure of vivax malaria by eliminating both exoerythrocytic and erythrocytic forms (thus preventing relapse). Primaquine also is active against the sexual forms (gametocytes) of plasmodia resulting in disruption of transmission of the disease by eliminating the reservoir from which the mosquito carrier is infected. Also used following termination of chloroquine phosphate suppression therapy where vivax malaria is endemic.

Contraindications: Very active forms of vivax and falciparum malaria. Use during pregnancy only if benefits outweigh risks. Concomitant use with quinacrine. In clients with rheumatoid arthritis or lupus erythematosis who are acutely ill or who have a tendency to develop granulocytopenia. Concomitant use with other bone marrow depressants or hemolytic drugs.

Special concerns: Use during pregnancy only when benefits outweigh risks.

Side Effects: *GI:* Abdominal cramps, epigastric distress, nausea, vomiting. *Hematologic:* Methemoglobinemia. Blacks and members of certain Mediterranean ethnic groups (Sardinians, Sephardic Jews, Greeks, Iranians) manifest a high incidence of glucose-6-phosphate dehydrogenase (G6PD) deficiency and as a result have a low tolerance for primaquine. These individuals manifest marked hemolytic anemia following primaquine administration. *Miscellaneous:* Headache, pruritus, interference with visual accommodation, cardiac arrhythmias, hypertension. *Symptoms of Overdose:* Abdominal cramps, burning and epigastric distress, cyanosis, methemoglobinemia, anemia, leukocytosis or leukopenia, CNS and cardiovascular disturbances. Granulocytopenia and acute hemolytic anemia in sensitive clients.

Drug Interactions

Bone marrow depressants, hemolytic drugs / Additive side effects

Quinacrine / Quinacrine interferes with metabolic degradation of primaquine and thus enhances its toxic side reactions. **Do not give**

primaquine to clients who are receiving or have received quinacrine within the past 3 months.

Dosage: Tablets: *Acute attack of vivax malaria, clients with parasitized red blood cells:* 15 mg (base) daily for 14 days together with chloroquine phosphate (to destroy erythrocytic parasites). *Suppression of malaria:* **Adults,** 26.3 mg (15 mg base) daily for 14 days or 78.9 mg once a week for 8 weeks; **children:** 0.68 mg/kg/day (0.5 mg/kg base) for 14 days.

NURSING CONSIDERATIONS

See also *General Nursing Considerations For All Anti-Infectives,* p. 83, and *4-Aminoquinolines,* p. 28.

Administration/Storage

1. Store in tightly closed containers.
2. For suppression therapy, initiate during the last 2 weeks of or after suppressive therapy with chloroquine or a similar drug.
3. *Treatment of Overdose:* Treat symptoms.

Assessment

1. Note any history of rheumatoid arthritis or lupus erythematosis.
2. List other medications currently prescribed.

Interventions

1. Monitor for indications to withdraw drug: dark urine that indicates hemolysis and a marked fall in hemoglobin or erythrocyte count.
2. Assess dark-skinned clients closely. Because of a possible inborn deficiency of G6PD, these clients are particularly

susceptible to hemolytic anemia while on primaquine.

Client/Family Teaching

1. For suppressive therapy, take drug on same day each week.
2. Take medication immediately before or after meal or with antacids, so as to minimize gastric irritation.
3. Monitor color of urine and report immediately any darkening or brown color.
4. Stress the importance of completing a full course of therapy for effective drug results.

Evaluation: Evaluate client for evidence of successful termination of acute malarial attacks and suppression of malarial symptoms.

Primidone

(PRIH-mih-dohn)
Apo-Primidone❉, Mysoline, PMS Primidone ❉, Sertan❉ (Rx)

Classification: Anticonvulsant, miscellaneous.

Action/Kinetics: Primidone is closely related to the barbiturates; however, the mechanism for its anticonvulsant effects is unknown. Primidone produces a greater sedative effect than barbiturates when used for seizure treatment. Side effects usually subside with use. **Peak plasma levels:** 3 hr. Primidone is converted in the liver to two active metabolites, phenobarbital and phenylethylmalonamide (PEMA). **Peak plasma levels (PEMA):** 7–8 hr. **t½ (primidone):** 3–24 hr; **t½ (PEMA):** 24–48 hr; **t½ (phenobarbital):** 72–144 hr. The appearance of phenobarbital in the plasma may be delayed several days after initiation of therapy. **Therapeutic plasma levels, primadone:** 5–12 mcg/ml; **phenobarbital,** 10–30 mcg/ml. Primidone and metabolites are excreted through the kidneys.

Uses: Psychomotor seizures, focal seizures, or refractory tonic-clonic seizures. May be used alone or with other drugs. Often reserved for client refractory to barbiturate-hydantoin regimen. *Investigational:* Benign familial tremor.

Contraindications: Porphyria. Hypersensitivity to phenobarbital. Lactation.

Special Concerns: Safe use during pregnancy has not been determined. Use during lactation may result in drowsiness in the neonate. Children and geriatric clients may react to primidone with restlessness and excitement. Due to differences in bioavailability, brand interchange is not recommended.

Side Effects: *CNS:* Drowsiness, ataxia, vertigo, irritability, general malaise, headache, fatigue, emotional disturbances, including mood changes and paranoia. *GI:* Nausea, vomiting, anorexia, painful gums. *Hematologic:* Megaloblastic anemia, leukopenia, thrombocytopenia. *Ophthalmologic:* Diplopia, nystagmus. *Miscellaneous:* Skin rash, edema of eyelids and legs, alopecia, impotence, morbilliform and maculopapular skin rashes. Occasionally has caused hyperexcitability, especially in children. Postpartum hemorrhage and hemorrhagic disease of the newborn. Symptoms of systemic lupus erythematosus.

Drug Interactions: See also *Barbiturates,* p. 101.
Acetazolamide / ↓ Effect of primidone
Carbamazepine / ↑ Plasma levels of primidone and phenobarbital and ↑ plasma levels of carbamazepine
Hydantoins / ↑ Plasma levels of primidone, phenobarbital, and phenylethylmalonamide
Isoniazid / ↑ Effect of primidone due to ↓ breakdown by liver
Nicotinamide / ↑ Effect of primidone due to ↓ rate of clearance from body
Succinimides / ↓ Plasma levels of primidone and phenobarbital

Dosage: Oral Suspension, Tablets. Adults and children over 8 years: initial, *in clients on no other anticonvulsant medication:* days 1–3, 100–125 mg at bedtime; days 4–6, 100–125 mg b.i.d.; days 7–9, 100–125 mg t.i.d.; **maintenance:** 250 mg t.i.d. (may be increased to 250 mg 5–6 times per day; daily dosage should not exceed 500 mg q.i.d.). **Children under 8 years: initial,** days 1–3, 50 mg at bedtime; days 4–6, 50 mg b.i.d.; days 7–9, 100 mg b.i.d.; **maintenance:** 125 mg b.i.d.–250 mg t.i.d. (10–25 mg/kg in divided doses). *If client receiving other anticonvulsants:* **initial,** 100–125 mg at bedtime; **then,** increase to maintenance levels as other drug is slowly withdrawn (transition should take at least 2 weeks).

NURSING CONSIDERATIONS

See also *Nursing Considerations* for *Anticonvulsants,* p. 63.

Client/Family Teaching

1. Review the goals of therapy and associated side effects of drug therapy. Instruct the client/family that the following conditions should be reported to the physician:
   • Hyperexcitability in children

- Excessive loss of hair
- Edema of eyelids and legs
- Impotence

2. Remind the pregnant client that the physician may order vitamin K during the last month of pregnancy. This is to prevent postpartum hemorrhage in the mother and hemorrhagic disease of the newborn.
3. May be taken with food if GI upset occurs.

Evaluation: Evaluate client for:
- Evidence of control of seizures
- Laboratory confirmation that serum drug levels are within therapeutic range (5–12 mcg/ml)

Probenecid
(proh-**BEN**-ih-sid)
Benemid, Benuryl✳, Probalan (Rx)

Classification: Antigout agent, uricosuric agent.

Action/Kinetics: Probenecid, a uricosuric agent, increases the excretion of uric acid by inhibiting the tubular reabsorption of uric acid; this action results in a decreased serum level of uric acid. Probenecid also inhibits the renal secretion of penicillins and cephalosporins; this effect is often taken advantage of in the treatment of infections because concomitant administration of probenecid will increase plasma levels of antibiotics. **Peak plasma levels:** 2–4 hr. **Time to peak effect, uricosuric:** 0.5 hr; **for suppression of penicillin excretion:** 2 hr. **Therapeutic plasma levels for inhibition of antibiotic secretion:** 40–60 mcg/ ml; **therapeutic plasma levels for uricosuric effect:** 100–200 mcg/ml. **t½:** approximately 5–8 hr. **Duration for inhibition of penicillin excretion:** 8 hr. Probenecid is metabolized in the liver to active metabolites and is excreted in urine (5%–10% unchanged). Excretion is increased in alkaline urine.

Uses: Hyperuricemia in chronic gout and gouty arthritis. Adjunct in therapy with penicillins or cephalosporins to elevate and prolong plasma antibiotic levels.

Contraindications: Hypersensitivity to drug, blood dyscrasias, uric acid, and kidney stones. Use for hyperuricemia in neoplastic disease or its treatment. Not recommended for use in children less than 2 years of age.

Special Concerns: Use during pregnancy only if benefits clearly outweigh risks. Administer with caution to clients with renal disease. Use with caution in porphyria, glucose-6-phosphate dehydrogenase (G6PD) deficiency, and peptic ulcer.

Side Effects: *CNS:* Headaches, dizziness. *GI:* Anorexia, nausea, vomiting, diarrhea, constipation, and abdominal discomfort. *Allergic:* Skin rash or drug fever, and rarely anaphylactoid reactions. *GU:* Nephrotic syndrome, uric acid stones with or without hematuria, urinary frequency, renal colic. *Miscellaneous:* Hypersensitivity reactions (dermatitis, pruritus, fever, anaphylaxis), flushing, hemolytic anemia, sore gums, hepatic necrosis, aplastic anemia, costovertebral pain.

Initially, the drug may increase frequency of acute gout attacks due to mobilization of uric acid.

Drug Interactions

Acyclovir / Probenecid ↓ renal excretion of acyclovir

Allopurinol / Additive effects to ↓ uric acid serum levels

Aminosalicylic acid (PAS) / ↑ Effects of PAS due to ↓ excretion by kidney

Captopril / ↑ Effect of captopril due to ↓ excretion by kidney

Cephalosporins / ↑ Effect of cephalosporins due to ↓ excretion by kidney

Ciprofloxacin / 50% ↑ in systemic levels of ciprofloxacin

Clofibrate / ↑ Effect of clofibrate due to ↓ excretion and ↓ plasma protein binding

Dapsone / ↑ Effect of dapsone

Dyphylline / ↑ Effect of dyphylline due to ↓ excretion by kidney

Indomethacin / ↑ Effect of indomethacin due to ↓ excretion by kidney

Methotrexate / ↑ Effect of methotrexate due to ↓ excretion by kidney

Nonsteroidal anti-inflammatory drugs / ↑ Effect of NSAIDs due to ↓ excretion by kidney

Penicillins / ↑ Effect of penicillins due to ↓ excretion by kidney

Pyrazinamide / Probenecid inhibits hyperuricemia produced by pyrazinamide

Rifampin / ↑ Effect of rifampin due to ↓ excretion by kidney

Salicylates / Salicylates inhibit uricosuric activity of probenecid

Sulfinpyrazone / ↑ Effect of sulfinpyrazone due to ↓ excretion by kidney

Sulfonamides / ↑ Effect of sulfonamides due to ↓ plasma protein binding

Sulfonylureas, oral / ↑ Action of sulfonylureas → hypoglycemia

Thiopental / ↑ Effect of thiopental

Zidovudine / ↑ Bioavailability of zidovudine

Dosage: Tablets. Adults: *Gout,* **PO, initial:** 250 mg b.i.d. for 1 week. **Maintenance:** 500 mg b.i.d. Dosage may have to be increased further (by 500 mg daily q 4 weeks to maximum of 2 g) until urate excretion is less than 700 mg in 24 hr. *Adjunct to penicillin or cephalosporin therapy:* 500 mg q.i.d. Dosage is decreased for elderly clients with renal damage. **Pediatric, 2–14 years, initial:** 25 mg/kg (or 700 mg/m^2); **maintenance,** 10 mg/kg q.i.d. (or 300 mg/m^2 q.i.d.). **For children 50 kg or more:** give adult dosage. Colbenemid, a combination tablet containing colchicine (0.5 mg) and probenecid (500 mg), is available. *Gonorrhea:* **Adults:** 1 g (as a single dose) 30 min before 4.8 million units of penicillin G procaine aqueous; **pediatric, less than 45 kg:** 25 mg/kg (up to a maximum of 1 g) with appropriate antibiotic therapy.

NURSING CONSIDERATIONS

Assessment

1. Note if the client has diabetes mellitus. There may be false + urine tests if cupric sulfate reagents such as Benedict's Qualitative Reagent are used.

2. Determine any evidence of peptic ulcer disease or G6PD deficiency.

Interventions

1. Anticipate that sodium bicarbonate may be used to maintain an alkaline urine to prevent urates from crystallizing and forming kidney stones.

2. Use a glucose oxidase method (Tes-Tape or Keto-Diastix) for

urine glucose determinations in clients with diabetes mellitus; finger sticks may be more accurate.

3. Promptly report any gastric intolerance so that dosage may be corrected without loss of therapeutic effect.

4. Be alert to hypersensitivity reactions that occur more frequently with intermittent therapy.

5. Assess for toxic plasma levels in clients whose excretion is inhibited by probenecid. Make appropriate dosage adjustments.

6. Observe client for skin rash, flushing or client complaints of increased sweating, headaches, or dizziness. Document and report to the physician.

7. Monitor CBC, liver and renal function studies on a regular basis. Report any abnormal findings to the physician.

Client/Family Teaching

1. Take the drug with food or milk to minimize gastric irritation.

2. Take a liberal amount of fluid (3 qt/day) to prevent the formation of sodium urate stones.

3. Note if there is any increase in the number of acute attacks of gout at the initiation of therapy. The physician may decide to add colchicine to the regimen.

4. Continue to take probenecid during acute attacks along with colchicine, as ordered, unless specifically told by the physician to discontinue the use of probenecid.

5. Do not take salicylates or use alcohol during uricosuric therapy. Acetaminophen preparations may be used for analgesic purposes.

6. Report any unexplained fever, fatigue, skin rash, or persistent GI upset to the physician.

Evaluation: Evaluate client for:

- Laboratory evidence of decreased serum uric acid level
- Reports of a reduction in joint pain and swelling associated with gout and gouty arthritis
- Any evidence of elevated and prolonged plasma antibiotic (penicillins or cephalosporins) levels
- Laboratory confirmation that serum drug levels are within desired range for designated effect

Probucol
(**PROH**-byou-kohl)
Lorelco (Rx)

Classification: Antihyperlipidemic.

Action/Kinetics: Mechanism for alteration of cholesterol metabolism unknown, although the drug increases excretion of fecal bile acids, inhibits early stages of cholesterol synthesis, and slightly inhibits absorption of cholesterol from the diet. Decreases LDL cholesterol, and HDL; produces no change in triglycerides and either does not change or increases VLDL levels. After prolonged administration, the drug becomes deposited in the adipose tissues, and after discontinuation persists in the body for up to 6 months. Absorption from the GI tract is variable (usually less than 10%). Food increases peak blood levels. **$t\frac{1}{2}$ (biphasic): initial** 24 hr; **final:** 20 days. **Therapeutic onset:** 2–4 weeks; maximum: 20–

50 days. Excreted through the feces and the urine (mainly unchanged).

Uses: Primary hypercholesterolemia, especially of type IIa, not responding to diet or weight control and clients who have a significant risk of coronary artery disease.

Contraindications: Hypersensitivity. Serious ventricular arrhythmias, unexplained syncope or syncope of cardiovascular origin, recent or progressive myocardial damage. In situations where the QT interval at an observed heart rate is more than 15% above the upper limit of normal (see package insert). Should not be used in treatment of elevated blood lipids to prevent coronary heart disease.

Special Concerns: Safe use during pregnancy (category: B) and lactation and in childhood has not been established.

Side Effects: *CV:* Prolongation of the QT interval on the ECG, syncope, ventricular arrhythmias; sudden death may occur. *GI:* Most common: diarrhea, anorexia, indigestion, flatulence, GI bleeding, abdominal pain, nausea, vomiting. *Ophthalmic:* Blurred vision, tearing, conjunctivitis. *CNS:* Headache, dizziness, insomnia, paresthesia. *Hematologic:* Thrombocytopenia, eosinophilia, low hemoglobin, low hematocrit. *Dermatologic:* Rash, pruritus, hyperhidrosis, fetid sweat, petechiae, ecchymosis. *Miscellaneous:* Angioneurotic edema, decreased taste and smell sensations, enlargement of multinodular goiter, tinnitus, peripheral neuritis.

During the beginning of therapy certain clients have manifested an idiosyncratic reaction including dizziness, syncope, nausea, vomiting, palpitations, and chest pain.

Laboratory Test Interferences: Transient ↑ AST, ALT, alkaline phosphatase, uric acid, bilirubin, creatine phosphatase, alkaline phosphatase, blood glucose, BUN.

Dosage: Tablets. Adults only: 500 mg b.i.d. with morning and evening meals. In some clients, 500 mg once daily may be as effective as giving the drug b.i.d.

NURSING CONSIDERATIONS

Administration/Storage

1. To be taken with morning and evening meals because food seems to increase absorption from the GI tract.
2. Clofibrate and probucol should not be given together because the combination may cause a significant decrease of HDL.
3. Store in a dry place, in light-resistant containers away from excessive heat.

Client/Family Teaching

1. Take with food, as directed, to enhance absorption. Continue to follow the prescribed dietary restrictions.
2. If diarrhea occurs, it is usually transient. Roughage should be eliminated until diarrhea stops.
3. Report any bothersome or persistent GI symptoms to physician.
4. Stress the importance of reporting any unexplained bruising or bleeding.
5. Clients may develop insomnia, dizziness, and/or headaches. These should be reported and a record kept of the frequency of occur rences.
6. If blurred vision occurs or if dizziness develops, client should avoid driving or using heavy equipment. The effects

of the medication need to be reevaluated.

7. Nocturia and impotence may occur. Discuss this when therapy is initiated. Report these developments at once because another medication may be necessary. Offer emotional support.

Evaluation: Evaluate client for:
- Laboratory evidence of a reduction in serum cholesterol levels
- Freedom from complications of adverse drug effects

Procainamide hydrochloride
(proh-**KAYN**-ah-myd)
Procan SR, Promine, Pronestyl, Pronestyl-SR (Rx)

See also *Antiarrhythmic Drugs*, p. 51.

Classification: Antiarrhythmic, type IA.

Action/Kinetics: Procainamide produces a direct cardiac effect to prolong the refractory period of the heart and depress the conduction of the cardiac impulse. Large doses may cause AV block. It has some anticholinergic and local anesthetic effects. **Onset: PO,** 30 min; **IV,** 1–5 min. **Time to peak effect, PO:** 60–90 min; **IM,** 15–60 min; **IV,** immediate. **Duration:** 3 hr. **t½:** 2.5–4.5 hr. **Therapeutic serum level:** 4–8 mcg/ml. **Protein binding:** 15%. From 50%–60% excreted unchanged.

Uses: Ventricular tachycardia, atrial fibrillation, resistant paroxysmal atrial tachycardia. Emergency treatment of ventricular tachycardia, digitalis intoxication, prophylactic control of tachycardia for clients at risk during anesthesia or undergoing thoracic surgery.

Contraindications: Hypersensitivity to drug, complete AV heart block, second- or third-degree AV heart block, myasthenia gravis, or blood dyscrasias.

Special Concerns: Safe use during pregnancy (category: C) and lactation has not been established. Use with extreme caution in clients for whom a sudden drop in BP could be detrimental, in clients with liver or kidney dysfunction, and in those with bronchial asthma or other respiratory disorders. Procainamide may cause more hypotension in geriatric clients; also, in this population, the dose may have to be decreased due to age-related decreases in renal function.

Side Effects: *CV:* Following IV use: Hypotension, ventricular asystole or fibrillation, partial or complete heart block. *GI:* Nausea, vomiting, diarrhea, anorexia, bitter taste, abdominal pain. *Hematologic:* Thrombocytopenia, agranulocytosis. *Allergic:* Urticaria, pruritus, angioneurotic edema, maculopapular rash. *CNS:* Depression, giddiness, psychoses, hallucinations. *Other:* Lupus erythematosus-like syndrome, especially in those on maintenance therapy. Also, granulomatous hepatitis, weakness, fever, chills.

Symptoms of Overdose: Nausea, vomiting, confusion, lethargy, oliguria, severe hypotension, junctional tachycardia, ECG changes, ventricular fibrillation.

Drug Interactions

Acetazolamide / ↑ Effect of procainamide due to ↓ excretion by kidney

Anticholinergic agents, atropine / Additive anticholinergic effects

Antihypertensive agents / Additive hypotensive effect

Cholinergic agents / Anticholinergic activity of procainamide antagonizes effect of cholinergic drugs

Cimetidine / ↑ Effect of procainamide due to ↓ excretion by kidney

Ethanol / ↓ Effect of procainamide due to ↑ rate of breakdown by liver

Kanamycin / Procainamide ↑ muscle relaxation produced by kanamycin

Lidocaine / Additive neurologic side effects

Magnesium salts / Procainamide ↑ muscle relaxation produced by magnesium salts

Neomycin / Procainamide ↑ muscle relaxation produced by neomycin

Sodium bicarbonate / ↑ Effect of procainamide due to ↓ excretion by the kidney

Succinylcholine / Procainamide ↑ muscle relaxation produced by succinylcholine

Laboratory Test Interferences: May affect liver function tests. False + ↑ serum alkaline phosphatase.

Dosage: Capsules / Tablets. Adults, initial: *Atrial arrhythmias:* **initial,** 1.25 g followed in 1 hr by 0.75 g; **then,** if no ECG changes, 0.5–1.0 g q 2 hr until arrhythmia stopped. **Maintenance:** 0.5–1.0 g q 4–6 hr. *Premature ventricular contractions:* 50 mg/kg daily in divided doses q 3 hr. *Ventricular tachycardia:* **initial,** 1.0 g; **then,** 6 mg/kg q 3 hr. **Pediatric,** *antiarrhythmic:* l2.5 mg/kg (375 mg/m²) q.i.d.

Sustained-release Tablets: Not recommended for initial therapy. **Maintenance:** *Atrial arrhythmias,* 1 g/6 hr. **Maintenance:** *ventricular arrhythmias,* 50 mg/kg/day in divided doses q 6 hr.

IM: Adults, 0.5–1.0 g q 4–8 hr until PO therapy possible. *Arrhythmias associated with surgery or anesthesia:* 0.1–0.5 g IM.

Direct IV use: 100 mg q 5 min by slow IV injection at a rate not to exceed 25–50 mg/min; give until arrhythmia stops or until 0.5 g is administered; **maintenance:** IV infusion, 2–6 mg/min. **IV infusion: initial,** 500–600 mg over 25–30 min; **then,** 2–6 mg/min. Switch to PO therapy as soon as possible, but wait at least 3–4 hr after the last IV dose.

NURSING CONSIDERATIONS

See also *Nursing Considerations* for *Antiarrhythmic Drugs,* p. 52.

Administration / Storage

1. IV use should be reserved for emergency situations.
2. For IV initial therapy, the drug should be diluted with 5% dextrose solution and administered slowly to minimize side effects.
3. For IV solutions, dose is usually 2–6 mg/min. Drug solutions should be administered with an electronic infusion device for safety and accuracy.
4. Discard solutions of drug that are darker than light amber or otherwise colored. Solutions that have turned slightly yellow on standing may be used. Consult with pharmacist for clarification.
5. Extended-release tablets are not recommended for use in children.

6. *Treatment of Overdose:*
   - Induce emesis or perform gastric lavage followed by administration of activated charcoal.
   - To treat hypotension, give IV fluids and/or a vasopressor (dopamine, phenylephrine, or norepinephrine).
   - Infusion of 1/6 molar sodium lactate IV reduces the cardiotoxic effects.
   - Hemodialysis (but not peritoneal dialysis) is effective in reducing serum levels.
   - Renal clearance can be enhanced by acidification of the urine and with high flow rates.
   - A ventricular pacing electrode can be inserted as a precaution in the event AV block develops.

Interventions

1. Place client in a monitored environment during IV administration. Have emergency drugs and equipment readily available.
2. Place client in a supine position during IV infusion and monitor BP frequently. Be prepared to discontinue infusion if BP falls 15 mm Hg or more during administration or if increased SA or AV block is noted on ECG and notify physician.
3. Assess clients on oral drug maintenance for symptoms of lupus erythematosus, as manifested by polyarthralgia, arthritis, pleuritic pain, fever, myalgia, and skin lesions.
4. Weigh clients and assess GI symptoms. If severe and persistent the physician may permit the client to take the medication with meals or with a snack to ensure compliance with drug therapy.
5. Monitor CBC, antinuclear antibody titers, and procainamide levels throughout therapy.

Client/Family Teaching

1. Review the anticipated results of therapy.
2. Take the medication with a full glass of water to lessen GI symptoms. The drug should be taken either 1 hr before or 2 hr after meals unless otherwise ordered by the physician.
3. Take medication only as directed. Set an alarm clock to awaken through the night to take the drug as ordered, if necessary.
4. If prescribed sustained-release preparations, they should be swallowed whole. They should not be crushed, broken, or chewed. The wax matrix of sustained-release tablets may be evident in the stool and is considered normal.
5. Report any sore throat, fever, rash, chills, bruising or diarrhea.
6. Stress the importance of reporting for scheduled laboratory studies.
7. Do not take any OTC drugs without physician approval.

Evaluation: Evaluate client for:
- ECG evidence of successful termination of cardiac arrhythmia
- Laboratory confirmation that serum drug levels are within therapeutic range (4–8 mcg/ml)

Procarbazine hydrochloride

(pro-**KAR**-bah-zeen)
Matulane, MIH, N-Methylhydrazine, Natulan✹ (Abbreviation: PCB) (Rx)

See also *Antineoplastic Agents,* p. 85.

Classification: Antineoplastic, miscellaneous.

Action/Kinetics: Procarbazine is both an alkylating agent and an inhibitor of MAO. The drug is cell-cycle specific for the S phase of cell division. It inhibits synthesis of protein, RNA, and DNA, possibly because of autooxidation (production of hydrogen peroxide). Well absorbed from GI tract. Drug equilibrates between plasma and CSF (peak levels occur within 30–90 min). **$t^{1/2}$, after IV:** 10 min. About 70% eliminated in urine, mostly as metabolites, after 24 hr. Procarbazine is mostly used in combination with other drugs (MOPP therapy).

Use: As an adjunct in the treatment of Hodgkin's disease (stage III and stage IV). *Investigational:* Non-Hodgkin's lymphomas, malignant melanoma, primary brain tumors, lung cancer, multiple myeloma, polycythemia vera.

Additional Contraindications: Hypersensitivity to drug. Depressed bone marrow. Low WBC and RBC or platelet counts. Lactation.

Special Concerns: Pregnancy category: D. Use with caution in impaired kidney or liver function.

Additional Side Effects: *GI:* Dysphagia, constipation or diarrhea.

CNS: Psychosis, manic reactions, insomnia, nightmares, foot drop, decreased reflexes, tremors, coma, delirium, convulsions. *Dermatologic:* Hyperpigmentation, photosensitivity. *Miscellaneous:* Petechiae, purpura, arthralgia, hemolysis, acute myelocytic leukemia, malignant myelosclerosis, azoospermia. In geriatric clients, the MAO inhibitor effects may cause increased vascular accidents and increased sensitivity to hypotensive effects.

Symptoms of Overdose: Nausea, vomiting, diarrhea, enteritis, hypotension, tremors, seizures, coma, hematologic and hepatic toxicity.

Drug Interactions

Alcohol / Antabuse-like reaction
Antihistamines / Additive CNS depression
Antihypertensive drugs / Additive CNS depression
Barbiturates / Additive CNS depression
Digoxin / ↓ Digoxin plasma levels if combination therapy used
Guanethidine / Excitation and hypertension
Hypoglycemic agents, oral / ↑ Hypoglycemic effect
Insulin / ↑ Hypoglycemic effect
Levodopa / Flushing and hypertension
MAO inhibitors / Possibility of hypertensive crisis
Methyldopa / Excitation and hypertension
Narcotics / Additive CNS depression
Phenothiazines / Additive CNS depression; also, possibility of hypertensive crisis
Reserpine / Excitation and hypertension
Sympathomimetics / Possibility of hypertensive crisis

P

Tricyclic antidepressants /
Possibility of hypertensive crisis
Tyramine-containing foods /
Possibility of hypertensive crisis

Dosage: Capsules. Adults: 2–4 mg/kg daily for first week; **then,** 4–6 mg/kg/day until leukocyte count falls below 4,000/mm³ or platelet count falls below 100,000/mm³. If toxic symptoms appear, discontinue drug and resume treatment at rate of 1–2 mg/kg/day; **maintenance:** 1–2 mg/kg/day. **Children:** *highly individualized,* 50 mg/m²/day for first week; then 100 mg/m² (to nearest 50 mg) until maximum response obtained.

NURSING CONSIDERATIONS

See also *Nursing Considerations* for *Antineoplastic Agents,* p. 88.

Administration/Storage: *Treatment of Overdose:* Induce vomiting or undertake gastric lavage. IV fluids. Frequent blood counts and liver function tests should be performed.

Client/Family Teaching

1. Unless approved by the physician, other prescription drugs should not be used.
2. Contraception should be practiced by both men and women.
3. Observe and report adverse CNS effects that may necessitate withdrawal of the drug, as noted under *Additional Side Effects.*
4. Do not drink alcohol because a disulfiram-type reaction may occur.
5. Consult physician before taking any other medication because procarbazine has MAO inhibitory activity. The use of sympathomimetic drugs and foods with a high tyramine content (yeasts, yogurt, caffeine, choco-

late, aged cheese, liver, smoked or pickled fish, fermented sausage, etc.) is contraindicated during therapy and for 2 weeks after discontinuing therapy. Ingestion of these products may precipitate a hypertensive crisis.
6. For clients with diabetes, procarbazine increases effect of insulin and oral hypoglycemics. Hypoglycemic symptoms should be reported to physician because adjustment of antidiabetic medication may be necessary.
7. Avoid exposure to sun or to ultraviolet rays because a photosensitive skin reaction may occur. Wear a sunscreen, sunglasses, and protective clothing if exposure is necessary.
8. Do not drive or perform tasks that require mental alertness until drug effects are realized.

Evaluation: Evaluate client for evidence of control of the size and spread of malignant tissue in Hodgkin's disease.

Prochlorperazine
(proh-klor-**PAIR**-ah-zeen)
Compazine, Prorazin✴, Stemetil✿ (Rx)

Prochlorperazine edisylate
(proh-klor-**PAIR**-ah-zeen)
Compazine Edisylate (Rx)

Prochlorperazine maleate
(proh-klor-**PAIR**-ah-zeen)
Compazine Maleate, PMS Prochlorperazine✴, Stemetil✿ (Rx)

See also *Phenothiazines,* p. 201.

Classification: Antipsychotic, antiemetic, piperazine-type phenothiazine.

Action/Kinetics: Prochlorperazine causes a high incidence of extrapyramidal and antiemetic effects, moderate sedative effects, and a low incidence of anticholinergic effects and orthostatic hypotension. It also possesses significant antiemetic effects.

Uses: Psychoneuroses. Postoperative nausea and vomiting, radiation sickness, vomiting due to toxins. Generally not used for clients who weigh less than 44 kg or who are under 2 years of age. Severe nausea and vomiting.

Special Concerns: Safe use during pregnancy has not been established. Dosage has not been established in children less than 2 years of age or 9.1 kg body weight. Geriatric, emaciated, and debilitated clients usually require a lower initial dose.

Dosage: Edisylate Syrup, Maleate Extended-release Capsules, Tablets. *Psychotic disorders:* **Adults and adolescents,** 5–10 mg (base) t.i.d.–q.i.d. (dose can be increased gradually q 2–3 days as needed and tolerated). For extended-release capsules, up to 100–150 mg daily can be given. **Pediatric, 2–12 years:** 2.5 mg (base) b.i.d.–t.i.d. *Nausea and vomiting:* **Adults and adolescents,** 5–10 mg (base) t.i.d.–q.i.d. (up to 40 mg daily). For extended-release capsules, the dose is 15–30 mg once daily in the morning (or 10 mg q 12 hr, up to 40 mg daily). **Pediatric, 18–39 kg:** 2.5 mg (base) t.i.d. (or 5 mg b.i.d.), not to exceed 15 mg daily; **14–17 kg:** 2.5 mg (base) b.i.d.–t.i.d., not to exceed 10 mg daily; **9–13 kg:** 2.5 mg (base) 1–2 times daily, not to exceed 7.5 mg daily. The total daily dose for children should not exceed 10 mg the first day; on subsequent days, the total daily dose should not exceed 20 mg for children 2–5 years of age or 25 mg for children 6–12 years of age. *Anxiety:* **Adults and adolescents,** 5 mg (base) t.i.d.–q.i.d. up to 20 mg daily for no longer than 12 weeks.

IM. Edisylate Injection. *Psychotic disorders, for immediate control of severely disturbed clients:* **Adults and adolescents:** 10–20 mg (base); dose can be repeated q 2–4 hr as needed (usually up to 3 or 4 doses). **Maintenance:** 10–20 mg (base) q 4–6 hr. **Pediatric:** 0.132 mg/kg. *Anxiety:* **Adults and adolescents,** 5–10 mg (base); dose can be repeated q 2–4 hr as needed. *Nausea and vomiting:* **Adults and adolescents,** 5–10 mg with the dose repeated q 3–4 hr as needed. **Pediatric, 2–12 years:** 0.132 mg/kg. *Nausea and vomiting during surgery:* **Adults and adolescents,** 5–10 mg (base) 1–2 hr before induction of anesthesia; to control symptoms during or after surgery, the dose can be repeated once after 30 min.

IV. Edisylate Injection. *Nausea and vomiting:* **Adults and adolescents,** 2.5–10 mg as a slow injection or infusion (rate should not exceed 5 mg/min up to 40 mg daily). *Nausea and vomiting during surgery:* **Adults and adolescents,** 5–10 mg (base) given as a slow injection or infusion 15–30 min before induction of anesthesia; to control symptoms during or after surgery the dose can be repeated once. The rate of infusion should not exceed 5 mg/ml/min.

Rectal Suppositories. Pediatric, 2–12 years: 2.5 mg b.i.d.–t.i.d.

with no more than 10 mg given on the first day. No more than 20 mg daily for children 2–5 years and 25 mg daily for children 6–12 years of age.

NURSING CONSIDERATIONS

See also *Nursing Considerations* for *Phenothiazines,* p. 205.

Administration/Storage

1. Store all forms of the drug in tight-closing amber-colored bottles; store the suppositories below 37°C (98.6°F).
2. Add the desired dosage of concentrate to 60 ml of beverage (e.g., tomato or fruit juice, milk, soup) or semisolid food just before administration to disguise the taste.
3. Drug should not be administered SC due to local irritation.
4. Prochlorperazine should not be mixed with other agents in a syringe.
5. Prochlorperazine should not be diluted with any material containing the preservative parabens.
6. When given IM to children for nausea and vomiting, the duration of action may be 12 hr.
7. Parenteral prescribing limits are 20 mg daily for children 2–5 years of age and 25 mg daily for children 6–12 years of age.

Interventions

1. Have emergency equipment and drugs available when treating an overdose.
2. Monitor vital signs and incorporate safety precautions during the treatment of an overdose.
3. If the client was taking span-

sules, continue the treatment until all signs of overdosage are no longer evident.
4. In treating clients for an overdosage, anticipate that saline laxatives may be used to hasten the evacuation of pellets that have not yet released their medication.

Client/Family Teaching

1. Advise parents not to exceed the prescribed dose of drug.
2. If the child shows signs of restlessness and excitement, withhold the medication and notify the physician.
3. Do not drive or operate machinery until drug effects are realized because drowsiness or dizziness may occur.
4. Review symptoms of extrapyramidal effects and tardive dyskinesia and advise to report immediately if evident.

Evaluation: Evaluate client for:
- Reports of a decreased incidence of nausea and vomiting
- Evidence of behavioral changes (such as ↓ excitability, ↓ paranoia, or ↓ withdrawn behavior) that indicate a positive response to drug therapy

---

Procyclidine hydrochloride

(proh-**SYE**-klih-deen)

Kemadrin, PMS Procyclidine✱, Procyclid✱ (Rx)

See also *Cholinergic Blocking Agents,* p. 136.

Classification: Antiparkinson agent, synthetic anticholinergic.

Action/Kinetics: Procyclidine, a synthetic anticholinergic, appears to be better tolerated by younger clients. It also possesses direct antispasmodic effects on smooth muscle. This drug is often more effective in relieving rigidity than tremor. **Onset:** 30–45 min. **Time to peak levels:** 1–2 hr. **Peak levels:** 80 mcg/L. **t½:** 11.5–12.6 hr. **Duration:** 4–6 hr.

Uses: Treatment of all types of parkinsonism. Drug-induced extrapyramidal symptoms. Control of sialorrhea following neuroleptic drug use.

Special Concerns: Pregnancy category: C.

Additional Drug Interaction: ↑ Effectiveness of levodopa if used together; such combined use not recommended in clients with psychoses.

Dosage: Elixir, Tablets. *Parkinsonism (for clients on no other therapy):* **initial,** 2.5 mg t.i.d. after meals; dose may be increased slowly to 4–5 mg t.i.d. and, if necessary, before bedtime.
Parkinsonism (transferring from other therapy): substitute 2.5 mg t.i.d.; slowly increase dose of procyclidine and decrease dose of other drug to appropriate maintenance levels. *Drug-induced extrapyramidal symptoms:* **initial,** 2.5 mg t.i.d.; increase to maintenance dose of 10–20 mg/day.

NURSING CONSIDERATIONS

See *Nursing Considerations* for *Cholinergic Blocking Agents,* p. 138.

Evaluation: Evaluate client for:
- Reports of ↓ muscle spasm and rigidity

- Evidence of a reduction in drug-induced extrapyramidal effects

Promazine hydrochloride
(PROH-mah-zeen)
Prozine-50, Sparine (Rx)

See also *Phenothiazines,* p. 201.

Classification: Antipsychotic, dimethylaminopropyl-type phenothiazine.

Action/Kinetics: The use of promazine is accompanied by significant anticholinergic, sedative, and hypotensive effects; moderate antiemetic effect; and, weak extrapyramidal effects. This drug is ineffective in reducing destructive behavior in acutely agitated psychotic clients.

Uses: Psychotic disorders.

Special Concerns: Safe use during pregnancy has not been established. Dosage has not been established in children less than 12 years of age. Geriatric, emaciated, and debilitated clients may require a lower initial dosage.

Dosage: Tablets. *Psychotic disorders:* **Adults:** 10–200 mg q 4–6 hr; adjust dose as needed and tolerated. Total daily dose should not exceed 1,000 mg. **Pediatric, 12 years and older:** 10–25 mg q 4–6 hr; adjust dose as needed and tolerated.
   IM. *Psychotic disorders, severe and moderate agitation:* **Adults, initial:** 50–150 mg; adjust dose if necessary after 30 min. **Maintenance:** 10–200 mg q 4–6 hr as needed and tolerated. Switch to PO therapy as soon as possible. **Pedi-**

atric over 12 years: 10–25 mg q 4–6 hr for chronic psychotic disorders (maximum dose: 1 g daily). The dose may be given IV.

NURSING CONSIDERATIONS

See also *Nursing Considerations for Phenothiazines,* p. 205.

Administration/Storage

1. Dilute concentrate as directed on bottle. Taste can be disguised when given with citrus fruit juice, milk, or flavored drinks.
2. IM injections should be given in the gluteal region.
3. IV doses should be diluted to 25 mg/ml with 0.9% sodium chloride injection and given slowly.

Evaluation: Evaluate client for clinical evidence and reports of improved behavior patterns with a reduction in paranoia, excitable or withdrawn behaviors.

Promethazine hydrochloride

(proh-METH-ah-zeen)

Syrup, Tablets: Phenergan Fortis, Phenergan Plain, PMS Promethazine ✱, Prothazine Plain. **Parenteral:** Anergan 25 and 50, K-Phen, Mallergan, Pentazine, Phenazine 25 and 50, Phencen-50, Phenergan, Phenoject-50, Pro-50, Prometh-25 and -50, Prorex-25 and -50, Prothazine, V-Gan-25 and -50. **Rectal:** Phenergan, Promethagan **(Rx)**

See also *Antihistamines,* p. 71, and *Antiemetics,* p. 70.

Classification: Antihistamine, phenothiazine-type.

Action/Kinetics: Promethazine is a potent antihistamine with prolonged action. It may cause severe drowsiness. The antiemetic effects are likely due to inhibition of the chemoreceptor trigger zone. The drug is effective in vertigo by its central anticholinergic effect which inhibits the vestibular apparatus and the integrative vomiting center as well as the chemoreceptor trigger zone. **Onset, PO, IM, rectal:** 20 min; **IV:** 3–5 min. **Duration, antihistaminic:** 6–12 hr; **sedative:** 2–8 hr. Slowly eliminated through urine and feces.

Uses: Treatment and prophylaxis of motion sickness. Nausea and vomiting due to anesthesia or surgery. Pre- or postoperative sedative, obstetric sedative. Treatment of pruritus, urticaria, angioedema, dermographism, nasal and ophthalmic allergies. Adjunct in the treatment of anaphylaxis or anaphylactoid reactions. Adjunct to analgesics for postoperative pain. IV with meperidine or other narcotics in special surgical procedures as bronchoscopy, ophthalmic surgery, or in poor-risk clients.

Contraindications: Lactation. Children up to 2 years of age.

Special Concerns: Safe use during pregnancy has not been established. Use in children may cause paradoxical hyperexcitability and nightmares. Injection not recommended for children less than 2 years of age. Geriatric clients are more likely to experience confusion, dizziness, hypotension, and sedation.

Additional Side Effects: Leukopenia and agranulocytosis (especially if used with cytotoxic agents).

Dosage: Syrup, Tablets. *Antihistaminic:* **Adults,** 12.5 mg q.i.d. before meals and at bedtime (or 25 mg at bedtime if needed). **Pediatric,** 0.125 mg/kg (3.75 mg/m²) q 4–6 hr; 0.5 mg/kg (15 mg/m²) at bedtime if needed; or, 6.26–12.6 mg t.i.d. (or 25 mg at bedtime if needed). *Anivertigo:* **Adults,** 25 mg b.i.d.; **pediatric,** 0.5 mg/kg (15 mg/m²) q 12 hr or 12.5–25 mg b.i.d. *Antiemetic:* **Adults,** 25 mg b.i.d. as needed; **pediatric,** 0.25–0.5 mg/kg (7.5–15 mg/m²) q 4–6 hr as needed (or 12.5–25 mg 4–6 hr). *Sedative-Hypnotic:* **Adults,** 25–50 mg; **pediatric,** 0.5–1 mg/kg (15–30 mg/m²) or 12.5–25 mg as needed.

Injectable, Suppositories. *Antihistaminic:* **Adults, IM, IV, Rectal,** 25 mg repeated in 2 hr if needed; **pediatric, IM, Rectal,** 0.125 mg/kg q 4–6 hr (or 0.5 mg/kg at bedtime). *Antiemetic:* **Adults, IM, IV, Rectal,** 12.5–25 mg q 4 hr; **pediatric, IM, Rectal,** 0.25–0.5 mg/kg q 4–6 hr (or 12.5–25 mg q 4–6 hr). *Sedative-Hypnotic:* **Adults, IM, IV, Rectal,** 25–50 mg; **pediatric, IM, Rectal,** 0.5–1 mg/kg (or 12.5–25 mg). *Antivertigo:* **Adults, Rectal,** 25 mg b.i.d.; **pediatric, Rectal,** 0.5 mg/kg q 12 hr (or 12.5–25 mg b.i.d.)

NURSING CONSIDERATIONS

See also *Nursing Considerations for Antihistamines,* p. 74, and *Antiemetics,* p. 71.

Administration/Storage

1. Drug may be taken with food or milk to lessen GI irritation.
2. Dosage should be decreased in dehydrated clients or those with oliguria.
3. When used to prevent motion sickness, the medication should be taken 30 min, and preferably 1–2 hr, before travel.

Evaluation: Evaluate client for:
- Reports of effective treatment and control of symptoms of motion sickness
- Evidence of control of nausea and vomiting R/T surgical anesthesia
- Evidence of desired level of sedation
- The control of symptoms R/T nasal and ophthalmic allergic manifestations

Propafenone hydrochloride
(proh-pah-FEN-ohn)
Rythmol (Rx)

Classification: Antiarrhythmic, type IC.

Action/Kinetics: Propafenone manifests local anesthetic effects and a direct stabilizing action on the myocardium. The drug reduces upstroke velocity (Phase O) of the monophasic action potential, reduces the fast inward current carried by sodium ions in the Purkinje fibers, increases diastolic excitability threshold, and prolongs the effective refractory period. Also, spontaneous activity is decreased. The drug has slight beta-adrenergic blocking activity. **Peak plasma levels:** 3.5 hr. **Therapeutic plasma levels:** 0.5–3 mcg/ml. Significant first-pass effect. Most clients metabolize propafenone rapidly. **t½:** 2–10 hr to two active metabolites: 5-hydroxypropafenone and N-depropylpropafenone. However, approximately 10% of clients (as well as those taking quinidine) metabolize the drug more slowly

($t\frac{1}{2}$: 10–32 hr). However, because the 5-hydroxy metabolite is not formed in slow metabolizers and because steady-state levels are reached after 4–5 days in all clients, the recommended dosing regimen is the same for all clients.

Uses: Sustained ventricular tachycardia that is life-threatening.

Contraindications: Uncontrolled congestive heart failure, cardiogenic shock, sick sinus node syndrome or atrioventricular block in the absence of an artificial pacemaker, bradycardia, marked hypotension, bronchospastic disorders, manifest electrolyte disorders, hypersensitivity to the drug. Myocardial infarction more than 6 days but less than 2 years previously.

Special Concerns: Use during pregnancy (category: C) only if benefits clearly outweigh the risks. Use with caution during labor, delivery, and lactation. The safety and effectiveness have not been determined in children. Use with caution in clients with impaired hepatic or renal function.

Side Effects: *CV:* First-degree AV block, intraventricular conduction delay, palpitations, premature ventricular contractions, proarrhythmia, bradycardia, atrial fibrillation, angina, syncope, congestive heart failure, ventricular tachycardia, second-degree AV block, increased QRS duration, chest pain, hypotension, bundle branch block. Less commonly, atrial flutter, AV dissociation, flushing, hot flashes, sick sinus syndrome, sinus pause or arrest, supraventricular tachycardia, cardiac arrest. *CNS:* Dizziness, headache, anxiety, drowsiness, loss of balance, ataxia, insomnia. Less commonly, abnormal speech, abnormal dreams, abnormal vision, confusion, depression, memory loss, apnea, psychosis/mania, seizures, vertigo, coma. *GI:* Unusual taste, constipation, nausea and/or vomiting, dry mouth, anorexia, flatulence, abdominal pain, cramps, diarrhea, dyspepsia, liver abnormalities (cholestasis, hepatitis, elevated enzymes). *Hematologic:* Agranulocytosis, increased bleeding time, anemia, granulocytopenia, bruising, leukopenia, purpura, thrombocytopenia. *Miscellaneous:* Blurred vision, dyspnea, weakness, rash, edema, tremors, diaphoresis, joint pain, possible decrease in spermatogenesis. Less commonly, tinnitus, unusual smell sensation, apnea, alopecia, eye irritation, hyponatremia, impotence, increased glucose, kidney failure, lupus erythematosus, muscle cramps or weakness, nephrotic syndrome, pain, pruritus.

Symptoms of Overdose: Bradycardia, hypotension, intra-arterial and intraventricular conduction disturbances, somnolence. Rarely, high-grade ventricular arrhythmias and seizures.

Drug Interactions

Cimetidine / Cimetidine ↓ plasma levels of propafenone
Digoxin / Propafenone ↑ plasma levels of digoxin necessitating a ↓ in the dose of digoxin
Local anesthetics / May ↑ risk of CNS side effects
Metoprolol / Propafenone ↑ plasma levels of metoprolol due to inhibition of metabolism
Propranolol / Propafenone ↑ plasma levels of propranolol due to inhibition of metabolism
Warfarin / Propafenone may ↑ plasma levels of warfarin necessitating a ↓ in the dose of warfarin

Dosage: PO, initial: 150 mg q 8 hr; dose may be increased at a minimum of q 3–4 days to 225 mg q 8 hr and, if necessary, to 300 mg q 8 hr.

NURSING CONSIDERATIONS

See also *Nursing Considerations* for *Antiarrhythmic Drugs,* p. 52.

Administration/Storage

1. Initiation of propafenone therapy should always be undertaken in a hospital setting.
2. The effectiveness and safety of doses exceeding 900 mg daily have not been determined.
3. There is no evidence that the use of propafenone will affect the survival or incidence of sudden death in clients with recent myocardial infarction or supraventricular tachycardia.
4. *Treatment of Overdose:* To control blood pressure and cardiac rhythm, defibrillation and infusion of dopamine or isoproterenol. If seizures occur, diazepam, IV, can be given. External cardiac massage and mechanical respiratory assistance may be required.

Assessment

1. Assess ECG and note any client history of cardiac problems.
2. Determine if there is any history of renal or hepatic disease. Propafenone must be used with caution in these clients.

Interventions

1. The dose of propafenone should be titrated in each client on the basis of response and tolerance.
2. Propafenone may induce new or worsened arrhythmias. Doc-

ument with rhythm strips and monitor client response closely.
3. Notify physician and anticipate reduction of dosage in clients who develop significant widening of the QRS complex or second- or third-degree AV block.
4. Anticipate that the dose of propafenone will be increased more gradually in elderly clients as well as in clients with previous myocardial damage.
5. Monitor liver and renal function studies. Anticipate reduced dosage in clients with impaired liver or kidney function.
6. Evaluate hematologic studies during drug therapy to determine the presence of anemia, agranulocytosis, leukopenia, thrombocytopenia, or altered prothrombin and coagulation times.
7. Weigh client and place on strict I&O.
8. Client may complain of an unusual taste in the mouth. This may interfere with eating and nutrition so observe closely.

Client/Family Teaching

1. Drink adequate quantities of fluid (2–3 L/day) and maintain adequate bulk in the diet to avoid constipation.
2. Report any incidence of increased or unusual bruising or bleeding.
3. Observe for indications of hepatic dysfunction such as yellow sclera, dark yellow urine, or yellow pigmentation of the skin and report.
4. Report any evidence of urinary tract problems such as decreased urinary output.

Evaluation: Evaluate client for ECG evidence of termination of life-threatening ventricular tachycardia.

Propantheline bromide
(proh-**PAN**-thih-leen)
Banlin✿, Norpanth, Novo–Propanthil✿, Pro-Banthine, Propanthel✿ (Rx)

See also *Cholinergic Blocking Agents,* p. 136.

Classification: Anticholinergic, antispasmodic (quaternary ammonium compound).

Action/Kinetics: Duration: 6 hr. Metabolized in the liver and excreted through the urine.

Uses: Adjunct in peptic ulcer therapy. Spastic and inflammatory disease of GI and urinary tracts. Control of salivation and enuresis. Duodenography. Urinary incontinence.

Special Concerns: Pregnancy category: C. Safety and effectiveness for use in children with peptic ulcer have not been established.

Dosage: Tablets. Adults: 15 mg 30 min before meals and 30 mg at bedtime. Reduce dose to 7.5 mg t.i.d. for mild symptoms, geriatric clients, or clients of small stature. **Pediatric:** 0.375 mg/kg (10 mg/m²) q.i.d. with dose being adjusted as needed.

NURSING CONSIDERATIONS

See also *Nursing Considerations for Cholinergic Blocking Agents,* p. 138.

Interventions

1. A liquid diet is recommended during initiation of therapy in clients with edematous duodenal ulcer.

2. Monitor I&O. Observe for urinary retention and constipation.

Client/Family Teaching

1. Drug may cause drowsiness or dizziness. Do not drive or operate equipment until drug effects are realized.
2. Visual acuity may be impaired; dark glasses may be necessary.
3. Increase fluid intake and fiber in diet to minimize the constipating effects of drug therapy.

Evaluation: Evaluate client for:
- Reports of symptomatic improvement with GI pain and discomfort
- Reports of ↓ salivation and enuresis
- Evidence of control of urinary incontinence

Propiomazine hydrochloride
(proh-pee-**OH**-may-zeen)
Largon (Rx)

Classification: Nonbarbiturate sedative, phenothiazine.

Action/Kinetics: At therapeutic dosages, this phenothiazine drug has sedative, antiemetic, antihistaminic, and anticholinergic effects. **Peak sedative effects: IV,** 15–30 min; **IM,** 40–60 min. **Time to peak serum levels:** 1–3 hr (following IM). **Duration** 3–6 hr. **t½, IV:** about 8 hr; **IM,** about 11 hr.

Uses: Preoperatively to reduce anxiety and during surgery to decrease emesis. Adjunct to narcotic analgesia during labor to relieve restlessness and apprehension.

Contraindications: Intra-arterial injection.

Special Concerns: Use with caution in pregnancy.

Side Effects: *GI:* Dry mouth, GI upset. *CNS:* Dizziness and confusion in the elderly. Transient restlessness. *CV:* Increase in blood pressure (may be desirable), hypotension, tachycardia. *Other:* Skin rashes, respiratory depression, altered respiratory pattern. Irritation and thrombophlebitis at injection site.

Dosage: IM and IV. Adults: *Preoperative sedation,* **usual,** 20 mg (up to 40 mg) with meperidine, 50 mg. *Obstetrics:* 20–40 mg in the early stages of labor; **then,** 20–40 mg given with meperidine, 25–75 mg. Doses may be repeated q 3 hr. *Sedation with local anesthesia:* 10–20 mg. **Pediatric.** *Pre- and postoperatively:* **children weighing less than 27 kg:** 0.55–1.1 mg/kg. *Alternative dosing:* **children, 2–4 years of age:** 10 mg; **4–6 years of age:** 15 mg; **6–12 years of age:** 25 mg.

NURSING CONSIDERATIONS

Administration/Storage

1. Inject into large, undamaged vein.
2. Avoid extravasation.
3. Never administer subcutaneously or intra-arterially.
4. Do not use solutions that are cloudy or contain precipitate.
5. Aqueous solutions are incompatible with barbiturate salts or alkaline solutions.
6. Store at 15°C–30°C (59°F–86°F) and protect from light.
7. If used with propiomazine, the dose of barbiturates should be reduced by at least ½; the dose of meperidine, morphine, or analgesic depressants should be reduced by ¼–½ if used with propiomazine.

Interventions

1. Anticipate reduction of dose by ¼–½ in strength of other sedatives administered concomitantly with propiomazine.
2. Anticipate that if vasopressor drugs are administered with propiomazine, norepinephrine should be used rather than epinephrine.
3. Provide mouth care to relieve xerostomia except for clients scheduled for surgery, for whom a dry mouth is desirable.
4. Monitor BP frequently after IM or IV administration because medication may have a hypotensive effect up to 5 hr.
5. Monitor and assess clients for any side effects (blood dyscrasias, hepatotoxicity, extrapyramidal symptoms, reactivation of psychotic processes, cardiac arrest, endocrine disturbances, dermatologic disorders, ocular changes, and hypersensitivity reactions) associated with long-term use of phenothiazines.
6. Provide a safe environment for elderly clients experiencing dizziness, confusion, or amnesia after administration of the drug.
7. Assess the client carefully because the antiemetic effect of propiomazine may be masking other pathology, such as toxicity to other drugs, intestinal obstruction, or brain lesions.

Evaluation: Evaluate client for:
- Reports of ↓ anxiety preoperatively

- Evidence of a reduction of emesis intraoperatively

Propoxyphene hydrochloride

(proh-**POX**-ih-feen)

642 Tablets✱, Darvon, Dolene, Doraphen, Doxaphene, Novo–Propoxyn✱, Profene, Pro Pox, Propoxycon (C-IV) (Rx)

Propoxyphene napsylate

(proh-**POX**-ih-feen)

Darvon-N (C-IV) (Rx)

Classification: Analgesic, narcotic, miscellaneous.

Action/Kinetics: Propoxyphene resembles the narcotics with respect to its mechanism and analgesic effect; it is one-half to one-third as potent as codeine. It is devoid of antitussive, anti-inflammatory, or antipyretic activity. When taken in excessive doses for long periods, psychologic dependence, and occasionally physical dependence and tolerance, will be manifested. **Peak plasma levels:** *hydrochloride:* 2–2.5 hr; *napsylate:* 3–4 hr. **Analgesic onset:** up to 1 hr. **Peak analgesic effect:** 2 hr. **Duration:** 4–6 hr. **Therapeutic serum levels:** 0.05–0.12 mcg/ml. **t½, propoxyphene:** 6–12 hr; **norpropoxyphene:** 30–36 hr. Extensive first-pass effect; metabolites are excreted in the urine.

Propoxyphene is often prescribed in combination with salicylates. In such instances, the information on salicylates should also be consulted. Propoxyphene hydrochloride is found in Darvon Compound and Wygesic, while propoxyphene napsylate is found in Darvocet-N.

Uses: To relieve mild to moderate pain. Propoxyphene napsylate has been used experimentally to suppress the withdrawal syndrome from narcotics.

Contraindications: Hypersensitivity to drug.

Special Concerns: Safe use during pregnancy has not been established. Use with caution during lactation. Safety and efficacy have not been established in children.

Side Effects: *GI:* Nausea, vomiting, constipation, abdominal pain. *CNS:* Sedation, dizziness, lightheadedness, headache, weakness, euphoria, dysphoria. *Other:* Skin rashes, visual disturbances. Propoxyphene can produce psychologic dependence, as well as physical dependence and tolerance.

Symptoms of Overdose: Stupor, respiratory depression, apnea, hypotension, pulmonary edema, circulatory collapse, cardiac arrhythmias, conduction abnormalities, coma, seizures, respiratory-metabolic acidosis.

Drug Interactions

Alcohol, Antianxiety drugs, Antipsychotic agents, Narcotics, Sedative-hypnotics / Concomitant use may lead to drowsiness, lethargy, stupor, respiratory, depression, and coma

Carbamazepine / ↑ Effect of carbamazepine due to ↓ breakdown by liver

CNS depressants / Additive CNS depression

Orphenadrine / Concomitant use may lead to confusion, anxiety, and tremors

Phenobarbital / ↑ Effect of phenobarbital due to ↓ breakdown by liver

Skeletal muscle relaxants /
Additive respiratory depression
Warfarin /
↑ Hypoprothrombinemic effects
of warfarin

Dosage: Capsules: (Hydrochloride). Adults, 65 mg q 4 hr, not to exceed 390 mg/day.
Oral Suspension, Tablets: (Napsylate). Adults, 100 mg q 4 hr, not to exceed 600 mg/day. Dose of propoxyphene should be reduced in clients with renal or hepatic impairment. **Not recommended for use in children.**

NURSING CONSIDERATIONS

See also *Nursing Considerations for Narcotic Analgesics,* p. 177.

Administration/Storage: *Treatment of Overdose:* Maintain an adequate airway, artificial respiration, and naloxone, 0.4–2 mg IV (repeat at 2–3-min intervals) to combat respiratory depression. Gastric lavage or administration of activated charcoal may be helpful. Correct acidosis and electrolyte imbalance. Acidosis due to lactic acid may require IV sodium bicarbonate.

Assessment

1. Note any history of opiate or alcohol dependency.
2. Obtain baseline liver and renal function studies.

Interventions

1. Anticipate reduced dose with renal and liver dysfunction.
2. Smoking reduces drug effect by increasing metabolism.

Evaluation: Evaluate client for:
- Reports of effective control of pain

- Evidence of suppression of narcotic withdrawal symptoms

Propranolol hydrochloride

(proh-**PRAN**-oh-lohl)
Apo-Propranolol✹, Detensol✹, Inderal, Inderal 10, 20, 40, 60, 80, and 90, Inderal LA, Novo–Pranol✹, PMS Propranolol✹, Propranolol Intensol (Rx)

See also *Beta-Adrenergic Blocking Agents,* p. 113.

Classification: Beta-adrenergic blocking agent; antiarrhythmic (type II).

Action/Kinetics: Propranolol manifests both beta-1 and beta-2 adrenergic blocking activity. The antiarrhythmic action results from both beta-adrenergic receptor blockade and from a direct membrane-stabilizing action on the cardiac cell. Propranolol has no intrinsic sympathomimetic activity and has high lipid solubility. **PO: Onset,** 30 min. **Maximum effect:** 1–1.5 hr. **Duration:** 3–6 hr. **t½:** 3–5 hr (8–11 hr for long-acting). Onset after IV administration is almost immediate. Completely metabolized by liver and excreted in urine. Although food increases bioavailability of the drug, absorption may be decreased.

Uses: Hypertension (alone or in combination with other antihypertensive agents). Angina pectoris, hypertrophic subaortic stenosis, prophylaxis of myocardial infarction, pheochromocytoma, prophylaxis of migraine, essential tremor. Cardiac arrhythmias including ventricular tachycardias and arrhythmias, tachycardias due to digitalis intoxication, supraventricular arrhythmias, premature ventricular contractions (PVCs), resistant tachyarrhythmias due to anesthesia/catecholamines.

Investigational: Schizophrenia, tremors due to parkinsonism, aggressive behavior, antipsychotic-induced akathisia, rebleeding due to esophageal varices, situational anxiety, acute panic attacks, gastric bleeding in portal hypertension, vaginal contraceptive, anxiety, alcohol withdrawal syndrome.

Special Concerns: Pregnancy category: C.

Additional Side Effects: Psoriasis-like eruptions, skin necrosis, systemic lupus erythematosus (rare).

Additional Drug Interactions

Haloperidol / Severe hypotension
Hydralazine / ↑ Effect of both agents
Methimazole / May ↑ effects of propranolol
Phenobarbital / ↓ Effect of propranolol due to ↑ breakdown by liver
Propylthiouracil / May ↑ the effects of propranolol
Rifampin / ↓ Effect of propranolol due to ↑ breakdown by liver
Smoking / ↓ Serum levels and ↑ clearance of propranolol

Laboratory Test Interferences: ↑ Blood urea, serum transaminase, alkaline phosphatase, LDH. Interference with glaucoma screening test.

Dosage: Tablets, Long-acting Capsules, Oral Solution. *Hypertension:* **initial,** 40 mg b.i.d. or 80 mg of sustained-release/day; **then,** increase dose to maintenance level of 120–240 mg daily given in 2–3 divided doses or 120–160 mg of sustained-release medication once daily. Maximum daily dose should not exceed 640 mg. *Angina, prophylaxis:* **initial,** 10–20 mg t.i.d.–q.i.d. or 80 mg of sustained-release once daily; **then,** increase dose gradually to maintenance level of 160 mg/day of sustained-release capsule. The maximum daily dose should not exceed 320 mg. *Arrhythmias:* 10–30 mg t.i.d.–q.i.d. given after meals and at bedtime. *Hypertrophic subaortic stenosis:* 20–40 mg t.i.d.–q.i.d. before meals and at bedtime or 80–160 mg of sustained-release medication given once daily. *Myocardial infarction prophylaxis:* 180–240 mg daily given in 2–3 divided doses. Total daily dose should not exceed 240 mg. *Pheochromocytoma, preoperatively:* 60 mg daily for 3 days before surgery, given concomitantly with an alpha-adrenergic blocking agent. *Inoperable tumors:* 30 mg/day in divided doses. *Migraine:* **initial,** 80 mg sustained-release medication given once daily; **then,** increase dose gradually to maintenance of 160–240 mg daily. If a satisfactory response has not been observed after 4–6 weeks, the drug should be discontinued and withdrawn gradually. *Essential tremor:* **initial,** 40 mg b.i.d.; **then,** 120 mg daily up to a maximum of 320 mg daily.

IV. *Life-threatening arrhythmias:* 1–3 mg not to exceed 1 mg/min; a second dose may be given after 2 min, with subsequent doses q 4 hr. Clients should begin PO therapy as soon as possible.

Pediatric. *Hypertension:* **PO, initial,** 1 mg/kg daily in divided doses (e.g., 0.5 mg/kg b.i.d.). May be increased at 3–5 day intervals to a maximum of 2 mg/kg daily. The dosage range should be calculated by weight and not by body surface area.

Investigational uses. Aggressive behavior: 80–300 mg daily. *Antipsychotic-induced akathisia:* 20–80 mg daily. *Tremors associated with parkinsonism:* 160 mg daily. *Rebleeding due to esophageal varices:* 20–180 mg daily. *Situational anxiety:* 40 mg. *Schizophrenia:* 300–5,000 mg daily. *Acute panic symptoms:* 40–320 mg daily. *Anxiety:* 80–320 mg daily. *Gastric bleeding in portal hypertension:* 24–480 mg daily.

NURSING CONSIDERATIONS

See also *Nursing Considerations* for *Beta-Adrenergic Blocking Agents,* p. 116.

Administration/Storage

1. Do not administer for a minimum of 2 weeks after client has received MAO inhibitor drugs.
2. If signs of serious myocardial depression occur following propranolol administration, isoproterenol (Isuprel) should be slowly infused IV.
3. After IV administration, have available emergency drugs and equipment to combat hypotension or circulatory collapse.

Interventions

1. Observe client for evidence of a rash, fever, and/or purpura. These may be symptoms of a hypersensitivity reaction.
2. Monitor intake and output. Observe for signs and symptoms of congestive heart failure, (e.g., shortness of breath, rales, edema and weight gain).

Client/Family Teaching

1. Do not smoke. Smoking decreases serum levels of the drug and interferes with drug clearance.
2. In clients with diabetes, drug may mask most symptoms of hypoglycemia. Monitor finger sticks carefully.
3. Instruct client to check BP and heart rate weekly and to report if any significant changes are noted.
4. Do not stop drug abruptly as this could precipitate hypertension, myocardial ischemia, or cardiac arrhythmias.

Evaluation: Evaluate client for:
- Evidence of a ↓ blood pressure
- Reports of ↓ frequency and intensity of angina episodes
- Reports of effective migraine prophylaxis
- ECG evidence of control of cardiac arrhythmia

—— *COMBINATION DRUG* ——
Propranolol and Hydrochlorothiazide
(proh-**PRAN**-oh-lohl, hy-droh-**klor**-oh-**THIGH**-ah-zyd)
Inderide 40/25, Inderide 80/25, Inderide LA 80/50, Inderide LA 120/50, Inderide LA 160/50 (Rx)

See also *Propranolol,* p. 1101, and *Hydrochlorothiazide,* p. 718.

Classification/Content: *Antihypertensive/diuretic:* Hydrochlorothiazide, 25 mg (Inderide) or 50 mg (Inderide LA).

Beta-adrenergic blocking agent: Propranolol HCl, 40 or 80 mg (Inderide) or 80, 120, or 160 mg (Inderide LA).

Also see information on individual components.

Uses: Hypertension (not indicated for initial therapy).

Special Concerns: Pregnancy category: C. Use with caution during lactation. Safety and effectiveness have not been established in children. The risk of hypothermia is increased in geriatric clients.

Dosage: PO. Individualized. *Inderide:* 1–2 tablets b.i.d. up to 320 mg propranolol HCl daily. *Inderide LA:* 1 capsule once daily.

NURSING CONSIDERATIONS

See also *Nursing Considerations* for individual components.

Administration/Storage

1. Because of side effects from hydrochlorothiazide, Inderide should not be used if propranolol must be given in excess of 320 mg daily.
2. If another antihypertensive agent is required, initial dosage should be one-half the usual recommended dose to prevent an excessive drop in blood pressure.
3. Inderide LA should not be considered a milligram-to-milligram substitute for Inderide because the LA produces lower blood levels.

Propylthiouracil

(proh-pill-thigh-oh-**YOUR**-ah-sill)
Propyl-Thyracil ✿ (Rx)

See also *Antithyroid Drugs,* p. 99.

Classification: Antithyroid preparation.

Action/Kinetics: May be preferred for treatment of thyroid storm as the drug inhibits peripheral conversion of thyroxine to triio-

dothyronine. Rapidly absorbed from the GI tract. **Duration:** 2–3 hr. **t½:** 1–2 hr. **Onset:** 10–20 days. **Time to peak effect:** 2–10 weeks. Eighty percent is protein bound. Metabolized by the liver and excreted through the kidneys.

Special Concerns: Incidence of vasculitis is increased.

Drug Interactions: Propylthiouracil may produce hypoprothrombinemia, adding to the effect of anticoagulants.

Dosage: Tablets. *Hyperthyroidism:* **Adults, initial:** 300 mg/day (up to 900 mg/day may be required in some clients with severe hyperthyroidism) given as 1–4 divided doses; **maintenance, usual:** 100–150 mg/day. **Pediatric, 6–10 years, initial:** 50–150 mg/day in 1–4 divided doses; **over 10 years, initial:** 150–300 mg/day in 1–4 divided doses. Maintenance for all pediatric use is based on response. **Alternative dose for children, initial:** 5–7 mg/kg/day (150–200 mg/m²/day) in divided doses q 8 hr; **maintenance:** ⅓–⅔ the initial dose when the client is euthyroid. *Thyrotoxic crisis:* **Adults,** 200–400 mg q 4 hr during the first day as an adjunct to other treatments. *Neonatal thyrotoxicosis:* 10 mg/kg daily in divided doses.

NURSING CONSIDERATIONS

See also *Nursing Considerations* for *Antithyroid Drugs,* p. 100.

Client/Family Teaching

1. Report any evidence of unusual bruising or bleeding.
2. Any fever, sore throat, or rash should be reported to the physician.
3. Review dietary sources of

iodine (shellfish, iodized salt) that should be avoided.

Evaluation: Evaluate client for:
- The control of symptoms of hyperthyroidism with evidence of weight gain and ↓ heart rate
- Laboratory evidence that serum thyroid levels are within desired range

---

Protamine sulfate
(PROH-tah-meen)
(Rx)

Classification: Heparin antagonist.

Action/Kinetics: Protamine sulfate is a strongly basic polypeptide that complexes with strongly acidic heparin to form an inactive stable salt. The complex has no anticoagulant activity. **Onset:** 30–60 sec. **Duration:** 2 hr (but depends on body temperature). Upon metabolism, the complex may liberate heparin (heparin rebound).

Use: Only for treatment of heparin overdose resulting in hemorrhage. Administration of whole blood or fresh frozen plasma may also be needed if hemorrhage is severe.

Contraindications: Previous intolerance to protamine. Not suitable for treating spontaneous hemorrhage, postpartum hemorrhage, menorrhagia, or uterine bleeding.

Special Concerns: Pregnancy category: C. Use with caution during lactation. Safety and efficacy have not been determined in children.

Side Effects: *CV:* Sudden fall in blood pressure, bradycardia, transitory flushing, warm feeling. *GI:* Nausea, vomiting. *CNS:* Lassitude. *Other:* Anaphylaxis, dyspnea.

Dosage: Slow IV. No more than 50 mg of protamine sulfate should be given in any 10-min period. One mg protamine sulfate can neutralize about 90 USP units of heparin derived from lung tissue or about 115 USP units of heparin derived from intestinal mucosa. **Note:** The dose of protamine sulfate depends on the amount of time that has elapsed since IV heparin administration. For example, if 30 min has elapsed, one-half the usual dose of protamine sulfate may be sufficient because heparin is cleared rapidly from the circulation.

NURSING CONSIDERATIONS
Administration/Storage
1. Protamine sulfate is incompatible with several penicillins and with cephalosporins.
2. If dilution of the product is required, use either dextrose 5% or normal saline. After reconstitution, the solution may be stored in the refrigerator for 24 hr.

Assessment: Note any history of previous intolerance to protamine.

Interventions
1. To minimize side effects, give protamine sulfate slowly over 1–3 min.
2. When administering heparin infusions, anticipate potential for heparin overdose and have protamine sulfate readily available.
3. Observe client closely in a monitored environment. Note any sudden fall in BP, bradycardia, dyspnea, transitory flushing, or client complaint of a sensation of warmth.
4. Coagulation studies should be performed 5–15 min after protamine sulfate has been ad-

P

ministered to evaluate its effectiveness. Repeat in 2–8 hr to assess for heparin rebound.

5. Observe client closely for increased bleeding, lowered BP, and/or shock. These are signs of heparin rebound and should be reported immediately as repeated doses of protamine sulfate may be indicated.

6. Record vital signs and intake and output, assess closely for sudden variations.

Evaluation: Evaluate client for:
- Evidence of successful control of heparin-induced hemorrhage
- Laboratory confirmation of the return of coagulation studies to preheparin therapy normal levels

---

Protriptyline hydrochloride

(proh-**TRIP**-tih-leen)

Triptil ✽, Vivactil (Rx)

See also *Tricyclic Antidepressants*, p. 239.

Classification: Antidepressant, tricyclic.

Action/Kinetics: Significant anticholinergic effects but low sedative and orthostatic hypotensive effects. **Effective plasma levels:** 100–200 ng/ml. **t½:** Approximately 67–89 hr.

Uses: Symptoms of depression. Withdrawn and anergic clients. Obstructive sleep apnea. Has also been used with amphetamines to treat cataplexy associated with narcolepsy and to relieve symptoms of attention deficit disorders in some children over 6 years of age with or without hyperactivity.

Special Concerns: Use with caution during pregnancy. Administer with caution to clients with myocardial insufficiency and those in whom tachycardia or a drop in blood pressure might lead to serious complications. Safety and efficacy for treating depression have not been determined in children.

Dosage: Tablets. Adults: *Antidepressant,* **individualized,** 15–40 mg daily in 3–4 divided doses. Up to 60 mg daily (maximum) may be given. **Elderly clients, adolescents: initial,** 5 mg t.i.d.; increase dose slowly. Monitor cardiovascular system closely if dose exceeds 20 mg/day in the elderly. **Not recommended for children.** *Anticataleptic:* 15–20 mg daily at bedtime.

NURSING CONSIDERATIONS

See also *Nursing Considerations* for *Tricyclic Antidepressants*, p. 242.

Administration/Storage: If drug causes insomnia, give last dose no less than 8 hr before bedtime.

Interventions: Assess vital signs at least b.i.d. during initiation of therapy.

Evaluation: Evaluate client for:
- Evidence of ↓ depression and ↓ withdrawn behaviors
- Reports of improved attention span (in attention deficit disorder)

Pseudoephedrine hydrochloride

(soo-doh-eh-**FED**-rin)

Balminil Decongestant Syrup✽, Benylin Decongestant✽, Cenafed, Children's Sudafed Liquid, Congestac N.D.

Caplets ✹, Decofed, DeFed 60, Dorcol Children's Decongestant Liquid, Eltor 120 ✹, Genaphed, Halofed, Halofed Adult Strength, Maxenal ✹, Myfedrine, NeoFed, Novafed, Ornex Cold ✹, Otrivin Nasal Decongestant ✹, PediaCare Infants' Oral Decongestant Drops, Pseudo, Pseudofrin ✹, Pseudogest, Robidrine ✹, Sudafed, Sudafed 12 Hour, Sudafed 60, Sudrin, Sufedrin (OTC)

Pseudoephedrine sulfate

(soo-doh-eh-**FED**-rin)
Afrinol (OTC)

See also *Sympathomimetic Drugs*, p. 218.

Classification: Direct- and indirect-acting sympathomimetic, nasal decongestant.

Action/Kinetics: Pseudoephedrine produces direct stimulation of both alpha-(pronounced) as well as beta-adrenergic receptors, as well as indirect stimulation through release of norepinephrine from storage sites. These actions produce a decongestant effect on the nasal mucosa. Systemic administration eliminates possible damage to the nasal mucosa. **Onset:** 15–30 min. **Time to peak effect:** 30–60 min. **Duration:** 3–4 hr. **Extended-release: duration,** 8–12 hr. Urinary excretion slowed by alkalinization, causing reabsorption of drug.

Pseudoephedrine is also found in Actifed, Chlor-Trimeton, and Drixoral.

Uses: Nasal congestion associated with sinus conditions, otitis, allergies.

Additional Contraindications: Lactation.

Special Concerns: Use during pregnancy only if benefits clearly outweigh risks (pregnancy category: B). Use with caution in newborn and premature infants due to a higher risk of side effects. Geriatric clients may be more prone to age-related prostatic hypertrophy.

Dosage: Hydrochloride: Capsules, Oral Solution, Syrup, Tablets. Adults: 60 mg q 4–6 hr not to exceed 240 mg in 24 hr. **Pediatric, 6–12 years:** 30 mg using the oral solution or syrup q 4–6 hr not to exceed 120 mg in 24 hr; **2–6 years:** 15 mg using the oral solution or syrup q 4–6 hr not to exceed 60 mg in 24 hr. For children less than 2 years of age, the dose must be individualized.

Hydrochloride: Extended-release Capsules. Adults and children over 12 years: 120 mg q 12 hr or 240 mg q 24 hr. Use is not recommended for children less than 12 years of age.

Sulfate: Extended-release Tablets. Adults and children over 12 years: 120 mg q 12 hr or 240 mg q 24 hr. Use is not recommended for children less than 12 years of age.

NURSING CONSIDERATIONS

See also *Nursing Considerations* for *Sympathomimetic Drugs*, p. 220.

Client/Family Teaching

1. Avoid taking the drug at bedtime. Pseudoephedrine causes stimulation that can produce insomnia.
2. If clients have hypertension, advise them to report to the physician symptoms such as headache or dizziness. These symptoms may be drug-related and could indicate an elevation of blood pressure.

Evaluation: Evaluate client for reports of a reduction in nasal, sinus, or eustachian tube congestion and their associated allergic manifestations.

Psyllium hydrophilic muciloid

(**SILL**-ee-um hi-droh-**FILL**-ik)
Effer-syllium, Fiberall Natural Flavor, Fiberall Orange Flavor, Fiberall Wafers, Fibrepur✿, Hydrocil Instant, Karacil✿, Konsyl, Konsyl-D, Metamucil, Metamucil Lemon-Lime Flavor, Metamucil Orange Flavor, Metamucil Sugar Free, Metamucil Sugar Free Orange Flavor, Modane Bulk, Natural Vegetable, Novo–Mucilax✿, Perdiem Fiber, Prodiem Plain✿, Reguloid Natural, Reguloid Orange, Reguloid Sugar Free Orange, Reguloid Sugar Free Regular, Serutan, Siblin, Syllact, V-Lax (OTC)

See also *Laxatives,* p. 171.

Classification: Laxative, bulk-forming.

Action/Kinetics: This drug is obtained from the fruit of various species of plantago. The powder forms a gelatinous mass with water, which adds bulk to the stools and stimulates peristalsis. It also has a demulcent effect on an inflamed intestinal mucosa. These preparations may also contain dextrose, sodium bicarbonate, monobasic potassium phosphate, citric acid, and benzyl benzoate. Dependence may occur.

Uses: Prophylaxis of constipation in clients who should not strain during defecation. Short-term treatment of constipation; useful in geriatric clients with diminished colonic motor response and during pregnancy and postpartum to reestablish normal bowel function. To soften feces during fecal impaction.

Contraindications: Severe abdominal pain or intestinal obstruction.

Side Effects: Obstruction of the esophagus, stomach, small intestine, and rectum.

Drug Interactions: Psyllium should not be used concomitantly with salicylates, nitrofurantoin, or cardiac glycosides (e.g., digitalis).

Dosage: Dose depends on the product. General information on adult dosage follows. **Granules/ Flakes:** 1–2 teaspoons 1–3 times/ day spread on food or with a glass of water. **Powder:** 1 rounded teaspoon in 8 oz of liquid 1–3 times/ day. **Effervescent powder:** 1 packet in water 1–3 times/day. **Chewable pieces:** 2 pieces followed by a glass of water 1–3 times/day.

NURSING CONSIDERATIONS

See *Nursing Considerations* for *Laxatives,* p. 172.

Administration/Storage

1. Laxative effects usually occur in 12–24 hr. The full effect may take 2–3 days.
2. The powder may be noxious and irritating to some personnel when removing from the packets or canister. Perform in a well-ventilated area and avoid inhaling particulate matter.
3. Mix powder with liquid just prior to administering; otherwise, the mixture may become thick and difficult to drink.

Evaluation: Evaluate client for:

- Evidence of effective constipation prophylaxis
- Reports of relief of constipation with evacuation of a soft, formed stool

---

Pyrantel pamoate
(pie-**RAN**-tell)
Antiminth, Combantrin✶, Reese's Pinworm (Rx)

See also *Anthelmintics,* p. 40.

Classification: Anthelmintic.

Action/Kinetics: The anthelmintic effect is attributed to the neuromuscular blocking effect of this agent, which paralyzes the helminth, allowing it to be expelled through the feces. It is poorly absorbed from GI tract. **Peak plasma levels:** 0.05–0.13 mcg/ml after 1–3 hr. Partially metabolized in liver. Fifty percent is excreted unchanged in feces and less than 15% excreted unchanged in urine.

Uses: Pinworm (enterobiasis) and roundworm (ascariasis) infestations. Multiple helminth infections.

Contraindications: Pregnancy. Hepatic disease.

Special Concerns: Use with caution in presence of liver dysfunction. Safe use in children less than 2 years of age has not been established.

Side Effects: *GI* (most frequent): Anorexia, nausea, vomiting, cramps, diarrhea. *Hepatic:* Transient elevation of AST. *CNS:* Headache, dizziness, drowsiness, insomnia. *Miscellaneous:* Skin rashes.

Drug Interactions: Use with piperazine for ascariasis results in antagonism of the effect of both drugs.

Dosage: Liquid Oral Suspension. Adults and children: 1 dose of 11 mg/kg (maximum). **Maximum total dose:** 1.0 g.

NURSING CONSIDERATIONS

See also *Nursing Considerations* for *Anthelmintics,* p. 42.

Client/Family Teaching

1. Drug may be taken without regard to food intake.
2. Purging is not necessary prior to or during treatment.
3. Drug may be taken with milk or fruit juice.
4. Provide a printed list of drug side effects, stressing those that require immediate physician notification.

Evaluation: Evaluate client for evidence of negative stool examinations and perianal swabs.

Pyridostigmine bromide
(peer-id-oh-**STIG**-meen)
Mestinon, Regonol (Rx)

For all information, see also *Neostigmine,* p. 926.

Classification: Indirectly acting cholinergic-acetylcholinesterase inhibitor.

Action/Kinetics: Has a slower onset, longer duration of action, and fewer side effects than neostigmine. **Onset, PO:** 30–45 min for syrup and tablets and 30–60 min for extended-release tablets; **IM:** 15 min; **IV:** 2–5 min. **Duration, PO:** 3–6 hr for syrup and tablets and 6–12 hr for extended-release tablets; **IM, IV:** 2–4 hr. Poorly absorbed from the GI tract; excreted in urine up to 72 hr after administration.

Uses: Myasthenia gravis. Antidote for nondepolarizing muscle relaxants (e.g., tubocurarine).

Additional Contraindications: Sensitivity to bromides.

Special Concerns: Safe use during pregnancy and during lactation has not been established. May cause uterine irritability and premature labor if given IV to pregnant women near term. In geriatric clients, the duration of action may be increased.

Additional Side Effects: Skin rash. Thrombophlebitis after IV use. *Symptoms of Overdose:* Abdominal cramps, vomiting, diarrhea, epigastric distress, excessive salivation, cold sweating, pallor, blurred vision, urinary urgency, fasciculation and paralysis of voluntary muscles (including the tongue), miosis, increased blood pressure (may be accompanied by bradycardia), sensation of internal trembling, panic, severe anxiety.

Dosage: Syrup, Tablets. *Myasthenia gravis:* **Adults:** 60–120 mg q 3–4 hr with dosage adjusted to patient response. **Maintenance:** 600 mg daily (range: 60 mg–1.5 g). **Pediatric:** 7 mg/kg (200 mg/m²) daily in 5–6 divided doses. **Sustained-release Tablets. Adults:** 180–540 mg 1–2 times daily with at least 6 hr between doses. Extended-release tablets not recommended for use in children.

IM, IV. *Myasthenia gravis:* **Adults, IM, IV,** 2 mg (about ¹⁄₃₀ the adult dose) q 2–3 hr. *Antidote for nondepolarizing drugs:* **Adults, IV,** 10–20 mg with 0.6–1.2 mg atropine sulfate given IV. *Myasthenia gravis:* **Neonates of myasthenic mothers, IM,** 0.05–0.15 mg/kg q 4–6 hr.

NURSING CONSIDERATIONS

See also *Nursing Considerations* for *Neostigmine,* p. 928.

Administration/Storage

1. During dosage adjustment, administer the drug to the client in a closely monitored environment.
2. Parenteral medication dosage is ¹⁄₃₀ of the oral dose.
3. After oral administration, onset of action occurs in 30–45 min and lasts for 3–6 hr. When administered IM, the onset of action occurs within 15 min. When administered IV, the onset of action occurs within 2–5 min.
4. *Treatment of Overdose:* Discontinue medication temporarily. Give atropine, 0.5–1 mg IV (up to 5–10 mg or more may be needed to get heart rate to 80 beats/min). Supportive treatment including artificial respiration and oxygen.

Interventions

1. Observe the client for toxic reactions demonstrated by generalized cholinergic stimulation.
2. Assess the client for muscular weakness. This may be a sign of impending myasthenic crisis and cholinergic overdose.
3. Work with the client to determine the best individualized medication administration schedule.

Client/Family Teaching

1. Explain how extended-release tablets work. Caution clients not to crush them and not to take these tablets more often than every 6 hr.

2. If ordered by the physician, extended-release tablets may be taken with conventional tablets.

3. Explain how to recognize symptoms of toxic reaction and myasthenic crisis.

4. Stress the importance of taking medication as prescribed since too early administration may result in cholinergic crisis, whereas too late administration may result in myasthenic crisis.

5. Provide with printed instructions and a list of toxic side effects that should be reported to the physician.

6. Clients may develop resistance to the drug. Explain the importance of close medical supervision as well as the prompt reporting of all side effects so that drug therapy can be evaluated.

7. Provide the names and addresses of local support groups that may assist the client and family to understand and cope with the disease.

Evaluation: Evaluate client for:

- Reports of control of the symptoms of myasthenia gravis
- Evidence of successful reversal of nondepolarizing muscle relaxants

---

Pyridoxine hydrochloride (Vitamin B₆)

(peer-ih-**DOX**-een)

Beesix, Hexa-Betalin✹, Nestrex (Rx: Injection; OTC: Tablets)

Classification: Vitamin B complex.

Action/Kinetics: Pyridoxine hydrochloride is a water-soluble, heat-resistant vitamin that is destroyed by light. It is prepared synthetically. It acts as a coenzyme in the metabolism of protein, carbohydrates, and fat. As the amount of protein increases in the diet, the pyridoxine requirement increases. However, pyridoxine deficiency alone is rare. **t½:** 2–3 weeks. Metabolized in the liver and excreted through the urine.

Uses: Pyridoxine deficiency including poor diet, drug-induced (e.g., oral contraceptives, isoniazid), and inborn errors of metabolism. *Investigational:* Hydrazine poisoning, premenstrual syndrome, high urine oxalate levels, nausea and vomiting due to pregnancy.

Special Concerns: Pregnancy category: A. Safety and effectiveness have not been established in children.

Side Effects: *CNS:* Unstable gait; decreased sensation to touch, temperature, and vibration; paresthesia, sleepiness, numbness of feet, awkwardness of hands, perioral numbness. **Note:** Abuse and dependence have been noted in adults administered 200 mg/day.

Symptoms of Overdose: Ataxia, severe sensory neuropathy.

Drug Interactions

Chloramphenicol / ↑ Pyridoxine requirements
Contraceptives, oral / ↑ Pyridoxine requirements
Cycloserine / ↑ Pyridoxine requirements
Ethionamide / ↑ Pyridoxine requirements
Hydralazine / ↑ Pyridoxine requirements

Immunosuppressants /
  ↑ Pyridoxine requirements
Isoniazid / ↑ Pyridoxine
  requirements
Levodopa / Daily doses exceeding
  5 mg pyridoxine antagonize the
  therapeutic effect of levodopa
Penicillamine / ↑ Pyridoxine
  requirements
Phenobarbital / Pyridoxine ↓
  serum levels of phenobarbital
Phenytoin / Pyridoxine ↓ serum
  levels of phenytoin

Dosage: Extended-release Capsules, Tablets. *Dietary supplement:* **Adults,** 10–20 mg daily for 2 weeks; **then,** 2–5 mg daily as part of a multivitamin preparation for several weeks. **Pediatric,** 2.5–10 mg daily for 3 weeks; **then,** 2–5 mg daily as part of a multivitamin preparation for several weeks. *Pyridoxine dependency syndrome:* **Adults and children, initial,** 30–600 mg daily; **maintenance,** 30 mg daily for life. **Infants, maintenance:** 2–10 mg daily for life. *Drug-induced deficiency:* **Adults, prophylaxis,** 10–50 mg daily for penicillamine or 100–300 mg daily for cycloserine, hydralazine, or isoniazid. **Adults, treatment,** 50–200 mg daily for 3 weeks followed by 25–100 mg daily to prevent relapse. **Adults, alcoholism,** 50 mg daily for 2–4 weeks; if anemia responds, continue pyridoxine indefinitely. *Hereditary sideroblastic anemia:* **Adults,** 200–600 mg daily for 1–2 months; **then,** 30–50 mg daily for life.

  IM, IV. *Pyridoxine dependency syndrome:* **Adults,** 30–600 mg daily. **Pediatric:** 10–100 mg. *Drug-induced deficiency:* **Adults,** 50–200 mg daily for 3 weeks followed by 25–100 mg daily as needed. *Cycloserine poisoning:* **Adults,** 300 mg daily. *Isoniazid poisoning:* **Adults,** 1 g for each gram of isoniazid taken.

NURSING CONSIDERATIONS

Administration/Storage

1. If the client is also receiving levodopa, preparations of vitamins containing vitamin B_6 should be avoided because vitamin B_6 decreases the availability of levodopa to the brain.
2. *Treatment of Overdose:* Discontinue pyridoxine; allow up to 6 months for CNS sensation to return.

Assessment: Take a complete drug history. If the client is taking cycloserine, isoniazid, or oral contraceptives, consult with the physician before administering vitamin B_6. These drugs increase pyridoxine requirements.

Interventions: Observe the client for changes in dermatitis around the eyes, nose, and mouth and document. These could indicate an appropriate response to the drug therapy.

Client/Family Teaching

1. Provide the client with a printed list of foods high in vitamin B_6 (e.g., potatoes, lima beans, bananas, meats, whole-grain cereals). Explain that well-balanced diets are the best source of vitamins and refer to dietitican as needed.
2. If the client is taking levodopa, avoid taking vitamin supplements containing vitamin B_6. More than 5 mg of the vitamin antagonizes the effect of levodopa. At the same time, concomitant administration of carbidopa will prevent the effect of vitamin B_6 on levodopa.

3. If the client is also taking phenobarbital and/or phenytoin, advise the client to report for serum levels on a routine basis since pyridoxine alters serum concentrations of these drugs.

4. If the client is a nursing mother, advise her that pyridoxine may inhibit lactation.

Evaluation: Evaluate client for evidence of a reduction in the symptoms of pyridoxine deficiency.

Quazepam

(KWAY-zeh-pam)
Doral (Rx, C-IV)

See also *Benzodiazepines,* p. 108.

Classification: Benzodiazepine, hypnotic.

Action/Kinetics: The drug will improve sleep induction time, duration of sleep, number of nocturnal awakenings, occurrence of early morning awakening, and sleep quality without producing an effect on REM sleep. Hangover effects are minimal. **Peak plasma levels:** 2 hr. Quazepam and two of its metabolites (2-oxoquazepam and N-desalkyl-2-oxoquazepam) are active on the CNS. **$t\frac{1}{2}$, quazepam and 2-oxoquazepam:** 39 hr; **$t\frac{1}{2}$, N-desalkyl-2-oxoquazepam:** 73 hr. Significantly (95%) bound to plasma protein.

Uses: Insomnia characterized by difficulty in falling asleep, frequent nocturnal awakenings, and/or early morning awakenings.

Contraindications: Clients with established sleep apnea. Pregnancy (category: X), lactation.

Special Concerns: Use with caution in clients with impaired renal or hepatic function, in chronic pulmonary insufficiency, and in depression. Safety and effectiveness have not been established in children less than 18 years of age. Use during lactation may cause sedation and feeding problems in the infant. Geriatric and debilitated clients may be more sensitive to the effects of quazepam.

Side Effects: *CNS:* Daytime drowsiness (most common), headache, dizziness, fatigue, irritability, slurred speech, paradoxical stimulation, agitation, sleep disturbances, hallucinations. *GI:* Dry mouth, dyspepsia. *Miscellaneous:* Incontinence, urinary retention, jaundice, dysarthria, dystonia, changes in libido, menstrual irregularities. **Note:** Rapid withdrawal after continued use may cause signs and symptoms of withdrawal from CNS depressant drugs.

Drug Interactions: Additive CNS depressant effects when taken with antihistamines, ethanol, antipsychotics, anticonvulsants, and other drugs producing depression of the CNS.

Dosage: Tablets. Adults, initial: 15 mg until individual response has been determined. The dose may be

Q

reduced to 7.5 mg in some clients (especially in geriatric or debilitated clients).

NURSING CONSIDERATIONS

See also *Nursing Considerations* for *Benzodiazepines,* p. 111.

Client/Family Teaching

1. Do not use alcohol or any other drugs having CNS depressant effects while taking quazepam.
2. Do not drive a car or operate potentially dangerous machinery until the sedative effects of the drug are known.
3. The drug may produce daytime sedation even for several days after it has been discontinued.
4. Do not increase the dose of quazepam without first consulting with the physician.
5. Do not stop taking the drug abruptly following prolonged and regular use.
6. Explore sleeping habits and offer alternative methods to induce sleep and ensure adequate rest such as relaxation techniques or white noise simulators.

Evaluation: Evaluate client for reports of improved sleeping patterns with less frequent awakenings.

Quinapril hydrochloride
(**KWIN**-ah-prill)
Accupril (Rx)

See also *Angiotensin-Converting Enzyme (ACE) Inhibitors,* p. 33.

Classification: Angiotensin-converting enzyme (ACE) inhibitor.

Action/Kinetics: Onset: 1 hr. **Time to peak serum levels:** 1 hr. The peak reduction of blood pressure occurs within 2–4 hr after dosing. Quinapril is metabolized to quinaprilat, the active metabolite. $t\frac{1}{2}$, **quinaprilat:** 2 hr. **Duration:** 24 hr. The drug is metabolized with approximately 60% excreted through the urine and 37% excreted in the feces.

Uses: Alone or in combination with a thiazide diuretic for the treatment of hypertension. *Investigational:* Congestive heart failure.

Special Concerns: Pregnancy category: D. Use with caution during lactation. Safety and effectiveness have not been determined in children. Geriatric clients may be more sensitive to the effects of quinapril.

Side Effects: *Dermatologic:* Angioedema of the lips, tongue, glottis, and larynx; sweating, pruritus, exfoliative dermatitis, photosensitivity. *CV:* Vasodilation, tachycardia, heart failure, palpitation, myocardial infarction, cerebrovascular accident, hypertensive crisis, angina pectoris, orthostatic hypotension, cardiac rhythm disturbances. *Body as a whole:* Malaise, back pain. *GI:* Dry mouth or throat, constipation, GI hemorrhage. *CNS:* Lightheadedness, syncope, somnolence, vertigo, nervousness, depression. *Hematologic:* Agranulocytosis, neutropenia, bone marrow depression, thrombocytopenia. *GU:* Oliguria and/or progressive azotemia and rarely acute renal failure and/or death in severe heart failure. *Miscellaneous:* Oligohydramnios in fetuses exposed to the drug *in utero.* Abnormal liver function tests, pancreatitis, hyperkalemia, amblyopia, pharyngitis, sinusitis, bronchitis.

Drug Interactions

Potassium-containing salt substitutes / ↑ Risk of hyperkalemia
Potassium-sparing diuretics / ↑ Risk of hyperkalemia
Potassium supplements / ↑ Risk of hyperkalemia
Tetracyclines / ↓ Absorption of tetracycline

Dosage: Tablets. Initial: 10 mg once daily; **then,** adjust dosage based on blood pressure response at peak (2–6 hr) and trough (predose) blood levels. The dose should be adjusted at 2-week intervals. **Maintenance:** 20, 40, or 80 mg daily as a single dose or in two equally divided doses. In clients with impaired renal function, the initial dose should be 10 mg if the creatinine clearance is greater than 60 ml/min, 5 mg if the creatinine clearance is between 30 and 60 ml/min, and 2.5 mg if the creatinine clearance is between 10 and 30 ml/min.

NURSING CONSIDERATIONS

See also *Angiotensin-Converting Enzyme Inhibitors,* p. 35.

Administration/Storage

1. If the client is taking a diuretic, the diuretic should be discontinued 2–3 days prior to beginning quinapril therapy. If the blood pressure is not controlled, the diuretic should be reinstituted. If the diuretic cannot be discontinued, an initial dose of quinapril should be 1.25 mg.
2. If the antihypertensive effect decreases at the end of the dosing interval in clients taking the medication once daily, either twice daily administra-tion should be considered or the dose should be increased.
3. The antihypertensive effect may not be observed for 1–2 weeks.

Interventions

1. Monitor vital signs, I&O, and weights.
2. Obtain baseline electrolytes, CBC, and renal function studies and monitor throughout therapy. Agranulocytosis and bone marrow depression are seen more often in clients with renal impairment, especially if they also have a collagen vascular disease (e.g., systemic lupus erythematosus, scleroderma).
3. Clients with unilateral or bilateral renal artery stenosis may manifest ↑ BUN and serum creatinine if given quinapril. Thus, renal function should be monitored closely the first few weeks of therapy.
4. If angioedema occurs, the drug should be discontinued immediately and the client observed until the swelling disappears. Antihistamines may be useful in relieving symptoms.
5. Infants exposed to quinapril *in utero* should be closely observed for the development of hypotension, oliguria, and hyperkalemia. Treat symptomatically.

Evaluation: Evaluate client for evidence of successful control of hypertension with a minimum of drug side effects.

Quinidine bisulfate

(KWIN-ih-deen)
Bioquin Durules ✿ (Rx)

Quinidine gluconate
(KWIN-ih-deen)
Duraquin, Quinaglute, Quinalan,
Quinate✲ (Rx)

Quinidine polygalacturonate
(KWIN-ih-deen)
Cardioquin (Rx)

Quinidine sulfate
(KWIN-ih-deen)
Apo-Quinidine✲, Cin-Quin,
Novo–Quinidin✲, Quinidex,
Quinora (Rx)

See also *Antiarrhythmic Drugs*, p. 51.

Classification: Antiarrhythmic, type IA.

Action/Kinetics: Quinidine reduces the excitability of the heart and increases the refractory period by decreasing potassium efflux from cardiac fibers. It also decreases cardiac output and possesses anticholinergic, antimalarial, antipyretic, and oxytocic properties. **PO: Onset:** 0.5–3 hr. **Duration:** 6–8 hr for tablets/capsules and 12 hr for extended-release tablets. $t\frac{1}{2}$: 6–7 hr. **Time to peak levels, PO:** 3–4 hr for gluconate salt and 1–1.5 hr for sulfate salt; **IM:** 1 hr. **Therapeutic serum levels:** 2–6 mcg/ml. **Protein binding:** 60%–80%. **Duration:** 6–8 hr for tablets/capsules and 12 hr for extended-release tablets. Metabolized by liver. Rate of urinary excretion (10%–50% excreted unchanged) is affected by urinary pH.

Uses: Treatment and control of atrial flutter, established atrial fibrillation, paroxysmal atrial fibrillation and tachycardia, paroxysmal AV junctional rhythm, paroxysmal ventricular tachycardia not associated with complete heart block, premature atrial and ventricular contractions. Often the drug of choice for atrial fibrillation and atrial and ventricular arrhythmias. Not indicated for prophylaxis during surgery.

Contraindications: Hypersensitivity to drug or other cinchona drugs.

Special Concerns: Safety for use during pregnancy (category: C) and lactation and in children has not been established. Quinidine should be used with extreme caution in clients in whom a sudden change in blood pressure might be detrimental or in those suffering from extensive myocardial damage, subacute endocarditis, bradycardia, coronary occlusion, disturbances in impulse conduction, chronic valvular disease, considerable cardiac enlargement, frank congestive heart failure, arrhythmias due to digitalis toxicity, renal disease. Cautious use is also recommended in clients with acute infections, hyperthyroidism, myasthenia gravis, muscular weakness, respiratory distress, and bronchial asthma. The dose in geriatric clients may have to be reduced due to age-related changes in renal function.

Side Effects: *CV:* Widening of QRS complex, hypotension, asystole, ectopic ventricular beats, ventricular tachycardia or fibrillation, arterial embolism, circulatory collapse, bradycardia, congestive heart failure, partial or total heart block. *GI:* Nausea, vomiting, abdominal pain, colic, anorexia, diarrhea, urge to defecate as well as urinate. *CNS:* Syncope, headache, confusion, excitement, vertigo, apprehension, tinnitus, decreased hearing acuity.

Dermatologic: Skin eruptions, urticaria, exfoliative dermatitis, photosensitivity, flushing. *Allergic:* Acute asthma, angioneurotic edema, respiratory paralysis, dyspnea, fever, vascular collapse. *Hematologic:* Hypoprothrombinemia, acute hemolytic anemia, thrombocytopenic purpura, agranulocytosis. *Ophthalmologic:* Blurred vision, mydriasis, alterations in color perception, decreased field of vision, double vision, photophobia, optic neuritis, night blindness, scotomata. *Other:* Liver toxicity including hepatitis, lupus erythematosus (rare).

Symptoms of Overdose: CNS symptoms include lethargy, confusion, coma, seizures, and respiratory arrest. Also, vomiting, diarrhea, abdominal pain, hypokalemia, cinchonism, sinus tachycardia, ventricular tachycardia or fibrillation, torsade de pointes, depressed automaticity and conduction (including bundle branch block, sinus bradycardia, SA block, prolongation of QRS and QT, sinus arrest, AV block). Hypotension due to decreased conduction and cardiac output and vasodilation.

Drug Interactions

Acetazolamide, Antacids / ↑ Effect of quinidine due to ↓ renal excretion
Anticholinergic agents, Atropine / Additive effect on blockade of vagus nerve action
Anticoagulants, oral / Additive hypoprothrombinemia
Barbiturates / ↓ Effect of quinidine due to ↑ breakdown by liver
Cholinergic agents / Quinidine antagonizes effect of cholinergic drugs
Cimetidine / ↑ Effect of quinidine due to ↓ breakdown by liver
Digoxin, Digitoxin / ↑ Symptoms of digoxin toxicity
Guanethidine / Additive hypotensive effect
Methyldopa / Additive hypotensive effect
Neuromuscular blocking agents / ↑ Respiratory depression
Phenobarbital, Phenytoin / ↓ Effect of quinidine by ↑ rate of metabolism in liver
Phenothiazines / Additive cardiac depressant effect
Potassium / ↑ Effect of quinidine
Propranolol / Both drugs produce a negative inotropic effect on the heart
Reserpine / Additive cardiac depressant effects
Rifampin / ↓ Effect of quinidine due to ↑ breakdown by liver
Skeletal muscle relaxants / ↑ Skeletal muscle relaxation
Sodium bicarbonate / ↑ Effect of quinidine due to ↓ renal excretion
Thiazide diuretics / ↑ Effect of quinidine due to ↓ renal excretion
Verapamil / Hypotension in clients with hypertrophic cardiomyopathy

Q

Laboratory Test Interferences: False + or ↑ PSP, 17-ketosteroids, prothrombin time.

Dosage: Quinidine Gluconate Extended-Release Tablets. Adults, maintenance: 324–660 mg q 6–12 hr as needed. Use not recommended for children. **Quinidine Polygalacturonate Tablets. Adults, initial:** 275–825 mg q 3–4 hr for 3–4 doses; **then,** increase by 137.5–275 mg q third or fourth dose until rhythm is restored. **Maintenance:** 275 mg b.i.d.–t.i.d. as needed. **Pediatric:** 8.25 mg/kg (247.5 mg/m^2) 5 times a day.

Quinidine Sulfate Capsules/Tablets. Adults, *premature atrial and ventricular contractions:* 200–300 mg t.i.d.–q.i.d. *Paroxysmal supraventricular tachycardias:* 400–600 mg q 2–3 hr until beneficial effect noted. *Conversion of atrial fibrillation:* 200 mg q 2–3 hr for 5–8 doses; dose may be increased daily as needed and tolerated. **Maintenance:** 200–300 mg t.i.d.–q.i.d. as needed. **Pediatric,** *antiarrhythmic:* 6 mg/kg (180 mg/m²) five times daily. **Quinidine Sulfate Extended-release Tablets.** 300–600 mg q 8–12 hr as needed. Use not recommended in children.

Quinidine Gluconate Injection. IM, initial: 600 mg; **then,** 400 mg repeated as frequently as q 2 hr if needed. **IV:** 800 mg in 40 ml of 5% dextrose injection at a rate of 1 ml/min.

Quinidine Sulfate Injection. IV, 600 mg in 40 ml of 5% dextrose injection at a rate of 1 ml/min.

NURSING CONSIDERATIONS

See also *Nursing Considerations* for *Antiarrhythmic Drugs,* p. 52.

Administration/Storage

1. A preliminary test dose may be given before instituting quinidine therapy. **Adults:** 200 mg quinidine sulfate or quinidine gluconate administered PO or IM. **Children:** Test dose of 2 mg of quinidine sulfate per kilogram of body weight.
2. IV solution can be prepared by diluting 10 ml of quinidine gluconate injection with 50 ml of 5% glucose solution; this should be given at a rate of 1 ml/min.
3. Use only colorless clear solution for injection because light may cause quinidine to crystallize, which turns solution brownish.
4. *Treatment of Overdose:*
   - Perform gastric lavage, induce vomiting, and administer activated charcoal if ingestion is recent.
   - Monitor ECG and blood pressure.
   - Institute cardiac pacing, if necessary.
   - Acidify the urine.
   - Use artificial respiration and other supportive measures.
   - Infusions of ⅙ molar sodium lactate IV may decrease the cardiotoxic effects.
   - Treat hypotension with metaraminol or norepinephrine after fluid volume replacement.
   - Hemodialysis is effective but not often required.

Assessment

1. Note any history of allergic reactions to antiarrhythmic drugs or tartrazine which is found in some formulations.
2. Determine that pretreatment lab tests including blood glucose, CBC, liver and renal function studies have been performed.
3. Obtain vital signs and ECG and auscultate heart sounds to determine baseline information against which to measure postmedication responses.

Interventions

1. Evaluate ECG and report any evidence of increased AV block, cardiac irritability or suppression during IV administration.
2. Observe client for hypersensitivity reactions.
3. Monitor I&O and vital signs;

observe closely for evidence of hypotension. The drug induces urinary alkalization.

4. Observe clients for neurologic deficits or sensory impairment and report if evident.

5. Monitor serum electrolytes, CBC, liver and renal function studies during prolonged therapy with quinidine. Report any persistent diarrhea.

6. Among the elderly, there is a higher risk of toxicity, reduced cardiac output, and unpredictable effects from drug therapy.

7. Clients with long-standing atrial fibrillation or CHF with atrial fibrillation run a risk of embolization from mural thrombi when converting to sinus rhythm.

Client/Family Teaching

1. Administer with food to minimize GI effects.

2. Take only as directed and notify physician of any persistent bothersome side effects.

3. Drug may cause dizziness or blurred vision. Activities that require mental alertness should be avoided until drug effects are realized.

4. Wear dark glasses if photophobia is experienced.

5. Incorporate fruit and grain in the diet. A high intake of fruits and vegetables (alkaline-ash foods) may prolong the half-life of quinidine.

6. Palpitations or faintness may indicate quinidine-induced ventricular arrhythmias and should be reported immediately.

7. If any of the following symptoms occur, advise the client to call the physician:
   • Severe skin rash, hives or itching

• Severe headache
• Unexplained fever
• Ringing in the ears, buzzing, or hearing loss
• Unusual bruising or bleeding
• Blurred vision
• Irregular heart beat
• Continued diarrhea

8. Stress the importance of reporting for laboratory studies and follow-up appointments as scheduled.

Evaluation: Evaluate client for:
• ECG evidence of effective control of cardiac arrhythmia
• Laboratory confirmation that serum drug levels are within therapeutic range (2–6 mcg/ml)

Quinine sulfate
(KWYE-nine)
Formula Q, Legatrim, M-KYA, Novo–Quinine ✿, Quinamm, Quiphile, Q-vel, (Rx)

Classification: Antimalarial.

Action/Kinetics: This drug is a natural alkaloid obtained from the bark of the cinchona tree. In addition to its antimalarial properties, it has antipyretic, analgesic, and oxytocic properties similar to those of the salicylates. It relieves muscle spasms and is used as a diagnostic agent for myasthenia gravis. Quinine has been used increasingly in the last several years since resistant forms of vivax and falciparum were observed in Southeast Asia. No resistant forms of the parasite have been found for quinine.

The precise antimalarial mechanism of action is not known; quinine does affect DNA replication.

The drug may also act to raise intracellular pH. The drug eradicates the erythrocytic stages of plasmodia. Quinine also increases the refractory period of skeletal muscle and decreases the excitability of the motor end-plate region, making it useful for nocturnal leg cramps. Quinine is rapidly and completely absorbed from the GI tract and is widely distributed in body tissues. **Peak plasma levels:** 1–3 hr **t½:.** 4–5 hr. The drug is highly bound to protein (70%–85%) and about 5% is excreted unchanged in urine. Small amounts of the drug are found in saliva, bile, feces, and gastric juice. Acidifying the urine increases the rate of excretion.

Uses: In combination with pyrimethamine and a sulfonamide or a tetracycline for resistant forms of *Plasmodium falciparum.* Chloroquine sensitive stains of *P. falciparum, P. malariae, P. ovale,* and *P. vivax.* Nocturnal leg cramps.

Contraindications: Clients with tinnitus. Glucose-6-phosphate dehydrogenase deficiency, optic neuritis, history of blackwater fever, and thrombocytopenia purpura associated with previous use of quinine. Pregnancy (category X) as the drug is oxytocic and may cause congenital malformations.

Special Concerns: Use with caution in clients with cardiac arrhythmias. Use with caution during lactation.

Side Effects: Use of quinine may result in a syndrome referred to as *cinchonism.* Mild cinchonism is characterized by tinnitus, headache, nausea, slight visual disturbances. Larger doses, however, may cause severe CNS, cardiovascular, GI, or dermatologic effects.

Allergic: Flushing, rashes, fever, facial edema, pruritus, dyspnea, tinnitus, gastric upset. *GI:* Nausea, vomiting, gastric pain. *Ophthalmologic:* Blurred vision, photophobia, diplopia, night blindness, decreased visual fields, impaired color perception. *CNS:* Headache, confusion, restlessness, vertigo, syncope, fever. *Hematologic:* Thrombocytopenia, hypoprothrombinemia. *CV:* Symptoms of angina, ventricular tachycardia, conduction disturbances. *Miscellaneous:* Sweating.

Symptoms of Overdose: Dizziness, intestinal cramping, skin rash, tinnitus. With higher doses, symptoms include apprehension, confusion, fever, headache, vomiting, and seizures.

Drug Interactions

Acetazolamide / ↑ Effect of quinine due to ↓ rate of elimination

Aluminum-containing antacids / ↓ Or delay absorption of quinine

Anticoagulants, oral / Additive hypoprothrombinemia due to ↓ synthesis of vitamin K-dependent clotting factors

Cimetidine / ↑ Effect of quinine due to ↓ rate of excretion

Digoxin / Quinine ↑ effect of digoxin

Heparin / Effect ↓ by quinine

Mefloquine / ↑ Risk of ECG abnormalities or cardiac arrest. **Do not use together.**

Pyrimethamine / ↑ Effect of quinine due to ↓ in plasma protein binding

Skeletal muscle relaxants (surgical) / ↑ Respiratory depression and apnea

Sodium bicarbonate / ↑ Effect of quinine due to ↓ rate of elimination

Dosage: Capsules, Tablets. *Chloroquine-resistant malaria:* **Adults,** 650 mg q 8 hr for at least 3 days (7 days in Southeast Asia) along with pyrimethamine, 25 mg b.i.d. for the first 3 days and sulfadiazine, 2 g daily for the first 5 days. There are two alternative regimens: (1) quinine, 650 mg q 8 hr for at least 3 days (7 days in Southeast Asia) along with a tetracycline, 250 mg q 6 hr for 10 days or (2) quinine, 650 mg q 8 hr for 3 days with sulfadoxine, 1.5 g and pyrimethamine, 75 mg as a single dose. *Chloroquine-sensitive malaria:* **Adults,** 600 mg q 8 hr for 5–7 days. **Pediatric,** 10 mg/kg q 8 hr for 5–7 days. *Nocturnal leg cramps:* 200–300 mg at bedtime; an additional 260–300 mg may be taken after the evening meal.

NURSING CONSIDERATIONS

See also *General Nursing Considerations For All Anti-Infectives,* p. 83.

Administration/Storage: *Treatment of Overdose:*
- Induce vomiting or undertake gastric lavage.
- Maintain blood pressure and renal function.
- If necessary, provide artificial respiration.
- Sedatives, oxygen, and other supportive measures may be required.
- Give IV fluids to maintain fluid and electrolyte balance.
- Treat angioedema or asthma with epinephrine, corticosteroids, and antihistamines.
- Urinary acidification will hasten excretion; however, in the presence of hemoglobinuria, acidification of the urine will increase renal blockade.

Assessment
1. Note any history or evidence of cardiac arrhythmias.
2. Obtain baseline CBC and ophthalmic exam and monitor throughout drug therapy.

Client/Family Teaching
1. Do not take medication with antacids. Take with or immediately after meals to reduce GI upset.
2. If also taking cimetidine or digoxin, report any side effects immediately because dosage may need to be adjusted.
3. Report any ringing of the ears, blurring of vision, and headache, which may be followed by digestive disturbances, impairment of hearing and sight, confusion, and delirium. This may indicate intolerance or overdosage and requires immediate medical intervention.
4. Drug may cause dizziness or blurred vision. Do not drive a car or operate machinery until drug effects are realized.
5. If female and of childbearing age, advise to use birth control because drug may harm fetus.

Evaluation: Evaluate client for:
- Evidence of termination of acute malarial attack and control of symptoms of malaria
- Reports of ↓ frequency and intensity of nocturnal leg cramps

R

Ramipril
(**RAM**-ih-prill)
Altace (Rx)

See also *Angiotensin-Converting Enzyme (ACE) Inhibitors,* p. 33.

Classification: Angiotensin-converting enzyme inhibitor.

Action/Kinetics: Onset: 1–2 hr. **Time to peak serum levels:** 1 hr (1–2 hr for ramiprilat, the active metabolite). Ramiprilat has approximately six times the ACE inhibitory activity than ramipril. **t½:** 1–2 hr (prolonged in impaired renal function). **Duration:** 24 hr. Metabolized in the liver with 60% excreted through the urine and 40% in the feces.

Uses: Alone or in combination with other antihypertensive agents (especially thiazide diuretics) for the treatment of hypertension. *Investigational:* Used with digoxin and diuretics to treat congestive heart failure.

Contraindications: Use during lactation.

Special Concerns: Pregnancy category: D.

Side Effects: *CV:* Hypotension, chest pain, palpitations, angina pectoris, arrhythmias. *GI:* Nausea, vomiting, abdominal pain, diarrhea, dysgeusia, anorexia, constipation, dry mouth, dyspepsia, enzyme changes suggesting pancreatitis, dysphagia, gastroenteritis, increased salivation. *CNS:* Headache, dizziness, fatigue, insomnia, sleep disturbances, somnolence, depression, nervousness, malaise, vertigo, anxiety, amnesia, convulsions, tremor. *Respiratory:* Cough, dyspnea, upper respiratory tract infection. *Hematologic:* Leukopenia, eosinophila, proteinuria. *Dermatologic:* Diaphoresis, photosensitivity, pruritus, rash, dermatitis, purpura. *Body as a whole:* Paresthesias, angioedema, asthenia, syncope, fever, muscle cramps, myalgia, arthralgia, arthritis, neuralgia, neuropathy, tremor, influenza, edema. *Miscellaneous:* Impotence, paresthesias, tinnitus, hearing loss, vision disturbances, epistaxis, weight gain.

Laboratory Test Interferences: ↓ Hemoglobin, hematocrit.

Dosage: Capsules. Initial: 2.5 mg once daily in clients not taking a diuretic; **maintenance:** 2.5–20 mg daily as a single dose or two equally divided doses. *Clients taking diuretics or who have a creatinine clearance less than 40 ml/min/1.73 m²:* initially 1.25 mg once daily; dose may then be increased to a maximum of 5 mg daily.

NURSING CONSIDERATIONS

See also *Nursing Considerations for Angiotensin-Converting Enzyme Inhibitors,* p. 35.

Administration/Storage

1. If the antihypertensive effect decreases at the end of the dosing interval in clients taking the medication once daily, either twice daily administration should be considered or the dose should be increased.
2. If the client is taking a diuretic, the diuretic should be discontinued 2–3 days prior to beginning ramipril therapy. If the

blood pressure is not controlled, the diuretic should be reinstituted. If the diuretic cannot be discontinued, an initial dose of ramipril should be 1.25 mg.

Evaluation: Evaluate client for successful control of hypertension with a minimum of drug side effects.

Ranitidine hydrochloride
(rah-**NIH**-tih-deen)
Apo-Ranitidine✷, Novo–Ranidine✷, Nu-Ranit✷, Zantac, Zantac-C✷ (Rx)

Classification: H$_2$-receptor antagonist.

Action/Kinetics: Ranitidine competitively inhibits gastric acid secretion by blocking the effect of histamine on histamine H$_2$ receptors. Both daytime and nocturnal basal gastric acid secretion, as well as food- and pentagastrin-stimulated gastric acid are inhibited. It is a weak inhibitor of cytochrome P-450 (drug-metabolizing enzymes); thus, drug interactions involving inhibition of hepatic metabolism are not expected to occur. Food increases the bioavailability. **Peak effect: PO,** 1–3 hr; **IM, IV,** 15 min. t½: 2.5–3 hr. **Duration, nocturnal:** 13 hr; **basal:** 4 hr. **Serum level to inhibit 50% stimulated gastric acid secretion:** 36–94 ng/ml. Excreted in urine.

Uses: Short-term (4–8 weeks) and maintenance treatment of duodenal ulcer. Pathologic hypersecretory conditions such as Zollinger-Ellison syndrome and systemic mastocytosis. Active, benign gastric ulcers, reflux esophagitis. *Investigational:* Prophylaxis of pulmonary aspiration of acid during anesthesia, prevent gastric damage from NSAIDs, prevent stress ulcers, acute upper GI bleeding.

Contraindications: Cirrhosis of the liver, impaired renal or hepatic function.

Special Concerns: Use with caution during pregnancy (category: B) and lactation and in clients with decreased hepatic or renal function. Safety and efficacy not established in children.

Side Effects: *GI:* Constipation, nausea, vomiting, diarrhea, abdominal pain, pancreatitis (rare). *CNS:* Headache, dizziness, malaise, insomnia, vertigo, confusion, anxiety, agitation, depression, fatigue, somnolence, hallucinations. *CV:* Bradycardia or tachycardia, premature ventricular beats. *Hematologic:* Thrombocytopenia, granulocytopenia, leukopenia, pancytopenia, agranulocytosis, aplastic anemia, autoimmune hemolytic anemia. *Hepatic:* Hepatotoxicity, jaundice, hepatitis, increase in ALT. *Dermatologic:* Pruritus, urticaria, erythema multiforme, rash, alopecia. *Allergic:* Bronchospasm, rashes, fever, eosinophilia. *Other:* Arthralgia, gynecomastia, impotence, loss of libido, blurred vision, angioneurotic edema, pain at injection site, local burning or itching following IV use.

Drug Interactions

Antacids / Antacids may ↓ the absorption of ranitidine
Glipizide / Ranitidine ↑ effect of glipizide
Procainamide / Ranitidine ↓ excretion of procainamide → possible ↑ effect
Theophylline / Possible ↑ effect of theophylline

R

Warfarin / Ranitidine may ↑ hypoprothrombinemic effects of warfarin

Laboratory Test Interference: False + test for urine protein using Multistix.

Dosage: Syrup, Tablets. Adults: *Duodenal ulcer:* 150 mg b.i.d. or 300 mg at bedtime to heal ulcer, although 100 mg b.i.d. will inhibit acid secretion. **Maintenance:** 150 mg at bedtime. *Hypersecretory conditions:* 150 mg b.i.d. (up to 6 g/day has been used in severe cases). *Gastroesophageal reflux, benign gastric ulcer:* 150 mg b.i.d. In impaired renal function (creatinine clearance less than 50 ml/min): **PO,** 150 mg/day; **IM, IV.** *All uses:* **Adults, IM,** 50 mg q 6–8 hr. **Intermittent IV injection or infusion:** 50 mg q 6–8 hr, not to exceed 400 mg daily.

NURSING CONSIDERATIONS

Administration/Storage

1. Antacids should be given concomitantly for gastric pain although they may interfere with absorption of ranitidine.
2. About one-half of clients may heal completely within 2 weeks; thus, endoscopy may show no need for further treatment.
3. No dilution is required for IM use. For IV injection, 50 mg should be diluted with 0.9% sodium chloride injection to a total volume of 20 ml. The diluted solution should be given over 5 min or more. For intermittent IV infusion, dilute 50 mg in 100 ml 5% dextrose injection and give over 15–20 min.
4. May be used for continuous infusion.

Assessment

1. Note any evidence of renal or liver disease and obtain baseline studies.
2. When working with sexually active female clients, determine the potential of an existing pregnancy. The drug should be used cautiously in these instances.
3. Assess for any evidence of infections. Have a CBC with differential conducted routinely to detect any potential increased risk of infection.

Client/Family Teaching

1. Take with or immediately following meals. Wait 1 hr before taking an antacid.
2. Do not drive a car or operate machinery until drug effects are realized; dizziness or drowsiness may occur.
3. Avoid alcohol and beverages that contain caffeine (tea, cola, coffee) because these tend to increase stomach acid.
4. Encourage the client not to smoke because smoking may interfere with the healing of duodenal ulcers and decreases the drug's effectiveness.
5. Report any evidence of diarrhea and maintain adequate hydration.
6. Advise that the development of any confusion or disorientation should be immediately reported.
7. Explain to the client with symptoms that breast tenderness will usually disappear after several weeks. If it persists, the physician should be notified because the drug therapy may need to be discontinued.
8. Report for scheduled visits so

physician can determine the extent of healing and when the drug can be safely discontinued.

Evaluation: Evaluate client for:
- Evidence of a decrease in gastric acidity and subjective reports of symptomatic improvement in abdominal pain and discomfort
- Endoscopic or radiographic evidence of duodenal ulcer healing

—— *COMBINATION DRUG* ——
Reserpine and Chlorothiazide
(reh-**SIR**-peen, klor-oh-**THIGH**-ah-zyd)
Diupres, Diurigen with Reserpine (Rx)

See also *Chlorothiazide*, p. 432.

Classification/Content: *Antihypertensive:* Reserpine, 0.125 mg. *Antihypertensive/diuretic:* Chlorothiazide, 250 or 500 mg.

Uses: Hypertension—not to be used for initial treatment.

Contraindications: Pregnancy, lactation, anuria. Reserpine is contraindicated in active peptic ulcer, ulcerative colitis, active mental depression, and in clients with suicidal tendencies.

Special Concerns: Pregnancy category: C. Safety and effectiveness have not been determined in children. Use with caution in severe renal disease, in impaired hepatic function, and progressive liver disease. Geriatric clients may be more sensitive to the usual adult dose.

Dosage: PO: 1–2 tablets 1–2 times daily.

NURSING CONSIDERATIONS

See also *Nursing Considerations* for *Thiazide Diuretics*, p. 233, and *Antihypertensive Agents*, p. 78.

Administration/Storage
1. Monitor BP carefully if Diupres is used with other antihypertensive agents.
2. Administer with or after meals.

Evaluation: Evaluate client for evidence of control of hypertension.

—— *COMBINATION DRUG* ——
Reserpine, Hydralazine, and Hydrochlorothiazide
(reh-**SIR**-peen, hy-**DRAL**-ah-zeen, hy-droh-**klor**-oh-**THIGH**-ah-zyd)
Cam-Ap-Es, Cherapas, Ser-A-Gen, Seralazide, Ser-Ap-Es, Serpazide, Tri-Hydroserpine, Unipres (Rx)

See also *Hydralazine*, p. 716, and *Hydrochlorothiazide*, p. 718.

Classification/Content: *Antihypertensive:* Hydralazine, 25 mg. *Antihypertensive:* Reserpine, 0.1 mg. *Antihypertensive/diuretic:* Hydrochlorothiazide, 15 mg.

Uses: Treatment of hypertension (not to be used for initial therapy).

Contraindications: Pregnancy, lactation, anuria. Reserpine is contraindicated in active peptic ulcer, ulcerative colitis, active mental depression, in clients with suicidal tendencies or in those receiving electroconvulsive shock therapy, coronary artery disease, mitral valvular rheumatic heart disease.

Special Concerns: Pregnancy category: C. Safety and effectiveness

R

have not been determined in children. Geriatric clients may be more sensitive to the adult dose.

Dosage: PO. Individualized. Usual: 1–2 tablets t.i.d.

NURSING CONSIDERATIONS

See also *Nursing Considerations* for *Hydralazine,* p. 717, *Hydrochlorothiazide,* p. 718, and *Antihypertensive Agents,* p. 78.

Administration/Storage

1. It may take up to 2 weeks to manifest the maximum effect on blood pressure reduction.
2. Clients should be maintained on the lowest dose possible (requires titration).
3. If additional antihypertensive medication is necessary, initial doses should be 50% of the usual recommended dose.

Assessment

1. Note any history of mental depression or electroshock therapy.
2. Determine presence of ulcerative colitis or peptic ulcer disease.

R

Evaluation: Evaluate client for evidence of control of hypertension.

Ribavirin

(rye-bah-**VYE**-rin)

Virazole, Virazole (Lyophilized) ✱ **(Rx)**

Classification: Antiviral agent.

Action/Kinetics: Although the precise mechanism is not known, ribavirin may act as a competitive inhibitor of cellular enzymes that act on guanosine and xanthosine. Ribavirin is distributed to the plasma, respiratory tract, and red blood cells and is rapidly taken up by cells. **t½:** 9.5 hr. Eliminated through both the urine and feces.

Uses: Hospitalized pediatric clients (including infants) with severe lower respiratory tract infections (viral pneumonia including bronchiolitis) due to respiratory syncytial virus (RSV). Ribavirin is intended to be used along with standard treatment (including fluid management) for such clients with severe lower respiratory tract infections. *Investigational:* Ribavirin aerosol has been used against influenza A and B. Oral ribavirin has been used against herpes genitalis, acute and chronic hepatitis, measles, and Lassa fever.

Contraindications: Infants requiring artificial respiration (the drug may precipitate in the equipment and interfere with appropriate ventilation of the client). Children with mild RSV lower respiratory tract infections who require a shorter hospital stay than required for a full course of ribavirin therapy. Pregnancy or women who may become pregnant during drug therapy (the drug may cause fetal harm and is known to be teratogenic). Lactation.

Special Concerns: Pregnancy category: X. Use with caution in adults with asthma or chronic obstructive lung disease (deterioration of respiratory function may occur).

Side Effects: *Pulmonary:* Worsening of respiration, pneumothorax, apnea, bacterial pneumonia, dependence on ventilator. *CV:* Hypotension, cardiac arrest, manifestations of digitalis toxicity. *Other:* Anemia (with IV or oral ribavirin); conjunctivitis and rash (with the aerosol).

Dosage: Aerosol only, to an infant oxygen hood using the Small Particle Aerosol Generator-2 (SPAG-2): The concentration administered is 20 mg/ml and the average aerosol concentration for a 12-hr period is 190 mcg/L of air. See *Administration/Storage.*

NURSING CONSIDERATIONS

Administration/Storage

1. Administration of the drug should be carried out for 12–18 hr/day for 3 (minimum)–7 (maximum) days.
2. Treatment is most effective if initiated within the first 3 days of the respiratory syncytial virus, which causes lower respiratory tract infections.
3. Ribavirin aerosol should only be administered using the SPAG-2 aerosol generator.
4. Therapy should *not* be instituted in clients requiring artificial respiration.
5. No other aerosolized medications should be given if ribavirin aerosol is being used.
6. The drug may be solubilized with sterile water (USP) for injection or inhalation in the 100-ml vial. The solution is then transferred to the SPAG-2 reservoir utilizing a sterilized 500 ml wide mouth Erlenmeyer flask and further diluted to a final volume of 300 ml with sterile water.
7. Solutions in the SPAG-2 reservoir should be replaced daily. Also, if the liquid level is low, it should be discarded before new drug solution is added.
8. Reconstituted solutions of ribavirin may be stored at room temperature for 24 hr.

9. Drug is not to be administered by women of childbearing age. Also, post this advisement so they do not come in contact with the drug.

Interventions

1. It is essential that constant monitoring be undertaken for both the fluid and respiratory status of the client.
2. Assess frequently for evidence of respiratory distress; stop therapy and call physician if distress occurs.
3. Monitor and record vital signs and I&O.
4. Anticipate limited use in infants and adults with chronic obstructive pulmonary disease or asthma.
5. With prolonged therapy (more than 7 days), observe for signs and symptoms of anemia; monitor CBC values.

Evaluation: Evaluate client for:
- Auscultatory and radiographic evidence of improved airway exchange
- Clinical evidence of resolution of RSV pneumonia

R

Riboflavin (Vitamin B₂)

(**RYE**-boh-flay-vin)
(OTC)

Classification: Vitamin B complex.

Action/Kinetics: Riboflavin is a water-soluble, heat-resistant substance that is sensitive to light. Riboflavin acts as a coenzyme as flavin adenine dinucleotide (FAD) and flavin mononucleotide (FMN), which are required for various respiration systems in tissues. Riboflavin deficiency is characterized by characteristic lesions of the tongue, lips and face, photophobia, itching, burning and keratosis of the eyes. Riboflavin deficiency often accompanies pellagra.

Uses: Prophylaxis or treatment of riboflavin deficiency. Adjunct, with niacin, in the treatment of pellagra.

Side Effects: Large doses may cause urine to have a yellow discoloration.

Drug Interactions

Alcohol / Impairs absorption of riboflavin
Antidepressants, tricyclic / ↑ Requirements of riboflavin
Chloramphenicol / Riboflavin may counteract bone marrow depression and optic neuritis due to chloramphenicol
Phenothiazines / ↑ Requirements for riboflavin
Probenecid / ↑ Requirements for riboflavin
Tetracyclines / Antibiotic activity ↓ by riboflavin

Dosage: Tablets. *Deficiency states:* 5–25 mg daily for several days; **then,** 1–4 mg daily. *Recommended dietary allowances:* **Adults, males:** 1.4–1.8 mg daily; **females:** 1.2–1.3 mg daily.

NURSING CONSIDERATIONS

Client/Family Teaching

1. Review dietary sources of riboflavin (dairy products, green leafy vegetables, nuts, meats, and enriched flours) and refer client to dietitian for assistance in meal planning and preparation.
2. Advise client that drug may cause urine to appear bright yellow and not to be alarmed.
3. Avoid alcohol as this impairs riboflavin absorption.

Evaluation: Evaluate client with riboflavin deficiency for effective prophylaxis or evidence of symptom improvement.

Rifampin

(rih-**FAM**-pin)
Rifadin, Rimactane, Rofact✤ (Rx)

Classification: First-line antitubercular agent.

Action/Kinetics: Semisynthetic antibiotic derived from *Streptomyces mediterranei*. Rifampin suppresses RNA synthesis by binding to the beta subunit of DNA-dependent RNA polymerase. This prevents attachment of the enzyme to DNA and blockade of RNA transcription. The drug is both bacteriostatic and bactericidal and is most active against rapidly replicating organisms. The drug is well absorbed from the GI tract and is widely distributed in body tissues. **Peak plasma concentration:** 4–32 mcg/ml after 2–4 hr. **t½:** 1.5–5 hr; (higher in clients with hepatic impairment). In normal clients t½ decreases with usage. The drug is metabolized in liver; 60% is excreted in feces.

Uses: All types of tuberculosis. Must be used in conjunction with at least one other tuberculostatic drug (such as isoniazid, ethambutol, pyrazinamide) but is the drug of choice for retreatment. Also for treatment of asymptomatic meningococcal carriers to eliminate *Neisseria meningitidis*. *Investigational:* Used in combination for infections due to *Staphylococcus aureus* and *S. epidermidis* (endocarditis, osteomyelitis, prostatitis); Legionnaire's disease; in combination with dapsone for leprosy; prophylaxis of meningitis due to *Haemophilus influenzae* and gram-negative bacteremia in infants.

Contraindications: Hypersensitivity; not recommended for intermittent therapy.

Special Concerns: Safe use during lactation has not been established. Use during pregnancy only if benefits clearly outweigh risks (pregnancy category: C). Safety and effectiveness not determined in children less than 5 years of age. Use with extreme caution in clients with hepatic dysfunction.

Side Effects: *GI:* Nausea, vomiting, diarrhea, anorexia, gas, pseudomembranous colitis, pancreatitis, sore mouth and tongue, cramps, heartburn, flatulence. *CNS:* Headache, drowsiness, fatigue, ataxia, dizziness, confusion, generalized numbness, fever, difficulty in concentrating. *Hepatic:* Jaundice, hepatitis. Increases in AST, ALT, bilirubin, alkaline phosphatase. *Hematologic:* Thrombocytopenia, eosinophilia, hemolysis, leukopenia, hemolytic anemia. *Allergic:* Flu-like symptoms, dyspnea, wheezing, shortness of breath, purpura, pruritus, urticaria, skin rashes, sore mouth and tongue, conjunctivitis. *Renal:* Hematuria, hemoglobinuria, renal insufficiency, acute renal failure. *Miscellaneous:* Visual disturbances, muscle weakness or pain, arthralgia, decreased blood pressure, osteomalacia, menstrual disturbances, edema of face and extremities, adrenocortical insufficiency, increases in BUN and serum uric acid. **Note:** Body fluids and feces may be red-orange.

Symptoms of Overdose: Shortly after ingestion, nausea, vomiting, and lethargy will occur. Followed by severe hepatic involvement (liver enlargement with tenderness, increased direct and total bilirubin, change in hepatic enzymes) with unconsciousness. Also, brownish red or orange discoloration of urine, saliva, tears, sweat, skin, and feces.

Drug Interactions

Acetaminophen / ↓ Effect of acetaminophen due to ↑ breakdown by liver
Aminophylline / ↓ Effect of aminophylline due to ↑ breakdown by liver
Anticoagulants, oral / ↓ Effect of anticoagulants due to ↑ breakdown by liver
Antidiabetics, oral / ↓ Effect of oral antidiabetic due to ↑ breakdown by liver
Barbiturates / ↓ Effect of barbiturates due to ↑ breakdown by liver
Benzodiazepines / ↓ Effect of benzodiazepines due to ↑ breakdown by liver
Beta-adrenergic blocking agents / ↓ Effect of beta-blocking agents due to ↑ breakdown by liver
Chloramphenicol / ↓ Effect of chloramphenicol due to ↑ breakdown by liver
Clofibrate / ↓ Effect of clofibrate due to ↑ breakdown by liver
Contraceptives, oral / ↓ Effect of oral contraceptives due to ↑ breakdown by liver
Corticosteroids / ↓ Effect of corticosteroids due to ↑ breakdown by liver
Cyclosporine / ↓ Effect of cyclosporine due to ↑ breakdown by liver
Digitoxin / ↓ Effect of digitoxin due to ↑ breakdown by liver
Digoxin / ↓ Serum levels of digoxin

R

Disopyramide / ↓ Effect of disopyramide due to ↑ breakdown by liver

Estrogens / ↓ Effect of estrogens due to ↑ breakdown by liver

Halothane / ↑ Risk of hepatotoxicity and hepatic encephalopathy

Hydantoins / ↓ Effect of hydantoins due to ↑ breakdown by liver

Isoniazid / ↑ Risk of hepatotoxicity

Ketoconazole / ↓ Effect of either ketoconazole or rifampin

Methadone / ↓ Effect of methadone due to ↑ breakdown by liver

Mexiletine / ↓ Effect of mexiletine due to ↑ breakdown by liver

Quinidine / ↓ Effect of quinidine due to ↑ breakdown by liver

Sulfones / ↓ Effect of sulfones due to ↑ breakdown by liver

Theophylline / ↓ Effect of theophylline due to ↑ breakdown by liver

Tocainide / ↓ Effect of tocainide due to ↑ breakdown by liver

Verapamil / ↓ Effect of verapamil due to ↑ breakdown by liver

Laboratory Test Interferences: ↑ AST, ALT, alkaline phosphatase, BUN, bilirubin, uric acid, BSP retention values. False + Coombs' test.

Dosage: Capsules. *Pulmonary tuberculosis:* **Adults:** single dose of 600 mg daily; **children over 5 years:** 10–20 mg/kg daily, not to exceed 600 mg/day. *Meningococcal carriers:* 600 mg daily for 4 days; **children:** 10–20 mg/kg q 12 hr for 4 doses. Dosage should not exceed 600 mg/day.

NURSING CONSIDERATIONS

See also *General Nursing Considerations For All Anti-Infectives,* p. 83.

Administration/Storage

1. Administer once daily 1 hr before or 2 hr after meals to ensure maximum absorption.
2. Check to be sure that there is a desiccant in the bottle containing capsules of rifampin because these are relatively moisture sensitive.
3. If administered concomitantly with PAS, drugs should be given 8–12 hr apart because the acid interferes with the absorption of rifampin.
4. When used for tuberculosis, therapy should continue for 6–9 months.
5. *Treatment of Overdose:* Gastric lavage followed by activated charcoal slurry introduced into the stomach. Antiemetics to control nausea and vomiting. Forced diuresis to enhance excretion. If hepatic function is seriously impaired, bile drainage may be required. Extracorporeal hemodialysis may be necessary.

Assessment

1. Obtain appropriate baseline laboratory studies. Evaluate for impaired renal function, blood dyscrasias, and liver dysfunction.
2. Assess for GI disturbance and auditory nerve impairment; document and notify physician.
3. Auscultate and document lung sounds and evaluate characteristics of sputum produced.

Client/Family Teaching

1. Take drug on an empty stomach 1 hr before or 2 hr after meals. If GI upset occurs, report to physician.

2. Rifampin may impart a red-or-ange color to urine, feces, saliva, sputum, and tears; contact lenses may become *permanently* discolored.
3. Symptoms such as headache, drowsiness, confusion, fever, and muscle and joint aches may occur during the first few weeks of therapy. If symptoms persist or increase in intensity, report to physician.
4. Women of childbearing age on the pill should practice alternative birth control since birth control pills may not be effective. Advise that drug has teratogenic properties.
5. Explain the necessity of taking this medication for months to treat TB.
6. Advise not to stop taking medication or skip doses without notifying physician.
7. Avoid alcohol as this increases the risk of liver toxicity.

Evaluation: Evaluate for:
- Effectiveness as a combination agent in treating TB based on radiographic and laboratory reports
- Prophylaxis of meningitis due to *H. influenzae* and gram-negative bacteremia in infants

―――― COMBINATION DRUG ――――
Rifampin and Isoniazid
(rih-**FAM**-pin, eye-so-**NYE**-ah-zid)
Rifamate (Rx)

See also *Isoniazid,* p. 762, and *Rifampin,* p. 1128.

Classification/Content: First-line antitubercular drugs. Each capsule contains: rifampin, 300 mg and isoniazid, 150 mg.

Uses: Pulmonary tuberculosis after the client has been titrated on the individual drugs and the drugs are known to be effective. Not intended for initial therapy or for preventive therapy.

Contraindications: This product is not recommended for use in children.

Dosage: Capsules. Adults/adolescents: 600 mg rifampin and 300 mg isoniazid once daily given either 1 hr before or 2 hr after a meal.

NURSING CONSIDERATIONS

See *Nursing Considerations* for *Rifampin,* p. 1130, and *Isoniazid,* p. 763.

―――― COMBINATION DRUG ――――
Robitussin-AC
(roh-bih-**TUS**-in)
(C-V) (Rx)

Classification/Content: *Expectorant:* Guaifenesin, 100 mg/5 ml. *Antitussive:* Codeine phosphate, 10 mg/5 ml. The product helps loosen mucus and thins bronchial secretions making coughs more productive.

See also information on individual components.

Uses: Coughs associated with bronchitis, the common cold, laryngitis, pharyngitis, pertussis, tracheitis, flu, and measles.

Contraindications: Chronic or persistent coughs. Children less than 2 years of age.

Laboratory Test Interferences: Guaifenesin may interfere with determination of 5-hydroxyindoleacetic acid (5-HIAA) or vanillylmandelic acid (VMA).

R

Dosage: Syrup. Adults and children over 12 years: 10 ml q 4 hr, not to exceed 60 ml daily; **pediatric, 6–12 years:** 5 ml q 4 hr, not to exceed 30 ml daily; **pediatric, 2–6 years:** 2.5 ml q 4 hr, not to exceed 15 ml daily.

NURSING CONSIDERATIONS

See also *Nursing Considerations for Narcotic Analgesics,* p. 177.

Assessment: Review the client history. If the cough is chronic, the drug is contraindicated.

Client/Family Teaching

1. Instruct the client to take only as directed and to notify the physician if symptoms persist or intensify.
2. Constipation may occur with drug therapy. Advise the client to drink between 2,500 and 3,000 ml of fluid per day and to increase intake of fruits, grains, and other high-fiber foods. If the problem persists a stool softener may be recommended. If the stool softener is not effective, report to the physician. Other reasons for the constipation may then need to be ruled out.
3. Advise the client that the drug may be habit-forming.

Evaluation: Evaluate client for control of cough with reports of less frequent cough-induced awakenings at rest.

—— *COMBINATION DRUG* ——
Robitussin-CF
(roh-bih-**TUSS**-in)
(OTC)

Robitussin-DM
(roh-bih-**TUSS**-in)
(OTC)

Robitussin-PE
(roh-bih-**TUSS**-in)
(OTC)

Classification/Content: Robitussin-CF. *Expectorant:* Guaifenesin, 100 mg/5 ml; *Decongestant:* Phenylpropanolamine HCl, 12.5 mg/5 ml; and, *Antitussive:* Dextromethorphan HBr, 10 mg/5 ml.

   Robitussin-DM. *Expectorant:* Guaifenesin, 100 mg/5 ml and *Antitussive:* Dextromethorphan HBr, 15 mg/5 ml.

   Robitussin-PE. *Expectorant:* Guaifenesin, 100 mg/5 ml and *Decongestant:* Pseudoephedrine HCl, 30 mg/5 ml.

   See also information on individual components.

Uses: Coughs associated with bronchitis, laryngitis, pharyngitis, the common cold, flu, pertussis, tracheitis, and measles. Robitussin-CF is indicated for coughs with congestion and irritating cough; Robitussin-DM is indicated for irritating coughs; and Robitussin-PE is indicated for coughs with congestion.

Contraindications: Products containing sympathomimetic decongestants should be used with caution in clients with hypertension, diabetes, cardiac disorders, peripheral vascular disease, glaucoma, prostatic hypertrophy.

Laboratory Test Interferences: Guaifenesin may interfere with determination of 5-hydroxyindoleacetic acid (5-HIAA) and vanillylmandelic acid (VMA).

Dosage: Robitussin-CF Syrup. Adults and children over 12 years: 10 ml q 4 hr, not to exceed 60 ml daily; **pediatric, 6–12 years:** 5 ml q 4 hr, not to exceed 30 ml daily; **pediatric, 2–6 years:** 2.5 ml q 4 hr, not to exceed 15 ml daily.

Robitussin-DM Syrup. Adults and children over 12 years: 10 ml q 6–8 hr, not to exceed 40 ml daily; **pediatric, 6–12 years:** 5 ml q 6–8 hr, not to exceed 20 ml daily; **pediatric, 2–6 years:** 2.5 ml q 6–8 hr, not to exceed 10 ml daily.

Robitussin-PE Syrup. Adults and children over 12 years: 10 ml q 4 hr, not to exceed 40 ml daily; **pediatric, 6–12 years:** 5 ml q 4 hr, not to exceed 20 ml daily; **pediatric, 2–6 years:** 2.5 ml q 4 hr, not to exceed 10 ml daily.

None of these products should be used in children under 2 years of age.

NURSING CONSIDERATIONS

See also *Nursing Considerations* for *Sympathomimetic Drugs,* p. 220, *Dextromethorphan,* p. 525, and *Robitussin-AC,* p. 1132.

Assessment

1. Note if the client has a history of hypertension, cardiac disease or peripheral vascular disorders. The drug is contraindicated in these conditions.
2. Determine if the client has diabetes mellitus and document. Syrups and other drugs in this class may upset blood sugar levels and alter the amount of hypoglycemic agent required for adequate control.
3. When working with elderly male clients, discuss any possible problems they may have with urinary output or any knowledge the client may have of prostatic hypertrophy and document.

Evaluation: Evaluate client for control of cough and reports of symptomatic improvement.

—— *COMBINATION DRUG* ——
Robitussin-DAC (C-V)
(roh-bih-**TUSS**-in)
(Rx)

Classification/Content: *Antitussive:* Codeine phosphate, 10 mg/5 ml. *Expectorant:* Guaifenesin, 100 mg/5 ml. *Decongestant:* Pseudoephedrine hydrochloride, 30 mg/5 ml. See also information on individual components.

Uses: To relieve nasal congestion and cough due to minor throat and bronchial irritation occurring with the common cold or inhaled irritants.

Contraindicationsn: Use in chronic pulmonary disease, shortness of breath, hypertension, heart disease, diabetes, thyroid disease. Children taking other drugs. Use of codeine in children less than 2 years of age. Clients taking medication for hypertension or depression.

Special Concerns: Use with caution in children less than 6 years of age.

Side Effects: Exceeding the recommended dose will result in dizziness, nervousness, or insomnia. Use with caution in clients with persistent or chronic cough.

Laboratory Test Interference: Guaifenesin may interfere with the determination of 5-hydroxyindole-acetic acid (5-HIAA) and vanillylmandelic acid (VMA).

Dosage: Syrup. Adults and children over 12 years of age: 10 ml q 4 hr, not to exceed 40 ml in a 24-hr period. **Children, 6–12 years of age:** 5 ml q 4 hr, not to exceed 20 ml in a 24-hr period.

R

NURSING CONSIDERATIONS

See also *Nursing Considerations* for *Narcotic Analgesics,* p. 177, *Pseudoephedrine hydrochloride,* p. 1107, and *Guaifenesin,* p. 697.

Administration/Storage: For children under 6 years of age, a special measuring device should be used to ensure accuracy.

Assessment

1. Document any history of lung, thyroid, or heart disease, diabetes, and hypertension.
2. Note any medications currently prescribed that may interact unfavorably with drug.

Evaluation: Evaluate for effective relief of cough and nasal congestion in clients with a cold or respiratory irritation.

―――― COMBINATION DRUG ――――

Rondec-DM Oral Drops

(**RON**-deck)

(Rx)

Rondec-DM Syrup

(**RON**-deck)

(Rx)

Classification/Content: *Antitussive:* Dextromethorphan HBr, 4 mg/ml Oral Drops or 15 mg/5 ml Syrup. *Decongestant:* Pseudoephedrine HCl, 25 mg/ml Oral Drops or 60 mg/5 ml Syrup. *Antihistamine:* Carbinoxamine maleate, 2 mg/ml Oral Drops or 4 mg/5 ml Syrup.

See also information on individual components.

Uses: Treatment of coughs, nasal congestion, and other upper respiratory tract symptoms due to the common cold or allergy.

Special Concerns: Safe use during pregnancy has not been established. Use with caution in hypertension, ischemic heart disease, in clients over 60 years of age, and during lactation.

Dosage: Syrup. Adults and children over 6 years: 5 ml q.i.d.; **children 18 months–6 years:** 2.5 ml q.i.d. **Oral Drops. Pediatric, 9–18 months:** 1 ml q.i.d.; **6–9 months:** 0.75 ml q.i.d.; **3–6 months:** 0.5 ml q.i.d.; **1–3 months:** 0.25 ml q.i.d.

NURSING CONSIDERATIONS

See also *Nursing Considerations* for *Antihistamines,* p. 74, *Dextromethorphan,* p. 525, and *Sympathomimetics,* p. 220.

Assessment: If female, sexually active, and of childbearing age, determine if pregnant. Safe use of drug during pregnancy has not been established.

Evaluation: Evaluate client for effective control of cough and reports of symptomatic improvement.

―――― COMBINATION DRUG ――――

Rynatan

(**RYE**-nah-tan)

(Rx)

Classification/Content: *Antihistamine:* Chlorpheniramine tannate, 8 mg (tablet) or 2 mg (per 5 ml suspension). *Antihistamine:* Pyrilamine tannate, 25 mg (tablet) or 12.5 mg (per 5 ml suspension). *Decongestant:* Phenylephrine tannate, 25 mg (tablet) or 5 mg (per 5 ml suspension).

See also information on individual components.

Uses: Nasal congestion and runny nose due to upper respiratory tract conditions including the common cold, allergic rhinitis, sinusitis, and other respiratory tract conditions.

Contraindications: Use during lactation and in newborns.

Special Concerns: Pregnancy category: C. Use with caution in hypertension, hyperthyroidism, cardiovascular disease, narrow angle glaucoma, diabetes, and prostatic hypertrophy. Use with caution (or avoid use) in clients taking MAO inhibitors.

Drug Interactions: Additive CNS depression if used with alcohol, sedative-hypnotics, antianxiety agents, or other drugs producing CNS depression.

Dosage: Oral Suspension, Tablets. Adults: 1–2 tablets q 12 hr. **Pediatric, over 6 years:** 5–10 ml of the suspension q 12 hr; **pediatric, 2–6 years:** 2.5–5 ml of the suspension q 12 hr. The dose should be carefully individualized in children under 2 years of age.

NURSING CONSIDERATIONS

See *Nursing Considerations* for *Antihistamines,* p. 74, and *Sympathomimetics,* p. 220.

Evaluation: Evaluate client for reports of symptomatic improvement of nasal congestion and allergic respiratory manifestations.

S

Sargramostim
(sar-**GRAM**-oh-stim)
Leukine, Prokine (Rx)

Classification: Colony-stimulating factor.

Action/Kinetics: Sargramostim is a granulocyte-macrophage colony-stimulating factor (rhu GM-CSF) that is produced by recombinant DNA technology in a yeast expression system. GM-CSF stimulates the proliferation and differentiation of hematopoietic progenitor cells. It stimulates partially committed progenitor cells to divide and differentiate in the granulocyte-macrophage pathways. Division, maturation, and activation are induced through GM-CSF binding to specific receptors located on the surface of target cells. GM-CSF can also activate mature granulocytes and macrophages. Sargramostim increases the cytotoxicity of monocytes toward certain neoplastic cell lines as well as activates polymorphonuclear neutrophils, thus inhibiting the growth of tumor cells. Sargramostim differs from the naturally occurring GM-CSF by one amino acid and by a different carbohydrate moiety. **Peak levels:** 2 hr. **t½, alpha half-life:** 12–17 min; **beta half-life:** 2 hr. Neutralizing antibodies have been detected in a small number of clients.

Uses: Increased myeloid recovery in clients with non-Hodgkin's lymphoma, acute lymphoblastic leukemia, and Hodgkin's disease undergoing autologous bone marrow transplantation. *Investigational:* To increase white blood counts in clients with myelodysplastic syndrome and in AIDS clients taking zidovudine; to correct neutropenia in clients with aplastic anemia; to decrease the nadir of leukopenia secondary to myelosuppressive chemotherapy and to decrease myelosuppression in preleukemic clients; and to decrease organ system damage following transplantation, especially in the liver and kidney.

Contraindications: More than 10% leukemic myeloid blasts in the bone marrow or peripheral blood. Known hypersensitivity to GM-CSF, yeast-derived products, or any component of the product. Use within 24 hr preceding or following chemotherapy or within 12 hr preceding or following radiotherapy.

Special Concerns: Pregnancy category: C. Use with caution in clients with preexisting cardiac disease, hypoxia, and during lactation. Safety and effectiveness have not been determined in children although it appears the drug is no more toxic in children than in adults. Insufficient data are available to support the effectiveness of sargramostim in increasing myeloid recovery after peripheral blood stem cell transplantation. It is possible that sargramostim can act as a growth factor for any tumor type, especially myeloid malignancies; thus, use with caution in any malignancy with myeloid characteristics.

Side Effects: *CV:* Transient supraventricular arrhythmia; fluid retention in presence of preexisting peripheral edema or pleural or pericardial effusion. *Musculoskeletal:* Asthenia, bone pain, myalgia. *Body as a whole:* Malaise, headache, fever, chills. *Miscellaneous:* Transient rashes, reactions at injection site, diarrhea, urinary tract disorder.

Symptoms of Overdose: Dyspnea, malaise, nausea, fever, rash, sinus tachycardia, chills, headache.

Drug Interactions: Drugs such as corticosteroids and lithium may ↑ the myeloproliferative effects of sargramostim.

Dosage: IV infusion. *Myeloid reconstitution after autologous bone marrow transplantation:* 250 mcg/m²/day for 21 days.

NURSING CONSIDERATIONS

Administration/Storage

1. Daily dosage should be given as a 2-hr IV infusion beginning 2–4 hr after the autologous bone marrow infusion making sure at least 24 hr have elapsed after the last dose of chemotherapy and 12 hr have elapsed since the last dose of radiotherapy.

2. The dose should be reduced or temporarily terminated if severe adverse reactions occur; therapy may be continued once the reactions abate.

3. The lyophilized powder is reconstituted with 1 ml of sterile water for injection without preservatives. The sterile water should be directed at the side of the vial, followed by a gentle swirling of the contents to avoid foaming. Excessive or vigorous agitation should be avoided.

4. Reconstituted solutions are clear, colorless, and isotonic with a pH of 7.4.

5. The vial should not be reentered or reused and any unused portion should be discarded.

6. Dilution for IV infusion should be with 0.9% sodium chloride injection. If the final concentration is less than 10 mcg/ml, human albumin should be added at a final concentration of 0.1% to the saline before sargramostim is added, to prevent adsorption to the components of the drug delivery system.

7. Since sargramostim contains no preservatives, it should be given as soon as possible, but within 6 hr, following reconstitution or dilution for IV infusion. Solutions can be stored in the refrigerator at 2°–6°C (36°–46°F).

8. Other drugs should not be added to infusion solutions containing sargramostim.

9. *Treatment of Overdose:* Discontinue therapy. Monitor for increases in white blood cells and for respiratory symptoms.

Assessment

1. Determine any sensitivity to yeast-derived products.
2. Obtain baseline CBC, liver and renal function studies.
3. Note any history of cardiac disease.
4. Document any therapy with chemotherapy or radiation. Drug should *not* be administered 24 hr preceding or following chemotherapy or within 12 hr preceding or following radiation therapy.

Interventions

1. Monitor I&O, vital signs, and weight. Observe for evidence of fluid retention or edema.
2. Observe for any evidence of dyspnea during IV administration. Carefully monitor respiratory symptoms during or immediately following infusion, especially in clients with preexisting lung disease. In the event of dyspnea during administration, the rate of infusion should be reduced by one-half.

3. Carefully monitor CBC and platelet count. The hematologic response to sargramostim can be detected by a CBC with differential undertaken twice weekly. If the absolute neutrophil count (ANC) exceeds 20,000 /mm³ or if the platelet count exceeds 500,000 /mm³, therapy should be stopped and the dose reduced by one-half. The decision to reduce the dose should be based on the clinical condition of the client. Excessive blood counts have returned to normal levels within 3–7 days following termination of therapy.

4. Renal and hepatic function should be monitored every 2 weeks in clients who have hepatic or renal dysfunction.

5. Drug effectiveness may be limited in clients who, before autologous bone marrow transplantation, received extensive radiotherapy in the chest or abdomen to treat the primary disease; effectiveness is also limited in clients who have received multiple myelotoxic agents such as antimetabolites, alkylating agents, or anthracycline antibiotics.

Evaluation: Evaluate client for:
- Clinical evidence of control of the spread of malignant disease
- Laboratory evidence of improved hematologic parameters

Scopolamine hydrobromide

(scoh-**POLL**-ah-meen)

Hyoscine Hydrobromide, Isopto Hyoscine Ophthalmic, Triptone (Rx)

Scopolamine transdermal therapeutic system

(scoh-**POLL**-ah-meen)

Transderm-Scop (Rx)

See also *Cholinergic Blocking Agents,* p. 136.

Classification: Anticholinergic, antiemetic.

Action/Kinetics: Scopolamine is an anticholinergic with CNS depressant effects. It produces amnesia when given with morphine or meperidine. In the presence of pain, delirium may be produced. Scopolamine dilates the pupil and paralyzes the muscle required to accommodate for close vision (cycloplegia). This enables the physician to examine the inner structure of the eye including the retina as well as to examine refractive errors of the lens without automatic accommodation by the client. Tolerance may develop if scopolamine is used alone. When used for refraction: **onset,** 25–75 min; **duration:** 24 hr. Recovery time can be reduced by using 1–2 gtt pilocarpine (1% or 2%). To reduce absorption, pressure should be applied over the nasolacrimal sac for 2–3 min.

The transdermal therapeutic system contains 1.5 mg scopolamine, which is slowly released from a mineral oil–polyisobutylene matrix. Approximately 0.5 mg is released from the system per day.

Uses: Parenteral: Antiemetic. Preanesthetic sedation and obstetric amnesia. **Ophthalmic:** Diagnostic ophthalmic examination and refraction in children; pre- and postoperative mydriasis during eye surgery; anterior uveitis; and iridocyclitis either pre- or postoperatively. **Transdermal:** Antiemetic. Prevention of motion sickness.

Additional Contraindications: For transdermal therapeutic system: Children, lactating women. Ophthalmic use contraindicated in glaucoma, infants less than three months of age.

Special Concerns: Pregnancy category: C. Use with caution in children, infants, geriatric clients, diabetes, hypo- or hyperthyroidism, narrow anterior chamber angle. Use for prophylaxis of excess secretions is not recommended for children less than 4 months of age. The transdermal system is not recommended for children.

Additional Side Effects: Disorientation, delirium, increased heart rate, decreased respiratory rate. *Ophthalmologic:* Blurred vision, stinging, increased intraocular pressure. Long-term use may cause irritation, photophobia, conjunctivitis, hyperemia, or edema.

Dosage: Ophthalmic Solution. *Refraction:* **Adults,** 1 gtt of the 0.25% solution 1 hr prior to refraction; **children:** 1 drop of the 0.25% solution b.i.d. for 2 days prior to refraction. *Uveitis:* 1 drop of the 0.25% solution 1–3 times daily. *Treatment of posterior synechiae:* 1 drop of the 0.25% solution q min for 5 min. (1 drop of either a 2.5% or 10% solution of phenylephrine instilled q min for 3 min will enhance the effect of scopolamine.)

Postoperative mydriasis: 1 drop of the 0.25% solution once daily. *Pre- or postoperative iridocyclitis:* 1 drop of the 0.25% solution 1–4 times daily as required.

IM, IV, SC. *Anticholinergic, antiemetic:* **Adults,** 0.3–0.6 mg (single dose). **Pediatric:** 0.006 mg/kg (0.2 mg/m²) as a single dose. *Prophylaxis of excessive salivation and respiratory tract secretions:* **Adults,** 0.2–0.6 mg 30–60 min before induction of anesthesia. **Pediatric (given IM): 8–12 years:** 0.3 mg; **3–8 years:** 0.2 mg; **7 months–3 years:** 0.15 mg; **4–7 months:** 0.1 mg. *Adjunct to anesthesia, sedative-hypnotic:* **Adults,** 0.6 mg t.i.d–q.i.d. *Adjunct to anesthesia, amnesia:* **Adults,** 0.32–0.65 mg.

Transdermal system. *Antiemetic, antivertigo:* **Adults,** 1 transdermal system placed on the postauricular skin to deliver 0.5 mg over 3 days (apply at least 4 hr before antiemetic effect is required).

NURSING CONSIDERATIONS

See also *Nursing Considerations* for *Cholinergic Blocking Agents,* p. 138.

Administration/Storage

1. Drops are instilled into the conjunctival sac.
2. Scopolamine should not be administered alone for pain because it may cause delirium. Use an analgesic or sedative in this event.
3. With the transdermal system:
   - Wash hands before and after application
   - Apply at least 4 hr before desired effect
   - Apply to a clean, non-hairy site, behind the ear.

- Use pressure to apply the patch to ensure contact with the skin
- Replace with a new system if patch becomes dislodged
- System is water-proof so bathing and swimming are permitted
- System effects last for 3 days

Assessment

1. Assess for additional side effects and for tolerance after a long course of therapy.
2. Before administering eye-drops, check whether client has a history of angle-closure glaucoma because the drug may precipitate an acute glaucoma crisis.

Interventions

1. Observe closely during initial therapy. Some clients experience toxic delirium with therapeutic doses. Have physostigmine available to reverse drug effects.
2. Orient and reassure client who experiences amnesia after receiving the drug.
3. Monitor I&O. Observe for evidence of urinary retention and constipation. Increase fluids and bulk in diet to prevent constipation.

Client/Family Teaching

1. Review appropriate method of administration and advise to take only as directed.
2. Advise not to drive a car or operate dangerous machinery because the drug may cause drowsiness, confusion, disorientation, and mydriasis (when used ophthalmologically).
3. Warn that scopolamine may

S

temporarily impair vision when instilled in the eye. Advise to wear dark glasses if photosensitivity occurs.
4. Provide a printed list of side effects that require reporting to the physician.
5. Use gum, sugarless candies, and frequent mouth rinses to alleviate symptoms of dry mouth.
6. Avoid alcohol and any other CNS depressants during drug therapy.

Evaluation: Evaluate client for:
- Reports of effective control of vomiting
- Evidence of effective preoperative sedation; postoperative amnesia
- Evidence of the desired amount of mydriasis
- The prevention of motion sickness

Secobarbital
(see-koh-**BAR**-bih-tal)
Seconal (C-II, Rx)

Secobarbital sodium
(see-koh-**BAR**-bih-tal)
Novo-Secobarb✿, Seconal Sodium (C-II, Rx)

See also *Barbiturates,* p. 101.

Classification: Sedative-hypnotic, barbiturate type.

Action/Kinetics: Short-acting. Distributed quickly as it has the highest lipid solubility of the barbiturates. **t½:** 15–40 hr. Is 46%–70% protein bound.

Uses: Short-term treatment of insomnia. Sedative to relieve anxiety, tension, and apprehension. Preoperative sedative. May be used parenterally as an anticonvulsant in tetanus.

Special Concerns: Pregnancy category: D.

Dosage: Capsules. *Hypnotic:* **Adults:** 100 mg at bedtime. *Preoperative sedation:* **Adults:** 200–300 mg 1–2 hr before surgery; **pediatric:** 2–6 mg/kg (up to a maximum of 100 mg) 1–2 hr before surgery. *Daytime sedation:* **Adults:** 30–50 mg t.i.d.–q.i.d. **Pediatric:** 2 mg/kg (60 mg/m²) t.i.d. **Rectal suppositories:** *Hypnotic:* **Adults:** 200 mg. *Daytime sedation:* **Adults,** 200 mg daily in 3 divided doses. Suppositories are not for use in children. **Rectal solution.** *Hypnotic:* **Pediatric, up to 40 kg:** 5 mg/kg; **over 40 kg:** 4 mg/kg. **IM, IV.** *Anticonvulsant in tetanus:* **Adults:** 5.5 mg/kg q 3–4 hr as needed. **Pediatric:** 3–5 mg/kg (125 mg/m²) per dose. **IM.** *Hypnotic:* **Adults:** 100–200 mg. **Pediatric:** 3–5 mg/kg (125 mg/m²) up to a maximum of 100 mg per dose. *Preoperative sedative:* **Pediatric:** 4–5 mg/kg. *Sedative for dentistry:* **Adults,** 1.1–2.2 mg/kg 10–15 min prior to procedure. **IV.** *Nerve block for dentistry:* **Adults:** 100–150 mg.

NURSING CONSIDERATIONS

See also *Nursing Considerations* for *Barbiturates,* p. 104.

Administration/Storage

1. For adults, the aqueous parenteral solution is preferred to polyethylene glycol, which may be irritating to the kidneys, especially in clients with signs of renal insufficiency.
2. Aqueous solutions for injection should be freshly prepared from dry-packed ampules.

Interventions

1. Rapid IV administration may precipitate hypotension, respiratory depression, laryngospasm or apnea; do not exceed recommended rate (50 mg/15 sec).
2. Following prolonged use, taper dosage and withdraw drug slowly to prevent precipitating withdrawal symptoms.

Evaluation: Evaluate client for:
- Reports of improved sleeping patterns with less frequent awakenings
- Evidence of effective sedation

Selegiline hydrochloride (Deprenyl)
(seh-**LEH**-jih-leen)
Eldepryl (Rx)

Classification: Antiparkinson agent.

Action/Kinetics: Although the precise mechanism of action is not known, selegiline is known to inhibit MAO, type B. Also, selegiline may act through other mechanisms to increase dopaminergic activity.

Uses: Adjunct in the treatment of Parkinson's disease in clients being treated with levodopa/carbidopa who have manifested a decreased response to this therapy. **Note:** There is no evidence that selegiline is effective in clients not taking levodopa.

Contraindications: Hypersensitivity to the drug. Doses greater than 10 mg daily.

Special Concerns: Pregnancy category: C. Use with caution during lactation. Safety and efficacy in children have not been established.

Side Effects: *CNS:* Dizziness, lightheadedness, fainting, confusion, hallucinations, vivid dreams/nightmares, headache, anxiety, drowsiness, depression, mood changes, delusions, fatigue, disorientation, apathy, malaise, vertigo, overstimulation, sleep disturbance, transient irritability, weakness. *Skeletal Muscle:* Tremor, chorea, loss of balance, blepharospasm, increased bradykinesia, facial grimace, dystonic symptoms, tardive dyskinesia, dyskinesia, involuntary movements, muscle cramps, heavy leg, falling down, stiff neck, freezing, festination, increased apraxia. *Altered Sensations/pain:* Headache, tinnitus, migraine, back or leg pain, supraorbital pain, burning throat, chills, numbness of fingers/toes, taste disturbance, generalized aches. *CV:* Orthostatic hypotension, hypertension, arrhythmia, angina pectoris, palpitations, hypotension, tachycardia, syncope, peripheral edema, sinus bradycardia. *GI:* Nausea, vomiting, constipation, anorexia, weight loss, dry mouth, poor appetite, dysphagia, diarrhea, rectal bleeding, heartburn. *GU:* Nocturia, slow urination, urinary hesitancy or retention, prostatic hypertrophy, urinary frequency. *Miscellaneous:* Blurred vision, sexual dysfunction, increased sweating, diaphoresis, facial hair, hair loss, rash, photosensitivity, hematoma, asthma, diplopia, shortness of breath, speech affected. *Symptoms of Overdose:* Hypotension, psychomotor agitation. Also, symptoms from overdose of nonselective MAO inhibitors (e.g., isocarboxazid, phenelzine, tranylcypromine).

Drug Interactions: Drugs inhibiting MAO are often contraindicated for use with meperidine or other opioids.

Dosage: Tablets. Adults: 5 mg taken at breakfast and lunch, not to exceed 10 mg daily.

NURSING CONSIDERATIONS

Administration/Storage

1. No evidence exists that doses higher than 10 mg daily will result in additional beneficial effects.
2. Following 2 or 3 days of selegiline therapy, attempts may be made to decrease the dose of levodopa/carbidopa (10%–30%).
3. *Treatment of Overdose:* IV fluids and a dilute pressor agent to treat hypotension and vascular collapse. Treat symptoms.

Client/Family Teaching

1. Selegiline is to be taken concurrently with prescribed dose of levodopa/carbidopa.
2. Do not exceed prescribed daily dose. Take with breakfast and lunch.
3. Review list of side effects associated with drug therapy and instruct client and family to report any bothersome and/or persistent symptoms.
4. Rise slowly from a sitting or lying position to minimize the hypotensive effects of drug therapy.
5. Do not drive or operate hazardous machinery until drug effects are realized.
6. Avoid tyramine-containing foods as they may precipitate a hypertensive crisis.

Evaluation: Evaluate for evidence of an improved response in clients with Parkinson's disease being treated with carbidopa/levodopa.

Senna
(SEN-nah)
Black-Draught Lax-Senna, Dr. Caldwell Senna Laxative, Fletcher's Castoria for Children, Senexon, Senokot, Senolax, X-Prep Liquid (OTC)

Sennosides A and B, Calcium Salts
(SEN-noh-syd)
Gentle Nature, Glysennid✹, Mucinum-Herbal✹, Nytilax (OTC)

Classification: Stimulant laxative.

Action/Kinetics: Senna is prepared from the dried leaf or fruit of the *Cassia acutifolia* or *Cassia angustifolia* tree. Senna is similar to cascara although it is more potent. It increases peristalsis of the colon by stimulating the intestinal mucosa and the myenteric plexus; it also alters electrolyte secretion. **Onset:** 6–10 hr.

Uses: Constipation, preoperative and prediagnostic procedures involving the GI tract.

Contraindications: Irritable colon, nausea, vomiting, abdominal pain, and appendicitis or possibility thereof.

Special Concerns: Administer with caution to nursing mothers.

Side Effects: Abdominal pain, colic, and diarrhea. Senna colors alkaline urine pink, red, or violet and acid urine yellow-brown.

Dosage: *Senna.* **Tablets: Adults,** 2 at bedtime; **pediatric, over 27.3 kg:** 1 tablet at bedtime. **Supposito-**

ries: **Adults,** 1 at bedtime; **pediatric, over 27.3 kg:** ½ suppository at bedtime. **Black-Draught Granules: Adults,** ¼–½ level teaspoon with water (not recommended for children). **Senokot Granules: Adults,** 1 teaspoon; **pediatric, over 27.3 kg:** ½ teaspoon. Taken at bedtime. **Senokot Syrup: Adults,** 10–15 ml at bedtime; **pediatric, 1–12 months:** 1.25–2.5 ml at bedtime; **pediatric, 1–5 years:** 2.5–5 ml; **5–15 years:** 5–10 ml. **Dr. Caldwell Senna Laxative: Adults,** 15–30 ml with or after meals or at bedtime; **pediatric, 6–15 years:** 10–15 ml at bedtime; **1–5 years:** 5–10 ml at bedtime. **Fletcher's Castoria for Children, 6–12 years:** 10–15 ml; **1–5 years:** 5–10 ml; **7–12 months:** 2.5–5 ml; **1–6 months:** 1.25–2.5 ml. *Sennosides A and B.* **Gentle Nature, Adults,** 1–2 tablets at bedtime taken with water; **children 6 years and older:** 1 tablet at bedtime. **Nytilax, Adults:** 12–36 mg (1–3 tablets) at bedtime.

NURSING CONSIDERATIONS

See also *Nursing Considerations* for *Laxatives,* p. 172.

Client/Family Teaching

1. Gripping pain may be a symptom of overdosage. Omit drug when this occurs and notify physician.
2. Explain that the drug causes acid urine to have a yellowish-brown color. Alkaline urine will develop a reddish color.

Evaluation: Evaluate client for:
- Reports of effective relief of constipation
- Evidence of the evacuation of a soft, formed stool

Simethicone
(sye-**METH**-ih-kohn)
Extra-Strength Gas-X, Gas-X, Mylicon, Mylicon-80, Mylicon-125, Ovol❃, Ovol-40 and -80❃, Phazyme, Phazyme 55❃, Phazyme 95 and 125, Silain (OTC)

Classification: Antiflatulent.

Action/Kinetics: Simethicone acts as a defoamant, which decreases surface tension of gas bubbles, thus facilitating their coalescence and expulsion as flatus or belching. It also prevents the accumulation of mucus-enclosed pockets of gas. Excreted in feces unchanged.

Uses: Relief of pain caused by excess gas in digestive tract. Adjunct in the treatment of postoperative gaseous distention, air swallowing, functional dyspepsia, peptic ulcer, spastic irritable colon, or diverticulitis. *Investigational:* Adjunct during gastroscopy to increase visualization and prior to radiography to reduce gas shadows in the bowel.

Dosage: Tablets: 50–100 mg after each meal and at bedtime (up to a maximum of 500 mg daily if used OTC). **Chewable Tablets:** 40–125 mg q.i.d. after each meal and at bedtime (up to 480 mg daily if used OTC). **Capsules:** 125 mg after each meal and at bedtime. **Oral Suspension:** 40 mg q.i.d. after meals and at bedtime. Also, for *gastroscopy, radiography of the bowel:* 67 mg in 2.5 ml water as a single dose.

NURSING CONSIDERATIONS
Administration/Storage

1. Tablets should be chewed thoroughly or dissolved in mouth.

2. Use calibrated dropper to administer medication.
3. Suspension should be shaken well before using.

Interventions

1. Assess bowel sounds periodically during therapy.
2. Question client concerning the effectiveness of prescribed therapy because dosage may need to be adjusted.

Evaluation: Evaluate client for:

- Evidence of decreased tympany and decreased abdominal distention
- Reports of symptomatic improvement in abdominal pain and discomfort with successful passing of flatus

---

Sodium benzoate and Sodium phenylacetate

(**SO**-dee-um **BEN**-zoh-ayt, fen-ill-**AH**-seh-tayt)

Ucephan (Rx)

Classification: Drug for hyperammonemia.

Action/Kinetics: In clients with urea cycle enzymopathies, there is a deficiency (either partial or complete) of argininosucciante synthetase, carbamylphosphate synthetase, and ornithine transcarbamylase. This leads to elevated blood ammonia levels, which is fatal in nearly 80% of clients. Sodium benzoate and sodium phenylacetate lower elevated blood ammonia levels by decreasing ammonia formation, thus substituting for the defective enzymes in these individuals.

Uses: Prophylaxis and chronic treatment of hyperammonemia in clients with urea cycle enzymopathies.

Contraindications: Hypersensitivity to sodium benzoate or sodium phenylacetate. The sodium ions in this product should be used with care (if at all) in congestive heart failure, edema due to sodium retention, and renal insufficiency.

Special Concerns: Pregnancy category: C. Use with caution during lactation and in neonates with hyperbilirubinemia.

Side Effects: *GI:* Nausea, vomiting, worsening of peptic ulcers. *Respiratory:* Respiratory alkalosis and hyperventilation. *Symptoms of Overdose:* Vomiting, irritability, metabolic acidosis, circulatory collapse.

Drug Interactions

Penicillin / ↑ Renal tubular secretion due to competition from sodium benzoate and sodium phenylacetate

Probenecid / ↓ Renal excretion of conjugation products of sodium benzoate and sodium phenylacetate

Dosage: Oral Solution. Adults: 2.5 ml/kg daily (250 mg each of sodium benzoate and sodium phenylacetate) in 3–6 equally divided doses. Total daily dose should not exceed 100 ml (i.e., 10 g each of sodium benzoate and sodium phenylacetate).

NURSING CONSIDERATIONS

Administration/Storage

1. This product must be diluted in 4–8 oz of milk (or infant formula) and given with meals. Acidic liquids should not be used since the drug may precipitate in an acid medium. The mixture should be visually in-

spected for compatibility before it is administered.

2. Sodium benzoate and sodium phenylacetate should be considered as adjunctive therapy for urea cycle enzymopathies.

3. For optimum results, combine with a low-protein diet and amino acid supplements.

4. Care should be exercised when mixing and administering sodium phenylacetate since contact with the skin and clothing will result in a lingering odor.

5. The product should be stored at room temperature; excess heat should be avoided.

6. *Treatment of Overdose:* Discontinue the drug and treat symptoms. It may be necessary to treat for metabolic acidosis and circulatory collapse. Hemodialysis or peritoneal dialysis may be helpful.

Interventions: Monitor electrolyte levels, pH, and serum ammonia levels throughout therapy.

Client/Family Teaching

1. Follow a low-protein diet. Refer to a dietitian for assistance with the diet and meal planning.

2. Provide written guidelines for the correct dilution and administration of the drug.

3. Instruct the client in keeping an accurate record of weight and advise client to report any significant changes to the physician.

4. Teach the client how to assess for edema and to report if evident.

5. Explain the importance of reporting for follow-up visits to the physician and for sched-

uled laboratory studies so that the effectiveness of the drug therapy can be evaluated.

6. Provide a printed list of adverse side effects. Discuss the importance of reporting to the physician any adverse effects and/or changes in mental attitude.

Evaluation: Evaluate client for laboratory evidence of a reduction of elevated serum ammonia levels.

Sodium bicarbonate

(SO-dee-um bye-KAR-bon-ayt)
Arm and Hammer Pure Baking Soda, Bell/ans, Citrocarbonate, Neut, Soda Mint (Rx and OTC)

Classification: Alkalinizing agent, antacid, electrolyte.

Action/Kinetics: The antacid action is due to neutralization of hydrochloric acid by forming sodium chloride and carbon dioxide (1 g of sodium bicarbonate neutralizes 12 mEq of acid). Provides temporary relief of peptic ulcer pain and of discomfort associated with indigestion. Although widely used by the public, sodium bicarbonate is rarely prescribed as an antacid because of its high sodium content, short duration of action, and ability to cause alkalosis (sometimes desired). Sodium bicarbonate is also a systemic and urinary alkalinizer by increasing plasma and urinary bicarbonate, respectively.

Uses: Treatment of hyperacidity, severe diarrhea (where there is loss of bicarbonate), nonspecific treatment of drug toxicity (e.g., barbiturates, salicylates, methanol). Treatment of acute mild to moderate metabolic acidosis due to shock, severe dehydration, renal disease,

S

cardiac arrest, severe primary lactic acidosis. Prophylaxis of renal calculi in gout. During sulfonamide therapy to prevent renal calculi and nephrotoxicity. *Investigational:* Sickle cell anemia.

Contraindications: Renal impairment, congestive heart failure, pyloric obstruction, clients on restricted-sodium diet, edema, cirrhosis of the liver, metabolic or respiratory alkalosis, toxemia of pregnancy. Do not use as an antidote for strong mineral acids because carbon dioxide is formed, which may cause discomfort and even perforation. Children less than 6 years of age.

Special Concerns: Pregnancy category: C. Use with extreme caution in clients losing chloride through vomiting or continuous GI suction and in those in whom diuretics produce hypochloremic alkalosis. Use with caution in clients with edema and cirrhosis.

Side Effects: *GI:* Acid rebound, gastric distention. *Milk-alkali syndrome:* Hypercalcemia, metabolic alkalosis (dizziness, cramps, thirst, anorexia, nausea, vomiting, hyperexcitability, tetany, diminished breathing, seizures), renal dysfunction. Extravasation following IV use may manifest ulceration, sloughing, cellulitis, or tissue necrosis at the site of injection. *Symptoms of Overdose:* Severe alkalosis that may be accompanied by tetany or hyperirritability.

Drug Interactions

Amphetamines / ↑ Effect of amphetamines by ↑ renal tubular reabsorption

Antidepressants, tricyclic / ↑ Effect of tricyclics by ↑ renal tubular reabsorption

Benzodiazepines / ↓ Effect due to ↑ alkalinity of urine

Ephedrine / ↑ Effect of ephedrine by ↑ renal tubular reabsorption

Erythromycin / ↑ Effect of erythromycin in urine due to ↑ alkalinity of urine

Flecainide / ↑ Effect due to ↑ alkalinity of urine

Iron products / ↓ Effect due to ↑ alkalinity of urine

Ketoconazole / ↓ Effect due to ↑ alkalinity of urine

Lithium carbonate / Excretion of lithium is proportional to amount of sodium ingested. If client on sodium-free diet, may develop lithium toxicity because less lithium is excreted

Methenamine compounds / ↓ Effect of methenamine due to ↑ alkalinity of urine

Nitrofurantoin / ↓ Effect of nitrofurantoin due to ↑ alkalinity of urine

Procainamide / ↑ Effect of procainamide due to ↓ excretion by kidney

Pseudoephedrine / ↑ Effect of pseudoephedrine due to ↑ tubular reabsorption

Quinidine / ↑ Effect of quinidine by ↑ renal tubular reabsorption

Salicylates / ↓ Effect due to ↑ alkalinity of urine

Sulfonylureas / ↓ Effect due to ↑ alkalinity of urine

Tetracyclines / ↓ Effect of tetracyclines due to ↑ excretion by kidney

Dosage: Effervescent Powder. *Antacid:* **Adults,** 3.9–10 g in a glass of cold water after meals. **Geriatric and pediatric, 6–12 years:** 1.9–3.9 g after meals. **Oral Powder.** *Antacid:* **Adults,** ½ teaspoonful in a glass of water q 2 hr; adjust dosage as required. *Urinary alkalinizer:* **Adults,** 1 teaspoonful in a glass of water q 4 hr; adjust dosage as required. Dosage not established for this form for children. **Tablets.** *Antacid:* **Adults,** 0.325–2 g 1–4 times daily; **pediatric, 6–12 years:** 520 mg; may be repeated once after 30 min. *Urinary alkalinizer:* **Adults, initial,** 4 g; **then,** 1–2 g q 4 hr. **Pediatric,** 23–230 mg/kg daily; adjust dosage as needed. **Injection.** *Systemic alkalizer, cardiac arrest:* **Adults, IV, initial,** 1 mEq/kg; **then,** 0.5 mEq/kg may be repeated q 10 min of continued arrest. **Pediatric, IV, initial:** 1 mEq/kg; **then,** 0.5 mEq/kg q 10 min of continued arrest. *Systemic alkalinizer, less severe metabolic acidosis:* **Adults and older children, IV infusion,** 2–5 mEq/kg given over 4–8 hr. *Urinary alkalinizer:* **Adults and children, IV,** 2–5 mEq/kg over 4–8 hr.

NURSING CONSIDERATIONS

Administration/Storage

1. Hypertonic solutions must be administered by trained personnel. Avoid extravasation as tissue irritation or cellulitis may result.
2. IV dose should be determined by arterial blood pH, pCO_2, and base deficit.
3. Isotonic solutions should be administered slowly as ordered. Too-rapid administration may result in death due to cellular acidity. Therefore, check rate of flow frequently.
4. If only the 7.5% or 8.4% solution is available, it should be diluted 1:1 with 5% dextrose in water when used in infants for cardiac arrest.
5. Have available a parenteral solution of calcium gluconate and 2.14% solution of ammonium chloride in the event of severe alkalosis or tetany.

6. *Treatment of Overdose:* Discontinue sodium bicarbonate. Symptoms of alkalosis can be reversed by rebreathing expired air from a paper bag or using a rebreathing mask. An IV infusion of ammonium chloride solution, 2.14%, can be used to control severe cases. Hypokalemia may be treated by IV sodium chloride or potassium chloride. Calcium gluconate will control tetany.

Assessment

1. Note any client history of renal impairment, congestive heart failure or if the client is on a sodium-restricted diet.
2. Assess the client for evidence of edema that may indicate the inability to utilize sodium bicarbonate.
3. If the client is on low continuous or intermittent NG suctioning or is vomiting, assess for evidence of excessive loss of chloride.
4. Note if the client is taking other medications. List and determine what their potential interactive effect may be.
5. If the client is to receive sodium bicarbonate to counteract metabolic acidosis, obtain arterial blood for pH, pCO_2, and HCO_3, and other designated electrolytes, as baseline data.

Interventions

1. Record I&O. Observe the client for dry skin and mucous membranes, polydipsia, polyuria, and air hunger. These are indications of a reversal of symptoms of metabolic acidosis and need to be documented and reported to the physician.

2. Compare the pH and electrolytes with the values taken prior to administering sodium bicarbonate to ensure that the client is not developing an alkalosis. If there is evidence of alkalosis, notify the physician and be prepared to have the client breathe in and out of a paper bag.
3. Periodically assess the client's serum pH during the therapy.
4. Assess the client with acidosis who is being treated with sodium bicarbonate for the relief of dyspnea and hyperpnea. Relief of these symptoms indicates that the drug may be discontinued.
5. Observe if the client being treated for acidosis develops edema. Report to the physician and anticipate the order will be changed to potassium bicarbonate since the sodium content of the drug is 27%.
6. At intervals during the day, test the client's urine with nitrazine paper to determine if the urine is becoming alkaline. Adjust the dosage of sodium bicarbonate accordingly.

Client/Family Teaching

1. Warn clients taking excessive oral preparations of sodium bicarbonate routinely to relieve gastric distress that there may be a rebound reaction resulting either in an increased acid secretion or systemic alkalosis. Remind them to consult a physician with persistent symptoms of gastric distress and that drug is not to be used routinely.
2. Also, advise the client taking sodium bicarbonate on a routine basis of the danger of forming phosphate crystals in the kidney and fluid retention.
3. Explain that if clients take sodium bicarbonate with milk or calcium, a milk-alkali syndrome may result. Clients may develop anorexia, nausea, and vomiting when this occurs. They may also become mentally confused. The physician should be notified immediately if these symptoms occur.
4. Explain to the client the need to avoid OTC preparations such as Alka-Seltzer or Fizrin that contain sodium bicarbonate.

Evaluation: Evaluate client for:
- Laboratory confirmation of a reversal of metabolic acidosis
- Laboratory evidence of ↑ urinary and serum pH
- Reports of a reduction in gastric discomfort

Sodium chloride
(**SO**-dee-um **KLOR**-eyed)
Tablets: Slo-Salt. **Topical: Ayr Saline, HuMIST Saline Nasal, NaSal Saline Nasal, Ocean Mist, Otrivin Saline✹, Salinex Nasal Mist. Ophthalmic: Adsorbonac Ophthalmic, AK-NaCl, Cordema✹, Hypersal 5%, Muro-128 Ophthalmic, Parenteral: Sodium Chloride IV Infusions (0.2%, 0.45%, 0.9%, 3%, 5%), Sodium Chloride Injection for Admixtures (50, 100, 625 mEq/vial), Sodium Chloride Diluent (0.9%), Concentrated Sodium Chloride Diluents (14.6%, 23.4%) (Parenteral is Rx; Topical and ophthalmic are OTC)**

Classification: Electrolyte.

Action/Kinetics: Sodium is the major cation of the body's extracellular fluid. It plays a crucial role in maintaining the fluid and electrolyte balance. Excess retention of sodium results in overhydration (edema, hypervolemia), which is often treated with diuretics. Abnormally low levels of sodium result in dehydration. Normally, the plasma contains 136–145 mEq sodium/L and 98–106 mEq chloride/L. The average daily requirement of salt is approximately 5 g.

Uses: PO: Prophylaxis of heat prostration or muscle cramps, chloride deficiency due to diuresis or salt restriction. **Parenteral:** Fluid and electrolyte replacement. **Topical:** Relief of inflamed, dry, or crusted nasal membranes; irrigating solution. **Ophthalmic:** Use hypertonic solutions to decrease corneal edema due to bullous keratitis; as an aid to facilitate ophthalmoscopic examination in gonioscopy, biomicroscopy, and funduscopy.

Contraindications: Congestive heart failure, severely impaired renal function. Administer with caution to clients with cardiovascular, cirrhotic, or renal disease, in presence of hyperproteinemia, and in clients receiving corticosteroids or corticotropin.

Special Concerns: Pregnancy category: C.

Side Effects: Hypernatremia, postoperative intolerance of sodium chloride characterized by cellular dehydration, asthenia, disorientation, anorexia, nausea, oliguria, and increased BUN levels.

Dosage: Tablets (including extended-release and enteric-coated): *Heat cramps/dehydra-*
tion: 0.5–1 g with 8 oz water up to 10 times/day; total daily dose should not exceed 4.8 g. **IV:** *Individualized* as required. *Hypotonic* (0.11%–0.45% NaCl) solutions are used when fluid losses exceed electrolyte depletion. *Isotonic* (0.9% NaCl) provides approximately physiologic concentrations of sodium and chloride ions. *Hypertonic* (3% or 5%) when sodium loss exceeds fluid loss. **Ophthalmic.** *Solution:* 1–2 gtt in eye q 3–4 hr. *Ointment:* Instill once (or more often, if necessary) daily.

NURSING CONSIDERATIONS

Administration/Storage: Hypertonic injections of NaCl must be given slowly and cautiously in an amount not to exceed 100 ml/hr. Plasma electrolyte levels should be determined before additional sodium chloride is given.

Interventions

1. Observe the client for flushed skin, elevated temperature, rough dry tongue, and edema. These are symptoms of hypernatremia; document and report to the physician.
2. Monitor vital signs for evidence of hypertension, hypotension, or tachycardia. Record I&O.
3. Monitor urine specific gravity and serum sodium levels. If the urine specific gravity is above 1.02, and if the serum sodium level is above 146 mEq/L, report to the physician and anticipate that the drug will be discontinued.
4. Monitor electrolyte levels and hepatic and renal function studies.
5. Note level of consciousness and periodically assess heart sounds.

S

Evaluation: Evaluate client for:
- Evidence of prophylaxis of heat prostration during exposure to high temperatures or during increased activity
- The prevention of chloride deficiency R/T excessive diuresis or salt restriction or excessive sweating
- Laboratory evidence of replacement of serum sodium and chloride electrolytes to desired levels

---

Sodium polystyrene sulfonate

(**SO**-dee-um pol-ee-**STY**-reen **SUL**-fon-ayt)

Kayexalate, PMS Sodium Polystyrene Sulfonate✿, SPS (Rx)

Classification: Potassium ion exchange resin.

Action/Kinetics: Sodium polystyrene sulfonate is a resin that exchanges sodium ions for potassium ions primarily in the large intestine. Thus, excess amounts of potassium (as well as calcium and magnesium) may be removed. Therapy is governed by daily monitoring of serum potassium levels. Discontinue therapy when serum potassium levels have reached 4–5 mEq/L. Clients should also be monitored for serum calcium and magnesium levels. **Onset, PO:** 2–12 hr.

Uses: Hyperkalemia.

Special Concerns: Use with caution in geriatric clients because they are more likely to develop fecal impaction. Use with caution in clients sensitive to sodium overload (e.g., in cardiovascular disease) or

for those receiving digitalis preparations because the action of these agents is potentiated by hypokalemia.

Side Effects: *GI:* Nausea, vomiting, constipation, anorexia, gastric irritation, diarrhea (rarely). Fecal impaction in geriatric clients. *Electrolyte:* Sodium retention, hypokalemia, hypocalcemia, hypomagnesemia. *Other:* Overhydration, pulmonary edema.

Drug Interactions

Aluminum hydroxide / ↑ Risk of intestinal obstruction
Calcium- or magnesium-containing antacids or laxatives / ↑ Risk of metabolic alkalosis

Dosage: Powder for Suspension, Suspension. Adults, PO: 15 g resin suspended in 20–100 ml water or syrup (to increase palatability) 1–4 times daily. Up to 40 g daily have been used. **Pediatric:** To calculate dose, use an exchange ratio of 1 mEq potassium/g resin (usually, 1 g/kg per dose). **Enema:** 25–100 g suspended in 100 ml sorbitol or 20% dextrose in water q 6 hr.

NURSING CONSIDERATIONS

Administration/Storage

1. To treat or to prevent constipation, 10–20 ml of 70% sorbitol may be given PO q 2 hr (or as necessary) to produce 1–2 watery stools each day.
2. For oral administration, give the resin suspended in water or syrup (3–4 ml/g resin). If necessary, the resin can be administered through a nasogastric tube, either as an

aqueous suspension, mixed with dextrose, or as a peanut or olive oil emulsion.

3. Rectal administration:
   - First, administer a cleansing enema.
   - To administer medication, insert a large-size rubber tube (e.g., French 28) into the rectum for a distance of 20 cm until it is well into the sigmoid colon and tape in place.
   - Suspend resin in appropriate vehicle (see *Dosage*) at body temperature. Administer by gravity while stirring suspension.
   - Flush suspension that remains in the container with 50–100 ml fluid, clamp the tube, and leave in place.
   - Elevate client's hips or ask the client to assume a knee-chest position, for a short time if there is back-leakage.
   - The enema should be kept in the colon as long as possible (3–4 hr).
   - Resin is removed by colonic irrigation with 2 quarts of a *nonsodium*-containing solution warmed to body temperature. Returns are drained constantly through a Y tube.

4. Retention enemas of the resin are less effective than oral administration.

5. Use freshly prepared solutions within 24 hr. Do not heat resin.

6. Oral suspension products contain sorbitol and sodium.

7. Orders for the drug should designate the grams of powder and the percent sorbitol and volume to be used or the amount of premixed suspension. The frequency and route of administration should also be specified.

8. Avoid inhaling the powder for suspension when admixing.

Assessment: Determine if the client has a history of cardiovascular disease and/or is taking digitalis preparations. These clients are at risk for having digitalis toxicity potentiated by this drug.

Interventions

1. Monitor renal function studies and the level of serum potassium, sodium, magnesium, and calcium. Observe the client for any signs of electrolyte imbalance.

2. Observe clients on sodium restrictions closely; drug contains 100 mg Na/g.

3. The administration of calcium- or magnesium-containing antacids during oral administration of sodium polystyrene sulfonate may predispose the client to metabolic alkalosis. Therefore, administer antacids cautiously.

4. Monitor vital signs and intake and output. If the client has an increase in urinary output or becomes constipated report to the physician.

5. Encourage clients receiving the medication rectally to retain the medication for several hours to ensure effectiveness of drug therapy.

Evaluation: Evaluate client for laboratory confirmation that serum potassium levels are within desired range (4.0–5.0 mEq/L).

———— COMBINATION DRUG ————
Soma Compound
(SO-mah)
(Rx)

Soma Compound with Codeine
(SO-mah, KOH-deen)
(Rx, C-III)

Classification/Content: Soma Compound contains: *Nonnarcotic analgesic:* Aspirin, 325 mg. *Centrally acting skeletal muscle relaxant:* Carisoprodol, 200 mg. In addition to the above, Soma Compound with Codeine contains: *Narcotic analgesic:* Codeine phosphate, 16 mg. See also information on individual components.

Uses: As an adjunct to rest and physical therapy for the relief of acute, painful musculoskeletal conditions including muscle spasm, pain, and conditions leading to limited mobility.

Contraindication: Acute intermittent porphyria, bleeding disorders, lactation. Use in children less than 12 years of age.

Special Concerns: Pregnancy category: C. Use with caution in clients with impaired hepatic or renal function, in elderly or debilitated clients, in clients with a history of gastritis or peptic ulcer, in those on anticoagulant therapy, and in individuals prone to addiction.

Dosage: Tablets: Soma Compound and Soma Compound with Codeine: Adults, 1–2 tablets q.i.d.

NURSING CONSIDERATIONS

See *Nursing Considerations* for *Aspirin,* p. 264, and *Narcotic Analgesics,* p. 177.

Evaluation: Evaluate client for reports of effective control of musculoskeletal pain.

Somatrem
(SO-mah-trem)
Protropin (Rx)

Somatropin
(so-mah-TROH-pin)
Humatrope (Rx)

Classification: Growth hormone.

Action/Kinetics: Both somatrem and somatropin are derived from recombinant DNA technology. Somatrem contains the same sequence of amino acids (191) as human growth hormone derived from the pituitary gland plus one additional amino acid (methionine). Somatropin, on the other hand, has the identical sequence of amino acids as does human growth hormone of pituitary origin. These agents stimulate linear growth by increasing somatomedin-C serum levels, which, in turn, increases the incorporation of sulfate into proteoglycans thereby stimulating skeletal growth. These hormones also increase the number and size of muscle cells, increase synthesis of collagen, increase protein synthesis, and increase internal organ size. Serum insulin levels increase (indicative of insulin resistance), and there is acute mobilization of lipid.

Uses: Stimulate linear growth of children who suffer from lack of adequate levels of endogenous growth hormone.

Contraindications: In clients in whom epiphyses have closed. Active intracranial lesions, sensitivity to benzyl alcohol (somatrem); sensitivity to m-cresol or glycerin (somatropin). **Note:** Hypothyroidism (which may be induced by the drug) decreases the response to somatrem.

Special Concerns: Concomitant use of glucocorticoids may decrease the response to growth hormone.

Side Effects: Development of persistent antibodies to growth hormone (30%–40% of clients taking somatrem and 2% of clients taking somatropin). Development of insulin resistance. Adults have experienced headache, weakness, glucosuria, muscle pain, edema. Leukemia has developed in a small number of children. *Symptoms of Overdose:* Acute overdose can cause hypoglycemia followed by hyperglycemia. Long-term overdose can result in signs and symptoms of acromegaly.

Drug Interactions: Glucocorticoids inhibit the effect of somatrem on growth.

Dosage: Somatrem. IM. Individualized. Usual: Up to 0.1 mg/kg (0.2 IU/kg) 3 times weekly. The incidence of side effects increases if the dose is greater than 0.1 mg/kg.
Somatropin. IM, SC. Individualized. Usual: Up to 0.06 mg/kg (0.16 IU/kg) 3 times weekly. Side effects increase if the dose exceeds 0.06 mg/kg.

NURSING CONSIDERATIONS

Administration/Storage

1. Somatrem should be administered only by a physician experienced in the diagnosis and treatment of pituitary disorders.
2. Due to the development of insulin resistance, clients should be evaluated for possible glucose intolerance.
3. The powder for injection for somatrem should be reconstituted *only* with bacteriostatic water for injection (benzyl alcohol preserved).
4. If somatrem is to be used in newborns, it should be reconstituted with water for injection because benzyl alcohol can be toxic to newborns.
5. Somatropin should be reconstituted only with the diluent provided; if sensitivity occurs, sterile water for injection can be used.
6. If somatropin is reconstituted with sterile water for injection, the following guidelines must be followed.
   • Use only one dose per reconstituted vial.
   • The solutions should be refrigerated if not used immediately after reconstitution.
   • The reconstituted dose should be used within 24 hr.
   • After the dose is administered, any unused portion should be discarded.
7. When reconstituting somatrem or somatropin, the vial should not be shaken. Rather, it should be swirled with a gentle rotary motion.
8. Only reconstituted somatrem solution that is clear and without particulate matter should be injected.
9. The needle used for injection should be at least 1 inch or greater in length to ensure that the injection reaches the muscle layer.
10. Reconstituted somatrem should be used within 7 days and should not be frozen.

Assessment

1. Determine that x-ray evidence of bone growth has been conducted.
2. Note if the client is receiving glucocorticoids. These inhibit the effect of somatrem on growth.

Interventions

1. Measure the client's height and weight monthly and record.
2. Monitor thyroid function studies routinely for evidence of hypothyroidism.
3. Routinely assess clients with diabetes for evidence of hyperglycemia and acidosis.
4. Note any limps or knee/hip pain because a slipped capital epiphysis may occur.

Evaluation

1. Measure growth hormone levels and compare skeletal height records with baseline measurements to determine evidence of growth.
2. Evaluate client for freedom from complications of drug therapy.

S Spectinomycin hydrochloride

(speck-tin-oh-**MY**-sin)

Trobicin (Rx)

See also *Anti-Infectives,* p. 80.

Classification: Antibiotic, miscellaneous.

Action/Kinetics: Spectinomycin is produced by *Streptomyces spectabilis*. It inhibits bacterial protein synthesis by binding to ribosomes (30S subunit), thereby interfering with transmission of genetic information crucial to life of microorganism. Spectinomycin is mainly bacteriostatic. It is not absorbed from GI tract and is only given IM. **Peak plasma concentration:** 100 mcg/ml after 1 hr. **t½:** 1.2–2.8 hr. Not significantly bound to protein. Excreted in urine.

Uses: Acute gonorrhea in infections resistant to penicillin or in clients allergic to penicillin. It is ineffective against syphilis, and thus is a poor drug to choose when mixed infections are present.

Contraindications: Sensitivity to drug.

Special Concerns: Safe use during pregnancy has not been established.

Side Effects: A single dose of spectinomycin has caused soreness at the site of injection, urticaria, dizziness, nausea, chills, fever, and insomnia. Multiple doses have caused a decrease in hemoglobin, hematocrit, and creatinine clearance and an increase in alkaline phosphatase, BUN, and ALT.

Dosage: IM only: 2 g. In areas where antibiotic resistance is known to be prevalent, give 4 g divided between two gluteal injection sites.

NURSING CONSIDERATIONS

See also *General Nursing Considerations For All Anti-Infectives,* p. 83.

Administration/Storage

1. Powder is stable for 3 years.
2. Use reconstituted solution within 24 hr.
3. Inject deeply into the upper, outer quadrant of the gluteus muscle.
4. Injections may be made in two

sites for clients requiring 4 g. Rotate and document injection sites.

Client/Family Teaching

1. Advise clients taking spectinomycin, who are suspected to have syphilis, to return for serologic tests monthly for at least 3 months.
2. Refer clients for counseling and encourage their sexual partners to receive treatment.
3. Advise to abstain from sex until infection is resolved. Review safe sex practices to prevent reinfection.

Evaluation: Evaluate client for:

- Laboratory confirmation of negative serologic test results
- Clinical evidence and reports of improvement in symptoms of gonorrheal urethritis

---

Spironolactone

(speer-oh-no-**LAK**-tohn)

Aldactone, Novospiroton✲ (Rx)

See also *Diuretics,* p. 140.

Classification: Diuretic, potassium-sparing.

Action/Kinetics: Spironolactone is a mild diuretic that acts on the distal tubule to inhibit sodium exchange for potassium which results in increased secretion of sodium and water and conservation of potassium. It is also an aldosterone antagonist. The drug manifests a slight antihypertensive effect. It also interferes with synthesis of testosterone and may increase formation of estradiol from testosterone thus leading to endocrine abnormalities.

Onset: Urine output increases over 1–2 days. **Peak:** 2–3 days. **Duration:** 2–3 days, and declines thereafter. It is metabolized to an active metabolite (canrenone). **t½:** 13–24 hr for canrenone. The drug is almost completely bound to plasma protein. Spironolactone is also found in Aldactazide.

Uses: Edema due to congestive heart failure, cirrhosis of the liver, nephrotic syndrome. Primary hyperaldosteronism, essential hypertension, hypokalemia (especially in clients taking digitalis). Frequently used as adjunct with potassium-losing diuretics when it is important to avoid hypokalemia. *Investigational:* Polycystic ovary syndrome.

Contraindications: Acute renal insufficiency, progressive renal failure, hyperkalemia, and anuria. Clients receiving potassium supplements.

Special Concerns: Use during pregnancy only if benefits clearly outweigh risks. Use with caution in impaired renal function. Geriatric clients may be more sensitive to the usual adult dose.

Side Effects: *Electrolyte:* Hyperkalemia, hyponatremia (characterized by lethargy, dry mouth, thirst, tiredness). *GI:* Diarrhea, cramps, ulcers, gastritis, gastric bleeding, vomiting. *CNS:* Drowsiness, ataxia, lethargy, confusion, headache. *Endocrine:* Gynecomastia, menstrual irregularities, impotence, bleeding in postmenopausal women, deepening of voice, hirsutism. *Miscellaneous:* Skin rashes, drug fever, urticaria, breast carcinoma, hyperchloremic metabolic acidosis in hepatic cirrhosis (decompensated), agranulocytosis. **Note:** Spironolactone has been shown to be tumorigenic in chronic rodent studies.

Drug Interactions

Anesthetics, general / Additive hypotension

Angiotensin-converting enzyme inhibitors / Significant hyperkalemia

Anticoagulants, oral / Inhibited by spironolactone

Antihypertensives / Potentiation of hypotensive effect of both agents. Reduce dosage, especially of ganglionic blockers, by one-half

Captopril / ↑ Risk of significant hyperkalemia

Digitalis / The potassium-conserving effect of spironolactone may decrease effectiveness of digitalis. Though severe consequences have occurred in clients with impaired kidney function, drugs are often given concomitantly. Monitor closely

Diuretics, others / Often administered concurrently because of potassium-sparing effect of spironolactone. Severe hyponatremia may occur. Monitor closely

Lithium / ↑ Chance of lithium toxicity due to ↓ renal clearance

Norepinephrine / ↓ Responsiveness to norepinephrine

Potassium salts / Since spironolactone conserves potassium excessively, hyperkalemia may result. Rarely used together

Salicylates / Large doses may ↓ effects of spironolactone

Triamterene / Hazardous hyperkalemia may result from combination

Laboratory Test Interference: Interference with radioimmunoassay for digoxin. False + plasma cortisol (as determined by fluorometric assay of Mattingly).

Dosage: Tablets.   *Diuretic:* Adults, initial, 100 mg/day (range: 25–200 mg/day) in 2–4 divided doses for at least 5 days; **maintenance:** 75–400 mg daily in 2–4 divided doses. **Pediatric:** 1–3 mg/kg/day as a single dose or as 2–4 divided doses. *Antihypertensive:* **Adults, initial,** 50–100 mg/day as a single dose or as 2–4 divided doses—give for at least 2 weeks; **maintenance:** adjust to individual response. **Pediatric:** 1–3 mg/kg in a single dose or in 2–4 divided doses. *Treat hypokalemia:* **Adults,** 25–100 mg/day as a single dose or 2–4 divided doses. *Diagnosis of primary hyperaldosteronism:* **Adults,** 400 mg/day for either 4 days or 3–4 weeks (depending on test used). *Hyperaldosteronism, prior to surgery:* 100–400 mg/day in 2–4 doses prior to surgery.

NURSING CONSIDERATIONS

See also *Nursing Considerations* for *Diuretics,* p. 141.

Administration/Storage

1. When used as the sole drug to treat edema, the initial dose should continue for at least 5 days. After that, adjustments may be made. If the dosage is not effective, a second diuretic may be added, especially one that acts in the proximal tubules.
2. When administered to small children, the tablets may be crushed and given as a suspension in cherry syrup.
3. Food may increase the absorption of spironolactone.
4. Protect the drug from light.

Assessment: Obtain baseline ECG and serum electrolyte levels prior to starting therapy. If the client's potassium level is greater than 5.5 mEq/L, withhold the medication and notify the physician.

Interventions

1. Monitor the client's serum electrolytes, liver and renal function studies and arterial blood gases. Compare with the baseline data and report any abnormalities.
2. Note if the client develops deep, rapid respirations, complains of headaches, or appears to be slower mentally. This may indicate the development of metabolic acidosis. Document and report these findings to the physician.
3. Record vital signs, I&O and weight.
4. Note if the client develops dysuria, urinary frequency, or renal spasm. Take a urine culture, check for sensitivity, request a urinalysis, and consult with the physician. It may be necessary to stop the medication.
5. Assess the client for tolerance to the drug, which may be characterized by edema and reduced urine output.
6. If the client has a history of cardiac disease, be alert to cardiac side effects.
7. If the client develops jaundice or tremors or appears mentally confused, report to the physician. If hepatic disease already exists, clients may develop hepatic encephalopathy.
8. Administer the drug with a snack or meals to relieve the symptoms of gastric distress. If nausea, bloating, anorexia, vomiting or diarrhea persist, notify the physician. The dosage of drug may need to be changed or the drug may need to be discontinued.

Client/Family Teaching

1. Take with food to minimize GI upset.
2. Instruct the client in how to take BP and assist to develop a method to maintain a written record for review by the physician.
3. Avoid foods or salt substitutes high in potassium because spironolactone is potassium-sparing.
4. Record weight twice a week. Report any evidence of edema or weight gain of more than 2 lbs/wk to the physician.
5. Caution clients taking large doses of medication not to drive a car and not to operate dangerous machinery until drug effects become apparent because drowsiness or ataxia may occur.

Evaluation: Evaluate client for:
- Effective control of edema
- Evidence of a reduction of blood pressure
- Successful treatment of primary hyperaldosteronism
- The prevention of hypokalemia in those taking digitalis and/or other diuretics

Streptokinase

(strep-toe-**KYE**-nayz)

Kabikinase, Streptase (Rx)

Classification: Thrombolytic agent.

Action/Kinetics: Most clients have a natural resistance to streptokinase that must be overcome with the loading dose before the drug becomes effective. Thrombin time and streptokinase resistance should be determined before initiation of the therapy. Streptokinase acts with plasminogen to produce an "activator complex," which enhances the conversion of plasminogen to plasmin. Plasmin then breaks down fibrinogen, fibrin clots, and other plasma proteins. Thus, the drug promotes the dissolution (lysis) of the insoluble fibrin trapped in intravascular emboli and thrombi. Also, inhibitors of streptokinase, such as alpha-2-macroglobulin, are rapidly inactivated by streptokinase. **Onset:** rapid; **duration:** 12 hr. **t½, activator complex:** 23 min.

Uses: Deep vein thrombosis; arterial thrombosis and embolism; acute evolving transmural myocardial infarction. Also, clearing of occluded arteriovenous and IV cannulae.

Contraindications: Any condition presenting a risk of hemorrhage, such as recent surgery or biopsies, delivery within 10 days, ulcerative disease. Arterial emboli originating from the left side of the heart. Also, hepatic or renal insufficiency, TB, recent cerebral embolism, thrombosis, hemorrhage, subacute bacterial endocarditis, rheumatic valvular disease, thrombocytopenia. Streptokinase resistance in excess of 1 million IU.

Special Concerns: Pregnancy category: C. The use of streptokinase in septic thrombophlebitis may be hazardous. History of significant allergic response. Safety in children has not been established.

Side Effects: *CV:* Superficial bleeding, severe internal bleeding. *Allergic:* Nausea, headache, breathing difficulties, bronchospasm, angioneurotic edema, urticaria, flushing, musculoskeletal pain, vasculitis, interstitial nephritis, periorbital swelling. *Other:* Fever, possible development of Guillain-Barre syndrome, development of antistreptokinase antibody (i.e., streptokinase may be ineffective if administered between 5 days and 6 months following prior use of streptokinase or following streptococcal infections).

Drug Interactions: The following drugs ↑ the chance of bleeding when given concomitantly with streptokinase: Anticoagulants, aspirin, heparin, indomethacin, and phenylbutazone.

Laboratory Test Interferences: ↓ Fibrinogen, plasminogen. ↑ Thrombin time, prothrombin time, and activated partial thromboplastin time.

Dosage: *Venous or arterial thrombosis, arterial or pulmonary embolism.* **IV infusion, initial,** 250,000 IU over 30 min (use the 1,500,000 IU vial diluted to 90 ml); **maintenance:** 100,000 IU/hr for 24–72 hr for arterial thrombosis or embolism, 72 hr for deep vein thrombosis, and 24 hr for pulmonary embolism. **Intracoronary infusion:** Same dose as IV infusion; however, the 1,500,000 IU vial should be diluted to 45 ml with a rate of infusion of 15 ml/hr for the loading dose and 3 ml/hr for maintenance doses. May be followed by continuous IV heparin infusion to prevent recurrent thrombosis (start only after thrombin time has decreased to less than twice the normal control value, usually 3–4 hr). *Acute evolving transmural myocardial infarction.* **IV infusion:** 1,500,000 IU within 60 min (use the 1,500,000 IU vial diluted to a total of 45 ml). **Intracoronary infusion,** 20,000 IU by bolus; **then,** 2,000 IU/min for 60 min (total dose of 140,000 IU). Use the 250,000 IU vial diluted to 125 ml. *Arteriovenous cannula occlusion:* 250,000 IU in 2-ml IV solution into each occluded limb of cannula; **then,** after 2 hr aspirate cannula limbs, flush with saline, and reconnect cannula.

NURSING CONSIDERATIONS

See also *Nursing Considerations* for *Alteplase, Recombinant,* p. 285.

Administration/Storage

1. Sodium chloride injection USP or 5% dextrose injection is the preferred diluent for IV use.
2. For AV cannulae, dilute 250,000 units with 2 ml of sodium chloride injection or 5% dextrose injection.
3. Reconstitute gently, as directed by manufacturer, without shaking vial.
4. Use within 24 hr after reconstitution.
5. Use an electronic infusion device to administer streptokinase and do not add any other medications to the line.
6. Have emergency drugs and equipment available. Have corticosteroids and aminocaproic acid available in the event bleeding is excessive.

Assessment

1. Ensure that baseline bleeding studies, type, and cross match have been completed prior to initiation of therapy.

2. Identify other drugs the client may be taking such as aspirin or similar products that could increase bleeding times.
3. During the nursing history, note any history of prior conditions that might contraindicate the use of streptokinase. (e.g., TB, SBE, ulcerative disease, recent surgery).
4. Determine from client or family any history or evidence of bleeding tendencies.
5. Note any evidence of heart disease and/or allergic reaction to any drugs.
6. Clients with high allergy potential or high streptokinase antibody titer may benefit by skin testing prior to administering therapy.

Interventions

1. Ensure that the client understands the purpose of the therapy and possible side effects.
2. Check that the client has had blood typed and cross matched before initiating thrombolytic therapy and ensure that blood is available in case of hemorrhage.
3. Review all contraindications before initiating therapy.
4. Clients receiving therapy should be observed in a closely monitored environment.
5. When administering thrombolytic agents, monitor plasma thrombin time q 4–12 hr. Thrombin time values should be 2–5 times higher than the normal control values.
6. Check access sites for evidence of bleeding. Check stools for evidence of occult blood.
7. During IV therapy, arterial sticks require 30 min of manual pressure followed by application of a pressure dressing.

8. To prevent bruising, avoid unnecessary handling of client.

9. If an IM injection is necessary, apply pressure after withdrawing the needle to prevent a hematoma and bleeding from the puncture site.

10. If excessive bleeding develops from an invasive procedure, discontinue therapy and call for packed RBCs and plasma expanders *other than dextran*.

11. To prevent new thrombus formation, or rethrombosis, anticipate the use of IV heparin and oral anticoagulants when the thrombolytic therapy is concluded.

12. Geriatric clients have an increased risk of bleeding during therapy.

13. Monitor BP and pulse. Have atropine available for hypotension and bradycardia.

14. Observe injection sites and postoperative wounds for bleeding during thrombolytic therapy. Document and report.

15. Note evidence of allergic reactions, ranging from anaphylaxis to moderate and mild reactions. These usually can be controlled with antihistamines and corticosteroids.

16. Note any redness and/or pain at the site of infusion. It may be necessary to further dilute the solution to prevent phlebitis.

17. Anticipate concomitant administration with aspirin.

18. Provide symptomatic treatment for fever reaction.

19. Following recanalization of an occluded coronary artery, clients may develop reperfusion reactions; these may include:
    - Reperfusion arrhythmias, usually of short duration. These may include accelerated idioventricular rhythm and sinus bradycardia.
    - A reduction of chest pain.
    - A return of the elevated ST segment to near baseline levels.

Client/Family Teaching

1. Review the inherent benefits and risks of drug therapy.
2. Answer all questions and assist to decrease anxiety levels.
3. Stress that to be effective, the therapy should be instituted within 4–6 hr of onset of symptoms of acute myocardial infarction.
4. Explain the importance of reporting any symptoms or side effects to the nurse immediately.

Evaluation: Evaluate client for:
- Evidence of successful lysis of emboli and thrombi with restoration of normal blood flow
- Evidence of catheter patency in previously occluded AV or IV cannulae

---

Streptomycin sulfate
(strep-toe-**MY**-sin)
(Rx)

See also *Aminoglycosides,* p. 23.

Classification: Antibiotic, aminoglycoside.

Action/Kinetics: Like other aminoglycoside antibiotics, streptomycin is distributed rapidly throughout most tissues and body fluids, including necrotic tubercular lesions. **Therapeutic serum levels: IM,** 25 mcg/ml. **$t^{1/2}$:** 2–3 hr.

Additional Uses: Tuberculosis in conjunction with other antitubercular agents. Emergence of resistant strains has greatly reduced the usefulness of streptomycin. Also used for tularemia, glanders (*Actinobacillus mallei*), bubonic plague (*Pasteurella pestis*), brucellosis, cholera, and bacterial endocarditis caused by *Hemophilus influenzae*.

Additional Contraindications: Hypersensitivity, contact dermatitis, and exfoliative dermatitis. Do not give to clients with myasthenia gravis.

Special Concerns: Use during pregnancy only if benefits clearly outweigh risks.

Additional Laboratory Test Interference: False urine glucose determinations with Benedict's solution and Clinitest.

Dosage: IM only. *Tuberculosis (adjunct):* **initial,** 1 g daily with other tuberculostatic drugs; **then,** reduce streptomycin dosage to 1 g 2–3 times/week for minimum of 1 year. **Pediatric:** in combination with other drugs, 20–40 mg/kg once daily (not to exceed 1 g/day). Older, debilitated clients should receive lower dosages. *Bacterial endocarditis due to penicillin-sensitive alpha-hemolytic and nonhemolytic streptococci (with penicillin):* 1 g b.i.d. for 1 week; **then,** 0.5 g b.i.d. for second week. *Enterococcal endocarditis (with penicillin):* 1 g b.i.d. for 2 weeks; **then,** 0.5 g b.i.d. for 4 weeks. *Plague:* 0.5–1 g q 6 hr until client has no fever for 3 days. *Tularemia:* 0.25–0.5 g q 6 hr for 7–10 days. *Other infections:* **Adults, IM,** 1–4 g/day in divided doses q 6–12 hr, depending on severity of infections; **pediatric:** 20–40 mg/kg/day in divided doses q 6–12 hr.

NURSING CONSIDERATIONS

See also *Nursing Considerations* for *Aminoglycosides,* p. 25.

Administration/Storage

1. Protect hands when preparing drug. Wear gloves if drug is prepared often because it is irritating.
2. In a dry form, the drug is stable for at least 2 years at room temperature.
3. Aqueous solutions prepared without preservatives are stable for at least 1 week at room temperature and for at least 3 months under refrigeration.
4. Use only solutions prepared freshly from dry powder for intrathecal, subarachnoid, and intrapleural administration because commercially prepared solutions contain preservatives harmful to tissues of the CNS and pleural cavity.
5. Commercially prepared, ready-to-inject solutions are for IM use only. These solutions are prepared with phenol and are stable at room temperature for prolonged periods of time.
6. Administer deep into muscle mass to minimize pain and local irritation.
7. Solutions may darken after exposure to light, but this does not necessarily cause a loss in potency. Check with pharmacist if unsure of potency.
8. When injection into the subarachnoid space is required for treatment of meningitis, only solutions made freshly from the dry powder should be used. Commercial solutions may contain preservatives toxic to the CNS.
9. *Treatment of Overdose/Toxicity:* Hemodialysis (preferred) or peritoneal dialysis.

S

Interventions

1. Use Tes-Tape for urine glucose test because Benedict's solution and Fehling's solution can give false + reactions. For more specific results, follow blood sugars with finger sticks.
2. Increase fluid intake to 2–3 L/day. Monitor I&O, weight, and renal function studies.
3. Monitor for evidence of hearing loss or vestibular dysfunction. High peak streptomycin levels may precipitate eighth cranial nerve dysfunction.

Client/Family Teaching

1. Solution is malodorous; inform client that this is normal.
2. Report any persistent or bothersome side effects as well as lack of response to drug therapy.

Evaluation: Evaluate client for:

- Laboratory evidence of negative culture results
- Clinical evidence and reports of symptomatic improvement

Streptozocin

(strep-toe-**ZOH**-sin)
Zanosar (Rx)

See also *Antineoplastic Agents,* p. 85, and *Alkylating Agents,* p. 20.

Classification: Antineoplastic, alkylating agent.

Action/Kinetics: Streptozocin is cell-cycle nonspecific although it does inhibit progression out of the G_2 phase of cell division. The drug forms methylcarbonium ions which alkylate or bind with intracellular substances such as nucleic acids. It is also cytotoxic by virtue of cross-linking of DNA strands resulting in inhibition of DNA synthesis. It may also cause hyperglycemia. Streptozocin does not penetrate the blood-brain barrier well although within 2 hr after administration, metabolites do and produce levels similar to those in plasma. **t½, unchanged drug, initial,** 35 min. **t½, metabolites, initial:** 6 min; **intermediate:** 3.5 hr; **terminal:** 40 hr. Unchanged drug and metabolites excreted in urine.

Uses: Metastatic islet cell pancreatic carcinomas (functional and nonfunctional) in clients with symptomatic or progressive metastases. *Investigational:* Malignant carcinoid tumors.

Contraindications: Use during lactation.

Special Concerns: Pregnancy category: C. Dosage has not been determined for children.

Additional Side Effects: Renal toxicity (up to two-thirds of clients) manifested by anuria, azotemia, glycosuria, hypophosphatemia, and renal tubular acidosis. Toxicity is dose-related and cumulative and may be fatal. Glucose intolerance (reversible) or insulin shock with hypoglycemia, depression.

Dosage: IV: *Daily schedule:* 500 mg/m² for 5 consecutive days every 6 weeks (until maximum benefit is achieved or toxicity occurs). Dose should not be increased. *Weekly schedule:* **Initial,** 1,000 mg/m² weekly for 2 weeks; **then,** if no response or no toxicity, dose can be increased, not to exceed a single dose of 1,500 mg/m². Response should be seen in 17–35 days.

NURSING CONSIDERATIONS

See also *Nursing Considerations* for *Antineoplastic Agents,* p. 88.

Administration/Storage

1. Drug should be reconstituted with dextrose injection or 0.9% sodium chloride injection. Reconstituted solution is pale gold in color.
2. No preservatives are found in the product; thus, total storage time for reconstituted drug is 12 hr. The ampule is not considered to be multiple dose.
3. Caution should be observed (wear gloves) in handling the drug.
4. Drug is a vesicant. Infiltration may result in tissue ulceration and necrosis.

Interventions

1. Measure fluid intake and urine output. Encourage 3 L of fluids per day to reduce the risk of renal damage. If urine output decreases, report to physician because streptozocin can cause anuria.
2. Perform finger sticks or test urine for glucose levels at least once a day and observe for symptoms of hypoglycemia.
3. Monitor blood sugar levels, CBC, and renal function studies during therapy.

Evaluation: Evaluate client for evidence of a reduction in tumor size and spread.

Succimer

(**SUCK**-sih-mer)

Chemet (Rx)

Classification: Chelating agent.

Action/Kinetics: Succimer acts to form water-soluble chelates, thus promoting the urinary excretion of lead. After oral administration, absorption is rapid but variable. **Peak blood levels:** 1–2 hr. **t½, elimination:** About 2 days. Approximately one-half of a dose is excreted, mainly through the feces with small amounts in the urine and as carbon dioxide through the lungs.

Uses: To treat lead poisoning in children with blood levels greater than 45 mcg/dl. *Investigational:* Heavy metal poisoning by mercury or arsenic.

Contraindications: Allergy to the drug. Use for prophylaxis of lead poisoning in a lead-containing environment. Use of succimer with other chelating agents (e.g., EDTA).

Special Concerns: Pregnancy category: C. Use with caution, if at all, during lactation. Use with caution in impaired renal function and in children less than one year of age. The drug is not a substitute for identification and removal of the source of the lead poisoning.

Side Effects: *GI:* Nausea, vomiting, diarrhea, loss of appetite, loose stools, metallic taste in mouth, abdominal cramps, hemorrhoidal symptoms. *CNS:* Drowsiness, dizziness, sleepiness, paresthesia, sensorimotor neuropathy. *Dermatologic:* Papular rash, herpetic rash, rash, pruritus, mucocutaneous eruptions. *Respiratory:* Cough, sore throat, nasal congestion, rhinorrhea. *Body as a whole:* Pain in back, stomach, head, rib, flank; chills, fever, flu-like symptoms, tired feeling, heavy head, head cold, headache, moniliasis. *Ophthalmic:* Cloudy film in eye, watery eyes. *GU:* Decreased urination, difficulty in voiding. *Miscellaneous:* Otitis media, ears plugged, arrhythmia, intermittent eosinophilia, kneecap pain, leg pains.

Laboratory Test Interferences: False + for urinary ketones using nitroprusside reagents (e.g., Ketostix). False−serum uric acid and CPK. ↑ Serum transaminases, AST, ALT, alkaline phosphatase, serum cholesterol, platelet count, proteinuria.

Dosage: Capsules. Initial: 10 mg/kg (350 mg/m^2) q 8 hr for 5 days; **then,** reduce frequency of dose to 10 mg/kg q 12 hr for an additional 2 weeks of therapy. A course of treatment lasts 19 days. Pediatric dosing is as follows: **8−15 kg:** 100 mg/dose; **16−23 kg:** 200 mg/dose; **24−34 kg:** 300 mg/dose; **35−44 kg:** 400 mg/dose; **over 45 kg:** 500 mg/dose.

NURSING CONSIDERATIONS

Administration/Storage

1. Uninterrupted drug therapy for more than 3 weeks is not recommended. A minimum of a 2-week rest period is recommended between courses of therapy unless blood lead levels indicate the need for more prompt treatment.
2. If a young child is not able to swallow capsules, the contents of the capsule can be given in a small amount of soft food or on a spoon followed by a fruit drink.
3. An interval of 4 weeks is recommended before starting succimer therapy in clients who have received EDTA with or without BAL.

Assessment

1. Document baseline pretreatment serum lead levels.
2. Identify the source of lead exposure.
3. Obtain baseline liver and renal function studies.
4. Note if client has received EDTA.

Interventions

1. Monitor I&O and ensure adequate hydration during therapy.
2. Monitor serum transaminases prior to therapy and weekly during therapy. Carefully monitor clients with a history of liver disease.
3. Carefully monitor client for rebound lead levels weekly following therapy until levels are stable.

Client/Family Teaching

1. Advise that elevated blood lead levels and symptoms of toxicity may return after discontinuing therapy due to redistribution of lead from bone stores to soft tissues and blood. Therefore, weekly blood levels should be performed.
2. Stress the importance of consuming at least 2 L of fluids/day to maintain adequate hydration.
3. Assist client in identifying source of lead exposure and appropriate resources to assist in its removal, if necessary.

Evaluation: Evaluate client for laboratory evidence of a reduction of serum lead levels.

Succinylcholine chloride

(suck-sin-ill-**KOH**-leen)

Anectine, Anectine Flo-Pack, Quelicin, Succinylcholine Chloride Min-I-Mix, Sucostrin High Potency (Rx)

See also *Neuromuscular Blocking Agents,* p. 183.

Classification: Depolarizing neuromuscular blocking agent.

Action/Kinetics: Succinylcholine initially excites skeletal muscle by combining with cholinergic receptors preferentially to acetylcholine. Subsequently, it prevents the muscle from contracting by prolonging the time during which the receptors at the neuromuscular junction cannot respond to acetylcholine. Short-acting. It has no effect on pain threshold, cerebration, or consciousness; thus, it should be used with sufficient anesthesia. Effects are not blocked by anticholinesterase drugs and may even be enhanced by them. **IV: onset,** 1 min; **duration:** 4–6 min; **recovery:** 8–10 min. **IM: Onset,** 3 min; **duration:** 10–30 min. Metabolized by plasma pseudocholinesterase to succinylmonocholine, which is a nondepolarizing muscle relaxant. About 10% succinylcholine is excreted unchanged in the urine.

Uses: Muscle relaxant during surgery, endotracheal intubation, endoscopy, and short manipulative procedures. *Investigational:* Reduce intensity of electrically induced seizures or seizures due to drugs.

Special Concerns: Safe use during pregnancy (category: C) not established. Use with caution during lactation. Pediatric clients may be especially prone to myoglobinemia, myoglobinuria, and cardiac effects. Use of IV infusion is not recommended in children due to the risk of malignant hyperpyrexia. Use with caution in clients with severe liver disease, severe anemia, malnutrition, impaired cholinesterase activity, genetic disorders of plasma pseudocholinesterase, myopathies associated with increased creatine phosphokinase, acute narrow-angle glaucoma, history of malignant hyperthermia, penetrating eye injuries, fractures. Also, in cardiovascular, pulmonary, renal, or metabolic diseases.

Side Effects: *Skeletal muscle:* May cause severe, persistent respiratory depression or apnea. Muscle fasciculations, postoperative muscle pain. *CV:* Bradycardia or tachycardia, blood pressure changes, arrhythmias, cardiac arrest. *Respiratory:* Apnea, respiratory depression. *Other:* Fever, malignant hyperthermia, salivation, hyperkalemia, postoperative muscle pain, anaphylaxis, myoglobinemia, myoglobinuria, skin rashes, increased intraocular pressure. Repeated doses may cause tachyphylaxis.

Drug Interactions

Aminoglycoside antibiotics / Additive skeletal muscle blockade

Amphotericin B / ↑ Effect of succinylcholine

Antibiotics, nonpenicillin / Additive skeletal muscle blockade

Anticholinesterases / Additive skeletal muscle blockade

Beta-adrenergic blocking agents / Additive skeletal muscle blockade

S

Chloroquine / Additive skeletal muscle blockade

Clindamycin / Additive skeletal muscle blockade

Cyclophosphamide / ↑ Effect of succinylcholine by ↓ breakdown of drug in plasma by pseudocholinesterase

Diazepam / ↓ Effect of succinylcholine

Digitalis glycosides / ↑ Chance of cardiac arrhythmias

Echothiophate iodide / ↑ Effect of succinylcholine by ↓ breakdown of drug in plasma by pseudocholinesterase

Furosemide / ↑ Action of succinylcholine

Isoflurane / Additive skeletal muscle blockade

Lidocaine / Additive skeletal muscle blockade

Lincomycin / Additive skeletal muscle blockade

Lithium / ↑ Effect of succinylcholine

Magnesium salts / Additive skeletal muscle blockade

Narcotics / ↑ Risk of bradycardia and sinus arrest

Oxytocin / ↑ Effect of succinylcholine

Phenelzine / ↑ Effect of succinylcholine

Phenothiazines / ↑ Effect of succinylcholine

Polymyxin / Additive skeletal muscle blockade

Procainamide / ↑ Effect of succinylcholine

Procaine / ↑ Effect of succinylcholine by inhibiting plasma pseudocholinesterase activity

Promazine / ↑ Effect of succinylcholine

Quinidine / Additive skeletal muscle blockade

Quinine / Additive skeletal muscle blockade

Thiotepa / ↑ Effect of succinylcholine by ↓ breakdown of drug in plasma by pseudocholinesterase

Trimethaphan / ↑ Effect of succinylcholine by inhibiting plasma pseudocholinesterase activity

Dosage: IM, IV. *Short or prolonged surgical procedures:* **Adults, IV: initially,** 0.3–1.1 mg/kg; **then,** repeated doses can be given based on client response. **Adults, IM:** 3–4 mg/kg not to exceed a total dose of 150 mg. *Prolonged surgical procedures, IV infusion (preferred),* 0.1%–0.2% solution in 5% dextrose, sodium chloride injection, or other diluent given at a rate of 0.5–10 mg/min depending on client response and degree of relaxation desired, for up to 1 hr. *Electroshock therapy:* **Adults, IV:** 10–30 mg given 1 min prior to the shock (individualize dosage). **IM:** Up to 2.5 mg/kg, not to exceed a total dose of 150 mg. *Endotracheal intubation:* **Pediatric, IV:** 1–2 mg/kg; if necessary, dose can be repeated. **IM:** Up to 2.5 mg/kg, not to exceed a total dose of 150 mg.

NURSING CONSIDERATIONS

See also *Nursing Considerations* for *Neuromuscular Blocking Agents,* p. 184.

Administration/Storage

1. An initial test dose of 0.1 mg/kg should be given to assess sensitivity and recovery time.
2. Review the drugs with which succinylcholine interacts.
3. Do not mix with anesthetic.
4. For IV infusion, use 1 or 2 mg/ml solution of drug in 5% dextrose injection, 0.9% sodium chloride, or other suitable

IV solution. Succinylcholine is not compatible with alkaline solutions.

5. Alter the degree of relaxation by altering the rate of flow.

6. To reduce salivation, premedication with atropine or scopolamine is recommended.

7. A low dose of a nondepolarizing agent may be given to reduce the severity of muscle fasciculations.

8. Store the drug in the refrigerator.

Assessment

1. Note if the client is taking digitalis products. These clients are sensitive to the release of intracellular potassium.

2. Assess clients with low plasma pseudocholinesterase levels. They are sensitive to the effects of succinylcholine and require lower doses.

3. Note any evidence of a history of malignant hyperthermia.

Interventions

1. A peripheral nerve stimulator should be used intraoperatively to assess the client's neuromuscular response.

2. Monitor the client's BP and pulse. Succinylcholine can cause vagal stimulation resulting in bradycardia, hypotension and cardiac arrhythmias.

3. Observe the client for excessive, transient increase in intraocular pressure. This can be dangerous to the eye. Document and report to the physician.

4. Muscle fasciculations may cause the client to be sore after recovery. Administer prescribed nondepolarizing agent

and reassure the client that the soreness is likely caused by the drug.

5. Monitor closely for any evidence of malignant hyperthermia, unresponsive tachycardia, jaw spasm, or lack of laryngeal relaxation. Stop infusion and report to the physician. Temperature elevations are a late sign of this condition.

6. Document the length of time the client is taking the drug. It should be used only on a short-term basis and in a continuously monitored environment.

Evaluation: Evaluate client for effective muscle relaxation as evidenced by suppression of the twitch response when tested with a peripheral nerve stimulator intraoperatively or evidence of muscle paralysis.

Sucralfate
(sue-**KRAL**-fayt)
Carafate, Sulcrate✽ (Rx)

Action/Kinetics: Sucralfate is the aluminum salt of a sulfurated disaccharide. It is thought to form an ulcer-adherent complex with albumin and fibrinogen at the site of the ulcer protecting it from further damage by gastric acid. It may also form a viscous, adhesive barrier on the surface of the gastric mucosa and duodenum. The drug adsorbs pepsin thus inhibiting its activity. May be used in conjunction with antacids. Approximately 90% excreted in the feces. **Duration:** 5 hr.

Use: Short-term treatment (up to 8 weeks) of duodenal ulcers. Maintenance for duodenal ulcer at decreased dosage after healing of

S

acute ulcers. *Investigational:* Hasten healing of gastric ulcers, chronic treatment of gastric or duodenal ulcers. Treatment of oral and esophageal ulcers due to chemotherapy, radiation, or sclerotherapy (suspension used). Treatment of aspirin- and NSAID-induced GI symptoms; prevention of stress ulcers and GI bleeding in critically ill clients.

Special Concerns: Safety for use in children and during pregnancy (category: B) and lactation has not been fully established. A successful course resulting in healing of ulcers will not alter post-healing frequency or severity of duodenal ulceration.

Side Effects: *GI:* Constipation (most common); also, nausea, diarrhea, indigestion, dry mouth, gastric discomfort. *Miscellaneous:* Back pain, dizziness, drowsiness, vertigo, rash, pruritus.

Drug Interactions

Antacids containing aluminum / ↑ Total body burden of aluminum
Cimetidine / ↓ Absorption of cimetidine due to binding to sucralfate
Ciprofloxacin / ↓ Absorption of ciprofloxacin due to binding to sucralfate
Digoxin / ↓ Absorption of digoxin due to binding to sucralfate
Norfloxacin / ↓ Absorption of norfloxacin due to binding to sucralfate
Phenytoin / ↓ Absorption of phenytoin due to binding to sucralfate
Rantidine / ↓ Absorption of rantidine due to binding to sucralfate
Tetracycline / ↓ Absorption of tetracycline due to binding to sucralfate
Theophylline / ↓ Absorption of theophylline due to binding to sucralfate

Dosage: Tablets. Adults: usual: 1 g q.i.d. 1 hr before meals and at bedtime (it may also be taken 2 hr after meals). The drug should be taken for 4–8 weeks unless x-ray films or endoscopy have indicated significant healing. **Maintenance:** 1 g b.i.d.

NURSING CONSIDERATIONS

Administration/Storage

1. If antacids are used, they should be taken 30 min before or after sucralfate.
2. Even though healing of ulcers may result, the frequency or severity of subsequent attacks is not altered.
3. Do not crush or chew tablets. If NG tube administration is necessary, consult with pharmacist for a diluent as sucralfate is fairly insoluble and may form a bezoar.

Client/Family Teaching

1. Stress the importance of taking the medication exactly as prescribed.
2. Take on an empty stomach 1 hr before or 2 hr after meals. Wait 30 min before or after dose before taking antacids.
3. Review and advise to report any bothersome side effects to the physician.
4. Drug may cause constipation. Advise client to increase fluids and bulk in the diet and to exercise as prescribed.
5. Avoid smoking as this may

assist to prevent a recurrence of duodenal ulcers.

Evaluation: Evaluate client for:
- Evidence of a reduction in signs and symptoms of duodenal ulcers as well as reports of symptomatic improvement in abdominal pain and discomfort
- Endoscopic or radiographic evidence of healing of duodenal ulcers

Sufentanil

(soo-**FEN**-tah-nil)
Sufenta (Rx)

See also *Narcotic Analgesics,* p. 174.

Classification: Narcotic analgesic.

Action/Kinetics: Onset, IV: 1.3–8 min. **Anesthetic blood concentration:** 8–30 mcg/kg. **t½:** 2.5 hr. Allows appropriate oxygenation of the heart and brain during prolonged surgical procedures. May be used in children.

Uses: Narcotic analgesic used as an adjunct to maintain balanced general anesthesia. To induce and maintain general anesthesia (with 100% oxygen), especially in neurosurgery or cardiovascular surgery.

Additional Contraindications: Use during labor.

Special Concerns: Pregnancy category: C. Dosage must be decreased in the obese, elderly, or debilitated client.

Additional Side Effects: Erythema, chills, intraoperative muscle movement. Extended postoperative respiratory depression.

Dosage: IV, individualized, adults, usual initial: 1–2 mcg/kg with oxygen and nitrous oxide; **maintenance:** 10–25 mcg as required. *For complicated surgery:* 2–8 mcg/kg with oxygen and nitrous oxide; **maintenance:** 10–50 mcg. *To induce and maintain general anesthesia:* 8–30 mcg/kg with 100% oxygen and a muscle relaxant; **maintenance:** 25–50 mcg. **Pediatric, less than 12 years:** *To induce and maintain general anesthesia:* 10–25 mcg/kg with 100% oxygen; **maintenance:** 25–50 mcg. *Induction and maintenance of general anesthesia in children less than 12 years of age undergoing cardiovascular surgery:* 10–25 mcg/kg with 100% oxygen; **maintenance:** 25–50 mcg.

NURSING CONSIDERATIONS

See also *Nursing Considerations* for *Narcotic Analgesics,* p. 177.

Administration/Storage
1. Dose should be reduced in the debilitated or elderly client.
2. The dose should be calculated based on lean body weight.

Client/Family Teaching
1. Advise to avoid activities that require mental alertness for at least 24 hr following surgery.
2. Instruct client to call for assistance with ambulation and transfers.
3. Avoid alcohol and any other CNS depressants for 24 hr following outpatient surgery.

Evaluation: Evaluate client for evidence of effective induction of anesthesia with pronounced analgesia.

Sulconazole nitrate
(sul-**KON**-ah-zohl)
Exelderm (Rx)

Classification: Antifungal, topical.

Action/Kinetics: This broad-spectrum antifungal and antiyeast agent inhibits growth of *Trichophyton mentagrophytes, Epidermophyton floccosum, Microsporum canis,* and *Malassezia fufur* as well as certain gram-positive bacteria.

Uses: Treatment of tinea cruris (jock itch), tinea corporis (ringworm), and tinea versicolor. Efficacy has not been demonstrated for tinea pedis (athlete's foot).

Contraindications: Ophthalmic use.

Special Concerns: Pregnancy category: C. Use with caution during lactation. Safety and efficacy have not been demonstrated in children.

Side Effects: *Dermatologic:* Burning, itching, stinging, redness.

Dosage: Cream, Solution: A small amount of the 1% cream or solution is gently massaged into the affected area and surrounding skin once or twice daily.

NURSING CONSIDERATIONS

Client/Family Teaching

1. Demonstrate how to apply medication and advise to use only as directed.
2. Advise that the drug is for external use only.
3. Contact with the eyes should be avoided.
4. Relief of symptoms usually occurs within a few days of initiating treatment, with clinical improvement occurring within 1 week. If symptoms do not improve after 4–6 weeks, an alternate diagnosis should be considered.
5. To reduce the chance of recurrent tinea cruris, tinea corporis, and tinea versicolor client should be treated for 3 weeks. Clients with tinea pedis should be treated for 4 weeks.

Evaluation: Evaluate client for:
- Reports of a reduction in skin irritation
- Clinical evidence and reports of symptomatic improvement

Sulfacetamide sodium
(sul-fah-**SEAT**-ah-myd)
AK-Sulf, Balsulph✤, Bleph-10, Cetamide, Isopto-Cetamide, I-Sulfacet, Ocu-Sul-10, Ocu-Sul-15, Ocu-Sul-30, Ocusulf-10, Ophthacet, Ophtho-Sulf✤, Sebizon, Sodium Sulamyd, Spectro-Sulf, Steri-Units Sulfacetamide, Sulf-10, Sulfacetamide Minims✤, Sulfair, Sulfair 10, Sulfair 15, Sulfair Forte, Sulfamide, Sulfex✤, Sulten-10 (Rx)

See also *Sulfonamides,* p. 213.

Classification: Sulfonamide, topical.

Uses: Topically for ophthalmic infections including trachoma, seborrheic dermatitis, dandruff, and cutaneous bacterial infections.

Special Concerns: Safe use during pregnancy, lactation, or in children less than 12 years of age has not been established. Use with caution in clients with dry eye syndrome.

Side Effects: *Topical:* Itching, redness, swelling, irritation. *Symptoms* *of Overdose:* If taken orally, nausea, vomiting, hematuria, crystalluria, and renal shutdown (due to precipitation of sulfa crystals) may occur.

Drug Interactions: Preparations containing silver are incompatible with sulfacetamide sodium.

Dosage: Ophthalmic Solution: 1–3 drops of 10%, 15%, or 30% solution in conjunctival sac q 2–3 hr. **Ophthalmic Ointment (10%):** Apply 1–4 times daily and at bedtime in conjunctival sac. *For cutaneous infections:* Apply **locally** (10%) to affected area b.i.d.– q.i.d. **Lotion.** *Seborrheic dermatitis:* Apply 1–2 times daily (for mild cases, apply overnight). *Cutaneous bacterial infections:* Apply b.i.d.– q.i.d. until infection clears.

NURSING CONSIDERATIONS

See also *Sulfonamides,* p. 213, and *General Nursing Considerations For All Anti-Infectives,* p. 83.

Administration/Storage: *Treatment of Overdose:* Client should ingest large amounts of fluid. Mannitol infusions may help if oliguria is present. Administration of bicarbonate may prevent crystallization in the kidney.

Assessment: Note any allergy to sulfa drugs.

Client/Family Teaching

1. When used for seborrheic dermatitis of the scalp, medication should be applied at bedtime and allowed to remain overnight. The hair and scalp may be washed the following morning, if desired. Hair should be washed at least once a week. The medication should be applied for 8–10 nights.
2. If hair and scalp are oily or if

there is debris, shampoo scalp before application.
3. Ophthalmic use may cause sensitivity to bright light; this can be minimized by wearing sunglasses.
4. Report any purulent eye drainage to the physician as this inactivates sulfacetamide.
5. If client is prescribed additional eye drops, advise to wait 5 min after sulfacetamide instillation.
6. Do not wear contact lenses until infection is resolved.

Evaluation: Evaluate client for clinical evidence and reports of improvement in symptoms of infection.

Sulfacytine
(sul-fah-**SIGH**-teen)
Renoquid (Rx)

See also *Sulfonamides,* p. 213.

Classification: Sulfonamide.

Special Concerns: Safe use during pregnancy has not been established. Not recommended for use in children less than 14 years of age. Reduced dosage may be necessary in clients with impaired renal function.

Dosage: Tablets. Adults and children over 14 years, initially: 500 mg; **maintenance:** 250 mg q.i.d. for 10 days. Not indicated for children less than 14 years of age.

NURSING CONSIDERATIONS

See also *General Nursing Considerations For All Anti-Infectives,* p. 83, and for *Sulfonamides,* p. 216.

Assessment: Obtain baseline CBC and renal function studies to determine any evidence of dysfunction as dosage may require adjustment.

Sulfadiazine
(sul-fah-**DYE**-ah-zeen)
Microsulfon (Rx)

Sulfadiazine sodium
(sul-fah-**DYE**-ah-zeen)
(Rx)

See also *Sulfonamides*, p. 213.

Classification: Sulfonamide.

Action/Kinetics: Short-acting, and often combined with other anti-infectives.

Uses: Urinary tract infections, bacillary dysentery, rheumatic fever prophylaxis.

Special Concerns: Safe use during pregnancy has not been established. Should not be used in infants less than 2 months of age unless combined with pyrimethamine to treat congenital toxoplasmosis.

Dosage: Tablets. Adults, initial: 2–4 g; **maintenance:** 4–8 g daily in 4–6 divided doses; **infants over 2 months, initial:** 75 mg/kg/day (2 g/m²); **maintenance:** 120–150 mg/kg/day (4 g/m²/day) in 4–6 divided doses, not to exceed 6 g daily. *Rheumatic fever prophylaxis,* **under 30 kg:** 0.5 g/day; **over 30 kg:** 1 g daily. *As adjunct with pyrimethamine in congenital toxoplasmosis:* **Infants less than 2 months, initial:** 75–100 mg/kg; **maintenance:** 100–150 mg/kg daily in 4 divided doses.

NURSING CONSIDERATIONS

See *General Nursing Considerations For All Anti-Infectives,* p. 83, and for *Sulfonamides,* p. 216.

Evaluation: Evaluate client for:
- Laboratory confirmation of negative culture reports
- Evidence of effective rheumatic fever prophylaxis during invasive procedures

—— *COMBINATION DRUG* ——
Sulfadoxine and Pyrimethamine
(sul-fah-**DOX**-een,
pie-rih-**METH**-ah-meen)
Fansidar (Rx)

See also *Sulfonamides,* p. 213.

Classification: Antimalarial.

Action/Kinetics: Sulfadoxine competes with para-aminobenzoic acid for biosynthesis of folic acid, whereas pyrimethamine inhibits the formation of tetrahydrofolate from dihydrofolate. These reactions are necessary for one-carbon transfer reactions in the synthesis of nucleic acids. Well absorbed following oral use and is widely distributed throughout the body. Each tablet contains sulfadoxine, 500 mg, and pyrimethamine, 25 mg. **Peak plasma levels:** sulfadoxine, 2.5–6 hr; pyrimethamine, 1.5–8 hr. Both drugs are long-acting with a $t^{1/2}$ of 170 hr for sulfadoxine and 110 hr for pyrimethamine. Both drugs are excreted through the urine with about 20%–30% of pyrimethamine excreted unchanged.

Uses: Prophylaxis and treatment of falciparum malaria, especially chloroquine-resistant strains. *Investigational:* Prophylaxis of *Pneumocystis carinii* pneumonia in AIDS clients (second-line agents).

Contraindications: Megaloblastic anemia. Infants less than 2 months old. Pregnancy (near term) and lactation. Significant liver parenchymal disease, renal insufficiency, in presence of blood dyscrasias.

Special Concerns: Pregnancy category: C. Use with caution in severe allergy, folate deficiency, bronchial asthma, and in clients with glucose-6-phosphate dehydrogenase deficiency. Fatalities have resulted due to Stevens-Johnson syndrome and toxic epidermal necrolysis.

Side Effects: See *Sulfonamides,* p. 213. Stevens-Johnson syndrome, toxic epidermal necrolysis.

Drug Interactions: Sulfonamides, including trimethoprim/sulfamethoxazole, will ↑ risk of folic acid deficiency if used with sulfadoxine, pyrimethamine, and methotrexate.

Dosage: Tablets: *Acute malaria (in combination with quinine):* **Adults,** 2–3 tablets as a single dose. **Pediatric, 9–14 years of age:** 2 tablets as a single dose; **4–8 years of age:** one tablet as a single dose; **under 4 years of age:** ½ tablet as a single dose. *Prophylaxis:* **Adults,** 1 tablet weekly or 2 tablets biweekly; **Pediatric, 9–14 years of age:** weekly, ¾ tablet; biweekly, 1½ tablets. **4–8 years of age:** weekly, ½ tablet; biweekly, 1 tablet. **Under 4 years of age:** weekly, ¼ tablet; biweekly, ½ tablet.

NURSING CONSIDERATIONS

See also *Nursing Considerations For All Anti-Infectives,* p. 83.

Administration

1. High intake of fluid should occur to prevent precipitation in the urine.
2. For prophylaxis, therapy should be initiated 1–2 days before the person enters the endemic area; therapy should continue during stay and for 4–6 weeks after leaving. Primaquine should be given.
3. If folic acid deficiency occurs, leucovorin can be given in a dose of 5–15 mg/day IM for 3 or more days.

Assessment

1. Assess labs for evidence of liver or renal dysfunction.
2. Determine any history or evidence of G-6-PDD.

Client/Family Teaching

1. Contact the physician immediately if fever, sore throat, purpura, jaundice, pallor, or glossitis is observed.
2. The drug should be discontinued immediately if erythema, rash, pruritus, orogenital lesions, or pharyngitis is noted.
3. Report as scheduled because blood counts and urinalyses should be performed periodically if chronic therapy is required.
4. Contraceptive measures should be used to prevent pregnancy while on this medication.
5. Breast-feeding should not be undertaken while on this medication.
6. Adequate fluids should be taken to prevent crystalluria and stone formation.

Evaluation: Evaluate for prevention of acute malarial attacks and a reduction in the severity of malarial symptoms.

Sulfamethizole
(sul-fah-**METH**-ih-zohl)
Thiosulfil Forte (Rx)

See also *Sulfonamides,* p. 213.

Classification: Sulfonamide, short-acting.

Use: Urinary tract infections.

Special Concerns: Safe use during pregnancy has not been established.

Additional Drug Interactions: Sulfamethizole ↑ effects of tolbutamide, phenytoin, and chlorpropamide due to ↓ breakdown by liver.

Dosage: Tablets. Adults, 0.5–1 g t.i.d.–q.i.d.; **infants over 2 months:** 30–45 mg/kg/day in 4 divided doses.

NURSING CONSIDERATIONS

See *General Nursing Considerations For All Anti-Infectives,* p. 83, and for *Sulfonamides,* p. 216.

Evaluation: Evaluate client for laboratory confirmation of negative urine culture results.

Sulfamethoxazole
(sul-fah-meth-**OX**-ah-zohl)
**Apo-Sulfamethoxazole✳,
Gantanol, Urobak (Rx)**

See also *Sulfonamides,* p. 213.

Classification: Sulfonamide, intermediate-acting.

Action/Kinetics: t½: 8.6 hr. Sulfamethoxazole is also a component of Bactrim, Bactrim DS, Septra, and Septra DS.

Uses: Urinary and upper respiratory tract infections; lymphogranuloma venereum.

Special Concerns: Pregnancy category: C (safe use during pregnancy has not been established). May be an increased risk of severe side effects in elderly clients.

Dosage: Oral Suspension, Tablets. Adults, initially: 2 g for mild to moderate infections; **then,** 1 g in morning and evening (for severe infections, give 2 g initially; then, 1 g t.i.d.). **Infants over 2 months, initial:** 50–60 mg/kg; **then,** 25–30 mg/kg in morning and evening, not to exceed 75 mg/kg/day. *Lymphogranuloma venereum:* 1 g b.i.d. for 2 weeks.

NURSING CONSIDERATIONS

See also *General Nursing Considerations For All Anti-Infectives,* p. 83, and for *Sulfonamides,* p. 216.

Client/Family Teaching

1. Drug may cause dizziness; assess response prior to any activity requiring mental alertness.
2. Advise the use of sunglasses, sunscreens, and protective clothing as a photosensitivity reaction may occur.

Evaluation: Evaluate client for clinical evidence and reports of symptomatic improvement.

—— *COMBINATION DRUG* ——
Sulfamethoxazole and Phenazopyridine
(sul-fah-meth-**OX**-ah-zohl,
fen-ay-zoh-**PEER**-ih-deen)
**Azo Gantanol, Azo
Sulfamethoxazole, Uro
Gantanol✳ (Rx)**

Classification/Content: *Sulfonamide:* sulfamethoxazole, 500 mg and *urinary analgesic:* phenazopyridine, 100 mg. See also *Sulfamethoxazole,* p. 1173, and *Phenazopyridine,* p. 1026.

Uses: Acute, painful phase of uncomplicated urinary tract infections due to susceptible strains of *Escherichia coli, Enterobacter, Klebsiella, Proteus mirabilis, Proteus vulgaris,* and *Staphylococcus aureus.*

Contraindications: Pregnancy at term, during lactation. Use in children less than 12 years of age. Glomerulonephritis, severe hepatitis, uremia, and pyelonephritis of pregnancy with GI disturbances.

Special Concerns: Pregnancy category: C. Use with caution in impaired hepatic or renal function, in severe allergy or bronchial asthma.

Dosage: Tablets. Adults and children over 12 years of age, initially: 2 g sulfamethoxazole and 400 mg phenazopyridine (4 tablets); **then,** 1 g sulfamethoxazole and 200 mg phenazopyridine (2 tablets) q 12 hr for 2 days.

NURSING CONSIDERATIONS

See also *General Nursing Considerations For All Anti-Infectives,* p. 83, and for *Sulfamethoxazole,* p. 1174.

Administration/Storage

1. Dose should be decreased in clients with impaired renal function.
2. Treatment should not exceed 2 days.

Client/Family Teaching

1. Fluid intake must be adequate for urine output to be at least 1,200–1,500 ml daily to prevent crystalluria and stone formation. Maintain record of I&O.
2. If GI upset occurs, the drug may be taken with or after meals.

Evaluation: Evaluate client for reports of a reduction in GU pain and discomfort.

Sulfasalazine
(sul-fah-**SAL**-ah-zeen)
Azulfidine, Azulfidine EN-Tabs, PMS Sulfasalazine✱, PMS Sulfasalazine E.C.✱, Salazopyrin✱, Salazopyrin-EN Tabs✱, S.A.S.✱, SAS-Enema✱, S.A.S. Enteric-500✱, SAS-500✱ (Rx)

See also *Sulfonamides,* p. 213.

Action/Kinetics: About one-third of the dose of sulfasalazine is absorbed from the small intestine while two-thirds passes to the colon, where it is split to 5-aminosalicylic acid and sulfapyradine. The drug does not affect the microflora.

Use: Ulcerative colitis.

Additional Contraindications: Children below 2 years, persons with marked sulfonamide and salicylate hypersensitivity.

Special Concerns: Pregnancy category: B.

Side Effects: Anorexia, vomiting, nausea.

Additional Drug Interactions

Digoxin / Sulfasalazine ↓ effect due to ↓ absorption from GI tract

Ferrous sulfate / Ferrous sulfate ↓ blood levels of sulfasalazine

Dosage: Oral Suspension, Enteric-coated Tablets, Tablets. Adults: initial, 3–4 g daily in divided doses (1–2 g daily may decrease side effects); **maintenance:** 500 mg q.i.d. **Pediatric, initial:** 40–60 mg/kg daily in 4–6 equally divided doses; **maintenance:** 20–30 mg/kg daily in 4 divided doses. *For desensitization* *to sulfasalazine:* Reinstitute at level of 50–250 mg daily; **then,** give double dose q 4–7 days until desired therapeutic level reached. Use oral suspension.

NURSING CONSIDERATIONS

See also *General Nursing Considerations For All Anti-Infectives,* p. 83, and for *Sulfonamides,* p. 216.

Assessment

1. Obtain baseline CBC and urinalysis.
2. Document frequency, quantity, and consistency of stool production as well as characteristics of abdominal pain.

Client/Family Teaching

1. Stress the importance of taking medication exactly as ordered because intermittent therapy (2 weeks on, 2 weeks off) is generally recom mended.
2. Take with food to reduce GI upset.
3. Drug may discolor urine or skin a yellow-orange color.
4. Take at least 2 qt/day of water to decrease incidence of crystalluria and stone formation.
5. Avoid prolonged exposure to sunlight because drug may increase sensitivity.

Evaluation: Evaluate client for reports of a decrease in the frequency of loose stools and a reduction in associated abdominal pain.

Sulfinpyrazone
(sul-fin-**PEER**-ah-zohn)
Anturane, Apo-Sulfinpyrazone ✤, Novo–Pyrazone ✤, (Rx)

Classification: Antigout agent, uricosuric.

Action/Kinetics: Sulfinpyrazone inhibits the tubular reabsorption of uric acid, thereby increasing its excretion. Sulfinpyrazone also manifests antithrombotic and platelet inhibitory actions. **Peak plasma levels:** 1–2 hr. **Therapeutic plasma levels:** Up to 160 mcg/ml following 800 mg daily for uricosuria. **Duration:** 4–6 hr (up to 10 hr in some). **t½:** 3–8 hr. Sulfinpyrazone is metabolized by the liver. Approximately 45% of the drug is excreted unchanged by the kidney, and a small amount is excreted in the feces.

Uses: Chronic gouty arthritis to reduce frequency and intensity of acute attacks of gout; hyperuricemia. Sulfinpyrazone is not effective during acute attacks of gout and may even increase the frequency of acute episodes during the initiation of therapy. However, the drug should not be discontinued during acute attacks. Concomitant administration of colchicine during initiation of therapy is recommended. *Investigational:* To decrease sudden death during first year after myocardial infarction.

Contraindications: Active peptic ulcer. Blood dyscrasias. Sensitivity to phenylbutazone or other pyrazoles.

Special Concerns: Use with caution in pregnant women. Dosage has not been established in children. Use with extreme caution in clients with impaired renal function and in those with a history of peptic ulcers.

Side Effects: *GI:* Nausea, vomiting, abdominal discomfort. May reactivate peptic ulcer. *Hematologic:* Leukopenia, agranulocytosis, anemia, thrombocytopenia, aplastic anemia. *Miscellaneous:* Skin rash (which usually disappears with usage), bronchoconstriction in aspirin-induced asthma. Acute attacks of gout may become more frequent during initial therapy. Give concomitantly with colchicine at this time. *Symptoms of Overdose:* Nausea, vomiting, diarrhea, epigastric pain, labored respiration, ataxia, seizures, coma.

Drug Interactions

Acetaminophen / ↑ Risk of acetaminophen hepatotoxicity; ↓ effect of acetaminophen

Anticoagulants / ↑ Effect of anticoagulants due to ↓ plasma protein binding

Insulin / Potentiation of hypoglycemic effect

Niacin / ↓ Uricosuric effect of sulfinpyrazone

Probenecid / ↑ Effect of sulfinpyrazone due to ↓ excretion by kidney

Salicylates / Inhibit uricosuric effect of sulfinpyrazone

Sulfonamides / ↑ Effect of sulfonamides by ↓ plasma protein binding

Sulfonylureas, oral / Potentiation of hypoglycemic effect

Theophylline / ↓ Effect of theophylline due to ↑ plasma clearance

Verapamil / ↓ Effect of verapamil due to ↑ plasma clearance

Dosage: Capsules, Tablets. Adults: initial, 200–400 mg/day in 2 divided doses with meals or milk. Clients who are transferred from other uricosuric agents can receive full dose at once. **Maintenance:** 100–400 mg b.i.d. Maintain full dosage without interruption even during acute attacks of gout. *Following myocardial infarction:* 300 mg q.i.d. or 400 mg b.i.d.

NURSING CONSIDERATIONS

Administration/Storage

1. At least 10–12 eight-ounce glasses of fluid should be taken daily.
2. If GI upset occurs, medication should be taken with food, milk, or antacids.
3. Acidification of the urine may cause formation of uric acid stones.
4. *Treatment of Overdose:* Supportive measures.

Client/Family Teaching

1. Take a liberal amount of fluid (2–3 L/day) to prevent the formation of uric acid stones.
2. Explain that sodium bicarbonate may be ordered to alkalinize the urine. This is to prevent urates from crystallizing in acid urine and forming kidney stones.
3. Take the drug with meals, milk, or an antacid to minimize gastric irritation.
4. Avoid alcohol and aspirin because they interfere with drug effectiveness.
5. Advise that during *acute* attacks of gout that concomitant administration of colchicine is indicated.

Evaluation: Evaluate client for:
- Reports of a decrease in the frequency and intensity of gout attacks
- Laboratory evidence of ↓ uric acid levels

Sulfisoxazole
(sul-fih-**SOX**-ah-zohl)
Gantrisin, Novo–Soxazole ✽ (Rx)

Sulfisoxazole acetyl
(sul-fih-**SOX**-ah-zohl)
Gantrisin, Lipo Gantrisin (Rx)

Sulfisoxazole diolamine
(sul-fih-**SOX**-ah-zohl)
Gantrisin Diolamine (Rx)

See also *Sulfonamides*, p. 213.

Classification: Sulfonamide, short-acting.

Action/Kinetics: $t^{1/2}$: 5.9 hr. Lipo Gantrisin contains sulfisoxazole acetyl in a homogenized vegetable oil mixture.

Uses: Urinary tract infections, topical and ophthalmic infections (including trachoma).

Special Concerns: Pregnancy category: C.

Additional Drug Interaction: Sulfisoxazole may ↑ effects of thiopental due to ↓ plasma protein binding.

Dosage: Oral Suspension, Extended-release Tablets, Syrup. Adults, initial: 2–4 g; **maintenance:** 1 g b.i.d.–t.i.d. depending on severity of the infection. **Infants over 2 months, initial:** 50–60 mg/kg/day; **maintenance:** 25–30 mg/kg in the morning and evening, not to exceed 75 mg/kg/day. Alternative dose: 50–60 mg/kg/day divided q 12 hr, not to exceed 3 g daily. **IM, IV (slow injection or drip), SC: Initially,** 50 mg/kg; **then,** 100 mg/kg in 2–4 divided doses. **Ophthalmic.** *Solution:* 1–2 gtt in conjunctival sac q 2–3 hr. *Ointment:* Small amount in con-

junctival sac 1–3 times during the day and at bedtime. *Diolamine.* **Ophthalmic solution (4%):** 1–2 gtt into conjunctival sac several times daily. **Ophthalmic ointment (4%):** Small amount in conjunctival sac 1–3 times daily and at bedtime.

NURSING CONSIDERATIONS

See also *General Nursing Considerations For All Anti-Infectives,* p. 83, and for *Sulfonamides,* p. 216.

Administration/Storage: For SC administration, dilute commercial solution containing 400 mg/ml with sterile water for injection, to obtain solution containing 50 mg/ml.

Evaluation: Evaluate client for:
- Laboratory evidence of negative culture reports
- Reports of symptomatic improvement

—— COMBINATION DRUG ——
Sulfisoxazole and Phenazopyridine
(sul-fih-**SOX**-ah-zohl,
fen-**ay**-zoh-**PEER**-ih-deen)
Azo-Cheragan, Azo Gantrisin, Axo-Sulfisoxazole, Azo-Truxazole, Sul-Azo (Rx)

Classification/Content: Each of the products contains sulfisoxazole (antibacterial), 500 mg and phenazopyridine (urinary analgesic), 50 mg. Also, see information on individual components.

Uses: For the first two days in treating uncomplicated urinary tract infections due to *Escherichia coli, Enterobacter, Klebsiella, Proteus mirabilis, Proteus vulgaris,* and *Staphylococcus aureus..* Sulfisoxazole can be used alone after the first two days.

Contraindications: Pregnancy at term, during lactation, and in children less than 12 years of age. Glomerulonephritis, severe hepatitis, uremia, and pyelonephritis of pregnancy with GI disturbances.

Special Concerns: Pregnancy category: C. Use with caution in impaired hepatic or renal function, in severe allergy or bronchial asthma.

Dosage: Tablets. Adults, initial: 4–6 tablets; **then,** 2 tablets q.i.d. for 2 days.

NURSING CONSIDERATIONS

See *General Nursing Considerations For All Anti-Infectives,* p. 83, and for *Sulfonamides,* p. 216.

Sulindac

(sul-**IN**-dak)

Apo-Sulin✸, Clinoril, Novo–Sundac✸ (Rx)

See also *Nonsteroidal Anti-Inflammatory Drugs,* p. 186.

Classification: Antirheumatic, analgesic.

Action/Kinetics: Sulindac is biotransformed in the liver to a sulfide, the active metabolite. **Peak plasma levels of sulfide:** after fasting, 2 hr; after food, 3–4 hr. **Onset, anti-inflammatory effect:** within 1 week; **duration, anti-inflammatory effect:** 1–2 wk. $t\frac{1}{2}$, of sulindac: 7.8 hr; of metabolite: 16.4 hr. Excreted in both urine and feces.

Uses: Acute and chronic treatment of rheumatoid arthritis, osteoarthritis, ankylosing spondylitis, acute gouty arthritis; acute, painful shoulder; tendinitis, bursitis. *Investigational:* Juvenile rheumatoid arthritis, sunburn.

Contraindications: Use with active GI lesions or a history of recurrent GI lesions.

Special Concerns: Safety and efficacy have not been established for children. Safe use during pregnancy has not been established. Use with caution during lactation.

Additional Side Effects: Hypersensitivity, pancreatitis, GI pain (common), maculopapular rash. Stupor, coma, hypotension, and diminished urine output.

Additional Drug Interactions: Sulindac ↑ effect of warfarin due to ↓ plasma protein binding.

Dosage: Tablets. Adults: *Osteoarthritis, rheumatoid arthritis, ankylosing spondylitis:* 150 mg b.i.d. *Acute painful shoulder, acute gouty arthritis:* 200 mg b.i.d. for 7–14 days. *Antigout:* 200 mg b.i.d. for 7 days.

NURSING CONSIDERATIONS

See also *Nursing Considerations* for *Nonsteroidal Anti-Inflammatory Drugs,* p. 189.

Administration/Storage

1. When used for arthritis, a favorable response usually occurs within one week.
2. For acute conditions, reduce dosage when satisfactory response is attained.
3. Should be given with food to decrease GI upset.

Assessment

1. If intake and output or laboratory studies indicate renal dysfunction, anticipate a reduction in dosage of drug.
2. Document baseline range of motion and a description of pain.

Client/Family Teaching

1. Do not take aspirin while taking sulindac. Plasma levels of sulindac will be reduced.
2. Report any incidence of unexplained bleeding such as oozing of blood from the gums, nosebleeds, or excessive bruising.
3. Drug may cause dizziness; assess response prior to any activity requiring mental alertness.

Evaluation: Evaluate client for evidence of improved joint mobility with reports of a reduction in joint pain.

Suprofen
(sue-**PROH**-fen)
Profenal (Rx)

See also *Nonsteroidal Anti-Inflammatory Drugs,* p. 186.

Classification: Nonsteroidal antiinflammatory drug, ophthalmic use.

Action/Kinetics: By inhibiting prostaglandin synthesis, suprofen reverses prostaglandin-induced vasodilation, leukocytosis, increased vascular permeability, and increased intraocular pressure. The drug also inhibits miosis, which occurs during cataract surgery.

Uses: Inhibition of intraoperative miosis.

Contraindications: Dendritic keratitis.

Special Concerns: Pregnancy category: C. Use with caution in clients sensitive to aspirin and other NSAIDs. Use with caution in surgical clients with a history of bleeding tendencies or who are on drugs that prolong bleeding time. Use with caution during lactation. Safety and efficacy have not been established in children.

Side Effects: *Ophthalmic:* Ocular irritation, transient burning, and stinging upon installation. Redness, itching, discomfort, pain, iritis, allergy, chemosis, photophobia, punctate epithelial staining.

Drug Interactions: Acetylcholine and carbachol may be ineffective if used in combination with suprofen.

Dosage: Ophthalmic. *Day before surgery:* 2 gtt into the conjunctival sac q 4 hr during waking hours. *Day of surgery:* 2 gtt into the conjunctival sac 3, 2, and 1 hr prior to surgery.

NURSING CONSIDERATIONS

See also *Nursing Considerations for Nonsteroidal Anti-Inflammatory Drugs,* p. 189.

Administration: For best results, follow administration guidelines carefully.

Evaluation: Evaluate client during surgery for evidence of successful miosis inhibition.

--- COMBINATION DRUG ---

Synalgos-DC
(sigh-**NAL**-gohs)
(C-III, Rx)

See also *Aspirin,* p. 260, *Narcotic Analgesics,* p. 174, and *Caffeine,* p. 377.

Classification/Content: *Nonnarcotic analgesic:* Aspirin, 356.4 mg. *Narcotic analgesic:* Dihydrocodeine bitartrate, 16 mg. *CNS stimulant:* Caffeine, 30 mg. See also information on individual components.

Uses: Relief of moderate to moderately severe pain.

Contraindications: Use in children less than 12 years of age.

Special Concerns: Safe use during pregnancy has not been established. Use with caution in presence of peptic ulcer or coagulation abnormalities and in geriatric and debilitated clients.

Dosage: Capsules. Individual- ized. **Adults, usual:** Two capsules q 4 hr as required for pain.

NURSING CONSIDERATIONS

See also *Nursing Considerations* for *Narcotic Analgesics,* p. 177, *Aspirin,* p. 264, and *Caffeine,* p. 378.

Administration/Storage: The dosage can be adjusted depending on the response of the client.

Evaluation: Evaluate client for reports of effective control of pain.

T

——— *COMBINATION DRUG* ———
Talwin Nx
(**TAL**-win)
(C-IV, Rx)

See also *Narcotic Analgesics,* p. 174, *Narcotic Antagonists,* p. 181, and *Pentazocine,* p. 1015.

Classification/Content: *Narcotic analgesic:* Pentazocine HCl, 50 mg (as the base). *Narcotic antagonist:* Naloxone HCl, 0.5 mg (as the base).

Action/Kinetics: When used orally, Talwin Nx is an effective analgesic. However, if the drug product is administered by injection (e.g., in an abuse situation), the presence of naloxone will prevent the effect of pentazocine.

Uses: Relief of moderate to severe pain.

Additional Contraindications: Children under 12 years of age. Parenteral use.

Special Concerns: Pregnancy category: C. Use with caution during lactation. This product is intended only for oral use. Potentially lethal effects may result by injecting this product.

Dosage: Tablets. Adults, initial: One tablet q 3–4 hr; **then,** dose may be increased to 2 tablets as needed, not to exceed 12 tablets daily.

NURSING CONSIDERATIONS

See also *Nursing Considerations* for *Narcotic Analgesics,* p. 177, *Narcotic Antagonists,* p. 181, and *Pentazocine,* p. 1015.

Administration/Storage

1. This product is intended only for oral use. Parenteral use may lead to severe (and possibly lethal) effects.
2. Aspirin may be given concomitantly with Talwin Nx if anti-inflammatory or antipyretic effects are necessary.
3. A severe reaction may occur if

this form is injected. A small amount of naloxone to eliminate abuse (with tripelennamine) is present.

Evaluation: Evaluate client for reports of effective pain relief.

Tamoxifen

(tah-**MOX**-ih-fen)
Alpha-Tamoxifen✳, Apo-Tamox✳, Nolvadex, Nolvadex-D✳, Novo–Tamoxifen✳, Tamofen✳, Tamone✳ (Rx)

See also *Antineoplastic Agents*, p. 85.

Classification: Antiestrogen.

Action/Kinetics: Antiestrogen is believed to occupy estrogen-binding sites in target tissue (breast). It also blocks uptake of estradiol. **Peak serum levels:** 0.06–0.14 mcg/ml attained after 7–14 hr. **t½, biphasic:** initial, 7–14 hr; distribution, 4 or more days. Metabolized to the equally active desmethyltamoxifen. Tamoxifen and metabolites are excreted mainly through the feces. Objective response may be delayed 4–10 weeks with bone metastases.

Uses: Palliative treatment of breast cancer in postmenopausal women, especially those with recent positive estrogen receptor tests. In premenopausal women with metastatic breast cancer, the drug is an alternative to oophorectomy or ovarian irradiation. *Investigational:* Mastalgia, gynecomastia (to treat pain and size).

Contraindications: Lactation.

Special Concerns: Pregnancy category: D. Use with caution in clients with leukopenia or thrombocytopenia.

Side Effects: *GI:* Nausea, vomiting, distaste for food, anorexia. *CV:* Peripheral edema, pulmonary embolism, thromboembolic disorders (especially when tamoxifen is combined with other cytotoxic agents). *CNS:* Depression, dizziness, lightheadedness, headache. *GU:* Hot flashes, vaginal bleeding and discharge, menstrual irregularities, pruritus vulvae. *Other:* Skin rash, hypercalcemia, increased bone and tumor pain, mild to moderate thrombocytopenia and leukopenia, ophthalmologic effects.

Laboratory Test Interference: ↑ Serum calcium (transient).

Dosage: Tablets: 10–20 mg b.i.d. (morning and evening). **Enteric-coated Tablets:** 10–20 mg once daily.

NURSING CONSIDERATIONS

See also *Nursing Considerations* for *Antineoplastic Agents*, p. 88.

Assessment

1. The effect of the steroid and osteolytic metastases may result in hypercalcemia. Assess routinely for symptoms of hypercalcemia: insomnia, lethargy, anorexia, nausea, vomiting, coma, and vascular collapse.
2. Obtain baseline CBC with differential and monitor periodically throughout therapy.

Interventions

1. Be certain that client with increased pain has adequate orders for analgesics; provide analgesics as needed.
2. Monitor for and report high serum calcium levels.
3. Encourage high fluid intake to minimize hypercalcemia.
4. Closely monitor clients who

resume therapy after drug-induced hypercalcemia is corrected.

Client/Family Teaching

1. Provide a printed list of side effects that should be reported to the physician; a reduction in dosage may be indicated.
2. Explain to client experiencing increased bone and lumbar pain or local disease flares that these symptoms may be associated with a good (tumor) response to medication. Advise to take prescribed analgesics as needed.
3. Have regular ophthalmologic examinations if doses of drug are much higher than those usually recommended for antihormonal antineoplastic agents.
4. Practice safe, non-hormonal methods of contraception during drug therapy and for one month following therapy.
5. Perform weights weekly and assess for edema. Report excessive weight gain or evidence of peripheral edema.
6. Advise that drug may cause "hot flashes."
7. Wear protective clothing, sunscreens, and sunglasses to prevent photosensitivity reactions.

Evaluation: Evaluate client for evidence of a decrease in breast tumor size and spread.

——— *COMBINATION DRUG* ———
Tavist-D
(TAV-ist)
(Rx)

Classification/Content: *Antihistamine:* Clemastine fumarate, 1.34 mg. *Decongestant:* Phenylpropanolamine HCl, 75 mg.

The clemastine is formulated in the outer shell of the tablet and is released immediately. The phenylpropanolamine component is incorporated into a sustained-release matrix, which releases the drug over a period of 12 hr; the slow release achieves blood levels equivalent to those achieved by giving 25 mg phenylpropanolamine q 4 hr for 3 doses.

See also information on individual components.

Uses: To treat symptoms of allergic rhinitis (i.e., hay fever) including nasal congestion; sneezing; itchy eyes, nose, or throat; runny nose or eyes.

Contraindications: Use in children less than 12 years of age and during lactation. To treat lower respiratory tract symptoms, including asthma. In clients taking MAO inhibitors or those with severe coronary artery disease or hypertension.

Special Concerns: Pregnancy category: B.

Dosage: Tablets. Adults and children over 12 years: One tablet (taken whole) q 12 hr.

NURSING CONSIDERATIONS

See also *Nursing Considerations* for *Antihistamines,* p. 74, and *Sympathomimetics,* p. 220.

Client/Family Teaching: Instruct the client not to break tablets or crush them, but to take tablets whole. This permits the specially designed release system to remain intact.

Evaluation: Evaluate client for evidence of ↓ nasal congestion and reports of improvement in symptoms of allergic responses.

—— COMBINATION DRUG ——
Tedral Elixir, Suspension, or Tablets
(TED-ral)
(OTC)

Tedral SA Tablets
(TED-ral)
(Rx)

Classification/Content: *Sympathomimetic bronchodilator:* Theophylline anhydrous, 29.5 mg/5 ml (Elixir), 59.1 mg/5 ml (Suspension), 118 mg (Tablets) or 180 mg (SA Tablets). *Sympathomimetic bronchodilator:* Ephedrine HCl, 6 mg/5 ml (Elixir), 12 mg/5 ml (Suspension), 24 mg (Tablets) or 48 mg (SA Tablets). *Sedative:* Phenobarbital, 2 mg/5 ml (Elixir), 4 mg/5 ml (Suspension), 8 mg (Tablets) or 25 mg (SA Tablets). Each tablet contains a portion of the drug in the immediate-release layer and a portion in the sustained-release layer.

See also information on individual components.

Uses: Adjunct in the treatment of bronchial asthma, asthmatic bronchitis, or other bronchial disorders. Prophylactically to prevent or minimize incidence of asthmatic attacks. Treatment of occasional, seasonal, or perennial asthma.

Contraindications: Porphyria. Use of SA tablets in children less than 12 years of age.

Special Concerns: Use with caution in cardiovascular disease, severe hypertension, prostatic hypertrophy, glaucoma, or hyperthyroidism.

Dosage: Elixir. Adults, 15–30 ml q 4 hr; **pediatric:** 5 ml/13.6 kg. body weight q 4–6 hr. **Suspension. Adults,** 10–20 ml q 4 hr;

pediatric: 5 ml/13.6 kg body weight q 4–6 hr. **Tablets. Adults:** 1–2 tablets q 4 hr; **pediatric (6–12 years:)** ½–1 tablet q 4 hr. **SA Tablets. Adults,** One tablet on arising and one 12 hr later.

NURSING CONSIDERATIONS

See also *Nursing Considerations* for *Sympathomimetic Drugs,* p. 220, *Theophylline,* p. 229, and *Barbiturates,* p. 104.

Administration/Storage

1. The Elixir and Suspension should be administered to children under 2 years of age with extreme caution.
2. Tablets should not be chewed.
3. If the medication is in suspension form, the container should be shaken well before administering.

Assessment: If the client is receiving the drug to treat asthma, note the extent and severity of asthma attacks. Also, document the compounds that have been used with positive clinical results prior to this drug therapy.

Evaluation: Evaluate client for:
- Evidence of improved airway exchange
- Reports of a decrease in frequency and intensity of asthmatic attacks

Temazepam
(teh-MAZ-eh-pam)
Restoril (C-IV, Rx)

See also *Benzodiazepines,* p. 108.

Classification: Benzodiazepine hypnotic.

Action/Kinetics: Temazepam is a

benzodiazepine derivative. Disturbed nocturnal sleep may occur the first one or two nights following discontinuance of the drug. Prolonged administration is not recommended because physical dependence and tolerance may develop. See also *Flurazepam,* p. 659. **Peak blood levels:** 2–4 hr. **t½, initial:** 0.4–0.6 hr; **final:** 10 hr. **Steady-state plasma levels:** 382 ng/ml (2.5 hr after 30-mg dose). Accumulation of the drug is minimal following multiple dosage. Significantly bound (98%) to plasma protein. The drug is metabolized in the liver to inactive metabolites.

Uses: Insomnia in clients unable to fall asleep, with frequent awakenings during the night and/or early morning awakenings.

Contraindications: Pregnancy (category: X).

Special Concerns: Use with caution in severely depressed clients. Use during lactation may cause sedation and feeding problems in the infant. Geriatric clients may be more sensitive to the effects of temazepam.

Side Effects: *CNS:* Drowsiness (after daytime use) and dizziness are common. Lethargy, confusion, euphoria, weakness, ataxia, lack of concentration, hallucinations. In some clients, paradoxical excitement (less than 0.5%), including stimulation and hyperactivity, occurs. *GI:* Anorexia, diarrhea. *Other:* Tremors, horizontal nystagmus, falling, palpitations. Rarely, blood dyscrasias.

Dosage: Capsules. Adults: usual, 15–30 mg at bedtime. **In elderly or debilitated clients: initial,** 15 mg; **then,** adjust dosage to response.

NURSING CONSIDERATIONS

See also *Nursing Considerations* for *Benzodiazepines,* p. 111.

Assessment: Assess client sleep patterns, attempting to identify factors that may cause insomnia and frequent awakenings.

Client/Family Teaching

1. Advise client to avoid alcohol and CNS depressants because they tend to increase feelings of depression.
2. Avoid cigarette smoking because this decreases drug's effect.
3. May cause daytime drowsiness so avoid activities that require mental alertness until drug effects are realized.
4. Advise not to increase dose as improvement may not be evident for several days.

Evaluation: Evaluate client for reports of improved sleeping patterns with less frequent awakenings.

Terazosin
(ter-**AY**-zoh-sin)
Hytrin (Rx)

Classification: Antihypertensive, alpha-1 adrenergic receptor blocking agent.

Action/Kinetics: Terazosin blocks postsynaptic alpha-1 adrenergic receptors, leading to a dilation of both arterioles and veins, and ultimately, a reduction in blood pressure. Both standing and supine blood pressure are lowered with no reflex tachycardia. Bioavailability is not affected by food. **Onset:** 15 min. **Peak plasma levels:** 1–2 hr. **t½:** 9–12 hr. **Duration:** 24 hr. Terazosin is excreted as unchanged drug and inactive metabolites in both the urine and feces.

Uses: Alone or in combination with diuretics or beta-adrenergic blocking agents to treat hypertension.

Special Concerns: Pregnancy category: C. Use with caution during lactation. Safety and efficacy have not been determined in children. Geriatric clients may be more sensitive to the hypotensive and hypothermic effects of terazosin.

Side Effects: *First-dose effect:* Marked postural hypotension and syncope. *CV:* Palpitations, tachycardia, postural hypotension, syncope, arrhythmias, vasodilation. *CNS:* Dizziness, headache, somnolence, nervousness, paresthesia, depression, anxiety, insomnia. *Respiratory:* Nasal congestion, dyspnea, sinusitis, epistaxis, bronchitis, cough, pharyngitis, rhinitis. *GI:* Nausea, constipation, diarrhea, dyspepsia, dry mouth, vomiting, flatulence. *Musculoskeletal:* Asthenia, arthritis, arthralgia, myalgia, joint disorders, back pain, pain in extremities, neck and shoulder pain. *Miscellaneous:* Peripheral edema, weight gain, blurred vision, impotence, chest pain, fever, gout, pruritus, rash, sweating, urinary frequency, tinnitus, conjunctivitis, abnormal vision. *Symptoms of Overdose:* Hypotension, drowsiness, shock.

Laboratory Test Interferences: ↓ Hematocrit, hemoglobin, white blood cells, albumin.

Dosage: Tablets. Individualized, initial: 1 mg at bedtime (this dose is not to be exceeded); **then,** increase dose slowly to obtain desired response. **Range:** 1–5 mg daily; doses as high as 20 mg may be required in some clients.

NURSING CONSIDERATIONS

See also *Nursing Considerations* for *Antihypertensive Agents,* p. 78.

Administration/Storage

1. The initial dosing regimen must be carefully observed to minimize severe hypotension.
2. Monitor BP 2–3 hr after dosing as well as at the end of the dosing interval to ensure BP control has been maintained.
3. An increase in dose or b.i.d. dosing should be considered if BP control is not maintained at 24-hr interval.
4. After the initial dose, the daily dose can be given in the morning.
5. If terazosin must be discontinued for more than a few days, the initial dosing regimen should be used if therapy is reinstituted.
6. Due to additive effects, caution must be exercised when terazosin is combined with other antihypertensive agents.
7. *Treatment of Overdose:* Restore blood pressure and heart rate. Client should be kept supine; vasopressors may be indicated. Volume expanders can be used to treat shock.

Client/Family Teaching

1. Use caution when performing activities that require mental alertness until drug effects are realized.
2. Do not drive or undertake hazardous tasks for 12 hr after the first dose and after increasing the dose or reinstituting therapy following an interruption of dosage.
3. Take medication at bedtime to minimize side effects.

4. Avoid symptoms of orthostatic hypotension associated with the medication by rising slowly from a sitting or lying position and waiting until symptoms subside.
5. Perform weights and report any evidence of weight gain or ankle edema.
6. Do not interrupt therapy without physician approval.
7. Report any persistent side effects so dosage may be evaluated and adjusted accordingly.

Evaluation: Evaluate client for evidence of control of hypertension.

Terbutaline sulfate

(ter-**BYOU**-tah-leen)
Brethaire, Brethine, Bricanyl (Rx)

See also *Sympathomimetic Drugs,* p. 218.

Classification: Direct-acting adrenergic agent, bronchodilator.

Action/Kinetics: Terbutaline is specific for stimulating beta-2 receptors, resulting in bronchodilation and relaxation of peripheral vasculature. Minimum beta-1 activity. Drug action resembles that of isoproterenol. **PO: Onset:** 60–120 min; **maximum effect:** 2–3 hr; **duration:** 4–8 hr. **SC: Onset,** 6–15 min; **maximum effect:** 30 min—1 hr; **duration:** 1.5–4 hr. **Inhalation: Onset,** 5–30 min; **time to peak effect:** 1–2 hr; **duration:** 3–6 hr.

Uses: Bronchodilator in asthma, bronchitis, emphysema, bronchiectasis, pulmonary obstructive disease, and other conditions associated with reversible bronchospasms. *Investigational:* Inhibit premature labor.

Special Concerns: Safe use during pregnancy (category: B) or in children less than 12 years of age not established. Use with caution during lactation.

Dosage: Tablets. *Bronchodilation:* **Adults,** 2.5–5 mg t.i.d. q 6 hr during waking hours, not to exceed 15 mg/24 hr. If disturbing side effects are observed, dose can be reduced to 2.5 mg t.i.d. without loss of beneficial effects. Anticipate use of other therapeutic measures if client fails to respond after second dose. **Children 12–15 years:** 2.5 mg t.i.d., not to exceed 7.5 mg/24 hr. *Premature labor:* 2.5 mg q 4–6 hr until term.

SC. *Bronchodilation:* **Adults,** 0.25 mg. May be repeated 1 time after 15–30 min if no significant clinical improvement is noted. Dose should not exceed 0.5 mg over 4 hr. *Premature labor:* **IV infusion,** 0.10 mg/min initially; **then,** increase rate by 0.005 mg/min q 10 min until contractions cease or a maximum dose of 0.08 mg/min is reached. The minimum effective dose should be continued for 4–8 hr after contractions cease.

Inhalation Aerosol. Adults and children over 12 years: 0.2–0.5 mg (1–2 inhalations) q 4–6 hr. Inhalations should be separated by 60-sec intervals. Dosage may be repeated q 4–6 hr.

NURSING CONSIDERATIONS

See also *Nursing Considerations* for *Sympathomimetic Drugs,* p. 220.

Assessment

1. Auscultate and document baseline lung findings.
2. Note evidence of preterm labor, documenting frequency and duration of contractions and fetal heart rate.

Interventions

1. Observe respiratory client for evidence of drug tolerance and rebound bronchospasm.
2. Observe mother for evidence of headache, tremor, anxiety, palpitations, and tachycardia. Monitor fetus for distress and report any increase in contractions.
3. Monitor mother and neonate for symptoms of hypoglycemia and mother for hypokalemia.

Client/Family Teaching

1. Report any bothersome side effects to the physician. The drug dose and administration times may need to be adjusted.
2. Take medication with meals to minimize GI upset.
3. Do not increase dose or frequency if symptoms are not relieved. Report to physician so dose can be reevaluated.
4. Advise to increase fluid intake to help liquefy secretions.
5. In clients with preterm labor, advise to notify physician immediately if labor resumes or unusual side effects are noted.

Evaluation: Evaluate client for:
- Evidence of improved airway exchange
- Successful inhibition of premature labor

Terconazole nitrate
(ter-**KON**-ah-zohl)
Terazol 3, Terazol 7 (Rx)

Classification: Antifungal, vaginal.

Action/Kinetics: Terconazole, a triazole derivative, is thought to exert its antifungal activity by disrupting cell membrane permeability leading to loss of essential intracellular materials. The drug also inhibits synthesis of triglycerides and phospholipids as well as inhibiting oxidative and peroxidative enzyme activity. When used for *Candida,* terconazole inhibits transformation of blastospores into the invasive mycelial form.

Uses: Vulvovaginitis caused by *Candida.* Ineffective in infections due to *Trichomonas* or *Hemophilus vaginalis.*

Special Concerns: Use in pregnancy only on advice of physician (pregnancy category: C). During lactation, consider discontinuing nursing or the drug. Safety and efficacy have not been established in children.

Side Effects: *GU:* Vulvovaginal burning, irritation, or itching. *Miscellaneous:* Headache (most common), body pain, photosensitivity.

Dosage: Topical, vaginal cream: One applicatorful (5 g) intravaginally, once daily at bedtime for 7 days. **Vaginal suppository:** One 80 mg suppository once daily at bedtime for 3 days.

NURSING CONSIDERATIONS
Assessment

1. Obtain a thorough nursing history because recurrent candidiasis may be caused by oral contraceptives, antibiotics, or diabetes.
2. Intractable candidiasis may be the result of undetected diabetes mellitus or reinfection. The client should be evaluated carefully.
3. Prior to a second course of therapy, the diagnosis should be confirmed to rule out other pathogens associated with vulvovaginitis.

Client/Family Teaching

1. Demonstrate the appropriate method for administration and cleansing (the cream should be inserted high into the vagina). Sitz baths and vaginal douches may also be ordered with this therapy.
2. Discontinue use and report if any burning, irritation, or pain occurs.
3. Medication may stain clothes; use sanitary napkins during therapy and change frequently because damp sanitary napkins may harbor infecting organisms.
4. To avoid reinfection, the client should refrain from sexual intercourse, or the partner should be advised to use a condom as medication may also irritate partner.
5. Continue to take medication for prescribed time frame even if symptoms subside.
6. The drug should continue to be used during menses to ensure a full course of therapy. Effectiveness is not altered by menstruation.

Evaluation: Evaluate client for:
- Laboratory confirmation of negative culture reports
- Reports of symptomatic improvement

Terfenadine
(ter-**FEN**-ah-deen)
**Contact Allergy Formula✿,
Seldane (Rx)**

See also *Antihistamines*, p. 71.

Classification: Antihistamine, piperidine type.

Action/Kinetics: Is said to manifest significantly less drowsiness

and anticholinergic effects than other antihistamines. **Onset:** 1–2 hr; **peak effect:** 3–4 hr; **peak plasma levels:** 2 hr. **t½:** About 20 hr. **Duration:** Over 12 hr. Metabolized in the liver and excreted in the urine and feces.

Additional Uses: *Investigational:* Histamine-induced bronchoconstriction in asthmatics; exercise and hyperventilation-induced bronchospasm.

Special Concerns: Pregnancy category: C. Safety and efficacy in children less than 12 years of age have not been established.

Dosage: Tablets. Adults and children over 12 years: 60 mg q 8–12 hr as needed.

NURSING CONSIDERATIONS

See also *Nursing Considerations* for *Antihistamines*, p. 74.

Client/Family Teaching

1. Take with food or milk to minimize GI upset.
2. Use caution as drug may cause drowsiness.

Evaluation: Evaluate client for:
- Evidence of improved airway exchange
- Reports of symptomatic improvement in allergic manifestations

—— *COMBINATION DRUG* ——
Terfenadine and Pseudoephedrine hydrochloride
(ter-**FEN**-ah-deen
soo-doh-eh-**FED**-rin)
Seldane-D (Rx)

Classification/Content: Each extended-release tablet contains: *Antihistamine:* Terfenadine, 60 mg, and *Decontestant:* Pseudoephedrine hydrochloride, 120 mg. Ten mg of the pseudoephedrine is in an outer coat for immediate release while 110 mg is in an extended-release core. **Onset of terfenadine:** 1–2 hr. **Maximum effect of terfenadine:** 3–4 hr. **t½, terfenadine:** 8.5 hr. **Duration of terfenadine:** 12 hr. See also individual components.

Uses: Relief of symptoms associated with seasonal allergic rhinitis including sneezing, pruritus, rhinorrhea, lacrimation, and nasal congestion.

Contraindications: During lactation, severe hypertension, coronary artery disease, individuals taking MAO inhibitors.

Special Concerns: Pregnancy category: C. Use with caution in diabetes, cardiovascular disease, hypertension, hyperreactivity to ephedrine. Clients with impaired hepatic function, or who are taking ketoconazole or troleandomycin, or who have conditions leading to QT prolongation may experience QT prolongation and/or ventricular tachycardia. Safety and effectiveness in children less than 12 years of age have not been determined.

Side Effects: See individual components.

Drug Interactions

Beta-adrenergic blocking agents / ↑ Effect of pseudoephedrine
Ketoconazole / Ketoconazole significantly alters the metabolism of terfenadine
MAO inhibitors / ↑ Effect of pseudoephedrine
Macrolide antibiotics / Macrolide antibiotics significantly alter the metabolism of terfenadine

Mecamylamine / Pseudoephedrine ↓ antihypertensive effect of mecamylamine
Methyldopa / Pseudoephedrine ↓ antihypertensive effect of methyldopa
Reserpine / Pseudoephedrine ↓ antihypertensive effect of reserpine

Dosage: Exended-release tablets. Adults and children over 12 years: 1 tablet morning and night.

NURSING CONSIDERATIONS

See also *Nursing Considerations* for *Terfenadine,* p. 1189, and *Pseudoephedrine hydrochloride,* p. 1107.

Administration/Storage

1. The tablets should be swallowed whole; they should not be crushed or chewed.
2. The medication should be stored in a tightly closed container in a cool, dry location away from heat, moisture, or direct sunlight.

Assessment: Note any client history of hypertension, diabetes, or coronary artery disease.

Evaluation: Evaluate client for reports of symptomatic improvement in congestion and allergic manifestations.

Teriparatide acetate
(ter-ih-**PAR**-ah-tyd)
Parathar (Rx)

Classification: Diagnostic agent, hypoparathyroidism.

Action/Kinetics: Teriparatide is a

synthetic hormone consisting of the 1–34 fragment of human parathyroid hormone. The drug will initially cause an increased rate of calcium release from bone into blood. The most sensitive indicator for determining the type of hypoparathyroidism is the change in urinary cyclic AMP during the 0–30-min postinfusion period. Clients with hypoparathyroidism will show up to a tenfold or greater increase over baseline of urinary cyclic AMP in the 0–30-min postinfusion period. Over 90% of these clients will also show a threefold or greater increase in urinary phosphate excretion in the 0–60-min postinfusion period. On the other hand, clients with pseudohypoparathyroidism will show less than a sixfold increase in urinary cyclic AMP excretion in the 0–30-min postinfusion period and less than a threefold increase in urinary phosphate excretion in the 0–60-min postinfusion period. **Time to peak excretion of AMP:** During the first 30 min after infusion; **time to peak excretion of phosphate:** during the second 30 min after infusion.

Uses: To determine the presence of either hypoparathyroidism or pseudohypoparathryoidism in clients manifesting hypocalcemia.

Special Concerns: Pregnancy category: C. Use with caution during lactation.

Side Effects: *Metabolic:* Hypercalcemia. *GI:* Nausea, diarrhea, abdominal cramps, urge to defecate. *Miscellaneous:* Metallic taste, tingling of extremities, pain at injection site (during or following infusion), allergic reactions.

Dosage: IV. **Adults:** 5 units/kg infused in 10 ml over 10 min up to a maximum of 200 units. **Pediatric, over 3 years of age:** 3 units/kg, not to exceed 200 units, infused over 10 min.

NURSING CONSIDERATIONS

Administration/Storage

1. The test will distinguish between hypoparathyroidism and pseudohypoparathyroidism but not between these conditions and normal parathyroid function.
2. Clients should be fasting when the drug is administered. To maintain an active urine output during the test, 200 ml water should be ingested per hr for 2 hr before the study as well as during the study.
3. A baseline urine collection should be made during the 60-min period preceding infusion of the drug. Following infusion of the drug, urine should be collected during the 0–30-, 30–60-, and 60–120-min postinfusion periods.
4. Accuracy of the test will be affected by adequate hydration and urine flow, as well as complete collection of urine samples.
5. The reconstituted solution should be used within 4 hr.
6. Have epinephrine 1:1,000 available in the event of an allergic reaction.

Assessment: Assess baseline urinary output. Document any history of renal dysfunction.

Interventions: Monitor the client's vital signs, especially the BP, during the test.

Client/Family Teaching

1. Instruct the client to fast for the test.

T

2. Provide printed guidelines for hydration and preparation for the test.
3. Explain that the client may experience a metallic taste in the mouth and pain at the site of the injection during administration of the drug.

Evaluation: Evaluate for appropriate differentiation of hypoparathyroidism (10 X or greater increase of urinary cyclic AMP in 0–30-min postinfusion period) or pseudohypoparathyroidism.

Terpin hydrate and Codeine Elixir

(TER-pin HY-drayt, KOH-deen)
(C-V, Rx or OTC)

See also *Codeine*, p. 476.

Classification: Antitussive and expectorant.

General Statement: Terpin hydrate is alleged to increase respiratory tract fluid secretion, liquefy sputum, and facilitate expectoration; however, the recommended doses probably do not cause this effect and the FDA does not recommend its use as an expectorant. Terpin hydrate is combined with codeine, a narcotic, which specifically depresses the cough reflex. Terpin hydrate and codeine elixir contains 40% alcohol, 85 mg terpin hydrate, and 10 mg codeine per 5 ml and is subject to federal narcotic regulations.

Use: Symptomatic treatment of cough.

Contraindications: Peptic ulcer and severe diabetes mellitus. Use in children less than 12 years of age due to the high alcohol content of the elixir.

Special Concerns: Use during pregnancy and during lactation only if benefits outweigh risks.

Side Effects: *CNS:* Drowsiness (due to alcohol). *GI:* Epigastric pain if taken on an empty stomach. Also, see *Codeine*, p. 476.

Dosage: Adults.. *Terpin hydrate and codeine elixir,* **PO:** 5 ml q 3–4 hr.

NURSING CONSIDERATIONS

Administration/Storage: Administer with a full glass of water to facilitate the loosening of mucus.

Assessment

1. In taking the client's history, note if the client has complaints that would suggest the presence of a peptic ulcer. This drug should not be given to these clients.
2. If the client has diabetes mellitus, note the severity of illness. Clients with severe diabetes should *not* be given this compound.
3. Note any evidence the client may present that would suggest an addiction to any medication, particularly opiates.
4. Note any history of alcohol addiction. Terpin hydrate elixirs have a high alcohol content.

Interventions

1. Observe the client for undue drowsiness. Document and report. Discuss the amount of drug the client is taking and the frequency because excessive use may lead to oversedation and possibly drug dependence.
2. If the client is hospitalized, do not leave the medication at the bedside. Those on the unit who are alcohol- or drug-dependent would have access to a medi-

cation that is contraindicated for them.

Client/Family Teaching

1. Warn the client that excessive use of this medication may lead to oversedation and prolonged use may lead to dependence.
2. Report any epigastric pain to the physician.
3. If purchasing any OTC preparations, check first with the physician, pharmacist, or nurse. Avoid drugs that have alcohol as a base.
4. To avoid constipation, increase fluids and bulk in diet.
5. Advise that coughs lasting more that a week or accompanied by persistent headache, fever, chest pain, or skin rash should be evaluated by a physician.

Evaluation

1. Evaluate client for reports of less frequent interruptions of sleep due to coughing and symptomatic improvement.
2. If symptoms are unrelieved after 7–10 days of therapy, further tests should be used to determine causative agent and to determine the need for more extensive treatment.

Testolactone

(tes-toe-**LACK**-tohn)

Teslac (Rx)

See also *Antineoplastic Agents,* p. 85.

Classification: Antineoplastic, androgen.

Action/Kinetics: Synthetic steroid related to testosterone. The drug may act to reduce synthesis of estrone from adrenal andro-stenedione by inhibiting steroid aromatase activity. The drug is well absorbed from the GI tract. It is metabolized in the liver and unchanged drug and metabolites are excreted through the urine. Does not cause virilization.

Uses: Palliative treatment of advanced or disseminated mammary cancer in postmenopausal women or in premenopausal ovariectomized clients. Is effective in only 15% of clients.

Additional Contraindications: Breast cancer in men; premenopausal women with intact ovaries. Lactation.

Special Concerns: Pregnancy category: C. Safety and efficacy have not been determined in children.

Additional Side Effects: *GI:* Nausea, vomiting, glossitis, anorexia. *CNS:* Numbness or tingling of fingers, toes, face. *Miscellaneous:* Inflammation and irritation at injection site; increases BP during parenteral administration. Hypercalcemia. Maculopapular erythema, alopecia, nail growth disturbances. See also *Testosterone,* p. 1194.

Drug Interactions: Testolactone may ↑ effect of oral anticoagulants.

Laboratory Test Interferences: ↑ Plasma calcium, urinary excretion of creatine (24 hr) and 17-ketosteroids. ↓ Estradiol levels using radioimmunoassays.

Dosage: Tablets: 250 mg q.i.d. Therapy usually should be continued for 3 months unless there is active progression of the disease.

NURSING CONSIDERATIONS

See also *Nursing Considerations* for *Antineoplastic Agents,* p. 88, and *Testosterone,* p. 1196.

Interventions

1. Anticipate a reduction in dose of anticoagulants if client is on concomitant therapy.
2. The effect of the steroid and osteolytic metastases may result in hypercalcemia. Thus, assess routinely for symptoms of hypercalcemia: insomnia, lethargy, anorexia, nausea, vomiting, coma, and vascular collapse.
3. Withhold drug and report high serum calcium levels.
4. Encourage high fluid intake to minimize hypercalcemia.
5. Closely monitor clients who resume therapy after drug-induced hypercalcemia is corrected.

Evaluation: Evaluate client for evidence of a reduction in tumor size and spread.

Testosterone aqueous suspension
(tess-**TOSS**-ter-ohn)
Andro 100, Histerone 50 and 100, Malogen✿, Testamone 100 (Rx)

Testosterone cypionate (in oil)
(tess-**TOSS**-ter-ohn)
Andro-Cyp 100 and 200, Andronate 100 and 200, dep-Andro 100 and 200, Depotest 100 and 200, Depo-Testosterone, Depo-Testosterone Cypionate✿, Duratest-100 and -200, Testred Cypionate 200 (Rx)

Testosterone enanthate (in oil)
(tess-**TOSS**-ter-ohn)
Andro L.A. 200, Andropository-200, Delatest, Delatestryl,

Durathate-200, Everone 100 and 200, Malogex✿, Testone LA 100 and 200, Testrin PA (Rx)

Testosterone propionate (in oil)
(tess-**TOSS**-ter-ohn)
Malogen in Oil✿, Testex (Rx)

Classification: Androgen, natural hormone and salts of natural hormone.

Action/Kinetics: Testosterone, its degradation products, and synthetic substitutes are collectively referred to as the *androgens* (from the Greek *andros,* man). Like the primary female hormones, estrogen and progesterone, the production of testosterone is controlled by the gonadotropins: follicle-stimulating hormone (FSH), and the interstitial cell-stimulating hormone (ICSH), both of which are produced by the anterior pituitary.

At puberty, these gonadotropins initiate the production of testosterone, which in turn stimulates the development of primary sex organs and secondary sexual characteristics. Testosterone also stimulates bone and skeletal muscle growth, increases the retention of dietary protein nitrogen (anabolism), and slows down the breakdown of body tissues (catabolism). The anabolic effect is due to stimulation of RNA polymerase activity and specific RNA synthesis, resulting in increased protein production. Androgens promote retention of sodium, potassium, nitrogen, and phosphorus and the excretion of calcium. Toward the end of puberty, testosterone hastens the conversion of cartilage into bone, thereby terminating linear growth.

Treatment with testosterone and

its congeners is complicated by the fact that the exogenous supply of the hormone may depress secretion of the natural hormone through inhibitory effects on the pituitary. Too large a dose may cause permanent damage. Treatment is usually associated with a feeling of well-being. In addition to testosterone and its various esters, several synthetic variants are available commercially.

Following oral use, 44% of testosterone is cleared by the liver in the first pass. Thus, the parenteral forms are used. **$t^{1/2}$, testosterone cypionate after IM:** 8 days. 90% is excreted through the urine as metabolites and 6% is excreted through the feces.

Uses: Replacement therapy in males for congenital or acquired primary hypogonadism, congenital or acquired hypogonadotropic hypogonadism, delayed puberty. In postmenopausal women to treat inoperable metastatic breast carcinoma or in premenopausal women following oophorectomy. Postpartum breast engorgement. Postpartum breast engorgement (evidence for effectiveness is lacking). *Investigational:* Male contraceptive (testosterone enanthate).

Contraindications: Prostatic or breast (males) carcinoma. Pregnancy (masculinization of female fetus) and lactation. Discontinue if hypercalcemia occurs.

Special Concerns: Pregnancy category: X. Use with caution in young males and females who have not completed their growth (because of premature epiphyseal closure). Androgens may also cause virilization in females or precocious sexual development in males. Geriatric

clients may manifest an increased risk of prostatic hypertrophy or prostatic carcinoma. Also use with caution in clients with cardiac, renal, or hepatic disorders (because of edema caused by androgen administration).

Side Effects: *Hepatic:* Liver toxicity is the most serious side effect. Jaundice, cholestasis, alterations in BSP retention, AST, and ALT. Rarely, hepatic necrosis, hepatocellular neoplasms, peliosis hepatis. *GI:* Nausea, vomiting, diarrhea, anorexia, symptoms of peptic ulcer. *CNS:* Headache, anxiety, increased or decreased libido, insomnia, excitation, paresthesias, sleep apnea syndrome, CNS hemorrhage, chills, choreiform movements, habituation, confusion (toxic doses). *GU:* Testicular atrophy with inhibition of testicular function, impotence, epididymitis, irritable bladder, prepubertal phallic enlargement. *Electrolyte:* Retention of sodium, chloride, calcium, potassium, phosphates. Edema. *Miscellaneous:* Acne, flushing, suppression of clotting factors (II, V, VII, X), polycythemia, leukopenia, rashes, dermatitis, anaphylaxis (rare), muscle cramps. Hypercalcemia, especially in immobilized clients or those with metastatic breast carcinoma.

In females, menstrual irregularities (including amenorrhea), virilization, clitoral enlargement, hirsutism, increased libido, baldness (male pattern), virilization of external genitalia of female fetus.

In males, decreased ejaculatory volume, oligospermia (high doses), gynecomastia, increased frequency and duration of penile erections.

In children, disturbances of growth, premature closure of epiphyses, precocious sexual development.

Buccal preparations may cause stomatitis. Inflammation and pain at site of IM or SC injection.

Note: Side effects of the cypionate and enanthate products are not readily reversible due to the long duration of action of these dosage forms.

Drug Interactions

Anticoagulants, oral / Anabolic steroids ↑ effect of anticoagulants
Antidiabetic agents / Additive hypoglycemia
Barbiturates / ↓ Effect of androgens due to ↑ breakdown by liver
Corticosteroids / ↑ Chance of edema
Phenylbutazone / Certain androgens ↑ effect of phenylbutazone

Laboratory Test Interferences:

Alter thyroid function tests. False + or ↑ BSP, alkaline phosphatase, bilirubin, cholesterol, and acid phosphatase (in women). Alteration of glucose tolerance tests.

Dosage: *Testosterone and testosterone propionate,* **IM only.** *Replacement therapy:* 25–50 mg 2–3 times/week. *Postpartum breast engorgement:* 25–50 mg daily for 3–4 days beginning at the time of delivery. *Breast cancer:* 50–100 mg 3 times/week. *Delayed puberty in males:* 12.5–25 mg 2–3 times a week for no more than 4–6 months. *Growth stimulation in Turner syndrome or constitutional delay of puberty:* 40–50 mg/m²/dose given monthly for 6 months.

Testosterone enanthate and cypionate, **IM only.** *Hypogonadism, replacement therapy, impotence:* 50–400 mg q 2–4 weeks. *Delayed puberty:* 50–200 mg q 2–4 weeks for no more than 4–6 months. *Breast cancer in women:* 200–400 mg q 2–4 weeks.

NURSING CONSIDERATIONS

Administration/Storage:

1. Crystals of testosterone enanthate or cypionate may be redissolved by warming and shaking the vial.
2. If the needle or syringe is wet, the product may become cloudy; this does not affect potency.
3. For IM oil-based suspensions, warm the unopened vial in warm water to decrease the viscosity of the oil. Vigorously rotate the vial to resuspend the medication in the oil. A film may appear on the sides of the vial. When no more suspended particles are observed on the bottom or sides of the vial, the drug has been suspended appropriately. Administer the needle deep into the muscle, and administer the medication slowly.
4. When parenteral injection is to be used, testosterone propionate is more effective than testosterone because it is released more slowly.
5. Continue the therapy for at least 2 months for a satisfactory response and for 5 months for an objective response.

Assessment

1. Review the client's general health history for evidence of existing cardiac, renal, or hepatic dysfunction.
2. Obtain baseline data concerning the client's neurologic status, BP, respirations, heart sounds, and GU function.

3. Note the client's hair distribution and skin texture.
4. Check the client's medication history for interacting drugs such as anticoagulants, hypoglycemic agents, and mineralocorticoids.
5. If the client is female, of childbearing age, and sexually active, note the potential for pregnancy.
6. Obtain a baseline CBC, serum glucose, cholesterol, and calcium levels, electrolyte levels and liver and renal function studies.

Interventions

1. Monitor the client for signs of mental depression such as insomnia, lack of interest in personal appearance, and a general withdrawal from social contacts.
2. Note any client complaints of tingling of the fingers and toes or complaint of loss of appetite. Document and report to the physician.
3. Monitor the client's weight, BP, pulse, and serum electrolytes. Auscultate the lung sounds and note distention of the jugular veins. Report any signs of edema to the physician because diuretics may be needed to control the edema.
4. Assess for relaxation of the skeletal muscles and note if client complains of pain deep in the bones. The discomfort in the bones is caused by a honeycombing of the bones. These complaints are often a first indication of an increase in the client's calcium levels and must be further investigated.
5. If client complains of flank pain, this may be caused by kidney stones, which may result from excessively high serum calcium levels.
6. Normal serum calcium levels are 4.5–5.5 mEq/L. If the client has a high serum calcium level, withdraw the drug, notify the physician and administer large amounts of fluids to prevent renal calculi. If the hypercalcemia is the result of metastases, other appropriate therapy should be instituted.
7. Observe the client for jaundice, malaise, complaints of right upper quadrant pain, pruritus, or a change in the color or consistency of the stools. Obtain liver function studies, document and report to the physician.
8. Observe the client for easy bruising, reports of bleeding, or client complaints of sore throat or the development of fever. Obtain a CBC to rule out polycythemia and leukopenia.
9. If the client is a child, monitor closely for growth retardation and development of precocious puberty.
   • Review the program of therapy with the parents. Often therapy will be intermittent to allow for periods of normal bone growth.
   • Discuss with the physician the advisability of regular x-rays of the wrists and hands to monitor the maturation of bone.
   • Monitor and record the child's height and weight.
10. If the client is female, report the onset of signs of virilization, such as deepening of the voice, unusual hair growth, menstrual irregularity, and clitoral enlargement.

11. Discuss with female clients any changes in libido. Provide emotional support and report this problem to the physician. Increased libido may be an early sign of serious drug toxicity.

12. Note the presence of acne and other skin changes. If the acne is severe, consult the physician. It may be necessary to change the dose of medication.

Client/Family Teaching

1. Report any unusual incidents of bleeding or bruising. Androgens suppress clotting factors and polycythemia and leukopenia may also occur.

2. If the client has received the drug via pellets, sloughing can occur. Notify the physician immediately if this occurs.

3. Discuss the potential for bladder irritation to occur. Review the symptoms that may result from this irritation and advise the client to report these findings to the physician.

4. Instruct parents of children receiving testosterone to weigh the child at least twice a week and to measure the child's length at least every 2–3 months. These measurements should be recorded and reported to the physician.

5. Discuss the importance of reporting to the laboratory for tests of serum calcium levels and serum cholesterol. If the serum cholesterol level is high, the physician may wish to change the dosage of drug. Also, discuss the need to follow a low-cholesterol diet and refer to a dietitian for further assistance in meal planning.

6. Reassure female clients that any growth in facial hair and the development of acne are reversible once the drug is withdrawn.

7. Explain to premenopausal female clients that the medication may cause irregularities in the menstrual cycle. In postmenopausal women the medication may cause withdrawal bleeding.
   - Advise women to keep a written record of their menstrual periods.
   - For sexually active women, discuss with them the advisability of consulting the physician regarding birth control measures during the first few weeks of androgen therapy and for several weeks after the androgen therapy has been withdrawn.
   - Advise women to notify the physician immediately if pregnancy is suspected. There is an increased risk of fetal abnormalities with this drug.

8. Instruct male clients to report priapism. The physician may withdraw the drug at least temporarily.

9. Unless contraindicated, recommend that the client follow a diet high in calories, proteins, vitamins, minerals, and other nutrients.

10. Advise clients with diabetes that hypoglycemia may occur as a result of drug therapy. Monitor finger sticks frequently and report because diet and/or dose of antidiabetic agents may require modification.

11. Discuss with young clients and their parents, if possible, the potential for drug abuse. Ex-

plain the long-term effects and the permanent physical damage that is caused by indiscriminate use of these agents.

Evaluation: Evaluate client for:
- Effective control and prevention of any S&S of androgen deficiency
- Evidence of a decrease in breast tumor size and spread

Tetracycline
(teh-trah-**SYE**-kleen)
Achromycin Ophthalmic Suspension (Rx)

Tetracycline hydrochloride
(teh-trah-**SYE**-kleen)
Achromycin IM and IV, Achromycin Ophthalmic Ointment, Achromycin Topical Ointment, Achromycin V, Ala-Tet, Apo-Tetra✳, Nor-Tet, Novo-Tetra✳, Nu-Tetra✳, Panmycin, Robitet, Robicaps, Sumycin 250 and 500, Sumycin Syrup, Teline, Teline-500, Tetracap, Tetracyn✳, Tetralan-250 and -500, Tetralan Syrup, Tetram (Rx)

See also *General Information* on *Tetracyclines,* p. 222.

Classification: Antibiotic, tetracycline.

Action/Kinetics: t½: 7–11 hr. From 40% to 70% excreted unchanged in urine; 65% bound to serum proteins. Dosage is always expressed as the hydrochloride salt.

Additional Uses: Superficial ophthalmic infections due to *Staphylococcus aureus, Streptococcus, Escherichia coli, Neisseria,* and *Bacteroides.* Prophylaxis of *Neisseria*

gonorrhoeae or *Chlamydia trachomatis* in newborns. **Topical:** Acne vulgaris, prophylaxis or treatment of infection following skin abrasions, minor cuts, wounds, or burns. *Investigational:* Pleural sclerosing agent in malignant pleural effusions (administered by chest tube); in combination with gentamicin for *V. vulnificus* infections due to wound infection after trauma or by eating contaminated seafood. Mouthwash (use suspension) to treat nonspecific mouth ulcerations, canker sores, aphthous ulcers. Possible drug of choice for stage I Lyme disease.

Contraindications: The topical ointment should not be used in or around the eyes. Ophthalmic products should not be used to treat fungal diseases of the eye, dendritic keratitis, vaccinia, varicella, mycobacterial eye infections, or following removal of a corneal foreign body.

Additional Side Effects: Dermatitis and photosensitivity following ophthalmic use.

Dosage: Capsules, Tablets. Adults: usual, *mild to moderate infections:* 500 mg b.i.d. or 250 mg q.i.d.; *severe infections:* 500 mg q.i.d. **Children over 8 years:** 25–50 mg/kg daily in 4 equal doses. *Brucellosis:* 500 mg q.i.d. for 3 weeks with 1 g streptomycin IM b.i.d. for first week and once daily the second week. *Syphilis:* Total of 30–40 g over 10–15 days. *Gonorrhea:* **initially,** 1.5 g; **then,** 500 mg q 6 hr until 9 g has been given. *Gonorrhea sensitive to penicillin:* **initially,** 1.5 g; **then,** 500 mg q 6 hr for 4 days (total: 9 g). *GU or rectal Chlamydia trachomatis infections:* 500 mg q.i.d. for minimum of 7 days. *Severe acne:* **initially,** 1 g

T

daily; **then,** 125–500 mg daily (long-term). **Note:** The Centers for Disease Control have established treatment schedules for sexually transmitted diseases.

IM. Adults: usual, 250 mg once daily or 300 mg/day in divided doses q 8–12 hr. Up to 800 mg daily may be used. **Children over 8 years:** 15–25 mg/kg up to maximum of 250 mg in single daily injection. The dose may be divided and given q 8–12 hr.

IV. Adults: 250–500 mg q 12 hr, not to exceed 500 mg q 6 hr. **Children over 8 years:** 12 mg/kg/day in 2 divided doses. Up to 20 mg/kg/day may be given if the disease is severe.

Ophthalmic. *Suspension. Acute infections:* **initially,** 1–2 gtt q 15–30 min; **then,** as infection improves, decrease frequency. *Moderate infections:* 1–2 gtt q 4 hr. *Trachoma:* 2 gtt in each eye b.i.d.–q.i.d. for up to 2 or more months (oral tetracycline may be given concomitantly). *Ointment. Acute infections:* ½ inch q 3–4 hr until improvement noted. *Mild to moderate infections:* ½ inch b.i.d.–t.i.d.

Topical. *Acne:* Apply topical solution to affected areas in the morning and at night, making sure that skin is completely wet after each application. *Infections:* Apply OTC ointment (3%) to affected areas 1–4 times daily. A sterile bandage may be used.

NURSING CONSIDERATIONS

See also *Nursing Considerations* for *Tetracyclines,* p. 224, and *General Nursing Considerations For All Anti-Infectives,* p. 83.

Administration/Storage

1. To reconstitute solutions for IV use, vials containing 250 or 500 mg should be diluted with 5 or 10 ml, respectively, of sterile water for injection. Further dilution (100–1,000 ml) can be done with sodium chloride injection, 5% dextrose injection, 5% dextrose and sodium chloride, Ringer's injection, and lactated Ringer's injection.
2. Except for Ringer's and lactated Ringer's injections, calcium-containing solutions should not be used to dilute tetracycline HCl.
3. For IM administration, inject into a large muscle mass.

Client/Family Teaching

1. Transient blurring of vision or stinging may occur when tetracycline is instilled into the eye.
2. Take oral form 1 hr before or 2 hr after meals.
3. Avoid dairy products, antacids, or iron preparations for 2 hr within ingestion of medication.
4. Drug may cause photosensitivity reaction. Avoid exposure to sunlight and wear protective clothing and sunscreen when exposure is necessary.
5. The topical ointment may stain clothing.
6. Drug may cause increased yellow-brown discoloration and softening of teeth and bones. *Not* advised for children under 8 years of age.

Evaluation: Evaluate client for:
- Laboratory confirmation of negative culture reports
- Reports of symptomatic improvement

Theophylline
(thee-**OFF**-ih-lin)
Immediate-release Capsules, Tablets, Liquid Products: Accurbron, Aerolate,

Aquaphyllin, Asmalix, Bronkodyl, Elixomin, Elixophyllin, Lanophyllin, Lixolin, PMS Theophylline ✿, Pulmophylline ✿, Quibron-T/ SR ✿, Quibron-T Dividose, Slo-Phyllin, Solu-Phyllin, Somnophyllin-T, Theo, Theoclear-80, Theolair, Theomar, Theostat-80, Truxophyllin. Timed-release Capsules and Tablets: Aerolate III, Aerolate Jr., Aerolate Sr., Constant-T, Elixophyllin SR, Quibron-T/SR Dividose, Respid, Slo-Bid Gyrocaps, Slo-Phyllin Gyrocaps, Somophyllin-12 ✿, Somophyllin-CRT, Sustaire, Theo-24, Theo 250, Theobid Duracaps, Theobid Jr Duracaps, Theoclear LA.-130 Cenules, Theoclear LA.-260 Cenules, Theocot, Theocron, Theo-Dur, Theo-Dur Sprinkle, Theo-SR ✿, Theolair-SR, Theospan-SR, Theo-Time, Theophylline SR, Theovent Long-Acting, Uniphyl (Rx)

See also *Theophylline Derivatives*, p. 226.

Classification: Antiasthmatic, bronchodilator.

Action/Kinetics: Time to peak serum levels, oral solution: 1 hr; **uncoated tablets:** 2 hr; **chewable tablets:** 1–1.5 hr; **enteric-coated tablets:** 5 hr; **extended-release capsules and tablets:** 4–7 hr. In healthy adults, about 60% is bound to plasma protein whereas in neonates 36% is bound to plasma protein.

Additional Uses: Oral liquid: Neonatal apnea as a respiratory stimulant. Theophylline and dextrose injection: Respiratory stimulant in neonatal apnea and Cheyne-Stokes respiration.

Dosage: Capsules, Elixir, Oral Solution, Oral Suspension, **Syrup, Tablets.** See *Dosage* for *Oral Solution, Tablets,* p. 299, under *Aminophylline.*

Extended-release Capsules, Extended-release Tablets. See *Dosage* for *Extended-release Tablets,* p. 300, under *Aminophylline. Bronchodilator, chronic therapy:* **9–12 years:** 20 mg/kg daily; **6–9 years:** 24 mg/kg daily.

Elixir, Oral Solution, Oral Suspension, Syrup. *Neonatal apnea,* **loading dose:** Using the equivalent of anhydrous theophylline administered by nasogastric tube, 5 mg/kg; **maintenance:** 2 mg/kg daily in 2–3 divided doses given by nasogastric tube.

NURSING CONSIDERATIONS

See also *Nursing Considerations* for *Theophylline Derivatives,* p. 229.

Administration/Storage

1. Dosage is individualized to maintain serum levels of 10–20 mcg/ml.
2. Dosage should be calculated based on lean body weight (theophylline does not distribute to body fat).
3. Serum theophylline levels should be monitored in chronic therapy, especially if the maximum maintenance doses are used or exceeded.
4. The extended-release tablets or capsules are not recommended for children less than 6 years of age. Dosage for once-a-day products has not been established in children less than 12 years of age.

Client/Family Teaching

1. Stress the importance of taking the drug only as prescribed by the physician.

2. Do not crush or break slow-release forms of the drug.
3. Avoid cigarette smoking because this decreases drug's effectiveness.
4. Take with food or milk to minimize GI upset.
5. Provide a printed list of side effects that require reporting to the physician.
6. Caffeine- and xanthine-containing beverages and foods (chocolate, coffee, colas) should be avoided because they tend to increase side effects of this drug.
7. Advise that fluid intake should be 2 L/day in order to decrease viscosity of secretions.

Evaluation: Evaluate client for:

- Evidence of improved airway exchange on auscultation
- Reports of ease in secretion removal and breathing
- Laboratory confirmation that drug levels are within therapeutic range (10–20 mcg/ml)

Thiabendazole
(thigh-ah-**BEN**-dah-zohl)
Mintezol (Rx)

See also *Anthelmintics*, p. 40.

Classification: Anthelmintic.

Action/Kinetics: The drug interferes with the enzyme fumarate reductase, which is specific to several helminths. It is readily absorbed from the GI tract. **Peak plasma levels:** 1–2 hr. **t½:** 0.9–2 hr. Most of the drug is excreted within 24 hr, mainly through the urine.

Uses: Primarily for threadworm infections, cutaneous larva migrans, visceral larva migrans. When pinworm occurs with the above infections. Use in the following infections only if specific therapy is not available or cannot be used or if a second drug is desirable: hookworm, whipworm, large roundworm. To reduce symptoms of trichinosis during the invasive phase.

Contraindications: Lactation. Use in mixed infections with ascaris as it may cause worms to migrate.

Special Concerns: Pregnancy category: C (safe use during pregnancy has not been established). Safety and efficacy not established in children less than 13.6 kg. Use with caution in clients with hepatic disease or impaired hepatic function.

Side Effects: *GI:* Nausea, vomiting, anorexia, diarrhea, epigastric distress. *CNS:* Dizziness, drowsiness, headache, irritability, seizures. *Allergic:* Pruritus, angioedema, flushing of face, chills, fever, skin rashes, Stevens-Johnson syndrome, anaphylaxis, lymphadenopathy. *Hepatic:* Jaundice, cholestasis, liver damage, transient increase in AST. *GU:* Crystalluria, hematuria, enuresis, foul odor of urine. *Miscellaneous:* Tinnitus, blurred vision, hypotension, collapse, hyperglycemia, leukopenia, perianal rash.

Symptoms of Overdose: Psychic changes, transient vision changes.

Drug Interactions: ↑ Serum levels of xanthines due to ↓ breakdown by liver.

Dosage: Oral Suspension, Chewable Tablets: Over 68 kg: 1.5 g/dose; **less than 68 kg:** 22 mg/kg/dose.

NURSING CONSIDERATIONS

See also *Nursing Considerations* for *Anthelmintics,* p. 42.

Administration/Storage

1. For strongyloidiasis, cutaneous larva migrans, hookworm, whipworm, or roundworm; 2 doses/day are given for 2 days. For trichinelliasis, give 2 doses/day for 2–4 days. For pinworm, give 2 doses for 1 day, repeat after 7–14 days.
2. *Treatment of Overdose:* Induce vomiting or perform gastric lavage. Treat symptoms.

Client/Family Teaching

1. Administer the drug after meals.
2. CNS disturbances (including muscular weakness and loss of mental alertness) may be caused by the drug.
3. The client should not operate hazardous machinery after taking the medication.

Evaluation: Evaluate client for laboratory evidence of negative culture reports and effective eradication of infestation.

Thiamine hydrochloride (Vitamin B₁)

(THIGH-ah-min)

Betaxin✶, Bewon✶, Biamine, Thiamilate (Rx: Injection; OTC: Tablets)

Action/Kinetics: Water-soluble vitamin, stable in acid solution. The vitamin is decomposed in neutral or acid solutions. Thiamine is re-

quired for the synthesis of thiamine pyrophosphate, a coenzyme required in carbohydrate metabolism. The maximum amount absorbed orally is 8–15 mg daily although absorption may be increased by giving in divided doses with food.

Uses: Prophylaxis and treatment of thiamine deficiency states and associated neurologic and cardiovascular symptoms. Prophylaxis and treatment of beriberi. Alcoholic neuritis, neuritis of pellagra, and neuritis of pregnancy. To correct anorexia due to thiamine insufficiency. *Investigational:* Treatment of subacute necrotizing encephalomyelopathy, maple syrup urine disease, pyruvate carboxylase deficiency, hyperalaninemia.

Special Concerns: Pregnancy category: A (parenteral use). Use with caution during lactation.

Side Effects: Serious hypersensitivity reactions can occur; thus, intradermal testing is recommended if sensitivity is suspected. *Dermatologic:* Pruritus, urticaria, sweating, feeling of warmth. *CNS:* Weakness, restlessness. *Other:* Nausea, tightness in throat, angioneurotic edema, cyanosis, hemorrhage into the GI tract, pulmonary edema, cardiovascular collapse. Death has been reported. *Following IM use:* Induration, tenderness.

Drug Interaction: Because vitamin B₁ is unstable in neutral or alkaline solutions, the vitamin should not be used with substances that yield alkaline solutions, such as citrates, barbiturates, carbonates, or erythromycin lactobionate IV.

Dosage: Tablets. *Mild beriberi or*

maintenance following severe beriberi: **Adults,** 5–10 mg daily (as part of a multivitamin product); **infants:** 10 mg daily. *Treatment of deficiency:* **Adults,** 5–10 mg daily; **pediatric:** 10–50 mg daily. *Alcohol-induced deficiency:* **Adults,** 40 mg daily. *Dietary supplement:* **Adults,** 1–2 mg daily; **pediatric:** 0.3–0.5 mg daily for infants and 0.5 mg daily for children. *Genetic enzyme deficiency disease:* 10–20 mg daily (up to 4 g daily has been used in some clients). **Slow IV.** *Wet beriberi with myocardial failure:* **Adults,** 10–30 mg t.i.d. **IM.** *Beriberi:* 10–20 mg t.i.d. for 2 weeks. An oral multivitamin product containing 5–10 mg thiamine daily should be given each day for 1 month to cause body saturation. *The recommended dietary allowance:* **males, adults,** 1.2–1.5 mg; **females, adults,** 1.1 mg.

NURSING CONSIDERATIONS

Administration/Storage: The drug may enhance the effects of neuromuscular blocking agents. Have epinephrine available to treat clients for anaphylactic shock if a large parenteral dose of thiamine is ordered.

Client/Family Teaching

1. Review dietary sources high in thiamine (enriched and whole grain cereals, meats, especially pork, and fresh vegetables) and refer to a dietitian for assistance in meal planning and preparation.
2. Provide a printed list of side effects that require reporting to the physician.

Evaluation: Evaluate client for evidence of effective prophylaxis and treatment of thiamine deficiency states.

Thioguanine
(thigh-oh-**GWON**-een)

**Lanvis✿, TG, 6-Thioguanine
(Abbreviation: 6-TG) (Rx)**

See also *Antineoplastic Agents,* p. 85.

Classification: Antimetabolite, purine analog.

Action/Kinetics: Purine antagonist that is cell-cycle specific for the S phase of cell division. Thioguanine is converted to 6-thioguanylic acid which, in turn, interferes with the synthesis of guanine nucleotides by competing with hypoxanthine and xanthine for the enzyme phosphoribosyltransferase (HGPRTase). Ultimately the synthesis of RNA and DNA is inhibited. Resistance to the drug may result from increased breakdown of 6-thioguanylic acid or loss of HGPRTase activity. Partially absorbed (30%) from GI tract. $t^{1/2}$: 80 min. Detoxified by liver and excreted in the urine. More effective in children than in adults. Cross-resistance with mercaptopurine. Perform platelet counts weekly; discontinue drug if abnormally large fall in blood count is noted, indicating severe bone marrow depression.

Uses: Acute and nonlymphocytic leukemias (usually in combination with other drugs such as cyclophosphamide, cytarabine, prednisone, vincristine). Chronic myelogenous leukemia (not first-line therapy).

Contraindications: Resistance to mercaptopurine or thioguanine.

Special Concerns: Pregnancy category: D. Use not recommended during lactation.

Additional Side Effects: Loss of

vibration sense, unsteadiness of gait. Hepatotoxicity myelosuppression (common), hyperuricemia. Adults tend to show a more rapid fall in WBC count than children. *Symptoms of Overdose:* Nausea, vomiting, hypertension, malaise, and diaphoresis may be seen immediately, which may be followed by myelosuppression and azotemia. Severe hematologic toxicity.

Laboratory Test Interference: ↑ Uric acid in blood and urine.

Dosage: Tablets: *Individualized* and determined by hematopoietic response; **adults and pediatric: initial:** 2 mg/kg daily (or 75–100 mg/m²) given at one time. From 2 to 4 weeks may elapse before beneficial results become apparent. Compute dose to nearest multiple of 20 mg. If no response, dosage may be increased to 3 mg/kg daily. **Usual maintenance dose** (even during remissions): 2–3 mg/kg daily (or 100 mg/m²). Dosage of thioguanine does not have to be decreased during administration of allopurinol (to inhibit uric acid production).

NURSING CONSIDERATIONS

See also *Nursing Considerations* for *Antineoplastic Agents*, p. 88.

Administration/Storage: *Treatment of Overdose:* Induce vomiting if client is seen immediately after an acute overdosage. Treat symptoms. Hematologic toxicity may be treated by platelet transfusions (for bleeding) and granulocyte transfusions. Antibiotics are indicated for sepsis.

Interventions

1. Provide assistance to ambulatory clients who may experience loss of vibration sense and thus have unsteady gait (these clients may be unable to rely on canes).
2. Encourage increased fluid intake (2 L/day) to minimize hyperuricemia and hyperuricosuria.
3. Monitor platelets, CBC, and liver function tests as a baseline before therapy is instituted and repeat platelets weekly and liver function tests monthly during course of therapy. Note any evidence of anemia and assess for evidence of fatigue or dyspnea.

Client/Family Teaching

1. Withhold drug and report if jaundice, ↓ urine output, diarrhea or extremity swelling occurs.
2. Emphasize to adult clients that contraceptive measures are advised with this drug.
3. Any sore throat, fever, or flu-like symptoms as well as increased bruising and bleeding tendencies require immediate physician notification.

Evaluation: Evaluate client for hematologic evidence of a remission of leukemia.

Thioridazine hydrochloride

(thigh-oh-**RID**-ah-zeen)
Apo-Thioridazine✶, Mellaril,Mellaril-S, Novo–Ridazine✶, PMS Thioridazine✶, Thioridazine HCl Intensol Oral (Rx)

See also *Phenothiazines*, p. 201.

Classification: Antipsychotic, piperidine-type phenothiazine.

Action/Kinetics: The use of thioridazine is accompanied by a high incidence of hypotensive effects; a moderate incidence of sedative and anticholinergic effects and weak antiemetic and extrapyramidal effects. Thioridazine can often be used in clients intolerant of other phenothiazines. It has little or no antiemetic effects. **Peak plasma levels** (after PO administration): 1–4 hr. Thioridazine may impair its own absorption at higher doses due to the strong anticholinergic effects. **t½:** 10 hr. Metabolized in the liver to both active and inactive metabolites.

Uses: Acute and chronic schizophrenia; moderate to marked depression with anxiety; sleep disturbances. *In children:* Treatment of hyperactivity in clients and those with retarded and behavior problems. Geriatric clients with organic brain syndrome. Alcohol withdrawal. Intractable pain.

Special Concerns: Safe use during pregnancy has not been established. Dosage has not been established in children less than 2 years of age. Geriatric, emaciated, or debilitated clients usually require a lower initial dose.

Additional Side Effects: More likely to cause pigmentary retinopathy than other phenothiazines.

Dosage: Oral Suspension, Oral Solution, Tablets. Highly individualized. *Neurosis, anxiety states, sleep disturbances, tension, alcohol withdrawal, senility,* **range:** 20–200 mg daily; **initial:** 25 mg t.i.d. **Maintenance,** mild cases: 10 mg b.i.d.–q.i.d.; severe cases: 50 mg t.i.d.–q.i.d. *Psychotic, severely disturbed hospitalized clients:* **initial,** 50–100 mg t.i.d. If necessary, increase to maximum of 200 mg q.i.d. When control is achieved, reduce gradually to minimum effective dosage. **Pediatric above 2 years:** 0.25–3.0 mg/kg daily. *Hospitalized psychotic children:* **initial,** 25 mg b.i.d.–t.i.d. *Moderate problems:* **initial,** 10 mg b.i.d.–t.i.d. Increase gradually if necessary. **Not recommended for children under 2 years of age.**

NURSING CONSIDERATIONS

See also *Nursing Considerations for Phenothiazines,* p. 205.

Administration/Storage: Dilute each dose just before administration with distilled water, acidified tap water, or suitable juices. Preparation and storage of bulk dilutions are not recommended.

Client/Family Teaching

1. Take only as directed and do not stop abruptly as withdrawal may activate nausea and vomiting, gastritis, dizziness, tachycardia, headache, and insomnia.
2. Use caution as drug may cause drowsiness.
3. Wear protective clothing and sunscreens to prevent a photosensitivity reaction.
4. Drug may impair body temperature regulation so avoid temperature extremes.

Evaluation: Evaluate client for:
- Evidence of improved behavioral patterns
- Reports of a reduction in anxiety levels with depression
- ↓ reports of sleep disturbances

Thiotepa

(thigh-oh-**TEP**-ah)
(Abbreviation: Thio) (Rx)

See also *Antineoplastic Agents,* p. 85, and *Alkylating Agents,* p. 20.

Classification: Antineoplastic, alkylating agent.

Action/Kinetics: Thiotepa is cell-cycle nonspecific; it is thought to act by causing the release of ethylenimmonium ions that bind or alkylate various intracellular substances such as nucleic acids. The drug is cytotoxic by virtue of cross-linking of DNA and RNA strands as well as by inhibition of protein synthesis. It is cleared rapidly from the plasma following IV use. Thiotepa may be significantly absorbed through the bladder mucosa. Approximately 85% is excreted through the urine, mainly as metabolites.

Uses: Adenocarcinoma of the breast or ovary. Control of serious effusions of pleural, pericardial, and peritoneal cavities. Superficial papillary carcinoma of the urinary bladder. Hodgkin's and non-Hodgkin's disease, lymphosarcoma, bronchogenic carcinoma. *Investigational:* Prevention of pterygium recurrences after surgery.

Contraindications: Use during lactation. Pregnancy. Renal, hepatic, or bone marrow damage. Acute leukemia. Use with other alkylating agents due to increased toxicity.

Special Concerns: Thiotepa is both carcinogenic and mutagenic.

Additional Side Effects: Anorexia or decreased spermatogenesis. Significant toxicity to the hematopoietic system. *Symptoms of Overdose:* Hematopoietic toxicity.

Drug Interaction: Thiotepa increases the pharmacologic and toxic effect of succinylcholine due to a decrease in breakdown by the liver.

Dosage: IV (may be rapid): 0.3–0.4 mg/kg at 1- to 4-week intervals or 0.2 mg/kg for 4–5 days q 2–4 weeks. **Intratumor or intracavitary administration:** 0.6–0.8 mg/kg q 1–4 weeks; **maintenance (intratumor):** 0.07–0.8 mg/kg at 1- to 4-week intervals, depending on condition of client. *Carcinoma of bladder:* 30–60 mg in 30–60 ml distilled water instilled into the bladder and retained for 2 hr. Give once a week for 4 weeks. May be repeated monthly, if necessary.

NURSING CONSIDERATIONS

See also *Nursing Considerations for Antineoplastic Agents,* p. 88.

Administration/Storage

1. Reconstitute with sterile water for injection (usually 1.5 ml to give a concentration of 5 mg/0.5 ml). The reconstituted solution can then be mixed with sodium chloride injection, dextrose injection, dextrose and sodium chloride injection, Ringer's injection, or lactated Ringer's injection (i.e., if a large volume is needed for intracavitary use, IV drip, or perfusion).
2. Minimize pain on injection and retard rate of absorption by simultaneous administration of local anesthetics. Drug may be mixed with procaine HCl 2% or epinephrine HCl 1:1,000, or both, upon order of the physician.
3. Store vials in the refrigerator. Reconstituted solutions may be stored for 5 days in the re-

frigerator without substantial loss of potency.

4. Since thiotepa is not a vesicant, it may be injected quickly and directly into the vein with the desired volume of sterile water. Usual amount of diluent is 1.5 ml.

5. Do not use normal saline as a diluent.

6. Discard solutions grossly opaque or with precipitate.

7. When used for bladder carcinoma, the client is dehydrated for 8–12 hr prior to each dose.

8. When used for intracavitary purposes, administer through the same tube used to remove fluid from the cavity.

9. *Treatment of Overdose:* To treat hematopoietic toxicity, transfusions of whole blood, platelets, or leukocytes have been used.

Interventions

1. Encourage clients who receive drug as bladder instillations to retain fluid for 2 hr.

2. Reposition client with a bladder instillation every 15 min to ensure maximum contact.

3. Stress importance of practicing contraception because drug is carcinogenic and mutagenic.

Evaluation: Evaluate client for evidence of control of tumor size and spread.

Thiothixene

(thigh-oh-**THICKS**-een)
Navane (Rx)

See also *Phenothiazines,* p. 201.

Classification: Antipsychotic, thioxanthine derivative.

Action/Kinetics: The antipsychotic action is due to blockade of postsynaptic dopamine receptors in the brain. Thiothixene causes significant extrapyramidal symptoms and antiemetic effects; minimal sedation, orthostatic hypotension, and anticholinergic effects. Its actions closely resemble those of chlorprothixene with respect to postural reflexes and motor coordination. The margin between a therapeutically effective dose and one that causes extrapyramidal symptoms is narrow. **Peak plasma levels, PO:** 1–3 hr. **t½:** 34 hr. **Therapeutic plasma levels** (during chronic treatment): 10–150 ng/ml.

Uses: Symptomatic treatment of acute and chronic schizophrenia, especially when condition is accompanied by florid symptoms.

Special Concerns: Safe use during pregnancy has not been established. Dosage has not been established for children under 12 years of age. Children are more prone to develop neuromuscular and extrapyramidal side effects (especially dystonias). Adolescents may experience a higher incidence of hypotensive and extrapyramidal reactions than adults. Geriatric clients may be more prone to orthostatic hypotension and manifest an increased sensitivity to tardive dyskinesia and Parkinson-like symptoms. Geriatric or debilitated clients usually require a lower starting dose.

Side Effects: See *Chlorprothixene,* p. 437.

Drug Interactions: See *Chlorprothixene,* p. 437.

Laboratory Test Interference: ↓ Serum uric acid.

Dosage: Capsules, Oral Solution. *Antipsychotic:* **Adults and**

adolescents, initial, 2 mg t.i.d. for mild conditions and 5 mg b.i.d. for severe conditions; can be increased gradually to usual maintenance dose of 20–30 mg/day, although some clients require 60 mg/day. **IM.** *Antipsychotic:* **Adults and adolescents:** 4 mg b.i.d.–q.i.d.; **usual maintenance:** 16–20 mg/day, although up to 30 mg/day may be required in some cases. Switch to **PO** form as soon as possible. **Not recommended for children under 12 years of age.**

NURSING CONSIDERATIONS

See also *Nursing Considerations* for *Phenothiazines,* p. 205.

Administration/Storage

1. The powder for injection can be reconstituted by adding 2.2 ml of sterile water for injection.
2. Thiothixene is well absorbed.

Client/Family Teaching: Review the purpose and goals of drug therapy. Discuss the responses client can anticipate, depending upon the method of administration:

- Advise and assess behavior for a therapeutic response in 1–6 hr after an IM injection.
- Oral medications will require several days to observe therapeutic effects.

Evaluation: Evaluate client for:

- Reports of a reduction in psychotic ideations
- Laboratory confirmation that drug levels are within desired range (10–150 ng/ml)

Thyroglobulin
(thigh-roh-**GLOB**-you-lin)
Proloid (Rx)

See also *Thyroid Drugs,* p. 235.

Classification: Thyroid preparation.

General Statement: Thyroid preparation containing levothyroxine (T_4) and liothyronine (T_3) in a ratio of 2.5 to 1. Drug is a natural product purified from hog thyroid glands. It has no clinical advantage over thyroid especially because the product contains varying amounts of the hormones. It has a slow onset of action that makes it unsuitable for the treatment of myxedematous coma.

Contraindications: Use for suppression therapy.

Dosage: Tablets. *Hypothyroidism without myxedema, pediatric hypothyroidism:* **Adults, children, initial,** 32 mg, increased gradually at 1- to 2-week intervals until control is established. **Usual maintenance:** 65–160 mg daily. Therapy is aimed at maintaining a level of 5–9 mcg/100 ml protein-bound iodine. *Myxedema or hypothyroidism with cardiovascular disease, cretinism or severe hypothyroidism:* **Adults, initial,** 16–32 mg daily; **then,** the dose can be doubled q 2 weeks until the desired effect is obtained. **Usual maintenance:** 65–160 mg daily. Transfer from and to sodium liothyronine should be made gradually.

NURSING CONSIDERATIONS

See *Nursing Considerations* for *Thyroid Drugs,* p. 237.

Thyroid, desiccated
(**THIGH**-royd)
Armour Thyroid, S-P-T, Thyrar, Thyroid Strong(Rx)

See also *Thyroid Drugs,* p. 235.

Classification: Thyroid preparation.

Action/Kinetics: These products are comprised of desiccated thyroid glands from bovine and porcine sources. Due to variable content of both levothyroxine and liothyronine in the product, fluctuations in plasma levels of these hormones will be observed. The drug has a slow onset of action that makes it unsuitable for the treatment of myxedematous coma. **Note:** Thyroid Strong is 50% stronger than thyroid USP (each grain is equivalent to 1.5 grains of thyroid USP).

Dosage: Tablets. *Hypothyroidism without myxedema, pediatric hypothyroidism:* **Adults, children, initial,** 30 mg daily; **then,** increase by 15 mg q 2–3 weeks until the desired effect is reached. **Usual maintenance:** 60–120 mg daily. *Myxedema, hypothyroidism with cardiovascular disease, cretinism or severe hypothyroidism:* **Adults, children, initial,** 15 mg daily; **then** increase to 30 mg after 2 weeks and to 60 mg daily after an additional 2 weeks. The client should be evaluated carefully after 30 and 60 days of treatment. If required, the dose can be further increased to 120 mg daily. **Usual maintenance:** 50–120 mg daily. *Congenital hypothyroidism:* **Over 12 years of age,** Over 90 mg/day (1.2–1.8 mg/kg/day); **6–12 years:** 60–90 mg/day (2.4–3 mg/kg/day); **1–5 years:** 45–60 mg/day (3–3.6 mg/kg/day); **6–12 months:** 30–45 mg/day (3.6–4.8 mg/kg/day); **up to 6 months:** 15–30 mg/day (4.8–6 mg/kg/day).

NURSING CONSIDERATIONS

See also *Nursing Considerations* for *Thyroid Drugs,* p. 237.

Administration/Storage

1. Store protected from moisture and light.
2. In geriatric clients, the initial dose should be 7.5–15 mg daily which can then be doubled q 6–8 weeks until desired effect has been attained.
3. Transfer from liothyronine: Start thyroid several days before withdrawal. When transferring from thyroid, discontinue thyroid before starting with low daily dose of replacement drug.

Evaluation: Evaluate client for:
- Evidence of a reduction in S&S of hypothyroidism as manifested by weight loss, ↑ heart rate, and energy levels and improved texture of skin and hair
- Laboratory evidence that T_3 and T_4 levels are within desired range

Thyrotropin
(thigh-roh-**TROH**-pin)
Thytropar, Thyroid Stimulating Hormone, TSH (Rx)

Classification: Thyroid preparation.

Action/Kinetics: Highly purified thyroid-stimulating hormone from bovine pituitary glands. Thyrotropin administration results in increased iodine uptake by the thyroid gland and increased formation and release of thyroid hormone. **Onset:** Within a few minutes. **Peak effect:** 1–2 days. **Duration:** Drug effects are terminated after the drug is withdrawn.

Uses: Diagnostic agent to evaluate thyroid function.

Contraindications: Untreated Addison's disease, coronary thrombosis.

Special Concerns: Safe use in pregnancy (category: C), lactation, or children has not been established. Use with caution in clients with cardiac disease who cannot withstand stress.

Side Effects: *CV:* Tachycardia, hypotension. *GI:* Nausea, vomiting. *Miscellaneous:* Swelling of thyroid gland, urticaria, headache, anaphylaxis.

Dosage: IM, SC: Administer 10 IU daily for 1–3 days followed by radioiodine uptake study within 24 hours. **Note:** No response will occur if there is thyroid failure; however, a significant response will result in pituitary failure.

NURSING CONSIDERATIONS

See also *Nursing Considerations* for *Thyroid Drugs,* p. 237.

Administration/Storage: The reconstituted solution may be stored in the refrigerator but for no longer than 2 weeks.

Assessment

1. Note any client history of coronary heart disease and document.
2. Assess for any history or evidence of hypopituitarism or untreated Addison's disease as drug would be contraindicated in this instance.

Interventions

1. Monitor vital signs and observe closely for evidence of allergic reactions.
2. Document and report immediately any evidence of urticaria,

swelling of the thyroid gland, client complaint of headaches, and symptoms of anaphylaxis.
3. Normal thyroid tissue responds to thyrotropin by ↑ uptake of iodine and by releasing thyroxine and triiodothyronine. This drug therefore tests the ability of the thyroid to respond to appropriate stimulation.

Evaluation: Assess for effective thyroid function evaluation and the diagnosis of hypothyroidism.

Ticarcillin disodium
(tie-kar-**SILL**-in)
Ticar (Rx)

See also *Anti-Infectives,* p. 80, and *Penicillins,* p. 197.

Classification: Antibiotic, penicillin.

Action/Kinetics: This drug is a parenteral, semisynthetic antibiotic with an antibacterial spectrum of activity resembling that of carbenicillin. Primarily suitable for treatment of gram-negative organisms, but also effective for mixed infections. Combined therapy with gentamicin or tobramycin is sometimes indicated for treatment of *Pseudomonas* infections. *The drugs should not be mixed during administration because of gradual mutual inactivation.* **Peak plasma levels: IM,** 25–35 mcg/ml after 1 hr; **IV,** 15 min. **t½:** 70 min. Elimination complete after 6 hr.

Uses: Bacterial septicemia, skin and soft tissue infections, acute and chronic respiratory tract infections caused by susceptible strains of *Pseudomonas aeruginosa, Proteus,*

Escherichia coli, and other gram-negative organisms. GU tract infections caused by above organisms and by *Enterobacter* and *Streptococcus faecalis.* Anaerobic bacteria causing empyema, anaerobic pneumonitis, lung abscess, bacterial septicemia, peritonitis, intra-abdominal abscess, skin and soft tissue infections, salpingitis, endometritis, pelvic inflammatory disease, pelvic abscess. Ticarcillin may be used in infections in which protective mechanisms are impaired such as during use of oncolytic or immunosuppressive drugs or in clients with acute leukemia. Clients seriously ill should receive higher doses such as in serious urinary tract and systemic infections.

Additional Contraindications: Pregnancy.

Special Concerns: Use with caution in presence of impaired renal function and for clients on restricted salt diets.

Additional Side Effects: Neurotoxicity and neuromuscular excitability, especially in clients with impaired renal function. Elevated alkaline phosphatase, AST, and ALT values.

Additional Drug Interactions: Effect of carbenicillin may be enhanced when used in combination with gentamicin or tobramycin for *Pseudomonas* infections.

Dosage: IV infusion, direct IV, IM. *Bacterial septicemia, intra-abdominal infections, skin and soft tissue infections, infections of the female genital system and pelvis, respiratory tract infections:* **Adults,** 200–300 mg/kg daily by IV infusion in divided doses q 3, 4, or 6 hr, depending on the severity of the infection; **pediatric, less than 40 kg,** 200–300 mg/kg daily by IV infusion q 4 or 6 hr (daily dose should not exceed the adult dose). *Urinary tract infections, uncomplicated:* **Adults,** 1 g IM or direct IV q 6 hr; **pediatric, less than 40 kg,** 50–100 mg/kg daily IM or direct IV in divided doses q 6 or 8 hr. *Urinary tract infections, complicated:* 150–200 mg/kg daily by IV infusion in divided doses q 4 or 6 hr (usual dose is 3 g q.i.d. for a 70-kg client). *Neonates with sepsis due to Pseudomonas, Proteus, or E. coli:* **less than 7 days of age and less than 2 kg,** 75 mg/kg q 12 hr; **more than 7 days of age and less than 2 kg,** 75 mg/kg q 8 hr; **less than 7 days of age and more than 2 kg,** 75 mg/kg q 8 hr; **more than 7 days of age and more than 2 kg,** 100 mg/kg q 8 hr. Can be given IM or by IV infusion over 10–20 min. Clients with renal insufficiency should receive a loading dose of 3 g **IV,** and subsequent doses, as indicated by creatinine clearance.

NURSING CONSIDERATIONS

See also *Nursing Considerations* for *Penicillins,* p. 200.

Administration/Storage

1. Discard unused reconstituted solutions after 24 hr when stored at room temperature and after 72 hr when refrigerated.
2. For IM use, reconstitute each g with 2 ml sterile water for injection, sodium chloride injection, or 1% lidocaine HCl (without epinephrine) to prevent pain and induration. The

reconstituted solution should be used quickly and should be injected well into a large muscle.

3. For IV use, reconstitute each g with 4 ml of the desired solution. Administer slowly to prevent vein irritation and phlebitis. A dilution of 1 g/20 ml (or more) will decrease the chance of vein irritation.

4. For an IV infusion, use 50 ml or 100 ml *ADD-Vantage* container of either 5% dextrose in water or sodium chloride injection and give by intermittent infusion over 30–120 min in equally divided doses.

5. Do not administer more than 2 g of the drug in each IM site.

6. Children weighing over 40 kg should receive the adult dose.

7. Ticarcillin should not be mixed together with amikacin, gentamicin, or tobramycin due to the gradual inactivation of these aminoglycosides.

8. Anticipate reduced dose with liver or renal dysfunction.

Interventions

1. Note client on high doses of drug for signs of electrolyte imbalance, especially sodium and potassium levels.

2. Assess bleeding times, liver and renal function studies, which should be monitored during therapy.

Client/Family Teaching

1. Report any symptoms of bleeding abnormalities, such as petechiae, ecchymosis, or frank bleeding.

2. Observe for edema, weight gain, or respiratory distress and report. This may be precipitated by large sodium content in the drug.

3. Provide a printed list of drug side effects that should be reported to the physician should they occur.

Evaluation: Evaluate client for:
- Laboratory evidence of negative culture reports
- Clinical evidence and reports of symptomatic improvement

―――― *COMBINATION DRUG* ――――
Ticarcillin disodium and Clavulanate potassium
(tie-kar-**SILL**-in, klav-you-**LAN**-ate poe-**TASS**-ee-um)
Timentin (Rx)

See also *Ticarcillin,* p. 1211, and *Penicillins,* p. 197.

Classification: Antibiotic, penicillin.

Action/Kinetics: This preparation contains clavulanic acid, which protects the breakdown of ticarcillin by beta-lactamase enzymes, thus ensuring appropriate blood levels of ticarcillin.

Uses: Complicated and uncomplicated urinary tract infections; infections of the bones and joints, lower respiratory tract, skin and skin structures; gynecologic infections, bacterial septicemia. In combination with an aminoglycoside for certain *Pseudomonas aeruginosa* infections.

Dosage: IV infusion. *Systemic and urinary tract infections:* **Adults more than 60 kg:** 3.1 g (containing 0.1 g clavulanic acid) q 4–6 hr for 10–14 days. **Adults less than 60 kg:** 200–300 mg ticarcillin/kg daily in divided doses q 4–6 hr for 10–14 days. *Gynecologic infections:* **Adults more than 60 kg, moderate infections:** 200 mg/kg/day in divided doses q 6 hr; **severe infections:** 300 mg/kg/day in divided doses q 4 hr. *In renal insufficiency,* **initially,** loading dose of 3.1 g ticarcillin and 0.1 g clavulanic acid; **then,** dose based on creatinine clearance (see package insert).

NURSING CONSIDERATIONS

See also *Nursing Considerations* for *Penicillins,* p. 200, and *Ticarcillin disodium,* p. 1212.

Administration/Storage

1. To attain the appropriate dilution for 3.1 g ticarcillin and 0.1 g clavulanic acid, dilute with 13 ml of either sodium chloride injection or sterile water for injection. Further dilutions, if necessary, can be undertaken with 5% dextrose injection, lactated Ringer's injection, or sodium chloride injection.
2. The drugs should be administered over a period of 30 min, either through a Y-type IV infusion or by direct infusion.
3. This product is incompatible with sodium bicarbonate.
4. Dilutions with sodium chloride injection or lactated Ringer's injection may be stored at room temperature for 24 hr or refrigerated for 7 days. Dilutions with 5% dextrose injection are stable at room temperature for 12 hr or for 3 days if refrigerated.
5. If used with another anti-infective agent (e.g., an aminoglyco-

side), each drug should be given separately.

Ticlopidine hydrochloride
(tie-**KLOH**pih-deen)
Ticlid (Rx)

Classification: Platelet aggregation inhibitor.

Action/Kinetics: Ticlopidine irreversibly inhibits ADP-induced platelet-fibrinogen binding and subsequent platelet-platelet interactions. This results in inhibition of both platelet aggregation and release of platelet granule constituents as well as prolongation of bleeding time. **Peak plasma levels:** 2 hr. **Maximum platelet inhibition:** 8–11 days after 250 mg b.i.d. **Steady-state plasma levels:** 14–21 days. **$t^{1}/_{2}$, elimination:** 4–5 days. After discontinuing therapy, bleeding time and other platelet function tests return to normal within 14 days. The drug is rapidly absorbed; bioavailability is increased by food. Highly bound (98%) to plasma proteins. Extensively metabolized by the liver with approximately 60% excreted through the kidneys; 23% is excreted in the feces (with one-third excreted unchanged). Clearance of the drug decreases with age.

Uses: To reduce the risk of fatal or nonfatal thrombotic stroke in clients who have manifested precursors of stroke or who have had a completed thrombotic stroke. Due to the risk of neutropenia or agranulocytosis, use should be reserved for clients who are intolerant to aspirin therapy. *Investigational:* Chronic arterial occlusion, coronary artery bypass grafts, intermittent claudication, open heart surgery, primary glomerulonephritis, subarachnoid hemorrhage, sickle cell disease, uremic clients with AV shunts or fistulas.

Contraindications: In the presence of neutropenia and thrombocytopenia, hemostatic disorder, or active pathologic bleeding such as bleeding peptic ulcer or intracranial bleeding. Severe liver impairment. Lactation.

Special Concerns: Pregnancy category: B. Use with caution in clients with ulcers (i.e., where there is a propensity for bleeding). Reduced dosage should be considered in impaired renal function. Geriatric clients may be more sensitive to the effects of the drug. Safety and effectiveness have not been established in children less than 18 years of age.

Side Effects: *Hematologic:* Neutropenia, agranulocytosis, thrombocytopenia, pancytopenia, thrombotic thrombocytopenia purpura, immune thrombocytopenia, hemolytic anemia with recticulocytosis. *GI:* Diarrhea, nausea, vomiting, GI pain, dyspepsia, flatulence, anorexia, GI fullness. *Bleeding complications:* Ecchymosis, hematuria, epistaxis, conjunctival hemorrhage, GI bleeding, perioperataive bleeding, intracerebral bleeding (rare). *Dermatologic:* Maculopapular or urticarial rash, pruritus, urticaria. *CNS:* Dizziness, headache. *Neuromuscular:* Asthenia, systemic lupus erythematosus, peripheral neuropathy, arthropathy, myositis. *Miscellaneous:* Tinnitus, pain, allergic pneumonitis, vasculitis, hepatitis, cholestatic jaundice, nephrotic syndrome, hyponatremia, serum sickness.

Drug Interactions

Antacids / ↓ Plasma levels of ticlopidine
Aspirin / Ticlopidine ↑ the effect of aspirin on collagen-induced platelet aggregation
Cimetidine / ↓ Clearance of ticlopidine probably due to ↓ breakdown by liver
Digoxin / Slight ↓ in digoxin plasma levels
Theophylline / ↑ Plasma levels of theophylline due to ↓ clearance

Laboratory Test Interferences: ↑ Alkaline phosphatase, ALT, AST, serum cholesterol, and triglycerides.

Dosage: Tablets: 250 mg b.i.d.

NURSING CONSIDERATIONS

Administration/Storage

1. To increase bioavailability and decrease GI discomfort, ticlopidine should be taken with food or just after eating.
2. If a client is switched from an anticoagulant or fibrinolytic drug to ticlopidine, the former drug should be discontinued before initiation of ticlopidine therapy.
3. IV methylprednisolone (20 mg) may normalize prolonged bleeding times, usually within 2 hr.

Assessment

1. Note any history of liver disease, bleeding disorders, or ulcer disease.
2. Determine baseline CBC, PT, and PTT.

Client/Family Teaching

1. Take with food or after meals to minimize GI upset.
2. Advise that it may take clients

on ticlopidine longer than usual to stop bleeding; unusual bleeding should be reported to the physician. Clients should inform their physician and dentist they are taking ticlopidine.

3. Advise clients to brush their teeth with a soft bristle tooth brush, to use an electric razor for shaving, and to use caution and avoid injury as bleeding times may be prolonged.

4. During the first 3 months of therapy, neutropenia can occur, resulting in an increased risk of infection. Advise to report for scheduled blood tests to monitor. Instruct clients to contact their physician if any symptoms of infection occur (e.g., fever, chills, sore throat).

5. Report promptly to the physician any severe or persistent diarrhea, subcutaneous bleeding, skin rashes, or any evidence of cholestasis (e.g., yellow skin or sclera, dark urine, light-colored stools).

Evaluation: Evaluate client for evidence of successful pharmacologic prevention of a complete or recurrent cerebral thrombotic event.

Timolol maleate
(TIE-moh-lohl)
Apo-Timol✹, Apo-Timop✹, Blocadren, Timoptic, Timoptic in Acudose (Rx)

See also *Beta-Adrenergic Blocking Agents,* p. 113.

Classification: Ophthalmic agent, beta-adrenergic blocking agent.

Action/Kinetics: Timolol exerts both beta-1 and beta-2 adrenergic blocking activity. Timolol has minimal sympathomimetic effects, direct myocardial depressant effects, and local anesthetic action. It does not cause pupillary constriction or night blindness. The mechanism of the protective effect in myocardial infarction is not known. **Peak plasma levels:** 1–2 hr. **t½:** 4 hr. Metabolized in the liver. Metabolites and unchanged drug excreted through the kidney.

Timolol also reduces both elevated and normal intraocular pressure, whether or not glaucoma is present; it is thought to act by reducing aqueous humor formation and/or by slightly increasing outflow of aqueous humor. The drug does not affect pupil size or visual acuity. For use in eye: **Onset:** 30 min. **Maximum effect:** 1–2 hr. **Duration:** 24 hr.

Uses: **Tablets:** Hypertension (alone or in combination with other antihypertensives such as thiazide diuretics). Within 1–4 weeks of myocardial infarction to reduce risk of reinfarction. Prophylaxis of migraine. *Investigational:* Ventricular arrhythmias and tachycardias, essential tremors.

Ophthalmic solution: Chronic open-angle glaucoma, selected cases of secondary glaucoma, ocular hypertension, aphakic (no lens) clients with glaucoma.

Contraindications: Hypersensitivity to drug.

Special Concerns: Use ophthalmic preparation with caution in clients for whom systemic beta-adrenergic blocking agents are contraindicated. Safe use during pregnancy (category: C) and in children not established.

Side Effects: *Systemic following use of tablets:* See *Beta-Adrenergic Blocking Agents,* p. 113.

Following use of ophthalmic product: Few. Occasionally, ocular irritation, local hypersensitivity reactions, slight decrease in resting heart rate.

Drug Interactions: When used ophthalmically, possible potentiation with systemically administered beta-adrenergic blocking agents.

Laboratory Test Interferences: ↑ BUN, serum potassium, and uric acid. ↓ Hemoglobin and hematocrit.

Dosage: Tablets. *Hypertension:* **initial,** 10 mg b.i.d. alone or with a diuretic; **maintenance:** 20–40 mg/day (up to 80 mg/day in 2 doses may be required), depending on blood pressure and heart rate. If dosage increase is necessary, wait 7 days. *Myocardial infarction prophylaxis:* 10 mg b.i.d. *Migraine prophylaxis:* **initially,** 10 mg b.i.d. **Maintenance,** 20 mg daily given as a single dose; total daily dose may be increased to 30 mg in divided doses or decreased to 10 mg, depending on the response and client tolerance. If a satisfactory response for migraine prophylaxis is not obtained within 6–8 weeks using the maximum daily dose, the drug should be discontinued. *Glaucoma:* One drop of 0.25%–0.50% solution in each eye b.i.d.

NURSING CONSIDERATIONS

See also *Nursing Considerations* for *Beta-Adrenergic Blocking Agents,* p. 116, and *Antihypertensive Agents,* p. 78.

Administration/Storage

Ophthalmic Solution

1. When client is transferred from another antiglaucoma agent, continue old medication on day 1 of timolol therapy (one drop of 0.25% solution). Thereafter, discontinue former therapy. Initiate with 0.25% solution. Increase to 0.50% solution if response is insufficient. Further increases in dosage are ineffective.

2. When client is transferred from several antiglaucoma agents, the dose must be individualized. If one of the agents is a beta-adrenergic blocking agent, it should be discontinued before starting timolol. Dosage adjustments should involve one drug at a time at one week intervals. The antiglaucoma drugs should be continued with the addition of timolol, 1 gtt of 0.25% solution b.i.d. (if response is inadequate, 1 gtt of 0.5% solution may be used b.i.d.). The following day, one of the other antiglaucoma agents should be discontinued while the remaining agents should be continued or discontinued based on client response.

Client/Family Teaching

1. Review the appropriate procedure for ophthalmic administration. Have client or person administering therapy return demonstrate.

2. Instruct client to apply finger lightly to lacrimal sac for 1 min following administration.

3. Stress the importance of continued regular intraocular measurements by an ophthalmologist because ocular hypertension may recur and/or progress without overt signs or symptoms.

4. When timolol tablets are used for long-term prophylaxis

T

against myocardial infarction, do not interrupt therapy without consulting with the prescribing physician. Abrupt withdrawal may precipitate re-infarction. Advise to report any evidence of rash, dizziness, heart palpitations, or depression.

5. Drug may cause dizziness. Do not perform tasks such as driving or operating machinery until drug effects are realized.

6. Clients with diabetes should be advised that drug may mask some symptoms of hypoglycemia so careful monitoring of glucose levels is imperative.

7. Drug may cause increased sensitivity to cold; advise to dress appropriately.

Evaluation: Evaluate client for:
- Evidence of a reduction in blood pressure
- Successful prevention of re-infarction following a heart attack
- Reports of prophylaxis of migraine
- Evidence of ↓ intraocular pressure (ophthalmic solution)

Tioconazole
(tie-oh-**KON**-ah-zohl)
Vagistat (Rx)

Classification: Antifungal, vaginal.

Action/Kinetics: The antifungal activity of tioconazole is thought to be due to alteration of the permeability of the cell membrane of the fungus, causing leakage of essential intracellular compounds. The systemic absorption of the drug in nonpregnant clients is negligible.

Uses: Local treatment of *Candida albicans* infections of the vulva and vagina. Also effective against *Torulopsis glabrata*.

Contraindications: Use of a vaginal applicator during pregnancy may be contraindicated.

Special Concerns: Pregnancy category: C. Safety and effectiveness have not been determined during lactation or in children.

Side Effects: *GU:* Burning, itching, irritation, vulvar edema and swelling, discharge, vaginal pain, dysuria, dyspareunia, nocturia, desquamation, dryness of vaginal secretions.

Dosage: Vaginal Ointment, 6.5%. One applicatorful (about 5 g) should be inserted intravaginally at bedtime for 3 days. If needed, the treatment period can be extended to 6 days.

NURSING CONSIDERATIONS

Assessment

1. Obtain a thorough nursing history. Clients who do not respond to treatment may have unrecognized diabetes mellitus. Urine and blood glucose studies should be undertaken.

2. *Any persistent resistant infection may be due to reinfection; therefore the sources of infection should be carefully evaluated.*

Interventions: Obtain appropriate lab studies as ordered, prior to initiating therapy.

Client/Family Teaching

1. Demonstrate the appropriate method for administration (the cream should be inserted high into the vagina).

2. Use the medication just prior to bedtime.
3. Report if any burning, irritation, or pain occurs.
4. Medication may stain clothes; use sanitary napkins during therapy and change frequently because damp sanitary napkins may harbor infecting organisms.
5. To avoid reinfection, the client should refrain from sexual intercourse, or the partner should be advised to use a condom.
6. Continue to take medication for prescribed time frame even if symptoms subside.
7. The drug should continue to be used during menses to ensure a full course of therapy. Effectiveness is not altered by menstruation.

Evaluation

1. Obtain appropriate lab data to evaluate response to treatment and to determine the need to extend therapy.
2. Evaluate client for reports of symptomatic improvement.

Tiopronin
(tie-oh-**PROH**-nin)
Thiola (Rx)

Classification: Prevention of cystinuria.

Action/Kinetics: Tiopronin undergoes thiol-disulfide exchange with cystine to form a tiopronin-cystine complex, thus reducing the levels of cystine, which is only sparingly soluble. Reducing cystine levels maintains cystine concentrations below the solubility limit in the urine, thus preventing formation of stones. Up to 48% of the

drug will appear in the urine in the first 4 hr following administration and up to 78% by 72 hr.

Uses: Prophylaxis of cystine stone formation. Usually reserved for clients with urinary cystine levels greater than 500 mg/day; those who are resistant to treatment with high fluid intake, alkali and diet modification; and, those who show adverse effects to d-penicillamine.

Contraindications: History of drug-induced agranulocytosis, aplastic anemia, or thrombocytopenia. Lactation.

Special Concerns: Use during pregnancy only if the benefits outweigh the potential risks (pregnancy category: C). Safety and efficacy have not been established in children less than 9 years of age.

Side Effects: *Dermatologic:* Generalized rash—erythematous, maculopapular, morabilliform—accompanied by pruritus. Wrinkling and friability of skin. *Miscellaneous:* Drug fever, lupus erythematosus-like reaction, hypogeusia, vitamin B_6 deficiency.

Dosage: Tablets. Adults, initial, 800 mg daily in clients with cystine stones; **children,** 15 mg/kg/day. **Maintenance:** Depends on urinary cystine levels and should be based on the dosage required to decrease urinary cystine levels to below its solubility limit (usually <250 mg/ L).

NURSING CONSIDERATIONS

Administration/Storage

1. A conservative program including large amounts of fluid and a modest amount of alkali (to maintain urinary pH from 6.5–7) in the diet should be tried prior to initiating tiopronin therapy.

2. Maintenance dosage should be given t.i.d. at least 1 hr before or 2 hr after meals.

Assessment

1. Note urinary pH and cystine level prior to initiating therapy.
2. Obtain baseline CBC and liver function studies.

Interventions

1. Monitor and record urinary pH during drug therapy.
2. Measure I&O and promote a high fluid intake.
3. Urinary cystine should be measured 1 month after initiation of therapy and every 3 months thereafter.

Client/Family Teaching

1. Take tiopronin only as prescribed on an empty stomach 1 hr before or 2 hr after meals.
2. Stress the importance of reporting for follow-up lab studies because the dose of drug may need to be adjusted by the physician.
3. Provide a printed list and advise the client to report any adverse side effects. Symptoms such as fever, chills, sore throat, or excessive bleeding and bruising may necessitate the discontinuation of drug therapy.
4. Drink plenty of fluids (2 L/day) during drug therapy. Encourage client to maintain a record of I&O and daily urine pH levels to share with the physician.

Evaluation: Evaluate client for:
• Laboratory confirmation of a significant decrease in urinary cystine levels

• Successful prevention of cystine stone formation
• Freedom from complications of adverse drug side effects

Tobramycin sulfate
(toe-brah-**MY**-sin)
Nebcin, Tobrex Ophthalmic (Rx)

See also *Aminoglycosides,* p. 23.

Classification: Antibiotic, aminoglycoside.

Action/Kinetics: This aminoglycoside is similar to gentamicin and can be used concurrently with carbenicillin. **Therapeutic serum levels: IM,** 4–8 mcg/ml. **t½:** 2–2.5 hr.

Additional Uses: Meningitis; neonatal sepsis. **Ophthalmic:** Eye infections due to *Staphylococcus, Streptococcus, Escherichia coli, Hemophilus aegyptius, Hemophilus influenzae, Klebsiella pneumoniae, Neisseria, Proteus, Acinetobacter calcoaceticus, Enterobacter aerogenes, Moraxella lacunata,* and *Pseudomonas aeruginosa.* Corneal ulcers.

Contraindications: Ophthalmically to treat dendritic keratitis, vaccinia, varicella, fungal or mycobacterial eye infections, after removal of a corneal foreign body. Lactation.

Special Concerns: Pregnancy category: D. Use with caution in premature infants and neonates. Ophthalmic ointment may retard corneal epithelial healing.

Additional Side Effects: *Symptoms of overdose when used ophthalmically:* Edema, lid itching, punctate keratitis, erythema, lacrimation.

T

Additional Drug Interactions:
With carbenicillin or ticarcillin, tobramycin may have an increased effect when used for *Pseudomonas* infections.

Dosage: IM, IV. Adults: 3 mg/kg/day in 3 equally divided doses q 8 hr; *for life-threatening infections:* up to 5 mg/kg/day in 3 or 4 equal doses. **Pediatric:** Either 2–2.5 mg/kg q 8 hr or 1.5–1.9 mg/kg q 6 hr; **neonates 1 week of age or less:** up to 4 mg/kg/day in 2 equal doses q 12 hr. *Impaired renal function:* **initially,** 1 mg/kg; **then,** maintenance dose calculated according to information supplied by manufacturer.
   Ophthalmic Solution. *Acute infections:* **initial,** 1–2 gtt q 15–30 min until improvement noted; **then,** reduce dosage gradually. *Moderate infections:* 1–2 gtt 2–6 times/day. **Ophthalmic Ointment.** *Acute infections:* 0.5-inch ribbon q 3–4 hr until improvement is noted. *Mild to moderate infections:* 0.5-inch ribbon b.i.d.–t.i.d.

NURSING CONSIDERATIONS

See also *Nursing Considerations* for *Aminoglycosides,* p. 25.

Administration/Storage

1. Prepare IV solution by diluting calculated dose of tobramycin with 50–100 ml of IV solution.
2. Infuse over 20–60 min.
3. Use proportionately less diluent for children than for adults.
4. Do not mix with other drugs for parenteral administration.
5. Store drug at room temperature—no longer than 2 years.
6. Discard solution of drug containing up to 1 mg/ml after 24 hr at room temperature.

Client/Family Teaching

1. Provide a printed list of side effects that require reporting to the physician should they occur.
2. Drink plenty of fluids (2–3 L/day) during parenteral drug therapy.
3. With eye infections, avoid wearing contact lenses until infection is cleared and physician approves.
4. If symptoms do not improve or if they worsen after 3 days of therapy notify physician.

Evaluation: Evaluate client for:
- Laboratory evidence of negative culture reports
- Reports of symptomatic improvement

Tocainide hydrochloride
(toe-**KAY**-nyd)
Tonocard (Rx)

See also *Antiarrhythmic Drugs,* p. 51.

Classification: Antiarrhythmic, type IB.

Action/Kinetics: Tocainide, which is similar to lidocaine, decreases the excitability of cells in the myocardium. Tocainide increases pulmonary and aortic arterial pressure and slightly increases peripheral resistance. Is effective in both digitalized and nondigitalized clients. **Peak plasma levels:** 0.5–2 hr. **t½:** 15 hr. **Therapeutic serum levels:** 4–10 mcg/ml. **Duration:** 8 hr. Approximately 10% is bound to plasma protein. Forty percent is excreted unchanged in the urine.

Uses: Ventricular arrhythmias including premature ventricular contractions, unifocal or multifocal couplets, and ventricular tachycardia.

Contraindications: Allergy to amide-type local anesthetics, second- or third-degree AV block in the absence of artificial ventricular pacemaker.

Special Concerns: Safety during pregnancy (category: C) and lactation and in children has not been established. Geriatric clients may have an increased risk of dizziness and hypotension; the dose may have to be reduced in these clients due to age-related impaired renal function.

Side Effects: *CV:* Increased arrhythmias, increased ventricular rate, congestive heart failure, tachycardia, hypotension, conduction disturbances, bradycardia, chest pain, left ventricular failure. *CNS:* Lightheadedness, dizziness, vertigo, giddiness, headache, tremors, restlessness, confusion, disorientation, hallucinations, ataxia, paresthesias, numbness, nystagmus, drowsiness. *GI:* Nausea, vomiting, anorexia, diarrhea. *Hematologic:* Leukopenia, agranulocytosis, hypoplastic anemia, thrombocytopenia. *Other:* Pulmonary fibrosis, blurred vision, tinnitus, hearing loss, sweating, arthritis, myalgia, lupus-like syndrome.

Symptoms of Overdose: Initially are CNS symptoms including tremor (see above). GI symptoms may follow (see above).

Drug Interactions: Use with metaprolol may result in additive effects.

Dosage: Tablets. Adults, individualized, initial: 400 mg q 8 hr,

up to a maximum of 2,400 mg/day; **maintenance:** 1,200–1,800 mg daily in divided doses. Total daily dose of 1,200 mg may be adequate in clients with liver or kidney disease.

NURSING CONSIDERATIONS

See also *Nursing Considerations* for *Antiarrhythmic Drugs,* p. 52.

Administration/Storage: *Treatment of Overdose:* In the event of respiratory depression or arrest or seizures, maintain airway and provide artificial ventilation. An IV anticonvulsant may be required if seizures are persistent.

Client/Family Teaching

1. Take medication with meals or food to minimize GI upset.
2. Report any evidence of bruising, bleeding, or signs of infection such as fever, sore throat, or chills. These symptoms may indicate a blood dyscrasia.
3. Stress the importance of reporting for scheduled laboratory tests (CBC, hepatic and renal function) and follow-up visits.
4. Pulmonary symptoms such as wheezing, coughing, or dyspnea, should be reported immediately. These may indicate pulmonary fibrosis and in this case the drug must be discontinued.
5. Drug may cause drowsiness or dizziness. Do not drive or operate machinery until drug effects are realized.

Evaluation: Evaluate client for:
- ECG evidence of a decreased frequency of ventricular arrhythmias
- Laboratory confirmation that

serum drug levels are within therapeutic range (4–10 mcg/ml)

Tolazamide
(toll-**AZ**-ah-myd)
Tolamide, Tolinase (Rx)

See also *Antidiabetic Agents, Oral*, p. 65.

Classification: First-generation sulfonylurea.

Action/Kinetics: Drug is effective in some clients with a history of coma or ketoacidosis. Also, it may be effective in clients who do not respond well to other oral antidiabetic agents. Use with insulin is not recommended for maintenance. **Onset:** 4–6 hr. **t½:** 7 hr. **Time to peak levels:** 3–4 hr. **Duration:** 10 hr. Metabolized in liver to metabolites with minor hypoglycemic activity. Excreted through the kidneys (85%) and feces (7%).

Additional Contraindication: Renal glycosuria.

Special Concerns: Pregnancy category: C.

Additional Drug Interaction: Concomitant use of alcohol and tolazamide may → photosensitivity.

Dosage: PO. Adults, initial: 100 mg daily if fasting blood sugar is less than 200 mg/100 ml, or 250 mg daily if fasting blood sugar is greater than 200 mg/100 ml. Adjust dose to response not to exceed 1 g daily. If more than 500 mg daily is required, the dose should be given in 2 divided doses, usually before the morning and evening meals. **Elderly or debilitated clients:** 100 mg daily with breakfast, adjusting dose by increments of 50 mg daily each week. Doses greater than 1 g daily will probably not improve control.

NURSING CONSIDERATIONS

See also *Nursing Considerations* for *Antidiabetic Agents, Oral*, p. 68.

Client/Family Teaching

1. Avoid alcohol as a disulfiram-like reaction may occur.
2. Use caution as drug may cause dizziness.
3. Use a nonhormonal form of contraception.
4. Wear protective clothing and a sunscreen to prevent a photosensitivity reaction.

Evaluation: Evaluate client for laboratory evidence of control of serum glucose levels.

Tolbutamide
(toll-**BYOU**-tah-myd)
**APO-Tolbutamide ✚,
Mobenol ✚, Novo–Butamide ✚,
Oramide, Orinase (Rx)**

Tolbutamide sodium
(toll-**BYOU**-tah-myd)
Orinase Diagnostic (Rx)

See also *Antidiabetic Agents, Oral*, p. 65.

Classification: First-generation sulfonylurea.

Action/Kinetics: Onset: 1 hr. **t½:** 4.5–6.5 hr. **Time to peak levels:** 3–4 hr. **Duration:** 6–12 hr. Changed in liver to inactive metabolites. Excreted through the kidney (75%) and feces (9%).

Additional Uses: Most useful for clients with poor general physical status who should receive a short-acting compound.

Tolbutamide sodium is used to diagnose pancreatic islet cell tumors. It causes blood glucose, in the presence of a tumor, to drop quickly after IV administration and remain low for 3 hr.

Special Concerns: Pregnancy category: C.

Additional Side Effects: Melena (dark, bloody stools) in some clients with a history of peptic ulcer. Relapse or secondary failure may occur a few months after therapy has been started. May cause hyponatremia and a mild goiter.

Additional Drug Interactions

Alcohol / Photosensitivity reactions
Sulfinpyrazone / ↑ Effect of tolbutamide due to ↓ breakdown by liver

Dosage: PO. Adults, initial: 0.5–2 g/day; adjust dosage depending on response (usual maintenance: 0.25–3 g/day). Maximum daily dose should not exceed 3 g.

NURSING CONSIDERATIONS

See also *Nursing Considerations* for *Antidiabetic Agents, Oral,* p. 68.

Administration/Storage: Administered as a single dose before breakfast or as divided doses before the morning and evening meals.

Client/Family Teaching

1. Provide a printed list of adverse drug effects that require immediate reporting to the physician.
2. Avoid alcohol and OTC medication.
3. Drug may cause a photosensitivity reaction. Wear protective clothing and sunscreen when exposure to sunlight is necessary.
4. Use a nonhormonal form of birth control.

Evaluation: Evaluate client for laboratory evidence that blood sugar levels are within desired range.

Tolmetin sodium

(TOLL-met-in)

Tolectin✤, Tolectin 200, Tolectin 600, Tolectin DS (Rx)

See also *Nonsteroidal Anti-Inflammatory Drugs,* p. 186.

Classification: Nonsteroidal, anti-inflammatory, analgesic.

Action/Kinetics: Peak plasma levels: 30–60 min. **t½:** 1 hr. **Therapeutic plasma levels:** 40 mcg/ml. **Onset, anti-inflammatory effect:** within 1 week; **duration, anti-inflammatory effect:** 1–2 weeks. Inactivated in liver and excreted in urine.

Uses: Acute and chronic treatment of rheumatoid arthritis and osteoarthritis. Juvenile rheumatoid arthritis. *Investigational:* Sunburn.

Special Concerns: Pregnancy category: C. Use with caution during lactation. Dosage has not been determined in children less than 2 years of age.

Laboratory Test Interference: Tolmetin metabolites give a false + test for proteinuria using sulfosalicylic acid.

Dosage: Capsules, Tablets. Adults: *Rheumatoid arthritis, osteoarthritis:* **Adults:** 400 mg t.i.d. (one dose on arising and one at bedtime); adjust dosage according to client response. **Maintenance:** *rheumatoid arthritis,* 600–1,800 mg daily in 3–4 divided doses; *osteoarthritis,* 600–1,600 mg daily in 3–4 divided doses. Doses larger than 1,800 mg/day for rheumatoid arthritis and osteoarthritis are not recommended. *Juvenile rheumatoid arthritis:* **2 years and older, initial:** 20 mg/kg/day in 3–4 divided doses to start; **then,** 15–30 mg/kg/day. Doses higher than 30 mg/kg daily are not recommended. Beneficial effects may not be observed for several days to a week.

NURSING CONSIDERATIONS

See also *Nursing Considerations for Nonsteroidal Anti-Inflammatory Drugs,* p. 189.

Administration/Storage

1. Doses of medication should be spaced so that one dose is taken in the morning upon arising, one during the day, and one at bedtime.
2. If the client develops symptoms of gastric irritation, administer the drug with meals, milk, a full glass of water, or antacids (other than sodium bicarbonate).
3. Elderly clients are particularly susceptible to gastric irritation. Therefore, they should receive their medication with milk, meals, or an antacid.
4. Never administer the medication with sodium bicarbonate.
5. Use caution as drug may cause dizziness or drowsiness.
6. Avoid alcohol and any OTC medications without physician approval.

Evaluation: Evaluate client for reports of improvement in joint pain and mobility.

Tolnaftate
(toll-**NAF**-tayt)

Aftate for Athlete's Foot, Aftate for Jock Itch, Genaspor, NP-27, Pitrex✱, Quinsana Plus, Tinactin, Tinactin for Jock Itch, Ting, Zeasorb-AF (OTC)

See also *Anti-Infectives,* p. 80.

Classification: Topical antifungal.

Action/Kinetics: The exact mechanism is not known although the drug is thought to stunt mycelial growth causing a fungicidal effect.

Uses: Tinea pedis, tinea cruris, tinea corporis, and tinea versicolor. Fungal infections of moist skin areas.

Contraindications: Scalp and nail infections. *Avoid getting into eyes.*

Special Concerns: Should not be used in children less than 2 years of age.

Side Effects: Mild skin irritation.

Dosage: Topical: Aerosol Powder, Aerosol Solution, Cream, Gel, Powder, Solution. Spray Solution. Apply b.i.d. for 2–3 weeks although treatment for 4–6 weeks may be necessary in some instances.

NURSING CONSIDERATIONS

See also *General Nursing Considerations For All Anti-Infectives,* p. 83.

Interventions

1. The skin should be thoroughly cleaned and dried before the medication is applied.
2. Carefully inspect the source of infection and document because the choice of vehicle is important for effective therapy.
   • Powders are used in mild

conditions as adjunctive therapy.

- For primary therapy and prophylaxis, creams, liquids, or ointments are used, especially if the area is moist.
- Liquids and solutions are used if the area is hairy.

3. Obtain appropriate lab data because concomitant therapy should be used if bacterial or *Candida* infections are also present.

Client/Family Teaching

1. Demonstrate the appropriate technique for medication administration.
2. Use care when administering and do not inadvertently rub medication into eye.
3. Report any bothersome side effects; local relief of symptoms should be evident within the first 24–48 hr of therapy.
4. Continue to use as directed, despite improvement of symptoms.
5. Discontinue use if improvement is not noted within 10 days and notify physician.

Evaluation

1. Evaluate client for reports of improved skin lesions with evidence of healing.
2. Assess response to therapy and note any evidence of secondary infections that may necessitate additional treatment.

Tranexamic acid

(tran-ex-**AM**-ick)
Cyklokapron (Rx)

Classification: Hemostatic, systemic.

Action/Kinetics: Tranexamic acid acts by competitively inhibiting activation of plasminogen, thus decreasing the conversion of plasminogen to plasmin (the enzyme that breaks down fibrin clots). Up to 50% of an oral dose is absorbed from the GI tract; absorption is not affected by food. **Peak plasma levels:** 8 mg/L 3 hr after 1 g and 15 mg/L 3 hr after 2 g. **Effective tissue levels:** Maintained for 17 hr. **Effective serum levels:** Maintained for 7–8 hr. **t½:** 2 hr (after IV use of 1 g). Over 95% of the drug is excreted via the kidney unchanged.

Uses: Short-term (2–8 days) in hemophiliacs to reduce or prevent hemorrhage (and to decrease need for replacement therapy) during and following tooth extraction. *Investigational:* Postsurgical hemorrhage, hyperfibrinolysis-induced hemorrhage, hereditary angioedema.

Contraindications: Subarachnoid hemorrhage, acquired defective color vision.

Special Concerns: Pregnancy category: B (use during pregnancy only if necessary). Use with caution during lactation.

Side Effects: *GI:* Nausea, vomiting, diarrhea. *Ophthalmologic:* Visual abnormalities. *Other:* Hypotension following rapid IV injection, giddiness.

Dosage: *Hemophiliacs requiring tooth extraction:* **IV, immediately before surgery,** 10 mg/kg; **then, after surgery, tablets,** 25 mg/kg t.i.d.–q.i.d. for 2–8 days. **Alternative regimen: PO,** 25 mg/kg t.i.d.–q.i.d. one day prior to surgery. If client unable to take PO medication, give **IV,** 10 mg/kg t.i.d.–q.i.d.

NURSING CONSIDERATIONS

Administration/Storage

1. Tranexamic acid may be mixed with any of the following solutions for IV infusion: carbohydrate, amino acid, electrolyte, dextran.
2. The drug should *not* be mixed with either blood or penicillin.
3. The mixture should be prepared on the day of use.
4. Heparin may be added to the solution for injection.
5. To minimize hypotension, IV administration should not exceed 1 ml/min.
6. The dosage should be reduced in clients with moderately to severely impaired renal function according to information provided by the manufacturer.

Assessment

1. Determine client's blood pressure and pulse before starting IV infusion of drug to establish a baseline against which to measure findings during and after drug therapy.
2. Review client history and question client/family for evidence of defective color vision.
3. Assess for any evidence of nausea, vomiting, or diarrhea.
4. When working with female clients, check for potential pregnancy. With pregnancy, this drug should only be used if absolutely necessary.
5. Review appropriate baseline lab data, including CBC, PT/PTT, and blood factors.

Interventions

1. Monitor client frequently for hypotension during IV infusion, which indicates that the rate of infusion is too fast. Slow the rate of infusion and report to the physician.
2. Observe and report for signs and symptoms of thrombosis, such as leg pain, respiratory distress, or chest pain.
3. Anticipate reduced dosage in clients with impaired renal function.
4. Stress to client the importance of reporting for ophthalmologic examinations at regular intervals during drug therapy.

Evaluation: Evaluate client for:

- Clinical and laboratory evidence of control or prevention of hemorrhage
- Freedom from complications of drug therapy

Trazodone hydrochloride
(TRAYZ-oh-dohn)
Desyrel, Desyrel Dividose, Trazon, Trialodine (Rx)

Classification: Antidepressant, miscellaneous.

Action/Kinetics: Trazodone is a novel antidepressant that does not inhibit MAO and is also devoid of amphetamine-like effects. Response usually occurs after 2 weeks (75% of clients), with the remainder responding after 2–4 weeks. The drug may inhibit serotonin uptake by brain cells, therefore increasing serotonin concentrations in the synapse. It may also cause changes in binding of serotonin to receptors. The drug causes moderate sedative and orthostatic hypotensive effects and slight anticholinergic effects. **Peak plasma levels:** 1 hr (empty stomach). **t½:** initial, 3–6 hr; final, 5–9 hr. **Effective plasma**

T

levels: 800–1,600 ng/ml. Metabolized in liver and excreted through both the urine and feces.

Uses: Depression with or without accompanying anxiety. *Investigational:* In combination with tryptophan for treating aggressive behavior. Treatment of cocaine withdrawal. Chronic pain including diabetic neuropathy.

Contraindications: During the initial recovery period following myocardial infarction. Concurrently with electroshock therapy.

Special Concerns: Use with caution during pregnancy (category: C) and lactation. Safety and efficacy in children less than 18 years of age have not been established. Geriatric clients are more prone to the sedative and hypotensive effects.

Side Effects: *General:* Dermatitis, edema, blurred vision, constipation, dry mouth, nasal congestion, skeletal muscle aches and pains. *CV:* Hypertension or hypotension, syncope, palpitations, tachycardia, shortness of breath, chest pain. *GI:* Diarrhea, nausea, vomiting, bad taste in mouth, flatulence. *GU:* Delayed urine flow, priapism, hematuria, increased urinary frequency. *CNS:* Nightmares, confusion, anger, excitement, decreased ability to concentrate, dizziness, disorientation, drowsiness, lightheadedness, fatigue, insomnia, nervousness, impaired memory. Rarely, hallucinations, impaired speech, hypomania. *Other:* Incoordination, tremors, paresthesias, decreased libido, appetite disturbances, red eyes, sweating or clamminess, tinnitus, weight gain or loss, anemia, hypersalivation. Rarely, akathisia, muscle twitching, increased libido, impotence, retrograde ejaculation, early menses, missed periods.

Symptoms of Overdose: Respiratory arrest, seizures, ECG changes, hypotension, priapism as well as an increase in the incidence and severity of side effects noted above (vomiting and drowsiness are the most common).

Drug Interactions

Alcohol / ↑ Depressant effects of alcohol
Antihypertensives / Additive hypotension
Barbiturates / ↑ Depressant effects of barbiturates
Clonidine / Trazodone ↓ effect of clonidine
CNS depressants / ↑ CNS depression
Digoxin / Trazodone may ↑ serum digoxin levels
MAO inhibitors / Initiate therapy cautiously if trazodone is to be used together with MAO inhibitors
Phenytoin / Trazodone may ↑ serum phenytoin levels

Dosage: Tablets. Adults and adolescents, initial, 150 mg/day; **then,** increase by 50 mg/day every 3–4 days to maximum of 400 mg/day in divided doses (outpatients). Inpatients may require up to, but not exceeding, 600 mg/day in divided doses. **Maintenance:** Use lowest effective dose. **Geriatric clients:** 75 mg daily in divided doses; dose can then be increased, as needed and tolerated, at 3–4 day intervals.

NURSING CONSIDERATIONS

Administration/Storage

1. Dose should be initiated at the lowest possible level and increased gradually.
2. Beneficial effects may be observed within 1 week with

optimal effects in most clients seen within 2 weeks.

3. *Treatment of Overdose:* Treat symptoms (especially hypotension and sedation). Gastric lavage and forced diuresis to remove the drug from the body.

Assessment

1. Take a complete medication history, noting if the client is taking MAO inhibitors because trazodone could cause an unfavorable interaction.
2. Determine if the client is taking drugs to treat hypertension because trazodone may reduce the required dosage.
3. Note any history of recent myocardial infarction.
4. Obtain baseline CBC with differential and ECG with history of CV diseases.

Client/Family Teaching

1. Take with food to enhance absorption and minimize dizziness and/or lightheadedness.
2. To reduce side effects during the day, take major portion of dose at bedtime.
3. Use caution when driving or when performing other hazardous tasks because trazodone may cause drowsiness or dizziness.
4. Avoid alcohol and do not take any other depressant drugs during therapy with trazodone.
5. Encourage family to share responsibility for drug therapy to optimize treatment and to prevent overdosage.
6. Encourage family to observe closely for cues for suicide. Clients taking antidepressants and emerging from the deepest

phases of depression are more prone to suicide.
7. Inform physician if elective surgery is planned to minimize interaction of trazodone with anesthetic agent.
8. Provide a printed list of drug side effects. Advise client to report any persistent or bothersome side effects.
9. Advise client to use sugarless gum or candies and frequent mouth rinses to diminish the dry mouth effects.

Evaluation: Evaluate client for:
- Evidence of behaviors that reflect a decreased level of depression such as improved appetite, ability to sleep better, and increased social interactions
- Reports of symptomatic improvement

Tretinoin (Retinoic Acid, Vitamin A Acid)
(TRET-ih-noyn)
Retin—A, StieVAA ✱ (Rx)

Classification: Antiacne drug.

Action/Kinetics: Topical tretinoin is believed to decrease microcomedone formation by decreasing the cohesiveness of follicular epithelial cells. The drug is also believed to increase mitotic activity and increase turnover of follicular epithelial cells as well as decrease keratin synthesis. Some systemic absorption occurs (approximately 5% is recovered in the urine).

Uses: Acne vulgaris. *Investigational:* Lamellar ichthyosis, follicularis keratosis, verruca plana.

Contraindications: Eczema, sunburn.

Special Concerns: Use with caution during pregnancy (category: B) and lactation. Safety and effectiveness have not been determined in children.

Side Effects: *Dermatologic:* Red, edematous, crusted, or blistered skin; hyperpigmentation or hypopigmentation, increased susceptibility to sunlight.

Dosage: Apply cream, gel, or liquid lightly over the affected areas once daily at bedtime. Beneficial effects many not be seen for 2–6 weeks.

NURSING CONSIDERATIONS

Administration/Storage

1. The liquid should be applied carefully with the fingertip, cotton swab, or gauze pad only to affected areas.
2. Excessive amounts of the gel will cause a "pilling" effect.

Assessment: Note if the client is of childbearing age and sexually active. Determine if she is pregnant prior to initiating therapy.

Client/Family Teaching

1. Keep the medication away from mucous membranes, eyes, mouth, and the angles of the nose.
2. Explain that upon application there will be a transitory feeling of warmth and stinging. Advise that client may be more sensitive to wind and cold during therapy.
3. Explain that the client should expect dryness and peeling of skin from the affected areas.
4. Wash hands thoroughly before and immediately after applying tretinoin.
5. During the early weeks of therapy, the lesions may worsen. This is caused by the effect of the drug on deep lesions that had been previously undetected. If the lesions become severe, the client should notify the physician and anticipate that the drug will be discontinued until the integrity of the skin has been restored.
6. Advise women of childbearing age to practice some form of birth control while they are receiving drug therapy.
7. Avoid excessive exposure to sunlamps and to the sun. Persons who must be in sunlight while using the medication should be instructed to use a sunscreen or protective clothing over affected areas.

Evaluation: Evaluate client for:
- Reports of a reduction in the frequency and intensity of acne vulgaris eruptions
- Clinical evidence of healing and reports of symptomatic improvement

——— *COMBINATION DRUG* ———
Triavil
(TRY-ah-vill)
(Rx)

See also *Tricyclic Antidepressants,* p. 239, and *Phenothiazines,* p. 201.

Classification/Content: *Antidepressant:* Amitriptyline HCl, 10–50 mg. *Antipsychotic:* Perphenazine, 2–4 mg.

There are five different strengths of Triavil: Triavil 2–10, Triavil 2–25, Triavil 4–10, Triavil 4–25, and Triavil 4–50. **Note:** The first number refers to the number of milligrams of perphenazine and the second number refers to the number of milligrams of amitriptyline.

Uses: Moderate to severe anxiety and/or agitation and depressed mood. Depression where anxiety and/or agitation are severe. Depression and anxiety in association with chronic physical disease. Also schizophrenic clients with symptoms of depression.

Contraindications: Use during pregnancy and lactation and in children. CNS depression from drugs, in presence of bone marrow depression, use with MAO inhibitors, and during the acute recovery phase from myocardial infarction.

Dosage: Tablets. Adults, initial: One tablet of Triavil 2–25 or 4–25 t.i.d.–q.i.d. or one tablet of Triavil 4–50 b.i.d. Schizophrenic clients should receive an initial dose of two tablets of Triavil 4–25 t.i.d., with a fourth dose at bedtime, if necessary. Initial dosage for geriatric or adolescent clients in whom anxiety dominates is Triavil 4–10 t.i.d.–q.i.d., with dosage adjusted as required. **Maintenance:** One tablet Triavil 2–25 or 4–25 b.i.d.–q.i.d. or one tablet Triavil 4–50 b.i.d.

NURSING CONSIDERATIONS

See also *Nursing Considerations* for *Tricyclic Antidepressants,* p. 242, and *Phenothiazines,* p. 205.

Administration/Storage

1. Triavil is not recommended for children.
2. Total daily dosage of Triavil should not exceed four of the 4–50 tablets or eight tablets of all other dosage strengths.
3. The therapeutic effect may take up to several weeks to be manifested.
4. Once a satisfactory response has been observed, the dose should be reduced to the smallest amount required for relief of symptoms.

Evalation: Evaluate client for:
- Reports of a reduction in feelings of depression
- Evidence of behaviors that reflect a decreased level of anxiety and agitation in those with depression

―――― *COMBINATION DRUG* ――――
Tri-Levlen 21 Day and Tri-Levlen 28 Day
(try-**LEV**-len)
(Rx)

See also *Oral Contraceptives,* p. 192.

Classification: Triphasic combination oral contraceptive.

Components: Phase 1 (first 6 tablets): Each tablet of either Tri-Levlen 21 Day or 28 Day contains ethinyl estradiol, 30 mcg and levonorgestrel, 0.05 mg (brown tablets). Phase 2 (next 5 tablets): Each tablet contains ethinyl estradiol, 40 mcg and levonorgestrel, 0.075 mg (white tablets). Phase 3 (next 10 tablets): Each tablet contains ethinyl estradiol, 30 mcg and levonorgestrel, 0.125 mg (yellow tablets). Tri-Levlen 28 Day also contains 7 inert green tablets.

Special Concerns: Pregnancy category: X.

NURSING CONSIDERATIONS

See *Oral Contraceptives,* p. 192.

―――― *COMBINATION DRUG* ――――
Tri-Norinyl 21 Day and Tri-Norinyl 28 Day
(try-**NOR**-ih-nill)
(Rx)

See also *Oral Contraceptives,* p. 192.

Classification: Triphasic combination oral contraceptive.

Components: Phase 1 (first 7 tablets): Each tablet of either Tri-Norinyl 21 Day or 28 Day contains ethinyl estradiol, 35 mcg and norethindrone, 0.5 mg (blue tablets). Phase 2 (next 9 tablets): Each tablet contains ethinyl estradiol, 35 mcg and norethindrone, 1 mg (green tablets). Phase 3 (next 5 tablets): Each tablet contains ethinyl estradiol, 35 mcg and norethindrone, 0.5 mg (blue tablets). The 28s also contain 7 inert orange tablets.

Special Concerns: Pregnancy category: X.

NURSING CONSIDERATIONS

See *Oral Contraceptives,* p. 192.

Triamcinolone
(try-am-**SIN**-oh-lohn)
Dental Paste: Kenalog in Orabase, Oracort, Oralone (Rx).
Tablets: Aristocort, Atolone, Kenacort (Rx)

Triamcinolone acetonide
(try-am-**SIN**-oh-lohn)
Inhalation Aerosol: Azmacort, Nasacort (Rx). Parenteral: Cenocort A-40, Kenaject-40, Kenalog-10 and -40, Tac-3 and -40, Triam-A, Triamonide 40, Tri-Kort, Trilog (Rx). Topical Aerosol: Kenalog (Rx). Topical Cream: Aristocort, Aristocort A, Aristocort C✸, Aristocort D✸, Aristocort R✸, Delta-Tritex, Flutex, Kenac, Kenalog, Kenalog-H, Kenonel, Triacet, Triaderm✸, Trianide Mild, Trianide Regular, Triderm, Trymex (Rx). Topical Lotion: Kenalog, Kenonel (Rx). Topical

Ointment: Aristocort, Aristocort A, Aristocort D✸, Aristocort R✸, Kenac, Kenalog, Kenonel, Triaderm✸, Trymex (Rx)

Triamcinolone diacetate
(try-am-**SIN**-oh-lohn)
Parenteral: Amcort, Aristocort Forte, Aristocort Intralesional, Articulose LA., Cenocort Forte, Triam-Forte, Triamolone 40, Trilone, Tristoject (Rx). Kenacort Diacetate (Rx)

Triamcinolone hexacetonide
(try-am-**SIN**-oh-lohn)
Aristospan Intra-Articular, Aristospan Intralesional (Rx)

See also *Adrenocorticosteroids and Analogs,* p. 8.

Classification: Adrenocorticosteroid, synthetic.

Action/Kinetics: More potent than prednisone. Intermediate-acting. Has no mineralocorticoid activity. **Onset:** several hours. **Duration:** 1 or more weeks. **t½:** Over 200 min.

Additional Uses: Pulmonary emphysema accompanied by bronchospasm or bronchial edema. Diffuse interstitial pulmonary fibrosis. With diuretics to treat refractory CHF or cirrhosis of the liver with ascites. Multiple sclerosis. Inflammation following dental procedures. Triamcinolone hexacetonide is restricted to intra-articular or intralesional treatment of rheumatoid arthritis and osteoarthritis.

Special Concerns: Use during pregnancy only if benefits clearly outweigh risks. Use with special caution in clients who have decreased renal function or renal disease.

Additional Side Effects: Intra-articular, intrasynovial, or intrabursal administration may cause transient flushing, dizziness, local depigmentation, and, rarely, local irritation. Exacerbation of symptoms has also been reported. A marked increase in swelling and pain and further restricted joint movement may indicate septic arthritis. Intradermal injection may cause local vesicular ulceration and persistent scarring.

Syncope and anaphylactoid reactions have been reported with triamcinolone regardless of route of administration.

Dosage: *Highly individualized. Triamcinolone.* **Tablets.** *Adrenocortical insufficiency (with mineralocorticoid therapy):* 4–12 mg/day. *Acute leukemias (children):* 1–2 mg/kg. *Acute leukemia or lymphoma (adults):* 16–40 mg daily (up to 100 mg daily may be necessary for leukemia). *Edema:* 16–20 mg (up to 48 mg may be required). *Tuberculosis meningitis:* 32–48 mg daily. *Rheumatic disease, dermatologic disorders, bronchial asthma:* 8–16 mg daily. *Systemic lupus erythematosus:* 20–32 mg daily. *Allergies:* 8–12 mg daily. *Hematologic disorders:* 16–60 mg daily. *Ophthalmologic diseases:* 12–40 mg daily. *Respiratory diseases:* 16–48 mg.

Triamcinolone acetonide. **IM only (not for IV use):** *Systemic,* 2.5–60 mg daily, depending on the disease and its severity. **Intra-articular, intrabursal, tendon sheaths:** 2.5–5 mg for smaller joints and 5–15 mg for larger joints, although up to 40 mg has been used. **Intradermal:** 1 mg/injection site (use 3 mg/ml or 10 mg/ml suspension only). **Topical** (0.025%, 0.1%, 0.5% ointment or cream; 0.025%, 0.1% lotion; aerosol—to deliver 0.2 mg): Apply sparingly to affected area b.i.d.–q.i.d. and rub in lightly. **Respiratory inhalant. Adults, usual:** 2 inhalations (about 200 mcg) t.i.d.–q.i.d., not to exceed 1,600 mcg daily. High initial doses (1,200–1,600 mcg/day) may be needed in some clients with severe asthma. **Pediatric, 6–12 years:** 1–2 inhalations (100–200 mcg) t.i.d.–q.i.d., not to exceed 1,200 mcg daily. Use in children less than 6 years of age has not been determined. **Respiratory Spray.** *Seasonal and perennial allergic rhinitis:* **Adults and children over 12 years of age,** 2 sprays (110 mcg) into each nostril once a day (i.e., for a total dose of 220 mcg/day). The dose may be increased to 440 mcg daily given either once daily or q.i.d. (1 spray/nostril).

Triamcinolone diacetate. **IM only,** 40 mg weekly. **Intra-articular/intrasynovial:** 5–40 mg. **Intralesional/sublesional:** 5–48 mg (no more than 12.5 mg/injection site and 25 mg/lesion).

Triamcinolone hexacetonide. **Intra-articular:** 2–6 mg for small joints and 10–20 mg for large joints. **Intralesional/sublesional:** up to 0.5 mg/square inch of affected area. **Not for IV use.**

NURSING CONSIDERATIONS

See also *Nursing Considerations* for *Adrenocorticosteroids and Analogs,* p. 15.

Administration/Storage

1. Initially the aerosol should be used concomitantly with systemic steroid. After 1 week, a gradual withdrawal of systemic

steroid should be initiated. The next reduction should be made after 1–2 weeks, depending on the response. If symptoms of insufficiency occur, the dose of systemic steroid can be increased temporarily. Also, the dose of systemic steroid may need to be increased in times of stress or a severe asthmatic attack.

2. The acetonide products should not be used if they clump due to exposure to freezing temperatures.
3. A single IM dose of the diacetate provides control from 4–7 days up to 3–4 weeks.
4. Triamcinolone acetonide nasal spray for allergic rhinitis may be effective as soon as 12 hr after initiation of therapy. If improvement is not seen within 2–3 weeks, the client should be re-evaluated.

Client/Family Teaching

1. Ingest a liberal amount of protein because with this drug clients experience gradual weight loss, associated with anorexia, muscle wasting, and weakness. Refer to dietitian for assistance in meal planning and preparation.
2. Remind client to lie down if feeling faint. If syncopal episodes persist and interfere with daily activities, then report to physician.
3. Advise that drug may suppress reactions to skin allergy testing.
4. Report immediately any new onset of symptoms of depression as well as aggravation of existing symptoms.

Evaluation: Evaluate client for evidence of a reduction in immune and inflammatory responses in autoimmune disorders and allergic reactions.

Triamterene
(try-**AM**-ter-een)
Dyrenium (Rx)

See also *Diuretics,* p. 140.

Classification: Diuretic, potassium-sparing.

Action/Kinetics: Triamterene is a mild diuretic that acts directly on the distal tubule. It promotes the excretion of sodium—which is exchanged for potassium or hydrogen ions—bicarbonate, chloride, and fluid. The drug increases urinary pH. It is also a weak folic acid antagonist. **Onset:** 2–4 hr. **Peak effect:** 1 to several days. **Duration:** 7–9 hr. **t½:** 1.5–2 hr. From one-half to two-thirds of the drug is bound to plasma protein. About 20% is excreted unchanged through the urine. Triamterene is also found in Dyazide.

Uses: Edema due to congestive heart failure, hepatic cirrhosis, nephrotic syndrome, steroid therapy, secondary hyperaldosteronism. Also, idiopathic edema. May be used alone or with other diuretics. *Investigational:* Prophylaxis and treatment of hypokalemia, adjunct in the treatment of hypertension.

Contraindications: Hypersensitivity to drug, severe renal insufficiency, severe hepatic disease, anuria, hyperkalemia, hyperuricemia, gout, history of nephrolithiasis. Lactation.

Special Concerns: Pregnancy category: B. Safety and efficacy have not been determined in children.

Side Effects: *Electrolyte:* Hyperkalemia, electrolyte imbalance. *GI:* Nausea, vomiting (may also be indicative of electrolyte imbalance), diarrhea, dry mouth. *CNS:* Dizziness, drowsiness, fatigue, weakness, headache. *Hematologic:* Megaloblastic anemia, thrombocytopenia. *Miscellaneous:* Anaphylaxis, photosensitivity, hypokalemia, jaundice, muscle cramps, rash.

Symptoms of Overdose: Electrolyte imbalance, especially hyperkalemia. Also, nausea, vomiting, other GI disturbances, weakness, hypotension, reversible acute renal failure.

Drug Interactions

Amantadine / ↑ Toxic effects of amantadine due to ↓ renal excretion
Angiotensin-converting enzyme inhibitors / Significant hyperkalemia
Antihypertensives / Potentiated by triamterene
Captopril / ↑ Risk of significant hyperkalemia
Digitalis / Inhibited by triamterene
Indomethacin / ↑ Risk of nephrotoxicity
Lithium / ↑ Chance of lithium toxicity due to ↓ renal clearance
Potassium salts / Additive hyperkalemia
Spironolactone / Additive hyperkalemia

Laboratory Test Interference: Triamterene may impart blue fluorescence to urine, interfering with fluorometric assays (e.g., lactic dehydrogenase, quinidine).

Dosage: **Capsules, Tablets.** *Diuretic:* **Adults, initial:** 25–100 mg daily after meals; **maximum daily dose:** 300 mg. **Maintenance:** 100 mg q other day. **Pediatric:** 2–4 mg/kg (120 mg/m²) daily or on alternate days; **maintenance:** Up to 6 mg/kg daily to a maximum of 300 mg daily in divided doses.

NURSING CONSIDERATIONS

See also *Nursing Considerations* for *Diuretics,* p. 141.

Administration/Storage

1. Minimize nausea by giving the drug after meals.
2. Triamterene dosage is usually reduced by one-half when another diuretic is added to the regimen.
3. *Treatment of Overdose:* Immediately induce vomiting or perform gastric lavage. Electrolyte levels and fluid balance should be evaluated and treated if necessary. Dialysis may be beneficial.

Assessment

1. Take a complete drug history, noting drugs with which triamterene interacts.
2. Obtain baseline serum electrolytes, renal function studies, and uric acid levels before administering the drug.
3. Determine that a CBC with differential and an ECG have been performed prior to initiating therapy.

Interventions

1. Monitor serum electrolytes, BUN, uric acid, and CBC. Report any variations from the baseline studies to the physician.
2. If the client has a history of heart disease, obtain an ECG and be alert to the development of cardiac arrhythmias.
3. If the client has a history of alcoholism, megaloblastic ane-

T

mia may occur because triamterene is a weak antagonist of folic acid. Monitor the CBC and WBC differential periodically.

4. Observe for hyperkalemia; this is an indication to withdraw the drug because cardiac irregularities may result.

Client/Family Teaching

1. Take drug with food to minimize GI upset.
2. Report any symptoms of sore throat, rash, or fever. These may be signs of blood dyscrasias and may require the withdrawal of the drug.
3. Complaints of headache, drowsiness, vomiting, restlessness, mental wandering, lethargy, and foul breath should be reported immediately to the physician. These may be signs of uremia.
4. Avoid using potassium supplements, salt substitutes that contain potassium, and foods high in potassium because the drug is potassium-sparing.
5. Advise that urine may appear pale fluorescent blue and not to be alarmed.
6. Avoid direct sunlight for prolonged periods because drug may cause a photosensitivity reaction.

Evaluation: Evaluate client for:
- Evidence of ↓ edema
- Reports of ↑ diuresis

─── *COMBINATION DRUG* ───

Triamterene and Hydrochlorothiazide Capsules

(try-**AM**-ter-een, hy-droh-**klor**-oh-**THIGH**-ah-zyd)
Dyazide (Rx)

Triamterene and Hydrochlorothiazide Tablets

(try-**AM**-teh-reen, hy-droh-**kloh**-roh-**THIGH**-ah-zyd)
Apo-Triazide✲, Dyazide✲, Maxzide, Neo-Diurex✲, Novo-Triamzide✲ Nu-Triazide✲ (Rx)

See also *Triamterene,* p. 1234, and *Hydrochlorothiazide,* p. 718.

Classification/Content: Capsules. *Diuretic:* Hydrochlorothiazide, 25 or 50 mg. *Diuretic:* Triamterene, 50 or 100 mg. **Tablets.** *Diuretic:* Hydrochlorothiazide, 25 or 50 mg. *Diuretic:* Triamterene, 37.5 or 75 mg. (In Canada the tablets contain 25 mg of hydrochlorothiazide and 50 mg triamterene.)

Uses: To treat hypertension or edema in clients who manifest hypokalemia on hydrochlorothiazide alone. In clients requiring a diuretic and in whom hypokalemia cannot be risked (i.e., clients with cardiac arrhythmias or those taking digitalis). Usually not the first line of therapy, except for clients in whom hypokalemia should be avoided.

Contraindications: Clients receiving other potassium-sparing drugs such as amiloride and spironolactone. Use in anuria, acute or chronic renal insufficiency, significant renal impairment, pre-existing elevated serum potassium.

Special Concerns: Pregnancy category: C. Use with caution during lactation. Geriatric clients may be more sensitive to the hypotensive and electrolyte effects of this combination; also, age-related decreases in renal function may require a decrease in dosage.

Dosage: Capsules. Adults: 1–2 capsules b.i.d. determined by individual titration with the components. Some clients may be controlled using 1 capsule every day or every other day. No more than 4 capsules should be taken daily. **Tablets. Adults:** 1 tablet daily determined by individual titration with the components. In Canada, 1–2 tablets may be taken daily.

NURSING CONSIDERATIONS

See also *Nursing Considerations* for *Triamterene,* p. 1235, and *Hydrochlorothiazide,* p. 718.

Administration: Clients who are transferred from less bioavailable formulations of triamterene and hydrochlorothiazide should be monitored for serum potassium levels following the transfer.

Evaluation: Evaluate client for:
- Evidence of ↓ blood pressure
- Reports of ↓ edema with laboratory evidence that serum potassium levels are within desired range

---

Triazolam

(try-**AYZ**-oh-lam)

Halcion (C-IV, Rx)

See also *Benzodiazepines,* p. 108.

Classification: Benzodiazepine sedative-hypnotic.

Action/Kinetics: Triazolam decreases sleep latency, increases the duration of sleep, and decreases the number of awakenings. **Time to peak plasma levels:** 0.5–2 hr. **t½:** 1.5–5.5 hr. Metabolized in liver and inactive metabolites excreted in the urine.

Uses: Insomnia (short-term management, not to exceed 1 month). May be beneficial in preventing or treating transient insomnia from a sudden change in sleep schedule.

Contraindications: Pregnancy (category: X).

Special Concerns: Safety and efficacy in children under 18 years of age not established. Use during lactation may cause sedation and feeding problems in the infant. Geriatric clients may be more sensitive to the effects of triazolam.

Side Effects: *CNS:* Rebound insomnia, anterograde amnesia, headache, ataxia, decreased coordination. Psychologic and physical dependence. *GI:* Nausea, vomiting.

Dosage: Tablets. Adults: initial, 0.25–0.5 mg before bedtime. **Geriatric or debilitated clients, initial:** 0.125 mg; **then,** depending on response, 0.125–0.25 mg before bedtime.

NURSING CONSIDERATIONS

See also *Nursing Considerations* for *Benzodiazepines,* p. 111.

Interventions

1. Assess client for tolerance and for psychological and physical dependence. Evaluate and document sleep habits.
2. When client suffers from simple insomnia, try warm baths, warm milk, and other interventions to induce sleep, such as soft music, guided imagery, or progressive muscle relaxation.
3. Attempt to determine underlying cause of insomnia so that source may be removed.
4. Initiate safety precautions (i.e., side rails up, frequent observations) at bedtime, especially with elderly clients and confused clients.

5. Monitor closely for CNS toxic effects especially during prolonged therapy (longer than 2 weeks).

Client/Family Teaching

1. Avoid the use of alcoholic beverages and other CNS depressants.
2. Use caution when driving or in operating machinery until daytime sedative effects have been evaluated.
3. Try warm baths, warm milk, and other methods to induce sleep, such as guided imagery or progressive muscle relaxation rather than become dependent on drugs for insomnia.
4. Report immediately any unusual side effects including hallucinations, nightmares, depression, or periods of confusion.

Evaluation: Evaluate client for:
- Reports of improved sleeping patterns with relief from insomnia
- Any evidence of adverse effects from drug therapy that may necessitate discontinuation

---

Trientine hydrochloride
(TRY-en-teen)
Syprine (Rx)

Classification: Chelating agent.

Action/Kinetics: Trientine is a chelating agent that binds copper, thus facilitating its excretion from the body.

Uses: Individuals with Wilson's disease (a metabolic defect resulting in excess copper accumulation) who are intolerant of penicillamine.

Contraindications: Use in cystinuria, rheumatoid arthritis, biliary cirrhosis.

Special Concerns: Pregnancy category: C. Use with caution during lactation. Safety and effectiveness in children have not been determined although the drug has been used in children as young as 6 years of age.

Side Effects: Iron deficiency anemia, systemic lupus erythematosus.

Dosage: Capsules. Adults: initial, 750 mg–1.25 g daily in divided doses b.i.d., t.i.d., or q.i.d.; **then,** may increase to a maximum of 2 g daily. **Children less than 12 years of age: initial,** 500–750 mg daily in divided doses b.i.d., t.i.d., or q.i.d.; **then,** may increase to a maximum of 1.5 g daily.

NURSING CONSIDERATIONS

Administration/Storage

1. Trientine should be taken on an empty stomach at least 1 hr before meals or 2 hr after meals and at least 1 hr apart from any other drug, food, or milk.
2. Capsules should be swallowed whole with water; they should not be chewed or opened.
3. The daily dose should be increased only if the response is not adequate or the serum copper level is consistently greater than 20 mcg/dl.
4. At 6–12-month intervals, the optimal long-term maintenance dosage should be determined.
5. If the contents of the capsule come in contact with any site on the body, it should be promptly washed with water to avoid contact dermatitis.

6. Capsules should be stored at 2°–8°C (36°–46°F).

Assessment

1. Obtain baseline CBC and serum copper levels.
2. Note previous treatment regimens and their results.

Client/Family Teaching

1. Take only as directed and on an empty stomach.
2. Advise to avoid mineral supplements as they may interfere with the absorption of trientine.
3. Advise that iron deficiency anemia may develop in children, menstruating or pregnant women, or as a result of the low copper diet necessary to treat Wilson's disease. Iron may be given in such cases but allow 2 hr between administration of iron and trientine.
4. Instruct that body temperature should be taken and recorded nightly for the first month of treatment and any symptoms such as fever or skin eruption should be reported to the physician.
5. Report for all scheduled lab studies so that effectiveness of drug therapy can be assessed. Serum copper levels will be followed and periodically, clients may be monitored with a 24-hr urinary copper analysis (i.e., q 6–12 months).

Evaluation: Determination of free serum copper is the most reliable way to monitor the effectiveness of therapy. Clients who are responsive to therapy will have less than 10 mcg/dl of free copper in the serum.

Trifluoperazine
(try-**flew**-oh-**PER**-ah-zeen)
Novo-Flurazine✶, Solazine✶, Stelazine, (Rx)

See also *Phenothiazines*, p. 201.

Classification: Antipsychotic, antiemetic, piperazine-type phenothiazine.

Action/Kinetics: Trifluoperazine is accompanied by a high incidence of extrapyramidal symptoms and antiemetic effects and a low incidence of sedation, orthostatic hypotension, and anticholinergic side effects. Recommended only for hospitalized or well-supervised clients. **Maximum therapeutic effect:** Usually 2–3 weeks after initiation of therapy.

Uses: Schizophrenia. Suitable for clients with apathy or withdrawal. Anxiety, tension, agitation in neuroses.

Special Concerns: Use during pregnancy only when benefits clearly outweigh risks. Dosage has not been established in children less than 6 years of age. Geriatric, emaciated, or debilitated clients usually require a lower initial dose.

Dosage: Oral Solution, Tablets. *Psychoses:* **Adults and adolescents, initial** 2–5 mg (base) b.i.d.; **maintenance:** 15–20 mg daily in 2 or 3 divided doses. **Pediatric, 6–12 years:** 1 mg (base) 1–2 times daily; adjust dose as required and tolerated. *Anxiety/tension:* **Adults and adolescents,** 1–2 mg daily up to 6 mg daily. Not to be given for this purpose longer than 12 weeks. **IM.** *Pyschoses:* **Adults** 1–2 mg q 4–6 hr, not to exceed 10 mg daily. Switch to PO therapy as soon as possible. **Pediatric:** *Severe symptoms only:* 1 mg 1–2 times/day.

T

NURSING CONSIDERATIONS

See also *Nursing Considerations* for *Phenothiazines,* p. 205.

Administration/Storage

1. Dilute concentrate with 60 ml of juice (tomato or fruit), carbonated drinks, water, milk, orange or simple syrup, coffee, tea, or semisolid foods (e.g., applesauce, pudding, soup).
2. Dilute just before administration.
3. Protect liquid forms from light.
4. Discard strongly colored solutions.
5. Avoid skin contact with liquid form to prevent contact dermatitis.
6. To prevent cumulative effects, at least 4 hr should elapse between IM injections.

Evaluation: Evaluate client for:
- Evidence of a reduction in paranoid, excitable, or withdrawn behaviors
- Reports of a decrease in levels of anxiety, agitation, and tension in those with neuroses

---

Triflupromazine hydrochloride

(try-flew-**PROH**-mah-zeen)

T **Vesprin (Rx)**

See also *Phenothiazines,* p. 201.

Classification: Antipsychotic, dimethylaminopropyl-type phenothiazine.

Action/Kinetics: This drug produces significant anticholinergic and antiemetic effects; moderate to strong extrapyramidal and sedative effects; and moderate hypotensive effects.

Uses: Severe nausea and vomiting. Psychotic disorders (should not be used for psychotic disorders with depression).

Special Concerns: Use during pregnancy only if benefits clearly outweigh risks. Dosage has not been established for children less than 30 months of age. IV use not recommended for children because of hypotension and rapid onset of extrapyramidal side effects. Geriatric, emaciated, or debilitated clients may require a lower initial dose.

Dosage: IM. *Psychoses.* **Adults and adolescents,** 60 mg up to maximum of 150 mg/day. **Pediatric,** 0.2–0.25 mg/kg to maximum of 10 mg/day. *Nausea and vomiting.* **Adults and adolescents,** 5–15 mg as single dose repeated q 4 hr up to maximum of 60 mg/day (for elderly or debilitated clients: 2.5 mg up to maximum of 15 mg/day). **Pediatric, over 2½ years:** 0.2–0.25 mg/kg up to maximum of 10 mg/day. **IV.** *Psychoses.* **Adults and adolescents,** 1 mg as required, up to a maximum of 3 mg daily.

NURSING CONSIDERATIONS

See also *Nursing Considerations* for *Phenothiazines,* p. 205.

Administration/Storage

1. Avoid excessive heat and freezing.
2. Store in amber-colored containers.
3. Do not use discolored (darker than light amber) solutions.
4. Avoid skin contact with liquid form to prevent contact dermatitis.
5. When used in children for nausea and vomiting, the duration may be 12 hr.

Evaluation: Evaluate client for:
- Reports of control of nausea and vomiting
- Evidence of a reduction in psychotic ideations

Trifluridine
(try-**FLUR**-ih-deen)
Viroptic (Rx)

See also *Anti-Infectives*, p. 80.

Classification: Antiviral, ophthalmic.

Action/Kinetics: Trifluridine closely resembles thymidine; the drug inhibits thymidylic phosphorylase and specific DNA polymerases necessary for incorporation of thymidine into viral DNA. Trifluridine, instead of thymidine, is incorporated into viral DNA, resulting in faulty DNA and the ability to infect or reproduce in tissue. Trifluridine is also incorporated into mammalian DNA. **t½:** 12–18 min.

Uses: Primary keratoconjunctivitis and recurrent epithelial keratitis caused by herpes simplex virus types 1 and 2. Epithelial keratitis resistant to idoxuridine. Is especially indicated for infections resistant to idoxuridine or vidarabine.

Contraindications: Hypersensitivity or chemical intolerance to drug.

Special Concerns: Safe use during pregnancy not established.

Side Effects: *Ophthalmic:* Local, usually transient; irritation of conjunctiva and cornea, including burning or stinging and edema of eyelids. Increased intraocular pressure. *Other:* Superficial punctate keratopathy, epithelial keratopathy, hypersensitivity, stromal edema, irritation, keratitis sicca, hyperemia.

Dosage: Solution, 1%. One drop of solution q 2 hr onto cornea, up to maximum of 9 drops/eye/day during acute stage (presence of corneal ulcer). Following reepithelialization, decrease dosage to 1 drop q 4 hr (or minimum of 5 drops/eye/day) for 7 days. Do not use for more than 21 days.

NURSING CONSIDERATIONS

See also *General Nursing Considerations For All Anti-Infectives*, p. 83.

Administration/Storage

1. May be used concomitantly in the eye with antibiotics (chloramphenicol, bacitracin, polymyxin B sulfate, erythromycin, neomycin, gentamicin, tetracycline, sulfacetamide sodium), corticosteroids, anticholinergics, epinephrine HCl, and sodium chloride.
2. Drug is heat-sensitive. *Store in refrigerator* at 2°C–8°C (35.6°F–46.4°F).

Client/Family Teaching

1. Instill drop onto cornea. Apply finger pressure lightly to lacrimal sac for 1 min after instillation.
2. A mild, transient burning sensation may occur on instillation.
3. Report any bothersome side effects to physician but do not stop medication without specific instructions to do so.
4. Arrange for regular examination by an ophthalmologist.
5. Improvement usually occurs within 7 days and healing takes place within 14 days. There-

T

after, 7 more days of therapy are necessary to prevent recurrence.

6. Report to physician if no improvement is noted within 7 days.
7. Do not administer drug for more than 21 days because toxicity may occur (remaining medication should be discarded after 21 days).
8. Keep medication in the refrigerator.

Evaluation: Evaluate client for evidence of successful reepithelialization of herpetic eye lesions.

Trihexyphenidyl hydrochloride

(try-hex-ee-**FEN**-ih-dill)

APO-Trihex✳, Artane, Artane Sequels, Novo–Hexidyl✳, PMS Trihexyphenidyl✳, Trihexy-2 and -5 (Rx)

See also *Cholinergic Blocking Agents,* p. 136, and *Antiparkinson Agents,* p. 99.

Classification: Antiparkinson agent, anticholinergic.

Action/Kinetics: Synthetic anticholinergic, which relieves rigidity but has little effect on tremors. Causes a direct antispasmodic effect on smooth muscle. Has a high incidence of side effects. Small doses cause CNS depression, whereas larger doses may result in CNS excitation. **Onset, PO:** 60 min. **Duration, PO:** 6–12 hr.

Uses: Adjunct in the treatment of all types of parkinsonism (often used as adjunct with levodopa). Drug-induced extrapyramidal symptoms. Sustained-release medication is for maintenance dosage only.

Additional Contraindications: Arteriosclerosis and hypersensitivity to drug.

Special Concerns: Pregnancy category: C.

Additional Side Effects: Serious CNS stimulation (restlessness, insomnia, delirium, agitation) and psychotic manifestations.

Additional Drug Interaction: ↑ Effectiveness of levodopa if used together; such combined use not recommended in clients with psychoses.

Dosage: Elixir, Extended-release Capsules, Tablets. *Parkinsonism:* **initial (day 1),** 1–2 mg; **then,** increase by 2 mg q 3–5 days until daily dose is 6–10 mg given in divided doses. Some clients may require 12–15 mg daily (especially those with postencephalitic parkinsonism). *Adjunct with levodopa:* 3–6 mg/day in divided doses. *Drug-induced extrapyramidal reactions:* **initial,** 1 mg daily; **then,** increase as needed to total daily dose of 5–15 mg. **Maintenance: extended-release,** 5–10 mg 1–2 times daily.

NURSING CONSIDERATIONS

See also *Nursing Considerations* for *Cholinergic Blocking Agents,* p. 138, and *Antiparkinson Agents,* p. 99.

Interventions

1. This drug has a high incidence of side effects; early detection and intervention are imperative.
2. Determine any added adverse CNS reactions to the drug. Note any increase in restlessness, complaints of insomnia, agitation, or psychotic manifesta-

tions. Document and notify the physician because drug dosage may need to be adjusted.

3. Monitor and record I&O, noting any urinary retention or constipation.

Client/Family Teaching
1. Take with meals to minimize GI upset.
2. Increase fluids and bulk in diet to prevent constipation.
3. Provide a printed list of adverse drug effects, stressing those that require immediate reporting to the physician.

Evaluation: Evaluate client for:
- Evidence of control of symptoms of Parkinson's disease or drug-induced extrapyramidal symptoms
- Any evidence of adverse drug effects as drug dosage may require adjustment

---

Trimethobenzamide hydrochloride
(try-meth-oh-**BENZ**-ah-myd)
Arrestin, Hymetic, Tebamide, T-Gen, Ticon, Tigan, Tiject-20 (Rx)

Classification: Antiemetic.

Action/Kinetics: Trimethobenzamide is an antiemetic related to the antihistamines but with weak antihistaminic properties. The drug is less effective than the phenothiazines but has fewer side effects. Not suitable as sole agent for severe emesis. Can be used rectally. Trimethobenzamide appears to control vomiting by depressing the chemoreceptor trigger zone of the medulla. **Onset: PO and IM,** 10–40 min. **Duration:** 3–4 hr. 30%–

50% of drug excreted unchanged in urine in 48–72 hr.

Uses: Nausea and vomiting.

Contraindications: Hypersensitivity to drug, to benzocaine, or similar local anesthetics. Do not use suppositories for neonates; do not use IM in children.

Special Concerns: Use during pregnancy only if benefits outweigh risks. Use with caution during lactation.

Side Effects: *CNS:* Depression of mood, disorientation, headache, drowsiness, dizziness, seizures, coma, Parkinson-like symptoms, seizures. *Other:* Hypersensitivity reactions, hypotension, blood dyscrasias, jaundice, muscle cramps, opisthotonos, blurred vision, diarrhea, allergic skin reactions. *After IM injection:* Pain, burning, stinging, redness at injection site.

Drug Interactions: Concomitant use with atropine-like drugs and CNS depressants including alcohol should be avoided.

Dosage: Capsules. Adults: 250 mg t.i.d.–q.i.d.; **pediatric, 13.6–40.9 kg:** 100–200 mg t.i.d.–q.i.d. **Suppositories. Adults:** 200 mg t.i.d.–q.i.d.; **pediatric, under 13.6 kg:** 100 mg t.i.d.–q.i.d.; **13.6–40.9 kg:** 100–200 mg t.i.d.–q.i.d. **IM only. Adults:** 200 mg t.i.d.–q.i.d. (IM route not to be used in children.)

NURSING CONSIDERATIONS

See also *Nursing Considerations for Antiemetics,* p. 71.

Administration/Storage
1. Inject drug IM deeply into the upper, outer quadrant of the gluteus muscle. Be careful to

avoid escape of fluid from the needle so as to minimize local reaction.

2. Expect the onset of action to occur in 10–40 min after oral administration and to last 3–4 hr.
3. After IM injection, the action of the drug lasts 2–3 hr.
4. Do not administer suppositories to clients allergic to benzocaine or similar anesthetics.

Assessment

1. Note any history of sensitivity to benzocaine and document.
2. Ask if the client has experienced any local reaction to the suppositories and document.

Interventions: Observe the client for any evidence of skin reaction. This is the first sign of hypersensitivity to the drug.

Client/Family Teaching

1. Provide a printed list of adverse drug effects that require reporting to the physician.
2. Do not drive or operate machinery until drug effects are realized. Drug may cause drowsiness and dizziness.
3. Avoid the use of alcohol and any other CNS depressants.

Evaluation: Evaluate client for reports of effective control of nausea and vomiting.

—— *COMBINATION DRUG* ——
Trimethoprim and Sulfamethoxazole
(try-**METH**-oh-prim, sul-fah-meth-**OX**-ah-zohl)
Apo-Sulfatrim✿, Bactrim, Bactrim DS, Bactrim I.V., Bactrim Roche✿, Cotrim, Cotrim DS,

Cotrim Pediatric, Cotrim IV, Novo–Trimel✿, Novo–Trimel DS✿, Nu-Cotrimix✿, Roubac✿, Septra, Septra DS, Septra IV, Sulfamethoprim, Sulfatrim, Uroplus DS, Uroplus SS (Rx)

See also *Sulfonamides,* p. 213.

Classification/Content: These products contain the antibacterial agents sulfamethoxazole and trimethoprim. See also *Sulfamethoxazole,* p. 1173. **Oral Suspension:** Sulfamethoxazole, 200 mg and trimethoprim, 40 mg/5 ml. **Tablets:** Sulfamethoxazole, 400 mg and trimethoprim, 80 mg/tablet. **Double Strength (DS) Tablets:** Sulfamethoxazole, 800 mg and trimethoprim, 160 mg/tablet. **Concentrate for injection:** Sulfamethoxazole, 80 mg and trimethoprim, 16 mg/ml.

Uses: PO, Parenteral: Urinary tract infections due to *Escherichia coli, Klebsiella, Enterobacter, Pseudomonas mirabilis* and *vulgaris,* and *Morganella morganii.* Enteritis due to *Shigellosis flexneri* or *S. sonnei. Pneumocystis carinii* pneumonitis in children and adults. **PO:** Acute otitis media in children due to *Haemophilus influenzae* or *S. pneumoniae.* Acute worsening of chronic bronchitis in adults due to *H. influenzae* or *S. pneumoniae.* Traveler's diarrhea in adults due to *E. coli. Investigational:* Cholera, salmonella, nocardiosis, prophylaxis of recurrent urinary tract infections in women, prophylaxis of neutropenic clients with *P. carinii* infections or leukemia clients to decrease incidence of gram-negative rod bacteremia. Treatment of prostatitis. Decrease chance of urinary and blood infections in renal transplant clients.

Additional Contraindications: Infants under 2 months of age. During pregnancy at term. Megaloblastic anemia due to folate deficiency. Lactation.

Special Concerns: Pregnancy category: C. Use with caution in impaired liver or kidney function. AIDS clients may not tolerate or respond to this product. Use with caution in clients with possible folate deficiency.

Additional Drug Interactions

Cyclosporine / ↓ Effect of cyclosporine; ↑ risk of nephrotoxicity

Methotrexate / ↑ Risk of methotrexate toxicity due to displacement from plasma protein binding site

Phenytoin / ↑ Effect of phenytoin due to ↓ hepatic clearance

Thiazide diuretics / ↑ Risk of thrombocytopenia with purpura in geriatric clients

Warfarin / ↑ Prothrombin time

Laboratory Test Interferences: Jaffe alkaline picnate reaction overestimation of creatinine by 10%.

Dosage: *Urinary tract infections, shigellosis, bronchitis, acute otitis media.* **Adults:** One DS tablet, 2 tablets, or 4 teaspoonfuls of suspension q 12 hr for 10–14 days. **Pediatric:** Total daily dose of 8 mg/kg trimethoprim and 40 mg/kg sulfamethoxazole divided equally and given q 12 hr for 10–14 days (**Note:** For shigellosis, give adult or pediatric dose for 7 days.) **IV. Adults and children:** 8–10 mg/kg/day (based on trimethoprim) in 2–4 divided doses q 6, 8, 12 hr for up to 14 days for severe urinary tract infections or 5 days for shigellosis.

Chancroid: 1 DS tablet b.i.d. for at least 7 days (alternate therapy: 4 DS tablets in a single dose). *Pharyngeal gonococcal infection due to penicillinase-producing Neisseria gonorrhoeae:* 720 mg trimethoprim and 3,600 mg sulfamethoxazole once daily for 5 days. *P. carinii pneumonia:* **Adults and children:** Total daily dose of 20 mg/kg trimethoprim and 100 mg/kg sulfamethoxazole divided equally and given q 6 hr for 14 days. *Traveler's diarrhea:* **Adults,** one DS tablet q 12 hr for 5 days. *Prostatitis, acute bacterial:* One DS tablet b.i.d. until client is afebrile for 48 hr; treatment may be required for up to 30 days. *Prostatitis, chronic bacterial:* One DS tablet b.i.d. for 4–6 weeks.

NURSING CONSIDERATIONS

See also *General Nursing Considerations For All Anti-Infectives,* p. 83, and for *Sulfonamides,* p. 216.

Administration/Storage

1. The IV infusion must be administered over a period of 60–90 min.
2. Each 5 ml of the IV infusion must be diluted to 125 ml with 5% dextrose in water and used within 6 hr. If the amount of fluid should be restricted, each 5 ml can be diluted up to 75 ml with 5% dextrose in water and used within 2 hr. The diluted solution should not be refrigerated.
3. The IV infusion should not be mixed with any other drugs or solutions.
4. If the diluted IV infusion is cloudy or precipitates after mixing, it should be discarded and a new solution prepared.

T

Assessment

1. Obtain baseline lab data to evaluate liver and renal function.
2. Assess for anemia because megaloblastic anemia due to folate deficiency is a contraindication for this drug therapy.
3. Document, when known, if client is infected with AIDS virus as this may contraindicate therapy.

Evaluation: Evaluate client for:
- Laboratory evidence of negative culture results
- Clinical evidence and reports of symptomatic improvement

Trimipramine maleate
(try-**MIP**-rah-meen)
Apo-Trimip✶, Rhotrimune✶, Surmontil (Rx)

See also *Tricyclic Antidepressants,* p. 239.

Classification: Antidepressant, tricyclic.

Action/Kinetics: Trimipramine causes moderate anticholinergic and orthostatic hypotensive effects and significant sedative effects. **Effective plasma levels:** 180 ng/ml. **t¹/₂:** 7–30 hr. Seems more effective in endogenous depression than in other types of depression.

Uses: Treatment of symptoms of depression. Peptic ulcer disease.

Special Concerns: Pregnancy category: C. Not recommended for use in children less than 12 years of age.

Dosage: Capsules. Adults, outpatients: initial, 75 mg/day in divided doses up to 150 mg/day.

Daily dosage should not exceed 200 mg; **maintenance:** 50–150 mg/day. Total dose can be given at bedtime. **Adults, hospitalized: initial,** 100 mg/day in divided doses up to 200 mg/day. If no improvement in 2–3 weeks, increase to 250–300 mg/day. **Adolescent/geriatric clients: initial,** 50 mg/day up to 100 mg/day. Not recommended for children.

NURSING CONSIDERATIONS

See *Nursing Considerations* for *Tricyclic Antidepressants,* p. 242.

Evaluation: Evaluate client for evidence of behaviors that reflect a decreased level of depression such as improved appetite, ability to sleep better, and increased social interactions.

--- COMBINATION DRUG ---

Trinalin
(TRIN-al-in)

Classification/Content: *Antihistamine:* Azatadine maleate, 1 mg. *Decongestant:* Pseudoephedrine sulfate, 120 mg in a long-acting formulation.See also information on individual components.

Action/Kinetics: The tablet is formulated so that the azatadine and one-half of the pseudoephedrine are released immediately; the remaining one-half of the pseudoephedrine is released after several hours.

Uses: Symptoms of allergic rhinitis and perennial rhinitis, nasal and eustachian tube congestion.

Contraindications: Lactation. Children under 12 years of age. Use to treat lower respiratory tract symptoms, including asthma. Narrow angle glaucoma, urinary retention, clients taking MAO inhibitors, severe hypertension, severe coronary artery disease, hyperthyroidism, clients hypersensitive to adrenergic agents.

Special Concerns: Pregnancy category: C. Use with caution in clients with stenosing peptic ulcer, pyloroduodenal obstruction, urinary bladder obstruction due to prostatic hypertrophy or narrowing of the bladder neck, hypertension, ischemic heart disease, increased intraocular pressure, diabetes mellitus, in clients taking digitalis or oral anticoagulants.

Dosage: Tablets. Adults: One tablet b.i.d.

NURSING CONSIDERATIONS

See also *Nursing Considerations* for *Antihistamines,* p. 74, and *Sympathomimetic Drugs,* p. 220.

Administration/Storage

1. Trinalin may be used in conjunction with other analgesics and/or antibiotics.
2. Do not administer to children under 12 years of age.

Evaluation: Evaluate client for:
- Evidence of ↓ nasal and eustachian tube congestion
- Reports of symptomatic improvement in allergic manifestations

---

Tripelennamine hydrochloride
(try-pell-**EN**-ah-meen)
PBZ, PBZ-SR, Pelamine, Pyribenzamine✲ (Rx)

See also *Antihistamines,* p. 71.

Classification: Antihistamine, ethylenediamine derivative.

Action/Kinetics: GI effects more pronounced than other antihistamines. **Duration:** 4–6 hr.

Special Concerns: Safe use during pregnancy has not been established. Use is not recommended in neonates. Geriatric clients may be more sensitive to the usual adult dose.

Side Effects: Low incidence. Moderate sedation, mild GI distress, paradoxical excitation, hyperirritability.

Dosage: Elixir, Tablets. Adults: usual, 25–50 mg q 4–6 hr; **pediatric:** 1.25 mg/kg (37.5 mg/m²) q 6 hr as needed, not to exceed 300 mg daily. **Extended-release Tablets. Adults:** 100 mg q 8–12 hr as needed, up to a maximum of 600 mg daily. Do not use sustained-release form in children.

NURSING CONSIDERATIONS

See *Nursing Considerations* for *Antihistamines,* p. 74.

Evaluation: Evaluate client for reports of a reduction in allergic symptoms.

--- COMBINATION DRUG ---
Triphasil 21 Day and Triphasil 28 Day
(try-**FAY**-sill)
(Rx)

T

See also *Oral Contraceptives,* p. 192.

Classification: Triphasic combination oral contraceptives.

Components: Phase 1 (first 6 tablets): Each tablet of either Triphasil 21 Day or 28 Day contains ethinyl estradiol, 30 mcg and levonorgestrel, 0.05 mg (brown tablets). Phase 2 (next 5 tablets): Each tablet contains ethinyl estradiol, 40 mcg and levonorgestrel, 0.075 mg (white tablets). Phase 3 (next 10 tablets): Each tablet contains ethinyl estradiol, 30 mcg and levonorgestrel, 0.125 mg (yellow tablets). The 28s also have 7 inert green tablets.

Special Concerns: Pregnancy category: X.

NURSING CONSIDERATIONS

See *Oral Contraceptives,* p. 192.

Triprolidine hydrochloride
(try-**PROH**-lih-deen)
Actidil, Alleract, Myidyl (OTC and Rx)

See also *Antihistamines,* p. 71.

Classification: Antihistamine, alkylamine-type.

Action/Kinetics: Sedative effects less pronounced. **Time to peak effect:** 2–3 hr. $t^{1/2}$: 3–3.3 hr. **Duration:** 4–25 hr. Also found in Actifed and Actifed-C.

Special Concerns: Pregnancy category: B. Geriatric clients may be more susceptible to the usual adult dose.

Additional Side Effects: Low incidence of side effects. *CNS:* Drowsiness, dizziness, paradoxical excitement, hyperirritability. *GI:* GI distress.

Dosage: Syrup, Tablets. Adults: 2.5 mg q 4–6 hr. **Pediatric 6–12 years:** 1.25 mg q 6–8 hr; **4–6 years:** 0.937 mg q 6–8 hr; **2–4 years:** 0.625 mg q 6–8 hr; **4 months–2 years:** 0.312 mg q 6–8 hr.

NURSING CONSIDERATIONS

See *Nursing Considerations* for *Antihistamines,* p. 74.

Evaluation: Evaluate client for reports of symptomatic improvement in allergic manifestations.

Tromethamine
(troh-**METH**-ah-meen)
Tham, Tham-E (Rx)

Classification: Systemic alkalizing agent.

Action/Kinetics: Tromethamine, an organic amine, is a buffering and systemic alkalizing agent. It actively binds hydrogen ions, thereby decreasing and correcting acidosis. It promotes the excretion of acids, carbon dioxide, and electrolytes and is thought to be able to neutralize some intracellular acid. It acts as an osmotic diuretic, increasing urine flow. Seventy-five percent of the drug is eliminated within 8 hr, the remainder within 3 days.

Uses: Prevention and correction of systemic acidosis, especially that accompanying cardiac bypass surgery and cardiac arrest.

Contraindications: Uremia and anuria, pregnancy.

Special Concerns: Pregnancy category: C. Use with caution in newborns and infants. Administer with caution to clients with renal disorders.

Side Effects: *Respiratory:* Respiratory depression. *Other:* Fever, hypervolemia, transient decrease of blood glucose. *At injection site:* Extravasation, phlebitis, venous thrombosis, infection. *In newborn:* Hemorrhagic liver necrosis when given by umbilical vein. *Symptoms of Overdose:* Alkalosis, overhydration, hypoglycemia (severe and prolonged), solute overload.

Dosage: Slow IV. Minimum amount to correct acid-base imbalance. The amount of tromethamine can be estimated using the buffer base deficit of the extracellular fluid:ml of 0.3 M tromethamine solution required = body weight (kg)×base deficit (mEq/L)×1.1 **Dose of tromethamine without electrolyte.** *Acidosis in cardiac bypass surgery:* **Adults,** 500 ml (150 mEq). Severe cases may require 1,000 ml. *Acidosis in cardiac arrest* (given at the same time as other standard procedures are being applied): **if chest is open, Adults,** 65–185 ml (2–6 g) into the ventricular cavity (not into the cardiac muscle); **if chest closed,** 111–333 ml (3.6–10.8 g) into a large peripheral vein. *For acidity in acid citrate dextrose (ACD) blood:* 15–77 ml (0.5–2.5 g) added to each 500 ml of ACD blood. **Dose of tromethamine with electrolytes.** *Acidosis in cardiac bypass surgery:* **Adults, usual,** 694 ml (25 g) given at a rate of 0.14 ml/kg/min. *Acidosis in cardiac arrest* (given at the same time as other standard procedures are being applied): **if chest is open, Adults,** 55–165 ml (2–6 g) into the ventricular cavity (not into the cardiac muscle); **if chest closed, Adults,** 100–300 ml (3.6–10.8 g) into a large peripheral vein. *For acidity in acid citrate dextrose (ACD) blood:* 14–70 ml (0.5–2.5 g) added to each 500 ml of ACD blood.

NURSING CONSIDERATIONS

Administration/Storage

1. Tests on blood pH, pCO_2, bicarbonate, glucose, and electrolytes should be determined before, during, and after administration of tromethamine.
2. Concentration of solution administered *must not* exceed 0.3 M.
3. Prepare a 0.3-M solution of tromethamine by adding 1,000 ml of sterile water for injection to 36 g of lyophilized tromethamine.
4. Infuse slowly.
5. Administer into the largest antecubital vein through a large needle or indwelling catheter and elevate limb.
6. For treatment of cardiac arrest, the drug may be injected into the ventricular cavity if the chest is open. If the chest is not open, the drug may be injected into a large peripheral vein.
7. Do not administer longer than 1 day unless acute life-threatening situation exists.
8. Discontinue administration *immediately,* if extravasation occurs:
   • Administer 1% procaine hydrochloride with hyaluronidase to reduce venospasm and to dilute the drug in the tissues.
   • Phentolamine mesylate (Regitine) has been used for local infiltration for its adrenergic blocking properties.
   • If necessary, a nerve block of the autonomic fibers may be done.
9. *Treatment of Overdose:* Discontinue the infusion and treat symptoms.

Assessment

1. Note if the client has any history of urinary or bladder problems.

T

2. Obtain renal and hepatic function studies prior to administration of the medication to serve as baseline data against which to compare once medication therapy has been initiated.
3. Determine that pH, pCO_2, bicarbonate, glucose, and electrolytes have been analyzed before administering drug.
4. If the client is female and of childbearing age, check to determine if she is pregnant.

Interventions

1. Observe for respiratory depression and have mechanical ventilation equipment readily available.
2. Observe for complaints of weakness, the presence of moist pale skin, tremors, and a full bounding pulse. These are symptoms of hypoglycemia, which can occur after a rapid or high dose of the drug has been administered. Document and report immediately to the physician.
3. Assess the client for nausea, diarrhea, tachycardia, oliguria, weakness, numbness or tingling sensations. These are symptoms of hyperkalemia and are more likely to occur in clients with impaired renal function.
4. Maintain an accurate record of I&O.
5. Monitor serum electrolytes, blood glucose levels, pH, and hepatic and renal function studies periodically throughout drug therapy. Report any abnormal findings to the physician.
6. Observe the client closely for extravasation. The drug is extremely irritating to the vein.

Evaluation: Evaluate client for:
- Laboratory confirmation of return of serum pH to desired range
- Resolution of symptoms associated with serum acidosis

Tubocurarine chloride
(too-boh-kyour-**AR**-een)
Tubarine ✲ (Rx)

See also *Neuromuscular Blocking Agents,* p. 183.

Classification: Nondepolarizing neuromuscular blocking agent.

Action/Kinetics: Cumulative effects may occur. Most likely of the nondepolarizing drugs to cause histamine release. Narrow margin between therapeutic dose and toxic dose. Overdosage chiefly treated by artificial respiration, although neostigmine, atropine, and edrophonium chloride should also be on hand. **Onset, IV:** 1 min; **IM:** 15–25 min. **Time to peak effect, IV:** 2–5 min. **Duration, IV:** 20–40 min. $t^{1/2}$: 1–3 hr. About 43% excreted unchanged in urine.

Uses: Muscle relaxant during surgery or setting of fractures and dislocations; spasticity caused by injury to or disease of CNS. Treat seizures electrically induced or induced by drugs. Diagnosis of myasthenia gravis.

Additional Contraindications: Drug may cause excessive secretion and circulatory collapse. Clients in whom release of histamine is hazardous.

Special Concerns: Use with caution during pregnancy (category: C) and lactation and in children. If repeated doses are used before delivery, the newborn may manifest decreased skeletal muscle activity. Children up to 1 month of age may be more sensitive to the effects of tubocurarine. Use with extreme caution in clients with renal dysfunction, liver disease, or obstructive states.

Additional Side Effects: Allergic reactions.

Additional Drug Interactions

Acetylcholine / Acetylcholine antagonizes effect of tubocurarine
Anticholinesterases / Anticholinesterases antagonize effect of tubocurarine
Calcium salts / ↑ Effect of tubocurarine
Diazepam / Diazepam may cause malignant hyperthermia with tubocurarine
Potassium / Antagonizes effect of tubocurarine
Propranolol / ↑ Effect of tubocurarine
Quinine / ↑ Effect of tubocurarine
Succinylcholine chloride / ↑ Relaxant effect of both drugs
Trimethophan / ↑ Effect of tubocurarine

Dosage: IV, IM: *Adjunct to surgical anesthesia:* **Adults, IM, IV, initial,** 6–9 mg/kg; **then,** 3–4.5 mg in 3–5 min if needed. Supplemental doses of 3 mg can be given for prolonged procedures. Dosage can be calculated on the basis of 0.165 mg/kg. **Pediatric, up to 4 weeks of age, IV, initial:** 0.25–0.5 mg/kg; **then,** give subsequent doses in increments of ⅕–⅙ the initial dose. **Infants and children, IV:** 0.5 mg/kg. *Aid to controlled respiration:* **Adults, IV, initial,** 0.0165 mg/kg with additional doses adjusted as required. *Electroshock*

therapy: **Adults, IV,** 0.165 mg/kg given over 30–90 sec. It is recommended that the initial dose be 3 mg less than the calculated total dose. *Diagnosis of myasthenia gravis:* **Adults, IV,** 0.004–0.033 mg/kg. A test dose should be given within 2–3 min with IV neostigmine, 1.5 mg, to minimize prolonged respiratory paralysis.

NURSING CONSIDERATIONS

See also *Nursing Considerations* for *Neuromuscular Blocking Agents,* p. 184.

Administration/Storage

1. Review the drugs with which tubocurarine interacts.
2. Tubocurarine is incompatible with alkaline solutions and may form a precipitate when mixed with them (e.g., methohexital sodium or thiopental sodium).
3. After IV administration, expect the peak action to occur in 2–5 min and the effect to last 25–90 min.
4. Have neostigmine methylsulfate available as an antidote.

Evaluation: Evaluate client for:
- Evidence that the desired level of muscle relaxation is attained
- Evidence of the control of drug or electrically induced seizures
- Appropriate diagnosis of myasthenia gravis

—— COMBINATION DRUG ——
Tuss-Ornade Capsules or Liquid
(TUSS-OR-nayd)
(Rx)

Classification/Content: *Antihistamine:* Caramiphen edisylate, 40 mg (Capsule) or 6.7 mg/5 ml (Liquid). *Decongestant:* Phenylpropanolamine HCl, 75 mg (Capsule) or 12.5 mg/5 ml (Liquid). See also information on individual components.

Uses: Nasal congestion and cough due to the common cold.

Contraindications: Capsules in children less than 12 years of age. The liquid in children under 6.8 kg and less than 6 months of age. Severe hypertension, clients taking MAO inhibitors, coronary artery disease, bronchial asthma.

Special Concerns: Use during pregnancy only if benefits outweigh risks. Use with caution in cardiovascular disease, thyroid disease, prostatic hypertrophy, diabetes, or glaucoma.

Dosage: Capsules. Adults and children over 12 years, One capsule q 12 hr. **Liquid. Adults and children over 12 years of age:** 10 ml q 4 hr, not to exceed 60 ml in 24 hr; **pediatric, 6–12 years:** 5 ml q 4 hr, not to exceed 30 ml daily; **pediatric, 2–6 years:** 2.5 ml q 4 hr, not to exceed 15 ml daily.

NURSING CONSIDERATIONS

See also *Nursing Considerations* for *Antihistamines,* p. 74, and *Sympathomimetic Drugs,* p. 220.

Administration/Storage

1. The capsules should not be used in children who are under 12 years of age.
2. The liquid should not be used for children who are under 6 months of age or who weigh less than 6.8 kg.
3. Pregnant women should avoid using the drug.

Evaluation: Evaluate client for reports of effective control of nasal congestion and cough associated with a cold.

————— *COMBINATION DRUG* —————
Tussi-Organidin
[TUSS-ee-or-GAN-ih-din]
(C-V) (Rx)

Tussi-Organidin DM
[TUSS-ee-or-GAN-ih-din]
(Rx)

Classification/Content: Each 5 ml of Tussi-Organidin contains: *Mucolytic/expectorant:* Iodinated glycerol, 30 mg. *Narcotic antitussive:* Codeine phosphate, 10 mg. Each 5 ml of Tussi-Organidin DM contains: *Mucolytic/expectorant:* Iodinated glycerol, 30 mg. *Nonnarcotic antitussive:* Dextromethorphan, 10 mg. See also information on *Narcotic Analgesics,* p. 174, and *Dextromethorphan,* p. 525.

Uses: Relief of irritating, nonproductive cough due to a variety of respiratory tract problems including the common cold, chronic bronchitis, bronchial asthma, tracheobronchitis, laryngitis, pharyngitis, pertussis, emphysema, and croup.

Contraindications: History of hypersensitivity to inorganic iodides, pregnancy, lactation, use in newborns.

Special Concerns: Pregnancy category: X. Use with caution (or avoid use) in clients with a history of thyroid disease.

Dosage: Tussi-Organidin Liquid or Tussi-Organidin DM Liquid. Adults: 5–10 ml q 4 hr; **pediatric:** 2.5–5 ml q 4 hr.

NURSING CONSIDERATIONS

See also *Nursing Considerations* for *Narcotic Analgesics,* p. 177, and *Dextromethorphan,* p. 525.

Assessment

1. Tussi-Organidin contains codeine. Therefore, assess the client for any history of drug addiction.
2. Determine how long the client has had the cough, the length of time the upper respiratory tract infection has been present, and what the client has done to correct the problems.
3. Note any history of thyroid dysfunction.

Client/Family Teaching

1. Notify the physician if the symptoms persist beyond a week or 10 days and/or intensify.
2. Explain that the drug may be habit-forming and is not for long-term indiscriminate use.
3. Constipation may develop as a side effect of therapy. Drink 2,500–3,000 ml of fluid per day and increase intake of fruits, fruit juices, and grains as a preventive action.

Evaluation: Evaluate client for reports of symptomatic improvement in cough with uninterrupted periods of rest.

——— COMBINATION DRUG ———

Tussionex Extended-Release Suspension

(TUSS-ee-oh-nex)

(Rx) (C-III)

Classification/Content: Each 5

ml of the extended-release suspension contains: *Narcotic antitussive:* Hydrocodone polistirex, 5 mg (equivalent to 10 mg of hydrocodone bitartrate). *Antihistamine:* Chlorpheniramine polistirex, equivalent to 8 mg chlorpheniramine maleate. See also *Narcotic Analgesics,* p. 174.

Uses: Relief of cough and upper respiratory tract symptoms due to colds or allergy.

Contraindications: Lactation. Children less than 6 years of age.

Special Concerns: Pregnancy category: C. Safety and effectiveness for use in children less than 6 years of age have not been determined. Use with caution in narrow-angle glaucoma, prostatic hypertrophy, asthma, geriatric or debilitated clients, impaired renal or hepatic function, hypothyroidism, Addison's disease, or urethral stricture. Dependence can develop due to hydrocodone.

Dosage: Suspension. Adults: 5 ml q 12 hr, not to exceed 10 ml in 24 hr. **Pediatric, 6–12 years:** 2.5 ml q 12 hr, not to exceed 5 ml in 24 hr.

NURSING CONSIDERATIONS

See also *Nursing Considerations* for *Narcotic Analgesics,* p. 177.

Client/Family Teaching

1. Notify the physician if the symptoms persist or intensify.
2. Explain that the drug may be habit-forming if it is used for long periods of time.
3. Advise that the suspension should be well shaken before using.

T

Evaluation: Evaluate client for reports of effective control of cough and associated upper respiratory symptoms.

─── COMBINATION DRUG ───

Tylenol with Codeine Elixir or Tablets

(TIE-leh-noll, KOH-deen)

(Tablets are C-III and Elixir is C-V) (Rx)

See also *Acetaminophen,* p. 250, and *Narcotic Analgesics,* p. 174.

Classification/Content: *Nonnarcotic analgesic:* Acetaminophen 300 mg in each tablet and 120 mg/5 ml elixir. *Narcotic analgesic:* Codeine phosphate, 7.5 mg (No. 1 Tablets), 15 mg (No. 2 Tablets), 30 mg (No. 3 Tablets), 60 mg (No. 4 Tablets), and 12 mg/5 ml (Elixir).

Uses: The tablets are used for mild to moderately severe pain while the elixir is used for mild to moderate pain.

Special Concerns: Pregnancy category: C. Use with caution during lactation. Safety has not been determined in children less than 3 years of age. This product may be habit-forming due to the codeine component.

Dosage: Tablets. Adults, individualized, usual: 1–2 No. 1, No. 2, or No. 3 Tablets or No. 3 Capsules q 2–4 hr as needed for pain. Or, 1 No. 4 Tablet or Capsule q 4 hr as required. Maximum 24-hr dose is 360 mg codeine phosphate and 4,000 mg acetaminophen. **Pediatric:** Dosage equivalent to 0.5 mg/kg codeine. **Elixir. Adults, individualized, usual:** 15 ml q 4 hr as needed; **pediatric, 7–12 years:** 10 ml t.i.d.–q.i.d.; **3–6 years:** 5 ml t.i.d.–q.i.d. Dosage has not been established for children under 3 years of age.

NURSING CONSIDERATIONS

See also *Nursing Considerations* for *Narcotic Analgesics,* p. 177, and *Acetaminophen,* p. 252.

Administration/Storage

1. Dosage should be adjusted depending on the response of the client and the severity of the pain.
2. Doses of codeine greater than 60 mg do not provide additional analgesia but may lead to an increased incidence of side effects.

Client/Family Teaching

1. Take only as directed.
2. Report any loss of pain control because drug and/or dosage may need to be changed.

Evaluation: Evaluate client for reports of effective control of pain.

─── COMBINATION DRUG ───

Tylox

(TIE-lox)

(C-II, Rx)

See also *Acetaminophen,* p. 250, and *Narcotic Analgesics,* p. 174.

Classification/Content: Each capsule contains: *Nonnarcotic analgesic:* Acetaminophen, 500 mg. *Narcotic analgesic:* Oxycodone HCl, 5 mg.

Uses: Relief of moderate to moderately severe pain.

Special Concerns: Pregnancy category: C. Use with caution during lactation. Safety and effectiveness have not been determined in children. Drug dependence can develop due to the oxycodone component.

Dosage: Capsules. Individualized. Adults, usual: One capsule q 6 hr as required for pain.

NURSING CONSIDERATIONS

See also *Nursing Considerations* for *Narcotic Analgesics,* p. 177, and *Acetaminophen,* p. 252.

Administration/Storage

1. The dose should be adjusted depending on the response of the client and the severity of the pain.
2. As the dose of oxycodone is increased, the incidence of side effects increases. The drug should not be used in high doses for severe or intractable pain.

Evaluation: Evaluate client for reports of effective control of pain.

U

Uracil mustard

(YOUR-ah-sill)

(Rx)

See also *Antineoplastic Agents,* p. 85, and *Alkylating Agents,* p. 20.

Classification: Antineoplastic, alkylating agent.

Action/Kinetics: Uracil mustard is a bifunctional alkylating agent and is cell-cycle nonspecific. It is not a vesicant. The drug forms unstable ethylenimmonium ions which bind or alkylate various intracellular substances. The drug cross-links with DNA and interferes with the function of DNA and RNA. The drug is excreted through the kidneys.

Uses: Chronic lymphocytic leukemia, non-Hodgkin's lymphomas (of the lymphocytic or histiocytic type), chronic myelogenous leukemia. Palliative therapy for polycythemia vera and mycosis fungoides.

Contraindications: Pregnancy and lactation. Leukopenia, thrombocytopenia, aplastic anemia.

Additional Side Effects: During therapy significant decreases in leukocyte and platelet counts occur. Also, hepatotoxicity, amenorrhea, azoospermia.

Laboratory Test Interference: ↑ Serum uric acid levels.

Dosage: Capsules. Adults: 0.15 mg/kg once weekly for 4 weeks. **Pediatric:** 0.30 mg/kg once weekly for 4 weeks. If a response is obtained, the weekly dose should be continued until relapse is noted.

NURSING CONSIDERATIONS

See also *Nursing Considerations* for *Antineoplastic Agents,* p. 88.

Administration/Storage

1. Uracil mustard should not be administered until 2–3 weeks after the maximum effect of other cytotoxic drugs or x-ray therapy has been determined.
2. Uracil capsules contain tartrazine; note any sensitivity to compound.
3. Complete blood counts should be done once or twice weekly

during therapy and 1 month thereafter.

4. Effect of drug sometimes takes 3 months to become apparent, and drug should be given that long unless precluded by a toxicity reaction.

Client/Family Teaching

1. Encourage continuation with therapy because beneficial effect may take as long as 3 months to appear.
2. Warn client not to have immunizations with vaccines containing live virus during therapy with uracil mustard because vaccinia may result as a complication of immunosuppression.
3. Encourage intake of large amounts of fluid during therapy to prevent hyperuricemia.

Evaluation: Evaluate client for evidence of control of progression of leukemia with hematologic stabilization.

Urofollitropin for Injection
(**YOUR**-oh-foll-ee-**troh**-pin)
Metrodin (Rx)

Classification: Ovarian stimulant.

Action/Kinetics: Urofollitropin is prepared from the urine of postmenopausal women. The drug is a gonadotropin that stimulates follicular growth in the ovaries of women without primary ovarian failure. Because treatment with urofollitropin only causes growth and maturation of a follicle, human chorionic gonadotropin (HCG) must also be given to effect ovulation. **Time to peak effect:** 32–36 hr after HCG.

Uses: To cause ovulation in women with polycystic ovarian disease; such clients should have an elevated LH/FSH ratio and should have failed to respond to therapy with clomiphene. In conjunction with HCG to stimulate development of several ova in clients undergoing in vitro fertilization.

Contraindications: Primary ovarian failure (as indicated by high levels of both LH and FSH), renal dysfunction, thyroid dysfunction, pituitary tumor, abnormal uterine bleeding of unknown cause, ovarian cysts, enlarged ovaries (not as a result of polycystic disease), infertility due to causes other than failure to ovulate. Pregnancy.

Special Concerns: Pregnancy category: X. Use with caution in lactation.

Side Effects: *Ovarian:* Hyperstimulation resulting in ovarian enlargement, abdominal distention or pain, ascites, pleural effusion. *GI:* Nausea, vomiting, diarrhea, bloating, abdominal cramps. *Pyrogenic or allergic reaction:* Chills, fever, muscle aches or pains, fatigue, malaise. *Dermatologic:* Hives, dry skin, loss of hair, rash. *Other:* Headache, ectopic pregnancy, breast tenderness.

Symptoms of Overdose: Hyperstimulation of the ovary, multiple gestations.

Dosage: IM. *Polycystic ovary syndrome:* **Adults, initial,** 75 IU urofollitropin daily for 7–12 days followed by 5,000–10,000 IU HCG 24 hr after the last dose of urofollitropin. If ovulation has occurred but pregnancy has not resulted, this dosage regimen may be repeated for 2 more courses of therapy. If pregnancy still has not resulted, the dose of urofollitropin may be increased to 150 IU daily for 7–12 days followed by 5,000–10,000 IU HCG 24 hr after the last dose of urofollitropin. This regimen may be repeated for 2 additional courses if pregnancy has not occurred. *In vitro fertilization:* **Adults,** 150 IU once daily beginning on day 2 or 3 of the cycle followed by 5,000–10,000 IU of HCG 1 day after the last dose of urofollitropin. Treatment is usually limited to 10 days.

NURSING CONSIDERATIONS

Administration/Storage

1. The powder for injection should be reconstituted by dissolving in 1–2 ml of sterile saline immediately before use.
2. Any unused drug should be discarded.
3. Urofollitropin should be protected from light and stored at 37°F–77°F (3°C–25°C).

Assessment

1. A thorough gynecologic and endocrinologic evaluation and examination should be completed before initiating urofollitropin therapy.
2. Note any history of renal dysfunction, thyroid dysfunction, or abnormal uterine bleeding from an unknown cause.

Client/Family Teaching

1. Report any sudden abdominal pain or tenderness to the physician.
2. Explain that the treatment usually consists of daily injections for 7–12 days.
3. Advise the couple to engage in daily intercourse, beginning 1 day prior to the administration of HCG until ovulation occurs.

4. During the treatment and for 2 weeks thereafter, the client should be examined at least every other day for hyperstimulation of the ovaries. Explain that if evidence of hyperstimulation occurs, the drug will be stopped immediately by the physician.
5. Provide a list of symptoms of hyperstimulation of the ovaries and advise the client to avoid having intercourse if these symptoms occur. A rupture of an ovarian cyst could occur resulting in hemoperitoneum.
6. Explain that the use of this drug enhances the risk of multiple births.
7. Stress the importance of reporting all side effects to the physician and reporting for all examinations as scheduled.

Evaluation

1. Evaluate client for evidence of successful ovulation.
2. In combination with HCG therapy, drug will stimulate ova development.

Urokinase
(your-oh-**KYE**-nayz)
Abbokinase, Abbokinase Open-Cath (Rx)

Classification: Thrombolytic agent.

Action/Kinetics: Urokinase converts plasminogen to plasmin; plasmin then breaks down fibrin clots and fibrinogen. **Onset:** rapid; **duration:** 12 hr. **t½:** Less than 20 min, although effect on coagulation disappears after a few hours.

Uses: Acute pulmonary thromboembolism. To clear IV catheters that are blocked by fibrin or clotted blood. *Investigational:* Acute arterial thromboembolism, acute arterial thrombosis, acute arterial coronary thrombosis, to clear arteriovenous cannula.

Contraindications: Any condition presenting a risk of hemorrhage, such as recent surgery or biopsies, delivery within 10 days, pregnancy, ulcerative disease. Also hepatic or renal insufficiency, TB, recent cerebral embolism, thrombosis, hemorrhage, subacute bacterial endocarditis, rheumatic valvular disease, thrombocytopenia.

Special Concerns: Pregnancy category: B. The use of the drugs in septic thrombophlebitis may be hazardous. Use with caution during lactation. Safe use in children has not been established.

Side Effects: *CV:* Superficial bleeding, severe internal bleeding. *Allergic:* Rarely, skin rashes, bronchospasm. *Other:* Fever.

Drug Interactions: The following drugs ↑ the chance of bleeding when given concomitantly with urokinase: Anticoagulants, aspirin, heparin, indomethacin, and phenylbutazone.

Dosage: IV infusion only. *Acute pulmonary embolism:* **loading dose,** 4,400 IU/kg administered over 10 min at a rate of 90 ml/hr; **maintenance, IV:** 4,400 IU/kg administered continuously at a rate of 15 ml/hr for 12 hr. May be followed by continuous IV heparin infusion to prevent recurrent thrombosis (start only after thrombin time has decreased to less than twice the normal control value). *Coronary artery thrombi:* **Initial,** heparin, as a bolus of 2,500–10,000

units **IV; then,** begin infusion of urokinase at a rate of 6,000 IU/min (4 ml/min) for up to 2 hr (average total dose of urokinase may be 500,000 IU). Urokinase should be administered until the artery is opened maximally (15–30 min after initial opening although it has been given for up to 2 hr). *Clear IV catheter:* instill into the catheter 1–1.8 ml of a solution containing 5,000 IU/ml.

NURSING CONSIDERATIONS

See also *Nursing Considerations* for *Streptokinase,* p. 1159, and *Alteplase, Recombinant,* p. 285.

Administration/Storage

1. Reconstitute only with sterile water for injection without preservatives. Do not use bacteriostatic water.
2. The vial should be rolled and tilted, but not shaken, during reconstitution.
3. Reconstitute immediately before using.
4. Discard any unused portion.
5. Dilute reconstituted urokinase before IV administration in 0.9% normal saline or 5% dextrose injection.

Evaluation: Evaluate client for:
- Evidence of successful lysis of thrombi with restoration of blood flow
- Evidence of the restoration of catheter or cannula patency in previously occluded AV or IV cannulae

Ursodiol
(ur-so-**DYE**-ohl)
Actigall (Rx)

Classification: Gall stone solubilizer.

U

Action/Kinetics: Ursodiol is a naturally occurring bile acid which inhibits the hepatic synthesis and secretion of cholesterol; it also inhibits intestinal absorption of cholesterol. The drug acts to solubilize cholesterol in micelles and to cause dispersion of cholesterol as liquid crystals in aqueous media. The drug undergoes a significant first-pass effect where it is conjugated with either glycine or taurine and then secreted into hepatic bile ducts.

Uses: In clients with radiolucent, noncalcified gall stones (< 20 mm) in whom elective surgery would be risky.

Contraindications: Clients with calcified cholesterol stones, radio-opaque stones, or radiolucent bile pigment stones. Acute cholecystitis, cholangitis, biliary obstruction, gall-stone pancreatitis, biliary-gastrointestinal fistula, allergy to bile acids, chronic liver disease.

Special Concerns: Pregnancy category: B. Use with caution during lactation. Safety and efficacy have not been determined in children. Safety for use beyond 24 months is not known.

Side Effects: *GI:* Diarrhea, nausea, vomiting, dyspepsia, metallic taste, abdominal pain, biliary pain, cholecystitis, constipation, stomatitis, flatulence. *Skin:* Pruritus, rash, dry skin, urticaria. *CNS:* Headache, fatigue, anxiety, depression, sleep disorders. *Other:* Sweating, thinning of hair, back pain, arthralgia, myalgia, rhinitis, cough.
Symptom of Overdose: Diarrhea.

Drug Interactions

Antacids, aluminum-containing / ↓ Effect of ursodiol due to ↓ absorption from GI tract

Cholestyramine / ↓ Effect of ursodiol due to ↓ absorption from GI tract

Clofibrate / ↓ Effect of ursodiol by ↑ hepatic cholesterol secretion

Colestipol / ↓ Effect of ursodiol due to ↓ absorption from GI tract

Contraceptives, oral / ↓ Effect of ursodiol by ↑ hepatic cholesterol secretion

Estrogens / ↓ Effect of ursodiol by ↑ hepatic cholesterol secretion

Dosage: Capsules. Adults: 8–10 mg/kg daily in 2 or 3 divided doses, usually with meals.

NURSING CONSIDERATIONS
Administration/Storage

1. If partial stone dissolution is not observed within 12 months, the drug will probably not be effective.
2. For the first year of therapy, ultrasound of the gallbladder should be performed every 6 months to determine the response.
3. *Treatment of Overdose:* Treat with supportive measures.

Assessment

1. Obtain a baseline ultrasound of the gallbladder and order liver function studies to serve as a baseline against which to measure subsequent studies and evaluate response throughout drug therapy.
2. List the drugs the client is taking, noting those with which ursodiol interacts unfavorably.
3. If the client is female, determine the possibility of pregnancy.
4. In screening the client, note

U

that the drug is not indicated for calcified cholesterol stones, radiopaque stones, or radiolucent bile pigment stones.

Interventions

1. Note any client complaints of nausea, vomiting, diarrhea, abdominal pain or the presence of a metallic taste in the mouth. Document and report to the physician.
2. Observe the client for complaints of headache, anxiety, depression, and sleep disorders. Document and report.

Client/Family Teaching

1. Explain that the ursodiol therapy may take up to 24 months and that the drug will need to be taken 2–3 times a day.
2. Avoid taking antacids unless prescribed by the physician. Many antacids have an aluminum base, which adsorbs the drug.
3. Discuss with the client the fact that stones may recur after the dissolution of the current stones.
4. Provide a printed list of drug side effects. Explain the importance of reporting to the physician symptoms such as persistent nausea and vomiting, abdominal pain, headaches, itching, rash, or altered bowel function.
5. For women of childbearing age, discuss the need to practice birth control because pregnancy should be avoided during drug therapy. The use of estrogens and oral contraceptives may decrease the effectiveness of the drug; therefore, other forms of birth control are advisable.
6. Stress the importance of reporting for follow-up visits to the physician and for reporting for routine laboratory studies and ultrasonography to evaluate the effectiveness of the drug therapy.

Evaluation

1. Evaluate client for radiographic evidence of a decrease in the number or complete dissolution of gallstones.
2. Continue ursodiol therapy for 1–3 months following dissolution and reconfirm again with ultrasound.

V

Valproic acid

(val-PROH-ick)
Depakene (Rx)

Classification: Anticonvulsant, miscellaneous.

Action/Kinetics: The following information also applies to divalproex sodium. The precise anticonvulsant action is unknown, but activity is believed to be caused by increased brain levels of the neurotransmitter gamma-amino butyric acid (GABA). Other possibilities include acting on postsynaptic receptor sites to mimic or enhance the inhibitory effect of GABA, inhibiting an enzyme that catabolizes GABA, affecting the potassium channel, or directly affecting membrane stability. Absorption from the GI tract is more rapid following administration of the syrup (sodium salt) than capsules. **Peak serum levels, capsules and syrup:** 1–4 hr (delayed if the drug is taken with food); **peak serum levels, enteric-coated tablet (divalproex sodium):** 3–4 hr. **t½:** 6–16 hr. **Therapeutic serum levels:** 50–100 mcg/ml. The drug is approximately 90% bound to plasma protein. It is metabolized in the liver and inactive metabolites are excreted in the urine; small amounts of valproic acid are excreted in the feces.

Uses: Alone (preferred) or in combination with other anticonvulsants for treatment of epilepsy characterized by simple and complex absence seizures (petit mal). As an adjunct in mixed seizure patterns. *Investigational:* Alone or in combination to treat atypical absence, myoclonic, and grand mal seizures; also, atonic, complex partial, elementary partial, and infantile spasm seizures. Prophylaxis of febrile seizures in children, manic-depressive illness, and subchronically to treat minor incontinence after ileoanal anastomosis.

Contraindications: Liver disease or dysfunction.

Special Concerns: Safe use during pregnancy (category: D) and during lactation has not been established. Use with caution in children 2 years of age or less as they are at greater risk for developing fatal hepatotoxicity. Geriatric clients should receive a lower daily dose

because they may have increased free, unbound valproic acid levels in the serum.

Side Effects: *GI:* (most frequent): Nausea, vomiting, indigestion. Also, abdominal cramps, diarrhea, constipation, anorexia with weight loss or increased appetite with weight gain. *CNS:* Sedation, psychosis, depression, emotional upset, aggression, hyperactivity, deterioration of behavior, tremor, headache, dizziness, dysarthria, incoordination, coma (rare). *Ophthalmologic:* Nystagmus, diplopia, "spots before eyes." *Hematologic:* Thrombocytopenia, leukopenia, eosinophilia, anemia, bone marrow suppression, relative lymphocytosis, hypofibrinogenemia, myelodysplastic-type syndrome. *Dermatologic:* Transient alopecia, petechiae, erythema multiforme, skin rashes. photosensitivity, pruritus. *Hepatic:* **Hepatotoxicity.** Also, minor increases in AST, ALT, LDH, serum bilirubin, and serum alkaline phosphatase values. *Endocrine:* Menstrual irregularities, breast enlargement, galactorrhea, swelling of parotid gland, abnormal thyroid function tests. *Miscellaneous:* Also asterixis, weakness, bruising, hematoma formation, frank hemorrhage, acute pancreatitis, hyperammonemia, hyperglycinemia, hypocarnitinemia, edema of arms and legs, weakness.

Symptoms of Overdose: Motor restlessness, asterixis, visual hallucinations, deep coma.

Drug Interactions

Alcohol / ↑ Incidence of CNS depression

Aspirin / ↑ Effect of valproic acid due to ↓ plasma protein binding. Also, additive anticoagulant effect

V

Benzodiazepines / ↑ Effect of benzodiazepines due to ↓ breakdown by liver

Carbamazepine / Variable changes in levels of carbamazepine with possible loss of seizure control

Charcoal / ↓ Absorption of valproic acid from the GI tract

Chlorpromazine / ↓ Clearance and ↑ t½ of valproic acid → ↑ pharmacologic effects

Cimetidine / ↓ Clearance and ↑ t½ of valproic acid → ↑ pharmacologic effects

Clonazepam / ↑ Chance of absence seizures (petit mal) and ↑ toxicity due to clonazepam

CNS depressants / ↑ Incidence of CNS depression

Ethosuximide / ↑ or ↓ Effect of ethosuximide

Phenobarbital / ↑ Effect of phenobarbital due to ↓ breakdown by liver

Phenytoin / ↑ Effect of phenytoin due to ↓ breakdown by liver or ↓ effect of phenytoin due to ↓ total serum phenytoin

Primidone / ↑ Effect of primidone due to ↓ breakdown by liver

Warfarin sodium / ↑ Effect of valproic acid due to ↓ plasma protein binding. Also, additive anticoagulant effect

Laboratory Test Interference: False + for ketonuria. Altered thyroid function tests.

Dosage: Capsules, Syrup, Enteric-coated Tablets (Divalproex). Adults and adolescents: initial, monotherapy 15 mg/kg/day. Increase at 1-week intervals by 5–10 mg/kg/day; **maximum:** 60 mg/kg/day. If the total daily dose exceeds 250 mg, the dosage should be divided. **Pediatric, 1–12 years of age: initial, monotherapy:** 15–45 mg/kg daily; dose can be increased by 5–10 mg/kg daily at 1-week intervals. **Adults and adolescents: initial, polytherapy:** 10–30 mg/kg daily; dose can be increased by 5–10 mg/kg daily at 1-week intervals. **Pediatric, 1–12 years of age: initial, polytherapy:** 30–100 mg/kg daily; dose can be increased by 5–10 mg/kg daily at 1-week intervals.

NURSING CONSIDERATIONS

See also *Nursing Considerations for Anticonvulsants,* p. 63.

Administration/Storage

1. Divide daily dosage if it exceeds 250 mg/day.
2. Initiate at lower dosage level or give with food to clients who suffer from GI irritation.
3. Valproic acid capsules should be swallowed whole to avoid local irritation. However, divalproex sodium capsules can either be swallowed whole or the contents sprinkled on a teaspoonful of a soft food (e.g., applesauce, pudding) and swallowed immediately without chewing.
4. Depakote is enteric coated and may decrease GI upset.
5. Do not administer valproic acid syrup to clients whose *sodium* intake must be restricted. Consult physician if a sodium-restricted client is unable to swallow capsules.
6. In clients taking valproic acid, conversion to divalproex sodium can be undertaken at the same total daily dose and dosing schedule.
7. *Treatment of Overdose:* Per-

form gastric lavage if client is seen early enough (valproic acid is absorbed rapidly). Undertake general supportive measures making sure urinary output is maintained. Naloxone has been used to reverse the CNS depression (however, it could also reverse the anticonvulsant effect). Hemodialysis and hemoperfusion have been used with success.

Client/Family Teaching

1. Take drug as directed and with meals to minimize GI upset if evident.
2. Advise clients with diabetes that the drug may cause a false + urine test for ketones. Review some of the symptoms of ketoacidosis (dry mouth, thirst, and dry flushed skin) so that clients can determine if they are acidotic. Instruct to report the development of any of these symptoms to the physician.
3. Stress the importance of reporting for periodic CBC, serum ketones, and liver function studies as scheduled, throughout therapy with valproic acid.
4. Any unexplained fever, sore throat, skin rash, or unusual bruising or bleeding should be reported immediately to the physician.
5. Do not drive or perform activities that require mental alertness until drug effects realized and seizure control verified by the physician.
6. Take only as directed and do not stop suddenly without physician knowledge because seizures may occur.

Evaluation: Evaluate client for:
- Evidence of control of seizures
- Laboratory confirmation that serum drug levels are within therapeutic range (50–100 mcg/ml)

Vancomycin hydrochloride
(van-koh-**MY**-sin)
Diatracin✽, Lyphocin, Vancocin, Vancoled (Rx)

See also *Anti-Infectives,* p. 80.

Classification: Antibiotic, miscellaneous.

Action/Kinetics: This antibiotic, derived from *Streptomyces orientalis,* diffuses in pleural, pericardial, ascitic, and synovial fluids after parenteral administration. It appears to bind to bacterial cell wall, arresting its synthesis and lysing the cytoplasmic membrane by a mechanism that is different from that of penicillin. The drug is bactericidal for most organisms and bacteriostatic for enterococci. It is poorly absorbed from GI tract. **Peak plasma levels, IV:** 33 mcg/ml 5 min after 0.5-g dosage. **t½:** 4–8 hr for adults and 2–3 hr for children. The half-life is increased markedly in the presence of renal impairment (240 hr has been noted). Primarily excreted in urine unchanged. Auditory and renal function tests are indicated before and during therapy.

V

Uses: Agent should be reserved for treatment of life-threatening infections when other treatments have been ineffective. Clients with severe staphylococcal infections resistant to (or clients allergic to) penicillin or cephalosporins (e.g., endocarditis, osteomyelitis, pneumonia, and septicemia). Oral administration is useful in treatment of enterocolitis and pseudomembranous colitis.

Contraindications: Hypersensitivity to drug. Minor infections.

Special Concerns: Pregnancy category: C. Use with extreme caution in the presence of impaired renal function or previous hearing loss. Geriatric clients are at a greater risk of developing ototoxicity.

Side Effects: Ototoxicity (may lead to deafness), nephrotoxicity (may lead to uremia). *Red-neck syndrome:* Chills, erythema of neck and back, fever, paresthesias. *Dermatologic:* Urticaria, macular rashes. *Allergic:* Drug fever, hypersensitivity, anaphylaxis. *Miscellaneous:* Nausea, tinnitus, eosinophilia, neutropenia, hypotension (due to rapid administration). Thrombophlebitis at site of injection. Deafness may progress after drug is discontinued.

Drug Interactions: Never give with other ototoxic or nephrotoxic agents, especially aminoglycosides and polymyxins.

Dosage: Capsules, Oral Solution: Adults, 0.5 g q 6 hr or 1 g q 12 hr. *Pseudomembranous colitis:* **PO: Adults,** 0.5–2 g daily in 3–4 divided doses for 7–10 days; **pediatric,** 40 mg/kg daily in divided doses, not to exceed 2 g daily; **neonates,** 10 mg/kg daily in divided doses. **IV: Adults,** 0.5 g q 6 hr or 1 g q 12 hr; **pediatric,** 40 mg/kg daily in divided doses (add to IV fluids). **Neonates, initial:** 15 mg/kg; **then, up to 1 month of age:** 10 mg/kg q 12 hr and after 1 month of age, 10 mg/kg q 8 hr.

Prophylaxis of bacterial endocarditis, penicillin-sensitive clients undergoing upper respiratory tract surgery/instrumentation or dental procedures: **IV, Adults and children over 27 kg,** 1 g given slowly over 60 min before procedure; **IV, pediatric, less than 27 kg:** 20 mg/kg given slowly over 60 min before procedure. If client is at high risk, the dose can be repeated in 8–12 hr. *Prophylaxis of bacterial endocarditis, penicillin-sensitive clients undergoing GI or urinary tract instrumentation/surgery:* **IV, Adults and children over 27 kg,** 1 g given slowly over 60 min concurrently with gentamicin, 1.5 mg/kg, **IV or IM,** 60 min prior to procedure; **IV, pediatric, less than 27 kg:** 20 mg/kg given slowly over 60 min concurrently with gentamicin, 2 mg/kg, **IM or IV,** 60 min prior to procedure. If client is at high risk, the dose can be repeated in 8–12 hr. Dosage must be reduced in clients with renal disease.

NURSING CONSIDERATIONS

See also *General Nursing Considerations For All Anti-Infectives,* p. 83.

Administration/Storage

1. Mix as indicated on package insert.
2. Intermittent infusion is the preferred route, but continuous IV drip may be used.
3. Avoid rapid IV administration because this may result in nausea, warmth, and generalized tingling.
4. Avoid extravasation during injections.
5. Reduce risk of thrombophlebitis by rotating injection sites or adding additional diluent.
6. Parenteral form may be ad-

V

ministered orally. Dilute one 500-mg vial in 1 oz of water for oral administration. Client may drink solution or it may be administered by nasogastric tube.

7. Aqueous solution is stable for 2 weeks.

8. Once rubber stopper is punctured, ampule should be refrigerated to maintain stability.

Interventions

1. Anticipate reduced dose with renal dysfunction.

2. Monitor and record vital signs and I&O.

3. Assess for evidence of adverse drug effects, such as:

   • Ototoxicity, demonstrated by tinnitus, progressive hearing loss, dizziness, and/or nystagmus

   • Nephrotoxicity, demonstrated by albuminuria, hematuria, anuria, casts, edema, and uremia

Evaluation: Evaluate client for:

   • Laboratory evidence of negative culture reports

   • Clinical evidence and reports of symptomatic improvement

---

Vasopressin

(vay-so-**PRESS**-in)
Pitressin Synthetic, Pressyn ✳ (Rx)

Vasopressin Tannate Injection

(vay-so-**PRESS**-in)
Pitressin Tannate in Oil (Rx)

Classification: Pituitary (antidiuretic) hormone.

Action/Kinetics: The antidiuretic hormone ADH, more often referred to as vasopressin, is released from the anterior pituitary gland. The hormone regulates water conservation by promoting reabsorption of water by increasing the permeability of the collecting ducts in the kidney.

Insufficient output of ADH results in neurogenic or central diabetes insipidus, characterized by the excretion of large quantities of normal but dilute urine and excessive thirst. These symptoms result from primary (no organic lesion) or secondary (injury) malfunction of posterior pituitary. Vasopressin is effective in the treatment of the condition. It is ineffective when the diabetes insipidus is of renal origin (nephrogenic diabetes insipidus).

In addition to its diuretic properties, vasopressin also causes vasoconstriction (pressor effect) of the splanchnic and portal vessels (and to a lesser extent of peripheral, cerebral, pulmonary, and coronary vessels). Vasopressin also increases the smooth muscular activity of the bladder, GI tract, and uterus. *Vasopressin.* **IM, SC: Onset,** variable; **duration,** 2–8 hr. **t½:** 10–20 min. **Effective plasma levels:** 4.5–6 microunits. *Vasopressin tannate.* **Duration:** 24–96 hr. Hormone metabolized by the liver and kidney.

Use: Vasopressin: Neurogenic diabetes insipidus, relief of postoperative intestinal gaseous distention, to dispel gas shadows in abdominal roentgenography. *Investigational:* Bleeding esophageal varices. **Vasopressin tannate:** Neurogenic diabetes insipidus. *Investigational:* Diagnosis of diabetes insipidus, diagnosis of renal function.

Contraindications: Vascular disease, especially when involving coronary arteries; angina pectoris. Chronic nephritis until reasonable blood nitrogen levels are attained. Never give the tannate IV.

Special Concerns: Pregnancy category: C. Pediatric and geriatric clients have an increased risk of hyponatremia and water intoxication. Use caution in the presence of asthma, epilepsy, migraine, and congestive heart failure.

Side Effects: *GI:* Nausea, vomiting, increased intestinal activity (e.g., belching, cramps, urge to defecate), flatus. *Miscellaneous:* Facial pallor, tremor, sweating, allergic reactions, vertigo, bronchoconstriction, anaphylaxis, "pounding" in head, water intoxication (drowsiness, headache, coma, convulsions).

IV use of vasopressin may result in severe vasoconstriction; local tissue necrosis if extravasation occurs. IM use of tannate may cause pain and sterile abscesses at site of injection.
Symptom of Overdose: Water intoxication.

Drug Interactions: Carbamazepine, chlorpropamide, or clofibrate may ↑ antidiuretic effects of vasopressin.

Dosage: Vasopressin, IM, SC. *Diabetes insipidus.* **Adults,** 5–10 units b.i.d.–t.i.d.; **pediatric:** 2.5–10 units t.i.d.–q.i.d. *Abdominal distention.* **Adults, initial, IM,** 5 units; **then,** 10 units q 3–4 hr; **pediatric:** dose should be individualized (usual: 2.5–5 units). *Abdominal roentgenography.* **IM, SC:** 2 injections of 10 units each 2 hr and ½ hr before films exposed.
 Vasopressin tannate, IM only. *Diabetes insipidus.* **Adults,** 1.5–5 units q 1–3 days; **pediatric:** 1.25–2.5 units q 1–3 days. *Diagnosis of*

diabetes insipidus. **Adults,** 5 units during the evening followed by collection of urine samples for comparison of osmolality. *Diagnosis of renal function.* **Adults,** 5–10 units 2 hr before collecting urine samples for determination of specific gravity.

NURSING CONSIDERATIONS

Administration/Storage

1. Administration of 1–2 glasses of water prior to use for diabetes insipidus will reduce side effects such as nausea, cramps, and blanching of the skin.
2. Warm the vial of vasopressin tannate in oil in the hands and mix until the hormone is distributed throughout the solution before withdrawing the dose.
3. *Treatment of Overdose:* Withdraw vasopressin until polyuria occurs. If water intoxication is serious, administration of mannitol (i.e., an osmotic diuretic), hypertonic dextrose, or urea alone (or with furosemide) is indicated.

Assessment

1. Note any client history of vascular disease, especially any involving the coronary arteries.
2. Determine if the client has any history of asthma or migraine headaches and document.

Interventions

1. Monitor I&O to evaluate the client's response to therapy.
2. Check skin turgor, the condition of mucous membranes, and assess for the presence of thirst to determine if dehydration is present.
3. Take the BP at least 2 times/day

while the client is on a regimen of vasopressin, and report to the physician any adverse reactions, such as an excessive elevation of BP or lack of response to the drug as characterized by a lowering of BP.

4. Weigh the client daily and record. Report any rapid weight gain and assess for edema.

5. Perform urine specific gravity and report if less than 1.005 or greater than 1.030. Determine urine osmolarity.

Evaluation

1. Evaluate client for reports of increased continence, decreased urinary frequency, and laboratory evidence of increased urine osmolarity (in diabetes insipidus).

2. Evidence of bowel sounds, the passage of flatus, resumption of bowel movements, and a reduction in abdominal distention when used to improve peristalsis in the GI tract.

Vecuronium bromide

(vh-kyour-**OH**-nee-um)

Norcuron (Rx)

See also *Neuromuscular Blocking Agents,* p. 183.

Classification: Nondepolarizing neuromuscular blocking agent.

Action/Kinetics: Less likely than other agents to cause histamine release. Effects can be antagonized by anticholinesterase drugs. **Onset:** 2.5–3 min; **peak effect:** 3–5 min; **duration:** 25–30 min using balanced anesthesia. No cumulative effects noted after re-

peated administration. Metabolized in liver and excreted through the kidney and bile. Is bound to plasma protein.

Uses: To induce skeletal muscle relaxation during surgery or to assist in endotracheal intubation. As an adjunct to general anesthesia. *Investigational:* To treat electrically induced seizures or seizures induced by drugs.

Additional Contraindications: Use in neonates, obesity. Sensitivity to bromides.

Special Concerns: Pregnancy category: C. Pediatric clients from 7 weeks to 1 year of age are more sensitive to the effects of vecuronium leading to a recovery time up to 1½ times that for adults. The dose for children aged 1–10 years of age must be individualized and may, in fact, require a somewhat higher initial dose and a slightly more frequent supplemental dosing schedule than adults.

Additional Side Effects: Moderate to severe skeletal muscle weakness, which may require artificial respiration. Malignant hyperthermia.

Additional Drug Interaction: Succinylcholine ↑ effect of vecuronium.

Dosage: IV only. Adults and children over 10 years of age. *Intubation:* 0.08–0.1 mg/kg. *For use after succinylcholine-assisted endotracheal intubation:* 0.04–0.06 mg/kg for inhalation anesthesia and 0.05–0.06 mg/kg using balanced anesthesia. (**Note:** For halothane anesthesia, doses from 0.15–0.28 mg/kg may be given without adverse effects.) *For use during*

V

anesthesia with enflurane or iso-flurane after steady-state estab-lished: 0.06–0.085 mg/kg (about 15% less than the usual initial dose). *Supplemental use:* **IV:** 0.01–0.015 mg/kg given 25–40 min following the initial dose; **then,** given q 12–15 min as needed. **IV infusion:** Initiated after recovery from effects of initial IV dose of 0.08–0.1 mg/kg has started. Infusion rate: 0.0008–0.0012 mg/kg. After steady-state enflurane, isoflurane, and possibly halothane anesthesia has been established: IV infusion should be reduced by 25%–60%.

NURSING CONSIDERATIONS

See also *Nursing Considerations* for *Neuromuscular Blocking Agents,* p. 184.

Administration/Storage

1. Dosage must be individualized and depends on prior or concomitant use of anesthetics or succinylcholine.
2. Vecuronium may be mixed with saline, 5% dextrose alone or with saline, lactated Ringer's solution, and sterile water for injection.
3. Vecuronium should be used within 8 hr of reconstitution.
4. Anticipate the onset of action to occur within 1–5 min and the effect to last 20–40 min.
5. The drug should be refrigerated after reconstitution.

Evaluation: Evaluate client for:
- Attainment of the desired level of skeletal muscle relaxation
- Effective suppression of the twitch response when tested with a peripheral nerve stimulator

Verapamil

(ver-**AP**-ah-mil)
Apo-Verap✤, Calan, Calan SR, Isoptin, Isoptin Parenteral✤, Isoptin SR, Novo-Veramil✤, Nu-Verap✤, Verelan (Rx)

See also *Calcium Channel Blocking Agents,* p. 118.

Classification: Calcium channel blocking agent (antianginal, antiarrhythmic).

Action/Kinetics: Slows AV conduction and prolongs effective refractory period. IV doses may slightly increase left ventricular filling pressure. The drug moderately decreases myocardial contractility and peripheral vascular resistance. Worsening of heart failure may result if verapamil is given to clients with moderate to severe cardiac dysfunction. **Onset: PO,** 30 min; **IV,** 3–5 min. **Time to peak plasma levels (PO):** 1–2 hr (5–7 hr for extended-release). $t^{1/2}$, **PO:** 4.5–12 hr with repetitive dosing; **IV, initial:** 4 min; **final:** 2–5 hr. **Therapeutic serum levels:** 0.08–0.3 mcg/ml. **Duration: PO:** 8–10 hr (24 hr for extended-release); **IV,** 10–20 min for hemodynamic effect and 2 hr for antiarrhythmic effect. Verapamil is metabolized to norverapamil, which possesses 20% of the activity of verapamil.

Uses: PO: Angina pectoris due to coronary artery spasm (Prinzmetal's variant), chronic stable angina including angina due to increased effort, unstable angina (preinfarction, crescendo); with digitalis to control rapid ventricular rate in chronic atrial flutter or atrial fibrillation; essential hypertension. Sustained-release tablets are used to treat essential hypertension

(Step I therapy). **IV:** Supraventricular tachyarrhythmias. *Investigational:* Orally for prophylaxis of migraine, manic depression (alternate therapy), exercise-induced asthma, recumbent nocturnal leg cramps, treatment of PSVT, cardiomyopathy.

Contraindications: Severe hypotension, second- or third-degree AV block, cardiogenic shock, severe congestive heart failure, sick sinus syndrome (unless client has artificial pacemaker), severe left ventricular dysfunction. Cardiogenic shock and severe congestive heart failure unless secondary to supraventricular tachycardia which can be treated with verapamil. Lactation. Use of verapamil, IV, with beta-adrenergic blocking agents (as both depress myocardial contractility and AV conduction). Ventricular tachycardia.

Special Concerns: Use during pregnancy only if benefits outweigh risks (pregnancy category: C). Infants less than 6 months of age may not respond to verapamil. Use with caution in hypertrophic cardiomyopathy, impaired hepatic and renal function, and in the elderly.

Side Effects: *CV:* Congestive heart failure, AV block, bradycardia, asystole, premature ventricular contractions and tachycardia (after IV use), peripheral and pulmonary edema, hypotension, syncope, palpitations, myocardial infarction, atrioventricular dissociation, cerebrovascular accident. *GI:* Nausea, constipation, abdominal discomfort or cramps, dyspepsia, diarrhea, dry mouth. *CNS:* Dizziness, headache, sleep disturbances, depression, amnesia, paranoia, psychoses, hallucinations, jitteriness, confusion, drowsiness, vertigo. IV verapamil may increase intracranial pressure in clients with supratentorial tumors at the time of induction of anesthesia. *Dermatologic:* Rash, dermatitis, alopecia, urticaria, pruritus, erythema multiforme, Stevens-Johnson syndrome. *Respiratory:* Nasal or chest congestion, dyspnea, shortness of breath, wheezing. *Musculoskeletal:* Paresthesia, asthenia, muscle cramps or inflammation, decreased neuromuscular transmission in Duchenne's muscular dystrophy. *Other:* Blurred vision, equilibrium disturbances, sexual difficulties, spotty menstruation, sweating, rotary nystagmus, flushing, gingival hyperplasia, polyuria, nocturia, gynecomastia, claudication, hyperkeratosis, purpura, petechiae, bruising, hematomas, tachyphylaxis.

Additional Drug Interactions

Antihypertensive agents / Additive hypotensive effects

Calcium salts / ↓ Effect of verapamil

Carbamazepine / ↑ Effect of carbamazepine due to ↓ breakdown by liver

Cyclosporine / ↑ Plasma levels of cyclosporine possibly leading to renal toxicity

Digoxin / ↑ Risk of digoxin toxicity due to ↑ plasma levels

Disopyramide / Additive depressant effects on myocardial contractility and AV conduction

Etomidate / Anesthetic effect of etomidate may be ↑ with prolonged respiratory depression and apnea

Lithium / ↓ Lithium plasma levels

Muscle relaxants, nondepolarizing / ↑ Neuromuscular blockade due to effect of verapamil on calcium channels

Prazosin / Acute hypotensive effect

Quinidine / Effect of quinidine altered by verapamil

Rifampin / ↓ Effect of verapamil

Sulfinpyrazone / ↓ Clearance of verapamil

Theophyllines / ↑ Effect of theophyllines

Vitamin D / ↓ Effect of verapamil

Warfarin / Possible ↑ effect of either drug due to ↓ plasma protein binding

Note: Since verapamil is significantly bound to plasma proteins, interaction with other drugs bound to plasma protein may occur.

Laboratory Test Interferences: ↑ Alkaline phosphatase, transaminase.

Dosage: Tablets. *Angina.* **Individualized. Adults: initial,** 80–120 mg t.i.d. (40 mg t.i.d. if client is sensitive to verapamil); **then,** increase dose to total of 240–480 mg/day. *Arrhythmias.* Dosage range in digitalized clients with chronic atrial fibrillation: 240–320 mg daily. For prophylaxis of nondigitalized clients: 240–480 mg daily in divided doses t.i.d.–q.i.d. *Essential hypertension.* **Initial, when used alone:** 80 mg t.i.d. In the elderly or in people of small stature, initial dose should be 40 mg t.i.d. *Essential hypertension.* **Extended-release Tablets:** 180–240 mg daily (120 mg daily in the elderly or people of small stature). If response is inadequate, 240 mg may be given b.i.d. **IV, slow.** *Supraventricular tachyarrhythmias:* **Adults: initial,** 5–10 mg (0.075–0.15 mg/kg) given over 2 min (over 3 min in older clients); **then,** 10 mg (0.15 mg/kg) 30 min later if response is not adequate. **Infants, up to 1 year:** 0.1–0.2 mg/kg over 2 min; **1–15 years:** 0.1–0.3 mg/kg (not to exceed 5 mg total dose) over 2 min. If

response to initial dose is inadequate, it may be repeated after 30 min.

NURSING CONSIDERATIONS

See also *Nursing Considerations* for *Calcium Channel Blocking Agents,* p. 119.

Administration/Storage

1. Before administration, ampules should be inspected for particulate matter or discoloration.

2. IV dosage should be administered under continuous ECG monitoring with resuscitation equipment readily available.

3. Give as a slow IV bolus over 2 min (3 min to elderly clients) to minimize toxic effects.

4. Ampules should be stored at 15°C–30°C (59°F–86°F) and protected from light.

5. Do not give verapamil in an infusion line containing 0.45% sodium chloride with sodium bicarbonate because a crystalline precipitate will form.

6. Do not give verapamil by IV push in the same line used for nafcillin infusion because a milky white precipitate will form.

7. Verapamil should not be mixed with albumin, amphotericin B, hydralazine, trimethoprim/sulfamethoxazole, or diluted with sodium lactate in polyvinyl chloride bags.

8. Verapamil will precipitate in any solution with a pH greater than 6.

9. Dosage of verapamil in the elderly should always be individualized.

10. In the elderly, the pharmacologic effects are more pronounced and more prolonged.

11. The SR tablets (120 mg) may be useful for small stature and

elderly clients who require less medication.
12. *Treatment of Overdose:* Beta-adrenergics, IV calcium, vasopressors, pacing, and resuscitation.

Assessment: Check vital signs and note any presence of hypotension. Verapamil may lower BP to dangerously low levels if the client already has a low BP.

Interventions

1. If the drug is to be administered IV, have continuous ECG monitoring and emergency drugs and resuscitative equipment readily available.
2. Assess for bradycardia and hypotension, symptoms that may indicate overdosage.
3. *Do not* administer concurrently with IV beta-adrenergic blocking agents.
4. If disopyramide is to be used, do not administer for at least 48 hr before verapamil to 24 hr after verapamil administration.
5. Unless treating verapamil overdosage, withhold any medication that elevates serum calcium levels and check with physician.
6. Clients receiving concurrent digoxin therapy should be assessed for symptoms of toxicity and have digoxin levels checked periodically.
7. Anticipate reduced dosage for clients with hepatic or renal impairment.
8. Administer extended-release tablets with food to minimize fluctuations in serum levels.

Evaluation: Evaluate client for:
• Reports of a decrease in the frequency and severity of anginal attacks

• Evidence of a ↓ blood pressure
• ECG confirmation of a return to normal sinus rhythm, usually attained 10 min after IV administration
• Laboratory evidence that serum drug levels are within therapeutic range (0.08–0.3 mcg/ml)

——— *COMBINATION DRUG* ———
Vicodin
(VYE-koh-din)
(C-III, Rx)

See also *Acetaminophen,* p. 250, and *Narcotic Analgesics,* p. 174.

Classification/Content: Each tablet contains: *Nonnarcotic analgesic:* Acetaminophen, 500 mg. *Narcotic analgesic:* Hydrocodone bitartrate, 5 mg.

Uses: Moderate to moderately severe pain.

Contraindication: Lactation.

Special Concerns: Pregnancy category: C. May cause dependence due to hydrocodone. Safety and effectiveness have not been determined in children.

Dosage: Tablets. Adults, individualized, usual: 1–2 tablets q 4–6 hr as needed for pain, up to maximum of 8 tablets in 24 hr.

NURSING CONSIDERATIONS

See *Nursing Considerations* for *Acetaminophen,* p. 252, and *Narcotic Analgesics,* p. 177.

Administration/Storage: The dose should be adjusted depending on the response of the client and the severity of the pain.

Evaluation: Evaluate client for reports of effective control of pain.

Vidarabine
(vye-**DAIR**-ah-been)
Vira-A (Rx)

See also *Anti-Infectives,* p. 80.

Classification: Antiviral, ophthalmic.

Action/Kinetics: Vidarabine is phosphorylated in the cell to arabinosyl adenosine monophosphate (ara-AMP) or the triphosphate (ara-ATP). These compounds cause inhibition of viral DNA polymerase, inhibition of virus-induced ribonucleotide reductase, or inhibition of enzymes specific for viruses to synthesis of DNA. These effects prevent lengthening of the DNA chain. Vidarabine is rapidly metabolized to ara-HX, which has decreased antiviral activity. **Peak plasma levels:** Vidarabine, 0.2–0.4 mcg/ml; ara-HX, 3–6 mcg/ml. **t½:** **IV**, vidarabine, 1.5 hr; ara-HX, 3.3. hr. Drug and metabolites excreted by kidneys.

Uses: *Systemic:* Herpes simplex viral encephalitis. Neonatal herpes simplex viral infections including disseminated infection with encephalitis, visceral involvement, and infections of the eyes, mouth, and skin. Herpes zoster in immunocompromised clients. *Topical:* Primary keratoconjunctivitis and recurrent epithelial keratitis caused by herpes simplex virus types 1 and 2. Epithelial keratitis resistant to idoxuridine. It is more effective than idoxuridine for deep recurrent infections.

Contraindications: Hypersensitivity to drug. Concomitant use of adrenocorticosteroids usually contraindicated. Lactation.

Special Concerns: Safe use during pregnancy not established

(pregnancy category: C). *Systemic:* Use with caution in clients susceptible to fluid overload, cerebral edema, or with impaired renal or hepatic function. The drug may be carcinogenic and mutagenic. Early diagnosis and treatment of viral infections are essential.

Drug Interactions: Allopurinol may interfere with the metabolism of vidarabine.

Side Effects: Systemic. *GI:* Nausea, vomiting, diarrhea, hematemesis. *CNS:* Tremor, dizziness, ataxia, confusion, hallucinations, psychoses, encephalopathy (may be fatal). *Hematologic:* Decrease in reticulocytes, hemoglobin, and hematocrit. *Miscellaneous:* Weight loss, malaise, rash, pruritus, pain at injection site. *Topical:* Photophobia, lacrimation, conjunctival injection, foreign body sensation, temporal visual haze, burning, irritation, superficial punctate keratitis, pain, punctal occlusion, sensitivity.

Symptoms of Overdose: Bone marrow depression with thrombocytopenia and leukopenia.

Laboratory Test Interferences: ↑ Bilirubin, AST.

Dosage: IV infusion: *Herpes simplex viral encephalitis, neonatal herpes simplex viral infections:* 15 mg/kg/day for 10 days. *Herpes zoster:* 10/mg/kg/day for 5 days. **Ophthalmic ointment:** ½ inch of 3% ointment applied to lower conjunctival sac 5 times daily at 3-hr intervals. Continue therapy for 7 days after complete reepithelialization but at reduced dosage (e.g., twice daily).

NURSING CONSIDERATIONS

See also *General Nursing Considerations For All Anti-Infectives,* p. 83.

Administration/Storage

1. Systemic: slowly infuse total daily dose at constant rate over 12–24 hr.
2. A total of 2.2 ml of IV solution is required to dissolve 1 mg of medication. A maximum of 450 mg may be dissolved in 1 L. Should be used within 48 hr after dilution. Do not refrigerate solution.
3. Any carbohydrate or electrolyte solution is suitable as diluent. Do not use biologic or colloidal fluids.
4. Shake vidarabine vial well before withdrawing dosage. Add to prewarmed (35°C–40°C, 95°F–104°F) infusion solution. Shake mixture until completely clear.
5. For final filtration use an in-line filter (0.45 μm).
6. Dilute just before administration and use within 48 hr.
7. Due to insolubility, the drug may have to be given in a large fluid volume. Care should be exercised in administering such a volume to clients susceptible to fluid overloading or with cerebral edema (e.g., with CNS infections or renal impairment).
8. Topical corticosteroids or antibiotics may be used concomitantly with vidarabine, but benefits and risks must be assessed.
9. Wait 10 min before use of an additional topical ointment.
10. *Treatment of Overdose:* Monitor hematologic as well as liver and kidney function.

Interventions

1. Record I&O and observe client on systemic therapy for fluid overload.

2. Assess client for renal, liver, and hematologic dysfunction precipitated by vidarabine; monitor appropriate laboratory data.

Client/Family Teaching

1. Take only as directed and do not share medications.
2. Wash hands before and after applying ointment.
3. Ophthalmic ointment will cause a temporary haze after application. Avoid hazardous activities until vision clears.
4. Report any persistent or bothersome side effects.
5. Wear sunglasses outside and avoid bright lights because drug may cause photophobic reactions.
6. Do not wear contact lenses until infection clears.
7. Client must remain under close supervision of an ophthalmologist while receiving therapy for ophthalmic problem.

Evaluation: Evaluate client for:
- Laboratory confirmation of negative culture results
- Clinical evidence of effective treatment of herpetic encephalitis
- Evidence of successful reepithelialization of herpetic eye lesions with complete healing of eyes in 1–3 weeks

V

Vinblastine sulfate

(vin-**BLAS**-teen)

**Velban, Velbe ✳, Velsar
(Abbreviation: VLB) (Rx)**

See also *Antineoplastic Agents,* p. 85.

Classification: Antineoplastic, plant alkaloid.

Action/Kinetics: Alkaloid, isolated from the periwinkle plant, is believed to inhibit mitosis (metaphase in cell cycle). Rapidly cleared from plasma but poor penetration to the brain. About 75% bound to serum proteins. Almost completely metabolized in the liver after IV administration. $t^{1/2}$, **triphasic:** initial, 3.7 min; intermediate 1.6 hr; final, approximately 25 hr. Metabolites are excreted in the bile with smaller amounts in the urine. No cross-resistance with vincristine.

Uses: Palliative treatment of Hodgkin's disease, lymphocytic leukemia, mycosis fungoides, advanced carcinoma of testis, histiocytic lymphoma, Kaposi's sarcoma, Letterer-Siwe disease, trophoblastic tumors, and breast cancer (especially cancer unresponsive to other drugs or surgery). Usually administered in combination with other drugs. *Investigational:* Cancer of the head and neck, bladder, lung, kidney, chronic myelocytic leukemia, and ovarian germ cell tumors.

Contraindications: Leukopenia, granulocytopenia. Bacterial infections. Lactation.

Special Concerns: Pregnancy category: D.

Additional Side Effects: Toxicity is dose-related and more pronounced in clients over age 65 or in those suffering from cachexia (profound general ill health) or skin ulceration. *GI:* Ileus, rectal bleeding, hemorrhagic enterocolitis, vesiculation of the mouth, bleeding from a former ulcer. *Dermatologic:* Total epilation, skin vesiculation. *Neurologic:* Paresthesias, neuritis, mental depression, loss of deep tendon reflexes, seizures. Extravasation may result in phlebitis and cellulitis with sloughing.

Symptoms of Overdose: Exaggeration of side effects (see above). Neurotoxicity.

Drug Interactions

Bleomycin sulfate / Combination of bleomycin and vinblastine may produce signs of Raynaud's disease in clients with testicular cancer

Glutamic acid / Inhibits effect of vinblastine

Mitomycin C / Severe bronchospasm with shortness of breath

Phenytoin / ↓ Effect of phenytoin due to ↓ plasma levels

Tryptophan / Inhibits effect of vinblastine

Dosage: IV, *individualized, using WBC count as guide.* Vinblastine is administered once every 7 days. **Adults: initial,** 3.7 mg/m²; **then,** after 7 days, graded doses of 5.5, 7.4, 9.25, and 11.1 mg/m² at intervals of 7 days (maximum dose should not exceed 18.5 mg/m²). **Children: initial,** 2.5 mg/m²; **then,** after 7 days, graded doses of 3.75, 5.0, 6.25, and 7.5 mg/m² at intervals of 7 days (maximum dose should not exceed 12.5 mg/m²). **Maintenance** doses are calculated based on WBC count—at least 4,000/mm³.

NURSING CONSIDERATIONS

See also *Nursing Considerations* for *Antineoplastic Agents,* p. 88.

Administration/Storage

1. Dilute vinblastine with 10 ml of sodium chloride injection.
2. Inject into flowing infusion or directly into vein.

3. Remainder of solution may be stored in refrigerator for 30 days.
4. If the drug gets into the eye, immediately wash eye thoroughly with water to prevent irritation and ulceration.
5. To reconstitute, under a laminar flow hood, add 10 ml sodium chloride injection, which is preserved with either benzyl alcohol or phenol for a final concentration of 1 mg/ml.
6. The drug should not be reconstituted with solutions that raise or lower the pH from between 3.5 and 5.
7. *Treatment of Overdose:*
   - If ingestion is discovered early enough, oral activated charcoal slurry should be given followed by a cathartic.
   - Treat side effects due to inappropriate secretion of antidiuretic hormone.
   - Prevent ileus (e.g., enemas, cathartic).
   - Administer an anticonvulsant (e.g., phenobarbital), if necessary.
   - Monitor the cardiovascular system.
   - Monitor blood counts daily to determine risk of infection and whether blood transfusions are necessary.

Assessment

1. Take a thorough drug history.
2. Note any evidence of neuropathies prior to onset of therapy.
3. Obtain CBC with neutrophil and platelet counts before starting therapy as a baseline against which to measure once therapy has been initiated.

Interventions

1. Assess peripheral IV site for patency to prevent extravasation and local irritation and pain. If extravasation occurs, move infusion to another vein. Treat affected area with injection of hyaluronidase and application of moderate heat to decrease local reaction.
2. Observe client for cyanosis and pallor of extremities and for signs of Raynaud's disease if also receiving bleomycin.
3. Check clients for manifestations of neurotoxicity. Monitor neurologic toxicity by checking client reflexes and strength of hand grip. Report these findings and document accordingly because the dosage of drug may need to be adjusted.
4. Administer an antiemetic to control nausea and vomiting.
5. Monitor I&O. Encourage fluid intake of 2 L/day.
6. Observe for symptoms of gout. Assess need for adding allopurinol or for alkalization of urine to decrease uric acid levels.

Client/Family Teaching

1. Advise to report any signs of infection, fever, sore throat, unusual bruising or bleeding to the physician.
2. Instruct women and men undergoing therapy to practice barrier contraception.
3. To prevent constipation, eat a high fiber diet, increase intake of fluids, remain active, and take stool softeners as prescribed.
4. Wear protective clothing and a sunscreen if exposure to sunlight is necessary.

V

5. Advise that partial hair loss may occur and assist with planning for cosmetic replacement.
6. Report any evidence of jaw pain, numbness, tingling, and deep tendon loss as well as diminished reflexes in the lower extremities because this is an indication to discontinue drug therapy.

Evaluation: Evaluate client for evidence of control and/or regression of malignant process.

Vincristine sulfate
(vin-**KRIS**-teen)
Oncovin, Vincasar PFS, Vincrex (Abbreviation: VCR or LCR) (Rx)

See also *Antineoplastic Agents,* p. 85.

Classification: Antineoplastic, plant alkaloid.

Action/Kinetics: Vincristine is an alkaloid obtained from periwinkle. Vincristine inhibits mitosis at metaphase. The antineoplastic effect is due to interference with intracellular tubulin function by binding to microtubule and spindle proteins in the S phase. After IV use, drug is distributed within 15–30 min to tissues. Poorly penetrates blood-brain barrier. **t½, triphasic:** initial, 5 min; intermediate, 2.3 hr; final, 85 hr. Approximately 80% is excreted in the feces and up to 20% in the urine. No cross-resistance with vinblastine.

Uses: Frequently used in combination therapy. Acute lymphocytic leukemia in children. Hodgkin's and non-Hodgkin's lymphomas (lymphocytic, mixed-cell, histiocytic, undifferentiated, nodular, and diffuse). Wilms' tumor, neuroblastoma, lymphosarcoma, rhabdomyosarcoma, reticulum cell sarcoma. *Investigational:* Idiopathic thrombocytopenic purpura; cancer of the breast, ovary, cervix, lung, colorectal area; malignant melanoma, osteosarcoma, multiple myeloma, ovarian germ cell tumors, mycosis fungoides, chronic lymphocytic leukemia, chronic myelocytic leukemia. Kaposi's sarcoma.

Contraindications: Clients with demyelinating Charcot-Marie-Tooth syndrome. Lactation. Use during radiation therapy.

Special Concerns: Pregnancy category: D. Geriatric clients are more susceptible to the neurotoxic effects. Intrathecal use (may cause death).

Additional Side Effects: *Neurologic:* Paresthesias, depression of deep tendon reflexes, foot drop, seizures, difficulties in gait. *GI:* Intestinal necrosis or perforation. Constipation, paralytic ileus. *Renal:* Inappropriate antidiuretic hormone secretion (polyuria or dysuria). Acute uric acid nephropathy. *Ophthalmic:* Blindness, ptosis, diplopia, photophobia. *Miscellaneous:* CNS leukemia, leukopenia or complicating infection, bronchospasm, shortness of breath. Less bone marrow depression than vinblastine. Significant tissue irritation if leakage occurs during IV use.

Symptoms of Overdose: Exaggeration of side effects.

Drug Interactions

L-Asparaginase / Asparaginase ↓ liver clearance of vincristine
Calcium channel blocking drugs / ↑ Accumulation of vincristine in cells

Digoxin / Vincristine ↓ effect of digoxin

Glutamic acid / Inhibits effect of vincristine

Methotrexate / Combination may cause hypotension

Mitomycin C / Severe bronchospasm and acute shortness of breath

Phenytoin / ↓ Effect of phenytoin due to ↓ plasma levels

Dosage: IV only (direct, infusion), *individualized with extreme care as overdose can be fatal.* **Adults: usual, initial,** 0.4–1.4 mg/m² (or 0.01–0.03 mg/kg) 1 time a week; **children:** 1.5–2 mg/m² 1 time a week. **Children less than 10 kg or with body surface area less than 1 m²,** 0.05 mg/kg 1 time a week. *For hepatic insufficiency:* if serum bilirubin is 1.5–3, administer 50% of the dose; if serum bilirubin is more than 3.1 or AST is more than 180, dose should be omitted.

NURSING CONSIDERATIONS

See also *Nursing Considerations* for *Antineoplastic Agents,* p. 88, and *Vinblastine,* p. 1274.

Administration/Storage

1. Dissolve powder in sterile water or isotonic saline injection to a concentration ranging from 0.01 to 1 mg/ml.
2. Medication is injected either directly into a vein or into the tubing of a flowing IV infusion over a period of 1 min.
3. Store in refrigerator. Dry powder is stable for 6 months. Solutions are stable for 2 weeks under refrigeration.
4. Protect drug from exposure to light.
5. Vincristine should not be mixed with any solution that alters the pH outside the range of 3.5–5.5.

6. Should not be mixed with anything other than normal saline or glucose in water.
7. *Treatment of Overdose:*
   - Treat side effects due to inappropriate secretion of antidiuretic hormone.
   - Use an anticonvulsant (e.g., phenobarbital), if necessary.
   - Prevent ileus by use of enemas, cathartics, or decompression of the GI tract.
   - Monitor the cardiovascular system.
   - Monitor blood counts daily to determine risk of infection and whether blood transfusions are necessary.
   - Folinic acid, 100 mg IV q 3 hr for 24 hr and then q 6 hr for a minimum of 48 hr, may help with treating the symptoms of overdose.

Assessment: Assess for early signs and symptoms of neurologic and neuromuscular side effects (e.g., sensory impairment and paresthesias) before neuritic pain and motor difficulties are apparent because neuromuscular manifestations are irreversible.

Interventions

1. Prevent constipation by encouraging increased intake of fluids and a high-fiber diet.
2. Assess for absence of bowel sounds indicative of paralytic ileus, which requires symptomatic care as well as temporary discontinuation of vincristine therapy.
3. Be prepared with laxatives and high enemas to treat high colon impaction caused by vincristine.
4. If extravasation occurs, move

V

infusion to another vein. Treat affected area with injection of hyaluronidase and application of moderate heat to decrease local reaction.
5. Administer antiemetic to control nausea and vomiting.

6. Record I&O and assess adequacy of nutrition.

Evaluation: Evaluate client for evidence of control and/or regression of malignant process.

W

Warfarin sodium
(**WAR**-far-in)
Carfin, Coumadin, Panwarfin, Sofarin, Warfilone ✹ (Rx)

See also *Anticoagulants,* p. 54.

Classification: Anticoagulant.

Action/Kinetics: Well absorbed from the GI tract although food affects the rate (but not the extent) of absorption. Suitable for parenteral administration. **Onset:** 0.5–3 days; **duration:** 2–5 days. **t½:** 1.5–2.5 days. Response to drug more uniform than with other anticoagulants.

Additional Contraindications: Liver or kidney disease.

Dosage: Tablets, IM, IV. Adults: Doses are identical regardless of route. 10–15 mg/day for 2–4 days; **then,** 2–10 mg daily, depending on prothrombin times. Dosage has not been established for children.

NURSING CONSIDERATIONS

See also *Nursing Considerations* for *Anticoagulants,* p. 55.

Administration/Storage

1. Daily monitoring of prothrombin time is recommended during the first week of therapy and weekly thereafter.
2. After reconstitution, sodium warfarin injection may be stored for several days at 4°C (39.2°F). Discard solution if precipitate becomes noticeable. Store in light-resistant containers.
3. Client should not change brands of warfarin sodium. There may be differences in bioavailability.
4. If client is receiving anticoagulants, intramuscular injections should be avoided.

Assessment

1. Determine if client may be taking any of the drugs with which warfarin may interact unfavorably.
2. Note any history of bleeding tendencies.
3. When working with sexually active females check for pregnancy. Fetal malformations have been documented. In addition, there is danger of hemorrhage.
4. Obtain baseline liver and renal function studies prior to initiating therapy.
5. Monitor prothrombin times

and check the most recent laboratory findings prior to administering warfarin.

Interventions

1. Query physician and determine the accepted therapeutic range for client prothrombin time.
2. Monitor for evidence of occult blood in stool and urine.

Client/Family Teaching

1. Stress the importance of reporting as scheduled for lab studies to evaluate the effectiveness of therapy as dosage may need to be adjusted.
2. Take oral warfarin before meals as directed and at the same time each day.
3. Do not change brands of drug unless approved by physician because dosage may be altered.
4. Advise sexually active women to use birth control measures (or abstinence) because there is an added risk involved when pregnant women are taking anticoagulant drugs.
5. Remind clients to wear an identification band that states that they are on anticoagulant therapy.
6. Avoid activities that may cause injury or cuts and bruises. Use a soft toothbrush, an electric razor to shave, and a night light to avoid falls at night.
7. Carry vitamin K. The usual dosage is 5–20 mg, to be used in the event of excessive bleeding.
8. Provide a list of foods high in vitamin K (asparagus, broccoli, cabbage, brussels sprouts, spinach, turnips, milk, cheese, etc.) that should be avoided during drug therapy.
9. Clients should be made aware that they may develop skin eruptions as an allergic reaction and to notify physician in this event.
10. Menstruation may be prolonged and flow slightly increased. Report if excessive and unusual.

Evaluation: Evaluate client for:
- Laboratory confirmation that prothrombin times are within desired range (usually 1.5–2 times the control)
- Freedom from complications of therapy, such as excessive bleeding or allergic reactions

W

X

Xylometazoline hydrochloride

(zye-low-met-**AZ**-oh-leen)

Chlorohist-LA, Neo-Synephrine II Long Acting Spray or Drops, Otrivin Nasal Drops or Spray, Otrivin Pediatric Nasal Drops, Otrivin with M-D Pump✲, Sinutab Sinus Spray✲ (OTC)

See also *Nasal Decongestants*, p. 182.

Classification: Nasal decongestant.

Special Concerns: Use during pregnancy only if benefits clearly outweigh risks.

Dosage: Drops, Spray. Adults and children over 12 years: 2–3 gtt of 0.1% solution in each nostril or 1–2 inhalations of 0.1% spray q 8–10 hr; **pediatric (2–12 years):** 2–3 gtt of 0.05% solution in each nostril q 8–10 hr.

NURSING CONSIDERATIONS

See also *Nursing Considerations* for *Nasal Decongestants*, p. 182.

Administration

1. Available as a 0.1% solution for drops and spray or as a 0.05% pediatric solution.
2. Should not be used in atomizers made of aluminum.
3. The nasal spray is more effective and is more likely to cause systemic side effects.

Evaluation: Evaluate client for reports of improvement in symptoms of nasal congestion.

Z

Zidovudine (Azidothymidine, AZT)

(zye-**DOH**-vyou-deen, ah-**zee**-doh-**THIGH**-mih-deen)

Retrovir (Rx)

See also *Anti-Infectives*, p. 80.

Classification: Antiviral.

Action/Kinetics: The active form of the drug is zidovudine triphosphate, which is derived from zidovudine by cellular enzymes. Zidovudine triphosphate competes with thymidine triphosphate (the natural substrate) for incorporation into growing chains of viral DNA by retroviral reverse transcriptase. Once incorporated, zidovudine triphosphate causes premature termination of the growth of the DNA chain. Low concentrations of zidovudine also inhibit the activity of *Shigella, Klebsiella, Salmonella, Enterobacter, Escherichia coli,* and *Citrobacter,* although resistance develops rapidly. The drug is absorbed rapidly from the GI tract and is distributed to both plasma and CSF. **Peak serum levels:** 0.1–1.5 hr. **t½:** approximately 1 hr. The drug is metabolized rapidly by the liver and excreted through the urine.

Uses: Adults manifesting symptoms due to human immunodeficiency virus (HIV) (i.e., acquired immunodeficiency syndrome [AIDS] or AIDS-related complex [ARC]) and who have confirmed *Pneumocystis carinii* pneumonia or a peripheral blood T_4 helper/inducer lymphocyte count of less than 200/mm^3.

Note: Zidovudine syrup has been authorized for use in HIV-infected children from 3 months to 12 years of age who have either HIV-associated symptoms or a CD4 (T_4) cell count of less than 400.

Contraindications: Allergy to zidovudine or its components. Lactation.

Special Concerns: Use with caution in clients who have a hemoglobin level of less than 9.5 g/dl or a granulocyte count less than 1,000/mm^3. Use during pregnancy only if benefits clearly outweigh risks (pregnancy category: C).

Side Effects: *Hematologic:* Anemia, granulocytopenia. *GI:* Nausea, vomiting, diarrhea, anorexia, GI pain, dyspepsia. *CNS:* Dizziness, headache, malaise, sleepiness, insomnia, paresthesias. *Other:* Myalgia, asthenia, diaphoresis, dyspnea, rash, change in taste perception.
Symptoms of Overdose: Nausea and vomiting. Transient hematologic changes.

Drug Interactions

Acetaminophen / ↑ Risk of granulocytopenia
Adriamycin / ↑ Risk of cytotoxicity, nephrotoxicity, or hematologic toxicity
Amphotericin B / See *Adriamycin*
Dapsone / See *Adriamycin*
Flucytosine / See *Adriamycin*
Interferon / See *Adriamycin*
Pentamidine / See *Adriamycin*
Probenecid / ↓ Biotransformation or renal excretion of zidovudine
Vinblastine / See *Adriamycin*
Vincristine / See *Adriamycin*

Dosage: Capsules/Syrup. *Symptomatic HIV infections:* **Adults, initial,** 200 mg (two 100-mg capsules or 20 ml syrup) q 4 hr around the clock. After 1 month, the dose may be reduced to 100 mg q 4 hr. *Asymptomatic HIV infections:* **Adults,** 100 mg q 4 hr while awake (500 mg daily); **Pediatric, 3 months–12 years,** 180 mg/m^2 q 6 hr, not to exceed 200 mg q 6 hr. **IV. Initially:** 1–2 mg/kg infused over 1 hr. The IV dose is given q 4 hr around the clock only until oral therapy can be instituted. Dosage adjustment may be necessary due to hematologic toxicity.

NURSING CONSIDERATIONS

See also *General Nursing Considerations For All Anti-Infectives,* p. 83.

Administration/Storage

1. The nurse and client must be aware that zidovudine therapy is not a cure for HIV infections, and clients may continue to develop opportunistic infections and other complications due to AIDS or AIDS-related complex.
2. Blood counts should be performed at least every 2 weeks. If anemia or granulocytopenia is severe, the dose of zidovudine must be adjusted or discontinued. Epoetin alfa recombinant may be administered to stimulate RBC production. A blood transfusion may also be required.

X
Y
Z

3. Safety and effectiveness of chronic zidovudine therapy in adults are not known, especially in clients who have a less advanced form of disease.
4. Capsules and syrup should be protected from light.
5. Should not be mixed with blood products or protein solutions.
6. After dilution, the solution is stable at room temperature for 24 hr and if refrigerated (2°C–8°C, 35.6°F–46.4°F) for 48 hr. However, to ensure safety from microbial contamination, the solution should be given within 8 hr if stored at room temperature and 24 hr if refrigerated.
7. *Treatment of Overdose:* Treat symptoms. Hemodialysis will enhance the excretion of the primary metabolite of zidovudine.

Client/Family Teaching

1. Stress the importance of taking the medication around the clock as ordered; sleep must be interrupted to take medication.
2. Report for all laboratory studies, especially CBC because drug causes anemia and the client may require additional medications or a blood transfusion.
3. The early signs and symptoms of anemia, such as shortness of breath, weakness, lightheadedness, or palpitations and increased tiredness should be reported to the physician.
4. Avoid acetaminophen and any other nonprescribed drugs that may exacerbate the toxicity of zidovudine.
5. Remind clients/family that the medication is not a cure, but it alleviates the symptoms of HIV infections.
6. Clients should be advised not to share medication and not to exceed the recommended dose of zidovudine.
7. The risk of transmission of HIV to others through blood or sexual contact is not reduced in individuals on zidovudine therapy.
8. Local support groups may assist client/family to understand and cope with the disease.

Evaluation: Evaluate for:
- Control and treatment of symptoms of AIDS, ARC, and opportunistic infections in clients with HIV
- Freedom from complications of drug therapy; review lab data (CBC) for evidence of complications that may require dose adjustment, discontinuation of drug therapy, or the addition of epoetin to the regimen

APPENDIX ONE
Controlled Substances in the United States and Canada

Controlled Substances Act—United States

The U.S. Federal Controlled Substances Act of 1970 placed drugs controlled by the Act into five categories or schedules based on their potential to cause psychological and/or physical dependence as well as their potential for abuse. The schedules are defined as follows:

Schedule I: Includes substances for which there is a high abuse potential and no current approved medical use (e.g., heroin, marijuana, LSD, other hallucinogens, certain opiates and opium derivatives).

Schedule II: Includes drugs that have a high abuse potential, high ability to produce physical and/or psychological dependence, and for which there is a current approved or acceptable medical use.

Schedule III: Includes drugs for which there is less potential for abuse than drugs in Schedule II and for which there is a current approved medical use. Certain drugs in this category are preparations containing limited quantities of codeine. Also, anabolic steroids are classified in Schedule III.

Schedule IV: Includes drugs for which there is a relatively low abuse potential and for which there is a current approved medical use.

Schedule V: Drugs in this category consist mainly of preparations containing limited amounts of certain narcotic drugs for use as antitussives and antidiarrheals. Federal law provides that limited quantities of these drugs (e.g., codeine) may be bought without a prescription by an individual at least 18 years of age. The product must be purchased from a pharmacist who must keep appropriate records. However, state laws vary and in many states such products require a prescription.

Controlled Substances—Canada

In Canada, narcotics are governed by the Narcotics Control regulations and are designated by the letter N. Drugs that are considered subject to abuse, which have an approved medical use, and are not narcotics are designated by the letter C.

Drug	Drug Schedule United States	Canada
Alfentanil	II	N
Alprazolam	IV	*
Amobarbital	II	C
Amphetamine	II	Not available
Aprobarbital	III	*
Benzphetamine	III	Not available
Buprenorphine	V	*
Butabarbital	III	C
Butorphanol	*	C
Chloral hydrate	IV	*
Chlordiazepoxide	IV	*
Clonazepam	IV	*
Clorazepate	IV	*
Codeine	II	N
Dextroamphetamine	II	C
Diazepam	IV	*
Diethylpropion	IV	C
Ethchlorvynol	IV	*
Ethinamate	IV	*
Fenfluramine	IV	*
Fentanyl	II	N
Flurazepam	IV	*
Glutethimide	III	*
Halazepam	IV	*
Hydrocodone	Not available	N
Hydromorphone	II	N
Levorphanol	II	N
Lorazepam	IV	*
Mazindol	IV	*
Meperidine	II	N
Mephobarbital	IV	C
Meprobamate	IV	*
Methadone	II	N
Methamphetamine	II	Not available
Metharbital	III	C
Methylphenidate	II	C
Methyprylon	III	*
Morphine	II	N

Drug	Drug Schedule	
	United States	Canada
Nalbuphine	*	C
Opium	II	N
Oxazepam	IV	*
Oxycodone	II	N
Oxymorphone	II	N
Paraldehyde	IV	*
Pemoline	IV	*
Pentazocine	IV	N
Pentobarbital,		
PO, parenteral	II	C
Rectal	III	C
Phendimetrazine	III	Not available
Phenmetrazine	II	Not available
Phenobarbital	IV	C
Phentermine	IV	C
Prazepam	IV	*
Propoxyphene	IV	N
Secobarbital		
PO	II	C
Parenteral	II	*
Rectal	III	*
Talbutal	III	*
Temazepam	IV	*
Triazolam	IV	*

*Not controlled

APPENDIX TWO
Pregnancy Categories: FDA Assigned

A: Adequate and well-controlled studies have failed to demonstrate a risk to the fetus in the first trimester of pregnancy (and there is no evidence of risk in later trimesters).

B: Animal reproduction studies have failed to demonstrate a risk to the fetus and there are no adequate and well-controlled studies in pregnant women.

C: Animal reproduction studies have shown an adverse effect on the fetus and there are no adequate and well-controlled studies in humans, but potential benefits may warrant use of the drug in pregnant women despite potential risks.

D: There is positive evidence of human fetal risk based on adverse reaction data from investigational or marketing experience or studies in humans, but potential benefits may warrant use of the drug in pregnant women despite potential risks.

X: Studies in animals or humans have demonstrated fetal abnormalities and/or there is positive evidence of human fetal risk based on adverse reaction data from investigational or marketing experience and the risks involved in use of the drug in pregnant women clearly outweigh potential benefits.

APPENDIX THREE

Commonly Used Laboratory Test Values

Test	Range	Units	Conversion Factor	SI Range	Units
Alanine aminotransferase [ALT]	0–35	U/L	0.01667	0–0.58	μkat/L
Albumin, serum	4–6	g/dl	10	40–60	g/L
Alkaline phosphatase	30–120	U/L	0.01667	0.5–2	μkat/L
Aspartate aminotransferase [AST]	0–35	U/L	0.01667	0–0.58	μkat/L
Bilirubin, total (serum)	0.1–1	mg/dl	17.1	2–18	μmol/L
Bilirubin, conjugated	0–0.2	mg/dl	17.1	0–4	μmol/L
Calcium, serum	8.8–10.4	mg/dl	0.2495	2.2–2.58	mmol/L
Chloride, serum	95–110	mEq/L	1	95–110	mmol/L

Test	Range	Units	Conversion Factor	SI Range	Units
Cholesterol					
< 29 years	< 200	mg/dl	0.02586	< 5.2	mmol/L
30–39 years	< 225	mg/dl	0.02586	< 5.85	mmol/L
40–49 years	< 245	mg/dl	0.02586	< 6.35	mmol/L
> 50 years	< 265	mg/dl	0.02586	< 6.85	mmol/L
Cortisol, serum					
0800 hours	4–19	μg/L	27.59	110–520	nmol/L
1600 hours	2–15	μg/L	27.59	50–410	nmol/L
2400 hours	5	μg/L	27.59	140	nmol/L
Creatine kinase (CK)	0–130	U/L	0.01667	0–2.167	μkat/L
Isoenzymes					
MB fraction	> 5 in MI	%	0.01	> 0.05	1
Creatinine, serum	0.6–1.2	mg/dl	88.4	50–110	μmol/L
Creatinine clearance	75–125	ml/min	0.01667	1.24–2.08	ml/s
Erythrocyte count					
male	4.3–5.9	106/mm³	1	4.3–5.9	1012/L
female	3.5–5	106/mm³	1	3.5–5	1012/L
Erythrocyte sedimentation rate (ESR)					
male	0–20	mm/hr	1	0–20	mm/hr
female	0–30	mm/hr	1	0–30	mm/hr

Test	Conventional range	Conventional unit	Factor	SI range	SI unit
Gases, arterial blood					
pO2	75–105	mm Hg	0.1333	10–14	kPa
pCO2	33–44	mm Hg	0.1333	4.4–5.9	kPa
Gamma-glutamyltransferase (GGT)	0–30	U/L	0.01667	0–0.5	µkat/L
Glucose, plasma (fasting)	70–110	mg/dl	0.05551	3.9–6.1	mmol/L
Hematocrit					
male	39–49	%	0.01	0.39–0.49	1
female	33–43	%	0.01	0.33–0.43	1
Hemoglobin					
male	14–18	g/dl	10	140–180	g/L
female	11.5–15.5	g/dl	10	115–155	g/L
Iron, serum					
male	80–180	µg/dl	0.1791	14–32	µmol/L
female	60–160	µg/dl	0.1791	11–29	µmol/L
Iron binding capacity	250–460	µg/dl	0.1791	45–82	µmol/L
Lactic dehydrogenase	50–150	U/L	0.01667	0.82–2.66	µkat/L
Lipoproteins					
low density (LDL)	50–190	mg/dl	0.02586	1.3–4.9	mmol/L
high density (HDL) male	30–70	mg/dl	0.02586	0.8–1.8	mmol/L
female	30–90	mg/dl	0.02586	0.8–2.35	mmol/L
Leukocyte count	3200–9800	mm^3	0.001	3.2–9.8	10^9/L
differential		%	0.01		1
Magnesium, serum	1.8–3	mg/dl	0.4114	0.8–1.2	mmol/L
	1.6–2.4	mEq/L	0.5	0.8–1.2	mmol/L
Mean corpuscular hemoglobin (MCH)	27–33	pg	1	27–33	pg

Test	Range	Units	Conversion Factor	SI Range	Units
Mean corpuscular hemoglobin concentration (MCHC)	33–37	g/dl	10	330–370	g/L
Mean corpuscular volume (MCV)	76–100	μm^3	1	76–100	fL
Osmolality, plasma	280–330	mOsm/kg	1	280–330	mmol/kg
Osmolality, urine	50–1200	mOsm/kg	1	50–1200	mmol/kg
Phosphate, serum	2.5–5	mg/dl	0.3229	0.8–1.6	mmol/L
Platelet count	130–400,000	$10^3/mm^3$	1	130–400	10^9/L
Potassium, serum	3.5–5	mEq/L	1	3.5–5	mmol/L
Reticulocyte count	1–24	#/1000 RBC's	0.001	0.001–0.024	1
Sodium, serum	135–147	mEq/L	1	135–147	mmol/L
Thyroid stimulating hormone (TSH)	2–11	μU/ml	1	2–11	mU/L
Thyroxine (T_4)	4–11	μg/dl	12.87	51–142	nmol/L
Thyroid binding globulin (TBG)	12–28	μg/dl	12.87	150–360	nmol/L
Thyroxine, free serum	0.8–2.8	ng/dl	12.87	10–36	pmol/L
Triiodothyronine (T_3)	75–220	ng/dl	0.01536	1.2–3.4	nmol/L
T_3 uptake	25–35	%	0.01	0.25–0.35	1
Transferrin	170–370	mg/dl	0.01	1.7–3.7	g/L
Triglycerides	<160	mg/dl	0.01129	<1.8	mmol/L
Urea nitrogen	8–18	mg/dl	0.357	3–6.5	mmol/L
Zinc, serum	75–120	μg/dl	0.153	11.5–18.5	μmol/L

"SI units" is the abbreviation of *Système International d'Unités*. It is a uniform system of reporting numerical values permitting interchangeability of information among nations and between disciplines.

(From Young DS: Implementation of SI units for clinical laboratory data. *Annals of Internal Medicine* 106:114–129, 1987.) Courtesy American College of Physicians.

ADDITIONAL PHYSIOLOGIC VALUES

Identified normal values will vary depending on the laboratory, quality controls utilized, and methods used for assay. For clarification, check with the laboratory that performed the analysis.

HEMATOLOGY

White blood cells (leukocytes)	5,000–10,000/mm^3
Neutrophils	50%–70%
Segments	50%–65%
Bands	0%–5%
Basophils	0.25%–0.5%
Eosinophils	1%–3%
Lymphocytes	25%–35%
Monocytes	2%–6%
Bleeding time	1–3 min (Duke)
	1–5 min (Ivy)
Coagulation time (Lee White)	5–15 min
Prothrombin time	10–15 sec (same as control)
Thrombin time	Within 5 sec of control
Partial thromboplastin time (PTT)	60–70 sec
Activated partial thromboplastin time (APTT)	30–45 sec
Fibrinogen split products (FSP)	2–10 mcg/ml
Ceruloplasmin	27–37 mg/dl
Copper	100–200 mcg/dl

ENZYMES

Amylase	60–180 Somogyi U/dl 111–296 IU/L
Creatine phosphokinase (CPK)	5–35 mcg/dl; 15–120 IU/L
MB (+)	>5% of total CPK
Lipase	0–1.5 U/ml
Phosphatase, acid	0.5–2.0 units/dl (Bodansky units)
Proteins	
Total	6–8 g/dl
Fibrinogen	0.2–0.4 g/dl
Globulin	1.5–3.0 g/dl

OTHER CHEMISTRY

Acetone	0.3–2.0 mg/dl
Alpha-1-antitrypsin	159–400 mg/dl
Ammonia	3.2–4.5 g/dl
Nonprotein nitrogen (NPN)	15–35 mg/dl
Uric acid	Males: 3.5–7.8 mg/dl
	Females: 2.5–6.8 mg/dl
Lactic acid	0.5–2.2 mmol/L

SEROLOGY

Antinuclear antibodies (ANA)	Negative
Carcinoembryonic antigen (CEA)	<2.5 ng/ml
Cold agglutinins (CA)	1:8 antibody titer
Immunoglobulins (Ig)	900–2,200 mg/dl
IgG	600–1,900 mg/dl
IgA	60–330 mg/dl
IgM	45–145 mg/dl
IgD	0.5–3.0 mg/dl
IgE	10–506 units/ml
Rheumatoid Factor (RF)	<1:20 titer

CEREBROSPINAL FLUID (CSF)

Cell count	0–8/mm^3
Chloride	118–132 mEq/L
Culture	No organisms
Glucose	40–80 mg/dl
Pressure	75–175 cm water
Protein	15–45 mg/dl
Sodium	145–150 mg/dl

BLOOD GASES

Whole blood oxygen, capacity	17–24 vol %
Arterial	
Saturation	96%–100% of capacity
pCO$_2$	35–45 mm Hg
pO$_2$	75–100 mm Hg
pH	7.38–7.44
Bicarbonate, normal range	24–28 mEq/L
Base excess (BE)	+2 to −2 (± 2 mEq/L)
Venous	
Saturation	60%–85% capacity
pCO$_2$	40–54 mm Hg
pO$_2$	20–50 mm Hg
pH	7.36–7.41
Bicarbonate, normal range	22–28 mEq/L

URINALYSIS

Casts	Occasional hyaline
Electrolytes	
Calcium	7.4 mEq/24 hr
Chloride	70–250 mEq/24 hr
Magnesium	15–300 mg/24 hr
Phosphorus, inorganic	0.9–1.3 g/24 hr
Potassium	25–120 mEq/24 hr
Sodium	40–220 mEq/24 hr
Glucose	0
5-Hydroxyindoleacetic acid (HIAA)	2–10 mg/24 hr

Ketones	0
Nitrogenous constituents	
Ammonia	30–50 mEq/24 hr
Creatinine clearance	100–200 ml/min
Creatinine	Males: 20–26 mg/kg/24 hr
	Females: 14–22 mg/kg/24 hr
Protein	10–50 mg/24 hr
Urea	6–17 g/24 hr
Uric acid	0.25–0.75 g/24 hr
Osmolality	500–1,200 mOsm/L
pH	6.0 (average: 4.6–8.0)
Protein	2–8
Red blood cells	1–2/LPF (low power field)
Specific gravity	1.005–1.030
Steroids	
17-Hydroxycorticosteroids	Males: 5–15 mg/24 hr
	Females: 3–13 mg/24 hr
17-Ketosteroids	Males: 8–25 mg/24 hr
	Females: 5–15 mg/24 hr
Urobilinogen	0–4 mg/24 hr
Vanillylmandelic acid (VMA)	1.5–7.5 mg/24 hr
Volume	600–2,500 ml/24 hr
White blood cells	3–4

APPENDIX FOUR

Nomogram for Estimating Body Surface Area

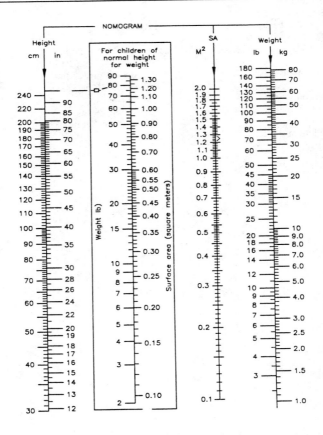

Reprinted with permission from Behrman, R.E. and Vaughan, V.C., *Nelson Textbook of Pediatrics,* 13th ed. (Philadelphia: W.B. Saunders Company, 1987.)

APPENDIX FIVE
Certified Poison Control Centers

The poison control centers in the following list are certified by the American Association of Poison Control Centers. To receive certification, each center must meet certain criteria. It must, for example, serve a large geographic area; it must be open 24 hours a day and provide direct dialing or toll-free access; it must be supervised by a medical director; and it must have registered pharmacists or nurses available to answer questions from the public.

Staff members of these centers are trained to resolve toxicity situations in the home of the caller, but, in some instances, hospital referrals are given.

The centers have a wide variety of toxicology resources, including a computer capability covering some 350,000 substances that are updated quarterly. They also offer a range of educational services to the public as well as to the health-care professional. In some states, these large centers exist side by side with smaller poison control centers that provide more limited information.

American Association of Poison Control Centers
Certified Regional Poison Centers, October 1991

ALABAMA

Children's Hospital of Alabama, Regional Poison Control Center
(205) 939-9201; (205) 933-4050; (800) 292-6678

ARIZONA

Arizona Poison & Drug Information Center Arizona Health Sciences Center
(602) 626-6016; (800) 362-0101 (AZ only)

Samaritan Regional Poison Center, Good Samaritan Medical Center
(602) 253-3334

CALIFORNIA

Fresno Regional Poison Control Center of Fresno Community Hospital and Medical Center
(800) 346-5922 (CA only)

Los Angeles County Medical Association Regional Poison Control Center
(213) 484-5151;

San Diego Regional Poison Center UCSD Medical Center
(619) 543-6000; (800) 876-4766

San Francisco Bay Area Regional Poison Control Center
San Francisco General Hospital
(415) 476-6300;
(800) 523-2222 (415, 707 only)

Santa Clara Valley Medical Center Regional Poison Center
(408) 299-5112;
(800) 662-9886

UCDMC Regional Poison Control Center
(916) 734-3392;
(800) 342-9293 (CA only)

COLORADO

Rocky Mountain Poison and Drug Center
(303) 629-1123;
(800) 332-3073 (CO only)

D.C.

National Capital Poison Center
Georgetown University Hospital
(202) 625-3333; (202) 784-4660 (TTY)

FLORIDA

Florida Poison Information Center at the Tampa General Hospital
(813) 253-4444;
(800) 282-3171 (FL only)

GEORGIA

Georgia Poison Control Center
Grady Memorial Hospital
(404) 589-4400;
(800) 282-5846 (GA only);
(404) 525-2823 (TTY)

INDIANA

Indiana Poison Center
Methodist Hospital of Indiana, Inc.
(800) 382-9097; (317) 929-2323

KENTUCKY

Kentucky Regional Poison Center of Kosair Children's Hospital
(502) 629-7275;
(800) 722-5725 (KY only)

MARYLAND

Maryland Poison Center
(301) 528-7701;
(800) 492-2414 (MD only)

National Capital Poison Center (D.C. suburbs only)
(202) 625-3333;
(202) 784-4660 (TTY)

MASSACHUSETTS

Massachusetts Poison Control System
(617) 232-2120;
(800) 682-9211 (MA only)

MICHIGAN

Blodgett Regional Poison Center
(800) 632-2727 (MI only);
(800) 356-3232 (TTY)

Poison Control Center, Children's Hospital of Michigan
(313) 745-5711;

MINNESOTA

Hennepin Regional Poison Center
Hennepin County Medical Center
(612) 347-3141;
(612) 337-7474 (TTY)

Minnesota Regional Poison Center
St. Paul-Ramsey Medical Center
 (612) 221-2113;

MISSOURI

Cardinal Glennon Children's Hospital Regional Poison Center
 (314) 772-5200;
 (800) 366-8888;

MONTANA

Rocky Mountain Poison and Drug Center
 (800) 525-5042 (MT only)

NEBRASKA

The Poison Center
 (402) 390-5555;
 (800) 955-9119;

NEW JERSEY

New Jersey Poison Information and Education System
 (800) 962-1253 (NJ only)

NEW MEXICO

New Mexico Poison and Drug Information Center
 (505) 843-2551;
 (800) 432-6866 (NM only)

NEW YORK

Long Island Regional Poison Control Center
Nassau County Medical Center
 (516) 542-2323

New York City Poison Control Center
 (212) 340-4494; (212) POISONS

OHIO

Central Ohio Poison Center
Columbus Children's Hospital
 (614) 228-1323;
 (800) 682-7625 (OH only);
 (614) 228-2272 (TTY)

Regional Poison Control System, Cincinnati Drug and Poison Information Center
 (513) 558-5111; (800) 872-5111

OREGON

Oregon Poison Center
Oregon Health Sciences University
 (503) 494-8968 (local);
 (800) 452-7165 (OR only)

PENNSYLVANIA

The Poison Control Center Serving the greater Philadelphia metropolitan area
 (215) 386-2100

Pittsburgh Poison Center
 (412) 681-6669

RHODE ISLAND

Rhode Island Poison Center – Rhode Island Hospital
 (401) 277-5727

TEXAS

North Texas Poison Center
 (214) 590-5000;
 (800) 441-0040 (TX only)

UTAH

Intermountain Regional Poison Control Center
 (801) 581-2151;
 (800) 456-7707 (UT only)

VIRGINIA

Blue Ridge Poison Center
UVA-Blue Ridge Hospital
  (604) 925-5543; (800) 451-1428

National Capital Poison
Center (Northern VA only)
Georgetown University
Hospital
  (202) 625-3333;
  (202) 784-4660 (TTY)

WEST VIRGINIA

West Virginia Poison Center
West Virginia University
Health Sciences Center/
Charleston Division
  (304) 348-4211;
  (800) 642-3625 (WV only)

WYOMING

The Poison Center
  (402) 390-5400

APPENDIX SIX
Drug Preview

The following drugs have been marketed subsequent to the submission of the manuscript for NDR-93. This appendix contains limited information for these drugs; a more complete profile will be included in next year's edition of this book.

Cefprozil
Cefzil (Rx)

See also *Cephalosporins,* p. 132.

Classification: Cephalosporin.

Uses: Pharyngitis and tonsillitis due to *Streptococcus pyogenes.* Otitis media caused by *S. pneumoniae, Hemophilus influenzae* and *Moraxella catarrhalis.* Uncomplicated skin and skin structure infections due to *Staphylococcus aureus* (including penicillinase-producing strains) and *S. pyogenes.* Secondary bacterial infection of acute bronchitis and acute bacterial exacerbation of chronic bronchitis due to *S. pneumoniae, H. influenzae* and *M. catarrhalis.*

Dosage: Suspension, Tablets.
Pharyngitis/tonsillitis: 500 mg daily for 10 days. *Secondary bacterial infection of acute bronchitis and acute bacterial exacerbation of chronic bronchitis:* 500 mg q 12 hr for 10 days. *Uncomplicated skin and skin structure infections:* Either 250 mg q 12 hr, 500 mg daily, or 500 mg q 12 hr (all for a duration of 10 days). **Infants and children, 6 months–12 years:** *otitis media,* 15 mg/kg q 12 hr for 10 days.

Flumazenil
Mazicon (Rx)

Classification: Benzodiazepine receptor antagonist.

Action/Kinetics: This drug competitively antagonizes the action of benzodiazepines on the CNS by inhibiting the effect on the GABA/benzodiazepine receptor site. **t½:** 54 min.

Uses: Reversal (complete or partial) of the sedative effects of benzodiazepines when these drugs have been used for induction or maintenance of general anesthesia, when sedation has been produced with benzodiazepines (i.e., for diagnostic and therapeutic purposes), and for the treatment of benzodiazepine overdose.

Special Concerns: Pregnancy category: C. Use of flumazenil has been associated with occurrence of seizures, especially in clients who have been on long-term benzodiazepines for sedation or in cases of overdose where clients are showing symptoms of serious cyclic antidepressant overdosage.

Dosage: IV only. *Reversal of conscious sedation or in general anesthesia:* 0.2 mg given over 15 seconds. A second dose of 0.2 mg may be given after 45 seconds if the desired level of consciousness was not reached. A further dose of 0.2 mg can be given at 60 second intervals if needed (up to a maximum of 4 additional times) The maximum total dose should not exceed 1 mg. *Suspected benzodiazepine overdose:* 0.2 mg given over 30 seconds; a further dose of 0.3 mg may be given over another 30 seconds if the desired level of consciousness is not reached. Further doses of 0.5 mg can be given over 30 seconds at 1 minute intervals to a maximum total dose of 3 mg.

NURSING CONSIDERATIONS

Administration/Storage

1. Administer the smallest amount of drug that is effective to high-risk clients. The one-minute interval between individual doses may be too short for high-risk clients as it takes 6–10 minutes for a single dose to reach full effects.
2. A major risk is re-sedation since the duration of effect of the benzodiazepine may exceed that of flumazenil.

Sertraline Hydrochloride
Zoloft (Rx)

Classification: Antidepressant.

Action/Kinetics: The antidepressant effect is believed to be due to inhibition of CNS neuronal uptake of serotonin. Steady state levels do not occur for about 1 week. The drug undergoes significant first-pass metabolism. $t^{1/2}$, **terminal elimination:** 26 hr.

Uses: Depression. *Investigational:* Obsessive-compulsive disorders.

Special Concerns: Pregnancy category: B. Due to the possibility of serious (and possibly fatal) side effects, sertraline should not be used in combination with a mono-amine oxidase inhibitor or within 14 days of discontinuing treatment with a MAO inhibitor. Close supervision of high-risk clients is necessary due to the possibility of suicide attempts in clients with depression. Use with caution in clients with hepatic or renal impairment.

Side Effects: A large number of side effects is possible. More common side effects (more than 1%) include dry mouth, increased sweating, palpitations, chest pain, headache, dizziness, tremor, paresthesia, hypoesthesia, twitching, hypertonia, confusion, rash, nausea, diarrhea, loose stools, constipation, dyspepsia, vomiting, flatulence, anorexia, abdominal pain, increased appetite, myalgia, insomnia, sexual dysfunction, somnolence, agitation, nervousness, anxiety, yawning, impaired concentration, menstrual disorders, rhinitis, pharyngitis, abnormal vision, tinnitus, taste changes, increased urination, urination disorders, fatigue, hot flashes, fever, back pain, thirst, asthenia.

Dosage: Tablets. Initial; 50 mg once daily. If a beneficial effect is not observed, the dose may be increased to a maximum of 200 mg daily.

NURSING CONSIDERATIONS

Administration/Storage

1. The drug should be given once daily, either in the morning or evening.
2. Several months of therapy may be required for a full beneficial effect.

Simvastatin
Zocor (Rx)

Classification: Antihyperlipidemic.

Action/Kinetics: Simvastatin inhibits 3-hydroxy-3-methylglutaryl-coenzyme A (HMG–CoA) reductase, the enzyme that catalyzes the early rate-limiting step in the conversion of HMG-CoA to mevalonate in the biosynthesis of cholesterol. This results in an increase of HDL cholesterol and a decrease in LDL cholesterol, VLDL cholesterol, and triglycerides.

Uses: Adjunct to diet in clients with primary hypercholesterolemia (Types IIa and IIb) when the response to diet and other nondrug measures has been inadequate.

Special Concerns: Pregnancy category: X. Use with caution in clients with a history of liver disease or who consume large quantities of ethanol.

Side Effects: Side effects are generally mild and include nausea, vomiting, diarrhea, abdominal pain, constipation, flatulence, dyspepsia, headache, asthenia, upper respiratory infection, myopathy, rhabdomyolysis, and arthralgias.

Dosage: Tablets. Initial: 5–10 mg once daily in the evening. For clients with LDL less than or equal to 190 mg/dl, the initial starting dose should be 5 mg/day; for clients with LDL greater than 190 mg/dl the initial starting dose is 10 mg/day. Dosage may be adjusted at intervals of 4 weeks up to a maximum daily dose of 40 mg given in the evening.

NURSING CONSIDERATIONS

Administration/Storage

1. May be given without regard to meals.
2. The client should be placed on a standard cholesterol-lowering diet for 3–6 months before starting simvastatin. The diet

should be continued during drug treatment.
3. The dosage of simvastatin should be reduced if cholesterol falls below the targeted range.

Temafloxacin hydrochloride
Omniflox (Rx)

See also *Fluoroquinolones,* p. 152.

Classification: Fluoroquinolone antibiotic.

Uses: Acute bacterial exacerbations of chronic bronchitis due to *Haemophilus influenzae, Moraxella catarrhalis,* or *Streptococcus pneumoniae.* Pneumonia due to *H. influenzae* or *S. pneumoniae.* Prostatitis due to *Escherichia coli, Enterococcus faecalis,* or *Proteus mirabilis.* Uncomplicated skin and skin structure infections. Uncomplicated urinary tract infections caused by *E. coli, P. mirabilis,* or *Staphylococcus epidermidis.* Complicated urinary tract infections due to *E. coli* or *Klebsiella pneumoniae.*

Special Concerns: Pregnancy category: C. Should not be used in children under 18 years of age, in pregnancy, and in lactating women.

Side Effects: Serious and possibly fatal hypersensitivity (anaphylactic) reactions. CNS stimulation manifested by seizures, tremors, restlessness, lightheadedness, confusion, and hallucinations. Pseudomembranous colitis, superinfection. The following side effects were observed in 1% or more of clients: nausea, diarrhea, dyspepsia, abdominal pain, constipation, vomiting, headache, dizziness, somnolence, asthenia, monilial vaginitis, rash, pruritus.

Dosage: Tablets. *Lower respiratory tract infections, skin and skin structure infections:* 600 mg q 12 hr. *Uncomplicated urinary tract infections:* 400 mg once daily. *Complicated urinary tract infections, prostatitis:* 400 mg b.i.d. Dosage should be modified in clients with impaired renal or hepatic function.

NURSING CONSIDERATIONS

Administration/Storage

1. May be taken without regard to food.
2. Fluids should be liberally consumed.
3. Vitamins with minerals or iron should not be taken within the 2-hr period before or after taking temafloxacin.
4. Hypersensitivity reactions may be manifested, even following the first dose.

APPENDIX SEVEN
Medic Alert Systems

WHO NEEDS MEDIC ALERT? Persons with any medical problem or condition that cannot be easily seen or recognized need the protection of Medic Alert. Heart conditions, diabetes, severe allergies and epilepsy are common problems. About one in every five persons has some special medical problem.

WHY MEDIC ALERT? Tragic or even fatal mistakes can be made in emergency medical treatment unless the special problem of the person is known. A diabetic could be neglected and die because he was thought to be intoxicated. A shot of penicillin could end the life of one who is allergic to it. Persons dependent on medications must continue to receive them at all times.

WHEN IS MEDIC ALERT IMPORTANT? Whenever a person cannot speak for himself — because of unconsciousness, shock, delirium, hysteria, loss of speech, etc. — the Medic Alert emblem speaks for him.

HOW DOES MEDIC ALERT WORK? The Medic Alert emblem —worn on the wrist or neck — is recognized the world over. On the back of the emblem is engraved the medical problem and the file number of the wearer, and the telephone number of Medic Alert's Central File. Doctors, police, or anyone giving aid can immediately get vital information — addresses of the personal physician and nearest relative, etc. — via collect telephone call (24 hours a day) to the Central File.

WHAT IS MEDIC ALERT? It is a charitable, nonprofit organization. Its services are maintained by a one-time-only membership fee and by voluntary contributions from friends, corporations and foundations. Additional services such as replacement of lost emblems and up-dating of records are charged to members at cost. Membership is tax deductible as a medical expense, and contributions are always deductible on income tax returns.

WHERE IS MEDIC ALERT? Medic Alert Foundation International was founded in Turlock, California in 1956, after a doctor's daughter almost died from reaction to a sensitivity test for tetanus antitoxin. The Foundation is endorsed by over 100 organizations including the American Academy of General Practice (and many more national and state medical organizations) the International Associations of Fire Chiefs, Police Chiefs, the National Sheriffs' Association, and the National Association of Life Underwriters.

For further information, write to:

Medic Alert Foundation International
Turlock, CA 95380
Phone (209) 632-2371.

John D. McPherson, President

Produced internally by Medic Alert Foundation

MEDIC ALERT EMBLEMS ARE
SHOWN IN ACTUAL SIZE

BRACELETS:

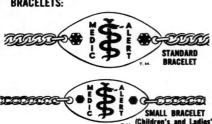

STANDARD
BRACELET

SMALL BRACELET
(Children's and Ladies')

DISC:

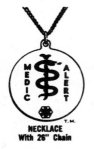

NECKLACE
With 26" Chain

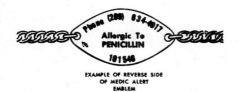

EXAMPLE OF REVERSE SIDE
OF MEDIC ALERT
EMBLEM

ALL MEMBERSHIP FEES AND DONATIONS ARE TAX-DEDUCTIBLE

Reprinted with permission from Medic Alert Foundation International, Turlock CA.

Index

Boldface = generic drug name
italics = therapeutic drug class
Regular type = trade names
CAPITALS = combination drugs

Boldface = generic drug name
italics = therapeutic drug class

Regular type = trade names
CAPITALS = combination drugs

Boldface = generic drug name
italics = therapeutic drug class

Regular type = trade names
CAPITALS = combination drugs

Boldface = generic drug name
italics = therapeutic drug class

Regular type = trade names
CAPITALS = combination drugs

Boldface = generic drug name
italics = therapeutic drug class

Regular type = trade names
CAPITALS = combination drugs

Boldface = generic drug name
italics = therapeutic drug class

Regular type = trade names
CAPITALS = combination drugs

Boldface = generic drug name   Regular type = trade names
italics = therapeutic drug class   CAPITALS = combination drugs

---

Boldface = generic drug name
italics = therapeutic drug class

Regular type = trade names
CAPITALS = combination drugs

Boldface = generic drug name
italics = therapeutic drug class

Regular type = trade names
CAPITALS = combination drugs

Boldface = generic drug name
italics = therapeutic drug class

Regular type = trade names
CAPITALS = combination drugs

Boldface = generic drug name
italics = therapeutic drug class

Regular type = trade names
CAPITALS = combination drugs

Boldface = generic drug name
italics = therapeutic drug class

Regular type = trade names
CAPITALS = combination drugs

Boldface = generic drug name
italics = therapeutic drug class

Regular type = trade names
CAPITALS = combination drugs

Boldface = generic drug name
italics = therapeutic drug class

Regular type = trade names
CAPITALS = combination drugs

Boldface = generic drug name
italics = therapeutic drug class

Regular type = trade names
CAPITALS = combination drugs

Boldface = generic drug name
italics = therapeutic drug class

Regular type = trade names
CAPITALS = combination drugs

Boldface = generic drug name
italics = therapeutic drug class

Regular type = trade names
CAPITALS = combination drugs

Boldface = generic drug name
italics = therapeutic drug class

Regular type = trade names
CAPITALS = combination drugs

Boldface = generic drug name
italics = therapeutic drug class

Regular type = trade names
CAPITALS = combination drugs

Boldface = generic drug name
italics = therapeutic drug class

Regular type = trade names
CAPITALS = combination drugs

Boldface = generic drug name
italics = therapeutic drug class

Regular type = trade names
CAPITALS ✦ = combination drugs

Boldface = generic drug name
italics = therapeutic drug class

Regular type = trade names
CAPITALS = combination drugs

Boldface = generic drug name
italics = therapeutic drug class

Regular type = trade names
CAPITALS = combination drugs

Boldface = generic drug name
italics = therapeutic drug class

Regular type = trade names
CAPITALS = combination drugs

Boldface = generic drug name
italics = therapeutic drug class

Regular type = trade names
CAPITALS = combination drugs

Boldface = generic drug name
italics = therapeutic drug class

Regular type = trade names
CAPITALS = combination drugs

Boldface = generic drug name
italics = therapeutic drug class

Regular type = trade names
CAPITALS = combination drugs

Boldface = generic drug name
italics = therapeutic drug class

Regular type = trade names
CAPITALS = combination drugs

Boldface = generic drug name
italics = therapeutic drug class

Regular type = trade names
CAPITALS = combination drugs

Boldface = generic drug name
italics = therapeutic drug class

Regular type = trade names
CAPITALS = combination drugs